Clinical Pharma
for Prescribing

Clinical Pharmacology for Prescribing

Dr Stevan R. Emmett, MBChB, BSc,
DPM, DPhil (Oxon), MRSB, MFPM
Principal Medical Officer, Defence Science and Technology Laboratories
Consultant Pharmaceutical Physician
Clinical Fellow in Emergency Medicine, Royal United Hospitals NHS Foundation Trust
Senior Research Fellow, Medical School, University of Bristol

Nicola L. Hill, BPharm, PgDip, MSc
Pharmacy Team Leader Portsmouth Hospitals NHS Trust

Dr Federico Dajas-Bailador, PhD, BSc
Assistant Professor, Faculty of Medicine & Health Sciences,
School of Life Sciences, University of Nottingham

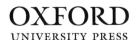

OXFORD
UNIVERSITY PRESS

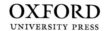

Great Clarendon Street, Oxford, OX2 6DP,
United Kingdom

Oxford University Press is a department of the University of Oxford.
It furthers the University's objective of excellence in research, scholarship,
and education by publishing worldwide. Oxford is a registered trade mark of
Oxford University Press in the UK and in certain other countries

Published in the United States of America by Oxford University Press
198 Madison Avenue, New York, NY 10016, United States of America

British Library Cataloguing in Publication Data

Data available

Library of Congress Control Number: 2019941441

ISBN 978–0–19–969493–8

Printed and bound by
CPI Group (UK) Ltd, Croydon, CR0 4YY

Illustrator

Dr Nick Love, PhD
Post-Sophomore Pathology Fellow
Stanford University School of Medicine

Acknowledgements

The authors would like to thank OUP for believing in the concept of this book from a very early stage, and for their continued support and enthusiasm in the editorial team through the years it has taken to turn it into a reality. We are also highly indebted to all those people that have contributed to the creation of this book and have freely given their time, effort, and knowledge to ensure its contents are relevant and up to date for the modern prescriber.

Steve Emmett is immeasurably appreciative of his wife, Kelly, and sons, Arthur and Albie, for their patience, understanding, and unswerving love and support over the long period of time it has taken to write this text from its original conception. Steve also wishes to express his sincere thanks to co-authors Nicky and Fed for their belief in this book and without whom it would have never progressed.

Nicola Hill would like to thank her husband, Martin, and their two children, Ethan and Isla, for their continued support and patience during the writing of this book.

Federico Dajas-Bailador would like to thank the constant support and understanding of his wife, Virginia, and their two children, Maia and Sienna, during the long process of researching and writing the many chapters of this book.

Contents

How to interpret the figures

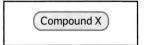

Figure 0.1 Drugs/ pharmaceutical compounds indicated in light blue ovals.

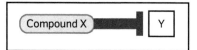

Figure 0.2 Inhibition/antagonism is indicated by a flat 'hammer', e.g. compound X inhibits Y.

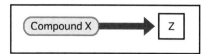

Figure 0.3 Activation/agonism is indicated by an arrow, e.g. compound X activates Z.

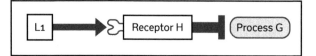

Figure 0.4 Molecular interactions, e.g. L1 activates receptor H, whose activity in turn antagonizes process G.

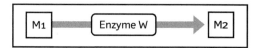

Figure 0.5 Chemical reactions can also be indicated by arrows, e.g. M1 is converted to M2 by enzyme W.

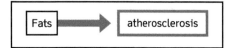

Figure 0.6 Pathological interactions are indicated in dark blue, e.g. fats contribute to atherosclerosis.

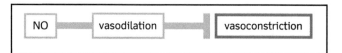

Figure 0.7 Therapeutic, antipathophysiological interactions or mediators are indicated in light blue, e.g. nitric oxide (NO) inhibits vasoconstriction via vasodilation.

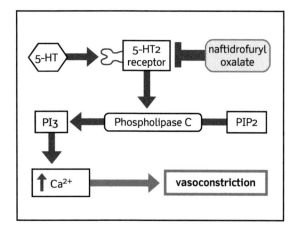

Figure 0.8 *Example 1*: 5-HT activates the 5-HT2 receptor, which then activates phospholipase C, an enzyme that catalyses the conversion of PIP2 to PI3. The PI3 molecule then functions to increase intracellular Ca^{2+}, which induces vasoconstriction. The drug naftidrofuryl oxalate inhibits 5-HT2 receptor function, and thereby reduces pathological vasoconstriction.

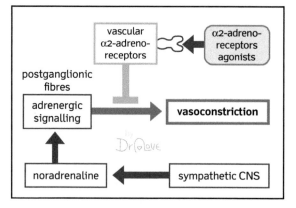

Figure 0.9 *Example 2*: sympathetic CNS outflow causes noradreline secretion from sympathetic post-ganglionic fibres, inducing adrenergic signalling pathways and thus vasoconstriction. Vascular α2-adrenoreceptors inhibit sympathetic noradrenaline activity, and thus, agonists cause a reduction in sympathetic outflow to the peripheral vasculature and reduce vasoconstriction.

Abbreviations

6-CIT	six-item cognitive impairment test
6-MP	6-mercaptopurine
6-TGN	6-thioguanine nucleotides
AA	arachidonic acid
AAS	anabolic-androgenic steroids
ABPA	allergic bronchopulmonary aspergillosis
ABPM	ambulatory
ABVD	adriamycin (doxorubicin), bleomycin, vinblastine dacarbazine
ACE	angiotensin-converting enzyme
ACh	acetylcholine
AChE	acetylcholinesterase
ACPA	anti-citrullinated protein antibodies
ACS	acute coronary syndrome
ACT	activated clotting time
ACTH	adrenocorticotropic hormone
AD	anti-arrhythmic drugs
ADCC	antibody-dependent cell-mediated cytotoxicity
ADH	antidiuretic hormone
ADME	absorption, distribution, metabolism, and excretion
ADP	adenosine diphosphate
ADR	adrenal receptor
AED	anti-epileptic drugs
AIH	autoimmune hepatitis
AIHA	autoimmune haemolytic anaemia
AIS	androgen insensitivity syndrome
AIT	autoimmune thyroiditis
AKI	acute kidney injury
ALD	Alzheimer's disease
ALF	acute liver failure
ALL	acute lymphoblastic leukaemia
ALP	alkaline phosphatase
ALPD	acute laryngopharyngeal dysthaesia
AML	acute myeloid leukaemia
AMP	adenosine monophosphate
AMPK	AMP-activated protein kinase
ANP	atrial natriuretic peptide
AP	activator protein
APC	antigen-presenting cells
APoE	apolipoprotein E
APP	amyloid precursor protein
AR	androgen receptors
ARB	angiotensin II receptor blocker
ARF	acute renal failure
ARNI	angiotensin II receptor neprilysin inhibitor
ARS	anticholinergic risk scores
ARV	antiretroviral drug
AS	ankylosing spondylitis
AT	antithrombin
ATN	acute tubular necrosis
ATP	adenosine triphosphate
AUDIT	Alcohol Use Disorders Identification Test
AV	atrioventricular
AVN	atrial ventricular node
AVP	arginine vasopressin
AZA	azathioprine
BD	twice daily
Bcl-2	B-cell lymphoma 2
BDNF	brain-derived neurotrophic factor
BDP	beclomethasone
BEACOPP	bleomycin, etoposide, adriamycin (doxorubicin), cyclophosphamide, oncovin (vincristine), procarbazine, prednisolone
BMD	bone mineral density
BNF	British National Formulary
BP	blood pressure
BPH	benign prostatic hyperplasia
BSA	body surface area
CABG	coronary artery bypass graft
CAH	congenital adrenal hyperplasia
CAIS	complete androgen insensitivity syndrome
cAMP	cyclic adenosine monophosphate
CaR	Ca^{2+} receptor
cART	combination antiretroviral therapy
CaSR	Ca^{2+}-sensing receptor
CBT	cognitive behavioural therapy
CCB	calcium channel blockers
CCF	congestive cardiac failure
CD	controlled drug
CDMS	clinically definite multiple sclerosis

CFTR	cystic fibrosis transmembrane conductance regulator
cGMP	guanosine 3',5'-cyclic monophosphate
ChAT	choline acetyltransferase
ChIVPP	chlorambucil, vinblastine, procarbazine, prednisolone
CINV	chemotherapy-induced nausea and vomiting
CIS	clinically isolated syndrome
CLL	chronic lymphocytic leukaemia
CML	chronic myeloid leukaemia
CMV	cytomegalovirus
CNS	central nervous system
COMT	catechol-O-methyltransferase
COPD	chronic obstructive pulmonary disease
COPDAC	cyclophosphamide, Oncovin® (vincristine), prednisolone, dacarbazine
COPP	cyclophosphamide, Oncovin® (vincristine), procarbazine, prednisolone
COX1	cyclo-oxygenase 1
CPAP	continuous positive airway pressure
CPE	carbapenemase-producing Enterobacteriaceae
CK	creatine kinase
CD	Crohn's disease
CREB	cAMP response element-binding protein
CRF	corticotrophin-releasing factor
CRH	corticotrophin-releasing hormone
CRP	C-reactive protein
CRPS	complex regional pain syndrome
CSF	cerebrospinal fluid
CT	computed tomography
CTPA	computed tomography pulmonary angiogram
CTZ	chemoreceptor trigger zone
CVD	cardiovascular disease
CXR	chest X-ray
D	drug
DA	dopamine
DAA	direct-acting antivirals
DAG	diacylglycerol
DAT	direct antiglobulin test
DBP	diastolic blood pressure
DCT	distal convoluted tubule
DGH	district general hospital
DHF	dihydrofolate
DHT	5α-dihydrotestosterone
DI	diabetes insipidus

DIT	diiodotyrosine
DKA	diabetic ketoacidosis
DLB	dementia with Lewy bodies
DLBCL	diffuse large B cell lymphoma
DM	diabetes mellitus
DM1	type 1 diabetes mellitus
DM2	type 2 diabetes mellitus
DMARD	disease-modifying anti-rheumatic drug
DMT	disease-modifying therapies
DOPA	3,4-dihydroxyphenylalanine
DR	drug–receptor interaction
DRESS	drug rash eosinophilia systemic symptoms
DVT	deep vein thrombosis
DXA	dual-energy X-ray absorptiometry
EAE	autoimmune encephalomyelitis
EBV	Epstein–Barr virus
EC$_{50}$	half maximal effective concentration
ECG	electrocardiogram
ECT	electroconvulsive therapy
ED	erectile dysfunction
EDRF	endothelium-derived relaxing factor
EEG	electroencephalogram
EF	ejection fraction
EGFR	vascular endothelial growth factor
EH	essential hypertension
EMA	European Medicines Agency
EMT	epithelial–mesenchymal transition
EPC	endothelial progenitor cell
EPO	erythropoietin
EPS	extrapyramidal side effects
ER	oestrogen
ESA	erythropoietin-stimulating agents
ESBL	extended-spectrum beta-lactamases
ESR	erythrocyte sedimentation rate
ESRD	end-stage renal disease
EWS	early warning scores
FBC	full blood count
FcεRI	high affinity immunoglobulin E receptor
FDA	Food and Drug Administration
FGA	first-generation antipsychotics
FH	familial hypercholesterolaemia
FSH	follicle-stimulating hormone
FVII	factor VII
GA	glatiramer acetate
GABA	gamma-amino-butyric acid
GAD	generalized anxiety disorder
GDP	guanosine diphosphate
GF	growth factor

GFR	glomerular filtration rate	**IDO**	idiopathic detrusor overactivity
GHR	growth hormone receptor	**IFIS**	intra-operative floppy iris syndrome
GI	gastrointestinal	**IFNAR**	interferon-α/β receptor
GLP-1	glucagon-like peptide 1	**IFRT**	involved field radiotherapy
GLP-1R	glucagon-like peptide 1 receptor	**IGE**	idiopathic generalized epilepsy
GLUT	glucose transporters	**IGF-1**	insulin-like growth factor
GMC	General Medical Council	**IL**	interleukins
GM-CSF	granulocyte-macrophage colony-stimulating factor	**ILAE**	International League Against Epilepsy
		IM	intramuscular
GnRH	gonadotropin-releasing hormone	**IMP**	investigational medicinal products
GORD	gastro-oesophageal reflux disease	**INI**	integrase inhibitor
GPhC	General Pharmaceutical Council	**INR**	international normalized ratio
GR	glucocorticoid receptor	**IRIS**	immune reconstitution inflammatory syndrome
GTC	generalized tonic–clonic seizure		
GTN	glyceryl trinitrate	**IRS**	insulin receptor substrate
GTP	guanosine triphosphate	**IT**	intrathecal chemotherapy
GWAS	genome-wide association studies	**ITP**	idiopathic thrombocytopenic purpura
HAART	highly active anti-retroviral therapy	**ITU**	intensive treatment unit
HAE	hereditary angioedema	**IUD**	intrauterine device
HAV	hepatitis A virus	**IV**	intravenous
HBeAg	hepatitis B surface antigen	**JC**	juxtaglomerular cells
HBPM	home blood pressure monitoring	**JVP**	jugular venous pressure
HBV	hepatitis B virus	**K**	equilibrium dissociation constant
HCC	hepatocellular carcinoma	**L**	ligand
HCV	hepatitis C virus	**LABA**	long-acting β2 agonist
HDL-C	high-density lipoprotein cholesterol	**LAMA**	long-acting muscarinic antagonist
HDU	high dependency unit	**LBBB**	left bundle branch block
HE	hepatic encephalopathy	**LC**	locus coeruleus
HF	heart failure	**LDH**	lactate dehydrogenase
HFpEF	heart failure preserved ejection fraction	**LDL**	low-density lipoprotein
HFrEF	heart failure reduced ejection fraction	**LDL-C**	low-density lipoprotein cholesterol
HHV	human herpes virus	**LFT**	liver function test
HPA	hypothalamic–pituitary axis	**LH**	luteinizing hormone
HRT	hormone replacement therapy	**LHRH**	luteinizing hormone-releasing hormone
HTN	hypertension	**LMWH**	low molecular weight heparin
HUS	haemolytic uraemic syndrome	**LNA**	locked nucleic acid
IA	intrinsic activity	**LRP5**	lipoprotein receptor-related protein 5
IBD	inflammatory bowel disease	**LTOT**	long-term oxygen therapy
IBS	irritable bowel syndrome	**LV**	left ventricular
IBS-C	IBS constipation-predominant	**LVEF**	left ventricular ejection fraction
IBS-D	IBS diarrhoea-predominant	**LVF**	left ventricular failure
IC$_{50}$	inhibitory concentration	**MAC**	minimum alveolar concentration
ICAM-1	intercellular adhesion molecule 1	**MACE**	amsacrine, cytarabine, and etoposide
ICD	impulse control disorder	**MAHA**	microangiopathic haemolytic anaemias
ICD-10	International Classification of Diseases-10	**MALT**	mucosa-associated lymphoid tissue
ICH	Intracerebral haemorrhage	**MAOA**	monoamine oxidase A
ICS	inhaled corticosteroid	**MAOB**	monoamine oxidase B
IDL	intermediate density lipoproteins	**MAOI**	monoamine oxidase inhibitors

MAP	mean arterial pressure	**NNRTI**	non-nucleoside reverse transcriptase inhibitor
MAPK	mitogen-activated protein kinase		
MBP	myelin basic protein	**NNT**	number needed to treat
mCRC	metastatic colorectal cancer	**NO**	nitric oxide
MDD	major depressive disorder	**NOAC**	novel oral anti-coagulants
MDI	metered dose inhaler	**NOS**	nitric oxide synthase
MDRD	Modification of Diet in Renal Disease	**NPC**	National Prescribing Centre
MET	mesenchymal–epithelial transition	**NPC1L1**	Niemann–Pick C1-like
MGUS	monoclonal gammopathy of unknown significance	**N-REM**	non-rapid eye movement
		NRI	NA re-uptake transporter
MHC	major histocompatibility complex	**NRT**	Nicotine replacement therapy
MHRA	Medicines and Healthcare products Regulatory Agency	**NSAID**	non-steroidal anti-inflammatory drugs
		NSTEMI	non-ST-elevation myocardial infarction
MI	myocardial infarction	**NYHA**	New York Heart Association
MIMs	Monthly Index of Medical Specialities	**OA**	osteoarthritis
MIT	monoiodotyrosine	**OAB**	overactive bladder syndrome
MMP	matrix metalloproteinases	**OCD**	obsessive compulsive disorder
MMR	measles, mumps, rubella vaccine	**OD**	once daily
MMSE	Mini Mental State Examination	**ODV**	O-desmethylvenlafaxine
MMX	multi-matrix	**OEPA**	Oncovin® (vincristine), etoposide, prednisolone, adriamycin (doxorubicin)
MoCA	Montreal Cognitive Assessment		
MODY	maturity onset diabetes of the young	**OP**	osteoporosis
MPTP	1-methyl-4-phenyl-1,2,3,6-tetrahydropyridine	**OPAT**	outpatient parenteral antibiotic therapy
MR	magnetic resonance	**OR**	oestrogen receptor
MRSA	meticillin-resistant *Staphylococcus aureus*	**ORS**	oral rehydration salts
MS	multiple sclerosis	**ORT**	oral rehydration therapy
MSU	midstream specimen of urine	**PAAP**	personalized asthma action plan
MTHFR	methylenetetrahydrofolate reductase	**PADH**	post-artesunate delayed haemolysis
NA	noradrenergic	**PAF**	paroxysmal atrial fibrillation
NA	nucleoside analogue	**PAIS**	partially androgen insensitivity syndrome
NAc	nucleus accumbens	**pANCA**	perinuclear anti-neutrophil cytoplasmic antibodies
NANC	non-adrenergic-non-cholinergic		
NaSSA	noradrenaline specific serotonin agonists	**PASD**	peripheral artery disease
NCE	new chemical entities	**PBC**	primary biliary cirrhosis
NDO	neurogenic detrusor overactivity	**PBP**	penicillin-binding proteins
NF	nuclear factor	**PCA**	patient-controlled analgesia
NFAT	nuclear factor of activated T cells	**PCI**	percutaneous coronary intervention
NG	nasogastric	**PCL**	plasma cell leukaemia
NGF	nerve growth factors	**PCOS**	polycystic ovary syndrome
NGS	next-generation sequencing	**PJP**	pneumocystis jiroveci pneumonia
NICE	National Institute for Health and Care Excellence	**PCT**	proximal convoluted tubule
		PD	Parkinson's disease
NIV	non-invasive ventilation	**PDA**	patent ductus arteriosis
NMAA	nitrogen mustard alkylating agents	**PDB**	Pagets disease of bone
NMC	Nursing and Midwifery Council	**PDD**	Parkinson's disease dementia
NMDA	N-methyl-D-asparate	**PDE**	phosphodiesterase
NMJ	neuromuscular junction	**PDE5**	phosphodiesterase type 5
NMS	neuroleptic malignant syndrome	**PDGF**	platelet-derived growth factor

PE	pulmonary embolism
PEF	peak expiratory flow
PEP	post-exposure prophylaxis
PET	positron emission tomography
PFC	prefrontal cortex
PG	prostaglandins
PGE	prostaglandin E
PHE	Public Health England
PI	protease inhibitor
Pi3-k	phosphatidylinositol 3-kinase
PIC	pre-integration complex
PIL	patient information leaflet
PKA	protein kinase A
PKC	protein kinase C
PLC	phospholipase C
PML	progressive multifocal leukoencephalopathy
PNH	paroxysmal nocturnal haemoglobinuria
PONV	post-operative nausea and vomiting
PORC	post-operative residual curarization
PP	paraprotein
PPAR-α	peroxisome proliferator activated receptor alpha
PPI	proton pump inhibitor
PPRE	peroxisome proliferator response elements
PR	progesterone receptor
PrEP	pre-exposure prophylaxis
PRH	prolactin hormone
PSA	prostate specific antigen
PSC	primary sclerosing cholangitis
PT	prothrombin time
PTH	parathyroid hormone
PTP	phosphotyrosine phosphatase
PTSD	post-traumatic stress disorder
PV	pharmacovigilance
PVD	peripheral vascular disease
PVL	panton-valentine leucocidin
QALY	quality-adjusted life-year
R	receptor
RA	rheumatoid arthritis
RANKL	receptor activator of nuclear factor kappa-B ligand
RBC	red blood cells
REM	rapid eye movement
RES	reticular endothelial system
RF	rheumatoid factor
RFA	radiofrequency ablation
RRMS	relapsing-remitting multiple sclerosis
RN	raphe nuclei

RPLS	reversible posterior leukoencephalopathy syndrome
RRT	renal replacement therapy
RSI	rapid sequence induction
RSV	respiratory syncitial virus
RVF	right ventricular failure
SA	sinoatrial
SABA	short-acting β2-adrenoceptor agonist
SAH	subarachnoid haemorrhage
SAMA	short acting muscarinic antagonist
SAN	sino-atrial node
SARI	serotonin antagonist and reuptake inhibitor
SBP	systolic blood pressure
SC	subcutaneous
SCD	sickle cell anaemia
SCID	severe combined immunodeficiency syndrome
SCN	suprachiasmatic nucleus
SERM	selective oestrogen receptor modulator
SERT	5-HT uptake transporter
SGA	second-generation antipsychotics
SGLT	sodium-glucose co-transporter
SHBG	sex-hormone-binding globulin
SIADH	syndrome of inappropriate anti-diuretic hormone
SLE	systemic lupus erythematosus
SMM	smouldering myeloma
SN	substantia nigra
SNc	substantia nigra pars compacta
SNRI	Serotonin-noradrenaline reuptake inhibitors
SORM	selective oestrogen-receptor modulator
SOS	sinusoidal obstruction syndrome
SPC	summary of product characteristics
SPECT	single-photon emission computed tomography
SPRM	Selective progesterone receptor modulator
SRI	serotonin re-uptake inhibitor
SSA	somatostatin analogues
SSRI	selective serotonin reuptake inhibitor
STEMI	ST-elevation myocardial infarction
STI	sexually transmitted infection
SUDEP	sudden unexpected death in epilepsy
SUI	stress urinary incontinence
SVR	sustained viral response
TBG	thyroxine-binding globulin
TCA	tricyclic antidepressants
TCR	T cell receptor
TDS	three times a day

TENS	transcutaneous electrical nerve stimulation		**TWOC**	trial without catheter
TF	tissue factor		**U&E**	urea & electrolytes
TFPI	tissue factor pathway inhibitor		**UA**	unstable angina
TFT	thyroid function test		**UC**	ulcerative colitis
TG	triglycerides		**UDCA**	ursodeoxycholic acid
TGF	transforming growth factor		**UFH**	unfractionated heparin
THF	tetrahydrofolate		**UTI**	urinary tract infections
TI	therapeutic index		**VAS**	visual analogue scale
TIA	transient ischaemic attack		**VCAM-1**	vascular-cell adhesion molecule 1
TIBC	total iron binding capacity		V_D	volume of distribution
TIPS	transjugular intrahepatic portosystemic shunt		**VEGF**	vascular endothelial growth factor
TPMT	thiopurine methyl transferase		**VIP**	vasoactive intestinal peptide
TMZ	temozolomide		**VLDL**	very low-density lipoproteins
TNF	tumour necrosis factor		**VOD**	veno-occlusive disease
TNFα	tumour necrosis factor-α		**VRE**	vancomycin-resistant *Enterococcus faecium*
t-PA	tissue plasminogen activator		**VT**	ventricular tachycardia
TPN	total parenteral nutrition		**VTA**	ventral tegmental area
TPO	thyroid peroxidase		**VTE**	venous thromboembolism
TRH	thyrotropin-releasing hormone		**vWF**	von Willebrand's factor
TSH	thyroid-stimulating hormone		**WPW**	Wolff–Parkinson–White
TTP	thrombotic thrombocytopenic purpura		**βhCG**	β-human chorionic gonadotrophin

Contributors

Dr Rob Adam (co-author of Topic 9.2, 'Epilepsy')

Dr Tomas-Paul Cusack (Topic 11.3, 'Viral infections')
Southampton University Hospital NHS Trust

Dr Alice Eyers (Questions for all sections)
Mann Cottage Surgery, Moreton in Marsh,
Gloucestershire

Dr Laurence Gray (Topic 13.1, 'Haemato-oncology and
malignancy')
Specialist Registrar, Clinical Pharmacology and
therapeutics, University Hospital Llandough, Penarth,
Cardiff

Dr John Jones (Topics 12.1, 'Anaemia', 12.2
'Haemoglobinopathies', Topic 13.1, 'Haemato-oncology
and malignancy')
Specialist Registrar, The Institute of Cancer Research,
London, UK. The Royal Marsden Hospital NHS
Foundation Trust, London

Dr Channarayapatna Krishna (Chapter 13, 'Haemato-
oncology and malignancy')
Consultant Physician, Clinical Pharmacologist and
Toxicologist, University Hospital Llandough, Penarth,
Cardiff

Dr Claudia Meyer (Topic 11.2, 'Fungal infections')
Specialist Registrar, Medical Microbiology, Portsmouth
Hospitals NHS Foundation Trust.

Dr Robert Owens (Topic 13.1, 'Haemato-oncology and
malignancy')
Specialist Registrar, Clinical Oncology, Churchill
Hospital, Oxford University Hospitals, Old Road,
Headington, Oxford

Dr Simon Page (Topic 13.1, 'Haemato-oncology and
malignancy', 'Management of lymphoma')

Adel Sheikh (Topic 11.1, 'Bacterial infection')
Pharmacist Microbiology, Portsmouth Hospital NHS Trust

Dr Manjeet Singh (Topic 13.1, 'Haemato-oncology and
malignancy')
Clinical Pharmacology and therapeutics, University
Hospital Llandough, Penarth, Cardiff

Dr Sarah Wyllie (Topic 11.4, 'Protozoal and helminth
infections')
Consultant Microbiologist, Portsmouth Hospital
NHS Trust

Publisher's acknowledgement

Thank you to the lecturers and clinicians who participated in our anonymous peer-review process and kindly gave their time to this project.

Advisers

Dr Mark Lythgoe (Chapter 1)
Imperial College London

Dr Chris Tham (Chapter 1)
Imperial College London

Dr Paul Brady (all sections of Chapter 2 except Topic 2.3, 'Dyslipidaemia' and Topic 2.8, 'Venous thromboembolism')
Royal United Hospitals NHS Foundation Trust

Dr Susan Fair (Topic 2.8, 'Venous thromboembolism')
Heart of England NHS Foundation Trust

Dr Sud Ramachandran (Topic 2.3, 'Dslipidaemia')
Heart of England NHS Foundation Trust

Dr Ben Green (Topic 3.2, 'Chronic obstructive pulmonary disease')
Portsmouth Hospital NHS Trust

Adel Sheikh (Topic 3.1, 'Asthma')
Portsmouth Hospitals NHS Trust

Dr Hitasha Rupani (Topic 3.1, 'Asthma')
Portsmouth Hospitals NHS Trust

Dr Dominic Hughes
Royal Brompton Hospital, London

Dr Partha Karr (Topic 4.5, 'Diabetes mellitus')
Portsmouth Hospital NHS Trust

Dr Mark Davey (Topic 4.6, 'Female reproduction')
Portsmouth Hospitals NHS Trust

Dr Vinoid Patel (all sections of Chapter 4 except Topic 4.5, 'Diabetes mellitus' and Topic 4.6, 'Female reproduction')
University of Warwick/George Eliot Hospital NHS Trust

Dr Andrew Stein (Topic 5.1, 'The kidney, drugs, and chronic kidney disease')
University of Warwick/University Hospital Coventry & Warwickshire NHS Trust

Dr Helen Cui (Topic 5.3, 'Disorders of micturition' and Topic 5.4, 'Erectile dysfunction')
Oxford University Hospitals NHS Foundation Trust

Dr Fergus Thorsby-Pelham (Chapter 6, 'Gastroenterology')
Portsmouth Hospital NHS Trust

Dr Martin Hill (Chapter 6, 'Gastroenterology')
Bosmere Medical Practice, Havant

Dr Fowell (Topic 6.7, 'Liver disease')
Portsmouth Hospitals NHS Trust

Dr Steven Young-Min (Chapter 7, 'Musculoskeletal medicine')
Portsmouth Hospital NHS Trust

Dr Luke Dyson (Chapter 8, 'Anaesthetics')
University Hospitals of Leicester

Dr Emily Henderson (all sections of Chapter 9 except Topic 9.2, 'Epilepsy')
Royal United Hospitals NHS foundation Trust and University of Bristol

Dr Rob Adam (Topic 9.2, 'Epilepsy')

Dr Paul Bentley (Topic 9.2, 'Epilepsy')
Imperial College London

Dr Andrew Drury (Chapter 10, 'Psychiatry')
South London and Maudseley NHS Foundation Trust

Dr Paul Russell (Chapter 11, 'Infectious disease')
Defence Science Technology Laboratories/Salisbury District NHS Trust

Dr John Jones (Topic 12.3, 'Allergy')
The Institute of Cancer Research, London, UK. The Royal Marsden Hospital NHS Foundation Trust, London, UK

Dr Tim Crevasse (Topic 12.2, 'Haemoglobinopathies')
Brighton and Sussex Medical School/Royal Sussex County Hospital

1 Principles of clinical pharmacology

1.1 Principles of clinical pharmacology

Pharmacology is defined as the study of the effects of drugs on the function of a living organism. It is an integrative discipline that tackles drug/compound behaviours in varied physiological systems and links these to cellular and molecular mechanisms of action.

As a scientific endeavour, pharmacology evolved from the early identification of therapeutic properties of natural compounds, with herbal medicines and relatively complex pharmacopoeias widely used in early cultures. Despite this, lack of understanding of the physiological, pathological, and chemical processes governing the human body prevented the early establishment of pharmacology as a scientific discipline. Since then, **pharmacology** has progressed to be considered a fully developed integrative science that employs techniques and theories from various disciplines, such as chemistry, biochemistry, genomics, medicinal chemistry, physiology, and cellular and molecular biology. Collectively, these are applied to study disease causality and the relevant mechanistic action of compounds, to establish new treatments.

In the last 100 years, the importance of clinical pharmacology has increased in line with the scientific and technological advances in biomedical research. Benefits gained from molecular and cellular approaches have enabled a more comprehensive analysis of drugs and their actions in functional context. Now, *clinical pharmacology and therapeutics* encompass the discovery, development, regulation, and application of drugs in a process that integrates scientific research with clinical practice to better treat illness and preserve health.

Part 1: principles of pharmacology

Within this textbook the principles of pharmacology are discussed by therapeutic area so that the reader can link disease pathophysiology, drug mechanism, and modern prescribing behaviours for conditions commonly seen in clinical practice. There are, however, fundamental concepts that are universal in understanding the interaction between drugs and their 'targets', including receptor pharmacology, genomic pharmacology, and pharmacokinetics.

Receptor pharmacology

The pharmacological receptor models preceded by many years the knowledge of the receptor as an entity. It was not until the last 150 years that a series of contributions from many notable biologists and chemists established the principles that founded modern day pharmacology. They produced a significant paradigm shift in therapeutics, where empirical descriptors of the activities observed (heating, cooling, moistening, emetic, etc.) were replaced by the concept of a 'target'. After more than a century, the basic receptor concept is still the foundation of biomedical research and drug discovery.

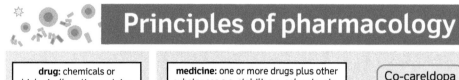
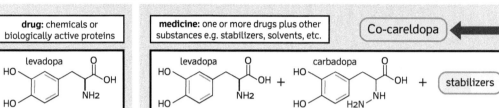

Figure 1.1 Drug or medicine.

Lock and key

The ground-breaking concept that all therapeutic agents act by targeting molecular entities comes from the work of Ehrlich and Langley in the early twentieth century, developing the 'lock and key' hypothesis for drug action. In this model, a drug/compound acts as a *ligand* (L) and interacts with a *receptive molecule* (R; drug target) in a reversible manner, forming a receptor–ligand complex (R/L), with a functional consequence that allows the modulation of cell function to preserve/restore tissue homeostasis (Figure 1.2).

Occupancy theory model

The improved understanding of receptor function, promoted the development of the occupancy theory model (Figure 1.2), in which a ligand acts as an *agonist* when it induces a tissue response that is a function of the number of receptors occupied. This concept assumed that the formation of an R/L complex was reversible, and that all receptors were functionally equivalent and had the ability to bind the ligand independently.

In this model, an *antagonist* is a ligand that can occupy the receptor/drug target site, but block the functional response of an agonist. When the functional effect of an antagonist could be overcome by increasing the concentration of the agonist, we define this as a *competitive antagonist*. The blockade of receptor function can also occur via *non-competitive antagonists*, which interact with the receptor at *allosteric sites* other than the site in the receptor that is recognized by the agonist (termed *orthosteric site*).

Intrinsic activity

To incorporate the concept that some agonists are not capable of producing a maximal response even at supramaximal concentrations, the occupancy theory incorporated the notion of *intrinsic activity* (IA) for a ligand. In this, a *full agonist* would have an IA value of 1.0, with zero given to an antagonist.

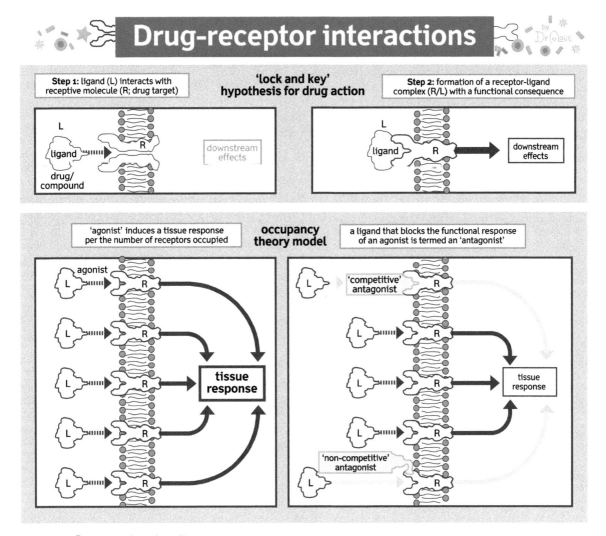

Figure 1.2 Drug–receptor interactions

When compounds that bind to the receptor are only capable of generating a fraction of the response observed with a full agonist, they are termed *partial agonists*, which by definition are also *partial antagonists* (since their receptor occupancy prevents a full agonist response). In the case of agonists that cause a response larger than the assumed 'gold standard' full agonist, these are referred to as *super agonists.*

Affinity

As part of this receptor–ligand theory a binding reaction occurs where free drug [D] and free receptor [R] interact to form a drug–receptor interaction [DR] in a reversible way that is dependent on concentration (Law of Mass Action). The ratio of the rate of the forward reaction and backward reaction define an affinity binding constant, the reciprocal of which is the equilibrium dissociation constant (K_A), which is expressed in mol/L, and is the concentration required to occupy 50% of the binding sites when equilibrium is achieved. When a drug has a low K_A it will have high affinity for its receptor.

$$D + R \rightleftharpoons DR$$
$$K_A = k-1/k+1$$

Efficacy

The concept of efficacy was initially introduced as a further refinement of the partial agonist model, where a maximal agonist response is observed with only a minor proportion of the total number of receptors occupied. In practice, efficacy has been used to define the magnitude of a response in relation to other compounds, such as agonists, partial agonists or super agonists.

Half maximal effective concentration (EC_{50}) vs effective dose (ED_{50})

In numerical terms, the effect of a drug in a given system can be expressed by the EC_{50}, which is used to describe the concentration at which 50% of maximal agonist effect is observed (Figure 1.3). The action of the ligand may be stimulatory or inhibitory, and generate a dose–response curve that is normally non-linear, but after plotting on a log scale can be transformed into sigmoidal. EC_{50} is generally used for receptor binding assays or cellular/tissue culture biological assays. It should not be confused with ED_{50}, the 'effective dose in 50% of the population'. The ED_{50} is useful to describe observations in experimental models, where the amount of drug at the receptors cannot be predicted (e.g. in vivo or in vitro perfusion studies).

The term IC_{50} (inhibitory concentration) has also been developed to describe the concentration at which a 50% reduction in agonist effect (inhibitory) is observed, after addition of an antagonist. It is often used in radio-ligand binding assays and denotes the functional strength of an antagonist, rather than true affinity.

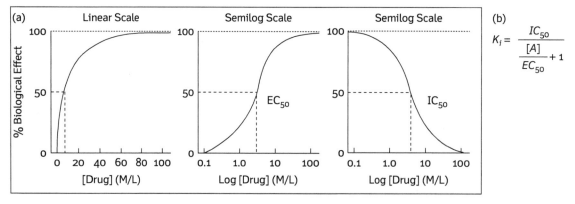

Figure 1.3 Dose–response curve. (a) The dose–response curve plotted on a linear scale (left panel); it is hyperbolic and is described by a Langmuir binding isotherm model (i.e. high concentrations lead to maximum drug effect). Right panel shows drug concentration expressed in logarithmic scale, which converts the plotted dose response from hyperbolic to sigmoid. In this way, the area between 25–75% of the maximum response will be linear and thus better for interpreting drug actions, e.g. EC_{50} and IC_{50}. (b) The inhibition constant (K_i) is an indication of how potent an inhibitor is. While the IC_{50} is more reflective of the functional strength of the inhibitor, the K_i is reflective of the binding affinity. In the equation depicted, [A] is fixed concentration of agonist, EC_{50} represents concentration of agonist resulting in half maximal activation of receptor. The IC_{50} can vary depending on experiment type and condition. K_i is an absolute value and is helpful in determining the likelihood that a particular drug is going to inhibit a particular target.

Therapeutic index

Beyond the therapeutic effect stated by the ED_{50} of a given drug, most drugs have toxic or unwanted side-effects that are dose-related (Type A adverse reactions). These properties can lead to a reluctance to develop and market the product, or non-compliance in the patient population. The therapeutic versus toxic effect can be defined as the therapeutic index (TI) and is indicative of a safety margin. In reality, TI is rarely quoted as a number, being clinically irrelevant because the ED_{50} is highly variable depending on what measures of effectiveness are used, while the LD_{50} (individual/lethal dose required to kill 50% of a population of test animals) does not reflect individual therapeutic toxicity.

$$TI = LD_{50} / ED_{50}$$

Despite this, such safety and efficacy considerations are paramount in the process of developing a drug, and the term 'narrow therapeutic index' is used generically to describe a drug with a narrow margin between effective and toxic levels.

Receptor activation

Two-state model

The concept that receptor activation by an agonist involved a conformational change in the receptor, was implicit in early pharmacological thinking. As such, the simplest theory to account for receptor activation assumes that a receptor exists in one of two conformational states, i.e. a *resting* (or closed) and an *active* (or open) state, with an equilibrium constant that determines the distribution of receptors between the two states. In the case of most receptors, this intrinsic equilibrium favours the inactive conformation and, therefore, receptors tend to be inactive in the absence of ligands.

In this model (Figure 1.4), an *agonist* is a ligand that preferentially binds to the active receptor conformation, using the free energy released to trap a fraction of the receptor molecules in the active state. When the drug has zero affinity for the inactive conformation, the active fraction will eventually exceed the ligand-bound fraction and this ligand is therefore a *full agonist* (e.g. the opioid **methadone**).

This model assumes that *antagonists* (e.g. α- and β-adrenergic blocking agents) bind selectively to the *resting* receptor conformation, shifting receptor equilibrium and thereby reducing receptor activity. This type of drug is also referred to as an *inverse agonist*. In the case of *partial agonists* (e.g. **buprenorphine** on opioid receptors), they should be able to bind to both the active and resting

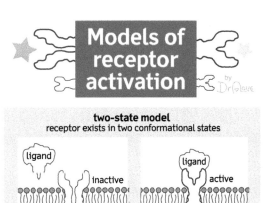

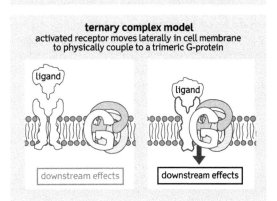

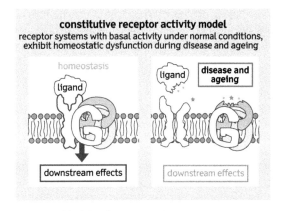

Figure 1.4 Models of receptor activation.

states, but achieve partial activation by having greater affinity for the active conformation. The mostly theoretical assumption of a ligand with perfectly equal affinities for active and resting states, would not change conformational equilibrium and receptor activity. These drugs are defined as *neutral antagonists*, since they could result in an antagonistic effect in the presence of an agonist.

The use of this type of model of receptor activation is central to the study of ligand-gated ion channels, and although this was not always the case for G protein–coupled receptors, it is now acknowledged that both these major families of receptors can observe the same, two-state mechanism of receptor activation.

Ternary complex model

Allosterism is a change in enzyme activity and conformation, following the binding of a ligand or protein at a site other than the active binding site. The model of allosterism was first defined for ion channels and enzymes, and was then used for receptors, leading to the model of the ternary complex for G protein–coupled receptors. Here, the activated receptor can move laterally in the cell membrane to physically couple to a trimeric G protein. In this mechanistic process the sensitivity of the system is dependent on the availability of an external component (i.e. a G protein). The three-component ternary complex model (Figure 1.4), establishes an equilibrium between the ligand-bound receptor and free G protein; and also among the receptor, ligand, and G protein complex.

Constitutive receptor activity model

This model was formulated to reflect the fact that receptors can also naturally form active complexes, resulting from interactions with other proteins in the absence of any ligand, an event denominated *constitutive activity*. This can occur with both G protein–coupled receptors and ion channels, and can reflect both the basal activity in a normally inactive system, as well as the homeostatic dysfunction observed in disease and ageing. Constitutive receptor activation is linked to allosteric transition in receptor states, where changes in the conformation of a receptor can happen through random thermal occurrences, leading to spontaneous activation.

It has now been suggested that receptors are generally in a constitutively active state that is regulated by other cellular factors in normal homeostatic conditions. This could explain why most drugs acting via receptors can function as antagonists.

Receptor types and drug targets

The receptor concept in its simplest form, i.e. a molecular entity capable of responding to the interaction with a ligand, has gradually expanded to incorporate different types of drug targets/receptors.

Transmembrane ion channels

These are pore-forming membrane proteins that gate the flow of ions across biological membranes (see Figure 1.5). Since phospholipid bilayers act as electrical insulators, ion channels constitute a high conducting, hydrophilic pathway across a membrane. This ion movement controls membrane potential and shapes many regulatory processes dependent on electrical signals and downstream Ca^{2+}.

Transmembrane ion channels have a prominent role in the function of neurons and synapses, making them common targets for organisms that want to arrest the nervous systems of predators and prey (e.g. **tetrodotoxin**, a potent neurotoxin). Their capacity to regulate ion conductance and membrane potential means they are also key components in various cellular processes, including muscle contraction, T-cell activation, pancreatic β-cell insulin release, and epithelial transport. These are frequent targets in drug development.

Hundreds of different ion channels have been identified, and are classified according to structure, gating mechanism, and ion permeability. The latter refers to the selective permeability to ions that is dependent on size and/or charge, producing a very high rate of transport through the channel. Since ions move down their electrochemical gradient (dependent on ion concentration and membrane potential), there is no required input of metabolic energy (as is the case in adenosine triphosphate (ATP)/active transport mechanisms, see 'Transporters').

Depending on the mechanism that triggers the conformational change required for channel gating (opening/closing), ion channels are classified into two main categories:

- *ligand-gated ion channels*, which open in response to ligand molecules binding to the extracellular domain.
- *voltage-gated ion channels*, which open following a conformational alteration triggered by changes in membrane potential.

In addition, *second messengers* can also activate ion channels from the intracellular side of the membrane, while *mechanosensitive* channels open under the influence of stretch, pressure, shear, or displacement, and *temperature-gated* channels can open in response to hot or cold temperatures.

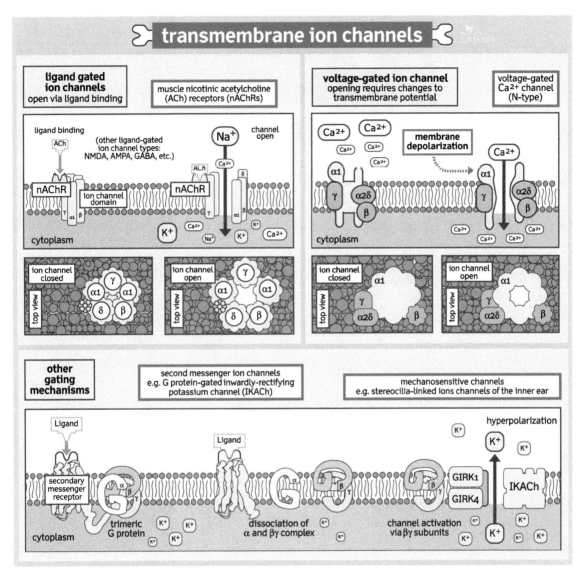

Figure 1.5 Transmembrane ion channels.

Transporters

This group includes membrane-spanning proteins that allow the movement of ions, peptides, small molecules and macromolecules across biological membranes (see Figure 1.6). They are distinguished from channels as the facilitation of movement occurs by physical binding and movement of the substance across the lipid bilayer. The action of transporters can be classified as either:

- *passive*: the transport of a molecule from high to low concentration areas;

- *active*: transport from an area of low to high concentration, which being thermodynamically unfavourable needs to be linked to the energy release of ATP hydrolysis and are thus referred to as ATPases.

Transporters are also classified based on the stoichiometry of the transport process across the membrane. In this way, *uniporters* transport a single molecule at a time, *symporters* transport two different molecules in the same direction simultaneously, and *antiporters* transport two different molecules in opposite directions.

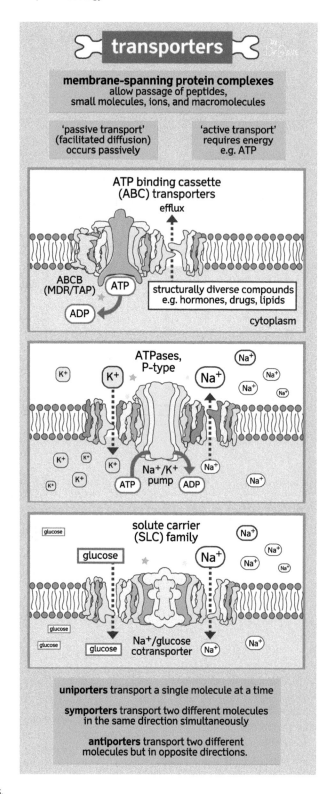

Figure 1.6 Transporters.

7-transmembrane heptahelical G protein–coupled receptors

This constitutes the largest and more diverse group of membrane receptors, with a vast number of functions in the body (see Figure 1.7). It is estimated that between 30 and 50% of drugs available in the market act by targeting this group of receptors. Structurally, they are made by a single polypeptide chain folded in a globular shape with seven segments spanning the entire membrane and intervening loops inside and outside the cell. Their cellular function is accomplished by the capacity to interact with G proteins in the plasma membrane. Binding of the receptor ligand causes a conformational change that triggers the interaction with G proteins.

These specialized heterotrimeric proteins have three different subunits (α, β, and γ), with two attached to the plasma membrane by lipid anchors. When inactive, a guanosine diphosphate (GDP) attaches to the α subunit and the G protein is bound to the receptor complex. The conformational change provoked by binding of the ligand to the receptor, activates the G protein so that a guanosine triphosphate (GTP) replaces the GDP bound to the α subunit. GTP binding leads to the dissociation of the G protein into the GTP-bound α subunit and the β–γ dimer, and both remain attached to the membrane. Membrane diffusion allows the active α subunit to interact with other membrane proteins and thus regulate signalling processes inside the cell. The hydrolysis of GTP back to GDP, promotes the reassembly of the heterotrimeric complex, which is then ready to bind an inactive transmembrane receptor complex.

Nuclear receptors

This includes a superfamily of ligand-activated transcription factors that can regulate the expression of specific genes; thus, controlling a variety of cellular processes in

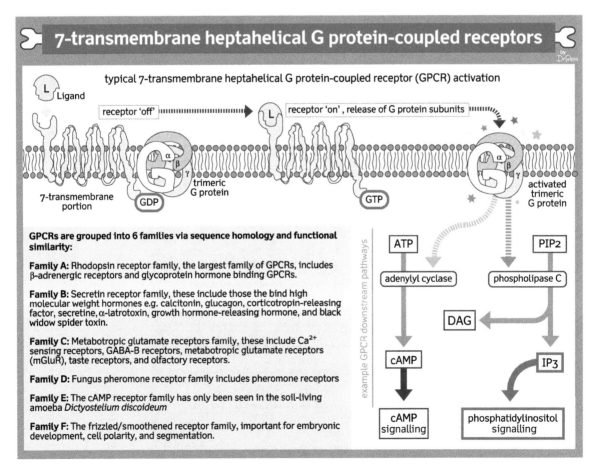

Figure 1.7 7-transmembrane heptahelical G protein-coupled receptors.

differentiation/development, proliferation, metabolism and cell homeostasis (see Figure 1.8). In structural terms, the superfamily is characterized by the presence of an N-terminal transactivation domain, a highly conserved DNA-binding domain, and a C-terminal ligand-binding domain. As well as being activated through ligand-binding, nuclear receptor activity can also be regulated by numerous signalling molecules that result in receptor phosphorylation or other post-translational modifications. These commonly target the transactivation domain in the N-terminus of the protein.

Nuclear receptors are found within the cells; therefore, ligands capable of binding and activating them are lipophilic substances, i.e. steroid hormones. Some of the members of this superfamily have no fully determined ligands, such as metabolic intermediates or xenobiotic endocrine disruptors.

The superfamily can be classified into two broad classes according to their mechanism of action and subcellular distribution when not bound to the ligand

- *Type I*: nuclear receptors bind to their ligands in the cytoplasmic compartment, resulting in dissociation

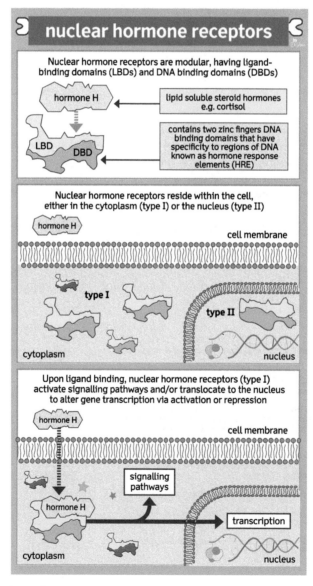

Figure 1.8 Nuclear hormone receptors.

from heat shock proteins, homodimerization, and trans-location into the nucleus. This class includes members such as androgen receptors, oestrogen receptors, and glucocorticoid receptors.

- *Type II*: are located in the nucleus, regardless of ligand-binding status, and bind to the DNA as heterodimers. Examples of receptors that belong to this group are the retinoic acid receptor and thyroid hormone receptor.

Catalytic receptors

These are membrane proteins, usually dimeric, composed of binding and functional domains in one polypeptide chain and includes the cytokine, receptor tyrosine kinase and phosphatase, receptor serine/threonine kinase, and tumour necrosis factor families. The *ligand-binding domain* is located on the extracellular side of the plasma membrane, with a transmembrane-spanning domain comprised of 20–25 amino acids that separates the *functional domain* on the intracellular side. This functional domain has catalytic activity or is capable of interacting with specific enzymes leading to the activation of signalling pathways.

The endogenous agonists are normally peptides or proteins that induce dimerization, which is the functional conformation of the receptor. Classification is based on the particular function of the enzymatic portion of the receptor, and this is depicted in Figure 1.9.

Enzymes

This group, which includes serine/threonine kinase super families, act as efficient catalysts of biochemical reactions by providing an alternative reaction pathway with lower energy of activation. Although they take part in the reaction, enzymes remain unchanged, only altering the rate of the reaction, not the direction of the equilibrium.

The molecular structure of enzymes makes them very specific catalysts for a wide range of reactions. In most cases, enzymes are associated with a non-protein part called a *co-factor*, which includes permanently bound organic groups (prosthetic groups), temporarily bound cations that provide positive charges to the active site and organic molecules. The latter are not permanently bound to the enzyme, but can facilitate its function by associating temporarily with the enzyme-substrate complex.

Enzymes have an *active site*, which has the shape and chemical groups to bind to the reacting molecule, or *substrate*. The catalytic activity of enzymes can be severely affected by changes in temperature and pH. A rise in the former, can increase kinetic energy and promote the

chances of successful collision of enzyme and substrate, thus increasing the reaction rate. Beyond this optimal temperature, intra- and intermolecular bonds can be broken and enzymes begin to denature. Changes in pH can also affect the molecular structure of the protein and thus each enzyme has a narrow range for optimal activity (optimal pH).

The block or distortions of the active site by substances can reduce/stop the catalytic activity of enzymes. These are called enzyme inhibitors and can be divided as *competitive* (active site–directed because they bind to the active site) or *non-competitive* (non-active site–directed because they interact with other parts of the enzyme molecule). Statins are a current example of competitive inhibitors that target HMG-CoA reductase controlling cholesterol biosynthesis. **Nifedipine**, on the contrary, acts as a non-competitive inhibitor of the CYP2C9 enzyme.

The type of binding also divides enzyme inhibitors into reversible or irreversible types. The latter usually changes the enzyme chemically (e.g. covalent bonds), modifying amino acids required for the enzymatic reaction. Reversible inhibitors bind non-covalently, whether to the enzyme, the enzyme-substrate complex or both.

Emerging drug targets

Although not technically grouped as a receptor type, biological research has started to incorporate a variety of new targets as potential options for therapy. These include messenger RNAs, micro- and short-interfering RNAs, non-coding functional elements in the DNA and antibodies. For example, there are many drug-discovery programmes that focus on miRNA-based therapeutics. This is based on numerous studies that show dramatic changes in miRNA populations in many pathological processes. As such, targeting specific miRNAs with modified oligonucleotides [i.e. locked nucleic acid (LNA)] could provide a viable option for therapy. In addition, monoclonal antibody therapy constitutes another emerging field in clinical research, used to specifically target proteins, either to directly block an abnormal function or to stimulate the patient's immune system. In recent years, the use of monoclonal antibodies for cancer therapy has evolved as a powerful new treatment option, with immunomodulatory antibodies also achieving remarkable clinical success. In particular, the development of molecular techniques that can alter antibody pharmacokinetics, effector function, size, and immunogenicity have emerged as crucial factors in the establishment of antibody-based therapies.

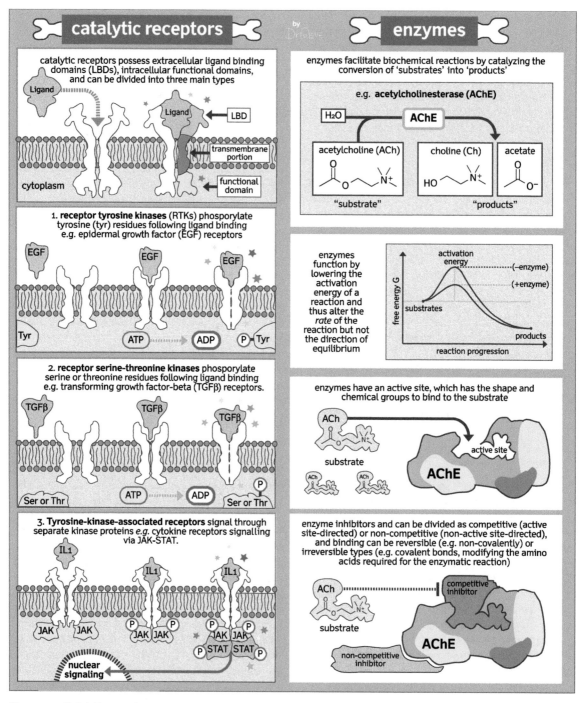

Figure 1.9 Catalytic receptors enzymes.

Receptor regulation

Receptors are subject to diverse regulatory mechanisms that can affect their specific function, location, and association with other proteins, and the degree of signalling coupling. All of which can determine the functional outcome of drug therapy.

Desensitization

The capacity of an agonist to activate a target can be subject to regulation via desensitization of the receptor, a process sometimes referred in the clinic as tachyphylaxis or tolerance (e.g. nitrates). It involves a series of cellular changes that lead to alterations in the receptor and/or its associated signalling pathways, which can weaken the magnitude/duration of signal. The cell can then enter a refractory/unresponsive state, which can result in the decrease/prevention of agonist response. In essence, the desensitization of a receptor is where ligand efficacy is a direct function of the state of the receptor and its previous exposure to agonist, a so-called state-dependent situation.

The mechanisms regulating this process are complex and can involve a variety of cellular processes, including a variety of post-translational modifications (i.e. phosphorylation) that can affect receptor function directly, or lead to its internalization and recycling.

Dimerization/oligomerization

Oligomerization can include both homo- and hetero-oligomeric interactions, i.e. proteins from the same target family or different receptor classes, such as adaptor, scaffold, or chaperone proteins. It has a fundamental role in the regulation of G protein–coupled receptors, receptor protein-tyrosine kinases, and enzymes, and can be ligand-dependent, allosteric, or arise in the absence of a ligand. The functional consequence of this process can be varied and include changes in receptor activation, modulation, and biogenesis, while also capable of affecting the translocation, and thus signalling environment of the target protein.

Endocytosis

The trafficking of a receptor (in its resting or occupied/activated state) away from the surface of the cell or its normal place of action, can directly modify its responsiveness to a ligand, and thus change the functional response. This can be used as a negative (preventing further stimulation) or a positive (interaction with intracellular activators) mechanism to affect the given properties of a particular cell/tissue.

Receptor complexes and allosteric modulation

In traditional receptor theory, it was presumed that affinity and efficacy were autonomous parameters, with no direct link between affinity and the capacity to elicit a full response. However, it has now been proposed that the inconsistent relation between occupancy and efficacy is possibly more indicative of the incapacity to measure receptor-mediated activity. In this scenario, all ligands are potentially capable of exhibiting certain type of efficacy if tested in the correct system, taking into consideration the presence of allosterism, constitutive activity and pluridimensional bias (see Useful definitions boxes).

Useful Definitions

Allosterism and allosteric ligands

An important property of a ligand is the capacity to interact with either the binding site for the endogenous ligand (orthosteric interaction), or a site on the receptor that is able to affect the endogenous ligand through a modification of conformation state (allosteric interaction). For receptors, an allosteric ligand affects the affinity of its related orthosteric counterpart by the allosteric ternary complex model, with the incorporation of a cooperativity factor that acts as a multiplier to modify the dissociation constant of the ligand at the orthosteric site.

In comparison with drugs that have an orthosteric interaction, allosteric modulators have three potential advantages:

- *Saturability*: an allosteric molecule will have a maximal asymptotic effect that occurs when allosteric sites are saturated. This limits the functional effect that can ensue.

- *Probe dependency/selectivity*: since the binding site is distinct from the endogenous ligand and the effect dependent on the degree of cooperativity between the two sites. Permissive actions on receptor function can happen such that different effects can be produced for diverse endogenous agonists.

- *Permissiveness of endogenous basal function*: the actions of an allosteric drug only occur in the presence of the endogenous ligand. As an allosteric modulator can be theoretically quiescent in the absence of the orthosteric ligand, it thus offers an ideal therapeutic option in disease states linked with sporadic or chronotropic receptor-mediated signalling dysfunction.

Useful Definitions

Pluridimensional bias

The pharmacological activity of a ligand is defined by the quantity and type of receptor conformations that the ligand stabilizes in conformational space. Receptors are beginning to be seen as information-processing units with promiscuous interactions, in which ligands can have the capacity to bias receptors towards behaviours/conformations that can have therapeutic applications. Efficacy then becomes dependent on the conformation of the receptor stabilized by a particular ligand and the associated signalling events that this particular conformation can trigger. This has major implications in drug development processes, where the efficacy resulting from the ligand–receptor interaction might be disease-dependent. In this scenario, the analysis of the effects of a drug in 'normal' tissue may lead to incorrect interpretation of therapeutic potential.

Genomic pharmacology

The elucidation of the human genome in 2004, prompted the idea that genome-wide association studies (GWAS) and next-generation (high throughput) sequencing (NGS), would promote the identification of disease-related genes as potential drug targets for the development of novel drugs and therapies. However, this optimism proved rather premature, and while the use of genome-wide technologies led to the association of thousands of loci for disease-related risk and causal genes in disease populations, their contribution to furthering our understanding of pathological mechanisms remains at an early stage.

It is now evident that the quantity and complexity of the accumulated data requires computationally based methods able to integrate and analyse multiple experimental sources into network-system approaches. Ultimately, it would be essential to incorporate the bioinformatics aspects of the networks approach into the armamentarium of disciplines that feed pharmacological sciences research, as was previously done with biochemistry and molecular biology.

Pharmacogenetics/pharmacogenomics

In recent years, these two terms have shown increasing overlap and are normally used to identify the study of genetic variations that influence an individual's response to drugs. A wide range of DNA mutations can affect the chains of chemical reactions that occur in every cell in the body. As such, the identification of genetic variants that can influence drug metabolism and its interaction with the specific drug targets are some of the main goals of pharmacogenetics/pharmacogenomics. The appeal of this approach is the possibility of personalized medicine, where information of an individual's genetic make-up would better enable physicians to define the nature of disease, thereby finding the most effective treatment with minimal side effects.

This is important in the context of a genetically variable population, where there is a higher probability of failure for biologicals drugs, since individuals may not express the precise amino-acid sequence that a ligand requires to bind (e.g. anti-TNF products). This is not the case for small molecules, which have a much more forgiving therapeutic index (TI). However, despite the relevance that should be assigned to genetic variations among human populations, it must not be ignored that environmental factors, together with diet, age, co-morbid disease, and lifestyle, can all influence the response of a patient to a drug treatment.

Pharmacokinetics

Although potency, efficacy, and selectivity are all key properties of a compound as a therapeutic option, for a chemical to become a drug it must be appropriately taken into the body, spread to the right tissue, metabolized without precluding its activity and eliminated in an appropriate manner (see Figure 1.10). In summary, failure to consider pharmacokinetics within the study of a compound/drug/NCE could have detrimental effects in the drug discovery process, clinical efficacy, and medical treatment. *Pharmacokinetics* encompasses four key processes—absorption, distribution, metabolism, and excretion.

Useful Definitions

- *Pharmacokinetics*: the analysis of the time course of the absorption, distribution, metabolism, and excretion (ADME) of a drug, compound, or NCE after administration to the body, i.e. what the body does to the drug.

- *Pharmacodynamics*: the study of the interaction between the concentration of a compound, drug, or NCE is the target site, the location of this therapeutic target, and the magnitude of the elicited response, i.e. what the drug does to the body.

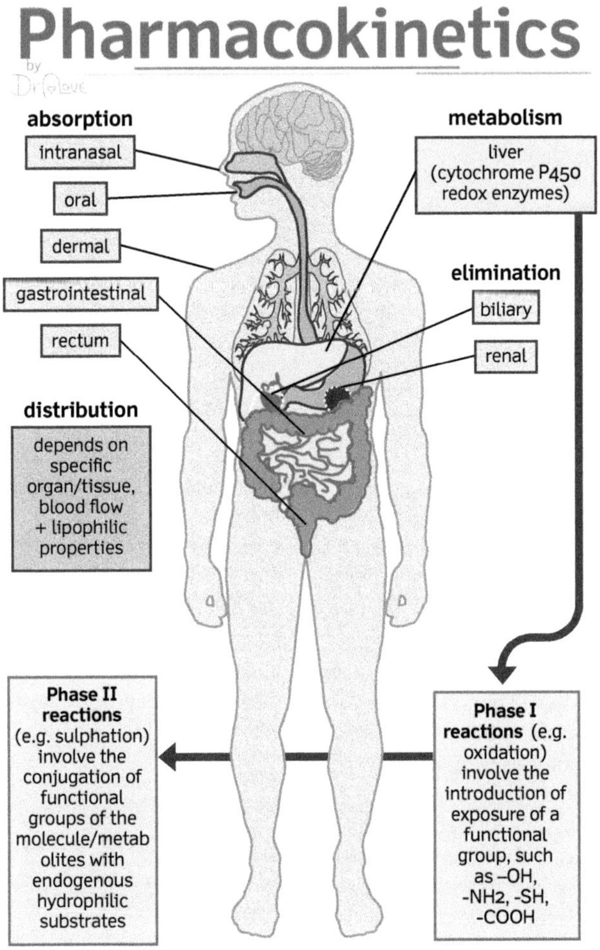

Pharmacokinetics

by
Dr Olove

absorption

- intranasal
- oral
- dermal
- gastrointestinal
- rectum

metabolism

- liver (cytochrome P450 redox enzymes)

elimination

- biliary
- renal

distribution

depends on specific organ/tissue, blood flow + lipophilic properties

Phase II reactions (e.g. sulphation) involve the conjugation of functional groups of the molecule/metabolites with endogenous hydrophilic substrates

Phase I reactions (e.g. oxidation) involve the introduction of exposure of a functional group, such as –OH, -NH2, -SH, -COOH

Figure 1.10 Pharmacokinetics overview.

Absorption

Absorption is the process by which a medicine moves from its site of administration to enter the systemic circulation. As most drugs are administered orally, absorption from the gastrointestinal (GI) tract is the most common mechanism. However, there are numerous sites from which a medication can be absorbed into the blood stream (see Box 1.1). *Bioavailability* is the proportion of unchanged drug that reaches the systemic circulation and can be influenced by drug properties, formulation, and specific patient factors.

In order for a compound to be absorbed it needs to permeate cellular membranes. In the case of orally administered solid forms, *disintegration* into a suspension must occur, followed by *dissolution* in the GI fluid. The process of disintegration is usually relatively fast, whereas *dissolution* or *permeability* tend to be rate-limiting steps. The rate of dissolution of a compound is a function of aqueous solubility, particle surface area, and the dissolution rate constant. These are all taken into consideration when medicines are formulated. In practical terms, dissolution rates can be improved by:

- increasing aqueous solubility through elevation in temperature or changing the pH in the case of ionizable compounds;
- decreasing particle size, thereby increasing the surface area to volume ratio available for solvation;
- augmenting the dissolution rate constant (e.g. by agitation of the medium).

The *permeability* of a compound is dependent on its lipophilicity (in order to partition into membranes from

Box 1.1 Sites of administration/drug absorption

- Gastrointestinal tract (oral; PO)
- Skin (topical)
- Cutaneous tissue (subcutaneous; SC)
- Nasal epithelium (intranasal; IN)
- Muscle (intramuscular; IM)
- Buccal cavity (buccal)
- Rectum (per rectum; PR)
- Vagina (per vagina; PV)
- Eye (topical, intraocular)
- Ear (topical)
- Peritoneum (intraperitoneum)
- Lung (inhaled)

an aqueous environment), molecular size, and charge. Patient factors, such as intestinal membrane permeability, the effective surface area of membrane available for permeation, and the concentration in the GI fluid will also influence permeation.

The absorption of drug into the systemic circulation can also be influenced by the extent of metabolism before it reaches the blood for general distribution, i.e. the gut (with digestive enzymes), the gut wall (with monoamine oxidase enzymes (see CYP, 'Metabolism')), and the liver can all metabolize a drug so that only a small proportion reaches target sites. This process of absorptive metabolism is termed first-pass metabolism. Importantly, some potent first-pass metabolism effects can be counteracted by using alternative sites of absorption, such as rectal, intramuscular, intravenous, or sublingual administration.

Useful Definitions

- *First-pass metabolism*: a process of drug metabolism where the concentration of a drug is reduced before it can enter the systemic circulation. It is defined by the intestinal and hepatic degradation/alteration of a drug or substance after absorption. Enzymes of the GI lumen, gut wall, bacteria, and/or liver can all affect first-pass metabolism.

Distribution

Distribution is the process by which a drug moves in and out of body tissues, having been absorbed into the systemic circulation. *Volume of distribution* (V_D) is the concentration of drug in the plasma relative to the total amount in the body and depends on the extent to which the drug is protein bound and degree of lipophilicity. Drugs that are highly protein bound (e.g. **doxycycline**) will tend to remain in the systemic circulation, whereas those that are highly lipophilic (e.g. **fluoxetine**) will diffuse more readily across cell membranes into tissue, and thus have a larger volume of distribution (i.e. $V_D > 15$ L). Substrates for active transporters are also more likely to have a large volume of distribution. When the V_D is < 5 L drugs will be highly retained in a person's vasculature; V_D can be calculated by the equation:

$$V_D = \text{Dose} / C_o,$$

which shows the calculation for volume of distribution (V_D) where C_o is the initial apparent plasma concentration.

Metabolism

For most drugs, metabolism is the main process of elimination. The intestine, kidney, lung, plasma, red blood cells, placenta, skin, and brain are all metabolic entities; however, the liver is the main organ that deals with the metabolism of xenobiotics via redox enzymes (e.g. cytochrome P450; CYP450). In general, drug metabolism involves an enzymatic process that converts a lipophilic compound into more hydrophilic metabolites, which facilitates their excretion in bile or urine. This is achieved by two main types of metabolic reactions:

- *Phase I reactions* (comprising reduction, oxidation, and hydrolysis): include the introduction or exposure of a functional group, such as –OH, -COOH, -SH, -NH2.
- *Phase II metabolism* (including N-acetylation, methylation, glutathione conjugation, amino acid conjugation, glucoronidation, sulphation): the conjugation of functional groups of the molecule/metabolites with endogenous hydrophilic substrates.

There is huge isoform diversity and population/species polymorphism in CYP450 enzymes, which presents a challenge for predicting pharmacokinetics (e.g. due to inter-individual variation in expression and drug interactions) and, hence, the outcome of drug development (i.e. preclinical to clinical species or regional population differences). Given that CYP450 isoenzymes are responsible for around 75% of drug metabolism processes, changes in expression and enzyme function can have a marked impact on drug pharmacokinetics. Moreover, drugs and natural compounds, like grapefruit juice, can modify CYP450 enzyme function, further influencing drug metabolism (see 'Drug interactions').

Importantly, metabolites should also be considered, as some are pharmacologically active and may be even more so than the parent drug. A *pro-drug* is a precursor chemical compound of a drug that is administered in its inactive or possibly less active form, and subsequently converted to its activated form via normal metabolic pathways. The list of pro-drugs is extensive, and includes drugs such as **valaciclovir**, **mercaptopurine**, **levodopa**, **carbamazepine**, **acetylsalicylate**, and many more. They are classified into two major groups based on the site of bioactivation, with Type I activated intracellularly, and Type II extracellularly. Pro-drugs are particularly useful when absorption is challenging, e.g. **dexamethasone phosphate**. They are normally designed to improve bioavailability, and may contribute to the avoidance of side effects and/or improve selectivity for target tissues.

Excretion

The excretion of a compound denotes its irreversible removal from the body. In pharmacokinetic terms, systemic clearance is expressed as the volume of blood or plasma cleared of a compound from the body per unit of time. There are two major routes of elimination—renal and biliary excretion.

Renal excretion is determined by glomerular filtration, active tubular secretion and reabsorption, and renal metabolism. Compounds eliminated by renal secretion have relatively low molecular weight, and are hydrophilic or are slowly transformed in the liver to be so (see phase I and phase II reactions above).

Hepatic clearance is the main way of excretion for blood-borne particles not undergoing renal clearance. After entering hepatocytes via endocytosis a compound undergoes metabolism and biliary excretion, which occurs through canalicular membranes surrounding the bile canaliculi of hepatocytes. The reticuloendothelial system in Kupffer cells can also produce independent degradation and intracellular removal of particles in the liver.

It is important to consider that large molecules, such as proteins and therapeutic antibodies, have different pharmacokinetic profiles to those of small molecules. In general, proteins are broken down into amino acids and re-utilized in endogenous protein synthesis. Therapeutic antibodies are excluded from renal filtration owing to their large molecular size, and are cleared slowly with long half-lives (7–23 days).

From the mathematical modelling perspective, plasma clearance is the sum of all clearance processes and the rate this occurs depends on the volume of plasma to be cleared per minute (CL), and the total voume that has to be cleared (V):

$$k = CL / V$$

Such that plasma half-life ($t_{1/2}$) can be calculated by:

$$t_{1/2} = 0.693 \, V / CL$$

where CL (mL/min) = rate of elimination (mg/min)/ [plasma concentration] (mg/mL).

The process of clearance is constant and characteristic for a given drug, so the greater the value, the more rapidly a drug is removed. For this to remain predictable, a drug must not saturate the system and follow first order kinetics, so that clearance occurs only from delivered plasma. Some drugs can remain in tissues; here, the volume of distribution is high and the elimination rate constant is therefore low.

Most drugs follow first-order elimination kinetic characteristics, a process that is concentration dependant, and exponential decay/loss over time as a *constant proportion* of drug is eliminated per unit of time. Intravenously administered drugs typically follow this pattern, but some drugs may follow a zero-order elimination profile, where drug loss occurs at a *constant rate* and is unaffected by concentration (Figure 1.11). Alcohol, salicylates, and **phenytoin** are examples of zero-order drugs, as enzymes

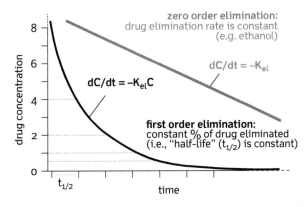

Figure 1.11 Zero first-order elimination. First-order and zero-order kinetic elimination profiles for circulating drugs. Drugs following first-order kinetics (e.g. diazepam) are characterized by exponential decay as a proportion of concentration. While drugs that follow zero-order elimination profiles (e.g. alcohol) saturate the metabolizing enzymes so decay is linear and independent of concentration.

responsible for their metabolism become saturated and they are no longer affected by drug concentration.

Part 2: Drug development and the healthcare marketplace

Drug development

The process of drug development starts when a new (e.g. synthesized molecule), or old but forgotten (e.g. plant extract) chemical entity is thought or shown experimentally to modify a disease process in a positive/beneficial way. This modification may be through any number of signalling mechanisms, enzyme action, chelation of toxic substances, or alterations in gene function, and this modulation may be with a chemical or biopharmaceutical compound (Table 1.1).

Clinical pharmacology (preclinical studies)

To become a licenced product, all drugs need to demonstrate clear efficacy, quality, and safety such that the

benefits of prescribing outweigh the risks (see Figure 1.12). Therefore, proof of concept studies provide important criteria for further development and dictate whether investors will support progress to the high expenditure areas of drug development progressing towards licencing and before first human studies.

The specific studies required, including the length of pre-clinical drug exposures and the in-depth assessment of specific organ systems, are heavily dependent on the proposed mechanisms of action and typically include toxicology, genotoxicology, and safety studies

Clinical development (clinical studies)

Human clinical trials aim to establish the pharmacology (PK and PD), adverse reactions, safety, and efficacy. Each phase of clinical studies have different goals in mind (e.g. Phase I studies include first in human, while Phase II studies are efficacy studies in patients who possess the clinical condition) designed across a developmental programme utilizing a benefit–risk-based approach.

Table 1.1 Differentiating chemical and biological drugs

Chemical medicines	Biopharmaceuticals
Low molecular weight (<1000 Dalton)	High molecular weight (>10 000 Dalton)
Produced by chemical synthesis	Produced by living cell cultures
Function predominantly intracellularly	Function predominantly extracellularly
Well-defined structure	Complex, heterogeneous structure
Mostly process-independent	Strongly process-dependent
Completely characterized	Impossible to fully characterize the molecular composition and heterogeneity
Stable	Unstable, sensitive to external conditions
Mostly non-immunogenic	Immunogenic
Oral administration	Parenteral administration
Cost of goods low	Coat of goods high
Hepatic metabolism/renal clearance	Degradation by plasma and tissue enzymes
Active in multiple species	Species restriction
Chemical toxicity	Potent pharmacological action

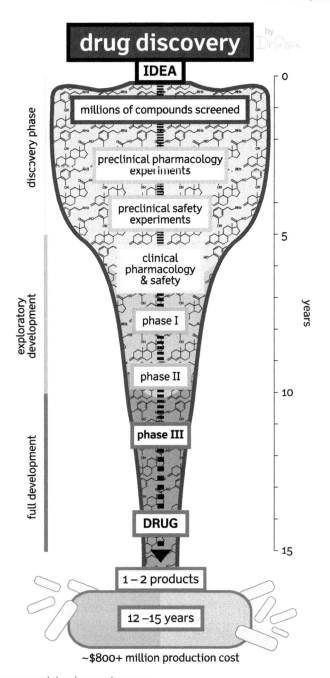

Figure 1.12 The drug discovery and development process.

License, marketing, and pharmacovigilance

For a drug to be licenced and available for mainstream prescribing, a marketing authorization application must first be submitted to a competent authority (e.g. Medicines and

Healthcare products Regulatory Agency; MHRA, European Medicines Agency; EMA, Food and Drug Administration; FDA), which will assess and review all submitted evidence, both non-clinical and clinical data, and make judgment. Licences are initially granted for 5 years. A key document is the summary of product characteristics (SPC) and includes chemical, clinical (including posology), pharma-cological and pharmaceutical properties (see http://www.medicines.org.uk/emc/).

Pharmacovigilance (PV) involves the detection of drug-related adverse events and their subsequent reporting. Most PV occurs during post-marketing and is a sensitive measure of 'real life' risk-benefit. From the healthcare pro-vider perspective there are three main methods by which significant PV issues can be raised. The most common spontaneous reporting system in the UK is the 'Yellow Card Scheme' where 'anyone' can submit ADR to the MHRA (some 25,000 submissions/year). Yellow cards (Figure 1.13) are in the British National Formulary (BNF), Monthly Index of Medical Specialities (MIMs) or online. Newer drugs (within 5 years of licencing) may also pos-sess a black triangle (▼) next to their name indicating 'additional monitoring'. Sporadic and spontaneous re-porting by healthcare professionals or consumers may also occur by unsolicited communications to a company, non-governmental organizations, or regulatory authority.

Part 3: Evidence-based prescribing

Prescribing

Prescribing is the act of authorizing the use of a medicine or medical device in someone for the purpose of treat-ment, usually in writing, or electronically, Before doing so, the prescriber must ensure that the medicine is being used appropriately, and that the benefits of giving out-weigh any risks. They must, therefore, ensure that their knowledge of the medicines they prescribe is up to date in order to justify any decision-making, as ultimate responsi-bility lies with the person signing the prescription. Where possible, the patient should be involved in any decisions made and thus consent obtained, verbally or otherwise. The prescription itself must comply with the law and rele-vant standards laid out by professional bodies such as the General Medical Council (GMC), National Prescribing Centre (NPC), Nursing and Midwifery Council; NMC and General Pharmaceutical Council (GPhC).

The clinical drug history

Medicines reconciliation

Medicines reconciliation is the gathering of accurate and reliable information of the medication(s) a patient is taking and should be carried out every time a patient is transferred between care settings. It is not simply a pro-cess of recording the patient's most recent medication list, but being aware of any changes or discrepancies that may exist, such as medicines discontinued for poor tolerance or verbal instructions to amend doses. Within secondary care a significant number of medication errors occur at admission and discharge, some of which have resulted in severe harm and even fatalities. Accurate medicines reconciliation is intended to reduce the risk of errors and therefore harm, and is based on the principle of right pa-tient, right drug, right dose, and right time. The process is divided into two stages.

- *Stage 1*: basic reconciliation is the complete and ac-curate documentation of a patient's current medication list to include both prescription and non-prescription medication, i.e. over the counter purchases and compli-mentary/alternative therapy. Documentation for each drug should include the approved name, form, route, dose, and frequency.

- *Stage 2*: full reconciliation is the identification and reso-lution of discrepancies between the current medication list, and what the patient is actually taking, clearly documented in the patient's notes.

Adverse drug reactions and allergies

Adverse drug reactions are defined by WHO as a nox-ious and unintended response to a drug that occurs at doses usually prescribed in humans. They are thought to occur in about 10–20% of hospital admissions, with the risk increased in the elderly or those with pre-existing morbidities. In 10–20% of cases reactions are severe, re-sulting in significant morbidity and mortality.

Reactions can be subdivided into type A (predictable and dose dependant) and type B (unpredictable and non-dose dependant) reactions, of which the latter includes allergies, defined by WHO as a hypersensitivity response known to be immunologically-mediated. Responses may be of B-cell or T-cell origin and most commonly result in cutaneous manifestations (in 80% of cases), although can affect any system, giving rise to reactions such as pneumonitis, nephritis, agranulocytosis, or thrombocyto-penia (see Table 1.2). Type B reactions occur less com-monly, accounting for less than 20% of all ADRs, but tend to be more severe.

Hypersensitivity reactions have historically been classi-fied according to the Gell–Coombs classification system (see Table 1.3), but may also be defined according to the major organ system involved or the rate of onset of symptoms.

YellowCard

It's easy to report online: www.mhra.gov.uk/yellowcard

MHRA

COMMISSION ON HUMAN MEDICINES (CHM)

SUSPECTED ADVERSE DRUG REACTIONS

If you suspect an adverse reaction may be related to one or more drugs/vaccines/complementary remedies, please complete this Yellow Card. See 'Adverse reactions to drugs' section in BNF or **www.mhra.gov.uk/yellowcard** for guidance. Do not be put off reporting because some details are not known.

PATIENT DETAILS   Patient Initials: _____ Sex: M / F   Ethnicity: _____   Weight if known (kg): _____

Age (at time of reaction):_____   Identification number (e.g. Your Practice or Hospital Ref): _____

SUSPECTED DRUG(S)/VACCINE(S)

Drug/Vaccine (Brand if known)	Batch	Route	Dosage	Date started	Date stopped	Prescribed for

SUSPECTED REACTION(S) Please describe the reaction(s) and any treatment given:

Outcome
Recovered ☐
Recovering ☐
Continuing ☐
Other ☐

Date reaction(s) started: _____   Date reaction(s) stopped: _____

Do you consider the reactions to be serious? Yes / No

If yes, please indicate why the reaction is considered to be serious (please tick all that apply):
Patient died due to reaction ☐   Involved or prolonged inpatient hospitalisation ☐
Life threatening ☐   Involved persistent or significant disability or incapacity ☐
Congenital abnormality ☐   Medically significant; please give details: _____

OTHER DRUG(S) (including self-medication and complementary remedies)

Did the patient take any other medicines/vaccines/complementary remedies in the last 3 months prior to the reaction? Yes / No
If yes, please give the following information if known:

Drug/Vaccine (Brand if known)	Batch	Route	Dosage	Date started	Date stopped	Prescribed for

Additional relevant information e.g. medical history, test results, known allergies, rechallenge (if performed), suspect drug interactions. For congenital abnormalities please state all other drugs taken during pregnancy and the last menstrual period.

Please list any medicines obtained from the internet:

REPORTER DETAILS
Name and Professional Address: _____

Postcode:_____ Tel No: _____
Email:_____
Speciality:_____
Signature:_____ Date:_____

CLINICIAN (if not the reporter)
Name and Professional Address: _____

Postcode:_____ Tel No: _____
Email:_____
Speciality:_____
Date:_____

Information on adverse drug reactions received by the MHRA can be downloaded at **www.mhra.gov.uk/daps**
Stay up-to-date on the latest advice for the safeuse of medicines with our monthly bulletin *Drug Safety Update* at **www.mhra.gov.uk/drugsafetyupdate**

Please attach additional pages if necessary. Send to: FREEPOST YELLOW CARD (no other address details required)

Figure 1.13 Yellow card of suspected adverse drug reaction.

Table 1.2 Drug allergies by system

System	Reaction	Examples of causative drugs
Cutaneous	Erythema multiforme	Sulfonamides, anti-convulsants, penicillins, anti-TB drugs
	Urticaria	Antibiotics
	Angioedema	Antibiotics
	Fixed drug eruptions	Allopurinol, anti-epileptics, antibiotics, NSAIDs, PPIs
	Stevens–Johnson	Allopurinol, anti-epileptics, antibiotics, NSAIDs, thiazide
	Toxic epidermal necrosis	Allopurinol, anti-epileptics, antibiotics, NSAIDs, thiazides
Pulmonary	Bronchospasm	NSAIDs, β-blockers
	Pneumonitis/pulmonary fibrosis	Amiodarone, nitrofurantoin, bleomycin
Haematological	Thrombocytopenia	Heparin, sulfonamides, gold, quinidine, procainamide, allopurinol
	Agranulocytosis	Clozapine, sulfonamides, carbimazole, rituximab
	Haemolytic anaemia	Penicillin, cephalosporins, amiodarone, NSAIDs, methyldopa
Renal	Interstitial nephritis	Antibiotics, NSAIDs, diuretics, allopurinol, anti-convulsants
	Nephrotic syndrome	NSAIDs, sulfonamides, gold, penicillamine
Hepatic	Hepatitis	Methyldopa, nitrofurantoin, diclofenac
	Cholestatic jaundice	Antibiotics, anti-TB, anti-convulsants, methyldopa

The most common drug hypersensitivity reactions occur with antibiotics (penicillins, cephalosporins, and sulfonamides), **aspirin**, and non-steroidal anti-inflammatory drugs (NSAIDs). However, although 1 in 10 patients report that they have a penicillin allergy, in reality about 90% of these may safely receive penicillin. It is, therefore, essential that both the allergen and nature of any allergic reaction is recorded.

PRACTICAL PRESCRIBING
Documenting allergies
- Over and under reporting of allergies is common.
- Patients commonly confuse adverse drug reactions for allergies.
- Incorrectly documenting a patient as being allergic to a medication could preclude the use of potentially life-saving treatment.
- Always document the allergen and the nature of reaction.
- Be aware of drugs that have cross-hypersensitivities, e.g. penicillins and cephalosporins.

Drug interactions

Drug interactions can be broadly divided into *pharmacodynamic* and *pharmacokinetic* interactions.

Pharmacodynamic interactions

Pharmacodynamic interactions occur as a result of two or more drugs interfering at their site of action, giving rise to additive or antagonistic effects, and can be predicted from an understanding of their mechanisms of action.

- *Additive effects*: when administered together, two drugs that induce the same pharmacological effect on the body, can lead to an increase in both the desired and unwanted effects. In some instances, this interaction may be intentional, for example, combining two anti-hypertensives when a single agent is inadequate. In other situations, however, particularly with unwanted effects, the outcome may be harmful, e.g. excessive sedation or profound hypotension. A good understanding of a drugs unwanted effects helps reduce the risk of doing harm.

Table 1.3 Gell–Coombs classification system

Gel–Coombs classification	Definition	Common causes
Type 1; IgE-mediated	Occur immediately after administration, e.g. anaphylaxis, urticarial, angioedema, bronchospasm	Most commonly occurs secondary to antibiotics
Type 2; Cytotoxic reactions	IgG-mediated cytotoxicity targeting erythrocytes, platelets, haematopoetic precursor cells, etc., resulting in cytopenias, vasculitis	Heparin, methyldopa, quinidine, penicillin
Type 3; Immune complex reactions	Formation of an immune complex, usually of no significance, but sometimes binds to endothelial cells, leading to deposition in small vessels, e.g. serum sickness, vasculitis	Thymoglobulin, penicillin, procainamide
Type 4; Cell-mediated reactions	T-cell mediated reactions that affect the skin (contact sensitivity) or cause systemic disease	Topical agents (neomycin, corticosteroids), sulfonamides and β-lactams

From Gell, P. and Coombs, R. (eds.) (1962). *Clinical Aspects of Immunology*. Oxford: Blackwell. Reproduced courtesy of John Wiley and Sons via PLS Clear.

- *Antagonistic effects*: drugs with opposing effects used concomitantly can lead to reduced efficacy and therapeutic failure if this is not accounted for when prescribing. For example, corticosteroids can induce hyperglycaemia and, therefore, reduce effectiveness of oral hypoglycaemics. Such interactions can be utilized to overcome adverse reactions, without affecting the desired therapeutic effects, e.g. the use of **domperidone** to antagonize the emetic effects of anti-Parkinson's therapy without affecting therapeutic effect, as it does not cross the blood–brain barrier.

Pharmacokinetic interactions

Pharmacokinetic interactions occur when one drug alters the way in which a second drug is handled by the body and can be predicted from an understanding of their absorption, distribution, metabolism, and excretion.

- *Absorption*: drug absorption can be enhanced or impaired when drugs are combined, either by binding directly, e.g. ion exchange resins (**colestyramine**) or by altering gastrointestinal GI pH. For many drugs, absorption is pH dependent, so that co-administration with drugs that alter pH can affect oral bioavailability, e.g. proton pump inhibitors.

- *Distribution*: drug interactions that occur as a result of altered drug distribution are uncommon, although there may be some impact from drugs that affect extracellular fluid or where highly protein-bound drugs compete for binding sites, thereby increasing the levels of free drugs. In patients with normal renal function, an increase in unbound drug is usually compensated for by an increase in renal clearance and is rarely associated with clinically significant interactions.

- *Metabolism*: altered metabolism accounts for the majority of clinically significant drug interactions and occurs as a result of altered enzyme activity, leading to enhanced or impaired metabolic function. Of these, the most clinically relevant are those that affect the cytochrome P450 enzyme system involved in phase I type reactions. The extent of the effect depends on a number of factors, such as the number of metabolic pathways involved, and also on the degree of inhibition or induction exerted by the affecting drug. Drugs that are metabolized by multiple pathways are therefore less likely to be significantly affected by enzyme inhibitors or inducers, compared to those reliant on a single pathway that has been modified. Table 1.4 gives examples of common substrates, inducers and inhibitors of the CYP 450 enzyme system, with potent inhibitors/inducers denoted by an asterisk (*).

- *Excretion*: the clearance of drugs normally excreted via the kidney can be affected when used in combination with a second drug that alters urinary pH or renal blood flow, or competes for the same active transport mechanism. Passive diffusion across the lipid membrane of the tubule occurs only when the drug is in its non-ionizable form, thus clearance of weakly acidic or basic drugs can be affected where a second drug changes

Table 1.4 Common substrates, inducers and inhibitors of the CYP450 enzyme system, with potent inhibitors/inducers denoted by an asterisk (*)

	Substrates	Inducers	Inhibitors
CYP1A2	Amitriptyline	Broccoli	Amiodarone*
	Caffeine	Brussel sprouts	Cimetidine*
	Clomipramine	Carbamazepine*	Fluvoxamine*
	Haloperidol	Omeprazole	Fluoroquinolones*
	Naproxen	Phenobarbital*	
	Olanzapine	Rifampicin*	
	Ondansetron	Tobacco*	
	Paracetamol		
	Propranolol		
	Theophylline		
	Verapamil		
	Warfarin		
CYP2B6	Cyclophosphamide	Phenobarbital	Ticlopidine
	Efavirenz	Rifampicin	
	Methadone		
CYP2C8	Paclitaxel	Rifampicin	Gemfibrozil
	Rapaglinide		Glitazones
			Montelukast
			Trimethoprim
CYP2C9	Amitriptyline	Carbamazepine*	Amiodarone*
	Celecoxib	Phenobarbital*	Fenofibrate
	Diclofenac	Phenytoin*	Fluconazole*
	Fluoxetine	Rifampicin*	Fluvastatin
	Fluvastatin		Isoniazid
	Glibenclaimide		Probenacid
	Glipizide		Ritonavir*
	Ibuprofen		Sertaline
	Irbesartan		Zafirlukast
	Losartan		
	Meloxicam		
	Naproxen		
	Phenytoin		
	Rosiglitazone		
	Tamoxifen		
	Warfarin		

Table 1.4 Continued

	Substrates	Inducers	Inhibitors
CYP2C19	Amitriptyline	Carbamazepine*	Chloramphenicol
	Chloramphenicol	Norethisterone	Cimetidine
	Citalopram	Phenytoin*	Fluoxetine
	Cyclophosphamide	Prednisolone	Fluvoxamine*
	Diazepam	Rifampicin*	Indometacin
	Imipramine		Isoniazid*
	Indometacin		Ketoconazole
	Lansoprazole		Lansoprazole
	Omeprazole		Omeprazole
	Pantoprazole		Oxcarbazepine
	Phenobarbital		Probenecid
	Phenytoin		Ritonavir*
	Rabeprazole		Topiramate
	Warfarin		
CYP2D6	Amitriptyline	Dexamethasone	Amiodarone*
	Carvedilol		Bupropion
	Chlorphenamine		Celecoxib
	Chlorpromazine		Chlorphenamine
	Clomipramine		Chlorpromazine
	Codeine		Cimetidine
	Duloxetine		Citalopram
	Flecainide		Duloxetine
	Fluoxetine		Escitalopram
	Haloperidol		Fluoxetine*
	Imipramine		H1 antagonists
	Lidocaine		Levomepromazine
	Metoclopramide		Methadone
	Nebivolol		Metoclopramide
	Ondansetron		Paroxetine*
	Oxycodone		Quinidine*
	Paroxetine		Ritonavir*
	Propranolol		Sertraline
	Risperidone		Terbinafine*
	Tamoxifen		Ticlopidine
	Tramadol		
	Venlafaxine		

(continued)

Table 1.4 Continued

	Substrates	Inducers	Inhibitors
CYP2E1	Enflurane	Ethanol	Disulfram
	Ethanol	Isoniazid	
	Haloflurane		
	Isoflurane		
	Paracetamol		
	Sevoflurane		
	Theophylline		
CYP3A4	Amlodipine	Carbamazepine*	Amiodarone
	Atorvastatin	Oxcarbazepine	Cimetidine
	Chlorphenamine	Phenobarbital*	Ciprofloxacin
	Ciclosporin	Phenytoin*	Clarithromycin*
	Clarithromycin	Piogltazone	Diltiazem*
	Dexamethasone	Rifabutin	Erythromycin*
	Diazepam	Rifampicin*	Fluvoxamine
	Diltiazem	St John's Wort*	Grapefruit juice*
	Domperidone	Troglitazone	Indinavir
	Erythromycin		Itraconazole*
	Felodipine		Ketoconazole*
	Fentanyl		Ritonavir*
	Finasteride		Verapamil*
	Haloperidol		
	Methadone		
	Midazolam		
	Nifedipine		
	Propranolol		
	Quetiapine		
	Risperidone		
	Ritonavir		
	Simvastatin		
	Tacrolimus		
	Tamoxifen		

urinary pH and the extent of ionization. In some scenarios urine is intentionally made more alkaline to facilitate excretion and therefore prevent toxicity, e.g. the use of **sodium bicarbonate** to prevent **methotrexate** toxicity when administered at high doses.

Administration of two drugs that compete for the same active transport system (e.g. methotrexate and penicillins) can impair clearance leading to increased toxicity, particularly when it involves drugs with a narrow therapeutic index.

The prescription

A prescription should be written in such a way that it is easily legible and not open to misinterpretation, meeting the legal requirements laid out in Box 1.2.

Box 1.2 Legal requirements for writing a prescription

- Legible
- Indelible ink
- Date
- Patient's name and address
- Prescriber's name and address
- Type of prescriber (doctor, dentist, non-medical)
- Age/date of birth—legal requirement if under 12 years
- Approved drug name (not generic or abbreviation)
- Preparation/route of administration (e.g. tablet, enema)
- Dose (avoid unnecessary decimal places)
- Units (do not abbreviate micrograms, units, nanograms)
- Frequency
- Quantity to supply or duration of therapy
- Prescriber's signature

Typically, rescriptions should state the approved generic drug name, although there are instances where a drug may be prescribed by brand, particularly where different brands of the same drug do not show bioequivalence, e.g. **tacrolimus**. Similarly, abbreviations may be used provided they are widely accepted (see Table 1.5 for examples).

Controlled drugs

The Misuse of Drugs Regulations 2001, lists the legal schedule of drugs susceptible to abuse and outlines the processes that must be followed for their storage and supply. Drugs are divided into five schedules, of which the first denotes drugs without medicinal benefit (e.g. cannabis, ecstasy, raw opium) and may not, therefore, be prescribed. Of the drugs that may be prescribed, the supply and storage must fulfil the pre-set criteria laid out within the schedule (see Table 1.6).

In addition to the requirements laid out in Table 1.6, prescriptions for controlled drugs must fulfil further legal requirements so as to include:

- Form and strength, where more than one strength exists.
- Total quantity to be supplied in words and figures.
- Handwritten signature (see exceptions below).
- 'For dental treatment only' if supplied by a dentist.
- Maximum of 30 days' supply.

Advanced electronic signatures will only be accepted for schedule 2 and 3 drugs where the Electronic Prescribing Service is used, the handwriting requirement for the rest of the prescription is no longer essential.

Table 1.5 Common prescribing abbreviations

	Abbreviation	Definition
Route	PO	Oral
	IV	Intravenous
Frequency	OD	Once a day
	BD	Twice a day
	TDS	Three times a day
	QDS	Four times a day
Timing	OM	In the morning
	NN	Noon
	ON	At night

Reproduced from Flockhart DA. Drug Interactions: Cytochrome P450 Drug Interaction Table. Indiana University School of Medicine (2007). https://drug-interactions.medicine.iu.edu

Other good practice points laid out by the NPC identifies the inclusion of patient's NHS number and prescriber details, such as registration numbers, full name, address, and contact details for the purpose of queries (Figure 1.14). Due to their potential for abuse, no more than 30 days of a controlled drug (CD) should be prescribed and the prescription must be dispensed within 28 days of it being written.

Monitoring

Monitoring is carried out to ensure the efficacy and tolerance of a given treatment. The intensity of monitoring depends on the balance of risk to benefit, so that drugs with a high tendency for adverse effects and a low tendency for being effective will require more intense monitoring. When monitoring for efficacy, consideration should be given to the desired effect and expected time to elicit a response (reach steady state), as well as making sure doses are titrated appropriately.

For some drugs toxicity, monitoring criteria is outlined in the SPC or by regulatory bodies such as the MHRA, e.g. LFTs with **tolvaptan**. This may include routine blood tests (full blood counts, liver function tests, and serum biochemistry) or imaging, in combination with patient counselling to enable prompt detection of potentially serious adverse effects. The efficacy of **warfarin** is assessed through monitoring INR.

Therapeutic drug monitoring is carried out for drugs with a *narrow therapeutic index*, where the margin between sub-therapeutic and toxic serum levels is small

Table 1.6 Legal requirements for controlled drugs

Schedule	Examples	Prescription requirements	Storage requirements	Register requirements
2	Opioids (e.g. diamorphine, morphine, fentanyl, pethidine), amfetamines, cocaine and secobarbital	Yes	Yes	Yes
3	Barbiturates (except secobarbital), buprenorphine, tramadol, midazolam, temazepam, pentazocine, gabapentin, and pregabalin	Yes (except temazepam)	Yes (except tramadol, phenobarbital, gabapentin, and pregabalin)	No
4	Part I: benzodiazepines (except midazolam and temazepam), z-drugs (e.g. zopiclone) Part II: androgenic and anabolic steroids (e.g. oxandrolone, nandrolone, stanzolol)	No	No	No
5	Weak oral opioids (e.g. codeine, dihydrocodeine, morphine 10 mg/5mL liquid)	No	No	No

(see Table 1.7 for examples). Monitoring drug levels can be of value where toxicity is suspected or to optimize efficacy, particularly when doses are changed or co-morbidities are thought to be affecting levels, e.g. renal impairment. To ensure accurate interpretation samples are taken once steady state has been achieved and timed to coincide with trough (immediately pre-dose) or peak levels, as recommended by local guidelines.

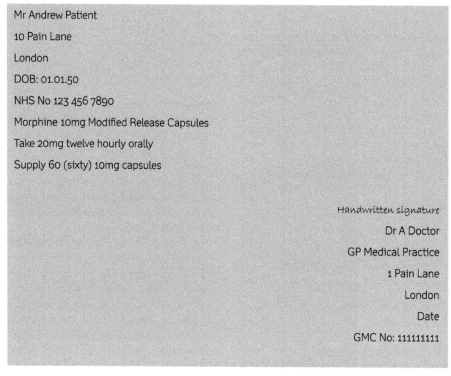

Mr Andrew Patient

10 Pain Lane

London

DOB: 01.01.50

NHS No 123 456 7890

Morphine 10mg Modified Release Capsules

Take 20mg twelve hourly orally

Supply 60 (sixty) 10mg capsules

Handwritten signature

Dr A Doctor

GP Medical Practice

1 Pain Lane

London

Date

GMC No: 111111111

Figure 1.14 Prescription form.

Table 1.7 Example of drugs where therapeutic, plasma level, monitoring is undertaken

Drugs suitable for therapeutic drug monitoring	Toxicity in overdose
Aminoglycosides (gentamicin, amikacin, tobramycin)	Nephrotoxicity, ototoxicity
Anti-convulsants (carbamazepine, phenytoin, phenobarbital, sodium valproate)	Neurological toxicity, but also cardiac and respiratory, etc.
Digoxin	Cardiac toxicity (bradycardia, heart block, cardiac arrest)
Lithium	Neurological and cardiac toxicity
Methylxanthines (aminophylline, theophylline)	Tachycardia, convulsions, gastrointestinal disturbances
Vancomycin	Nephrotoxicity, ototoxicity

Times of doses and sampling **must** also be recorded accurately.

Unlicensed/off-label medicines

All licensed medicines have a product license or marketing authorization that outlines its terms of use, including the way it should be administered, the indication for which it is licensed, side effects, and any criteria for whom it may or may not be used in, e.g. indications, cautions, contraindications, etc. (see SmPC).

Off-label refers to the use of a medicine outside of its product license, i.e. deviations from the SPC, e.g. different dose, patient group, indication, or administration. Examples of this may include the use of a medicine in children that only has a license for use in adults, or manipulation of a dosage form contrary to the SPC, e.g. crushing tablets or mixing with food or fluids. Patients must be made aware that the medicine is being used off-label and that the information in the patient information leaflet (PIL) may differ from what they have been advised. Where possible, a licensed medicine should always be prescribed in preference to a drug used off-label.

An unlicensed medicine is one that lacks a product license and, therefore, has not been subjected to the same scrutiny or intense monitoring as a licensed medicine. The prescriber, therefore, takes responsibility for its use and should only prescribe an unlicensed medicine where they believe it to be, based on evidence, in the best interest of the patient. As well as the safety and efficacy of the medication, the prescriber should take into consideration its quality, e.g. reproducibility of doses and the implication of any excipients within

the formulation. They are also responsible for making the patient aware that the medication they are being prescribed is unlicensed and the significance of this. An unlicensed drug should be reserved for use where a licensed medicine is not available and is the least favourable option.

Prescribing in patient groups

Elderly

With increasing age deterioration in renal and, to a lesser extent, hepatic function, leads to altered drug handling, so that drugs are eliminated more slowly and, therefore, more likely to accumulate. Renal clearance deteriorates at an average rate of about 1% a year beyond 40, although this can be significantly increased in the presence of co-morbidities, such as diabetes, heart failure, and hypertension. This is of particular relevance in the case of renally cleared drugs with a narrow therapeutic index, where more intense monitoring and careful dose adjustments are necessary. Similarly, decreased hepatic blood flow and liver mass results in delayed metabolism, especially with drugs cleared via the cytochrome P450 enzyme system. Other factors that can contribute to altered bioavailability in the elderly include reduced lean body mass and lower levels of circulating albumin.

As well as changes in pharmacokinetics, elderly patients demonstrate altered sensitivity to some drugs, in particular central nervous system (CNS) drugs (e.g. benzodiazepines), anti-cholinergics, and anti-hypertensives. The risk of toxicity is compounded by the high incidence of multiple co-morbidities and polypharmacy in this patient group, who are often on five or more medicines, even with appropriate prescribing. This may lead to increased drug inter-actions and cumulative toxicity. It is, therefore, essential that regular medication reviews are carried out, where the relative risk/benefits of any given treatment are assessed with consideration given to stopping or reducing doses. Guidance from the National Service Framework for older people recommends regular medication reviews in patients over 75; annually when taking less than four drugs, and 6-monthly in those taking four or more.

The Beers criteria compiled by an expert panel and last updated in 2019 provides a comprehensive list of medicines to avoid/use with caution in the elderly, since the risks of using are likely to outweigh the benefits (see Table 1.8). For some drugs, the age-appropriate doses must be adhered to, in order to prevent unnecessary toxicity.

More recently, the use of anti-psychotics in elderly patients with dementia has been widely reviewed, with warnings issued by the MHRA on the risk of stroke and increased mortality in this patient group. In the UK, **risperidone** is the only anti-psychotic licensed for use in dementia-related behavioural disturbances, for short-term use only and when other non-pharmacological measures have failed. Despite this, anti-psychotics are widely used in the elderly and infrequently reviewed.

PRACTICAL PRESCRIBING

Summary of points to consider when prescribing in the elderly

- Medication reviews should be carried out once or twice a year in patients over 75 years, depending on the number of medicines they take.
- Changes in renal and hepatic function can alter clearance.
- Elderly patients are more sensitive to the adverse effects of drugs, in particular sedatives, anticholinergics, and anti-hypertensives
- Anti-psychotics should not be routinely used in elderly patients with dementia due to increased risk of stroke and mortality.

Table 1.8 Examples of drugs known to be poorly tolerated in the elderly

Drug class	Associated risk
NSAIDs	Increased risk of gastrointestinal and renal toxicity especially with prolonged use
Benzodiazepines	Increased risk of confusion and falls
Anticholinergics	Increased risk of confusion, constipation, and urinary retention
Anti-psychotics	Increased risk of stroke and mortality
Sulfonylureas	Increased risk of hypoglycaemia, particularly with long-acting agents
α1-blockers	Increased risk of orthostatic hypotension
Antiparkinsonian agents	Increased risk of EPS with benztropine and trihexyphenidyl
Antispasmodics	Increased risk of anticholinergic toxicity, uncertain efficacy
Antithrombotics	Increased risk of orthostatic hypotension with short-acting dipyridamole
Anti-infectives	Increased risk of pulmonary toxicity with long-term use of nitrofurantoin
Digoxin	Increased risk of mortality, other more effective agents available first line
Antidepressants	Increased risk of anticholinergic effects/sedation with TCAs and paroxetine
Barbiturates	Increased risk of physical dependence
Metoclopramide	Increased risk of extrapyramidal side effects (EPS)
Proton pump inhibitors	Increased risk of *Clostridium difficile* and osteoporosis/ fractures

Children

Prescribing in children is complicated by the lack of licensed medicines and the paucity of clinical trials. As a result, many drugs used in children are done so off-label, with doses extrapolated from small studies or clinical practice (both paediatric and adult). Where dosing information is available, this is most commonly calculated based on body weight, or surface area and/or by age. Even then, the practicalities of administering the dose are frequently hampered by a lack of child-friendly formulations. Changes in EU legislation in 2007 were introduced to encourage drug companies to develop paediatric formulations and obtain paediatric licenses for both new and existing medicines.

Drug handling in children varies with age due to changes in body composition, as well as hepatic and renal maturation, and although these changes are more pronounced in the neonatal period, they are still evident in older children. Prescribing drugs off-label in paediatrics, therefore, carries the risk of under or overdosing, as well as putting patients at risk of side effects that are unique to children, either from the active ingredient or excipients. For example, alcohol is widely used as a solvent in liquid preparations licensed for use in adults, making them unsuitable for use in children, e.g. some **phenobarbital** liquid preparations.

Absorption

GI absorption is affected by factors including gastric pH, bowel length, gut motility, bile salt formation, and microbial flora; all of which show variations in neonates and children. For example, in the neonatal period gastric secretions tend to be reduced, therefore increasing the bioavailability of drugs that are normally destroyed in an acidic environment (e.g. penicillins). Gastric emptying and gut motility are decreased in the neonatal period, so that drugs normally absorbed in the small intestine will take longer to have an effect.

Absorption via non-enteral routes are affected by different body composition in paediatrics and neonates. Reduced muscle mass makes administration by intramuscular injections unreliable and unnecessarily painful, and is therefore best avoided. Transdermal administration can lead to increased systemic absorption and toxicity, due to increased surface area relative to weight and an immature stratum corneum, particularly in the neonates. Rectal administration is also less predictable in paediatrics and generally reserved for emergencies, e.g. rectal **diazepam** for status epilepticus.

Distribution

Body composition at birth is predominantly made up of water, accounting for between 70–80% of body weight and decreasing to approximately adult levels (about 60%) by the age of 1 year. Consequently, drugs that are largely water soluble with a large volume of distribution will need to be administered at relatively higher doses to overcome this. Conversely, protein levels are lower at birth, potentially leading to increases in 'free' levels of highly protein bound drugs.

Hepatic metabolism

Extent of hepatic metabolism in paediatrics is affected by hepatic blood flow and maturation of hepatic enzymes. From birth, enzyme systems develop at varying rates and as a result drugs metabolized via phase I or phase II reactions are affected. The cytochrome P450 enzymes responsible for phase I reactions, usually reach adult levels by the end of the first year of life, however, this varies between subsets of enzymes and some patients never reach full effect due to genetic polymorphism, e.g. CYP2D6 responsible for converting **codeine** to **morphine** is only evident in 47% of 3–12-year-olds. Although some subsets are present from birth, others are completely absent such as CYP3A4, instead neonates have high levels of CYP3A7, which is present only in low levels in adults. As CYP3A4 accounts for the metabolism of a large number of drugs, its relative absence in the first 1–2 years of life can increase the risk of toxicity for drugs metabolized by this route.

With regards to phase II reactions (glucoronidation, sulfation, acetylation, and glutathione conjugation) their activity also develops at different rates. In particular, glucoronidation has limited activity for the first few years of life, whereas enzymes responsible for sulfation and glutathione conjugation are present from birth. Consequently, some drugs administered to paediatrics are metabolized via different pathways to adults. For example, in adults **paracetamol** is metabolized via glucoronidation and sulfation at a ratio of 2:1, whereas neonates rely solely on sulfation and only achieve adult ratios by the age of about 12 years.

Renal excretion

As with hepatic function, renal function continues to develop postnatally. Although glomerular filtration rate (GFR) increases significantly in the first 2 weeks of life in term babies, it does not approximate to adult levels until 6 months of age. Renal tubular function takes even longer to mature, not reaching full maturation until 1 year of age. The combined effect of this is delayed clearance

of renally excreted drugs, so that drugs given to neonates and infants are often administered less frequently
in the day.

PRACTICAL PRESCRIBING

Summary of points to consider when prescribing in children

- Children should not be considered as small adults.
- When prescribing in children, a licensed medicine should always be considered first.
- Where an unlicensed drug or off-label drug is used the parent/carer should be made aware of this.
- For unlicensed specials, be aware of marked differences in product quality in terms of reproducibility and bioavailability.
- Consider the dosage form when prescribing for children and ensure the dose prescribed is measurable.
- Consider the presence of excipients in medicines, e.g. alcohol.

Renal impairment

The deficiency of renal function predictably leads to delayed
clearance of drugs that are excreted via the kidneys. The
clinical significance of this depends on the extent the drug
undergoes renal excretion, the margin between toxic and
therapeutic levels, and the severity of renal impairment. For
example, drugs that are solely cleared via the kidneys with
a narrow therapeutic index (see Table 1.9), are associated
with a higher risk of accumulation and toxicity. Possible
consequences of prescribing in renal impairment include:

- Exacerbation of pre-existing renal failure, e.g. NSAIDs.
- Increased sensitivity to the prescribed dose, e.g. anti-psychotics, **furosemide**.
- Increased toxic side effects due to decreased removal of drug/metabolites, so circulating volume remains high, e.g. opiates.

Most of the time, for the purpose of prescribing, GFR can
be estimated in adults using either eGFR (based on the
Modification of Diet in Renal Disease study—MDRD) or
the Cockcroft and Gault equation (see equation) which estimates creatinine clearance.

$$\text{Estimated creatinine clearance (mL/min)} = \frac{\{[140 - \text{Age (years)}] \times \text{Weight (kg)} \times n\}}{\text{Serum creatinine} (\mu m/L)}$$

where $n = 1.04$ (females) or 1.23 (males).

Table 1.9 Stages of renal impairment

Chronic kidney disease (CKD) stage	MDRD eGFR	Description
1	90 mL/min or greater	Normal
2	60–89 mL/min	Mild impairment
3	30–59 mL/min	Moderate impairment
4	15–29 mL/min	Severe impairment
5	Less than 15 mL/min	End stage renal impairment

Both methods provide only an estimate and become
less reliable at extremes of ages and weights, or in rapidly fluctuating renal function such as in acute kidney
injury (AKI). For many drugs, dose modifications in
the SPC are based on creatinine clearance and, thus,
estimation using Cockcroft and Gault is preferred.
Dose modifications in renal impairment may involve
dose reductions or an increase in dosing intervals,
so that drugs are administered less frequently. With
deteriorating renal function the use of some drugs is
contraindicated (Table 1.10).

For patients on renal dialysis, decisions on drug dosing
will depend on the type of dialysis and drug properties
that affect the extent it is dialysed, e.g. molecular size, extent of protein binding, and solubility/volume of distribution. Smaller drugs that are less protein bound and highly
water soluble, are therefore more likely to be eliminated by
dialysis and will require repeat doses. In all patients with
renal impairment, the use of drugs that are nephrotoxic or
cleared by renal elimination should only be considered in
the absence of suitable alternatives.

In certain circumstances where patients lie outside the
normal population (e.g. a cachectic cancer patient or grossly
oedematous heart failure patient), absolute GFR can be
calculated from body surface area (BSA) using height and
weight, to establish dosage adjustments required.

$$GFR_{ABS} = eGFR \times \frac{BSA}{1.73}$$

$$BSA = \sqrt{\frac{(\text{height (cm)} \times \text{weight (kg)})}{3600}}$$

Table 1.10 Child–Pugh Score

Measure	1 point	2 points	3 points	
Total bilirubin (micromol/L)	<34	34–50	>50	
Serum albumin (g/dL)	>3.5	2.8–3.5	<2.8	
INR or	<1.7	1.7–2.3	>2.3	
PT (seconds)	<4	4–6	>6	
Ascites	None	Mild	Moderate to severe	
Hepatic encephalopathy	None	Grade I–II	Grade III–IV (refractory)	

Points	Class	Definition	1-year survival	2-year survival
5–6	A	Well compensated	100%	85%
7–9	B	Significant functional compromise	81%	57%
10–15	C	Decompensated liver failure	45%	35%

Reproduced with permission from Pugh RN, Murray-Lyon IM, Dawson JL, Pietroni MC, Williams R, Transection of the oesophagus for bleeding oesophageal varices. *British Journal of Surgery*, Volume 60, Issue 8, pp. 646–9, Copyright © 1973 British Journal of Surgery Society Ltd. https://doi.org/10.1002/bjs.1800600817

PRACTICAL PRESCRIBING

Summary of points to consider when prescribing in renal impairment

- Where renal impairment is suspected, an estimated creatinine clearance using Cockcroft and Gault can be used to assess for dose adjustments of drugs that are cleared via the kidney.
- Estimates of creatinine clearance or GFR are less accurate at extremes of body weight and age, or where function is fluctuating.
- Where possible drugs that are not excreted via the kidney should be used preferentially.
- Drugs with a narrow therapeutic index will require regular monitoring in order to avoid toxicity.

Hepatic impairment

Unlike renal impairment, the impact of hepatic impairment on drug clearance is more difficult to predict, with no single test available to aid with dose adjustment calculations. In general, the risk of altered clearance is greater with chronic, rather than acute liver disease; however, in both instances patients will require careful monitoring for side effects and, where possible, serum drug levels.

In the absence of dosing calculations, consideration can be given to specific drug properties to help predict the impact of liver disease on drug handling. This includes:

- *Hepatic metabolism*: drugs that are primarily metabolized in the liver are predictably more prone to accumulation in liver disease due to reduced enzyme activity, e.g. in decompensated cirrhosis or reduced hepatic blood flow. This applies to both the drug and any active metabolites that may be generated in this way, e.g. via the cytochrome P450 enzyme system. Some drugs metabolized via one pathway, may be cleared by an alternative route once the first reaches saturation.
- *First pass metabolism*: drugs that undergo extensive first-pass metabolism demonstrate poor oral bioavailability in healthy patients. In cirrhosis, this effect is diminished, thereby increasing bioavailability and the risk of adverse effects.
- *Biliary excretion*: biliary excretion is reduced in cholestasis thus increasing the risk of toxicity.
- *Renal excretion*: in advanced disease, hepatic dysfunction often leads to renal impairment 'hepatorenal syndrome', leading to impaired clearance of renally excreted drugs. Furthermore, as hepatic disease is associated with reduced muscle mass, creatinine levels are also reduced, making creatinine clearance a less reliable indicator of renal function.
- *Enterohepatic recirculation*: as with biliary excretion, cholestasis leads to reduced clearance of drugs eliminated via enterohepatic recirculation.
- *Lipophilicity/hydrophilicity*: drugs that are highly lipid soluble (lipophilic) tend to rely on bile salts to promote

absorption, and hence, in cholestasis, drug absorption is likely to be impaired. Similarly, absorption of highly water-soluble (hydrophilic) drugs can be reduced in patients with ascites, as the drug can accumulate in ascitic fluid. These drugs may require higher loading doses.

- *Protein binding*: in hepatic impairment reduced serum albumin means that highly protein-bound drugs have the potential to be more available in their unbound state, leading to increased toxicity. In normal renal function this is compensated for by an increase in clearance of the unbound fraction. A high presence of bilirubin may agonize this effect by competing with the unbound drug for binding sites on albumin.

- *Pro-drugs*: drugs that are administered as pro-drugs requiring activation in the liver, will demonstrate reduced efficacy where hepatic enzyme activity is impaired.

- *Half-life*: the risk of accumulation in liver disease is more pronounced for drugs with a long half-life or with prolonged release preparations.

Understanding the nature and extent of liver disease is essential for predicting the impact on drug handling. The Childs Pugh score (see Table 1.10) can be useful in estimating the degree of hepatic impairment and is used by some drug manufacturers to determine dose reductions.

For some drugs, impaired hepatic function leads to altered pharmacodynamic effects, so that drug sensitivity is increased or decreased, although this is often difficult to distinguish from altered pharmacokinetics. For example, in cirrhosis, patients demonstrate an increased sensitivity to sedatives, such as benzodiazepines and opiates, thereby increasing the risk of hepatic encephalopathy. However, this may, in part, be due to increased CNS penetration across the blood–brain barrier, secondary to low albumin levels and increased unbound drug. Absorption of vitamin K as a fat soluble vitamin is also reduced in hepatic impairment, increasing the risk of bleeding and sensitivity to the effects of some anti-coagulants.

Drugs with reduced efficacy in liver disease include β-adrenoceptor antagonists, which is possibly explained by a reduced density of β-adrenoceptors on some cells. Similarly, the effects of loop diuretics, such as **furosemide**, are also reduced in cirrhosis, so that larger doses are required to achieve diuresis. Potassium losing diuretics increase the risk of precipitating hepatic encephalopathy secondary to hypokalaemia, and should not be used first line in hepatic dysfunction.

PRACTICAL PRESCRIBING

Summary of points to consider when prescribing in hepatic impairment

- No single test exists to calculate altered drug doses in hepatic impairment.
- When selecting a drug to use in a patient with hepatic impairment consider the route of elimination, lipophilicity, half-life, extent of protein binding, and existence of pro-drugs.
- CNS toxicity to benzodiazepines and opioids is likely to be increased in hepatic impairment, i.e. increased risk of hepatic encephalopathy.
- The risk of bleeding with anti-coagulants and anti-platelets is increased in hepatic impairment due to reduced vitamin K absorption in cholestatic disease.

Pregnancy

Any decision to use or not use a drug in a pregnant woman, should be made by balancing risks against benefits, and ensuring the woman is involved in the decision. The risks vary considerably between drugs but will also be affected by gestation, dose, and duration. This applies not only to prescription medicines, but also to over the counter and alternative therapies. To aid with decision-making, the teratogenicity of a drug is classified into risk categories (see Table 1.11), although more than 90% of drugs fall into class C where the safety is unknown. Furthermore, the class does not take into consideration any potential benefits.

Organogenesis occurs primarily in the first trimester, so that drugs administered in this period are more likely to result in foetal abnormalities, and with more than a third of pregnancies being unintended, the risk of exposure in this period is potentially high. The **thalidomide** scandal in the late 1950s, which saw babies born with severe limb malformation, is the most widely publicized example of drug-induced foetal abnormalities, and has resulted in huge changes in practice and legislation around medicine use.

The effects of drug exposure on the foetus in the second and third trimester can lead to toxicity, such as growth retardation, or withdrawal symptoms at birth, for example, with opioids or anti-depressants. NSAIDs are avoided in the third trimester due to the theoretical risk of premature closure of the patent ductus arteriosis (PDA). Some drugs may require caution due to their effects on the mother, who is at increased risk of complications such

Table 1.11 Tetrogenicity classification of drugs

Class	Definition
A	Adequate and well controlled trials have demonstrated no risk to the foetus
B	No evidence of risk to human foetus exists, although adequate and well-controlled studies have only been carried out in animals
C	Animal studies may show risk of harm, or there is a lack of adequate and controlled studies in animals or humans. However, the benefit of using may outweigh the risk.
D	Evidence of human risk does exist, either through studies or post-market research. The benefit of using may still outweigh the risks.
X	There is clear evidence of risk to the foetus and the risks of using outweighs the benefits. These drugs are contraindicated in pregnancy

as hyperglycaemia or hypertension during pregnancy, thereby indirectly affecting the foetus.

Ideally, any woman receiving medication for a chronic condition who is considering becoming pregnant, should seek specialist advice first so that consideration can be given to adjusting therapy. In reality, most present to the clinician once they are pregnant, by which time some have already discontinued chronic therapy, e.g. anti-depressants. The ultimate decision to continue, alter, or stop treatment should be made by the mother ensuring first that she has been adequately informed about the risks and benefits.

For those that do continue with chronic therapy, changes in maternal body composition and metabolic rate can have a significant effect on the serum levels of drugs, particularly those with a narrow therapeutic index. In particular, many anti-epileptics will need to have levels monitored during pregnancy, to prevent therapeutic failure, and into the post-partum period to avoid unintentional overdose when body composition reverts back to a pre-pregnancy state.

PRACTICAL PRESCRIBING

Summary of points to consider when prescribing in pregnancy

- When a medicine is prescribed in pregnancy, the risks and benefits should be clearly outlined to the mother.
- Where medication is deemed necessary, the drug with the lowest teratogenic risk should, where possible, be used first.
- The risk of foetal malformation, although greatest in, is not exclusive to, the first trimester.

- Some drugs used prior to birth can induce a state of withdrawal when the baby is born. At-risk babies should be closely monitored, e.g. for opioids, anti-depressants use.
- As pregnancy progresses and in the period post-partum, consider the affect changes in maternal body composition might have on serum levels of drugs, particularly those with a narrow therapeutic index.

Breast-feeding

It is widely recommended that babies are exclusively breastfed for the first 6 months of life and this should continue until the baby is weaned onto a solid diet. In reality, however, although about 78% of mothers breastfeed at birth, this rapidly declines to less than 50% by 6–8 weeks. That said, figures are improving and for those who do choose to breastfeed, it is essential they have access to good advice on the risks and benefits of taking medication should it be needed.

The properties that affect the extent that a drug diffuses into breastmilk are its molecular size, lipophilicity, and the degree of protein binding, as it is the drug in its free form that passes into breastmilk. Consequently, smaller, lipophilic drugs that are minimally protein-bound are most likely to be present in breastmilk (e.g. **nifedipine**), particularly in the early post-partum period, where the gaps between the mammary alveolar cells are larger. Drug concentrations may also be affected by half-life, as those with a shorter half-life are more rapidly cleared and less likely to accumulate in the breastmilk. Where a once daily drug is used, the dose should ideally be taken following a feed, preferably the feed that precedes the longest feed-free interval, to help minimize exposure. In general, medication that is applied topically, locally, or undergoes extensive first-pass metabolism in the mother is unlikely to be available in breastmilk.

Not all drugs that diffuse into breastmilk will go on to affect the infant, for example, drugs with poor oral bioavailability are unlikely to be absorbed. Conversely, drugs that do enter the breastmilk and are avoided in the neonatal period, should also be avoided during breastfeeding; this includes drugs that require clearance via metabolic pathways that are underdeveloped in infants.

PRACTICAL PRESCRIBING

Summary of points to consider when prescribing for breastfeeding mothers

- Drugs should only be prescribed in breastfeeding mothers where deemed absolutely necessary.
- Any decision to take a medication while breastfeeding should be made by the mother once she has been fully informed of the potential risks and benefits.
- Drug choice should be made based on those that are less likely to pass into the breastmilk, i.e.
  - large molecular size;
  - poor lipophilicity;
  - highly protein bound;
  - short half-life.
- Where a drug is known to pass into breastmilk, drugs with poor oral bioavailability, and a good safety profile in neonates should be used in preference.
- Where possible, topical or local treatments should be selected for maternal use, e.g. nasal sprays in hay fever instead of oral antihistamines.

Further reading

Alcorn J, McNamara PJ (2003) Pharmacokinetics in the newborn. *Advanced Drug Delivery Reviews* 55, 667–86.

Aster RH, Bougie DW (2007) Drug-induced immune thrombocytopenia. *New England Journal of Medicine* 357, 580–7.

Chun-Yu W, Tai-Ming K, Chen-Yang S, et al. (2012) A recent update of pharmacogenomics in drug-induced severe skin reactions. *Drug Metabolism and Pharmacokinetics* 27(1), 132–41.

Garbe E, Andersohn F, Bronder E, et al. (2011) Drug induced immune haemolytic anaemia in the Berlin Case-Control Surveilance Study. *British Journal of Haematology* 154(5), 644–53.

Jianghong Fan, Ines Lannoy (2014) Pharmacokinetics. *Biochemical Pharmacology* 87, 93–120.

Kenakin T, Williams M (2014) Defining and characterizing drug/compound function. *Biochemical Pharmacology* 87, 40–63.

Kilcoyne A, Ambery P, O'Connor D (Eds). (2013) *Pharmaceutical Medicine*. Oxford: Oxford University Press.

Lynch T, Price A (2007) The effect of cytochrome P450 metabolism on drug response, interactions, and adverse effects. *American Family Physician* 76(3), 391–6.

Mullane K, Winquist R, Williams M (2014) Translational paradigms in pharmacology and drug discovery. *Biochemical Pharmacology* 87, 189–210.

Rocchi F, Tomasi P (2011) The development of medicines for children. *Pharmacological Research* 64, 169–75.

Skinner A (2010) Neonatal pharmacology. *Anaesthesia and Intensive Care Medicine* 12(3), 79–84.

Sloss A, Kubler P (2009) Prescribing in liver disease. *Australian Prescriber* 32, 32–5.

Spencer JP, Gonzalez LS, Barnhart DJ (2001) Medications in the breast-feeding mother. *American Family Physician* 64 119–26

Tesfa D, Keisu M, Palmblad J (2009) Idiosyncratic drug-induced agranulocytosis: possible mechanisms and management. *American Journal of Hematology* 84, 428–34.

Verbeeck RK (2008) Pharmacokinetics and dosage adjustment in patients with hepatic dysfunction. *European Journal of Clinical Pharmacology* 64, 1147–61.

Wand L (2005) Epidemiology and prevention of adverse drug reactions in the elderly. *Journal of Geriatric Cardiology* 2(4), 248–53.

Winquist RJ, Mullane K, Williams M (2014) The fall and rise of pharmacology: (re)defining the discipline? *Biochemical Pharmacology* 87, 4–24.

Professional bodies

American Geriatrics Society (2019) Updated AGS beers criteria for potentially inappropriate medication use in older adults: the American Geriatrics Society 2019 Beers Criteria Update Expert Panel. *Journal of the American Geriatrics Society* 00:1–21, 2019.

Electronic Medicines Compendium http://www.medicines.org.uk/emc/ (accessed 14 March 2019).

EMA. Scientific guidelines. Available at: http://www.ema.europa.eu/ema/index.jsp?curl=pages/regulation/general/

general_content_000043.jsp&mid=WC0b01ac05800240cb (accessed 14 March 2019).

FDA. Drugs: guidance, compliance and regulatory information. Available at: http://www.fda.gov/Drugs/GuidanceComplianceRegulatoryInformation/default.htm (accessed 14 March 2019).

ICH official website. http://www.ich.org/ (accessed 14 March 2019).

National Service Framework for Older People (2001), DoH https://www.gov.uk/government/uploads/system/uploads/attachment_data/file/198033/National_Service_Framework_for_Older_People.pdf (accessed 14 March 2019).

UKMI (2012) Q&A 170.2a What pharmacokinetic and pharmacodynamic factors need to be considered when prescribing drugs for patients with liver disease?

2 Cardiovascular medicine

2.1 Hypertension

Hypertension (HTN) is the most common condition managed in primary care and a major risk factor for cardiovascular disease. Numerous randomized controlled trials have demonstrated that the use of antihypertensives to manage blood pressure (BP) helps reduce cardiovascular disease risk. Prevalence of HTN increases with age so that around 33% of men and 25% of women aged 45–54 years have a clinical diagnosis. It is generally defined as a raised blood pressure exceeding 140/90 mmHg, divided into two types:

- *Essential (or primary) hypertension*: accounts for 95% of cases and is where no secondary cause is identified.
- *Secondary hypertension*: the result of an underlying disease (e.g. renal, pulmonary, endocrine, or drug/toxin).

Pre-HTN is defined as systolic BP (SBP) 120–139 mmHg and diastolic BP (DBP) 80–89 mmHg.

Pathophysiology

BP is the product of cardiac output (heart stroke volume and heart rate) and the total peripheral resistance of vessels supplied by the heart. Thus, three main systems are responsible for generating BP: *the heart* (pumping pressure), *vessel tone* (being the systemic resistance), and the *kidney* (regulating intravascular volume).

Three main physiological systems regulate heart, vessels, and kidney with respect to blood pressure:

1. *The sympathetic nervous system*: changes in BP are sensed by a feedback mechanism mediated by baroreceptors in the walls of the aortic arch and carotid sinuses. Increasing BP causes firing of glossopharyngeal and vagus nerves, inhibiting sympathetic outflow via the medulla (tractus solitarius). This, in turn, leads to parasympathetic dominance and a reduction in peripheral resistance (vasodilation through β_1-adrenoceptors) and cardiac output (by reduced heart rate and reduced contractility through α_1-adrenoceptors). Centrally acting antihypertensive drugs act at the nucleus tractus solitarius (e.g. **clonidine/methyldopa**) or ventrolateral medulla (e.g. **moxonidine**).

2. *The renin-angiotensin-aldosterone system*: this system regulates blood volume and systemic vascular resistance, thus influencing cardiac output and arterial pressure. This feedback mechanism starts in the kidney with the release of renin into the peripheral circulation. Renin release, from juxtaglomerular cells (JC), is stimulated by sympathetic mechanisms (involving α_1-receptors on JC themselves), decreased afferent arteriole pressure (from systemic hypotension or renal artery stenosis) or declining Na^+ levels in the distal tubules of the kidney. Prostaglandins, such as PGE2 and PGI2 (prostacyclin), also cause release of renin secondary to reduced NaCl transport in the macular densa (see Topic 5.2 'Acute kidney injury').

Once released into the circulation, renin acts on angiotensinogen causing its cleavage into angiotensin I. Angiotensin-converting enzyme (ACE) in the vascular endothelium converts angiotensin I to angiotensin II, which has several important functions:

- Increases vascular resistance and arterial pressure by constricting resistance vessels (via [AT1] receptors).
- Causes noradrenaline release from sympathetic nerve endings and stops its re-uptake, thus enhancing sympathetic outflow.
- Acts on the adrenal cortex to release aldosterone, which in turn acts on the distal tubule of the kidneys to increase Na^+ and fluid retention, leading to increased BP.
- Stimulates release of vasopressin (antidiuretic hormone, ADH) from posterior pituitary gland, which

results in fluid retention at the collecting ducts of the kidney.

- Acts on atrial myocytes to cause release of atrial natriuretic peptide (ANP, see 'Atrial natriuretic peptide').

The thiazide diuretics used to treat HTN to reduce BP act by decreasing Na^+ uptake and, hence, water uptake via the Na^+/Cl^- co-transporter located at proximal distal convoluted tubules and collecting ducts of the nephron (see 'Thiazide diuretics', in drugs used in management).

3. *Endothelium-related vasoactive factors*: circulating or local hormones, like ANP, bradykinin, nitric oxide, endothelin, and adenosine, can regulate vascular tone and circulating volume. Of particular importance:

  - *Atrial natriuretic peptide*: ANP is released from atrial myocytes in response to atrial distension, α-adrenergic receptor stimulation, rising angiotensin II and endothelin levels. This peptide then acts via guanylyl cyclase linked receptors, ANP-R, located in the collecting duct of the kidney. Agonist activation of these receptors leads to a reduction in circulating volume and BP by:

    - Dilation of the afferent glomerular arteriole and constriction of the efferent glomerular arteriole, causing an increased glomerular capillary pressure and thus GFR, resulting in Na^+ and water loss.

    - Increased blood flow through the vasa recta, thereby washing solutes (NaCl and urea) out, thus lowering osmolarity of interstitium, causing less reabsorption of tubular fluid.

    - Reduces the absorption of Na^+ in the proximal convoluted tubule and cortical collecting duct of the nephron via guanosine 3',5'-cyclic monophosphate (cGMP) dependent phosphorylation of the epithelial sodium channel ENaC

    - Inhibits renin secretion (see '2. The renin-angiotensin-aldosterone system').

  - *Endothelin & bradykinin*: the relationship between endothelial cells and vascular smooth muscle is important for local regulation of vasoconstriction/dilation. Endothelins, potent vasoconstrictors, act via ETa receptors on smooth muscle cells, leading to retention of Na^+ and thus increasing BP. Action at ETb receptors, located on the endothelial cell, on the other hand, leads to release of nitric oxide, natriuresis, and diuresis, lowering BP; thus, the importance in local vascular haemostasis.

Bradykinin acts on endothelial cells through G protein–coupled receptors to enhance nitric oxide levels and cause smooth muscle vessel relaxation (Figure 2.1). Coincidentally, bradykinin is also cleaved into small peptides by ACE. This is responsible for some of important common side effects of ACE inhibitors (e.g. dry cough and angioedema).

As outlined above, nearly 95% of hypertensive patients have primary or essential hypertension (EH), where the mechanisms cannot easily be explained, although they are likely to involve one or more of the systems outlined previously. Essential hypertension is typically asymptomatic, yet remains a potent risk factor for cardiovascular disease. As symptoms are silent, yet increase the risk of cardiovascular disease, hypertension should be identified through active investigation (see 'Management').

The pathophysiological mechanisms of secondary hypertension are more clearly understood and are summarized in Table 2.1.

For a full summary of the relevant pathways and drug targets, see Figure 2.2.

Management

The underlying principle of hypertension management is to reduce arterial pressure by reducing cardiac output (i.e. heart rate and/or stroke volume) and/or by reducing systemic vascular resistance through vasculature dilation. In the case of secondary hypertension, any underlying pathology will also require management.

As the majority of patients with hypertension are asymptomatic, diagnosis is generally made during routine screening to assess risk factors and BP. This is carried out every 5 years in adults, or annually following a previous high–normal or raised result. Diagnosis is based on several elevated measurements, ideally through the use of ambulatory (ABPM) and home blood pressure monitoring (HBPM).

On diagnosis, all patients should be provided with advice on lifestyle modifications, as this can help reduce BP sufficiently to enable lower doses of anti-hypertensive drugs, or negate their need altogether (see Box 2.1). Patients with high-normal BP also benefit.

Once a diagnosis of hypertension has been made, the decision to treat is based on grade (see Table 2.2) and cardiovascular risk. Evidence and expert consensus suggests that target BPs vary with age, so that patients over 80 should aim for a SBP/DBP less than 150/90 mmHg, for those aged over 80 years, and 140/90 mmHg, for those under 60 years of age.

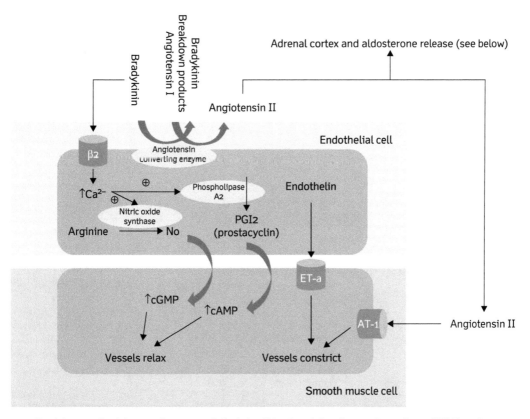

Figure 2.1 Bradykinin acts at β_2 receptors on endothelial cell to stimulate nitric oxide synthase (NOS) and phospholipase A2 to increase levels of nitric oxide and prostacyclin, respectively, to cause smooth muscle relaxation and thus decrease systemic vascular resistance.

Numerous tools exist to calculate cardiovascular risk that take into consideration factors such as age, sex, SBP, cholesterol, smoking, and diabetes. In the UK it is currently recommended that all patients under the age of 85 have their cardiovascular risk assessed using the online QRISK2 tool. This tool predicts the risk of a cardiovascular event in the next 10 years. At-risk patients are defined as those with a risk greater than 10%. Patients over 85 years and those with pre-existing cardiovascular disease, type 1 diabetes, chronic kidney disease, or familial hypercholesterolaemia are automatically considered to be at increased risk, without the need for using the QRISK2 tool. All at-risk patients will require further management, primarily to exclude secondary causes, followed by lifestyle advice and statin therapy where lifestyle modifications alone are inadequate.

For hypertension management, any of the available classes of anti-hypertensives *are* effective in reducing BP per se; however, efficacy, mechanism, and tolerance varies between drug classes and patients, and this forms the basis of international recommendations. Achieving control is done in a stepwise manner, optimizing treatment with any single agent before the addition of a second or further drugs (see Figure 2.3).

Consideration should be given to the patient's age, ethnic origin, allergies, and the presence of any pre-existing co-morbidities, all of which will influence the preferred choice of anti-hypertensives. For example, those of African/Caribbean descent are more likely to respond to calcium channel blockers (CCBs), whereas for patients with pre-existing heart failure a thiazide-like diuretic (**indapamide** or **chlortalidone**) would be the drug of choice. Similarly, when introducing a second agent, prescribers should take into consideration side effect profiles of the various agents; for example, the risk of impaired glucose tolerance is increased when using a β-blocker in combination with thiazide-like diuretic and so a CCB is preferred as add-on therapy.

Once stabilized, patients will require an annual review of BP to ensure adequate control. In some instances, this

Table 2.1 The pathophysiological mechanisms of secondary hypertension

Causes		Pathophysiology	Additional signs and symptoms
Renal	*Intrinsic renal disease:* ● Glomerulonephritis ● Diabetic nephropathy ● Polycystic kidney dysease	Interstitial damage causes rising Na^+ levels, followed by water, so circulating volume increases	● Renal failure, proteinuria ● Asymptomatic, poor DM control ● Loin pain, haematuria, stones
	Renovascular hypertension: ● Atheroma ● Fibromuscular dysplasia	Decreased renal blood flow decreases renal perfusion pressure cause a rise in renin	● Associated with angina, peripheral vascular disease ● Asymptomatic
Pulmonary	Sleep apnoea	Hypoxia and hypercapnoea can increase sympathetic drive Dysfunctional baro/chemoreceptors maintain hypertension	Daytime tiredness, poor concentration, morning headaches, depression
Endocrine	Conn's syndrome	Adrenal adenoma secreting aldosterone directly stimulating receptors of distal convoluted tubule and collecting duct; increased Na^+ uptake (hence, water) and K^+ loss	Weakness, muscle cramps, palpitations, polyuria/dipsia, hypokalaemia, hypernatraemia
	Cushing's disease: ACTH-dependent Cushing' syndrome	Anterior pituitary adenoma secreting ACTH-stimulating adrenal cortex to release cortisol; Na^+ retention	Trunk obesity, facial fullness, purple striae of skin, muscle wasting
	Phaeochromocytoma	Tumour secreting NA directly stimulating peripheral α-adrenoceptors	Asymptomatic or episodes of headaches, sweating, palpitations
Drugs	Oral contraceptive pill	Direct increase of hepatic synthesis of angiotensinogen	
	Corticosteroids: (Cushing's syndrome*)	● Overstimulation of mineralocorticoid receptor thus Na^+ retention ● Reduced production of prostaglandins via inhibition of phospholipase A ● Increased insulin resistance	As Cushing's disease

may lead to a reduction in therapy, particularly in the young following lifestyle changes, or in the elderly who can become increasingly sensitive to therapy.

A hypertensive crisis can be subdivided into hypertensive urgency and hypertensive emergency (malignant hypertension). Treatment of the former (a BP exceeding 180/110 mmHg), can invariably be managed at home with oral therapy to reduce BP over a period of 24 hours to achieve a diastolic <110 mmHg. Treatment options include **captopril**, **labetalol**, and **clonidine**, i.e. short-acting oral agents that possess a rapid onset of action. Treatment with **nifedipine** is not recommended, as onset is likely to be too rapid and can result in cerebral hypoperfusion.

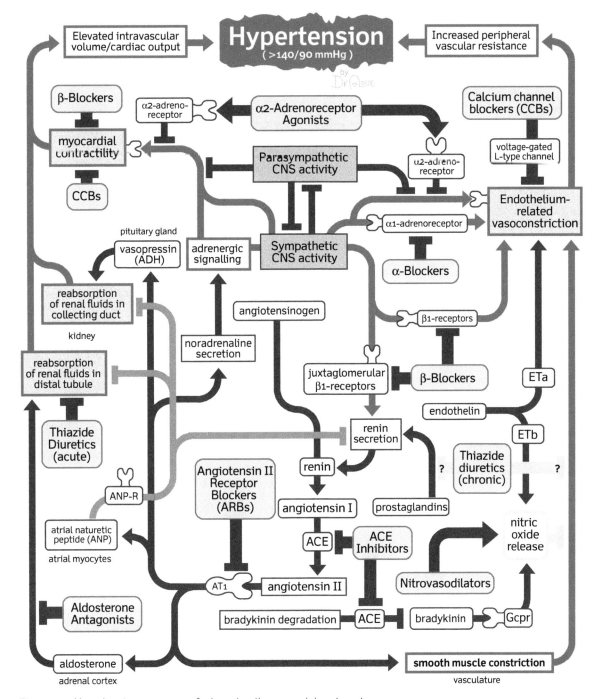

Figure 2.2 Hypertension: summary of relevant pathways and drug targets.

Malignant hypertension is a more severe form of hypertension associated with target organ damage. Patients present with BP in excess of 180/120 mmHg and evidence of end-organ dysfunction, e.g. retinal haemorrhages, renal dysfunction, and confusion. Malignant hypertension is always considered a medical emergency and is best managed in an intensive care setting to allow for administration of IV treatment, where

Box 2.1 Advice on lifestyle modifications in hypertension

- Maintain a normal BMI (<25 kg/m²)
- Restrict NaCl intake to <6 g/day
- Eat at least five portions of fruit and vegetables a day
- Restrict saturated and total fat
- Moderate alcohol consumption to <14 units per week for males and females
- Exercise for at least 30–60 minutes five times per week
- Try relaxation therapy, e.g. stress management, cognitive therapies, meditation
- Quit smoking (reduces cardiovascular disease (CVD) risk, rather than hypertension)

patients can be closely monitored. Rapid reversal is necessary where hypertension causes severe complications, such as dissecting aortic aneurysm, hypertensive encephalopathy, acute left ventricular failure, acute renal failure, myocardial infarction (MI), and eclampsia. In this instance, treatments of choice are those that can be administered intravenously with a rapid onset of action and are easy to titrate, such as **labetalol**, **nicardipine**, **fenoldopam**, and until recently, **sodium nitroprusside**. In intracranial haemorrhage, the aim is to achieve a mean arterial pressure of 130 mmHg and ensure a cerebral perfusion pressure > 70 mmHg.

Table 2.2 Classification of hypertension

Category	SBP (mmHg)	DBP (mmHg)
Optimal BP	<120	<80
Normal BP	<130	<85
High–normal BP	130–139	85–89
Grade 1 hypertension (mild)	140–159	90–99
Grade 2 hypertension (moderate)	160–179	100–109
Grade 3 hypertension (severe)	≥180	≥110
Isolated systolic hypertension (Grade 1)	140–159	<90
Isolated systolic hypertension (Grade 2)	≥160	<90

Drug classes used in management

ACE inhibitors

ACE inhibitors decrease the formation of vasoconstrictive angiotensin II and the degradation of vasodilatory bradykinin. Examples include captopril, enalapril, fosinopril, lisinopril, moexipril, perindopril, quinapril, ramipril, and trandolapril.

Mechanism of action

A membrane-bound bivalent dipeptidyl carboxyl metalopeptidase, the ACE (or kinase II) is found in endothelial, epithelial, or neuroepithelial cells, in the brain, lung, and as a soluble form in the blood. ACE cleaves the C-terminal dipeptide from angiotensin I, promoting its conversion into the angiotensin II peptide. ACE can also cleave and decrease levels of the vasodilator and natriuretic compound bradykinin. The inhibition of circulating and tissue-associated ACE ultimately leads to arterial dilation and, therefore, a reduction of BP.

Prescribing

There are numerous ACE inhibitors on the market with choice generally guided by local availability, cost, and frequency of administration. With the exception of **captopril**, all ACE inhibitors are administered once daily (OD) in hypertension. As many are also licensed for other indications, consideration should also be given to any co-morbidities such as heart failure or diabetic nephropathy when selecting an agent. In all instances, doses are started low and titrated according to response, ideally with the first dose given at night due to the risk of hypotension.

PRACTICAL PRESCRIBING

ACE inhibitors in hypertension

- All ACE inhibitors are indicated for hypertension with many also licensed for use in other indications, in particular heart failure.
- It should be noted that the recommended dose and frequency varies with indication.

Unwanted effects

In general, ACE inhibitors can be used safely in most patients and are well tolerated. First doses are commonly

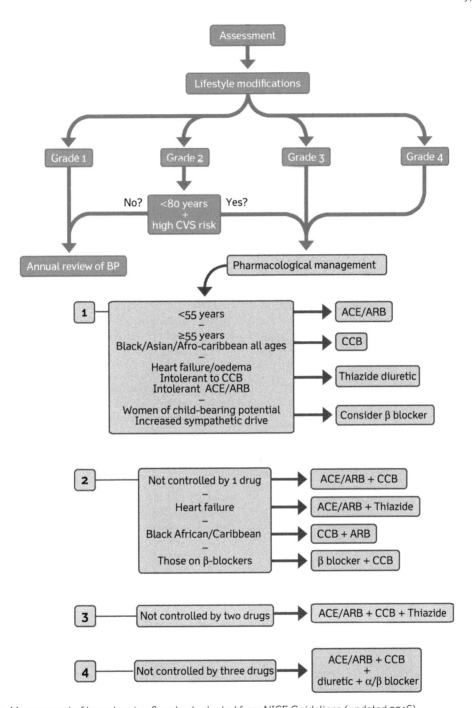

Figure 2.3 Management of hypertension flowchart adapted from NICE Guidelines (updated 2016).
Data from NICE 'Hypertension in adults: diagnosis and management'. Published 2011, updated 2016. https://www.nice.org.uk/guidance/cg127

associated with hypotension, particularly in patients taking concomitant diuretics who may be volume-depleted. Particular care is required in patients with ischaemic heart or cerebrovascular disease, where a sudden drop in BP may precipitate an MI or CVA, respectively.

The most widely recognized adverse effect to ACE inhibitors is a persistent dry cough thought to be caused by an increase in bradykinin levels. Patients who are affected may be switched to an angiotensin II receptor antagonist. Other common non-specific side effects include headache, fatigue, nausea and vomiting, and hypersensitivity reactions such as rash or, more rarely, anaphylaxis.

Most ACE inhibitors are primarily renally excreted. Furthermore, ACE inhibitors cause vasodilation of efferent arterioles, which supply blood to the glomerulus and can reduce the perfusion pressure across the glomerulus. It is, therefore, not uncommon for ACE inhibitors to result in renal dysfunction, and it is advisable to assess renal function prior to initiation and monitor patients while on treatment. In the case of moderate or severe impairment, dose reductions may be necessary and treatment may need to be held. Patients showing marked sensitivity to treatment or early signs of renal toxicity may have an underlying renovascular disease, and should be closely monitored. ACE inhibitors are best avoided in bilateral renal stenosis, as they can reduce or stop glomerular filtration leading to renal failure. Many of the ACE inhibitors are pro-drugs (e.g. **ramipril**, **perindopril**), requiring activation in the liver, thus, in theory, efficacy may be impaired in hepatic impairment. Furthermore, ACE inhibitors have been known to cause fulminant hepatic necrosis, which can be fatal.

ACE inhibitors should be avoided in pregnancy as they are known to cause oligohydramnios and may also adversely affect neonatal BP and renal function.

Drug interactions

Although ACE inhibitors can augment the hypotensive effects of other drugs known to cause hypotension, this is rarely of clinical significance. The exception to this is with diuretics, as patients with significant volume depletion can experience profound hypotension.

Caution is also required when taken with drugs whose renal clearance is affected by ACE inhibitors, leading to accumulation and toxicity, particularly with drugs possessing a narrow therapeutic index, e.g. **lithium**. Where ACE inhibitors are taken in combination with drugs known to cause hyperkalaemia, monitoring is advisable, e.g. **ciclosporin**, potassium sparing diuretics etc.

Angiotensin II receptor blockers

Angiotensin receptor blockers (ARBs) bind to the AT1 receptor with high affinity, inhibiting most of the biological effects of angiotensin II. Examples include candesartan, eprosartan, irbesartan, losartan, olmesartan, telmisartan, and valsartan.

Mechanism of action

Angiotensin II acts on two main receptors, AT_1 and AT_2, to exert its effect. The ARBs bind with high affinity to the AT_1 receptors and are largely more selective for AT_1 than AT_2 receptors. The AT_1 receptors mediate most of the known biological effects of angiotensin II and are widely distributed in adult tissues, including blood vessels, heart, liver, kidney, brain, and adrenal gland. They are cell-surface G protein receptors, involved in the regulation of central sympathetic nervous system activity and central osmocontrol. They activate phospholipase C to increase cytosolic Ca^{2+} concentrations via IP_3, which in turn can stimulate protein kinase C. Activation also leads to inhibition of adenylate cyclase. They promote aldosterone synthesis and secretion, vasoconstriction, vasopressin secretion, sodium reabsorption, cardiac hypertrophy and contractility, and the proliferation of vascular smooth cells. They also decrease renal blood flow and renal renin.

Angiotensin II can also promote inflammation, vascular remodelling, and thrombosis, all key components of the atherosclerotic process. As a result, the effects of ARBs are not limited to BP reduction, and they may confer an additional advantage in some hypertensive patients.

Prescribing

The angiotensin II receptor antagonists provide a useful alternative in patients who develop a cough with ACE inhibitors, as they are considered to be of equal efficacy. As with the ACE inhibitors, all ARBs are licensed for use in hypertension, but some also hold a license for heart failure, secondary prevention post-myocardial infarction, or diabetic nephropathy. All are taken OD as a tablet, although **losartan** is also available in a liquid formulation. Aside from this, choice may be influenced by any coexisting morbidities (including renal or hepatic impairment, see 'Unwanted effects').

Unwanted effects

Of the ARBs, **candesartan**, **eprosartan**, **losartan**, **olmesartan**, **telmisartan**, and **valsartan** are eliminated via the bile and are, therefore, contraindicated (or cautioned in the case of eprosartan or losartan) in severe hepatic impairment, biliary obstruction or cholestasis.

As with ACE inhibitors, caution is advised in renal artery stenosis, due to their effects on the renin-angiotensin-aldosterone pathway potentially impairing glomerular filtration. The doses of some ARBs, with the exception of losartan and **irbesartan**, require dose reductions in renal impairment.

ARBs should not be used in pregnancy as they can adversely affect foetal and neonatal BP, and where possible, women trying to become pregnant should be switched to an alternative. Use in breastfeeding should also be avoided.

Adverse effects to ARBs tend to be mild and self-limiting, with incidences comparable to placebo. The most widely reported affects are dizziness, headache, and less commonly hypotension. Although the risk of hypotension is greater with ACE inhibitors, any volume depletion secondary to diuretic therapy should be corrected prior to initiation of ARB therapy. Patients at greater risk of hypotension, including the elderly, should be started on a lower dose.

Drug interactions

Drug interactions with ARBs are as for ACE inhibitors as they both act on the renin–angiotensin–aldosterone pathway, affecting renal blood flow.

Calcium channel blockers

The diverse group of Ca^{2+} channel blockers have the capacity to lessen the rate of calcium ion entry through the voltage-gated L-type channel. Examples include amlodipine, diltiazem, felodipine, isradipine, lacidipine, lercanidipine, nicardipine, nifedipine, and verapamil.

Mechanism of action

CCBs are classified as dihydropyridines (the majority of CCBs) or non-dihydropyridines (**verapamil** and **diltiazem** only). All can decrease arterial pressure by lowering peripheral vascular resistance, decreasing both SBP and DBP. In addition, they improve myocardial oxygen demand by reducing venous returns and, therefore, are also used in the treatment of angina pectoris.

There are at least five different types of Ca^{2+} channels, but only two are found in cardiovascular tissues:

- *Voltage-gated T-type channels* are transient, low-threshold, fast-inactivated Ca^{2+} channels found in pacemaker cells and in vascular smooth muscle. None of the currently available Ca^{2+} channel blockers affect this type of receptor to any significant extent.

- *Voltage-gated L-type channels* are long-acting, high-threshold, slowly inactivated Ca^{2+} channels found in the cell membranes of a large number of excitable cells, including cardiac and vascular smooth muscle.

Calcium channel blockers limit Ca^{2+} entry through the channel by reducing channel opening rates; this action is specific for the voltage-gated mode of Ca^{2+} entry.

Each of the three prototypical Ca^{2+} channel blockers has its own particular binding site on the receptor, called the N (for dihydropyridines such as **nifedipine**), V (for

verapamil) and D (for **diltiazem**). The V receptor site is intracellular, while the N and D site have extracellular location. While verapamil and diltiazem exhibit frequency-dependent receptor binding and gain entry to the Ca^{2+} channel in its open state, the dihydropyridines bind preferentially to the channel in its inactivated state. Given that more Ca^{2+} channels are inactive in relaxed smooth muscle, these factors account for the relative vascular selectivity of dihydropyridines and the anti-arrhythmic properties of verapamil and diltiazem. In addition, although the α1 subunit of the Ca^{2+} channel of vascular smooth muscle is very similar to that of the heart, there are critical molecular differences that also help to explain why the dihydropyridines are vascular-selective.

Prescribing

Due to their vascular selectivity, the dihyropyridines (**nifedipine**, **lercanidipine**, **lacidipine**, **felodipine**, **nicardipine**, **isradipine**) are more suitable for use in hypertension, although **verapamil** and **diltiazem** are still licensed for this indication. Ultimately, the choice of agent comes down to ease of administration (OD), co-existing morbidities and cost.

Unwanted effects

CCBs vary in their affinity for vascular and cardiac smooth muscle, thereby influencing the patient groups they can be safely used in. In particular, the more pronounced negative inotropic effects associated with the non-dihydropyridines, **verapamil**, and to a lesser extent, **diltiazem**, preclude their use in conditions likely to be aggravated by this, e.g. heart failure, cardiogenic shock, severe bradycardia, AV block, and severe left ventricular dysfunction.

The dihydropyridines should be avoided in unstable angina, within 1 month of an MI, uncontrolled heart failure, and cardiogenic shock.

Many of the common side effects seen with dihydropyridines can be attributed to their vasodilatory effects, i.e. flushing, headaches, dizziness, hypotension, tachycardia, palpitations, and swollen ankles. These effects can, in part, be managed through the use of longer-acting drugs or slow-release preparations. Although verapamil and diltiazem are less likely to cause side effects associated with vasodilation, (flushing, dizziness, swollen ankle etc.), their use is associated with bradycardia and atrioventricular block. Less commonly erectile dysfunction has been reported with CCBs, although this occurs more commonly with non-selective β-blockers.

Drug interactions

CCBs interact with numerous drugs, particularly those known to cause hypotension (e.g. anti-hypertensives, some anaesthetics) and in the case of verapamil those known to cause bradycardia or AV block (e.g. **amiodarone**, **disopyramide**, and **flecainide**). **Verapamil** should *not*, therefore, be used in combination with a β-blocker, due to the risk of asystole.

As well as augmentation of pharmacological effects, many of the CCBs are metabolized through the cytochrome P450 enzyme system. Furthermore, **diltiazem** and verapamil are known inhibitors of CYP 3A4 and, as such, are known to increase levels of drugs including **ciclosporin**, **digoxin**, **simvastatin**, and **colchicine**. Patients requiring concomitant therapy should be closely monitored for signs of toxicity.

Thiazide diuretics

> The acute hypotensive effect of thiazides is due to depletion of salt and intracellular water. Direct vasodepressor influence is observed with chronic treatment, possibly due to ionic gradient changes in smooth-muscle cells and prostaglandin synthesis. Examples include bendroflumethiazide, chlortalidone, cyclopenthiazide, indapamide, metolazone, and xipamide.

Mechanism of action

The exact way by which thiazide-type diuretics manage to decrease blood pressure remains unclear (see Topic 5.2, 'Acute kidney injury'), but can be separated into three phases—acute (1–2 weeks), sub-acute (several weeks), and chronic (months). The initial response is produced by intravascular salt and water depletion, accompanied by a similar reduction in plasma volume, leading to BP loss. However, compensatory mechanisms due largely to stimulation of the renin–angiotensin–aldosterone system makes the effect on volume and cardiac output to decrease with time (sub-acute phase), so that plasma volume returns to levels close to pretreatment stage after a few weeks.

The vasodepressor effect of thiazide treatment occurs in the chronic phase, although the precise mechanism of vasodilation is not well understood. It has been suggested to result from the alteration of ion gradients across smooth muscle cells and/or activation of K^+ channels, possibly due to intracellular sodium depletion and reduced calcium entry into the smooth muscle cell of the arteriolar resistance vessel walls. A change in membrane-bound ATP activity and synthesis of vasodilator prostaglandins has also been reported.

Prescribing

Currently, the thiazide-like diuretics (**indapamide** and **chlortalidone**) are recommended in preference to conventional thiazide diuretics (**bendroflumethiazide** or **hydrochlorothiazide**) in the management of hypertension, as the evidence for their clinical benefit is more robust and up to date.

The recommended doses for hypertension are lower than those used to treat oedema and should not be exceeded (e.g. indapamide 2.5 mg daily), as higher doses are unlikely to be more effective in the management of hypertension, but will increase diuretic effects.

Unwanted effects

Due to their mechanism of action, electrolyte disturbances are common with thiazide treatment and they should, therefore, be avoided in patients with refractory hypokalaemia, hyponatraemia, hypercalcaemia, hyperuricaemia, or gout. While on treatment, it is essential to monitor electrolytes, particularly in the elderly, renal or hepatic impairment, and those on concomitant drugs also known to cause electrolyte disturbances (see 'Drug interactions' for this section).

As thiazides act within the kidneys, treatment is contraindicated in severe renal impairment (GFR <30 mL/min/1.73 m^2) and their efficacy likely to be impaired in moderate renal impairment.

Treatment is also associated with hyperglycaemia and can exacerbate diabetes, making it a less favourable treatment option in patients predisposed to high serum glucose levels. **Indapamide** as a sulfonamide is more likely to induce a hypersensitivity reaction than other drugs in the class and should be avoided in patients known to be hypersensitive to sulfonamides.

Drug interactions

Unsurprisingly, the hypotensive effects of thiazides are augmented in patients taking concurrent antihypertensive or other drugs known to reduce BP. Of greater clinical significance is their co-prescribing with drugs likely to cause electrolyte disturbances, such as hypokalaemia, thereby increasing the risk of ventricular arrhythmias and other cardiac toxicity, e.g. some antiarrhythmics (**disopyramide**, **flecainide**), **amisulpride**, and **digoxin**.

Thiazide electrolyte disturbances

- Hypokalaemia is particularly common within the first 2 weeks of initiating treatment.
- Severe hyponatraemia can be particularly troublesome (independent of ADH and water intake) in the elderly due to urinary Na^+ loss. Thiazide treatment should be stopped.

Due to their effects on renal excretion, thiazide diuretics can reduce the clearance of some renally excreted drugs, leading to toxic levels, particularly those with a narrow therapeutic index, such as **ciclosporin** and **lithium**.

Aldosterone antagonists

Prescribed mostly for their diuretic effects, aldosterone antagonists increase Na^+ and water excretion, and can be used in patients with resistant hypertension. For example, spironolactone, and eplenerone.

Mechanism of action

Unlike thiazides, aldosterone antagonists have a K^+-sparing effect. A synthetic 17-lactone steroid, **spironolactone** is a specific competitive antagonist of aldosterone. Its mechanism of action involves the binding of receptors at the aldosterone-dependent Na^+–K^+ exchange site that is present in the distal convoluted renal tube. This leads to the augmented excretion of Na^+ and water, with K^+ retention (see Topic 5.2, 'Acute kidney injury').

Prescribing

Aldosterone antagonists can be used as an alternative or in addition to thiazide therapy in patients with resistant hypertension. Within the class, **spironolactone** tends to be the drug of choice and is prescribed at an initial dose of 25 mg daily. As with other diuretics, doses are best taken in the morning to prevent diuresis overnight.

Unwanted effects

Caution and close monitoring is recommended in patients predisposed to hyperkalaemia, such as the elderly or those with renal impairment, and in those with refractory hyperkalaemia treatment is contraindicated.

As aldosterone is produced by the adrenal gland, spironolactone is contraindicated in Addison's disease, where adrenal function is already impaired.

Drug interactions

Aside from enhanced hypotensive effects when taken with other anti-hypertensives, care is recommended in patients taking concomitant therapy known to cause hyperkalaemia, in particular ACE inhibitors, ARBs, and other potassium sparing-diuretics (e.g. **amiloride**). **Spironolactone** has also been reported to increase serum **digoxin** levels.

β-blockers

Vasodilatory β-blockers reduce BP mainly by decreasing systemic vascular resistance (i.e. carvedilol, nebivolol), rather than by reducing the cardiac output, which is the observed mechanism for traditional, non-vasodilating β-blockers (i.e. atenolol). Examples include acebutolol, atenolol, bisoprolol, carvedilol, celiprolol, labetalol, metoprolol, nadolol, nebivolol, oxprenolol, pindolol, propranolol, and timolol.

Mechanism of action

β-blockers are a heterogeneous class of agents with varied pharmacological and physiological properties. Collectively, they reduce the effects of endogenous catecholamines, adrenaline, and noradrenaline, by acting as antagonists of β-adrenoceptors. These are G protein–coupled receptors, linked to adenylate cyclase and subsequent increase in the intracellular concentration of cAMP and activation of protein kinase A.

Conventional β-blockers (**metoprolol**, **atenolol,** and **propranolol**) decrease BP mainly through the reduction of heart rate and myocardial contractility. Still, the decreased cardiac output could promote compensatory peripheral vasoconstriction in order to sustain BP.

Newer vasodilating β-blockers (**labetalol** and **carvedilol**) seem to promote vasodilation through $β_1$-receptor blockade, decreasing BP in a more physiological way via the reduction of resistance in systemic vasculature, but maintaining cardiac output.

β-blockers can also reduce renin secretion by blocking renal juxtoglomerular $β_1$-adrenoceptors. Moreover, blockade of presynaptic β-adrenoceptors in sympathetic neurons regulating arteriolar resistance vessels may reduce noradrenaline release and attenuate reflex vasoconstriction.

Prescribing

Of the available oral β-blockers, all but **sotalol** are licensed for use in hypertension. However, their usage is now generally limited to patients with resistant disease or where other agents cannot be used. Evidence for their use as anti-hypertensives comes largely from **atenolol**, although their ability to lower BP is considered a class effect; choice of agent is, therefore, dictated by frequency of administration (ideally OD), licensed status, and any selective properties (see Table 2.3).

Labetalol and less commonly, **esmolol,** are both available for intravenous (IV) administration in the management of a hypertensive crisis. In both cases, an initial bolus dose is followed by an IV infusion.

Unwanted effects

Common side effects include dizziness (secondary to postural hypotension), bradycardia, cold extremities (secondary to peripheral vasoconstriction), impaired glucose control, and dyspnoea or bronchospasm. Prescribers should, therefore, avoid or use cautiously in patients with hypotension,

bradycardia, peripheral vascular disease, diabetes, or asthma, respectively. The β-blockers are also contraindicated in second- or third-degree heart block or cardiogenic shock. While undergoing treatment, patients commonly complain of sleep disturbances, headaches, and general fatigue.

Drug interactions

With their broad range of pharmacological effects, there is a large potential for interactions when taken concurrently with other drugs. In particular, those with similar cardiovascular effects, e.g. hypotension with anti-hypertensives/MAOIs, bradycardia with anti-arrhythmics, and heart block or heart failure with CCBs (**verapamil** and **diltiazem**). As β-blockers impair glucose control, doses of insulin or oral anti-diabetic therapy may need to be altered.

As a substrate and inhibitor of P-glycoprotein, **carvedilol** is more likely to interact with other drugs. Dose reductions are recommended for **ciclosporin** and **digoxin** when they are co-prescribed with carvedilol.

Table 2.3 Properties of β-blockers

Property	Significance	Examples
Cardioselectivity	Less likely to cause bronchospasm or peripheral vasoconstriction—may be useful in patients with respiratory disease or peripheral vascular disease	Atenolol, bisoprolol, metoprolol
Water solubility	Water soluble β-blockers are less likely to cross the blood–brain barrier so less likely to cause CNS toxicity, e.g. nightmares or sleep disturbances	Atenolol, nadolol, sotalol
	Conversely, fat soluble agents are preferred in essential tremor	Propranolol
Duration of action	β-blockers with longer duration of action can be administered OD to improve compliance	Atenolol, bisoprolol, carvedilol, celiprolol, nadolol, nebivolol (Metoprolol, oxprenolol and propranolol available in MR preparations)
Licensed in angina		Acebutolol, atenolol, bisoprolol, carvedilol, metoprolol, nadolol, oxprenolol, pindolol, propranolol, timolol
Licensed in heart failure		Bisoprolol, carvedilol, nebivolol
Licensed in arrhythymias		Atenolol, metoprolol, nadolol, oxprenolol, propranolol

α-blockers

Selective α1-adrenoceptor antagonists block post-synaptic α1-adrenoceptors on vascular smooth muscle, thus inhibiting the vasoconstrictor effect of catecholamines. Examples include doxazosin, indoramin, prazosin, and terazosin

Mechanism of action

The adrenergic receptors are metabotropic G protein-coupled receptors that are activated by adrenaline and noradrenaline in particular. The contraction of vascular smooth muscle by the α1 subtype of adrenoceptors is mediated by the second messengers IP_3 and diacylglycerol (DAG), leading to increases in myoplasmic Ca^{2+}.

The α-blockers act with varying potency in blocking α1 and α2 adrenoceptors; the agents with a higher affinity for α1 are more commonly used in essential hypertension. The blocking of α1 adrenoceptors has well-characterized haemodynamic actions in hypertension, leading to reduced tone in arteriolar resistance vessels, and lower peripheral resistance. In addition, they lower cardiac output by reduction of venous return through dilation of venous capacitance vessels.

Classic non-selective α-adrenoceptor antagonists failed as hypertensive agents due to the blockade of presynaptic α2-adrenoceptors on sympathetic nerve terminals, which function as inhibitors of catecholaminergic release attenuating reflex tachycardia.

Prescribing

Nowadays, α-blockers are reserved for add-on therapy in resistant hypertension, due to their poor tolerability compared with other anti-hypertensives. On initiation, treatment can lead to a profound drop in BP (postural hypotension) and, therefore, doses should be started low and gradually titrated up every 1–2 weeks, according to response and tolerance.

Unwanted effects

The most common side effects are predictable from the pharmacological effects of α-blockers, in particular, postural hypotension (often presenting as dizziness or syncope), and tachycardia or palpitations.

As potent vasodilators, care is advised in patients with cardiac conditions that may be aggravated by this, such as left ventricular heart failure and high output cardiac failure.

PRESCRIBING WARNING

Cataract surgery and α-blockers

Intra-operative floppy iris syndrome (IFIS) has been reported during cataract surgery in patients previously taking tamsulosin. This is potentially a class effect and, therefore, an ophthalmic surgeon should be made aware of any α-blocker usage prior to surgery.

Doses of all α-blockers (except **terazosin**) may need to be reduced in severe hepatic impairment, as excretion tends to be via hepatic metabolism. Dose reductions are also recommended for **prazosin** in renal impairment.

Drug interactions

The hypotensive effect of α-blockers is augmented when taken concurrently with other drugs known to cause hypotension. In particular, the use of phosphodiesterase inhibitors (**sildenafil**, **tadalafil**, and **vardenafil**) is only recommended in patients who have been stabilized on α-blockers.

α2-adrenoreceptor agonists

α2-adrenergic agonists are centrally acting antihypertensive agents, with peripheral activity being of marginal clinical significance. For example, clonidine and methyldopa.

Mechanism of action

Stimulation of α2-receptors and/or imadozoline receptors that are located on adrenergic neurons in the rostral ventrolateral medulla or nucleus tractus solitarius in the CNS can cause a reduction in sympathetic outflow together to the peripheral vasculature and heart. They decrease plasma catecholamine levels and reduce plasma renin activity.

α2-adrenoceptors are G protein–coupled receptors associated with the Gi heterotrimeric receptor that bind noradrenaline and adrenaline released by the adrenal medulla. Stimulation leads to inactivation of adenyl cyclase, decrease of intracellular cAMP, and reduced breakdown of glycogen.

Prescribing

Clonidine is reserved for use in severe hypertension, either orally or intravenously. Due to its short duration of action, it is administered three times a day, orally, and can be given as repeated IV doses in a hypertensive emergency. IV doses should be administered slowly over a period of 10–15 minutes to prevent a sudden drop in BP.

Methyldopa is only available for oral administration and has largely been succeeded in the management of hypertension with the exception of pregnancy-induced hypertension, where the body of evidence suggests it to be safe to use.

Unwanted effects

Due to their mechanism of action in reducing heart rate and vascular tone, combined with their rapid onset of action, treatment with these agents is commonly associated with profound postural hypotension, and symptoms such as dizziness and headaches. Monitoring is essential, particularly in patients with pre-existing bradycardia, where alternative treatment options may be necessary. Sedation is widely reported with both drugs, although this tends to be transient.

Due to the potency of **clonidine**, treatment should not be discontinued suddenly, particularly in patients on high doses due to the risk of a rebound in hypertension and the potential to induce a hypertensive crisis. In patients going for surgery, treatment should be continued during anaesthesia, either orally or, if necessary, intravenously.

Clonidine also causes peripheral vasoconstriction and is cautioned in peripheral vascular disease. With about 70% of the dose being excreted unchanged in the urine, the half-life of clonidine can be significantly extended in patients with renal impairment and, therefore, a dose reduction is necessary.

Drug interactions

The potential for pharmacodynamic interactions with **clonidine** and **methyldopa** is high. Concurrent use with other drugs known to cause hypotension, bradycardia, or sedation will predictably lead to an augmentation of this effect.

Of particular concern is the increased risk of a rebound in hypertension in patients taking concurrent β-blockers when clonidine is discontinued. β-blockers should be withdrawn first, then clonidine gradually after an interval of about a week. The combination of β-blockers with clonidine is also likely to increase the risk of 'cold extremities'.

Methyldopa in combination with **salbutamol** infusion has been reported to cause an acute hypotension.

Nitrovasodilators

The clinical effectiveness of organic nitrate esters, such as glyceryl trinitrate, is due to vasodilatory activity in large veins and arteries. For example, sodium nitroprusside

Mechanism of action

It is generally accepted that they act through the formation of the reactive free radical nitric oxide (NO). In endothelial cells, NO is formed from L-arginine by nitric oxide synthase, and rapidly diffuses to the underlying smooth muscle. Nitrovasodilators form NO directly via denitration by either enzymatic or non-enzymatic mechanisms, in a manner independent of endothelial cells. NO activates guanylyl cyclase, increasing the levels of cGMP and dependent kinases that lead to relaxation of vascular smooth muscle.

Prescribing

The duration of action of **sodium nitroprusside** is just 5 minutes and must, therefore, be administered by continuous IV infusion. Rates are started low and gradually increased at 5-minute intervals, ensuring reduction in BP is not overly rapid. In patients taking concurrent anti-hypertensives, lower doses may be necessary. Sodium nitroprusside infusions should be handled with care as solutions degrade when exposed to light and are vesicant. On the whole, its use has largely fallen out of favour.

Unwanted effects

Aside from profound hypotension and an increase in intracranial pressure, side effects associated with **sodium nitroprusside** therapy are largely attributed to accumulation of its toxic metabolites cyanide and thiocyanate. The risk of cyanide poisoning is increased with renal and hepatic impairment, and prolonged infusions. Symptoms include nausea and vomiting, dizziness, headache, sweating, palpitations, arrhythmias, and metabolic acidosis. To avoid the risk of toxicity treatment should be discontinued after 10 minutes if ineffective and a few hours where effective. Symptomatic patients should have treatment discontinued and require urgent treatment with oxygen and possibly **dicobalt edetate**.

Further reading

Barra S, Vitagliano A, Cuomo V, et al. (2009) Vascular and metabolic effects of angiotensin II receptor blockers. *Expert Opinions in Pharmacotherapy* 10(2), 173–89.

Eisenberg MJ, Brox A, Bestawros AN (2004) Calcium channel blockers: an update. *American Journal of Medicine* 116(1), 35–43.

Hanif K, Bid HK, Konwar R (2010) Reinventing ACE inhibitors: some old and new implications of ACE inhibition. *Hypertension Research* 33(1), 11–21.

Kurtz TW, Klein U (2009) Next generation multifunctional angiotensin receptor blockers. *Hypertension Research* 32(10), 826–34.

Oparil S, Zaman MA, Calhoun DA (2003) Pathogenesis of hypertension. *Annals of Internal Medicine* 139, 761–76.

O'Rourke MF (2002) From theory into practice. Arterial hemodynamics in clinical hypertension. *Journal of Hypertension* 20, 1901–15.

Ram CVS (2010) Beta-blockers in hypertension. *American Journal of Cardiology* 106(12), 1819–25.

Rhoades R, Planzer R. (1996) *Human Physiology*. Philadelphia, PA: Saunders College Publishing.

Smithburger PL, Kane-Gill SL, Nestor BL, Seybert AL (2010) Recent advances in the treatment of hypertensive emergencies. *Critical Care Nurse* 30(5), 24–30.

Varon J, Marik P (2003) Clinical review: the management of hypertensive crisis. *Critical Care* 7(5), 374–84.

Guidelines

Diao D, Wright JM, Cundiff DK, et al. (2012) Pharmacotherapy for mild hypertension. *Cochrane Database Systems Review* 18(8), CD006742.

European Society of Cardiology (2013) Guidelines for the management of arterial hypertension. https://academic.oup.com/eurheartj/article/39/33/3021/5079119 [accessed 22 March 2019]

James PA, Oparil S, Carter BL, et al. (2014) Evidence-based guidelines for the management of high blood pressure in adults; report from the panel members appointed to the Eighth Joint National Committee (JNC 8). *Journal of the American Medical Association* 311(5), 507–20.

NICE CG127 (2011) Hypertension; Clinical management of primary hypertension in adults (Updated 2016). https://www.nice.org.uk/guidance/cg127 [accessed 16 March 2019].

SIGN 149 (2017) Risk estimation and the prevention of cardiovascular disease. https://www.sign.ac.uk/assets/sign149.pdf [accessed 22 March 2019].

2.2 Peripheral vascular disease

Peripheral vascular disease (PVD), is a group of common conditions that occur secondary to insufficient perfusion of peripheral tissues and may be occlusive or vasospastic in nature. Occlusive disease is caused by atherosclerosis, possibly complicated by an embolus or thrombus, and may be acute or chronic in onset, e.g. critical limb ischaemia or intermittent claudication. PVD affects 12–14% of the population, with men and women equally implicated.

Raynaud's phenomenon is an exaggerated vasospastic response to cold or emotional stimuli affecting around 10% of the population and is invariably idiopathic in origin.

Pathophysiology

Occlusive peripheral artery disease

Atherosclerosis can affect multiple arterial territories, but predominantly involves coronary and cerebrovascular vessels. Peripheral artery disease (PAD) is mainly atherosclerotic (i.e. plaques of lipid, connective tissue, and inflammatory cells; see Topic 2.4, 'Stable angina') in origin, and tends to occur at arterial bifurcations or tapering vessels. Most symptomatic patients have involvement of femoral and popliteal arteries, while tibial and peroneal are also common locations. Around 90% of patients with PAD have concurrent coronary disease and 50% have cerebrovascular disease. The Fontaine classification system is used to stage PAD according to limb pain on exercise and presence of peripheral pulses (see Table 2.4).

Intermittent claudication (IC) (stages 1–2) occurs when atherosclerosis of vessels, and thus partial or complete occlusion, leads to failure of metabolic delivery to meet muscular demand. Men are twice as likely to have IC, particularly those at risk of atherosclerosis. Typically, IC is associated with single vessel disease (e.g. aorto-iliac, femoral or popliteal, or calf vessels), as collateral blood supply will help with oxygen delivery to tissues.

Critical limb ischaemia (stages 3–4) results in patients being symptomatic at rest and requiring management with analgesia, treatment of risk factors, and endovascular or surgical revascularization, otherwise amputation may be required. Ankle-brachial pressure index, duplex ultrasonography, and magnetic resonance (MR) or computed tomography (CT) angiography can help to confirm diagnosis.

Acute limb ischaemia is the sudden occlusion of a vessel secondary to a thrombus or embolus. About 60% of acute events are caused by a thrombus occluding an already atherosclerotic-stenosed vessel. This occurs in the presence of dehydration, hypotension, malignancy, or other prothrombotic conditions. Acute events from an embolus (30%) tend to be from a cardiac cause such as atrial fibrillation, myocardial infarction, or aneurysm, and are of rapid onset, resulting in complete distal vessel occlusion. Patients present clinically with the six 'P's' and 40% will have irreversible limb damage if not treated within 6 hours (see Table 2.5). Early assessment and considered use of heparin, to avoid thrombus propagation is essential unless undergoing surgery within 4 hours.

In addition to treating risk-modifiable factors (e.g. diabetes, hypertension, and smoking), pharmacological management with the 5-HT$_2$ receptor antagonist **naftidrofuryl** can increase blood flow to the distal limb via vascular smooth muscle vasodilation. Other less favourable options include phosphodiesterase inhibitors, like **cilostazol**, which inhibit platelet aggregation, cause vascular smooth muscle proliferation and promote

Table 2.4 The Fontaine classification system of occlusive peripheral arterial disease

Stage	Symptoms
Stage 1	No symptoms
Stage 2	Intermittent claudication subdivided into:
2a	without pain on resting, but with claudication at a distance of greater than 200 m
2b	without pain on resting, but with a claudication distance of less than 200 m
Stage 3	Nocturnal and/or resting pain
Stage 4	Necrosis (death of tissue) and/or gangrene in the limb

Reproduced from Fontaine R, Kim M, Kieny R; Kim; Kieny (1954). 'Die chirugische Behandlung der peripheren Durchblutungsstörungen. (Surgical treatment of peripheral circulation disorders)'. Helvetica Chirurgica Acta (in German). 21 (5/6): 499–533.

vasodilation, potentially slowing disease progression and reduce symptoms.

Vasospastic/Raynaud's phenomenon

Raynaud's phenomenon is characterized by an exaggerated vasospastic response to cold or emotion so that digits turn white (ischaemic), then blue (cyanotic), then red (reperfusion). Primary or idiopathic Raynaud's' disease accounts for 90% of cases, while secondary disease can be caused by other conditions (see Box 2.2); especially systemic sclerosis.

The pathophysiology in Raynaud's phenomenon is still poorly understood, but is a result of the dysregulation of neuroendothelial control mechanisms such that vasoconstriction predominates. Peripheral oxygen delivery is regulated by vascular, intravascular or neural factors.

Vascular factors include impaired endothelial vasodilation function (because of increased levels of vasoconstrictor endothelin-1) or reduced supply of vasodilators (e.g. nitric oxide or prostacyclin; see Topic 2.1, 'Hypertension'). Furthermore, higher levels of angiotensin II, a potent vasoconstrictor, have been found in those with systemic sclerosis, suggesting that ACE inhibitors may be beneficial.

Intravascular factors that may compromise microcirculation include:

Table 2.5 Symptoms and management of acute limb ischaemia

The six P's of acute limb ischaemia: pain, pallor, paralysis, pulseless, paraesthesia, perishingly cold (poikilothermia)		
	Symptoms and signs	Management options
Incomplete (viable limb)	Reduced pulses, Reduced capillary refill	Heparinization—prevent propagation of thrombus. Urgent imaging. Consider thrombolysis,* angioplasty, arterial surgery)
Complete (acutely threatened limb)	White limb, Cold limb, Pulseless limb	Thrombolysis* Angioplasty Embolectomy, or urgent arterial bypass
Irreversible (non-salvageable limb)	Mottling of skin, Petechial haemorrhages, Painful, wood hard muscles	Amputation

*Thrombolysis is used for acute thrombosis (see Topic 2.5, 'Acute coronary syndrome'), although this often fails in embolic causes of occlusion so interventional embolectomy or angioplasty is required.

- platelet activation, through increased levels of thromboxane;
- defective fibrinolysis, in the case of systemic sclerosis (e.g. through changes in tissue plasminogen activating factors);
- oxidative stress or increased blood viscosity, which is strongly associated with hand–arm vibration syndrome.

Neural factors are also involved in the form of dysfunction from sensory afferents that may result in abnormal peripheral nerve function. Post-junctional α2-adrenoceptors also predominate in Raynaud's disease above the normal α1 receptors function that regulate finger blood flow, prolonging vasoconstriction.

For a full summary of the relevant pathways and drug targets, see Figure 2.4.

Box 2.2 Secondary causes of Raynaud's syndrome

Rheumatology/autoimmune diseases

- Scleroderma
- Systemic lupus erythematosus
- Rheumatoid arthritis
- Sjögren's syndrome

Endocrine/metabolic disorders

- Carcinoid syndrome
- Phaeochromocytoma
- Hypothyroidism
- Diabetes

Malignant diseases

- Pulmonary neoplasm
- Ovarian carcinoma
- Other neoplasms/paraneoplastic syndromes
- Lymphoma

Arterial and vasospastic disorders

- Arteriosclerosis
- Buerger's disease (thromboangiitis obliterans)
- Prinzmetal angina
- Migraine

Mechanical/environmental causes

- Tobacco smoking
- Trauma
- Vibration (hand/arm vibration syndrome)
- Frostbite

Drugs

- β-blockers
- Ergot derivatives
- Combined oral contraceptive pill
- *Cytotoxics*: bleomycin, vinblastine, cisplatin

Management

Occlusive peripheral artery disease

The primary management of peripheral arterial disease is through the modification of risk factors, either by introducing lifestyle change or with drug therapy (Box 2.3). Supervised exercise programmes are recommended to gradually build up strength and enable patients to do exercise while remaining pain free.

In patients who remain symptomatic despite these measures, revascularization such as angioplasty or, less commonly, a bypass may be an option. In more severe cases of occlusive peripheral arterial disease, gangrenous limbs may require amputation.

The peripheral vasodilator, **naftidrofuryl**, provides symptomatic relief of intermittent claudication, but has no effect on disease progression. It is, therefore, reserved for patients where angioplasty is unsuitable, has failed or is about to be performed. Other treatment options, such as **pentoxifylline**, **inositol nicotinate**, and **cilostazol** are not currently recommended by NICE for treatment of intermittent claudication in PAD, as they have been shown to be inferior to naftidrofuryl with regards to pain-free walking distance, and improvement in maximum walking distance. They are also more expensive.

Vasospastic/Raynaud's phenomenon

Initial investigations and a full drug history may be carried out to exclude any underlying causes and any drugs known to cause 'cold extremities' should be discontinued, e.g. β-blockers. Although referral may be necessary for secondary disease, idiopathic disease is initially managed in primary care, with advice given on lifestyle changes that may help minimize symptoms (see Box 2.4).

Where lifestyle measures alone are inadequate, patients can be offered a trial of **nifedipine**, prescribed as either regular or intermittent therapy during cold exposure. Immediate release nifedipine is the only medication licensed for this, but in the three-quarters of patients that experience side effects, such as flushing or headaches, alternative off-label medication can be tried. Off-label options, and those used in secondary care for their peripheral dilation effects include nifedipine MR or other dihydropyridines, peripheral vasodilators (**naftidrofuryl oxalate** or **inositol nicotinate**), ACE inhibitors, or ARBs. SSRIs and α-adrenoceptor antagonists, like **prazosin** have been used, but evidence for their use is weak.

To avoid side effects from treatment, doses are started low, preferably taken at night, and increased every few days to the target dose. Each drug should be continued for at least 2 weeks to allow a response, with a washout period of at least 3 days given before trying an alternative therapy. Patients unresponsive to first or second-line treatment may require referral.

Prostaglandin treatments, such as **iloprost** and **epoprostenol**, are reserved for specialist treatment of severe episodes associated with underlying connective tissue disorders (e.g. scleroderma) and, therefore, administered under the supervision of a rheumatologist.

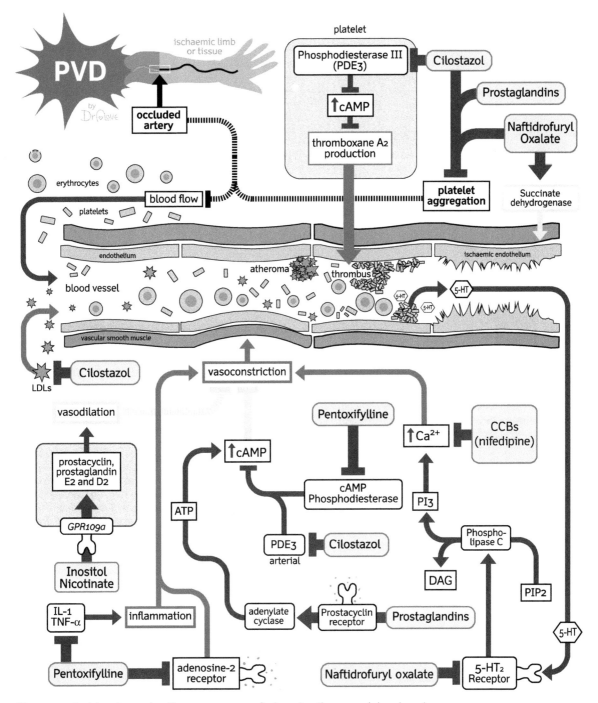

Figure 2.4 Peripheral vascular disease: summary of relevant pathways and drug targets.

Box 2.3 Modifiable risk factors for peripheral arterial disease

- Smoking cessation
- *Regular exercise*: ideally supervised exercise programmes
- Management of hypertension
- Lowering cholesterol
- Optimal management of diabetes mellitus (DM)
- Anti-platelet therapy

Drug classes used in management

Naftidrofuryl oxalate

Naftidrofuryl is a potent 5-hydroxytriptamine serotonergic antagonist, which can also activate succinic dehydrogenase.

Mechanism of action

The 5-HT_2 G protein–coupled receptors stimulate phospholipase C activity, leading to DAG and IP_3 release, which promotes an increase in intracellular Ca^{2+} and vascular smooth muscle contraction. The blocking actions of **naftidrofuryl** on 5-HT_2 receptors favours vasodilation, not only because it blocks the direct contraction of muscle cells by platelet-released serotonin, but also because it stops the amplifying effect that serotonin exerts on further platelet aggregation. It also enhances the release of endothelium-derived relaxing factors.

Naftidrofuryl also affects cellular metabolism by improving aerobic glucose utilization. It promotes the production of high-energy phosphates in ischaemic tissue by activating the enzyme succinic dehydrogenase. The

Box 2.4 Lifestyle measures in Raynaud's phenomenon

- Keep warm (applies to whole body, as well as hand and feet)
- Exercise regularly
- Smoking cessation
- Stress management if this is trigger

protective action of naftidrofuryl seems to occur first by preventing the endothelial cell mortality induced by prolonged ischaemia, and, in this way, it avoids blood elements from coming into contact with the underlying tissue. As a result, neither platelet aggregation and thrombus formation nor the smooth muscle cell contraction induced by circulating serotonin occurs.

Prescribing

Naftidrofuryl oxalate is the only peripheral vasodilator advocated by NICE for the management of intermittent claudication, where drug therapy is indicated. It is administered orally with food and plenty of water to ensure adequate diuresis and reduce the risk of developing kidney stones.

Unwanted effects

At recommended treatment doses side effects to **naftidrofuryl oxalate** are infrequent, but may include GI toxicity, such as nausea and diarrhoea, or central effects, including dizziness and difficulty in sleeping. In overdose, it can cause cardiac depression or convulsions, which should be treated with activated charcoal. It should be avoided in patients with a history of renal calcium stones due to the risk outlined above.

Cilostazol

The phosphodiesterase III inhibitor cilostazol has diverse pharmacological effects, including inhibition of platelet activation and aggregation, vasodilation, augmented limb blood flow, and improvement in serum lipids.

Mechanism of action

Cilostazol and its metabolites increase intracellular cAMP through inhibition of phosphodiesterase III (PDE III)-mediated hydrolysis. Intra-platelet cAMP inhibits phospholipase and cyclo-oxigenase activity, reducing thromboxane A_2 production and preventing platelet aggregation.

Increased cAMP also affects the vasomotor tone and smooth muscle relaxation, which leads to arteriolar vasodilation. The vasodilatory properties of cilostazol are more pronounced on femoral arteries than on vertebral, carotid, or superior mesenteric arteries, which might be a consequence of the differential abundance of PDE III in these tissues.

Cilostazol can have beneficial effects in slowing the progression of atherosclerosis by improving the serum lipid profile, decreasing serum triglycerides by the release of lipoprotein lipase from adipocytes and increasing high-density lipoprotein cholesterol (HDL-C).

Prescribing

Cilostazol is licensed for use in intermittent claudication in the absence of rest pain, Fontaine class 2. It is taken orally twice daily (BD) on an empty stomach as the presence of food can markedly increase plasma levels, thereby increasing adverse effects. An improvement in symptoms should be seen after 4–6 months (maybe as early as 4 weeks), and treatment should be discontinued if patients fail to respond after this time.

Unwanted effects

Side effects due to vasodilation are relatively common with **cilostazol**, leading to headache in more than 30% of patients, and less commonly dizziness, flushing, and palpitations, preventing its use in patients with some arrhythmias.

As cilostazol inhibits platelet aggregation the risk of haemorrhage and bruising is increased and should, therefore, be avoided in patients at high risk of bleeding, such as those undergoing surgery or with a history of haemorrhagic stroke or peptic ulcer disease.

Other common side effects reported with treatment include loose or abnormal stools, which affects more than 15% of patients.

Cilostazol is extensively metabolized in the liver and metabolites excreted via the kidney, therefore requiring dose reductions in severe renal and hepatic impairment.

Drug interactions

Cilostazol is metabolized via the cytochrome P450 enzyme system, making it susceptible to interaction with drugs known to induce or, more significantly, inhibit this enzyme. Potent inhibitors of CYP3A4 including **ketoconazole**, **omeprazole**, **diltiazem**, and **erythromycin**, can increase the effects of cilostazol by more than 100% and concurrent use is best avoided. The risk of interactions with other drugs known to cause vasodilation or prolong bleeding time, remains theoretical, although manufacturers advise caution.

Pentoxifylline

Pentoxifylline inhibits the cyclic nucleotide phosphodiesterases, acts as an antagonist at adenosine 2 receptors, and can inhibit the pro-inflammatory actions of IL-1 and TNF-α.

Mechanism of action

Pentoxifylline is a derivative of the methylxanthine theobromine that has been shown to decrease blood viscosity, develop red blood cell flexibility, and reduce the activity of platelets and hypercoagulability in patients who suffer from PVD.

It can suppress the pro-inflammatory action of IL-1 and TNF-α on neutrophil function, including degranulation, adhesion, migration, and superoxide production. The inhibition of TNF-α production by pentoxifylline seems to occur by the regulation of gene transcription, as it can decrease the levels of TNF-α mRNA in endotoxin-treated monocytes and macrophages.

The effects of pentoxifylline are ascribed to the inhibition of intracellular cAMP phosphodiesterase, leading to an increase in the concentration of cAMP inside the cell. This, in turn, acts on the cytokine network, to reduce phagocytic activity, superoxide anion production, and lysosomal enzyme release by polymorphonuclear cells. It is assumed that the induction of prostacyclin formation endogenously may contribute to the increase in cAMP, through stimulation of specific cyclo-oxygenases.

Prescribing

The use of **pentoxifylline** is largely outdated and no longer recommended, due to inferior efficacy. Where used, it is administered orally 2–3 times a day with food and plenty of water.

Unwanted effects

The frequency of side effects to **pentoxifylline** is comparable with placebo and tends to be non-specific GI side effects and headaches. As it impairs platelet function, it is contraindicated in cerebral and extensive retinal haemorrhage, as well as acutely following an MI.

Pentoxifylline is extensively metabolized by the liver before metabolites are excreted via the kidney; dose reductions are therefore recommended in severe renal or hepatic impairment.

Inositol nicotinate

Inositol nicotinate is made by the inositol esterification of niacin and acts as a vasodilator that has reduced reddening effects on epidermal tissues.

Mechanism of action

Niacin is a water-soluble vitamin of the B complex, required for the formation of coenzymes NAD and NADP. As a modified niacin derivative, **inositol nicotinate** is supposed to be broken down into the metabolites niacin and inositol at a lower rate, thus reducing or preventing the 'flushing' observed with other preparations. Unlike niacin, it seems that inositol nicotinate lacks any significant lipid lowering properties and there is no evidence to recommend it to treat dyslipidaemia.

Experimental evidence suggests that the prostanoids are involved in the vasodilatory properties of nicotinic acid administration, with increased levels of the prostanoids prostacyclin, prostaglandin E2 and D2 and their metabolites. Also, cutaneous blood flow was decreased in mice lacking the nicotinic acid receptor GPR109A, suggesting that it can also have a direct role in the vasodilatory effect.

Prescribing

Inositol nicotinate is no longer recommended for use in intermittent claudication due to its inferior efficacy and greater cost compared with **naftidofuryl**, but has been used in Raynaud's, albeit rarely. When taken orally, only small amounts are absorbed and large doses are therefore required, three times a day (TDS).

Unwanted effects

Side effects are uncommon, but where they do occur are secondary to vasodilation, i.e. flushing, dizziness, headache, and postural hypotension. It should be avoided acutely following an MI or cerebrovascular accident due to the risk of bleed.

Ca²⁺ channel blockers

Ca^{2+} channel blockers promote widespread vasodilation by acting on the voltage-gated Ca^{2+} channels of the plasma membrane. For example, nifedipine.

Mechanism of action

See dihydropyridine Ca^{2+} channel blockers (see Topic 2.1, 'Hypertension').

Prescribing

Although only immediate-release **nifedipine** is licensed for symptom relief in Raynaud's phenomenon, other dihydropyridines are used and slow-release nifedipine tends to be better tolerated. Treatment doses are started low and gradually increased as necessary, i.e. from 5 mg to 20 mg TDS.

Unwanted effects

The vasodilator-related toxicities associated with **nifedipine** treatment, are more pronounced with the immediate-release preparation, i.e. flushing, headaches, dizziness, etc. For more details see Topic 2.1, 'Hypertension'.

Prostaglandins

Prostaglandins, such as prostacyclin and its analogue, iloprost, activate adenylate cyclase, increasing cAMP levels and causing a potent vasodilatory action. For example, iloprost and epoprostenol.

Mechanism of action

Prostacyclin (prostaglandin I2) is a member of the prostaglandin family of lipid mediators and is the main product of arachidonic acid metabolism by endothelial cells. The deficiency in prostacyclin has been linked with the pathogenesis of PVD. The plasma membrane prostacyclin receptor is a member of the G protein–coupled receptor superfamily. The vasodilatory properties of prostacyclin are probably mediated through activation of adenylate cyclase and increase in cAMP.

Although a chemically unstable molecule, prostacyclin is available as a freeze-dried preparation, **epoprostenol**, which is used for IV administration. The two major pharmacological actions of epoprostenol are vasodilation of pulmonary and systemic vasculature and inhibition of platelet aggregation. **Iloprost**, a stable synthetic analogue of prostacyclin (prostaglandin I2), is a potent vasodilator and inhibitor of platelet aggregation. It binds with equal affinity to human prostacyclin and prostaglandin EP1 receptors.

Prescribing

Neither **iloprost** nor **epoprostenol** are licensed for use in Raynaud's phenomenon, although both these agents are widely used, administered IV in severe disease unresponsive to oral dihydropyridines. Iloprost, is also available orally, but only demonstrates a benefit for this indication when administered IV.

For either drug, the infusion is started slowly and gradually titrated up as tolerated. Patients should be monitored closely for a fall in BP, oxygen saturations, or a raised pulse. Poor oxygen saturations may be indicative of pulmonary oedema.

Unwanted effects

As potent vasodilators, side effects predictably include postural hypotension, headaches, dizziness, palpitations, and flushing; in part, this can be minimized by careful titration of infusion. Treatment should be avoided in patients at high risk of bleeding or in severe heart failure.

Further reading

Creager MA, Kaufman JA, Conte MS (2012) Clinical practice. Acute limb ischemia. *New England Journal of Medicine* 366(23), 2198–206.

Herrick AL (2005) Pathogenesis of Raynaud's phenomenon. *Rheumatology (Oxford)* 44(5), 587–96.

Pearce L, Ghosh J, Counsell A, et al. (2008) Cilostazol and peripheral arterial disease. *Expert Opinion in Pharmacotherapy* 9(15), 2683–90.

Spittell PC (2012) Peripheral vascular disease. In: Murphy JG, Lloyd MA (Eds) *Mayo Clinic Cardiology: Concise Textbook*, pp. 447–54. Oxford: Oxford University Press.

Vane J, Corin RE (2003) Prostacyclin: a vascular mediator. *European Journal of Vascular and Endovascular Surgery* 26(6), 571–8.

Guidelines

Hirsch AT, Haskal ZJ, Hertzer NR (2006) ACC/AHA 2005 guidelines for the management of patients with peripheral arterial disease. *Journal of the American College of Cardiology* 47, 1239–1312.

NICE CG147 (Aug 2012) Peripheral arterial disease: diagnosis and management. https://www.nice.org.uk/guidance/CG147/ [accessed 22 March 2019].

NICE QS52 (Jan 2014) Peripheral arterial disease. https://www.nice.org.uk/guidance/qs52 [accessed 16 March 2019].

NICE TA223 (May 2011) Cilostazol, naftidrofuryl, oxalate, pentoxifylline and inositol nicotinate for the treatment of intermittent claudication in people with peripheral arterial disease. https://www.nice.org.uk/guidance/ta223 [accessed 16 March 2019].

SIGN 129 (2012) Antithrombotics: indications and management. http://www.sign.ac.uk/guidelines/fulltext/129/index.html [accessed 22 March 2019].

2.3 Dyslipidaemias

Dyslipidaemia is an abnormal level of serum lipids including total cholesterol, high-density lipoprotein cholesterol (HDL-C), low-density lipoprotein cholesterol (LDL-C) or triglycerides (TG), and is usually associated with an augmented risk of cardiovascular disease. The UK population expresses one of the highest serum cholesterol levels worldwide. Reducing levels of LDL-C remains the key target for lipid lowering, hence current therapeutic strategies aim to reduce the rate of cholesterol biosynthesis (statins) or decrease the rate of absorption of cholesterol into the circulation (**ezetimibe**, bile acids).

Primary hyperlipidaemias, such as heterozygous familial hypercholesterolaemia (FH), are one of the most common familial conditions and have a prevalence of almost 1 in 500 (in heterozygous FH). Here, total cholesterol is typically above 7.5 mmol/L, and 50% of men and 30% of women will go on to develop coronary heart disease by the age of 50 and 60 years, respectively (see Broome and Welsh criteria, 'Primary hyperlipidaemias').

Pathophysiology

Lipids have a central role in initiation and deposition in atherosclerosis; ultimately leading to cardiovascular disease (be it angina, myocardial infarction, stroke, or intermittent claudication; see Topics 2.4, 'Stable angina', 2.5, 'Acute coronary syndrome', 9.1, 'Cerebrovascular disease', and 2.2, 'Peripheral vascular disease', respectively). In addition to lipid deposition, the inflammation of vessel walls is also a fundamental process in the pathogenesis of atherosclerosis (see Topic 2.4, 'Stable angina').

Lipoproteins are complex particles formed of multiple proteins that transport all lipids. There are four classes of lipoproteins, classified according to density (Table 2.6). In the absence of disease 70% of plasma cholesterol is bound up as low-density lipoprotein (LDL).

Cholesterol is important as a cellular membrane protein and as a precursor to many steroid hormones (e.g. cortisol). *De novo* synthesis occurs in liver hepatocytes from the reduction of acetyl coenzyme A by HMG-CoA reductase. Conversely, enzyme activity is reduced by an increase in intracellular cholesterol, available either through absorption from the gut (e.g. via the Niemann–Pick-like receptor) or from enterohepatic recycling of bile salts; the drug **ezetimibe** blocks the former causing a reduction in cholesterol absorption.

Triglycerides are stored as fat and during periods of fasting can be utilized as free fatty acids to act as an energy supply. When triglycerides are laid down for storage they are synthesized from esterification of free fatty acids with glycerol.

Lipoprotein particle metabolism is the handling of the lipoprotein particles within the body. Hydrophilic groups of the phospholipids, cholesterol, and apoproteins facing outward, while triglyceride fats and cholesteryl esters are carried internally, protected from the water. The capacity of the proteins that form the surface of the particles to interact with enzymes in the blood and with specific proteins on the surface of cells, can determine the triglycerides and cholesterol addition or removal from the transport particles.

The metabolism of lipoprotein particles can be divided into two pathways, which vary in the origin of the lipoprotein particles, either mainly from the diet (*exogenous*) or the liver (*endogenous*).

Exogenous metabolism: enterocytes absorb fatty acids and monoglycerides from the chymus. Inside enterocytes, the lipids (triacylglycerols, phospholipids, cholesterol, and cholesteryl esters) are assembled into large lipoproteins (chylomicrons) that allow passage through the lymphatic system into the blood.

Endogenous metabolism: hepatocytes can mediate the *de novo* synthesis of triacylglycerols, which after assembly with cholesteryl esters and apolipoprotein B-100

Table 2.6 Fat composition

Lipoproteins	Composition	Associated apolipoprotein	Source	Effect/role
Chylomicrons	95% triglycerides (TG), 5% cholesterol	APO A,B,B_{48},C,E	Intestine	Mobilize dietary lipids, deliver dietary triglycerides to adipose tissue and muscles, and dietary cholesterol to the liver
VLDL (very low-density lipoproteins)	80% TG, 20% cholesterol	APO B_{100},C,E	Liver	Transport triglycerols to extrahepatic tissues
IDL (intermediate density lipoproteins)	50% TG, 50% cholesterol	APO B_{100},E	Formed from VLDL in plasma	Either converted to LDL or taken up by the liver
LDL	10% TG, 90% cholesterol	APO B_{100}	VLDL	Principal plasma carrier of cholesterol for delivering to peripheral tissues
HDL (high-density lipoproteins)	5% TG, 95% cholesterol	APO A	Chylomicrons, VLDL, liver, intestine	Increases uptake of cholesterol by the liver

form nascent very low-density lipoproteins (VLDL) particles that are released into the circulation.

In the circulation, the triglycerides are hydrolysed 'off' by lipoprotein lipase in the presence of a cofactor (chylomicron-associated apolipoprotein C). This releases free fatty acids, which can then be used as energy in muscle or liver, or stored as energy (in fat). Any remaining lipoproteins enter the HDL pool, leaving behind the chylomicron remnants.

The chylomicron remnants bind to LDL-receptor-like proteins (e.g. Apo E receptor) on the hepatocytes, enabling their uptake. Any excess hepatic cholesterol and triglycerides form a complex with VLDL and, as such, re-enter the circulation where they are acted on by lipoprotein lipases, thereby releasing free fatty acids and intermediate density lipoproteins (IDL); triglycerides in IDL are, once again, hydrolysed to release further free fatty acids and LDL. Subsequently, about 75% of LDL is taken back into hepatocytes and removed from the circulation.

LDL particles deliver cholesterol to tissues so that an excess in LDL (e.g. through diet) or deficiency in receptor numbers, increases the deposition of cholesterol in arterial walls. The oxidation of LDL and subsequent formation of atheromatous plaques is dealt with elsewhere (see Topic 2.4, 'Stable angina').

Free cholesterol can be sequestered back to the liver by HDL, potentially protecting against atheroma formation. Free cholesterol bound to (Apo A1 taking up cholesterol via ABCA1 initially and the ABCG1) nascent HDL is esterified by lecithin-cholesterol acyltransferase to mature HDL particles, which can be removed directly via HDL receptors [e.g. scavenger receptor BI (SR-BI)]. The cholesteryl esters can be transferred to other lipoproteins (such as LDL and VLDL) with the aid of CETP (cholesteryl ester transfer protein) in exchange for triglycerides. These lipoproteins can be taken up by secreting unesterified cholesterol into the bile or by conversion of cholesterol to bile acids.

Types of hyperlipidaemias

Primary hyperlipidaemias

Around 70% of hyperlipidaemias are primary or familial in origin and are biochemically classified according to the Fredrickson classification (Table 2.7).

The most common familial hyperlipidaemia is heterozygous FH, an autosomal dominant condition resulting in many mutations of the LDL receptor. Receptor failure means *delayed clearance* of LDL from plasma resulting in raised total and LDL-C levels from early childhood. In the western world prevalence is approximately 1:500 (heterozygotes) and results in cholesterol levels of 6.5–10 mmol/L and TGs in excess of 2.3 mmol/L. Another common mutation in apolipoprotein (apoB) also reduces LDL uptake and results in a clinically indistinguishable condition; rarer

Table 2.7 The Fredrickson classification scheme organizes primary dyslipidaemias into several categories

Hyperlipoproteinaemia	Elevated lipoprotein(s)	Serum lipid pattern
Type I	Chylomicrons	Elevated triglycerides
Type IIa	LDL	Elevated cholesterol
Type IIb	LDL and VLDL	Elevated triglycerides and cholesterol
Type III	IDL and chylomicron remnants	Elevated triglycerides and cholesterol
Type IV	VLDL	Elevated triglycerides
Type V	Chylomicrons and VLDL	Elevated triglycerides and cholesterol

protein mutations also exist (see Table 2.8). Diagnosis of FH is made on the Simon Broome criteria:

- *Definite* FH:
  - Total cholesterol >7.5 mmol/L and LDL-C of >4.9 mmol/L (adult values)

  and
  - xanthomata or evidence of this in a first-degree or second-degree relative

  or
  - DNA evidence of an LDL receptor mutation, familial defective apo-B-100 or a PCSK9 mutation.

Diagnosis of possible FH can also be made with Simon Broome criteria (see NICE guidance). In adults with a LDL-C greater than 13mmol/L, a diagnosis of homozygous familial hypercholesterolaemia should be considered, a much rare condition affecting 1 in a million people.

There are other diagnostic classifications systems, such as Welsh or Dutch criteria (https://www.fhscore.eu), which score various aspects of clinical history, physical signs, cholesterol levels, DNA analysis, and family history of markers (e.g. 1st degree relative with premature coronary disease).

Recently, the role of mutations in the *PCSK9* gene has gained much clinical significance where polymorphism may lead to 'loss of function' in PCSK9, so affecting the ability to lower expression of LDL receptors in the liver, as a consequence circulating LDL-C levels are reduced with associated reductions in cardiovascular risk; prevalent in ~2% of the population. Conversely, 'gain of function' polymorphism is also seen where LDL receptor removal is increased resulting in higher levels of circulating LDL-C in the circulation, since it is not so efficiently cleared, resulting in early development of atherosclerosis and associated risks of cardiovascular disease.

Secondary hyperlipidaemias

Secondary hyperlipidaemias are those caused by a primary disorder (see Table 2.8). For a full summary of the relevant pathways and drug targets, see Figure 2.5.

Management

Primary hypercholesterolaemia

Lipid-lowering therapy with a high-intensity statin (see Table 2.9) is recommended for all adults diagnosed with familial hypercholesterolaemia with the aim of reducing the LDL-C by 50% from baseline levels (see NICE guidance). Doses should be titrated up to the maximum tolerated dose to achieve the desired effect and patients advised that treatment will be lifelong. Where a statin is not tolerated or contraindicated, monotherapy with **ezetimibe** is recommended. Alternatively ezetimibe can be added into statin therapy, where statin monotherapy is insufficient to achieve a 50% reduction in LDL-C from baseline levels. Treatment with bile acid sequestrants, such as **nicotinic acid** (but not modified release formulations) or fibrates (primarily reserved for treatment of VLDL cf. LDL-C) may be considered in patients intolerant of ezetimibe or statins, or where combination therapy is again insufficient. The use of these agents, however, should be under the direction of a specialist for monitoring and advice, as not all agents can be used in combination, e.g. **gemfibrozil** should not be given in combination with a statin (see VOYAGER Study).

Table 2.8 Common causes of secondary and associated hyperlipoproteinaemias

Diabetes mellitus	Mainly a hypertriglyceridaemia ± hypercholesterolaemia (decreased HDL cholesterol)
Thyroid disease	Hypothyroidism LDL-C is raised due to decreased receptor-mediated LDL uptake and decreased lipoprotein lipase activity
Obesity	High energy intake—raised LDL-C, triglycerides. and reduced HDL-C
Alcohol excess	Alcohol-induced hypertriglyceridaemia
β-adrenoreceptor blockers	Raise triglyceride levels and lower HDL
Thiazide diuretics	Increase triglycerides and cholesterol
Steroid hormones	Androgens raise levels of LDL-C, decrease triglycerides and HDL. Glucocorticoids increase LDL-C, triglycerides and HDL
Cholestasis	Hypercholesterolaemia (from an abnormal lipoprotein (lipoprotein X) production from spill-over of biliary phospholipids to circulation)
Hepatocellular dysfunction	Hypertriglyceridaemia (due to impaired hepatic lipoprotein clearance)

Certain monoclonal antibodies may also be available by specialist prescribing in the case of primary hypercholesterolaemia or mixed dyslipidaemia; NICE defines specific criteria. **Evolocumab** or **alirocumab** work by inhibiting PCSK9 (proprotein convertase subtilisin/kexin type 9), an enzyme that binds to the receptor for LDL, which transports 3000–6000 fat molecules (including cholesterol) per particle so promoting removal of LDL cholesterol from circulation.

Lipid modification in CVD

Cardiovascular disease, through MI or stroke, is the leading cause of death in the UK. Identification of modifiable risk factors like smoking, BP, and lipid profile can significantly reduce mortality; with the latter being the most important modifier. Current advice is to complete a risk assessment using the on-line QRISK2 tool to determine 10-year risk of a cardiovascular event in patients under 85 years. Where the 10-year risk is found to be greater than 10%, patients will require a full risk assessment and intervention measures, including lifestyle advice (diet, physical activity, moderate alcohol consumption, smoking cessation, and weight management), and lipid modification. Patients with known coronary heart disease, angina, stroke, peripheral vascular disease, or familial hyperlipidaemia, are considered higher risk, thus requiring lifestyle changes and lipid modification from the outset (NICE).

Lipid modification therapy is the mainstay of treatment to reduce the risk of coronary heart disease and the process of atherosclerosis. Prior to starting lipid modification therapy, a full lipid profile should be carried out to include total cholesterol, HDL, non-HDL, and TG concentrations. Measurement of non-HDL is currently thought to be a better predictor of CVD risk compared with LDL-C; being more accurate, cheaper, and not requiring a fasting level. Patients with a total cholesterol greater than 9 mmol/L, non-HDL greater than 7.5 mmol/L or triglyceride level greater than 20 mmol/L (or 10 mmol/L fasting, unrelated to excessive alcohol), will require referral to a lipid specialist for management (NICE).

Statins are the preferred agents for lipid modification and the only drug class known to reduce CVD risk. Choice depends on risk scores and any pre-existing CVD (see Table 2.10); however, **atorvastatin** has largely replaced **simvastatin** as the drug of choice, due to its superior efficacy to toxicity profile and some evidence of plaque regression. For those with primary hypercholesterolaemia in whom a statin is not tolerated or contraindicated, **ezetimibe** may be used, as monotherapy or add-on therapy where statin monotherapy is insufficient. Other lipid-modifying agents, such as bile sequestrants, fibrates, nicotinic acid derivatives, and omega-3 fatty acids, are not currently recommended for use by NICE, either alone or in combination for primary prevention, as although effective in improving lipid profile they are unlikely to have any benefit in reducing CVD risk. These are mentioned herein for historical and mechanistic value.

A stain should be offered to all patients with cardiovascular disease for secondary prevention, however, the ultimate decision to treat made following discussion between patient and clinician, once they have been fully informed of the risks and benefits.

Patients on statin therapy for primary or secondary prevention should have their non-HDL rechecked at 3 months to ensure a 40% or greater reduction from baseline level. Where there has been a smaller than 40% reduction, compliance with lifestyle measures and treatment should be assessed, and atorvastatin escalated to 80 mg in patients on lower doses. Response to statins can fluctuate as individual's synthesis and absorption ratios vary.

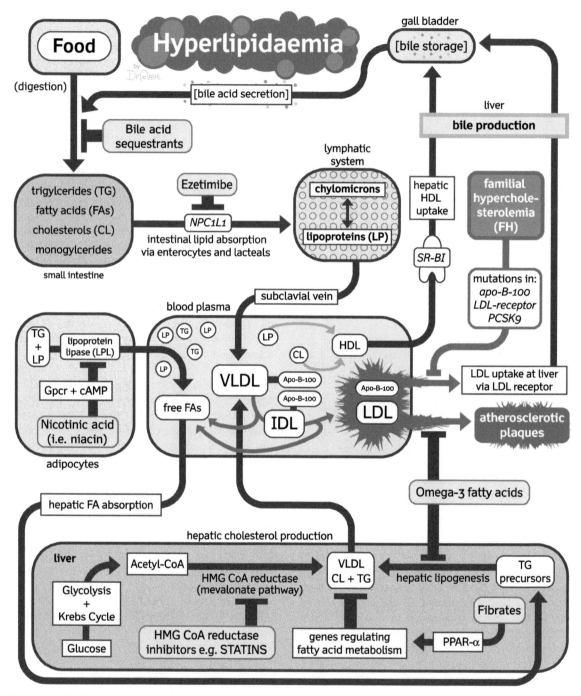

Figure 2.5 Dyslipidaemia: summary of relevant pathways and drug targets.

Table 2.9 Relative statin intensity

Intensity	Statin	Dose
High (greater than 40% reduction)	Atorvastatin	20, 40, 80 mg
	Rosuvastatin	10, 20, 40 mg
	Simvastatin	80 mg (not recommended)
Medium intensity (31–40% reduction)	Simvastatin	20, 40 mg
	Atorvastatin	10 mg
	Rosuvastatin	5 mg
	Fluvastatin	80 mg
Low intensity (20–30% reduction)	Simvastatin	10 mg
	Fluvastatin	20, 40 mg
	Pravastatin	10, 20, 40 mg

Drug classes used in management

HMG-CoA reductase inhibitors

Statins reduce cholesterol *de novo* synthesis through the inhibition of HMG-CoA reductase activity, the key enzyme in the cholesterol synthesis pathway catalysing the conversion of HMG-CoA in mevalonate. Examples include atorvastatin, pravastatin, fluvastatin, rosuvastatin, and simvastatin.

Mechanism of action

Statins have a β-hydroxy acid sequence within their chemical structure that is related to the structure of HMG-CoA. As a result, they competitively inhibit HMG-CoA reductase.

The lipid-altering effects of statins and the reduction of LDL-C in particular, reduces the formation of an atheromatous plaque associated with coronary heart disease. In addition, statins have pleiotropic properties independent of their effects on LDL levels, such as atherosclerotic plaque stabilization, anticoagulant effects, anti-inflammatory properties, nitric oxide-mediated improvement of endothelial dysfunction, and antioxidant effects.

Proportionally to doses, statins reduce LDL-C, while moderately increasing HDL-C (see VOYAGER) and decreasing TG.

Prescribing

Statins are the drug of choice for lipid modification, unless contraindicated, due to their superior efficacy in reducing LDL-C and the risk of CVD. Agents and doses are classified according to their potency, so that doses equivalent to **simvastatin** 80 mg are considered high intensity (e.g. **atorvastatin** 80 mg and **rosuvastatin** 40 mg). However, high-intensity doses are not recommended with simvastatin, as the risk of toxicity outweighs the benefits. Statin choice is dictated by the severity of hyperlipidaemia and patient tolerance.

Table 2.10 Choice of lipid therapy

Patient factors	Choice of therapy	Comments
≥10% risk of CVD in 10 years No CVD	Atorvastatin 20 mg	Consider higher dose in high risk patients based on co-morbidities, QRISK2 , or clinical judgment
Patients with CVD (secondary prevention)	Atorvastatin 80 mg	Use lower dose in the case of potential interactions, intolerance, or patient preference
Primary hypercholesterolaemia	High intensity statin	Increase to maximum tolerated dose
Primary hypercholesterolaemia where statin not tolerated/contraindicated	Ezetimibe 10 mg OD	
Primary hypercholesterolaemia where statin monotherapy ineffective	Atorvastatin 80 mg + ezetimibe 10 mg OD	
Primary hypercholesterolaemia intolerant of statin and ezetimibe	Bile acid sequestrant, nicotinic acid, fibrate	Initiated under the advice of a specialist

For optimal effects statins should be administered orally at night, as most cholesterol is synthesized when dietary intake is low. However, due to their relatively long half-life, atorvastatin, and rosuvastatin can be taken at any time of the day.

Unwanted effects

Side effects to statins are rare and comparable with placebo. Those most frequently reported are liver toxicity (raised transaminases), GI disturbances (nausea, diarrhoea), headache, dizziness, rash, insomnia, and muscle toxicity (myopathy and rhabdomyolysis).

As statins can cause hepatic toxicity and are predominantly hepatically cleared, they are contraindicated in active liver disease. While on treatment it is recommended that LFTs are measured at baseline and 3 months from starting treatment, where manufacturers advise that treatment is discontinued if levels exceed three times the upper limit of normal. That said, expert opinion in the UK and US suggests they may be used cautiously in patients with raised transaminases within three times the normal limit, providing liver enzymes remain static with regular monitoring.

Differential myalgia, myopathy, and rhabdomyolysis

The effects of statins on muscles is a widely publicized phenomena, although actually occurs very rarely; rhabdomyolysis affects approximately 3.4 in 100 000 patient years, and myopathy 11 in 100 000 patient years. Incidence is dose-related and increases when statins are co-prescribed with drugs that inhibit specific cytochrome P450 enzymes (see 'Drug interactions'). Where affected, the consequences can be severe; it is therefore essential that creatine kinase (CK) levels are the baseline levels measured on initiation in at-risk patients (elderly, renal impairment, family or personal history, interacting drugs, and uncontrolled hypothyroidism) and repeated in the event of muscle pain, weakness, or cramp. Levels should not be taken immediately following strenuous exercise as this may influence creatine kinase levels. Where levels are in excess of 5 × upper limit of normal (ULN), or in the event of severe muscle pain treatment should be discontinued. All patients receiving statins should be made aware of the potential for muscle toxicity, and advised to report any symptoms of muscle pain or weakness. CK can also be raised in hypothyroidism and certain ethnicities.

> ### PRESCRIBING WARNING
>
> **Simvastatin**
>
> Until 2011, simvastatin was prescribed at doses up to 80 mg, although due to an increased risk of myopathy (including rhabdomyolysis) compared with other statins used at equivocal LDL-lowering potencies, a maximum dose of 40 mg is now recommended unless a patient has been taking higher doses chronically with no adverse effects

Drug interactions

Simvastatin and **atorvastatin** are both substrates of CYP3A4, which is responsible for most of their interactions. In particular, guidance has been issued by the MHRA on co-administration of simvastatin with a number of drugs known to inhibit CYP 3A4 (see Table 2.11).

Although the level of risk associated with atorvastatin interactions is lower, close monitoring, temporary discontinuation, and dose reductions should be considered as they are for simvastatin. Caution is recommended when statins are co-prescribed with other drugs known to cause myopathy, in particular fibrates and **ezetimibe**.

Cholesterol absorption inhibitors (ezetimibe)

> Ezetimibe is a selective inhibitor of intestinal absorption of cholesterol and related phytosterols, leading to a reduction in one of the major routes for increasing cholesterol levels in the body.

Mechanism of action

Specific cholesterol absorption inhibitors lower cholesterol levels by acting at the brush border of the intestine, selectively binding to the transmembrane protein, Niemann–Pick C1-like (NPC1L1), which facilitates uptake of cholesterol from the GI tract into enterocytes on route to the liver. The reduction in cholesterol influx to the liver leads to a compensatory up-regulation of hepatic LDL receptors, which increases LDL clearance.

Prescribing

Ezetimibe is an oral therapy administered OD, either as adjunctive therapy with statins or an alternative in

Table 2.11 MHRA recommendations for interacting drugs known to increase risk of myopathy/rhabdomyolysis

Interacting drugs	Prescribing recommendations
Itraconazole, ketoconazole, posaconazole, erythromycin, clarithromycin, telithromycin, HIV protease inhibitors, nefazodone, ciclosporin, danazol, gemfibrozil	Contraindicated with simvastatin
Other fibrates	Do not exceed 10 mg simvastatin
Amiodarone, amlodipine, verapamil, diltiazem	Do not exceed 20 mg simvastatin daily
Fusidic acid	Monitor patients closely, consider stopping simvastatin temporarily
Grapefruit juice	Avoid grapefruit juice while taking simvastatin
Warfarin, coumarins	Monitor INR on initiation and during treatment in particular with dose changes

Reproduced from Medicines and Healthcare products Regulatory Agency, Simvastatin: updated advice on drug interactions (2012). Licensed under the Open Government Licence v3.0. https://www.gov.uk/drug-safety-update/simvastatin-updated-advice-on-drug-interactions

patients intolerant of or unable to take statins. In monotherapy, ezetimibe reduces plasma total cholesterol by about 15%, and LDL-C by about 20%, although it is not advocated first-line as, unlike with statins, studies have yet to demonstrate conclusively a reduction in cardiovascular morbidity or mortality when used alone. In combination ezetimibe acts synergistically with low-dose statin to significantly reduce LDL-C levels and improve cardiovascular outcomes.

Unwanted effects

Side effects to **ezetimibe** tend to be mild, transient, and non-specific, leading to GI symptoms and fatigue. The incidence of adverse effects increases when ezetimibe is co-administered with a statin, in particular, deranged LFTs, myalgia, and myopathy, although the latter has rarely been seen with ezetimibe monotherapy. Patients

are still advised to report any unexplained muscle pain or weakness.

Treatment can be safely administered in renal impairment, but should be avoided in moderate to severe hepatic impairment. It is also contraindicated in patients with persistently raised liver enzymes or active liver disease in combination with a statin.

Drug interactions

For a new drug, **ezetimibe** has been studied extensively in combination with other therapies, but as neither an inducer of, nor substrate for the cytochrome P450 enzyme system, the risk of interactions compared to statins is low. Ezetimibe in combination with **ciclosporin** has, however, been reported to significantly increase levels of both drugs. Monitoring of ciclosporin levels is, therefore, recommended where use of the two is unavoidable.

Bile acid sequestrants

Anion-exchange resins bind bile acids in the intestinal lumen and prevent their reabsorption. Examples include colesytramine, colestipol, and colesevelam

Mechanism of action

Bile acid sequestrants are large polymeric structures that exchange anions for bile acids, thus removing them from enterohepatic circulation. Bile acids are amphipathic, polar derivatives of cholesterol that are synthesized in the liver and secreted into the duodenum, where they are necessary for the digestion and absorption of cholesterol, fats, and fat-soluble vitamins. In the physiological process of enterohepatic circulation bile acids are reabsorbed in the terminal ileum and returned to the liver.

In the liver, bile acids inhibit the rate-limiting enzyme for bile acid synthesis from cholesterol. As a result, the rate of bile acids synthesis becomes maximal if resins interrupt their enterohepatic recycling. The increase in bile acid synthesis causes the depletion of intrahepatic cholesterol, and induces over-transcription of the LDL-receptor gene, increasing LDL-receptor activity. Hepatic LDL uptake is thus raised and clearance of circulating LDL-C increased. The increase in cholesterol synthesis often leads to an increase in VLDL secretion and small rise in plasma triglycerides. Moreover, resins promote apo-A1 synthesis and tend to raise HDL.

Prescribing

The bile acid sequestrants (**colestyramine**, **colesevelam**, and **colestipol**) are of limited value in lipid modification due to inferior efficacy and poor tolerability compared with other classes. They are generally reserved for use under specialist supervision, where other agents are ineffective alone or not tolerated; however, patients are frequently intolerant of their adverse effects (see 'Practical prescribing: colestyramine/ colestipol—improving concordance') and unaccepting of their poor palatability. Doses are taken orally either as sachets (colestyramine, colestipol) or multiple large tablets (colesevelam).

> **PRACTICAL PRESCRIBING**
>
> **Colestyramine/ colestipol—improving concordance**
>
> To improve the palatability of colestyramine and colestipol they may be mixed with fruit juices/pulp, thin soup, or skimmed milk. They should not be taken dry.

Unwanted effects

As the bile acid sequestrants remain within the gut lumen, GI side effects are common, i.e. constipation, bloating, nausea, and abdominal discomfort. As they impair fat absorption, bile acid-sequestrants impair absorption of fat soluble vitamins (A, D, E, and K), as well as some other medication. Accordingly, patients on other medication are advised to avoid taking these 1 hour before and 4–6 hours after taking a bile acid sequestrant. Drugs known to be affected include **digoxin**, **warfarin**, **levothyroxine**, **chlorthiazide**, and **propranolol**. The risk of impaired absorption of fat-soluble vitamins increases with prolonged treatment and at high doses.

Fibrates

> Fibrates are chemically related to fibric acids and exert their action by activating peroxisome proliferator-activated receptor alpha (PPAR-α). Examples include bezafibrate, ciprofibrate, fenofibrate, and gemfibrozil.

Mechanism of action

Peroxisome proliferator-activated receptors, PPAR-α (or NR1C1) receptors are part of the family of hormone-activated nuclear receptors that, upon activation, bind to the peroxisome proliferator response elements (PPREs) and induce the expression of target genes involved in fatty acid metabolism. PPARs are physiologically activated by natural agonists, such as eicosanoids (products of arachidonic acid metabolism) and fatty acids. Fibrates

predominantly activate the PPARα subtype of receptor, found mostly in organs such as the liver and muscle, leading to reduced atherosclerotic progression due to changes in lipid metabolism and inflammation; clinical benefit is clear in metabolic syndrome. In particular, PPARα is highly expressed in tissues that have high rates of fatty acid catabolism, and its activation can increase free fatty acid uptake and esterification in the liver; and fatty acid degradation through the peroxisomal and mitochondrial oxidation pathways and via ketone body synthesis. Moreover, PPARα activation inhibits the gene expression of apolipoprotein C-III, which functions by delaying the catabolism of TG-rich lipoproteins.

Prescribing

Fibrates are reserved for patients intolerant of statins, due to their inferior efficacy in reducing LDL-C and unlikely benefit in reducing the risk of CVD. There is little to distinguish between the four agents in the class in terms of ease of administration, as all are available as OD oral preparations (**bezafibrate** as a standard release product is taken TDS). Fibrates should be mainly reserved for treatment of VLDL as opposed to LDL.

Unwanted effects

Adverse effects to fibrates tend to be non-specific, i.e. GI effects, fatigue, headaches, and rash. They increase the lithogenic index of bile acids, thereby increasing the risk of gall stones, particularly in patients with history of cholelithiasis in whom use is best avoided.

Fibrates are contraindicated in severe renal and hepatic impairment as they are metabolized to varying extents prior to being excreted via the kidney. With **gemfibrozil** metabolism is via the cytochrome P450 enzyme system, making it more likely to interact with other drugs (see, 'Drug interactions').

Drug interactions

Interactions of clinical significance occur with drugs known to have similar toxicities, so that concurrent use with **ezetimibe** increases the risk of gallstones and the risk of myopathy is increased with statins. **Gemfibrozil** in particular should not be prescribed in combination with a statin.

As class fibrates increase the efficacy of antidiabetic therapy enhancing their hypoglycaemic effects. **Gemfibrozil** is contraindicated with **repaglinide** and caution advised with **rosiglitazone**.

Nicotinic acid

> Nicotinic acid inhibits lipoprotein lipase through a
> G-protein-coupled membrane receptor, decreasing
> triglyceride rich VLDL and cholesterol rich LDL levels
> and increasing HDL-C concentrations. For example,
> acipimox and nicotinic acid.

Mechanism of action

Nicotinic acid is a B-complex vitamin soluble in water
that is needed for the formation of coenzymes NAD
and NADP in the body, although this is unrelated to its
hypolipidaemic properties. It acts on adipocytes through
an inhibitory G protein–coupled membrane receptor, reducing intracellular generation of cAMP and inhibiting
lipoprotein lipase. This, in turn, decreases the release of
free fatty acids from adipose tissue and reduces free fatty
acid flux to the liver, which is required for the hepatic triglyceride synthesis necessary for the generation of VLDLs.

The synthetic derivative of nicotinic acid, **acipimox**,
has longer-acting effects, but is less effective in
lowering LDL-C.

Prescribing

Nicotinic acid is now only available in the UK as a combined slow release product together with **laropiprant**,
for the treatment of dyslipidaemias as adjunct to statin
therapy. Nicotinic acid as monotherapy was discontinued
due to the flushing associated with the high doses required for this indication. Laropiprant, a prostaglandin D2
receptor 1 antagonist inhibits this flushing effect. Doses
are increased after a 4-week interval to minimize toxicity
and patients off treatment for more than 7 consecutive
days should be restarted at the lower dose. In some countries a long-acting nicotinic acid preparation (Niaspan®)
has also been formulated to reduce liver side effects.

Acipimox, not used in the UK, is taken 2 or 3 times a
day for hyperlipidaemia, and like nicotinic acid, is best
taken with food to reduce side effects.

Unwanted effects

The most common side effects reported with the nicotinic
acid group are a consequence of prostaglandin-mediated
vasodilation (through activation of prostaglandin D2 receptors) presenting as flushing, itching, headaches, and
faintness. These tend to be transient and decrease with
use, but can be further reduced by slow titration of doses,
taking with food, and the use of combination products.

Conversely, effects may be enhanced in patients taking
other drugs known to cause vasodilation, e.g. nitrates
and CCBs.

Nicotinic acid should be avoided in severe hepatic impairment as it is extensively metabolized (before being
excreted in the urine) by the liver and known to cause hepatic toxicity ranging from deranged liver function tests to
fulminant hepatic necrosis. The risk is increased at higher
doses and with modified release preparations. Liver function tests are recommended 6–12-weekly for the first year
and periodically thereafter.

Both drugs are cautioned in renal impairment, with
delayed clearance potentially increasing the risk of
myopathy.

Omega-3 fatty acids

> Omega-3-fatty acids can potentially exert their
> beneficial effect through reduction of sympathetic over-
> activity, promoting nitric oxide vasodilation, reducing
> monocyte adhesion, and decreasing arachidonic acid
> mediators. Examples include omega-3-acid ethyl esters,
> omega-3-marine triglycerides

Mechanism of action

Omega-3-fatty acids are polyunsaturated acids with long
chains that can be found in high quantities in oily fish such
as mackerel and salmon. They have varied biological actions that include hypotriglyceridaemic, anti-aggregatory,
anti-inflammatory and anti-arrhythmic activity.

Their capacity to lower triglycerides is due to decreased
hepatic lipogenesis. As poor substrates for the enzymes
that synthesize triglycerides, they lead to the production
of triglyceride-poor LDL and reduce their plasma levels.
They also increase circulating HDL-C.

In platelet phospholipids, they reduce platelet aggregation, by substituting for arachidonic acid, which increases
production of thromboxane A3 instead of A2. The reduced
expression of endothelial adhesion molecules and anti-
inflammatory action also contributes to the retardation of
atherosclerotic plaques formation.

Prescribing

There are two omega-3 fatty acid preparations on the market
licensed for use in hyperlipidaemia; **omega-3-acid ethyl
esters** (Omacor®) and **omega-3-marine triglycerides**
(Maxepa®), both available for use in patients with raised
triglycerides as an alternative to fibrates, in combination

with a statin. Of the two Omacor® is also licensed for use adjunctively for secondary prevention in patients who have had an MI in the last 3 months at a dose of one capsule daily taken with food, however, the evidence is poor and they are not advocated for this indication by NICE or SIGN.

Unwanted effects

Side effects tend to be GI (nausea, dyspepsia) and less commonly taste disturbances. Hepatic toxicity is rare, however monitoring of liver function is recommended in patients with pre-existing impairment. Therapy with omega-3 fatty acids can lead to an increase in bleeding time and is, therefore, cautioned in haemorrhagic disorders or in patients who are anti-coagulated.

Further reading

Cannon CP, Blazing MA, Giugliano RP, et al. (2015) Ezetimibe added to statin therapy after acute coronary syndromes. *New England Journal of Medicine* 372(25), 2387–97.

Filippatos T, Milinois HJ (2008) Treatment of hyperlipidaemia with fenofibrate and related fibrates. *Expert Opinion on Investigational Drugs* 17(10), 1599–614.

Gille A, Bodor ET, Ahmed K, et al. (2008) Nicotinic acid: pharmacological effects and mechanisms of action. *Annual Review of Pharmacological Toxicology* 48, 79–106.

Jain KS, Kulkarni RR, Misal SH, et al. (2010) Current drug targets for antihyperlipidemic therapy. *Mini-Reviews in Medicinal Chemistry* 10(3), 232–62.

Last AR, Ference JD, Falleroni J, et al. (2011) Pharmacologic treatment of hyperlipidaemia. *American Family Physician* 84(5), 551–8.

Lee CH, Olson P, Evans RM (2003) Minireview: lipid metabolism, metabolic diseases, and peroxisome proliferator-activated receptors. *Endocrinology* 144(6), 2201–7.

Riccioni G, Sblendorio V (2012) Atherosclerosis: from biology to pharmacological treatment. *Journal of Geriatric Cardiology* 9, 305–17.

Toutouzas K, Drakopoulou M, Skoumas I, et al. (2010) Advancing therapy for hypercholesterolemia. *Expert Opinions in Pharmacotherapy* 11(10), 1659–72.

Guidelines

NICE CG67 (2010) Lipid modification: cardiovascular risk assessment and the modification of blood lipids for the primary and secondary prevention of cardiovascular disease. https://www.nice.org.uk/guidance/cg67?unlid=10669774532016415189 [accessed 18 March 2019].

NICE CG71 (Aug 2008). Familial hypercholesterolaemia: identification and management of familial hypercholesterolaemia. https://www.nice.org.uk/guidance/cg71?unlid=661145998201631392356 [accessed 18 March 2019].

NICE CG181 (July 2014) Cardiovascular disease: risk assessment and reduction, including lipid modification. http://www.nice.org.uk/guidance/cg181 [accessed 18 March 2019].

NICE Pathway: Familial hypercholsterolaemia overview (Jan 2016) http://pathways.nice.org.uk/pathways/familial-hypercholesterolaemia [accessed 18 March 2019].

NICE QS41 (2013) Familial hypercholesterolaemia. https://www.nice.org.uk/guidance/qs41 [accessed 22 March 2019].

NICE TA385 (Feb 2016) Ezetimibe for treating primary heterozygous-familial and non-familial hypercholesterolaemia http://www.nice.org.uk/guidance/ta385 [accessed 18 March 2019].

2.4 Stable angina

Stable angina is brought about by myocardial ischaemia when there is a mismatch between myocardial oxygen supply and demand, and usually occurs as a result of atheromatous plaque formation. Contributory factors to progression of atheromatous disease include smoking, hypertension, hyperlipidaemia, diabetes, and obesity. Typically, it presents clinically as chest tightness and is often described as a 'band across the chest', which is brought on by exercise and relived by rest. Patients may also experience symptoms following emotion, exposure to cold weather, or following heavy meals. It is estimated that 6–16% of men and 3–10% of women aged 65–74 years have experienced some form of angina and the lifetime risk in men after the age of 40 years is 49%. The incidence is around 1/1000 and more commonly affects men.

Unstable angina is defined as the occurrence of angina at rest, new onset severe angina (e.g. walking one flight of stairs or similar low level of exertion), or the presence of angina with increased severity and frequency. Acute coronary syndrome is an umbrella term that encompasses unstable angina, NSTEMI, and STEMI, which can all occur as a result of atheromatous plaque rupture, thrombosis or inflammation (see Topic 2.5, Acute coronary syndrome).

Pathophysiology

In the non-diseased heart, there is generally a continuous matching of oxygen demand of the myocardium with coronary arterial supply, in a balanced system. Numerous factors affect myocardial oxygen supply:

- *Perfusion pressure*: this is normally equivalent to aortic diastolic pressure and can be decreased by hypotension or aortic regurgitation leading to impaired oxygen supply.
- *Coronary vascular resistance*: this is affected by compressive forces and factors that affect intrinsic coronary

tone. In the heart, any increased oxygen demand must be met by an increased flow. This is accomplished by coronary vessel autoregulation. When oxygen demand outstrips supply, cellular hypoxia ensues and mitochondrial work is inhibited. Therefore, ATP cannot be regenerated. This, in turn, leads to an accumulation of adenosine diphosphate (ADP) and adenosine monophosphate (AMP) that are rapidly degraded to adenosine. Adenosine acts to reduce vascular smooth muscle uptake of Ca^{2+}, resulting in smooth muscle relaxation and enhanced blood flow. The endothelial cells of coronary vessels also regulate vascular tone via vasodilators, such as nitric oxide, prostacyclin, and endothelium-derived relaxing factor (EDRF).

In endothelial cells, platelet-derived factors, shear stress, acetylcholine (ACh), and cytokines stimulate the production of nitric oxide (NO) by activating nitric oxide synthase (NOS). NOS catalyses the reaction between L-arginine and oxygen to form NO and L-citrulline. NO being a small soluble molecule diffuses readily to adjacent smooth muscle cells where it activates guanylate cyclase. This, in turn, converts guanosine triphosphate (GTP) to cyclic guanine monophosphate (cGMP), which leads to muscle relaxation by reducing cytosolic Ca^{2+} levels. An exogenous supply of NO compounds can also activate the same smooth muscle relaxation.

Endothelial cells also release prostacyclin, arachidonic acid, and metabolites in response to hypoxia, sheer stress, ACh, and platelet products like 5-HT. Prostacyclin acts via a cyclic AMP-dependant mechanism to cause vasodilation.

Atheroma is the most common cause of angina; however, anaemia, aortic stenosis, hypertrophic cardiomyopathy, and arteritis can also cause symptoms of angina by causing an imbalance between oxygen supply and demand. For example, with aortic stenosis, muscle hypertrophy results in increased myocardial muscle oxygen

Box 2.5 Risk factors for angina

- Hypercholesterolemia
- Hypertension
- Smoking
- Diabetes
- Family history of premature coronary disease

demand thereby producing an imbalance in oxygen supply and demand leading to symptoms of angina. Furthermore, oxygen is delivered to the myocardium during diastole, so any process that interferes with this mechanism can also result in angina (e.g. tachyarrhythmia). A number of risk factors contribute to the formation of atherosclerosis Box 2.5).

Atherosclerosis is a complex inflammatory process, involving accumulation of lipid, macrophages, and smooth muscle cells of coronary vessels. It is an intimal disease, where mechanical sheer stresses from conditions like hypertension, high levels of LDL, diabetes, high levels of free radicals, e.g. smoking and inflammation, lead to endothelial dysfunction. Atherogenesis involves accumulation of lipids that modifies the lipoprotein make-up; accumulated oxidized lipoproteins recruit leukocytes and smooth muscle cells, causing deposition of an extracellular matrix. Macrophages become lipid laden leading to the formation of foam cells; seen macroscopically as fatty streaks. These fatty streaks progress within the endothelium to form a transitional plaque. Cytokines produced by monocytes, macrophages, and damaged endothelium, such as platelet-derived growth factor (PDGF) and transforming growth factor β (TGF-β), promote further accumulation of macrophages and smooth muscle cells (migration and proliferation). This smooth muscle proliferation covered by a collagen cap, leads to the formation of an advanced plaque, which encroaches on the lumen and can lead to reduced coronary flow. A reduction in lumen diameter of approximately 70% is sufficient to precipitate angina symptoms.

Nitrates can lead directly to vasodilation of coronary vessels and reduce venous return from the peripheral vascular bed, thereby relieving symptoms. Dihydropyridine CCBs (e.g. **nifedipine**) and K^+ channel openers (e.g. **nicorandil**) decrease arterial resistance to alleviate symptoms, while the other L-type Ca^{2+} channel antagonists (e.g. **verapamil**, **diltiazem**) have similar effects, but also are negative inotropes/chronotropes.

There are numerous presentations of angina relating to the pathophysiology:

- *Stable angina* is a tight, dull, or heavy chest discomfort that is associated with exertion or emotional stress. It results from oxygen delivery mismatch due to luminal occlusion. It is relieved within several minutes by rest, and can be characterized to four functional classes (Box 2.6).

- *Variant angina* also called prinzmetal angina, presents as pain at rest, due to a transient reduction in oxygen supply secondary to focal coronary artery spasm. The mechanism is not known, but may relate to early atherosclerosis and an abnormal response to endogenous vasodilators.

- *Syndrome X* is caused by microvascular dysfunction and presents as angina-like pain that occurs unpredictably (during rest or exercise), and is typically prolonged and unresponsive to GTN. Patients tend to be younger and on investigation often have normal coronary arteries.

- *Unstable angina,* which has three principle presentations:
  - *Rest angina*—occurring at rest and usually for less than 20 minutes, and occurring within 1 week of presentation.
  - *New-onset angina*—presenting as at least Class III severity (Box 2.6) with onset within 2 months of initial presentation.
  - *Increasing angina*—previously diagnosed angina that is distinctly more frequent, longer in duration, or lower in threshold (i.e. increased by at least 1 CCS class within 2 months to ≥Class III severity).

Box 2.6 Canadian Cardiovascular Society Classification of Angina

- *Class I: 'Ordinary activity does not cause angina':* angina with strenuous or rapid or prolonged exertion only
- *Class II: 'Slight limitation of ordinary activity':* angina on walking or climbing stairs rapidly, walking uphill, or exertion after meals, in cold weather, when under emotional stress, or only during the first few hours after awakening
- *Class III: 'Marked limitation of ordinary physical activity':* angina on walking one or two blocks on the level or one flight of stairs at a normal pace under normal conditions
- *Class IV: 'Inability to carry out any physical activity without discomfort' or 'angina at rest':* equivalent to 100–200 m.

Reprinted with permission from the Canadian Cardiovascular Society grading of angina pectoris. © Canadian Cardiovascular Society

In addition to symptoms there may be signs of hyper-lipaemia, e.g. xanthelasma, or corneal arcus lipidus and/or peripheral vascular disease (carotid bruise, absent/diminished foot pulses). There may also be cardiac and systemic pathologies that can cause or contribute to an-gina, e.g. the irregularly irregular pulse of atrial fibrillation, the murmur of aortic stenosis, the signs of cardiomyop-athy (apical heave or prominent a wave of jugular venous pressure (JVP)) or signs of anaemia. Thyroid status should also be assessed.

PRACTICAL PRESCRIBING

Acute coronary syndrome

Acute coronary syndrome (ACS) is a more likely diagnosis if:

- Chest pain and/or pain referred to other areas (arms, jaw) persists for > 15 minutes.
- Chest pain is associated with nausea and vomiting, sweating, or shortness of breath.
- There is new onset chest pain or worsening stable angina pain at rest or with minimal exertion.

Should ACS be suspected immediate referral to a rapid access chest pain clinic or Emergency Department should take place. See NICE CG95 for further information.

For a full summary of the relevant pathways and drug targets, see Figure 2.6.

Management

Stable angina is diagnosed primarily through clinical assessment, including a clinical history and physical examination. Additional diagnostic investigations are re-commended where the risk of coronary artery disease is considered to be less than 90% (see Table 2.12). Typical angina pain presents with the three following features:

- Constricting discomfort in the front of the chest, neck, shoulders, jaw, or arms.
- Precipitation by physical exertion.
- Relief by rest or **glyceryl trinitrate** (GTN) within about 5 minutes.

In atypical angina, however, patients present with only two of these symptoms, and in non-anginal pain, only one.

Typical angina is associated with the greatest risk of cor-onary artery disease (CAD), see Table 2.12.

In primary care, baseline investigations should be per-formed on initial presentation of stable chest pain, to confirm diagnosis, and assess for risk or precipitating factors:

- Full blood count (to exclude anaemia).
- HbA1C/Fasting plasma glucose (to exclude diabetes).
- Lipid profile (to exclude familial hypercholesterolemia and risk stratify).
- Thyroid function.
- Biochemistry profile (to assess renal function).

A resting 12-lead electrocardiogram (ECG) is recom-mended where a diagnosis of stable angina can be neither excluded nor confirmed, although a normal ECG, as seen in 50% of cases, *does not exclude* stable angina and re-sults should be considered alongside clinical assessment and patient risk factors. An ECG taken during an episode of chest pain may demonstrate ST-segment depression (i.e. ischaemia). Patients requiring diagnostic testing to confirm diagnosis, should have a secondary care referral for further invasive (e.g. coronary angiography) or non-invasive investigations, e.g. functional imaging such as stress echocardiography, MRI perfusion scan or anatom-ical imaging with computed tomography (CT) angiog-raphy. Patients with angina that have previously had a MI, coronary artery bypass graft, or percutaneous transluminal angioplasty, or have an ejection systolic murmur, should be referred early to secondary care.

Once diagnosed, there are two main aims in the man-agement of stable angina:

- enhancing quality of life by minimizing symptom frequency;
- improving patient survival/prognosis.

This can be achieved through modification of risk factors, drug therapy, and revascularization (see Figure 2.7).

- *Alteration of lifestyle*: stopping smoking, encouraging weight loss, dietary advice, and exercise (within pa-tients own limits).
- *Modification of risk factors*: monitor plasma cholesterols and reduce cholesterol; all patients with atheroma should receive a statin, management of hypertension, and optimization of diabetes control. All patients with proven coronary artery disease should be commenced on an antiplatelet as a secondary prevention strategy.

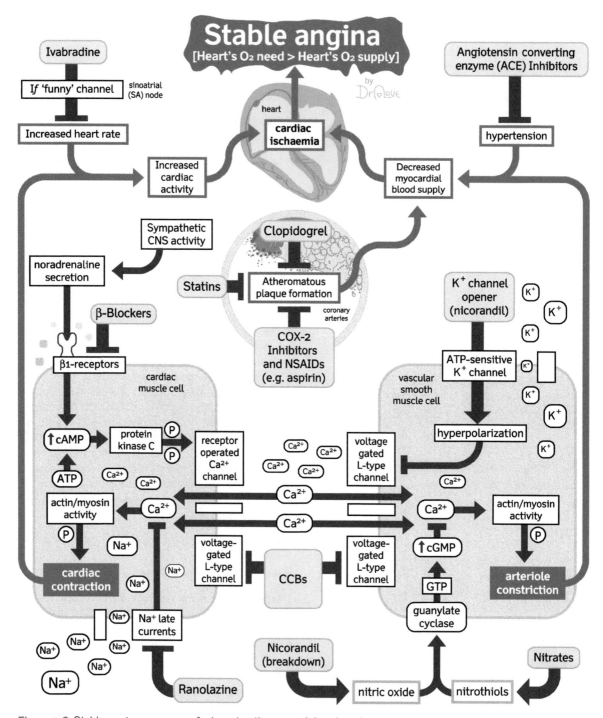

Figure 2.6 Stable angina: summary of relevant pathways and drug targets.

Table 2.12 Risk of CAD: Hi—high risk includes diabetes, smoking, and hyperlipidaemia; Lo—low risk is none of these

Age	Non-anginal chest pain				Atypical pain				Typical angina			
	Men		Women		Men		Women		Men		Women	
	Lo	Hi	Lo	Hi	Lo	Hi	Lo	Hi	Lo	Hi	Lo	Hi
35	3	35	1	19	8	59	2	39	30	88	10	78
45	9	17	2	22	21	70	5	43	51	92	20	79
55	23	59	4	25	45	79	10	47	80	95	38	82
65	49	69	9	29	71	86	20	51	93	97	56	84

- *Medical management of symptoms*: these can be treated in the short term in an acute setting with rapidly acting nitrates or minimized over a longer time frame with β–blockers and/or Ca^{2+} channel antagonists (see figure 2.7 Management of stable angina).

- *Surgical/interventional management of symptoms*: revascularization can be performed surgically by coronary artery bypass graft (CABG) or by interventional cardiologists, i.e. percutaneous coronary intervention (PCI). This should be considered in patients with stable

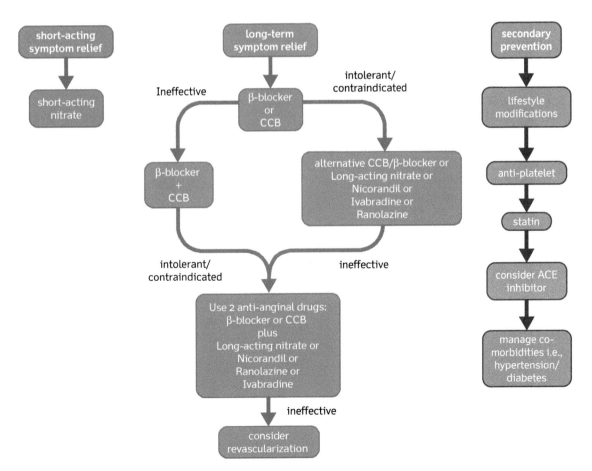

Figure 2.7 Management of stable angina.

angina where symptoms are not adequately controlled with optimal drug therapy. Surgery is often the preferred option in patients who are found to have severe coronary disease that is likely to have an unfavourable impact on prognosis.

All patients with stable angina should be offered a short-acting sublingual nitrate (e.g. **glyceryl trinitrate**) for immediate symptomatic relief. Furthermore, either a β-blocker or CCB (e.g. dihydropyridine group; **nifedipine** extended-release, **amlodipine**) should be commenced as first line therapy to reduce symptoms in the long term. β-blockers should be avoided in prinzmetal angina (vasospastic) where patients get pain at rest, as they may worsen vasospasm. In these patients, dihydropyridine CCBs should be used as first line, e.g. nifedipine. In patients where both a β-blocker and CCB are contraindicated or poorly tolerated, alternative treatment options include a long-acting nitrate (e.g. **isosorbide mononitrate**), K$^+$-channel activator (i.e. **nicorandil**) or under specialist advice, either **ranolazine** or **ivabradine**.

In all cases, treatment should be gradually titrated within the licensed doses in order to optimize symptom control in the absence of intolerable side effects. Patients should be assessed within 2–4 weeks of a dose change.

Where patients remain uncontrolled on optimal first line therapy, treatment may either be switched between first line therapy or both classes used together. However, a rate-controlling CCB (**diltiazem** or **verapamil**) should *not* be used in combination with β-blockers, due to their negative chronotropic effects and the increased risk of heart block. Similarly the non-dihydropyridines should not be used in patients with heart failure or pre-existing heart block.

In patients intolerant of either β-blockers or CCBS, alternative add-on therapies include long-acting nitrates, nicorandil, ivabradine, and ranolazine. As with β-blockers, ivabradine should not be prescribed in combination with verapamil or diltiazem.

If symptoms fail to improve despite dual therapy and 'tweaking' of doses, referral to a cardiologist for consideration of revascularization should be arranged. There is currently no evidence to support the use of a third anti-anginal agent, although it may be considered in patients who are unsuitable for, or awaiting revascularization.

As well as symptomatic treatment, patients will require interventions for secondary prevention of cardiovascular disease (CVD). Patients with atherosclerotic stable angina should be placed on **aspirin** (or **clopidogrel** where aspirin is unsuitable) and a statin (see Topic 2.3, 'Dyslipidaemia').

Controversy exists around the use of ACE inhibitors for angina, but they are of clear benefit in those with co-incidental cardiovascular conditions (i.e. hypertension, heart failure, left ventricular (LV) dysfunction, previous MI with LV dysfunction, or diabetes).

Drug classes used in management

Nitrates

Nitrates increase intracellular concentration of cGMP leading to smooth muscle relaxation. Examples include glyceryl trinitrate, isosorbide mononitrate, isosorbide dinitrate.

Mechanism of action

All nitrates are enzymatically broken down to nitrothiols. These species and the endogenous free-radical species nitric oxide (NO) activate guanylatecyclase and increase the synthesis of cGMP in smooth muscle and other tissues. cGMP leads to a reduction in intracellular Ca^{2+} and, as such, dephosphorylation of myosin light-chain occurs leading to smooth muscle relaxation. This mechanism means:

- Arterial dilation that lowers peripheral resistance and, therefore, reduces cardiac work and oxygen demand.
- Vasodilation reduces venous return so there is less left ventricle filling, thus decreasing work and oxygen demand.
- Relief of arterial vasospasm so blood can flow again.
- Improved perfusion to ischaemic areas via vessel dilation.

Prescribing

GTN is available as a spray, tablet, IV infusion, or transdermal patch, and has a short duration and rapid onset of action. Due to extensive first-pass metabolism and rapid absorption, sublingual administration is the preferred route, either in a spray or tablet form for use in acute attacks, as well as prophylactically, where patients anticipate that an acute attack is likely. Anti-anginal action occurs within minutes and last for half an hour.

GTN transdermal patches lasting 24 hours, or sustained release tablets are considered as long-acting nitrates. However, they are infrequently used, with **isosorbide** mononitrate or to a lesser extent isosorbide dinitrate, being the preferred agents in the class. The patches may, however, be of benefit in patients where oral administration is compromised. GTN tablets should be stored in dark containers as otherwise they lose efficacy over a period of months. Patients using patches that are free from attacks at night should be advised to remove patches prior to sleep to avoid tolerance (see 'Unwanted effects').

In practice isosorbide mononitrate is the preferred long-acting nitrate for preventing symptoms in angina. It is available orally in both standard release and modified release preparations, although in terms of compliance, the latter is generally preferred as it can be taken once a day.

Isosorbide dinitrate, like GTN, is active sublingually and can be used for treatment and prophylaxis, although sublingual preparations are not widely available. Onset of action is slower than GTN, but it is chemically more stable and, as such, may be beneficial in patients who require nitrates infrequently. Modified release preparations are licensed for use as prophylaxis, with a duration of action close to 12 hours. The action of isosorbide dinitrate may, in part, be prolonged because it is broken down to active metabolites including isosorbide mononitrate.

PRACTICAL PRESCRIBING

GTN spray: counselling points

- It can be used before anything you do that is likely to bring on pain or symptoms of angina.
- Keep your spray out of sunlight and store it in a cool place.
- You can buy GTN spray over the counter at the chemist.
- If you get an attack *sit down and stop*, hold the GTN spray upright and do not shake it.
- Spray once or twice under the tongue and *keep your mouth closed (very important)*.
- Wait 5 minutes, still resting. If you still have symptoms after this time, take *a second dose*.
- Wait 5 minutes, still resting. If the symptoms are still present, take a third dose.
- Wait 5 minutes, still resting. If the symptoms are still present then *dial emergency number for an ambulance*.
- *Do not wait more than 20 minutes for the symptoms to go away without seeking medical assistance.*

Unwanted effects

The vasodilatory effects of nitrates mean they should be used with caution in hypotensive conditions and avoided in those with hypertrophic cardiomyopathy, aortic stenosis, and marked anaemia. Because of their non-specific vasodilatory actions, many patients on nitrates complain of a throbbing headache, dizziness, flushing, and postural symptoms related to postural hypotension; this may, in part, be managed through the use of lower doses and delayed release preparations. Tolerance develops rapidly in many patients on long-acting or transdermal nitrates, which can be avoided by reducing blood-nitrate concentrations to low levels for 4–8 hours each day. If tolerance is suspected with transdermal patches, they should be left off for several consecutive hours in each 24 hours (usually overnight). In the case of BD tablet formulations of **isosorbide dinitrate** and **isosorbide mononitrate**, the second dose can be given after 8 hours rather than 12 hours. Conventional formulations of isosorbide mononitrate should only be given more frequently than BD when small doses are used; modified-release formulations of isosorbide mononitrate should only be given OD to avoid tolerance.

PRESCRIBING WARNING

Nitrates

- Ensure the patient knows to contact their GP should they require frequent daily doses of sublingual GTN or if they get rest symptoms.
- Anginal pain that does not respond to nitrates should be managed as a MI until proven otherwise.

Drug interactions

Due to their potent vasodilatory effects, nitrates are likely to enhance the effects of other anti-hypertensives and phosphodiesterase 5 (PDE5) inhibitors, such as **sildenafil**, leading to profound hypotension. This is likely to be more pronounced with short-acting agents.

Beta-adrenoceptor antagonists

β-blockers antagonize noradrenaline release via β_1 receptors reducing rate and contractility of heart. Examples include acebutolol, atenolol, bisporolol, carvedilol, metoprolol, nadolol, oxprenolol, pindolol, propranolol, sotalol, and timolol.

Mechanism of action

These drugs antagonize noradrenaline release from sympathetic nerve endings and slow the activation of cardiac tissue through β_1 receptors. The β_1 adrenergic receptor is a G protein–coupled receptor, associated with the Gs alpha subunit, which activates adenylate cyclase resulting in increased intracellular cAMP. This effect activates protein kinase A, causing phosphorylation of Ca^{2+} channels, which will leave the channels open for longer, thus increasing cardiac contraction. Furthermore, the β_1 receptors may also increase the contractility of the cells via troponin C, due to the increased amount of Ca^{2+} captured by the sarcoplasmic reticulum. As such the β-adrenoceptor antagonists:

- Reduce the heart rate and lengthen the time the heart is in diastole so more oxygen can be delivered to ischaemic tissues.
- Reduce the force of contraction so there is less oxygen demand placed upon the tissues.

Prescribing

Numerous β-blockers are licensed for the treatment of angina: **acebutolol, atenolol, bisoprolol, carvedilol, metoprolol, nadolol, oxprenolol, pindolol, propranolol**, and **timolol**. The APSIS and TIBET trials have shown that treatment with metoprolol in patients with stable angina both improves prognosis and reduces the chance of a subsequent cardiovascular event. There is, however, little evidence to suggest that one β-blocker is more effective than another and, therefore, certain drug properties should be taken into consideration when selecting which agent to prescribe:

- *Cardioselectivity*: these β-blockers are less likely to induce bronchospasm and are therefore useful in patients with respiratory disease such as chronic obstructive pulmonary disease (COPD). They are also less likely to cause peripheral vasoconstriction, so may be of use in patients with peripheral vascular disease, e.g. atenolol, bisoprolol, metoprolol.
- *Water solubility*: β-blockers that are more water than lipid soluble are less likely to cross the blood–brain barrier, and cause nightmares or sleep disturbance, e.g. atenolol, nadolol, sotalol.
- *Duration of action*: agents with longer duration of action require less frequent administration, which promotes adherence, e.g. atenolol, bisoprolol, and nadolol are all administered OD (carvedilol, BD). In some instances,

modified-release preparations can extend duration, e.g. metoprolol, oxprenolol, and propranolol.

- *Licensing*: some of the β-blockers licensed for use in angina are also licensed for prophylaxis post-MI and may therefore be useful in patients who have had a previous MI, e.g. atenolol, metoprolol, propranolol, and timolol.

Ideally, drug doses should be titrated to response in terms of symptoms and reduction in heart rate, with a resting heart rate of <60 bpm indicative of satisfactory blockade.

> ### PRESCRIBING WARNING
>
> **Discontinuing β-blockers**
> - Sudden withdrawal may cause an exacerbation of angina and, therefore, gradual reduction of dose is preferable when β-blockers are to be stopped.
> - β-blockers and verapamil must not be prescribed together because bradycardia, asystole, and heart failure can occur.

Unwanted effects

As can be predicted from their mechanism of action, β-blockers should be avoided in patients with severe bradycardia, atrioventricular (AV) block, sick sinus syndrome, decompensated heart failure, and asthma. Due to the bronchodilator effects of β-blockers, their use is contraindicated in severe asthma and COPD. That said, however, a growing body of evidence suggests that, in most patients with asthma, the use of a β-blocker is unlikely to adversely affect asthma control and in patients with COPD, the benefits of using a β-blocker in eligible patients is likely to outweigh the risks.

β-blockers also affect carbohydrate metabolism, so can cause hypo- or hyper- glycaemia (also interfering with metabolic and autonomic responses to hypoglycaemia) and should, therefore, be withheld in those diabetics who have frequent hypo-/hyperglycaemic episodes.

Cold extremities, paraesthesia, and numbness can occur, and in people with peripheral vascular disease β-blockers can worsen symptoms due to their vasoconstrictive effects; this effect is less pronounced with cardioselective β-blockers (such as **atenolol, bisoprolol**, and **metoprolol**). Sleep disturbance or nightmares tend to be more pronounced with the more lipophilic agents (e.g. **propranolol**) and fatigue has an incidence of about 18 per 1000 people per year. Sexual dysfunction (impotence and loss of libido) can affect approximately 5 in

1000 people. The high risk of side effects needs to be taken into account when prescribing for individuals and the options discussed with the patient to help ensure optimal compliance.

Drug interactions

β-blockers have the potential for numerous pharmacodynamic interactions when used with drugs known to have similar pharmacological properties, in particular, drugs with negative chronotropic or anti hypertensive effects. For this reason, use is ideally avoided in combination with the non-dihydropyridine CCBs (**verapamil** and **diltiazem**) due to the risk of heart block, and caution is required in combination with **digoxin** or class I anti-arrhythmics (such as **quinidine**, **disopyramide**, **flecainide**, and **lidocaine**). Concomitant use with other anti-hypertensives will increase their hypotensive effects, which may be of benefit to some patients.

Calcium channel blockers

In angina Ca²⁺-antagonists block L-type Ca²⁺ channels leading to the relaxation of arterioles and cardiac cells. Examples include amlodipine, felodipine, nifedipine, verapamil, and diltiazem.

Mechanism of action

This group of drugs has been shown to be beneficial for the improvement of symptoms, however, like β-blockers, have little direct effect on the longer-term prognosis of patients with stable angina. When compared with β-blockers, the CCBs have been shown to be equivalent with respect to symptom relief (angina episodes and exercise tolerance) and secondary prevention (long-term mortality and cardiovascular risk). Thus, NICE currently consider that either can be considered for first line use. Decision to use one class over another, however, may be influenced by the presence of other co-morbidities or contraindications.

There are numerous subtypes of Ca²⁺ channels of which two are mainly associated with cardiovascular tissues (see Topic 2.7, 'Arrhythmias'). The two cardiac types are both voltage -gated and include the long-acting (L-type) and the transient (T-type) channels. The most important Ca²⁺ channels in the pharmacology of angina are the L-type, which predominate in arteriolar vessels and myocardial cells. The concentration of intracellular Ca²⁺ is normally regulated by cellular surface and sarcoplasmic reticulum Ca²⁺channels. A rise in the level of intracellular Ca²⁺

results in phosphorylation of myosin via myosin light-chain kinase, and subsequent contraction of arterioles and myocardial cells. The Ca²⁺ channel blockers reduce this intracellular rise.

The dihydropyridine derived antagonists (e.g. **amlodipine**, **felodipine**) are the most potent vasodilators and act primarily by binding to the α1-subunit (extracellular) of the L-type channel allosterically blocking Ca²⁺ flux. This class of drugs act primarily peripherally to cause arterial dilation, thereby reducing total peripheral resistance and lessening myocardial work, to reduce oxygen demand. Furthermore, coronary artery dilation occurs, leading to improved myocardial blood flow, which reduces ischaemic pain. Any negative inotropic effects of this class are offset by sympathetic compensatory reflex tachycardia.

The phenylalkyamine (**verapamil**) and the benzothiazepine (**diltiazem**) act at distinct sites on the α1-subunit, intracellular and extracellular site, respectively, of the L-type channel, a location distinct to the dihydropyridine site. This different location means that they have preferential and intermediate action respectively on the heart, compared with the dihydropyridine antagonists; they are, therefore, to be avoided in heart failure. Verapamil in particular is contraindicated due to its negative inotropic and chronotropic effects. Diltiazem has mainly negative chronotropic effects, so that the reflex tachycardia as seen with dihydropyridines are hidden by its action. Interestingly, verapamil and diltiazem only gain access to binding sites when the channel is in the open state, i.e. frequency dependent action, demonstrating how their action is so important in treatment of cardiac arrhythmias (see Topic 2.7, 'Arrhythmias').

Prescribing

> **PRESCRIBING WARNING**
>
> Avoid verapamil and diltiazem in heart failure of AV block

Of the dihydropyridines, only **amlodipine**, **felodipine**, **nicardipine**, and **nifedipine** are licensed for use in stable angina. As a class, they are inactivated by hepatic metabolism and many have short half-lives so are preferentially prescribed as modified release preparation to ensure optimal cover. The short-acting preparations may also cause unwanted fluctuations in blood pressure and heart rate. **Amlodipine** and **felodipine** are longer-acting dihydropyridines that can be given once daily for prophylaxis in angina. Furthermore, they do not exacerbate heart failure. These two drugs, along with **nifedipine** (modified-release), are useful not only in stable angina but also variant angina. Nifedipine may rarely reduce myocardial contractility and can therefore contribute to heart failure. **Verapamil** and **diltiazem** should be avoided in patients with heart failure. In patients with good cardiac function, diltiazem may be used where β-blockers are ineffective or contraindicated (e.g. asthmatics). For treatment or prophylaxis, the standard or immediate preparations may be used, although longer-acting, modified-release preparations may be more beneficial in prophylaxis. When prescribing modified-release preparations of diltiazem, the brand name should be specified on prescriptions due to variations in oral bioavailability.

PRACTICAL PRESCRIBING

CCBs

- Warn patients that they may get side effects, such as facial flushing, headaches, swollen ankles, dizziness, tiredness, and skin rashes, but these should pass within a few days.
- Advise not to take grapefruit juice as this may overly affect their BP.
- Warn that verapamil commonly causes constipation, so advise eating more fibre and drinking eight cups of liquid per day.

Unwanted effects

Side-effects with the dihydropyridine CCBs are typically a result of widespread vasodilatation, i.e. flushing, headache (which becomes less obtrusive after a few days) and dizziness. Many patients complain of gravitational ankle swelling/oedema, which is more often than not unresponsive to diuretics. Some may also complain of palpitations and tachycardias. These reflex tachycardias are most commonly seen with the shorter-acting dihydropyridine antagonists (e.g. **nifedipine**) and thus can be managed through use of alternative agents or modified-release preparations. GI disturbances, nausea, and heartburn are also reported with the dihydropyridines.

As previously mentioned, the CCBs have variable effects on myocardial contractility; **amlodipine** has little or no effect; nifedipine may rarely reduce contractility; and **verapamil** has strong effects in reducing contractility. As such,

the latter may precipitate heart failure in those at risk and should, therefore, be avoided in those with unknown cardiac function. Verapamil and **diltiazem** can also cause bradycardias so must be used with caution in patients on other negative chronotropic drugs (see 'Drug interactions').

As a class, the CCBs are extensively metabolized in the liver, in most cases via CYP 3A4, with minimal renal excretion. Dose reductions are therefore more likely to be required in significant hepatic impairment.

Drug interactions

There are numerous drug interactions that involve CCBs, both pharmacodynamic (enhanced pharmacological effects) and pharmacokinetic (altered clearance as modifiers and substrates of the CYP P450 enzyme). Of particular significance is the increased risk of bradycardia and heart block when **verapamil** and **diltiazem** are used in combination with drugs such as β-blockers, **digoxin**, and other anti-arrhythmics.

Care is also recommended when CCBs are taken in combination with drugs known to be potent inhibitors or inducers of the CYP450 enzyme system, including grapefruit juice, as it increases the plasma concentration particularly of the dihydropyridine CCBs (i.e. **felodipine** and **nifedipine**) and verapamil.

K+ channel openers

These are ATP sensitive K$^+$ channel activators that are used for symptom control. For example, nicorandil.

Mechanism of action

The principal agent in this class of drugs used for angina is **nicorandil**. This has been shown to reduce the number of coronary events in those with stable angina and also improve ischaemic chest pain. Despite this, nicorandil is not believed to reduce the risk of cardiac death to below background levels in angina patients.

Nicorandil is an interesting drug in that it has a dual mechanism of action owing to its structure, containing a reactive nitrate moiety in addition to its K$^+$-channel binding site. There are numerous K$^+$ channels and these have a variety of slightly different jobs (see Topic 2.7, 'Arrhythmias'). Overall, the channels tend to be responsible for repolarizing cell membranes following depolarization. Nicorandil acts primarily at the ATP-sensitive K$^+$ channel, a ligand-gated channel, located in heart, muscle, pancreas, and mitochondria. The normal role of this channel is to open in times of ischaemia, when intracellular ATP is low, so cells hyperpolarize to protect them from damage. This hyperpolarization causes smooth muscle cells to relax because of closed L-type Ca^{2+} channels (which are voltage dependent), and inhibit release of Ca^{2+} from intracellular stores. Collectively, this reduced intracellular Ca^{2+} leads to vasodilation systemically, and in coronary arteries.

Nicorandil binds to the ATP-sensitive K^+ channel forcing the channel to stay open so cells become hyperpolarized. In addition to the action at ATP-sensitive K^+ channels the nitrate groups of unbound drug reacts to form NO, which binds to guanylate cyclase and causes vasodilation of smooth muscle cells in an identical way to the nitrates (see previously).

Prescribing

Nicorandil is rapid acting, almost completely absorbed from the GI tract and not significantly metabolized by the liver. Consequently, it has high oral bioavailability, but a short half-life (approximately 1 hour), with steady-state plasma concentrations reached after 100 hours of oral drug. Despite its short half-life, the biological effect of nicorandil lasts for 12 hours, making BD dosing a good option for treatment. Doses are started low and titrated according to response.

Unwanted effects

Clearly, those with cardiogenic shock or left heart failure should not be placed on **nicorandil** as it will contribute to their failure. Nicorandil should also be used with caution in patients with low BP, acute pulmonary oedema, and acute MI with left ventricular failure.

Like the nitrates, many patients (25–50%) complain of headache (especially on initiation, usually transient) due to vasodilation. This is often accompanied by flushing, nausea, vomiting, and dizziness. Less commonly, nicorandil may reduce BP and, hence, increase heart rate (reflex tachycardia) leading to some palpitations. As with most vasodilators, hypovolaemia may result, which can impair performance affecting a patient's ability to drive or operate machinery.

Drug interactions

As with nitrates, the hypotensive effects of **nicorandil** will enhance the effects of PDE5 inhibitors, e.g. **sildenafil**, and as such the two should be avoided concomitantly.

Ivabradine

Ivabradine acts to block the 'funny' channel (If) in the sinoatrial node, reducing heart rate.

Mechanism of action

Ivabradine is a novel medication that acts by blocking the I_f or 'funny' channel. The I_f channel has unique properties, in that It has mixed inward flux of Na^+ and K^+ activated by a hyperpolarized state. These channels are primarily located at the sinoatrial (SA) node and endogenously modulated by the autonomic nervous system. The I_f current is directly activated by intracellular cAMP through the hyperpolarization-activated cyclic nucleotide-gated family of ion channels, so adrenergic agonists activate adenylate cyclase, which increases cAMP, leading to increased cAMP binding to the I_f channel and opening. A closed channel is likely to slow heart rate. Ivabradine, acting from the intracellular side, blocks the I_f channel to reduce the firing rate of pacemaker cells, with no other effects on other ionic channels. As such, ivabradine reduces heart rate without affecting contractility. The reduction in rate reduces cardiac load, therefore, diminishing oxygen demand, leading to symptom relief. It is also probable that a reduced rate increases the coronary blood flow and oxygen supply by increasing diastolic time.

Prescribing

Ivabradine is licensed for the symptomatic treatment of angina pectoris. It is administered orally BD, initially at a low dose that is increased at 3–4 weeks if the patient remains symptomatic. Lower doses are recommended in elderly patients.

Unwanted effects

Due to its bradycardic effects, **ivabradine** should not be started in anyone with a heart rate <60 bpm, and is contraindicated in those with unstable angina or MI, hypotension, heart failure (NYHA III or IV), sinus node disease, or 3rd degree AV. Following initiation, it is important to monitor heart rate for the first few months since patients may become bradycardic and require dose modification or cessation; particularly in the elderly. Around 15% of people have visual disturbance and luminous phenomena, and experience difficulties with changing light intensities. Headache is common, but tends to resolve with time.

Drug interactions

As with the CCBs, **ivabradine** has a high potential for both pharmacokinetic and pharmacodynamic drug interactions. Concomitant administration with drugs that prolong the QT interval (e.g. some anti-arrhythmics, etc.) is best avoided. Similarly, care is recommended when taking with drugs known to be potent inhibitors of CPYP 3A4 (e.g. azole antifungals and macrolides), responsible for the metabolism of ivabradine; due to increased risk of toxicity being a substrate for this enzyme pathway.

Ranolazine

Ranolazine is thought to improve angina symptoms by promoting diastole relaxation.

Mechanism of action

The exact mechanism of action is poorly understood, but **ranolazine** seems to inhibit late Na^+ currents in cardiac cells (see Topic 2.7, 'Arrhythmias'); hence, reducing intracellular Na^+ and Ca^{2+}. The decreased Ca^{2+} load improves myocardial relaxation and, hence, lessen diastole stiffness; thereby improving angina symptoms. Unlike other anti-anginal drugs it does not alter heart rate or BP.

Prescribing

Ranolazine was licensed in the UK in 2009 as an adjuvant therapy for those who are inadequately controlled on, or intolerant to, first-line treatments in stable angina. Despite being advocated for use by NICE as a second-line option, many regional prescribing committees promote the use of other agents first on the basis of relative benefit for cost.

Unwanted effects

QT prolongation has been reported with **ranolazine** and is thought to occur due to inhibition of a K^+ rectifying current. Caution should be taken when prescribing in those with a family history of QT syndromes, low weight, or renal impairment. Ranolazine is extensively metabolized in the liver via cytochrome P450 3A4 and, as such, is contraindicated in moderate or severe hepatic impairment and in concomitant use with potent CYP3A4 inhibitors (e.g. **clarithromycin**). It should also be avoided in combination with anti-arrhythmics. In clinical trials, adverse events have been reported in 38% of ranolazine patients, so its overall usefulness may be limited.

Secondary prevention therapy

These include drugs that will improve prognosis in the long term—aspirin, clopidogrel, statins (e.g. atrorvastatin), ACE inhibitors (e.g. ramipril).

Antiplatelets

Antiplatelets such as **aspirin** are of great benefit, decreasing mortality in angina by 34%, as they stop platelet aggregation forming on atheromatous plaques. Patients with malignant hypertension should have their BP managed before commencing aspirin. Antiplatelet strategies are dealt with in Topics 2.3, 'Dyslipidaemia' & 2.5, 'Acute coronary syndrome'. **Clopidogrel**, an ADP-sensitive receptor inhibitor, should be considered in those unable to take aspirin.

Statins

There is no direct evidence that statins are of benefit in angina, but extrapolations can be made against cardiovascular disease risk factors and, hence, the European Society of Cardiology recommends all patients with stable angina receive a statin. For more details, see Topic 2.3, 'Dyslipidaemia'.

Angiotensin-converting enzyme inhibitors

All patients with angina should be considered for treatment with an ACE inhibitor, i.e. if known hypertension, heart failure, left ventricular dysfunction (± previous MI), or diabetes. ACE inhibitors are discussed in (Topic 2.1, 'Hypertension').

Further reading

Fihn SA, Blankenship JC, Alexandra KP, et al. (2014) 2014 ACC/AHA/AATS/PCNA/SCAI/STS focused update of the guideline for the diagnosis and management of patients with stable ischemic heart disease. *Circulation* **130**, 1749–67. http://circ.ahajournals.org/content/130/19/1749.full.pdf+html [accessed 19 March 2019].

Kumar A, Cannon P (2009) Acute coronary syndromes: diagnosis and management. *Mayo Clinic Proceedings* 84(10), 917–38.

Guidelines

European Society of Cardiology (ESC) guidelines on the management of stable coronary artery disease 2013 European Heart Journal 34 2949–3003: http://eurheartj.oxfordjournals.org/content/ehj/34/38/2949.full.pdf [accessed 19 March 2019].

NICE CG95 (2010) Chest pain of recent onset: https://www.nice.org.uk/guidance/cg95 [accessed 19 March 2019].

NICE CG126 (July 2011) Management of stable angina: https://www.nice.org.uk/guidance/cg126 [accessed 19 March 2019].

NICE Pathway (July 2015) Stable angina overview http://pathways.nice.org.uk/pathways/stable-angina [accessed 19 March 2019].

NICE QS21 (Aug 2012) Stable angina https://www.nice.org.uk/guidance/qs21/resources/stable-angina-2098540738501 [accessed 19 March 2019].

SIGN 96 Management of Stable Angina: a national guideline. https://www.sign.ac.uk/assets/sign96.pdf [accessed 22 March 2019].

2.5 Acute coronary syndrome

Acute coronary syndromes (ACS) encompass three clinical conditions, typically characterized by sudden-onset chest pain caused by a rapid reduction in blood flow (and oxygen) to the heart. This is usually the result of the rupture of an atherosclerotic plaque in the wall of the coronary artery.

Clinical conditions:

- Unstable angina (UA).
- ST-elevation myocardial infarction (STEMI).
- Non-ST-elevation myocardial infarction (NSTEMI).

Diagnosis can be made by the presence of ischaemic chest pain and can be differentiated by means of an ECG (identifying ST-elevation in the context of STEMI or new ischaemic changes, such as ST depression of T wave inversion in the context of NSTEMI and UA) and blood troponins. In approximately 50% of patients presenting to ED with chest pain, the cause will be non-cardiac. Of those that are cardiac, only 5–10% will be a STEMI, with 15–20% NSTEMI and 10% UA. Incidence of STEMI in the UK is approximately 1/5000 and nearly 50% of deaths occur within 2 hours of symptom onset; thus prompt management is paramount.

Pathophysiology

The development of an atheromatous plaque and its encroachment into vessel lumen, with the subsequent reduction in oxygen delivery to end organs, is key to the understanding of stable angina (see Topic 2.4, 'Stable angina'). The changes to the plaques collagenous fibrous cap dictates the stability of the deposit and confers tendency toward an acute coronary syndrome. The fibrous cap undergoes constant remodelling and can thin, leading to rupture and release of thrombogenic contents into the bloodstream. Vulnerability to disruption depends on the lipid burden within the core, the thickness of the fibrous cap, and the degree of inflammatory cell infiltrate. Mechanical stress or hydrostatic forces can cause the shoulder of plaques to lift off, leading to cap rupture, and ultimately the formation of occlusive thrombi with subsequent ACS. Overt plaque rupture with thrombus-lipid core interaction is estimated to be seen in 60% of ACS and it is the degree of disruption (ulceration or erosion), which determines thrombogenicity. It appears that certain patient groups are predisposed to plaque vulnerability, e.g. hypercoagulable states, systemic inflammation, and smokers.

Following plaque disruption, thrombogenic material (e.g. tissue factor) is released from the core and combines with factor VII/VIIa, activating factor IX and X, which through a cascade forms thrombin and fibrinogen (see Topic 2.8, 'Venous thromboembolism'). As the plaque ruptures the sub-endothelial exposed surface reveals Von Willebrands factor and collagen. The former causes a platelet monolayer to form over the site in an attempt to heal, while the latter causes the bound platelets to undergo conformational changes, and express GP IIb/IIIa receptors and release ADP, thromboxane A2, serotonin, and adrenaline. These products recruit further platelets, further occluding the lumen, while serotonin causes local vasoconstriction. The activated platelets, expressing GP IIb/IIIa receptors, bind with fibrinogen (in plasma) allowing platelets to clump together. More often than not, small fragments of thrombus break off and act as micro-emboli to distal vessels causing tissue ischaemia. As platelet aggregation continues, thrombin and circulating fibrinogen combine and stabilize the thrombus;

macrophages and red blood cells also become trapped. If this process is unchecked, complete vessel occlusion can occur causing tissue ischaemia with necrosis; presenting clinically as a STEMI. In the case of NSTEMI, ischaemia occurs as a result of persistent thrombotic or vasospastic occlusion, which spontaneously resolves or is limited by collateral vessels so the extent of tissue damage is limited. Unstable angina results when the thrombus is labile causing transient occlusion, the myocardial cells are stressed, but recover. In contrast to unstable angina, the death of myocardial cells that occurs in the case of NSTEMI or STEMI, mean structural proteins like creatine kinase and troponin are released into the circulation. These molecular fragments aid in the diagnosis and time course of ACS events.

For a full summary of the relevant pathways and drug targets, see Figure 2.8.

Management

In patients presenting with ACS within 12 hours of symptoms, a prompt diagnosis and early management is essential to improve prognosis and minimize complications. Typically, patients will present with chest pain lasting more than 15 minutes that radiates to the lower jaw, neck, or left arm, and may be accompanied by nausea/shortness of breath, sweating, or palpitations. Atypical presentation includes epigastric pain or isolated dyspepsia. This atypical presentation is seen more commonly in women, the elderly, and patients with chronic renal failure or diabetes (and has been termed a silent MI).

Early identification of ACS ensures that patients receive the most appropriate management in a timely way. Thus, initial management aims to obtain an accurate diagnosis, relieve symptoms, and reduce the likelihood of thrombus extension and embolization. All patients presenting with suspected ACS within 12 hours should, therefore, have:

- Pain relief:
  - **GTN**—sublingual/ buccal;
  - IV **morphine.**
- **Aspirin** (300 mg stat, chewed).
- Anti-emetic (e.g. **metoclopramide**).
- *Supplemental oxygen*: if oxygen saturations are less than 94%.
- Resting 12-lead ECG as soon as possible, ideally within 10 minutes of first medical contact.
- Vital signs monitored (heart rate/rhythm, BP).

- IV access and bloods taken for cardiac markers (e.g. troponins, CK), electrolytes, and FBC as soon as possible.

The 12-lead ECG is essential to facilitate an early diagnosis of a STEMI (see Box 2.7), so that, where indicated, *reperfusion therapy* can be carried out promptly, thereby minimizing cardiac myocyte death. Ideally, a diagnosis should be made within 10 minutes to prevent treatment delay. In contrast, serial troponins are required to support the diagnosis of NSTEMI and distinguish NSTEMI from UA (troponin is normal in UA). Following a diagnosis of MI, ECG monitoring should be initiated as soon as possible to identify any life-threatening arrhythmias that may require defibrillation.

Treatment immediately post-STEMI aims to:

- Restore perfusion either medically (thrombolysis) or mechanically (endovascular stent, PCI) to minimize damage to myocardium where necessary.
- Rebalance mismatch between oxygen supply and demand.
- Manage pain.
- Prevent any further complications.

The mismatch between oxygen supply and demand is addressed pharmacologically by decreasing myocardial oxygen demand and increasing oxygen supply.

- *Decreasing myocardial oxygen demand*: β-blockers achieve this by reducing heart rate, BP, preload, and contractility, thereby reducing the risk of mortality in the first 7 days post-MI. They also help reverse any life-threatening ventricular arrhythmias.
- *Increasing oxygen supply*: administration of oxygen, according to SpO_2 and the use of nitrates post-MI act to improve supply either directly, or by way of coronary vasodilation, respectively. GTN can be administered sublingually or, in the case of persistent symptoms, intravenously to relieve angina.

Early management of STEMI

STEMI patients presenting within 12 hours of symptoms starting, should be offered PCI as soon as possible, or within 120 minutes of when they could have received fibrinolysis (see Figure 2.9). Due to its superior efficacy, primary PCI is the reperfusion therapy of choice; however, where PCI remains unavailable or there is the potential for delay, fibrinolysis can be given, ideally within

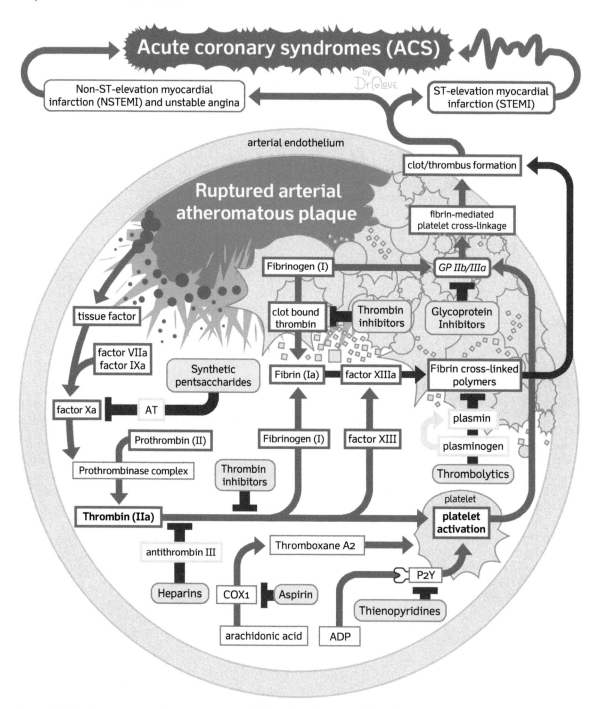

Figure 2.8 Acute coronary syndromes: summary of relevant pathways and drug targets.

30 minutes of presentation. Patients presenting beyond 12 hours of symptom onset, but with signs of ongoing ischaemia may still benefit from reperfusion with PCI. Prior to PCI, when patients arrive in the cardiac catheter lab, IV anticoagulants are commenced, for example, **bivalirudin** or **unfractionated heparin** (UFH).

Dual antiplatelet therapy should be initiated as early as possible in patients presenting with STEMI, with

Box 2.7 Universal definition of myocardial infarction

Universal definition of myocardial infarction

Fall and/or rise in biomarker values (preferably troponin) with at least one value above the 99th centile URL plus one of the following:

- Symptoms of ischaemia
- New (or presumed new) significant ST-T changes
- New left bundle branch block (LBBB)
- New pathological Q waves on ECG
- New loss of myocardium or regional wall motion abnormality on imaging
- Intracoronary thrombus identified by angiography or autopsy

Cardiac death with symptoms and ECG changes suggestive of MI, but death occurring prior to blood cardiac markers being available or increased.

Stent thrombosis associated with MI as detected by angiography or autopsy, with a rise and/or fall in biomarker values with at least one above the 99th centile URL.

aspirin plus an ADP inhibitor, preferably **prasugrel** or **ticagrelor**. Although less effective, **clopidogrel** may also be used if other ADP inhibitors are unavailable. Additional antiplatelet therapy with a GP IIb/IIIa inhibitor (e.g.

tirofiban) may be considered in some patients, such as in the presence of a large thrombus or possibly in high-risk patients requiring transfer for PCI. As a class, however, the use of a GP IIb/IIIa inhibitor is unlikely to confer any additional advantage in patients managed with bivalirudin, although it may do so where UFH or **enoxaparin** has been used for anti-coagulation.

Fibrinolysis may be used as an alternative to primary PCI, where PCI is unavailable or there is likely to be a significant delay before it can occur. Treatment of choice is with a fibrin-specific agent, i.e. **alteplase**, **tenecteplase**, or **reteplase**. However, although less effective, **streptokinase** may still be used as a second-line option. Following treatment, dual antiplatelets should be continued for 12 months, after which time aspirin alone is normally continued. In addition, patients will require anti-coagulation with enoxaparin or UFH for at least 48 hours following fibrinolysis, and up to 8 days if they remain hospitalized. The role of GP IIb/IIIa inhibitor has again not been established in this patient group. Following discharge, patients will probably require referral for angiography and revascularization.

Early management of NSTEMI/ unstable angina

Early management of NSTEMI or unstable angina is intended to reduce the risk of a further event. The GRACE (Global Registry of Acute Cardiac Events) score calculated

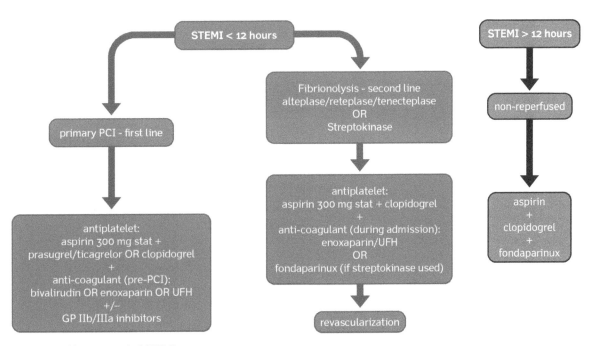

Figure 2.9 Management of STEMI.

using the GRACE-2 risk calculator, is the most accurate way to predict 6-month mortality (see Table 2.13), taking into consideration clinical history (previous PCI, coronary artery bypass graft; CABG), physical examination, Killip class, ECG findings, and blood results (including biomarkers). Regardless of score, all patients will require immediate treatment with antiplatelets and antithrombin therapy, ideally with **fondaparinux**, although **heparin** can be used. The need for dual antiplatelet therapy and GPIIb/IIIa inhibitors will depend on predicted 6-month mortality.

Coronary angiography should be offered within 96 hours of admission, to all patients who are at intermediate risk or higher of a future cardiovascular event, so that ischaemic damage can be minimized. Lower-risk patients should undergo ischaemia testing prior to discharge, as those with evidence of ischaemia should also be considered for coronary angiography. In the absence of ischaemia, patients can be managed conservatively.

The choice of revascularization strategy (CABG or PCI) will be determined by angiography findings, co-morbidities, and patient choice, for which they will need to be fully informed of the relevant risks and benefits. Prior to a CABG, **clopidogrel** should be withheld for 5 days due to the risk of bleeding. Following PCI, dual antiplatelets should be continued for up to 12 months. This time frame may be shorter, depending on the specific stent deployed during PCI.

Secondary prevention post-MI

Secondary prevention following an MI aims to reduce the risk of a second event through modification of risk factors. In addition to the usual lifestyle recommendations (diet, exercise, smoking, etc.), patients will require pharmacological therapy with:

- *Dual antiplatelet therapy*: aspirin should be continued lifelong following an MI, and a second agent (ADP inhibitor) taken for up to 12 months. Where **aspirin** is not tolerated, **clopidogrel** monotherapy could be considered.

- *β-blockers*: a β-blocker should be initiated orally once the patient has been stabilized to reduce workload on the heart. It should be continued long term to reduce the risk of mortality, although most studies demonstrating a benefit in this context, pre-date the use of modern reperfusion therapy.

- *Statins*: all patients should be offered a high-intensity statin (Topic 2.3, 'Dyslipidaemia') soon after an MI, ideally with **atorvastatin** 80 mg. Patients should be re-evaluated after 4–6 weeks to assess response.

- *ACE inhibitors*: it is generally accepted that all patients should receive an ACE inhibitor early post-MI, although the evidence is stronger in those with other co-morbidities, such as heart failure or an impaired ejection fraction. In patients unable to tolerate an ACE inhibitor, an ARB may be used, ideally **valsartan**.

Table 2.13 Initial antiplatelet management as per cardiovascular risk

Predicted 6-month mortality	Risk of future cardiovascular events	Antiplatelet management
1.5% or below	Lowest	Aspirin monotherapy (clopidogrel in case of aspirin hypersensitivity)
>1.5–3%	Low	Dual antiplatelet therapy: aspirin + clopidogrel/ticagrelor with initial loading dose
>3–6%	Intermediate	Dual antiplatelet therapy: aspirin + clopidogrel/ticagrelor with initial loading dose.
>6–9%	High	Consider GPIIb/IIIa if angiography scheduled within 96 hours of admission OR bivalirudin as an alternative to heparin + GPIIb/IIIa if angiography scheduled within 24 hours of admission
>9%	Highest	

- *Anti-coagulant*: this is only required in patients with a clear indication for anti-coagulation such as in AF (Topic 2.7, 'Arrhythmias').
- *Eplerenone*: this may be indicated in some patients with an impaired ejection fraction or heart failure, providing they have adequate renal function.

Prior to discharge, it is essential that patients are counselled on their treatment and the associated risks of not taking them, in order to optimize compliance in this high-risk population.

Drug classes used in management

Antiplatelets: aspirin

Aspirin blocks the synthesis of thromboxane A2 via the irreversible inhibition of cyclo-oxygenase 1, thus decreasing the aggregation of platelets.

Mechanism of action

Aspirin irreversibly acetylates Ser_{529} of cyclo-oxygenase 1 (COX1), the key enzyme in prostaglandin biosynthesis, leaving its catalytic site inaccessible to arachidonic acid, thus preventing the production of prostaglandin H2 and thromboxane A2. The inhibited release of thromboxane A2 from platelets stops platelet activation via thromboxane receptor.

Prescribing

Low-dose **aspirin** is available to take orally, as dispersible or enteric-coated tablets, both of which are available for purchase over the counter. Although intended to provide gastric protection, enteric-coated tablets are not recommended as there is no evidence of increased protection, while bioavailability is likely to be impaired. Patients at risk of GI bleeding should instead be prescribed gastroprotection ideally with a proton pump inhibitor. Doses vary internationally, based on available standard tablet strengths, although there is little to support doses greater than 75 mg (81 mg in the USA).

Despite its short half-life (15–20 minutes), aspirin is administered OD due to the irreversible nature of its antiplatelet effects, which continues for the lifetime of the platelet.

PRACTICAL PRESCRIBING
Enteric-coated aspirin
- Enteric-coated aspirin was developed to prevent gastric irritation, although as GI toxicity is secondary to both the local and systemic effects of aspirin, there is no evidence to suggest it is of any benefit.
- Pharmacodynamic studies suggest that enteric coating might impair bioavailability of aspirin.
- Enteric-coated aspirin is therefore not recommended and instead patients at risk of peptic ulcer disease should be prescribed a proton pump inhibitor.

Unwanted effects

Low-dose **aspirin** is associated with a very small increased risk of a major bleed and more commonly with GI side effects. The latter is thought to be caused by COX1 inhibition, both locally and systemically, resulting in damage to the gastric mucosa. It is therefore contraindicated in patients with active peptic ulcer disease or clotting disorders, and should be used with caution in patients at risk of peptic ulcer disease, where concurrent proton pump inhibitors are recommended.

Rarely, aspirin can precipitate bronchospasm in asthmatics, precluding further use. Aspirin use in patients under 16 years has been known to induce Reye's syndrome and should, therefore, only be used where the benefits outweigh the risks.

Drug interactions

Predictably, co-prescribing with other drugs known to affect bleeding times requires caution, i.e. anti-coagulants, thrombolytics, and other antiplatelets, although in many cases this combined action is intentional.

PRACTICAL PRESCRIBING
Aspirin and NSAIDS in STEMI patients
The European Cardiology Society recommends avoiding concomitant use of aspirin with other NSAIDS in STEMI patients due to the increased risk of reinfarction, cardiac rupture, and death.

Antiplatelets: thienopyridines

Thienopyridines act through an active metabolite preventing the action of ADP, an important platelet agonist in vivo. Examples include clopidogrel, prasugrel, and ticagrelor.

Mechanism of action

There are two types of receptors for the endogenous platelet agonist ADP in the platelet plasma membrane: P2Y1 and P2Y12. P2Y1 is a seven-transmembrane domain G protein–coupled receptor. Activation of this receptor by ADP results in Ca^{2+} mobilization, an alteration in platelet morphology, and rapid and reversible platelet aggregation. P2Y12 is also a seven transmembrane domain receptor, but it leads to decreased levels of cyclic AMP. As a result, its activation amplifies stable platelet aggregation and secretion.

Clopidogrel is a thienopyridine that is metabolized in the liver by cytochrome P450. Its active metabolite antagonizes the P2Y12 receptor, decreasing platelet activation and aggregation, reducing blood viscosity, and increasing bleeding time.

Prasugrel is another thienopyridine pro-drug metabolized in the liver, which irreversibly inhibits the P2Y12 receptor. Due to its efficient metabolism, it is a more rapid, potent, and consistent inhibitor of platelet function compared with clopidogrel.

Ticagrelor also inhibits the P2Y12 receptors, but its action is reversible and via an allosteric mechanism at a different site. Furthermore, ticagrelor is not a pro-drug, so may work well in those with genetic liver metabolism variations (e.g. CYP2C19).

Preliminary *in vitro* evidence has shown that some modified diadenosine tetraphosphonate derivatives (diadenosine P1, P4-tetraphosphate; P1, P4-dithio chloromethyl; dithio-chloromethyl), can synergistically inhibit platelet activation through both P2Y1 and P2Y12, thus offering some potential novel therapeutic options as antithrombotic agents.

Prescribing

Of the drugs in this class, **clopidogrel** has historically been the most widely used in ACS, having been available for longer. However, updates to national guidelines has seen a swing to the use of other agents in the class. More recently, a large randomized study (TRITON), comparing clopidogrel with **prasugrel** in the treatment of patients undergoing PCI, demonstrated superior efficacy of prasugrel in preventing non-fatal MI, but an increased risk of major bleeds. **Ticagrelor** has also been approved for use in ACS as a further alternative to clopidogrel. This is primarily based on the PLATO trial, where it demonstrated superior efficacy in reducing the risk of an MI or a vascular death, but not stroke.

Prasugrel has a faster onset of antiplatelet activity compared with clopidogrel and therefore, may be beneficial in STEMI patients requiring urgent PCI. It may also confer a greater benefit over clopidogrel in patients with DM having PCI.

Clopidogrel and prasugrel are administered OD, while ticagrelor is administered BD, in combination with aspirin for ACS, following an additional loading dose. Clopidogrel may be used as monotherapy in patients intolerant of aspirin.

Unwanted effects

Bleeding and GI toxicity are the most widely reported adverse effects to the thienopyridines, although the risk of bleeding is greater with **prasugrel** and **ticagrelor** than **clopidogrel**. There is no specific antidote to either therapy in case of a major bleed; however, affected patients will probably require platelet transfusions. Although very rare, thrombotic thrombocytopenic purpura (TTP) has been reported with thienopyridines, necessitating urgent treatment and future avoidance

Manufacturers of clopidogrel recommend avoiding in severe hepatic impairment as it is extensively metabolized in the liver, primarily to its active metabolite. Although prasugrel is also a pro-drug, it is hydrolysed in the intestine to its active metabolite and, therefore, does not requires dose adjustments in renal or hepatic impairment.

Drug interactions

As with **aspirin**, consideration should be given to prescribing with other drugs known to prolong bleeding times.

As **clopidogrel** is metabolized to its active metabolite via the cytochrome P450 enzyme (CYP2C19), it has demonstrated significantly lower levels of active metabolite when used concurrently with **omeprazole** (at a dose of 80 mg), which inhibits this enzyme. Other drugs known to inhibit this enzyme include **esomeprazole, voriconazole, fluconazole, ciprofloxacin, carbamazepine,** and **fluoxetine**. The same has not been shown with **prasugrel**. If gastric protection is required, **lansoprazole** is a good option.

Antiplatelets: glycoprotein inhibitors

Glycoprotein IIb/IIIa inhibitors act by disrupting the final common pathway of fibrinogen-mediated cross-linkage that leads to platelet aggregation. Examples include abciximab, eptifibatide, and tirofiban.

Mechanism of action

Developed following the finding that patients with an inherited defect in platelet aggregation were deficient in integrin αIIbβ3, antagonists for this protein were the first rationally designed antiplatelet therapy. Integrin αIIbβ3 (GPIIb/IIIa) supports the aggregation of platelets and thrombus formation that is mediated by fibrinogen. As a final shared component of pathways leading to platelet activation, it has become an ideal target for antiplatelet therapies.

Inhibition of platelet activation is not the central mechanism of action of integrin αIIbβ3 antagonists, it is instead the final stages of platelet-to-platelet aggregation, induced by fibrinogen binding to integrin αIIbβ3. In addition, inhibition of prothrombin binding to αIIbβ3 is part of the mechanism behind the anti-coagulant properties of αIIbβ3 antagonists, which leads to less thrombin generation and decrease in the formation of pro-coagulant platelet-derived microparticle.

- **Abciximab** is a murine human chimeric Fab fragment that was derived from the murine monoclonal antibody 7E3.

- **Eptifibatide** is a cyclic heptapeptide isolated from the venom of the southeastern pygmy rattlesnake (*Sistrurus miliarus barbouri*), and it is part of the arginine–glycine–aspartate–mimetics drug class, reversibly binding to platelets.

- **Tirofiban** is a non-peptide reversible antagonist of the integrin αIIbβ3 receptor.

Prescribing

Eptifibatide and **tirofiban** are licensed for use in the prevention of MI in patients with UA or NSTEMI, whereas **abciximab** is licensed for the prevention of ischaemic cardiac complications, in patients having PCI. More recent evidence suggests that they should not be used routinely in patients undergoing angiography, but instead a decision made based on risk of ischaemia versus risk of bleed.

All three drugs are administered as an IV infusion with short half-lives and rapid onset of action (within 15 minutes of starting treatment). With eptifibatide and tirofiban, normal platelet function returns within 4 and 8 hours, respectively, of the infusion stopping, whereas the effects of abciximab can persist for 24–48 hours.

Glycoprotein IIb/IIIa therapy is used in combination with **unfractionated heparin** and **aspirin** unless contraindicated, and should only be carried out in a hospital setting under specialist care. Increasingly, the treatment of choice is with eptifibatide or tirofiban based on their more favourable side effect profile and more rapid reversal on cessation.

Unwanted effects

Unsurprisingly, given their role as potent inhibitors of platelet aggregation, the greatest risk associated with therapy is major or even fatal bleeding. Use is therefore contraindicated in patients with active bleeding (GI, intracranial, etc.), intracranial disease (arteriovenous malformations, aneurysms), severe hypertension, thrombocytopenia, severe liver disease, and in those with a recent history of stroke or major surgery. Glycoprotein IIb/IIIa inhibitors rely, in part, on renal clearance and require dose reductions in severe impairment. Thrombocytopenia is also reported with treatment, occurring more commonly with **abciximab**.

Prior to, and within 6 hours of starting treatment, patients will require clotting studies and an FBC. These should be repeated at least daily during treatment and therapy discontinued if necessary.

Other side effects more commonly reported with abciximab include headaches, nausea and vomiting, chest pain, and hypersensitivity reactions; the latter is probably due to abciximab being derived from a recombinant monoclonal antibody.

Drug interactions

In theory, concomitant use with other drugs known to prolong bleeding time may be exacerbated with glycoprotein IIb/IIIa inhibitors; however, as they are only indicated for short-term use and patients on treatment require close monitoring, it is rarely of clinical significance.

Anti-coagulants: heparins

Heparins form a complex with antithrombin III, altering its conformation state and allowing the rapid inhibition of thrombin and other clotting factors. Examples include unfractionated heparin, enoxaparin, dalteparin, and tinzaparin.

Mechanism of action

Heparins are a diverse group of straight-chain anionic mucopolysaccharides (glycosaminoglycans), which have anticoagulant properties and are found in mast cells, basophils, and endothelium. The anti-coagulant effect requires anti-thrombin III (AT) as a plasma cofactor. **Heparin** binds to a lysine site on AT, producing a change in conformation at the arginine reactive site that transforms AT into a fast inhibitor of thrombin and factor Xa.

Heparin is available as an unfractionated preparation or as low molecular weight heparins (LMWHs), consisting of the heparin subfractions that have molecular weights less than 7000 Da. LMWHs-antithrombin complexes mainly inactivate factor Xa, while high molecular weight heparin complexes inactivate thrombin and factors IXa, Xa, Xia, and XIIa. Both the unfractionated and LMWHs induce the secretion of tissue factor pathway inhibitor (TFPI) by vascular endothelial cells. This decreases the pro-coagulant activity of tissue factor VIIa complex, which could be part of the antithrombotic actions. Platelet aggregation can also be inhibited by heparins, through binding to platelet factor 4 and the activation of lipoprotein lipase. This generates a reduction in platelet adhesiveness.

In addition to its anticoagulant effect, heparin augments the permeability of the vessel wall and inhibits the production of vascular smooth muscle cells. It can also suppress osteoblast formation while activating osteoclasts that can stimulate bone loss. In the circulation, heparin binds to various plasma proteins, which decreases its activity as an anticoagulant and explains the variability of therapeutic response.

Prescribing

The use of **unfractionated heparin** (UFH) has been largely superseded by **low molecular weight heparins** (LMWH), as the latter demonstrates a more predictable relationship between dose and effect, thereby requiring less monitoring. It is also more easily administered. However, in severe renal impairment and in patients requiring rapid reversal of anti-coagulation, e.g. pre-surgery, UFH is preferred. UFH is, therefore, the anti-coagulant of choice in the acute management of UA or NSTEMI, in patients planned to have coronary angiography within 24 hours, or in those with a creatinine clearance less than 20 mL/min.

UFH is administered IV as a bolus followed by a continuous infusion. The APTT must be measured at baseline and repeated at the same time each day throughout treatment, 4–6 hours after the start of the infusion, in order to maintain an APTT 1.5–2.5 times the normal range.

Of the LMWHs on the market only **enoxaparin** and **dalteparin** are licensed for use in unstable angina and NSTEMI. Enoxaparin also has a license for the treatment of acute STEMI. Enoxaparin can be used following an MI with persistent ST elevation, given initially as an IV bolus, followed immediately by a BD subcutaneous dose of 1 mg/kg. However, patient's undergoing primary PCI with successful stent deployment are commenced on prophylactic dose LMWH following this procedure. Dose adjustments are unnecessary in obese or underweight patients. Where enoxaparin or dalteparin are used in unstable angina or an NSTEMI (second-line to **fondaparinux**), the initial IV bolus dose is omitted.

> **PRESCRIBING WARNING**
>
> **LMWH**
>
> LMWHs are not interchangeable due to variations in dosing and specific anti-Xa activity.

Unwanted effects

As with all anti-coagulants, the use of heparins increase bleeding risk, particularly in high-risk patients with predisposing factors, such as active bleeding, recent haemorrhagic stroke, or thrombocytopenia, where treatment is contraindicated. Caution is also advised in elderly patients and those taking concomitant drugs known to increase bleeding, e.g. NSAIDs.

In patients requiring urgent reversal of heparin (**UFH** and **LMWH**), treatment with **protamine** may be necessary. The dose is calculated from the amount of heparin given in a period determined by the half-life of the heparin, i.e. the half-life of LMWH is considerably longer with effects lasting up to 24 hours from the last dose.

Heparin-induced thrombocytopenia is an immune-mediated reaction that can occur within 5–10 days of treatment requiring immediate cessation of therapy and is a contraindication to further use. It occurs more commonly with unfractionated heparin, however, all patients receiving a heparin should have platelet counts done at baseline and repeated regularly throughout treatment.

LMWHs are renally cleared, thereby requiring dose reductions in mild-moderate renal impairment. In more severe renal impairment (creatinine clearance less than 20 mL/minute), UFH is preferred as this is hepatically metabolized to inactive by-products that are renally excreted.

A small proportion of patients have a reduced response to heparin and are considered to be resistant, this is more common in severe illness or in those with underlying clotting disorders and should be picked up with routine monitoring.

As heparin can suppress adrenal secretion of aldosterone causing hyperkalaemia, potassium levels should be checked in at risk patients at baseline and monitored regularly when heparin therapy exceeds 7 days. At-risk patients include those with co-morbidities such as DM, acidosis, or chronic renal failure, or in those taking concurrent potassium sparing drugs or supplements.

Anti-coagulants: thrombin inhibitors

Direct thrombin inhibitors can inhibit clot-bound thrombin without the need of a cofactor. For example, bivalirudin.

Mechanism of action

Hirudin is a naturally occurring anticoagulant found in the salivary gland of the leech. The extended conformation of the three N-terminal hirudin residues lets the side chains of Ile1I (Val1I) and Tyr3I occupy regions that correspond approximately to the active site cleft of thrombin, thus blocking its function.

Bivalirudin is a synthetic hirudin peptidomimetic hirulog-1. It is a specific, reversible and direct inhibitor of thrombin that binds in a concentration-dependent manner to thrombin catalytic site and its substrate recognition site, affecting both circulating thrombin and fibrin bound thrombin.

Prescribing

Of the available thrombin inhibitors, only **bivalirudin** holds a license for use in ACS, where it is used in combination with **aspirin** and **clopidogrel** for patients undergoing percutaneous coronary intervention (PCI).

Doses are administered IV as a bolus (0.5 mg/kg), followed by an infusion administered throughout the PCI and continued for up to 4 hours after. At this point, the infusion can be continued at a reduced rate for 4–12 hours as required. Patients continuing to coronary by-pass surgery should have the infusion stopped 1 hour before and should be switched to unfractionated heparin.

Efficacy of bivalirudin can be assessed by monitoring activated clotting time (ACT), aiming for a value of greater than 225 seconds. This is of particular importance at initiation of therapy and in patients with renal impairment in whom clearance is impaired.

Unwanted effects

Predictably bleeding is the most commonly reported adverse effect to treatment and although the risk of a major bleed is less than with glycoprotein inhibitors, treatment is still, however, contraindicated in high-risk patients. Other reported adverse effects include local effects such as thrombosis and bruising, and less commonly allergic reactions or other non-specific toxicities, such as sickness and headache.

As **bivalirudin** is renally cleared, a dose reduction is necessary in moderate renal impairment and it should be avoided in severe impairment.

Anti-coagulants: synthetic pentsaccharides

The synthetic pentasaccharide fondaparinux enhances the innate ability of AT to inhibit factor Xa, a key enzyme in the coagulation cascade.

Mechanism of action

Fondaparinux contains a synthetic pentasaccharide analogue of the minimal binding sequence on antithrombin (AT). It accelerates the rate at which AT neutralizes factor Xa by inducing a conformational change, which increases its affinity. Unlike **heparin**, which interacts with many plasma components, fondaparinux binds selectively to AT, but it is unable to inactivate thrombin itself.

Prescribing

Fondaparinux is now favoured over heparin in the management of ACS, due to the ease of administration, greater efficacy, and superior tolerance. Doses are administered subcutaneously OD, due to its long half-life of 17 hours. Unlike **UFH** and **LMWH**, it is administered at a set dose of 2.5 mg for a maximum of 8 days, regardless of weight or APTT; therefore, monitoring is unnecessary.

Unwanted effects

Although **fondaparinux** treatment can cause major haemorrhage, the risk is considerably less than with **heparin**, due to its increased selectivity. It is, however, still contraindicated in active bleeding and cautioned in patients at high risk of major haemorrhage.

Fondaparinux is associated with a slight increased risk of thrombus on administration compared with **enoxaparin**, which can be prevented by pre-treating patients with a dose of **unfractionated heparin** prior to PCI.

Other side effects, including thrombocytopenia, are generally less common than with heparins.

Being predominantly excreted unchanged via the kidney, a dose reduction is necessary in patients with moderate renal impairment (20–50 mL/min/1.73 m²), and treatment is contraindicated in severe impairment. As elimination decreases with weight the risk of bleeding is increased in smaller patients, so caution is advised in patients less than 50 kg. Dose adjustments are unnecessary in hepatic impairment.

Drug interactions

Although the risk of bleeding is likely to be increased when taken concurrently with other drugs known to cause bleeding; studies have shown that **fondaparinux** does not affect the pharmacokinetics of antiplatelets, NSAIDS, or anti-coagulants so, for example, when taken with **warfarin** the INR is not affected.

Thrombolytics

Thrombolytics activate plasminogen to form the proteolytic enzyme plasmin, which degrades fibrin and contributes to dissolve blood clots. Examples include streptokinase, alteplase, reteplase, and tenecteplase

Mechanism of action

Thrombolysis is the breakdown of a clot or thrombus to clear the blockage of an artery and prevent any permanent damage resulting from poorly perfused tissue. It acts via the fibrinolytic system, which involves a plasminogen pro-enzyme converted to the active enzyme plasmin by plasminogen activators. This, in turn, digests fibrin to soluble degradation products.

Although free plasmin in the blood is rapidly inactivated by α2-antiplasmin, the plasmin that is generated at the fibrin surface is, at least in part, protected from inactivation. If the α2-antiplasmin becomes exhausted in the circulating blood, residual plasmin will degrade several plasma proteins and cause serious bleeding risks. Thrombolytics can be divided into fibrin-specific agents (**alteplase**, **reteplase**, **tenecteplase**), which act only on fibrin-bound plasminogen and those capable of also acting on circulating plasminogen, termed fibrin-non-specific agents (**streptokinase**).

Streptokinase, which is derived from various streptococci, rapidly converts endogenous plasminogen to its active form plasmin. As a non-specific thrombolytic, it affects both circulating, unbound plasminogen, as well as fibrin-bound plasminogen, and is therefore associated with life-threatening side effects, due to increased levels of circulating plasmin.

Alteplase is a recombinant glycosylated serine protease with fibrin-binding properties that also has proteolytic plasminogen-specific activities. It is a mainly single-chain form of the endogenous enzyme tissue plasminogen activator.

Reteplase is a plasminogen activator that mimics the endogenous tissue plasminogen activator (t-PA). This is a serine protease that converts plasminogen to plasmin and thus precipitates thrombolysis. It is a third-generation recombinant peptide that consists of the kringle 2 protein domain, and protease domains of human tissue-type plasminogen activator. It operates in the presence of fibrin.

Prescribing

Fibrinolytic therapy with **streptokinase**, **alteplase**, **reteplase**, and **tenecteplase** is an alternative to primary PCI, usually where PCI is not readily available. It should be initiated as soon as possible after the onset of symptoms in MI and within at least 6 hours for tenecteplase or 12 hours for the other fibrinolytics. Treatment of choice should ideally be with a fibrin-specific agent, i.e. not streptokinase.

All drugs are administered IV, although the administration of reteplase and tenecteplase is by one or two IV bolus doses compared with infusions required with streptokinase and alteplase.

Unwanted effects

As thrombolysis is commonly associated with bleeding major bleed is the greatest risk associated with therapy, in particular haemorrhagic stroke (0.5–1% of patients). As with other drugs associated with high bleeding risk they are contraindicated in active bleeding and compared with other drug classes are associated with a greater number of contraindications (see Table 2.14).

Side effects can occur as a result of reperfusion such as arrhythmias, oedema, hypotension, and angina. Other common adverse effects include nausea and vomiting, and allergic reactions that may first present as lower back pain. Where fibrinolytics are administered by infusion, slowing the rate of administration may help prevent some side effects including chills and fevers.

Table 2.14 Contraindications for fibrinolysis.

Absolute contraindications	Relative contraindications
Previous ICH or stroke of unknown origin	TIA in last 6 months
Ischaemic stroke in last 6 months	Oral anticoagulants
CNS trauma or neoplasm or AVM	Pregnancy or less than 1 week post-partum
Major trauma/surgery/head injury in last 3 weeks	Refractory hypertension
GI bleed in last month (incl. oesophageal varices)	Advanced liver disease
Bleeding disorder	Active peptic ulcer disease
Aortic dissection	Prolonged or traumatic resuscitation
Non compressible puncture in the last 24 hours, e.g. liver biopsy or LP	

Reproduced from Ibanez B, James S, Agewall S, et al; 2017 ESC Guidelines for the management of acute myocardial infarction in patients presenting with ST-segment elevation, *European Heart Journal* 2018; 39 (2): 119–177. Copyright © 2017, European Society of Cardiology. doi:10.1093/eurheartj/ehx393

Further reading

Fareed J, Thethi I, Hoppensteadt D (2012) Old versus new oral anticoagulants: focus on pharmacology. *Annual Review of Pharmacology and Toxicology* 52, 79–99.

Fuster V, Badimon L, Badimon JJ, et al. (1992) The pathogenesis of coronary artery disease and the acute coronary syndromes. *New England Journal of Medicine* 326(4), 242–50.

Grech E (2003) Pathophysiology and investigation of coronary artery disease. *British Journal of Medicine* 326, 1027–30.

Michelson AD (2010) Antiplatelet therapies for the treatment of cardiovascular disease. *Nature Reviews: Drug Discovery* 9(2), 154–69.

Wallentin L, Becker RC, Budaj A, et al. (2009) Ticagrelor versus clopidogrel in patients with acute coronary syndromes. *New England Journal of Medicine* 361, 1045–57.

Wiviott SD, Braunwald E, McCabe CH, et al. (2007) Prasugrel versus clopidogrel in patients with acute coronary syndrome. *New England Journal of Medicine* 357, 2001–15.

Guidelines

Amsterdam EA, Wenger NK, Brindis RG, et al. (2014) AHA/ACC Guideline for the Management of Patients with Non-ST Elevation Acute Coronary Syndromes: Executive Summary. *Journal of the American College of Cardiology* 64(24), e139–e228. https://www.sciencedirect.com/science/article/pii/S0735109714062792?via%3Dihub [accessed 22 March 2019].

NICE CG94 (2013): Unstable angina and NSTEMI: the early management of unstable angina and non-ST-segment-elevation myocardial infarction. https://www.nice.org.uk/guidance/cg94?unlid=90680432120161148181 [accessed 20 March 2019].

NICE CG167 (2013): Myocardial infarction with ST-segment elevation: the acute management. https://www.nice.org.uk/guidance/cg167?unlid=73734275201629122 [accessed 20 March 2019].

NICE Pathways (July 2015): Acute Coronary Syndromes Overview. http://pathways.nice.org.uk/pathways/acute-coronary-syndromes [accessed 20 March 2019].

NICE QS68 (Sept 2014) Acute coronary syndromes in adults. http://www.nice.org.uk/Guidance/QS68 [accessed 20 March 2019].

NICE TA230 (2011): Bivalirudin for the treatment of ST segment elevation myocardial infarction. https://www.nice.org.uk/Guidance/TA230 [accessed 20 March 2019].

NICE TA236 (2011): Ticagrelor for the treatment of acute coronary syndromes. https://www.nice.org.uk/guidance/TA236 [accessed 20 March 2019].

NICE TA317 (2014): Prasugrel with percutaneous coronary intervention for the treatment of acute coronary syndromes. http://www.nice.org.uk/guidance/ta317 [accessed 20 March 2019].

NICE TA420 (2016) Ticagrelor for preventing atherothrombotic events after myocardial infarction. https://www.nice.org.uk/guidance/ta420 [accessed 20 March 2019].

Roffi M, Patrano C, Collet J-P, et al. (2016) 2015 ESC Guidelines for the management of acute coronary syndromes in patients presenting without persistent ST-segment elevation. *European Heart Journal* 37, 267–315. http://eurheartj.oxfordjournals.org/content/ehj/37/3/267.full.pdf [accessed 20 March 2019].

SIGN 148: Acute coronary syndrome. https://www.sign.ac.uk/assets/sign148.pdf [accessed 22 March 2019].

Steg G, James SK, Atar D, et al. (2012) ESC Guidelines for the management of acute myocardial infarction in patients presenting with ST-segment elevation. *European Heart Journal* 33, 2569–619. http://eurheartj.oxfordjournals.org/content/ehj/33/20/2569.full.pdf [accessed 20 March 2019].

2.6 Heart failure

Heart failure (HF) is diagnosed where cardiac output, and thus oxygen delivery, is insufficient to meet the body's needs. Acute heart failure is characterized by a rapid onset of symptoms (e.g. breathlessness, ankle swelling, and fatigue) and signs (elevated JVP, pulmonary crackles, displaced apex beat) secondary to an event such as myocardial infarction, presenting either for the first time or as an acute decompensation of chronic failure. Conversely, chronic heart failure is gradual in progression, results typically from long-standing hypertension, coronary artery disease, or valvular disease, and presents as venous congestion with a maintained BP. Collectively, heart failure affects 1–3% of the population and around 10% of the elderly.

Pathophysiology

There are four key components that contribute to cardiac output:

- *Cardiac preload*: end-diastolic volume (related to venous return).
- *Heart rate*: modified by sympathetic nervous system and baroreceptors.
- *Cardiac contractility*: conforms to Frank–Starling phenomenon (figure 2.10).
- *Cardiac afterload*: resistance the ventricle needs to overcome to eject its contents.

These four factors are normally in a dynamic equilibrium, such that a decrease in preload would lead to an increase in heart rate to maintain end-organ perfusion. Likewise, as defined by the Frank–Starling phenomenon (Figure 2.10), an increase in preload dictates the efficiency of cardiac contraction. Loading the heart with fluid stretches cardiac tissues, so more blood will latterly be ejected. In the failing heart, cardiac ejection fraction (EF) is a key prognostic factor and important in diagnosis. It is calculated as the volume ejected by the heart (stroke volume-SV), divided by the volume of the filled heart (end-diastolic volume), and thus determines cardiac output.

Heart failure can, therefore, be defined according to whether or not ejection fraction has been preserved (HFpEF), or reduced (HFrEF). Essentially, reduced contractions mean reduced emptying, but the SV is maintained by an increased end-diastolic volume, i.e. a smaller fraction is ejected for an increasing volume.

Modification in any of the four key components listed above can result in symptomatic heart failure.

Systolic failure may occur where ventricles fail to contract efficiently; EF <40%, for example, secondary to ischaemic heart disease, MI, cardiomyopathy β-blockers, or negative inotropic drugs.

Diastolic failure occurs when ventricles fail to relax, leading to increased filling pressure and thus restricted filling; EF >50%. This is often caused by conditions that result in a chronically elevated afterload, e.g. aortic stenosis or hypertension.

Clinically, distinctions can be made between *left* (LVF) and *right* ventricular failure (RVF), and collectively, both sides '*congestive cardiac*' failure (CCF). If a particular side has predominant failure, logically, symptoms and signs relate to the associated venous drainage system (e.g. LVF—dyspnoea, orthopnoea, paroxysmal nocturnal dyspnoea; RVF—peripheral oedema and ascites). However, many of these symptoms are subtle, and most of the clinical signs result from sodium and water retention as a result of ongoing failure, i.e. pulmonary and peripheral oedema (see also Topic 2.1, 'Hypertension'). Reducing cardiac output as a result of HF leads to a decreased renal blood flow, which in turn causes renin release, followed by angiotensin II, and aldosterone release, ultimately elevating Na^+ (see Topic 5.2, 'Acute kidney injury') and resulting in fluid retention. This retention may then increase preload and further exacerbate poor cardiac output.

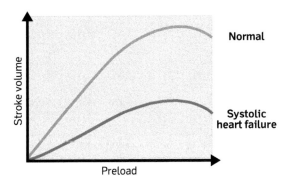

Figure 2.10 Frank–Starling demonstrating normal and impaired cardiac output in response to preload.

It is evident that numerous systems may be targeted to reduce 'stress' on the cardiac output by:

- Reducing preload and afterload with, ACE inhibitors, aldosterone antagonists, and diuretics.
- Controlling heart rate with **ivabradine** or **digoxin.**
- Improving cardiac contractility with β1 sympathomimetics or phosphodiesterase III inhibitors.

Given the diversity of systems involved in HF, consideration of patient co-morbidity is important as they may dictate restrictions in treatment (e.g. renin-angiotensin system inhibitors or aldosterone antagonists in those with renal failure). Atrial fibrillation is common in HF and may contribute to poor CO so should be managed along current guidance:

- identify and correct underlying or precipitating causes (e.g. hyperthyroidism, chest infection, or surgery);
- rate control with β-blocker ± digoxin;
- give thromboembolism prophylaxis (see Topic 2.8, 'Venous thromboembolism').

For a full summary of the relevant pathways and drug targets, see Figures 2.11 and 2.12.

Management

The primary aim of heart failure management is to improve symptoms and reduce the risk of hospitalization and mortality by slowing disease progression. At presentation patients should be provided with advice on lifestyle measures that address diet and exercise (see Table 2.15). Traditionally, patients have been encouraged to restrict their salt intake to less than 2 g/day; however, there

is conflicting evidence to support the long-term benefits. Recent SIGN guidance advocates intake be restricted to within the adult daily maximum levels. Patients should also be given advice on alcohol consumption and smoking cessation where relevant.

Where HF is suspected key investigations are the 12-lead ECG and echocardiogram, as collectively these give information on heart rate, rhythm, conduction pathways, chamber volume, ventricular and valve function, and cardiac wall thickness. Such information will dictate if anticoagulation, rate control, pacing, or interventions for ischaemia, valve dysfunction, or cardiomyopathies are required. Routine full blood count (FBC) and urea & electrolytes (U&Es) should be carried out to identify any precipitating factors such as anaemia, or to guide on treatment decisions, e.g. a poor GFR may preclude initiation of renin–angiotensin–aldosterone system blockade. A chest X-ray (CXR) should be performed to identify any pulmonary venous congestion or oedema in HF.

Natriuretic peptides, such as BNP or NT-proBNP, are members of a family of hormones that are secreted by the heart in response to increased myocardial wall stress, thus evidence of low levels can be used to exclude a diagnosis of heart failure. Furthermore, monitoring of levels has the potential to direct the titration of medication, as BNP levels will decrease with effective treatment.

Acute heart failure management

Acute HF requires urgent medical attention and invariably hospitalization. Treatment is, therefore, initiated in parallel with diagnostic work-up to improve symptoms and stabilize haemodynamics. On presentation, in patients with a suspected diagnosis of new-onset acute heart failure, measuring natriuretic peptide levels can be a useful screening tool in the diagnosis of HF (i.e. BNP <10 ng/L or NT-proBNP<300 ng/L), particularly for GPs where echocardiogram is not readily available. Where levels are raised above the threshold or if there is a high degree of suspicion for heart failure without a BNP level, patients will require a transthoracic echocardiogram to check for any cardiac structural abnormalities and help establish the aetiology of underlying heart failure.

Where a diagnosis of acute HF is confirmed, treatment is required to manage any precipitating factors, e.g. arrhythmias or acute coronary syndrome, and provide relief of symptoms.

Treatment strategies should include:

- ***Oxygen***, only recommended for use in patients with hypoxia (SpO_2< 94%), to reduce short-term mortality.

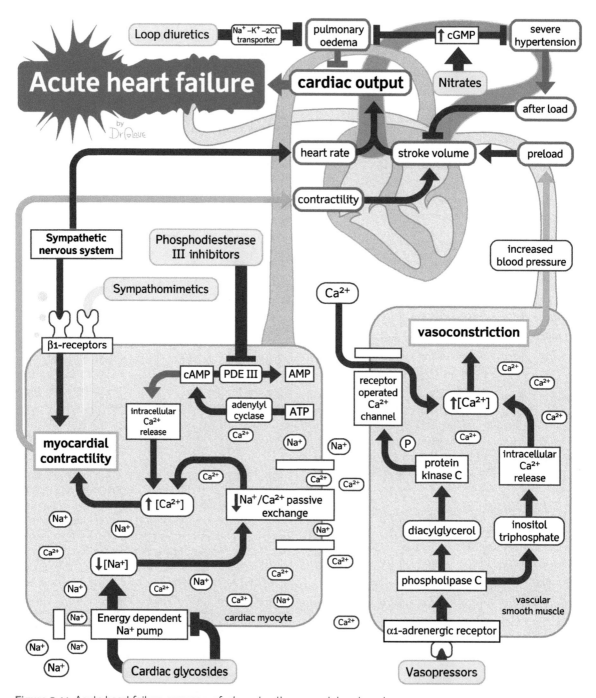

Figure 2.11 Acute heart failure: summary of relevant pathways and drug targets.

- **Diuretics** are used to treat oedema and dyspnoea, by promoting renal excretion of excess Na^+ and water. In acute severe disease, diuretics should be administered IV at high doses to optimize effects, either as intermittent bolus doses or continuous infusions.

Where patients remain resistant to monotherapy, they can be used in combination, e.g. **furosemide** and **metolazone**. In patients already on diuretics, dose increases may be necessary. Patients require close monitoring of weight, urine output, and U&Es to avoid over

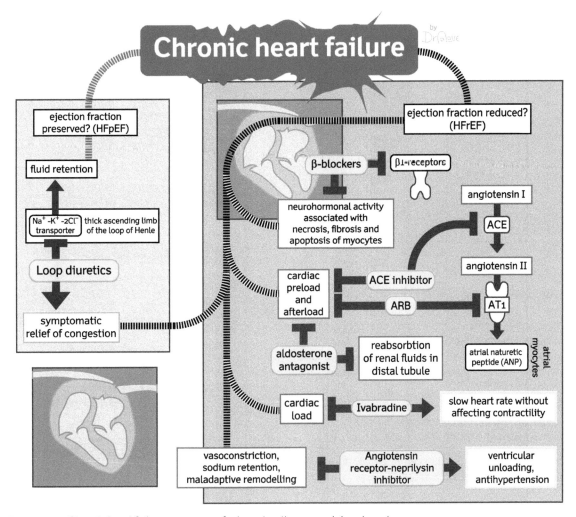

Figure 2.12 Chronic heart failure: summary of relevant pathways and drug targets.

diuresis, as well as to detect hypokalaemia or renal impairment.

- ***Vasodilators***, such as **glyceryl trinitrate**, are effective in reducing preload and afterload, and therefore can improve cardiac performance via the Frank–Starling phenomenon. However, hypotension is a major side effect which can reduce organ perfusion and thereby limit their use in patients with hypotension. They are, therefore, not recommended for routine use in acute HF, but may be of value in patients with severe hypertension and acute pulmonary oedema. They should be avoided in patients with a systolic pressure less than 110 mmHg.

- ***Opiates*** can help reduce anxiety and distress associated with dyspnoea, as well as potentially reducing preload through vasodilation. However, the balance of evidence suggests that their use is unlikely to be of clinical benefit and they may be associated with an increased risk of harm, i.e. increased need for mechanical ventilation and risk of in-hospital mortality. They are, therefore, not recommended for use in acute HF.

- The use of inotropes (e.g. **dobutamine**) in HF has been associated with an increase in mortality, due to increased myocardial oxygen consumption in a 'hibernating' myocardium, causing myocardial ischaemia and arrhythmias. Use is therefore restricted to patients with profound hypotension or shock, and in whom there is significant hypoperfusion of vital organs. While on treatment, patients will require close monitoring of BP and cardiac rhythm.

Table 2.15 Dietary and exercise advice in heart failure

Dietary advice	Exercise advice
Restrict dietary sodium intake to <6 g/day	Offer a moderate-intensity supervised exercise programme
Fluid restrict to 2 L/day with hyponatraemia	Encourage regular low intensity exercise in stable patients
Monitor daily weight for signs of fluid retention	Avoid heavy labour or intensive exercise
Avoid excessive alcohol consumption	Avoid exercise during acute exacerbations/ myocarditis

- **Vasopressors** (e.g. **noradrenaline**) may be used as an alternative to inotropes, where end-organ hypoperfusion persists in patients where cardiac filling pressures are adequate. They are, however, also associated with risks as they increase afterload and reduce cardiac output. **Dopamine** has both inotropic and vasopressor activity.
- **Phosphodiesterase III inhibitors** can be used to counteract the effects of β-blockers, but again their use is associated with an increased risk of mortality.

Once stabilized, patients will need to be considered for long-term treatment as outlined below.

Chronic heart failure

Management of chronic HF will depend on severity of symptoms and presence of any co-morbidities such as hypertension (Topic 2.1, 'Hypertension') or arrhythmias (Topic 2.7, ' Arrhythmias') (Figure 2.13). Clinical status can be assessed using the New York Heart Association (NYHA) functional class (Table 2.16) and ACC/AHA stage, which takes into consideration symptom severity (see Table 2.17). Arrhythmias are particularly common in HF and give a significantly poor prognosis (esp. ventricular) so pharmacotherapy (see Topic 2.7, 'Arrhythmias') or pacemaker/implantable cardioverter defibrillators may be required.

Long-term treatment strategies will depend on whether ejection fraction is preserved (HFpEF) or reduced (HFrEF). In those with HFpEF, treatment targets any underlying

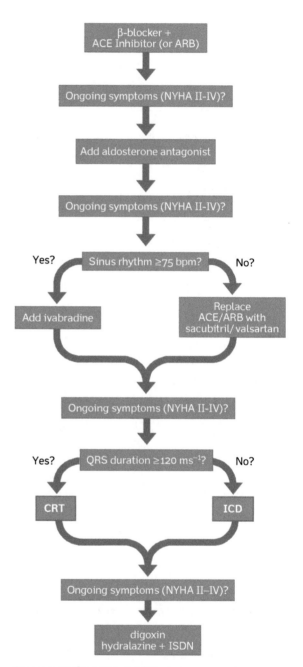

Figure 2.13 Chronic heart failure management.

Adapted from McMurray, John J.V. ESC Guidelines for the diagnosis and treatment of acute and chronic heart failure 2012: The Task Force for the Diagnosis and Treatment of Acute and Chronic Heart Failure 2012 of the European Society of Cardiology. Developed in collaboration with the Heart Failure Association (HFA) of the ESC. *European Heart Journal.* Volume 33, Issue 14, 1 July 2012, Pages 1787–1847. Copyright © 2012, by permission of the European Society of Cardiology. [https://doi.org/10.1093/eurheartj/ehs104].

Table 2.16 NYHA functional class

NYHA class	Symptoms
Class I	Ordinary physical activity does not cause undue fatigue, palpitations, dyspnoea, and/or angina
Class II	Ordinary physical activity does cause undue fatigue, palpitations, dyspnoea, and/or angina
Class III	Less than ordinary physical activity does cause undue fatigue, palpitations, dyspnoea, and/or angina
Class IV	Fatigue, palpitations, dyspnoea, and/or angina occurs at rest

Adapted with permission from The Criteria Committee of the New York Heart Association. Nomenclature and Criteria for Diagnosis of Diseases of the Heart and Great Vessels (9th ed.). Philadelphia, United States: Lippincott Williams and Wilkins.

co-morbidities, such as hypertension and AF, with diuretics used as needed. Patients with HFrEF, however, will require more extensive pharmacotherapy with disease-modifying agents (β-blockers, ACE inhibitors/ARBs and aldosterone antagonists, etc.) to reduce the risk of mortality (cardiovascular or secondary to HF), in addition to diuretics for symptomatic relief of congestion. Traditionally, dose escalations have been made, based on clinical symptoms and signs (fatigue, palpitations, oedema, dyspnoea, etc.), to determine response and efficacy. However, there is growing evidence to suggest that monitoring natriuretic peptide to guide decisions on treatment escalation, has a more marked effect on reducing mortality and hospitalization.

Table 2.17 ACC/AHA stages of heart failure

Class	Symptoms
A	At high risk of HF, but without structural heart disease or symptoms of HF
B	Structural heart disease, but without signs or symptoms of HF
C	Structural heart disease with prior or current symptoms of HF
D	Refractory HF requiring specialized interventions

Reproduced with permission from Yancy, C. et al. 2013 ACCF/AHA Guideline for the Management of Heart Failure A Report of the American College of Cardiology Foundation/American Heart Association Task Force on Practice Guidelines. *Circulation*. 2013;128:e240–e327. Copyright © 2013, Wolters Kluwer Health

The cost-benefit of using natriuretic peptide monitoring is only evident in patients 75 years of age or younger.

Diuretics, as with acute management, are used to control oedema and dyspnoea in patients with mild symptoms. Thiazides may be the preferred option, due to their delayed onset of action and less pronounced effect, whereas loop diuretics are of greater benefit in moderate to severe disease. Potassium sparing-diuretics may be considered in patients requiring additional diuresis and in whom hypokalaemia is a problem, although this effect may be offset anyway in combination with an ACE inhibitor or aldosterone antagonist. Diuretic doses should be titrated to control symptoms at the lowest possible dose.

β-blockers should be offered to all patients with a reduced ejection fraction unless contraindicated (see 'β-blockers'), as data from numerous studies have demonstrated that they are beneficial in the medium to long term in reducing mortality. In the short term, however, they can cause hypotension and decompensation, leading to worsening of heart failure. For this reason, treatment should only be initiated once the patient is haemodynamically stable, with doses started low and gradually titrated to optimal effective doses.

ACE inhibitors (or **ARBs** if intolerant) are recommended for use in all patients with a reduced ejection fraction, as they again have been shown to reduce the risk of mortality and hospitalization. Treatment should be started once the patient is stable, within 24–48 hours of an acute episode. Patients already on treatment may continue during an acute episode unless there is evidence of significant renal impairment.

An **aldosterone antagonist** can be added to treatment in patients that remain symptomatic despite optimal treatment with a β-blocker and ACE inhibitor (or ARB), to further reduce the risk of mortality. In general, this is with **spironolactone**, however, the risk of gynaecomastia is lower with **eplerenone**, so affected patients may need to be switched. For either drug, treatment is not recommended in moderate renal impairment or in patients with hyperkalaemia.

More recently, **sacubitril** (neprilysin inhibitor) in combination with **valsartan** has been licensed for use in chronic heart failure for symptom control, and is advocated for use by SIGN in patients that fail treatment with an aldosterone antagonist added in. It is indicated as an alternative to an ACE or ARB, which must be stopped for 36 hours first, to reduce the risk of angioedema.

Ivabradine should be added to treatment in patients with NYHA class II–IV and LVEF ≤35% that have required hospitalization for HF in the last 12 months, and persistently have a heart rate ≥75 bpm despite maximum tolerated β-blocker doses. As it works on the sinoatrial node, it is only effective in patients in sinus rhythm. In these patients, the use of ivabradine reduces the risk of death secondary to HF.

The role of **digoxin** in HF is less convincing as it has failed to show a survival benefit and has been associated with sudden death. It may, however, be beneficial in patients with AF for up-front use while patients are titrated onto a β-blocker, or as a last measure add on therapy where other treatment strategies have failed to reduce symptoms.

Isosorbide dinitrate and **hydralazine** can be used in combination either as add on therapy or as an alternative to an ACE or ARB, although the evidence base for this is considerably smaller. The evidence is marginally better in African-Americans with HF.

Certain drugs are known to have an adverse effect in HF and are, therefore, best avoided. NSAIDs and COX-2 inhibitors for example can aggravate sodium and water retention, as well as adversely affecting renal function. Most CCBs, in particular the non-dihydropyridines (e.g. **verapamil**, **diltiazem**), should be avoided as their negative inotropic effects can aggravate heart failure.

Drug classes used in management

Loop diuretics

> Loop diuretics block the luminal Na^+-K^+-$2Cl^-$ transporter in the thick ascending limb of the loop of Henle. Importantly, the level of diuretic effect is dependent on the functional integrity of the transporter. Examples include bumetanide, furosemide, and torasemide

Mechanism of action

The Na^+-K^+-$2Cl^-$ transporter has 12 putative membrane-spanning domains, with loop diuretics binding to portions of domains 11 and 12. Loop diuretics reach the transporter in the luminal membrane after being secreted into the urine at the proximal tube. Binding to albumin minimizes glomerular filtration. The inhibition of Na^+ and Cl^- reabsorption is achieved by competitive binding to the Cl^- binding site. Since the reabsorption of Mg^{2+} and Ca^{2+} is also dependent on Na^+ and Cl^-, the reabsorption of these electrolytes is also inhibited. This leads to a decrease in osmotic driving force for water, resulting in increased urine volume production (see Topic 5.2, 'Acute kidney injury').

Prescribing

As a class, the loop diuretics are highly effective in promoting fluid loss, thus require careful monitoring to prevent over diuresis and excessive electrolyte disturbances. Unlike other diuretics their rapid onset of action makes them unsuitable for the management of hypertension. **Furosemide**, the most widely used, can be administered orally or IV, but due to poor oral bioavailability, the oral dose is twice that of the IV dose. Alternative loop diuretics include **bumetanide**, which can be administered orally or IV, and **torasemide** for oral administration only. Unlike furosemide, both of these agents have good oral bioavailability, and no dose conversion is required when switching between oral or IV bumetanide. Due to their rapid onset of action, doses are best administered in the morning, so patients are not disturbed at night, with larger doses split so a second dose is given at lunch time.

Unwanted effects

As loop diuretics act to promote Na^+, K^+, and fluid loss, they are contraindicated in hypovolaemia, severe hypokalaemia or hyponatraemia. Patients should be monitored for the presence of electrolyte disturbances and treatment tailored to clinical need, with any underlying electrolyte disturbances corrected as appropriate. As well as hypokalaemia and hyponatraemia, excessive use can also cause magnesium and calcium loss, as well as hypotension secondary to hypovolaemia. The risk of toxicity is most pronounced with prolonged use, in patients with underlying hepatic disease or the elderly. Extra care is also required in patients on digoxin as the risk of digoxin toxicity is increased in the presence of hypokalaemia or hypomagnesemia. Patients should be advised to report symptoms suggestive of electrolyte disturbances such as cramps, headaches, dizziness, and confusion. Other effects of loop diuretics include increases in uric acid, glucose, and lipids.

Renal function should be monitored on treatment and in severe impairment treatment, less than 30 mL/min/1.73 m² loop diuretics should be used with caution. Treatment has also been associated with an increase in liver enzymes.

Drug interactions

Drug interactions with loop diuretics tend to be pharmacodynamic in nature, i.e. electrolyte loss may be either exaggerated or reversed in the presence of other diuretics and hypotensive effects enhanced in combination with anti-hypertensives. Some drugs that affect renal function, such as NSAIDs or **probenecid**, may alter the efficacy of loop diuretics by promoting their excretion.

Nitrates

> Nitrates increase intracellular concentration of cGMP leading to smooth muscle relaxation. Examples include sodium nitroprusside and glyceryl trinitrate.

Mechanism of action

See Topic 2.4, 'Stable angina'.

Prescribing

The nitrates like **glyceryl trinitrate** are used to provide rapid relief of symptoms associated with pulmonary oedema and severe hypertension, in patients showing an inadequate response to diuretic therapy.

The nitrates lower left ventricular filling pressure and provide symptomatic improvement in haemodynamically stable acute exacerbation of HF.

Sodium nitroprusside is administered as an IV infusion due to its rapid onset and short duration of action (1–10 minutes). While on treatment, BP and heart rate should be monitored, and treatment discontinued once the patient is normotensive. Treatment should be withdrawn gradually to prevent a rebound in BP. Infusions should be continued for a maximum of 3 days due to the risk of cyanide poisoning beyond this time.

Unwanted effects

See Topic 2.4, 'Stable angina'.

β-blockers

> β-blockers act to reduce cardiac output and decrease systemic vascular resistance. Examples include acebutolol, atenolol, bisoprolol, carvedilol, celiprolol, labetalol, metoprolol, nadolol, nebivolol, oxprenolol, pindolol, propranolol, and timolol.

Mechanism of action

In heart failure, β-blockers are thought to reduce mortality by inhibiting neurohormonal activity associated with necrosis, fibrosis, and apoptosis of myocytes. Inhibition of adrenergic drive within the myocardium

is, therefore, thought to reduce left ventricular damage and improve cardiac function. In addition, β-blockers act to improve contractility, particularly in ischaemic myocardium.

Prescribing

Of the available β-blockers, **atenolol**, **bisoprolol**, **carvedilol**, **metoprolol**, and **nebivolol** have the greatest evidence for use in chronic heart failure, although not all are licensed for this indication. In all instances, treatment should be initiated only once patients are considered to be haemodynamically stable following an acute event, starting with the lowest possible dose. Doses should be increased slowly to achieve symptom control. For more information on β-blockers in general, see Topic 2.1, 'Hypertension'.

Unwanted effects

See Topic 2.1, 'Hypertension'.

ACE inhibitors

> ACE inhibitors decrease the formation of vasoconstrictive Ang II and the degradation of vasodilatory bradykinin. Examples include captopril, enalopril, fosinopril, lisinopril, moexipril, perindopril, quinapril, ramipril, and trandolapril.

Mechanism of action

In heart failure, ACE inhibitors alter haemodynamics by reducing both cardiac preload and afterload. This, in turn, increases cardiac output without increasing heart rate in patients with systolic dysfunction. They act to inhibit the renin-angiotensin cascade and neurohormonal activation, responsible for left ventricular hypertrophy, collagen deposition, and ultimately dysfunction. As with β-blockers, their benefits are, therefore, evident with long-term use in slowing the rate of LV dysfunction and associated cardiovascular mortality. Furthermore, ACE inhibitors have some effect on LV remodelling. For general information on ACE inhibitors see Topic 2.1, 'Hypertension'.

Prescribing

The beneficial effects of ACE inhibitors are a class effect although not all are licensed for this indication. Doses should be started low once patients are haemodynamically stable following an acute event and gradually titrated to response. See also Topic 2.1, 'Hypertension'.

Unwanted effects

See Topic 2.1, 'Hypertension'

Angiotensin receptor blockers

Angiotensin receptor blockers bind to the AT1 receptor with high affinity, inhibiting the majority of the biological effects of angiotensin II. Examples include candesartan, eprosartan, irbesartan, losartan, olmesartan, telmisartan, and valsartan.

Mechanism of action

ARBs provide an alternative to ACE inhibitors in patients that are intolerant. Like ACE inhibitors they reduce cardiac preload and afterload, and inhibit sympathetic adrenergic activity, albeit by a different mechanism. See Topic 2.1, 'Hypertension'.

Prescribing

ARBs are generally considered as a second-line option to ACE inhibitors. As with other chronic therapy options, treatment should be started low and titrated to response. For more general information see Topic 2.1, 'Hypertension'.

Unwanted effects

See Topic 2.1, 'Hypertension'.

Angiotensin receptor neprilysin inhibitor

The neutral endopeptidase neprilysin degrades several endogenous vasoactive peptides, such as natriuretic peptides, bradykinin, and substance P. Its inhibition results in natriuretic, vasodilatory, and anti-proliferative effects. For example, sacubitril.

Mechanism of action

Inhibition of neprilysin causes an increase in the levels of vasoactive peptides that can counterbalance vasoconstriction, Na^+ retention, and maladaptive remodelling. These effects can produce a powerful ventricular unloading and antihypertensive response.

Although isolated neprilysin inhibitors have demonstrated only modest effects, drugs involving combined inhibition of neprilysin and renin-angiotensin-aldosterone system have been developed. **Sacubitril** is a first in class angiotensin II receptor neprilysin inhibitor (ARNI) that has shown hemodynamic and neurohormonal effects that were greater than those of an angiotensin receptor blocker alone.

Prescribing

Sacubitril is available in a combined preparation with the ARB **valsartan**, licensed for use in chronic heart failure in patients with an impaired ejection fraction. Doses are administered orally BD, initially at a low dose and titrated at 2–4-week intervals according to response and tolerance. Thirty-six hours prior to initiation, any ACE inhibitor or ARB should be discontinued due to the risk of angioedema. Treatment should be withheld in hyperkalaemia or in end-stage renal failure, and otherwise reduced in renal impairment.

Unwanted effects

Side effects to **sacubitril** are similar to those seen with ACE inhibitor or ARB therapy, in particular hypotension, renal impairment, and hyperkalaemia. The former can, in part, be managed by gradual dose titration.

Angioedema, although uncommon can be severe, and in some instances associated with life-threatening laryngeal oedema. Patients should be advised to seek immediate help if they experience swelling that affects the face, tongue, glottis, or larynx. Most cases can be managed with antihistamines, but treatment should be discontinued regardless.

Other common adverse effects include dizziness and headache, likely related to vasodilation, and non-specific GI toxicity (nausea, vomiting, diarrhoea, etc.).

Drug interactions

Interactions of clinical significance with **sacubitril** tend to be pharmacodynamic in nature, so that toxicity is enhanced in combination with other drugs known to cause hypotension, renal impairment, or hyperkalaemia. Of greatest significance is the need to avoid concomitant use with ACE inhibitors or ARBS, due to the increase risk of angioedema.

Other possible reactions include reduced clearance of statins and lithium leading to an increased risk of toxicity.

Sinus node inhibitor

> Ivabradine acts to block the 'funny' channel (If) in the sinoatrial node, reducing heart rate.

Mechanism of action

As in stable angina (see Topic 2.4, 'Stable angina'), the sinus node inhibitor **ivabradine** acts to slow heart rate without affecting contractility, leading to a reduction in cardiac load.

Prescribing

Ivabradine has demonstrated improved outcomes in patients with persistently raised heart rate (≥70 bpm) despite treatment optimization with β-blockers and ACE inhibitors. They are, therefore, only effective in patients in sinus rhythm. For more information see Topic 2.4, 'Stable angina'.

Unwanted effects

See Topic 2.4, 'Stable angina'.

Inotropes: cardiac glycosides

> Digitalis glycosides inhibit the Na^+–K^+-dependent membrane pump that is located in myocardial cells, increasing intracellular Ca^{2+} and contractility of the myocardial muscle (i.e. positive inotropic effect). For example, digoxin.

Mechanism of action

Digitalis glycosides inhibit the energy dependent Na^+ pump (Na^+/K^+-ATPase) in the myocyte membrane, lowering the concentration gradient for Na^+ across the membrane and decreasing the passive exchange of Na^+/Ca^{2+}. This leads to an increase in intracellular Ca^{2+}, enhancing myocardial contractility.

The Na^+/K^+-ATPase enzyme is a heterotrimer that contains α, β, and γ subunits. The α subunit has binding sites for Na^+, K^+ and ATP, and on its extra-cytoplasmic side the binding sites for digitalis glycosides. Levels of glycoside at the therapeutic range inhibit about 10–30% of this receptor enzyme, and more than 50% inhibition leads to toxic effects. Early intervention of the high affinity, low capacity α3 Na^+/K^+-ATPase isoform present in sympathetic nerve endings of cardiac muscle, leads

to extracellular noradrenaline accumulation. In turn, this elicits the primary effect-amplifying cAMP cascade, resulting in catecholamine inotropy. The low-affinity α1 Na^+/K^+-ATPase isoform in cardiac muscle plasma membrane is the one responsible for increasing intracellular Ca^{2+} and enhancing myocardial contractility.

Digitalis glycosides also have a negative chronotropic effect that is produced via direct influence on the sinus node, by increasing vagus and decreasing adrenal activity. In effect, inhibition of the Na^+/K^+ pump in non-myocardial cells could lead to sympatholytic effects, due to cardiac baroreceptor readjustment and suppression of renin secretion caused by decreased tubular Na^+ reabsorption.

Prescribing

Due to its prolonged elimination half-life (1.5–2 days) and slow onset of action, **digoxin** requires loading to achieve timely therapeutic levels, with the regimen dependent on the urgency of treatment. Doses can be administered orally (by tablet of liquid) or intravenously, although the two are not bioequivalent.

> **PRESCRIBING WARNING**
>
> **Digoxin liquids**
> Digoxin is available in oral preparations as a liquid or tablet, where 50 μg of liquid is equivalent to 62.5 μg given as tablet.

Unwanted effects

Side effects to **digoxin** are dose dependent and this risk is augmented by its narrow therapeutic index. Plasma monitoring and dose reductions may be necessary in certain at-risk patients; particularly, those with renal impairment and the elderly, where the half-life can be considerably prolonged. Digoxin distributes widely throughout the body, but has a high affinity for the myocardium, where it exerts much of its unwanted effects.

Due to its increased effects on myocardial excitability and automaticity, the risk of arrhythmias with treatment is high. This occurs due to the inhibition of the Na^+/K^+ pump, which makes the membrane potential less negative and closer to the depolarization threshold; combined with the spontaneous release of Ca^{2+} from the sarcoplasmic reticulum, which causes transient depolarization after an action potential. Treatment should be avoided with supraventricular arrhythmias, ventricular tachycardia, and ventricular fibrillation, and patients on treatment should be closely monitored for signs of toxicity. The risk of toxicity to digoxin is increased in hypokalaemia, hypomagnesaemia, and hypercalcaemia due to increased myocardial sensitivity.

In overdose, digoxin is highly toxic and at excessive levels (greater than 10 mg) can be fatal. Early signs of toxicity include nausea and vomiting, as well as supraventricular tachycardia and arrhythmias. Patients are also likely to experience neurological effects, such as headache, drowsiness, and agitation. Treatment can include steps to reduce gastric absorption such as charcoal, cardiac pacing or the use of digoxin antibodies to reverse the effects. In some instance, the use of the antidote, **DigiFab®** may be indicated, although not widely available.

Inotropes: sympathomimetics

Sympathomimetics act on β_1-adrenoceptors, mimicking the stimulation conveyed by adrenergic nerves of the sympathetic nervous system and thereby increasing the contractility of cardiac muscle, without affecting the rate. For example, dobutamine, dopamine, and dopexamine

Mechanism of action

Dobutamine is a synthetic catecholamine that has a positive inotropic effect in conjunction with reduction of both aortic impedance and systemic vascular resistance. These effects usually lead to a reduction in cardiac afterload and some increase in cardiac output, with little direct effect on vascular tone. It acts primarily by stimulating β_1-adrenoceptors, with minor effect on β_2 or α receptors. Unlike **dopamine**, it does not cause the release of endogenous noradrenaline.

Dopexamine, an N-substitute analogue of dopamine, is a synthetic catecholamine that was designed to combine and improve the desirable haemodynamic properties of dopamine and dobutamine. The chronotropic and inotropic effects of dopexamine are mediated by various mechanisms—direct agonist effect on β_2-adrenoceptors increasing heart rate and vasodilation, and the potentiation of neurally released noradrenaline, leading to indirect activation of β_1-adrenoceptors and a positive inotropic effect. The decrease in systemic vascular resistance appears to be mediated by β_2-adrenoceptors stimulation, and vascular DA_1 and DA_2 receptors. Unlike dopamine, it does not cause peripheral vasoconstriction at high doses.

Dopamine is a natural catecholamine derived from tyrosine and formed by decarboxylation of 3,4-dihydroxyphenylalanine (DOPA). It is a precursor to noradrenaline in noradrenergic terminals, and it is also a neurotransmitter in a few peripheral sympathetic sites and in particular areas of the CNS. Dopamine produces positive chronotropic and inotropic effects on the cardiac muscle, leading to an increase in cardiac contractility and heart rate. This is partly due to a direct action on β-adrenoceptors and an indirect increase in noradrenaline stimulation by causing its release from storage sites in sympathetic nerve terminals. The effects of dopamine are dose related, with moderate doses required for the β-adrenoceptor-mediated inotropic response, and low doses being responsible for peripheral DA receptors stimulation leading to arterial vasodilation. At high doses, activation of α-adrenoceptors produces peripheral vasoconstriction. Unfortunately, the doses that produce these effects differ widely among individuals.

Prescribing

Of the sympathomimetics, **dobutamine** and low dose **dopamine** are the most widely used. Treatment is administered as an intravenous infusion as both drugs possess a very short half-life (about 2 minutes) and are therefore rapidly cleared. During treatment heart rate, blood pressure, cardiac output and urine output should be closely monitored, and treatment discontinued in the case of symptomatic hypotension or worsening tachyarrhythmias.

In acute heart failure dobutamine is generally run at a rate of between 2.5- and 10 µg/kg/min, although higher rates have been used. With dopamine lower doses of 2–10 µg/kg/minute act directly to cause vasodilation of renal and mesenteric blood vessels, whereas higher doses of 10–20 µg/kg/minute have a vasoconstrictive effect, due to stimulation of α-adrenergic receptors.

Unwanted effects

Toxic effects seen with the sympathomimetics are commonly cardiovascular and directly related to their cardiac effects, i.e. ectopic heart beats, tachycardia, hypotension, and hypertension. Patients also commonly complain of headache, dyspnoea, and nausea and vomiting. Where necessary, hypovolaemia must be corrected prior to starting treatment with either drug.

As **dopamine** promotes the release of noradrenaline, a potent vasoconstrictor, treatment can aggravate peripheral vascular disease and, in severe cases, lead to gangrene. Patients with a history of PVD should be closely monitored for changes in skin colour or temperature.

Inotropes: phosphodiesterase III inhibitors

The inotropic effects of phosphodiesterase III inhibitors result from an increase in the intracellular levels of cAMP, leading to mobilization of intracellular Ca^{2+}; for example, enoximone and milrinone.

Mechanism of action

Adenylyl cyclase activity converts ATP to cyclic adenosine monophosphate (cAMP), by forming an intramolecular phosphodiester. The cyclic nucleotide phoshodiesterases are enzymes that attenuate these cyclic nucleotide signals by hydrolysing the phosphodiester bonds, converting cAMP to AMP.

The cAMP-mediated signalling is regulated specifically in functionally and spatially restricted intracellular compartments of cardiac myocytes. The compartmentalization of cAMP signalling permits different extracellular stimuli to specifically stimulate diverse functional responses. It appears that distinct phosphodiesterase isoforms are functionally coupled to discrete compartments in cardiac myocytes, and are capable of regulating cAMP-mediated signalling in these domains. In addition to increased contractility of the myocardial tissue, phosphodiesterase inhibition in vascular smooth muscle produces peripheral arterial vasodilation.

The use of PDE3 inhibitors in the treatment of heart failure follows the observation that decreased levels of cAMP and cAMP-mediated signalling are found in the failing myocardium, and this can be improved by PDE3 inhibition. However, taking into consideration the multiple actions of cAMP in cardiac myocytes, which includes energy metabolism, gene transcription, and mobilization of intracellular Ca^{2+}, it seems plausible that several molecular mechanism can be affected by phosphodiesterase inhibition.

Prescribing

The phosphodiesterase inhibitors **milrinone** and **enoximone** are both indicated in acute heart failure associated with poor cardiac output, despite conventional treatment, although they are only indicated for short-term use due to an increased risk of mortality.

Where indicated, treatment is administered IV as an infusion, preceded by a loading dose administered as a bolus dose (milrinone) or faster infusion (enoximone).

Unwanted effects

Many of the adverse effects seen with the phosphodiesterase type III inhibitors are similar to those seen with the sympathomimetics, i.e. ectopic beats, tachycardia, hypotension, headaches, and nausea and vomiting, due to their similar pharmacological effects on muscle contractility and vasodilation.

During treatment, patients will therefore require close monitoring of heart rate, BP, cardiac output, and fluid and electrolyte status. Dose reductions may be necessary in renal and hepatic impairment, although this should be detected with close monitoring.

Vasopressors

Vasopressors increase BP through vasoconstriction, secondary to stimulation of α-adrenoceptors, e.g. noradrenaline

Mechanism of action

Noradrenaline is the neurotransmitter found in the majority of sympathetic post-ganglionic neurons. It activates α-adrenoceptors, leading to positive chronotropism, inotropism, and vasoconstriction. The α_1-adrenoceptors are located on vascular smooth muscle cells and the heart, among other tissues. When stimulated with noradrenaline, G protein–coupled α_1-adrenoceptors activate phospholipase C, leading to the generation of inositol triphosphate (IP_3) and diacylglycerol. IP_3 activates Ca^{2+} ion channels from the intracellular endoplasmic reticulum leading to increase in cytoplasmic Ca^{2+}. Diacylglycerol activates protein kinase C, which is thought to phosphorylate ion channels, which promote the increase in cytoplasmic Ca^{2+} concentrations and contractile force.

Prescribing

Noradrenaline is licensed for the management of severe hypotension in an emergency situation. It is administered as an IV infusion via a central venous catheter, dosed according to weight, and titrated to achieve a systolic pressure between 100 and 120 mmHg. Due to its short half-life, the effects on BP reverse within 1–2 minutes of discontinuation.

Unwanted effects

Side effects are dose-dependent and are largely explained by its cardiac activity, i.e. hypertension, bradycardia, and arrhythmias. Patients also complain of anxiety, headache, and dyspnoea.

As a potent vasoconstrictor, **noradrenaline** should not be administered via a peripheral line due to the risk of ischaemia. Care should also be taken to monitor the injection site as it is a vesicant that can cause local tissue necrosis in case of extravasation.

During treatment, patients should receive adequate fluid and electrolytes in order to promote blood flow and adequate tissue perfusion, thereby reducing the risk of hypoxia and lactic acidosis.

Further reading

Chatterjee K. (2012) Pathophysiology of systolic and diastolic heart failure. *Medical Clinics of North America* 96(5), 891–9.

Kemp CD, Conte JV (2012) The pathophysiology of heart failure. *Cardiovascular Pathology* 21(5), 365–71.

Lee CS, Tckacs NC (2008) Current concepts of neurohormonal activation in heart failure. *Advances in Critical Care* 19(4), 364–85.

Metra M, Cotter G, Gheorghiade M, et al. (2012) The role of the kidney in heart failure. *European Heart Journal* 33(17), 2135–42.

Movsesian M, Stehlik J, Vandeput F, et al. (2009) Phosphodiesterase inhibition in heart failure. *Heart Failure Review* 14(4), 255–63.

Rathi S, Deedwania PC (2012) The epidemiology and pathophysiology of heart failure. *Medical Clinics of North America* 96(5), 881–90.

Yancy CW, Jessup M, Bozkurt B, et al. (2013) ACCF/AHA guideline for the management of heart failure: a report of the American College of Cardiology Foundation/American Heart Association Task Force on practice guidelines *Circulation* 128(16), e240–327.

Guidelines

McMurray JJV, Adamapoulos S, Anker SD, et al. ESC guidelines for the diagnosis and treatment of acute and chronic heart failure 2012: ESC Committee for Practice Guidelines (2012) *European Journal of Heart Failure* 33, 1787–847. http://www.escardio.org/guidelines-surveys/esc-guidelines/GuidelinesDocuments/Guidelines-Acute%20and%20Chronic-HF-FT.pdf [accessed 22 March 2019].

NICE CG106 (2018): Chronic heart failure in adults: diagnosis and management. https://www.nice.org.uk/guidance/NG106 [accessed 27 March 2019].

NICE TA267 (2012) Ivabradine for treating chronic heart failure. https://www.nice.org.uk/guidance/ta267 [accessed 22 March 2019].

SIGN 147 (2016) Management of chronic heart failure. https://www.sign.ac.uk/assets/sign147.pdf [accessed 22 March 2019].

2.7 Arrhythmias

Pathophysiology

The combined effects of anti-arrhythmic drugs (AD) are complex, so that no single classification system addresses the precise mode of action and efficacy of drugs for a specific indication (e.g. atrial fibrillation or ventricular tachycardia). Given this imperfect position, it is important to consider the overall cardiac conduction system of the heart and the electrophysiology of cardiac cells, i.e. pacemaker cells and cardiac myocytes.

Cardiac conduction pathway

The basic pathway of the cardiac conduction system is made up of five components:

1. *The sino-atrial node (SAN)*: located in the right atrium, these specialized cells possess regular spontaneous activity (automaticity), which triggers atrial myocardial contractility that propagates through and depolarizes the atria (i.e. P-wave on ECG), down a conductive pathway to the atrial ventricular node (AVN). The SAN normally sets the pace for the cardiac cycle.

2. *The atrioventricular node*: the signal from the SAN arrives at the AVN, located in the inferior–posterior region of the interarterial septum; here, conduction is slowed slightly, allowing the atria to pump all their blood into the ventricles. AVN cells also have their own intrinsic activity, but this is slower than that of the SAN.

3. *Bundle of His*: conduction continues from the AVN down the bundle of His where it branches into two main pathways.

4. *Left and right bundle branches*: the left bundle divides into two fascicles, creating a bifasicular system (one anterior and one posterior fascicle), while the right branch is singular and anteriorly placed. Both lead to systolic contraction of respective ventricles.

5. *Purkinje fibres*: the wave of conductive depolarization from the branches is distributed through Purkinje fibres to cause ventricular myocyte activation and ventricular contraction (i.e. QRS on ECG).

The automaticity of this conduction pathway is heavily influenced by the autonomic nervous system, primarily via the SAN (right vagal nerve) and the AVN (left vagal nerve). Sympathetic stimulation, via noradrenergic β-adrenoceptors located in the SAN increase heart rate (a positive chronotrope), have inotropic effects, and increase the speed of conduction through the pathway (hence, shortening P–R interval). Conversely, increased parasympathetic tone decreases SAN activity and slows conduction via cholinergic muscarinic receptors, which can result, if over stimulated, in heart block.

Electrophysiology of pacemaker cells

Most cells described previously are pacemaker cells (except the myocytes and Purkinje cells) and have a characteristic electrophysiology depending on their location. Most cells when they depolarize have a large-fast Na^+ influx. However, cardiac pacemaker cells also possess a slow-sustained Ca^{2+} current (via L-type Ca^{2+} channels), which drives depolarization with a subsequent repolarizing K^+ current. Unlike other electro-physiologically active cells, the action potential pacemaking nature of these cells is made up of three phases meaning that a stable resting membrane potential is absent in these cells (Figure 2.14):

- *Phase 4*: this is a spontaneous slow depolarizing current mediated through an I_f (funny) inward Na^+ current that when reaching −50 mV opens a transient Ca^{2+} channel $I_{ca(T)}$ further depolarizing the cell until moving into phase 0. The I_f current is mainly through hyperpolarization-activated cyclic nucleotide-gated channels.

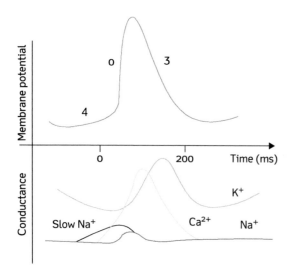

Figure 2.14 Action potentials and conductance changes at the SAN, Training in Anaesthesia Spoors, Kiff (2010).

- *Phase 0*: this is predominantly an L-type Ca^{2+} influx, which is triggered by the I_f and $I_{ca(T)}$ flux. These channels close as the $I_{ca(L)}$ takes over leading to full depolarization.
- *Phase 3*: as the membrane potential reaches 0 mV, repolarization occurs through the opening of K^+ channels with resulting K^+ efflux and also closure of the Ca^{2+} channel, which drives hyperpolarization. This strong hyperpolarized state to −60 mV determines the pacemaking nature of these cells.

These tightly controlled currents can be heavily influenced by hypoxia, ischaemia, and changes in autonomic innervation. Cholinergic stimulation decreases the rate of the depolarization, through an additional K^+ current that affects the slope of the pacemaker potential and, hence, slows heart rate. Conversely, β-adrenergic stimulation can increase heart rate by increasing the slope of the pacemaker potential (Figure 2.14).

Electrophysiology of non-pacemaker cells

Non-pacemaker cardiac cells include the myocytes, both atrial and ventricular, and the Purkinje cells. These cells, like most other electrophysiologically active cells have a true resting membrane potential, which is approximately −80 mV (diastole on the cardiac cycle; see Figure 2.15). This resting potential (phase 4) is maintained by an outward

flux of K^+ ions down a chemical gradient. Following stimulation, the cell rapidly depolarizes generating an 'action potential' via a fast Na^+ influx, associated with closure of K^+ channels, so reaching a 'depolarized' positive membrane potential; denoted as phase 0. At the generation of an action potential, a short-lived transient K^+ current (I_{TO}) starts and lasts 30–40 ms, resulting in transient repolarization and dictating the action potential duration (phase 1). This is quickly followed by a sustained slow inward Ca^{2+} flux (phase 2) through L-type channels, extending the plateau of the action potential. The balance between Ca^{2+} and K^+ is crucial in phase 2, as the latter produces repolarization [through I_{Kr} (rapid) and I_{Ks} currents] and modifies the QT interval. In the final phase (3) of repolarization the Ca^{2+} flux ceases and further outflow of K^+ (via I_{Kr} and I_{Ks}) leads to a resting membrane state again.

It is important to note that, during the action potential, the cell is unable to respond to further stimulation, i.e. it is in a refractory state. No adjacent cells can lead to further depolarization until it has returned to near phase 4. This electrochemical protective mechanism, means that cell-to-cell depolarization is propagated directionally through the myocardium during systole, and local cyclical circuits or retrograde contractions are avoided. In the structurally damaged heart or during periods of hypoxia, depolarization may occur at different thresholds and thus lead to arrhythmias. Alteration of these ion fluxes, alone or together, is the basis for many of the treatments used for cardiac arrhythmias. The modification of these net fluxes and the associated receptors with anti-arrhythmic drugs, have been classified by the Vaughan Williams system. It is important to note this drug classification system *does not* correspond cleanly to isolated ion fluxes or arrhythmia *per se*, but are associated with the phases of the overall electrophysiology response so can ameliorate unwanted arrhythmic activity.

For a full summary of the relevant pathways and drug targets, see Figure 2.16.

Management

Overview of arrhythmias

As would be expected from the physiology outlined previously, arrhythmias can cause changes in rate and/or rhythm, and tend to result from three sources:

- other or ectopic cells taking up pace making responsibilities (e.g. in hypoxia/ischaemia);

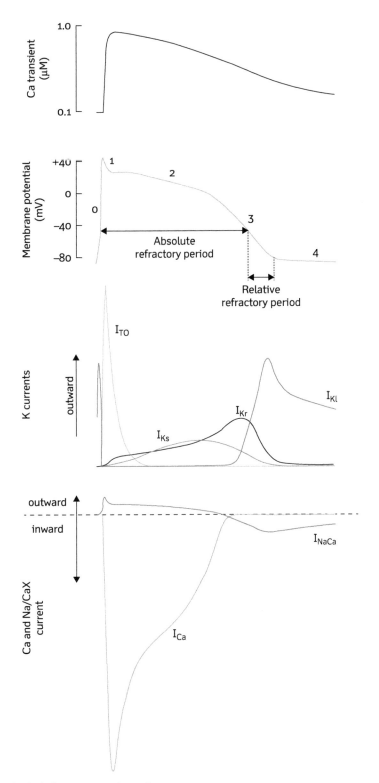

Figure 2.15 Action potential of non-pacemaker cells.

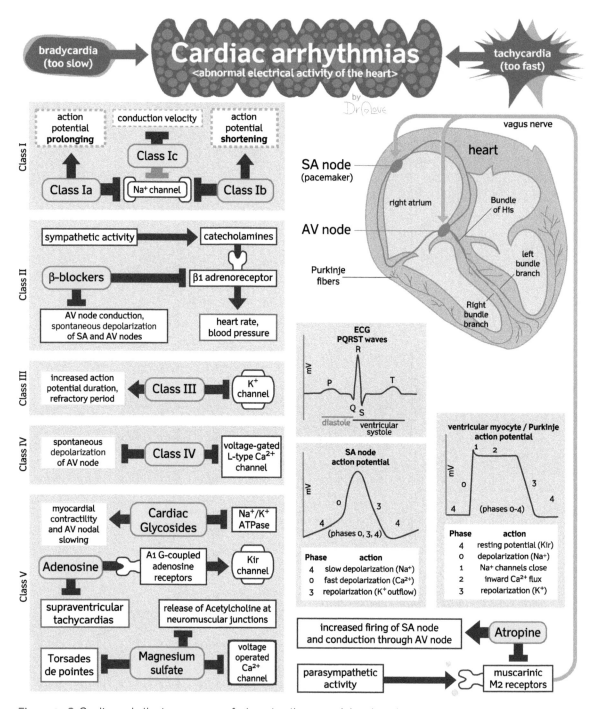

Figure 2.16 Cardiac arrhythmias: summary of relevant pathways and drug targets.

- changes in the normal conduction route (e.g. local circuits or retrograde conduction);
- early depolarizations.

The pathophysiology of the more common arrhythmias is set out below, focusing on the basis of electrophysiological alteration by drug classes as means to manage the condition.

Bradycardia and bradyarrythmias

These rhythms have, by definition, a rate of <60 bpm and may be caused by a number of disorders, including AV conduction block, i.e. heart block, sinoatrial disease, and sinus bradycardia. The latter may be a normal finding in an athlete, due to high vagal (cholinergic) tone, but can also be secondary to drugs (e.g. β-blockers and digoxin) or neurogenic causes. The symptomatic patient may have a reduced conscious level, fatigue, and in the event of haemodynamic compromise, can be treated initially with IV **atropine**.

Heart block is very common and may occur within the AVN or further down the conduction system in the His-Purkinje system. Typically in the elderly, fibrosis leads to delayed conduction transmission, so the P–R interval on ECG is prolonged to >200 ms. In first-degree block every

atrial contraction makes it to the ventricle, but is just delayed; it is often asymptomatic. In second-degree block (of which there are two types—Mobitz I and Mobitz II) there is intermittent failure of conduction from the atrium to the ventricle. While in third-degree or 'complete' block, there is complete dissociation from atrial and ventricular depolarization (see ECG Figure 2.17).

- *First-degree block*: prolongation of the PR interval >200 ms.
- *Second-degree block—Mobitz type 1* (AKA Wenckebach): the P–R interval gets progressively longer until eventually a QRS complex is dropped.
- *Second-degree block—Möbitz type 2*: intermittent non-conducted P waves without progressive prolongation of P–R interval.
- *Third-degree (complete) block*: complete dissociation between P waves and QRS complexes

Drugs such as **digoxin**, **verapamil**, **diltiazem,** or β-blockers can slow AV conduction. Verapamil and β-blockers are particularly dangerous in combination, as they can result in first, second, or third degree blocks. For symptomatic heart block (i.e. syncope or pre-syncope) or high degree AV blocks (e.g. Mobitz II or third-degree), pacing is the first line of treatment. If increase vagal tone

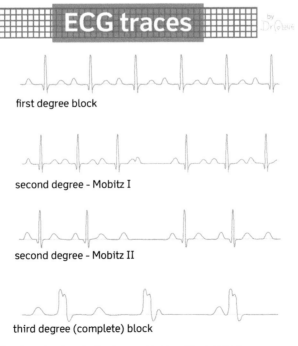

first degree block

second degree - Mobitz I

second degree - Mobitz II

third degree (complete) block

Figure 2.17 ECG examples of various bradyarrhythmias and types of heart block.

is responsible for the slow rate, **atropine** can be of benefit in the acute setting. In asystolic cardiac arrest, however, atropine is no longer recommended, but may be used when adverse features, such as shock, syncope, or heart failure are apparent; **isoprenaline** or IV **salbutamol** (off-label) can be used as alternatives.

Atropine acts by blocking muscarinic receptors (M_2) within the SAN and AVN, so rate suppressing cholinergic transmission is interrupted and there is an increased pacemaker cell activity that pushes up the ventricular rate (i.e. a positive chronotrope). Muscarinic receptors are Gi-protein-linked receptors, where ACh action decreases cAMP and the Gi-protein-linked activation of K_{ACh} channels. This activation increases K^+ efflux so cardiac cells hyperpolarize. Atropine antagonizes this so cells are more prone to depolarize. Isoprenaline was commonly used to treat bradycardia and blocks via its non-selective action as a β1/β2 agonist, causing positive chronotropic and inotropic effects.

Tachyarrythmias

As outlined previously, the tachyarrythmias generally stem from one of three sources:

- dysfunctional automaticity;
- triggered activity;
- re-entrant activity.

Narrow complex tachycardias are nearly always supraventricular in origin (see below), while wide complex tachycardia (QRS> 120 ms) may be supraventricular (e.g. in patients who also have a bundle branch block) *or* ventricular (e.g. VT) in origin (see ECG Figure 2.18).

Broad complex tachycardia

Broad complex tachycardia is generally poorly managed due to its complexity, considering there may be aberrant conduction pathways. Furthermore, there is a risk of misdiagnosis as patients may not be haemodynamically compromised, or have self-terminating episodes that are missed.

Ventricular tachycardia (VT) is three or more ventricular extra systoles in succession at a rate of >120 bpm, and is often associated with underlying heart abnormalities, cardiac ischaemia, or heart failure. If this rhythm is sustained, it may result in haemodynamic compromise and should be treated as a medical emergency. Patients may have a pulse or be pulseless (see ALS guidance, 'Guidelines', Resuscitation Council UK Guideline, 2010). VT can also be triggered by hypokalaemia, hypocalcaemia, or hypomagnesaemia. Symptoms typically include chest pain, palpitations, dyspnoea, and syncope. In stable VT, patients tend not to have haemodynamic compromise, but this can deteriorate so treatment with **lidocaine** (class

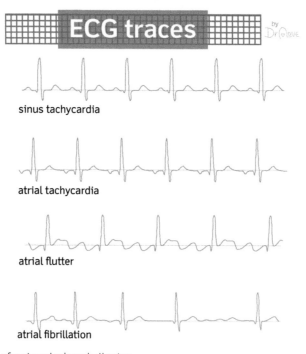

sinus tachycardia

atrial tachycardia

atrial flutter

atrial fibrillation

Figure 2.18 ECG examples of various tachyarrhythmias.

Ib), **amiodarone,** or cardioversion can be effective. The ALS algorithms recommend unsynchronized DC shock in pulseless VT and the use of amiodarone (class III) as the initial drug treatment of choice. Second-line drugs for the termination of ventricular tachycardia include lidocaine or, less commonly, **procainamide** or **disopyramide**. One variation of VT is polymorphic VT, which can degenerate into VF without treatment. This usually occurs secondary to toxicity, such as an electrolyte abnormality or is-chaemia, and is best managed by treating the underlying pathology.

Torsades de pointes is a distinctive polymorphic VT with variable amplitude QRS complexes, which possesses an undulating variable QRS. This condition is associated with prolonged QT interval and can present as sudden cardiac death. The QT syndromes may be congenital or acquired (e.g. MI, drugs; **erythromycin**, **ketoconazole**, tricyclic antidepressants, or electrolyte disturbances) and presents as episodes of palpitations or pre-syncope. In the acute situation, IV infusions of magnesium are most effective, while **isoprenaline** can accelerate the AV con-duction and decrease QT interval. In the chronic situation, β-blockers (type II) are first line in congenital—these *must* be avoided in acquired cases as they can cause a Torsade episode.

Another type of broad complex is from a narrow com-plex tachycardia, with an accessory conduction pathway (often termed 'supraventricular tachycardia with pre-excitation'). One example is the congenital condition *Wolff–Parkinson–White (WPW)* syndrome, where an accessory pathway may allow conduction of other ar-rhythmias like atrial fibrillation or atrial flutter; in this particular setting, this can produce life-threating arrhyth-mias. If atrial excitation finds the accessory pathways a re-entry tachycardia or pre-excited AF may result. First-line treatment is with radiofrequency ablation, although Ic or III drugs can be effective for prophylaxis. However, class Ic agents should not be given to patients with struc-tural heart disease.

In patients with Wolff–Parkinson–White (WPW) syn-drome, a more common and less serious acute arrhythmia can result from a narrow-complex AV re-entrant tachy-cardia. This may respond to vagal manoeuvres or **ad-enosine** IV. In the less common but more life threating case of atrial flutter/fibrillation in patients with WPW syn-drome, cardioversion is the best option as conventional drugs such as **digoxin**, β-blockers, or CCBs can increase the ventricular rate so risking ventricular fibrillation. IV **flecainide** or **amiodarone** can restore sinus rhythm through slowing anterograde conduction through the ac-cessory pathway.

Narrow complex tachycardia

Coronary artery disease, hypertensive heart disease, and congenital abnormalities are most commonly asso-ciated with the observation of atrial flutter, although it is also common in patients with lung disease and endur-ance athletes. In atrial flutter, the atrium beats rapidly at approximately 250–300 times per min with regular, but incomplete conduction of these beats to the ven-tricle (i.e. ≥2:1 block). Most often (type I) atrial flutter is initiated by a single re-entrant circuit with circus acti-vation around the right atrium; the underlying problem is probably anatomical in origin, such as the presence of scar tissue. Atrial flutter is supraventricular in origin and produces a characteristic 'sawtooth' pattern of the P wave on ECG (Figure 2.19). Patients present with symp-toms of sudden-onset palpitation, failing exercise tol-erance, dyspnoea, and presyncope due to decreases in cardiac output. If the ECG diagnosis is not clear, vagal manoeuvres or **adenosine**, which works to transiently block the AV node, can reveal the changes. Both these treatment options are also effective in terminating acute regular SVT.

First-line treatment for symptomatic atrial flutter is now considered to be with radiofrequency ablation (RFA). This has been proven to be superior to both rate and rhythm control by pharmacological therapy and also prevents the need for long-term anti-coagulation or anti-arrhythmics. That said, following successful RFA, patients are at an in-creased risk of AF and stroke; thus, cardiovascular risk should be assessed. Patients that are unsuitable for, or decline RFA, may be managed pharmacologically with therapy that slows AVN conduction, such as β-blockers or **verapamil/diltiazem**. Thromboprophylaxis is re-commended in these patients, particularly where atrial flutter persists beyond 48 hours (see 'Atrial fibrillation' in following paragraph). Prior to starting anticoagulation, bleeding risk should be assessed using HAS-BLED score (Table 2.18). Class Ia, Ic, and III agents are further op-tions for long-term management in patients unsuitable for ablation or where β-blockers or CCBs are contraindi-cated. **Flecainide** and **propafenone**, however, should be avoided in patients with structural heart defects due to the risk of pro-arrhythmia. Some agents with anticholin-ergic activity (e.g. the class 1a drug **disopyramide**) should be avoided, as they may exacerbate nodal con-duction of the flutter.

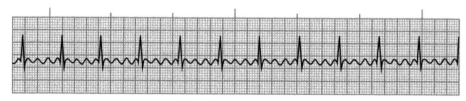

Figure 2.19 Characteristic 'sawtooth' P wave pattern seen with atrial flutter.

Atrial fibrillation (AF) occurs when atrial contraction is ineffective and uncoordinated, such that conduction is variable to the ventricle, causing an irregularly irregular ventricular response. On the ECG, there is replacement of consistent P waves by rapid oscillations or fibrillatory waves (350–600 discharges/min) that vary in amplitude, shape, and timing; P wave are, therefore, not visible. Many atrial fluctuations are not conducted to the ventricles as the AV node cell may be in a refractory state, so not all impulses are conducted. On average, a ventricular rate of 110–140 bpm with an irregularly irregular trace may be seen. With fast rates of ventricular conduction, there may be haemodynamic compromise due to inefficient pumping (compromised left ventricular filling and stroke volume), and this may present as hypotension, angina/ischaemia or heart failure. Approximately 90% of patients

Table 2.18 Bleeding risk classification defined as percentage bleeds per 100 patient-years

HAS-BLED risk	Score
Hypertension	1
Abnormal liver function	1
Abnormal renal function	1
Stroke	1
Bleeding	1
Labile INRs	1
Elderly (>65 years)	1
Drugs	1
Alcohol	1

Score 0–1; low risk (1.1%), score 2; intermediate risk (1.9%), score ≥ 3: high risk (4.9%).

Reprinted from Pisters, R. et al. A novel user-friendly score (HAS-BLED) to assess 1-year risk of major bleeding in patients with atrial fibrillation: the Euro Heart Survey. *Chest.* 138 (5): 1093–100. Copyright © 2010 The American College of Chest Physicians. Published by Elsevier Inc. All rights reserved. https://doi.org/10.1378/chest.10-0134.

do not present with haemodynamic compromise, but may experience shortness of breath, palpitations, dizziness, or angina. Due to blood stasis in the atria, there is a risk of thromboembolic events in AF so the management focuses around rate and rhythm control in combination with anticoagulation. Hypertension is the most common cause of AF, closely followed by ischaemic heart disease, while 30% of patients with heart failure or valve disease have AF. Should AF present acutely, it may have been triggered, or become exacerbated by acute MI, sepsis, or hyperthyroidism.

In acute presentation with life-threatening haemodynamic compromise, DC cardioversion should be performed immediately. If patient presents with onset of AF at more than 48 hours or an unknown period, and there is no haemodynamic compromise, attempts should be made to restore rate control by means of a β-blocker (other than **sotalol**), or a rate-limiting calcium channel blocker (e.g. **verapamil**). **Digoxin** may be an option in non-paroxysmal AF in patients with a sedentary lifestyle. Some patients may require dual therapy in order to achieve rate control. For those where the arrhythmia is less than 48 hours old, rhythm control/cardioversion with **flecainide** or **amiodarone** can be attempted, in the absence of structural abnormality or ischaemic heart disease. Subsequent rate control (as mentioned previously) should then be attempted if pharmacological cardioversion failed, ideally with a β-blocker (other than sotalol). Amiodarone should not be offered for long-term rate control, unless there is evidence of left ventricular impairment or heart failure. In paroxysmal AF, the 'pill-in-the-pocket' strategy may be considered using a β-blocker.

All patients must also be anticoagulated on the basis of CHA$_2$DS$_2$-VASc scoring (Table 2.19) balanced against individual bleeding risks, as assessed by HAS-BLED. Initial anticoagulation management can be with a low molecular weight heparin (**LMWH**). In the longer term, prevention of stroke and systemic embolism can be addressed by offering patients with a CHA2DS2-VASc score of 2 or more anticoagulation with **apixaban**, **dabigatran**, **rivaroxaban**, or **warfarin** (see Topic 2.8, 'Venous thromboembolism').

Table 2.19 CHA$_2$DS$_2$-VASc scoring

CHA$_2$DS$_2$-VASc scoring	Score
Congestive heart failure (inc. left ventricular dysfunction	1
Hypertension	1
Aged 75 years or older	2
Diabetes	1
Stroke/ TIA/thromboembolism	2
Vascular disease (previous MI, peripheral artery disease, aortic plaque)	1
Aged 65–74 years	1
Sex category: female	1

Reprinted from Lip, G.Y. et al. Refining clinical risk stratification for predicting stroke and thromboembolism in atrial fibrillation using a novel risk factor-based approach: the euro heart survey on atrial fibrillation. *Chest.* 137 (2): 263–72. Copyright © 2010 The American College of Chest Physicians. Published by Elsevier Inc. All rights reserved. https://doi.org/10.1378/chest.09-1584

Drug classes used in management

Anti-arrhythmic drugs have traditionally been classified into groups presumed to have common mechanisms of action on arrhythmias. In the last couple of decades, however, the classification most commonly used to categorize AD has been that created by Singh and Vaughan Williams in the 1970s. The most important aspect of this system is that it classifies anti-arrhythmic actions, not drugs. This is important because most drugs have multiple actions, and the pharmacology of each agent is more complex than a simple rigid classification. Moreover, many of the active metabolites of pharmacologically active drugs have actions that belong to a class other than that of the parent compound. Nonetheless, there has been a tendency to attempt to allocate individual drugs to each of these specific classes.

According to the Vaughan Williams classification, AD are divided into four main classes:

I. Na$^+$ channel blockers;

II. anti-sympathetic agents;

III. drugs that prolong the duration of action potentials;

IV. Ca^{2+} antagonists (see Table 2.20).

Class I drugs

Drugs with class I action are local anaesthetic-type agents that depress the fast inward depolarizing Na$^+$ current, and thus slow the rate of the rise of the action potential (phase 0). They are often called membrane stabilizers and reduce the excitability of the myocardial cells. They rapidly penetrate the lipid bilayer of the cell membrane, and bind to hydrophobic amino acids in the Na$^+$ channel.

Class I drugs are subdivided in accordance to their effects on the duration of the action potential i.e. *Ia* prolong, *Ib* shorten, and *Ic* have minimal effect on the action potential.

Class Ia

Class Ia anti-arrhythmic drugs have Na$^+$ channel blocking and action potential prolonging actions. Examples include disopyramide, procainamide, and quinidine.

Mechanism of action

The Ia ADs not only produce moderate Na$^+$ channel blockade that slows impulse conduction, but also block some K$^+$ channels, prolonging repolarization and the refractory period of isolated cardiac tissue. In clinical use, they may cause measurable increases in the QRS duration and the QT interval.

Disopyramide, as with all class Ia drugs, interferes directly with cardiac membrane depolarization and serves as a membrane-stabilizing agent; it is rarely used clinically, except in AF in hypertrophic cardiomyopathy. It also possesses some anti-cholinergic and local anaesthetic properties.

Procainamide, another Na$^+$ channel blocker, is hepatically metabolized to an active metabolite N-acetylprocainamide, which exhibits pure class III anti-arrhythmic activity. The rate of metabolism is genetically determined, limiting the value of measuring plasma levels. It is associated with a high incidence of adverse effects (GI disturbances, negative inotropic effects, and pro-arrhythmic effects) and, as a result, has been withdrawn from the market in most countries.

Quinidine, an optical isomer of **quinine**, was among the first drugs observed to have anti-arrhythmic properties. In addition to its action as Na$^+$ and K$^+$ channel blocker, quinidine also blocks muscarinic and α-adrenergic transmission. However, like procainamide, it has been largely withdrawn from the market worldwide.

Prescribing

Disopyramide is licensed for oral or IV administration in the treatment of a wide range of arrhythmias; however, it is

Table 2.20 Summary of anti-arrhythmic drugs.

Class	Site of action	Effect on action potential	Examples	Clinical use
Ia	Na+ channel blocker (intermediate association/dissociation)	Prolongs action potential	Disopyramide, procainamide, quinidine	Ventricular arrhythmias, prevention of recurrent atrial fibrillation
Ib	Na+ channel blocker (fast association/dissociation)	Shortens action potential	Lidocaine, mexiletine,	Ventricular tachycardia, atrial fibrillation. Use limited due to risk of asystole
Ic	Na+ channel blocker (slow association/dissociation)	No significant effect on action potential	encainide, flecainide, moricizine, propafenone	Paroxysmal atrial fibrillation, resistant tachyarrhythmias
II	β-blockers	Depress phase 4 rate of rise	Atenolol, bisoprolol, esmolol, metoprolol, propranolol, timolol	Prevent recurrence of tachyarrhythmias
III	K+ channel blockers	Prolong repolarization, increase action potential duration	Amiodarone*, bretylium, dofetilide, dronedarone, ibutilide, sotalol	Ventricular tachycardia, (atrial flutter, atrial fibrillation. Sotalol used in WPW syndrome
IV	Slow Ca2+ channel blockers	Depress phase 2 and 3	Diltiazem, verapamil	Prevent recurrence of paroxysmal supraventricular tachycardia, ventricular rate control in atrial fibrillation
V	N/A	N/A	Adenosine, digoxin, magnesium	Supraventricular arrhythmias. Magnesium also use in Torsades de Pointes

*Amiodarone also has class I, II and III activity.
Adapted with permission from Harrison, D.C. Current Classification of Antiarrhythmic Drugs as a Guide to Their Rational Clinical Use Drugs (1986) 31: 93. Copyright © 1986, ADIS Press Limited/Copyright © 1986, Springer Nature. https://doi.org/10.2165/00003495-198631020-00001.

rarely used clinically. Following IV administration, it has a rapid onset of action of 2–4 minutes (15 minutes following an MI) and should, therefore, be administered slowly over 5 minutes to reduce the risk of toxicity. Conversion should have occurred within 15 minutes if it is going to be effective.

Unwanted effects

Toxicity to **disopyramide** results mainly from its cardiovascular effects, i.e. strong negative inotropic effects and ability to prolong the QT interval; thereby, aggravating heart failure and inducing arrhythmias. It should,

therefore, not be used in second or third degree heart block, cardiogenic shock, or severe decompensated heart failure. In patients taking concomitant medication known to exert similar toxicities, the risk is increased, particularly with Torsades de Pointes.

Other non-cardiac side effects are attributable to its anti-muscarinic effects including dry mouth, blurred vision, confusion, and urinary retention.

About 25% of the drug is metabolized and the remainder excreted unchanged in the urine; dose reductions are therefore recommended in both renal and hepatic impairment.

Drug interactions

Drug interactions with **disopyramide** of clinical significance are frequent in combination with other drugs that
possess similar pharmacological effects. Drugs known to
prolong the QT interval increasing the risk of ventricular
arrhythmias, such as anti-psychotics, non-sedating
antihistamines, azoles; or those that possess negative
inotropic effects such as β-blockers and **verapamil**. Antimuscarinic side effects are augmented in combination
with other anti-muscarinics.

> ### PRACTICAL PRESCRIBING
> Disopyramide is an infrequently used anti-arrhythmic,
> generally reserved for patients where other treatment
> options have failed.

Class Ib

> Class Ib drugs have weak Na$^+$ channel blocking effects,
> but do not prolong the action potential; e.g. lidocaine,
> mexiletine.

Mechanism of action

Drugs with class Ib action are only moderately potent Na$^+$
channel blockers that slow impulse conduction, but only
in abnormal tissue (i.e. ischaemic myocardium), having
no effect in healthy tissue. Unlike class Ia agents, they do
not block K$^+$ channels and as a result have no effect on
repolarization, which normally shortens the duration of
action potentials. They therefore exert little effect on the
PR, QRS, or QT intervals.

Lidocaine has been used for many years as a highly
effective anti-arrhythmic drug, but it has poor systemic
bioavailability when taken orally. It undergoes extensive
first-pass metabolism to a potentially toxic metabolite
making oral administration impracticable and is further
metabolized by the liver, to compounds with little anti-
arrhythmic activity.

Mexiletine is a lidocaine analogue that is orally active and well absorbed from the GI tract. It is extensively
metabolized in the liver and has a half-life of 8–20 hours
(compared with 2 hours for lidocaine).

Prescribing

The class Ib anti-arrhythmics are generally reserved for
the management of life-threatening ventricular arrhythmias, particularly following a MI. Due to its poor oral

availability and short duration of action, **lidocaine** is
administered by continuous IV infusion, or in an emergency, as repeated injections. During the infusion ECG
monitoring is required and resuscitation facilities should
be available.

Mexiletine is only available in the UK as an import,
limiting its value. However, as an oral therapy it may
be useful in patients with an implantable cardioverter
defibrillator that remain in VT if they respond to
lidocaine.

Unwanted effects

Systemic toxicity with **lidocaine** is dose related and primarily affects the cardiovascular or nervous system. It
should not be used in patients with sino-atrial disorders
or AV block, due to its depressant effects, i.e. bradycardia,
hypotension, and myocardial depression. CNS toxicity
tends to also be depressant (drowsiness, confusion and
coma). Although excitatory reactions may also occur,
these tend not to be sustained.

As an analogue of lidocaine, **mexiletine** possesses
the same toxicities; however, being orally administered
there is a higher incidence of GI effects such as nausea,
vomiting, and dyspepsia.

Class Ic

> Class Ic compounds are very powerful blockers of the
> Na$^+$ channel and markedly reduce conduction velocity
> within the myocardium. Examples include flecainide
> and propafenone.

Mechanism of action

Class Ic anti-arrhythmics are potent Na$^+$ channel blockers
that slow conduction velocity. They are weak inhibitors of
the K$^+$ channels and as a result have minimal effect on
repolarization. They can also block inward Ca^{2+} channels,
and increase the PR and QRS intervals. The QT interval
is prolonged as well, but only to the extent that QRS prolongation is seen.

Flecainide and **propafenone**, the main agents in the
class, are very effective at eliminating ventricular ectopic activity, but also depress cardiac conduction and
contractility.

In addition to its class Ic action, propafenone has weak
β-adrenergic-blocking activity. It is almost completely
absorbed orally and undergoes hepatic metabolism,
producing two active metabolites with comparable anti-
arrhythmic activity.

Prescribing

In the absence of structural abnormalities or ischaemia, where pharmacological therapy is indicated, class Ic anti-arrhythmics may be used in the management of ventricular and supraventricular arrhythmias. Due to their good oral bioavailability, they can be used for long-term management (**flecainide** may also be administered IV). Treatment should be initiated cautiously, with doses gradually increased every 3–5 days, to establish the lowest effective dose. An ECG should be carried out within a few days of starting to assess efficacy.

Once patients have been stabilized on a dose of flecainide, they may be switched to a long-acting preparation, which has the advantage of OD dosing. In comparison, **propafenone** is administered 3 times a day, making it a less favourable option.

Unwanted effects

Flecainide and **propafenone** display negative inotropic effects and are therefore contraindicated in any patient demonstrating a cardiac abnormality, e.g. heart failure, conduction disorders, heart failure, or ischaemic heart disease. Use should also be avoided within 3 months of an MI. As propafenone has weak β-blocking effects, it should be used in caution in patients with asthma.

Unsurprisingly, the toxicities most commonly associated with the use of flecainide and propafenone are cardiac, in particular conduction disorders and palpitations. Other non-cardiac effects may include dizziness and headaches, as well as GI effects. In general, however, they are reasonably well tolerated and, as such, used as second line in paroxysmal atrial fibrillation (PAF).

Drug interactions

Interactions of clinical significance with **propafenone** and **flecainide** are also common. As relatively toxic drugs, augmentation of toxicity is likely when taken in combination with other drugs possessing similar properties, i.e. negative inotropes (β-blockers, CCBs) and pro-arrhythmics (antihistamines, antipsychotics).

The risk of interactions with propafenone is made greater by the fact that it is a substrate for various CYP 450 enzymes, including 2D6 and 3A4, which are commonly inhibited or induced by other drugs.

Class II: β-blockers

Arrhythmias are more frequently observed in the setting of enhanced sympathetic tone, resulting in both an increase in automaticity and a reduction in the refractory periods, which may enhance potential re-entrant circuits. As a result, it is not surprising that β-adrenergic blockers are used in the treatment of cardiac arrhythmias.

β-blockers

The ability to block β-adrenoceptors and prevent the action of catecholamines in the heart is what distinguish class II anti-arrhythmic agents. Examples include acebutolol, atenolol, esmolol, metoprolol, nadolol, oxprenolol, and propranolol.

Mechanism of action

Activation of β_1-adrenoceptors by catecholamines leads to increased heart rate and BP. In cardiac arrhythmias, β-blockers antagonize the effect of the sympathetic neurotransmitters by competing for receptor binding sites. They reduce the rate of spontaneous depolarization of SA and AV nodal tissue and reduce conduction through the AV node.

Acebutolol is a cardioselective $\beta_1$adrenoceptor antagonist with stabilizing and **quinidine**-like effects on cardiac rhythm, as well as weak inherent sympathomimetic action. It has less antagonistic effects on the peripheral vascular β_2-receptors than non-selective β-blockers. **Atenolol**, like other selective β_1-adrenoceptor antagonists, competitively blocks β_2-adrenergic-mediated responses in the bronchial and vascular smooth muscles at higher doses.

Prescribing

As the anti-arrhythmic properties of β-blockers are associated with β_1 activity, all drugs have the potential to be effective in arrhythmias; however, the β_1 selective drugs are preferred for this indication. As in hypertension, doses are started low and titrated up to achieve the minimum effective dose, although in general, doses required to maintain sinus rhythm tend to be higher.

Choice of drug will depend on the type of arrhythmia; **esmolol,** for example, is a very short-acting cardioselective β-blocker, which is indicated for short-term treatment of supraventricular arrhythmias and for tachycardia postoperatively. It can only be administered IV and is rapidly eliminated on discontinuation of infusion.

As most β-blockers are licensed in AF, the choice here tends to be determined by ease of administration, e.g. OD **atenolol**, and cost. **Sotalol**, although a β-blocker is considered as a class III agent and is *not* recommended for rate control in AF, however, may have a role in rhythm control. It is no longer available in the UK as an IV formulation.

Unwanted effects

See Topic 2.1, 'Hypertension'.

Class III

Class III drugs block K^+ channels involved in repolarization, lengthening the duration of the action potential and increasing the refractory period. Examples include amiodarone, dronedarone, and sotalol

The prolongation of the cardiac action potential and, hence, the refractory period, has a role as an anti-arrhythmic mechanism, in particular in the setting of a re-entrant arrhythmia. This effect can be achieved by blocking outward repolarizing potassium currents, and is what defines the class III anti-arrhythmic action.

Mechanism of action

The only agents in widespread clinical use as class III agents are **amiodarone**, **dronedarone**, and **sotalol**. Amiodarone is a drug with a complex pharmacological profile that is used in the treatment of a wide range of cardiac tachyarrhythmias, including ventricular and atrial arrhythmias. In addition to its ability to prolong the duration of the cardiac action potential, it is also a smooth muscle relaxant that can act on Na^+ channels (as class Ib drugs), block β-adrenoceptors (class II drugs), and Ca^{2+} channels (class IV). Its clinical use is complicated by very unusual pharmacokinetics. Incompletely absorbed orally, it undergoes significant uptake into adipose tissue and is extensively metabolized in the liver. Its major metabolite, desethylamiodarone also has anti-arrhythmic properties, and both have extremely long half-lives (50–60 days).

Dronedarone is a structural analogue of amiodarone, but it lacks the iodine content attributed to the significant toxicity seen with amiodarone. Although predominantly a class III agent due to its action on potassium channels, like amiodarone it also inhibits sodium channels (class Ib), calcium channels (class IV), and β activity (class II).

Sotalol is a non-cardioselective β-blocking agent with marked class III activity. Although it is primary active on β-adrenoceptors in the heart, it can also inhibit the inward K^+ current, which is particularly involved in phase 2 and 3 repolarization. It is most effective at slow rates of cell depolarization (bradycardia), as it has higher receptor binding when the channel is closed.

Prescribing

Despite its poor tolerability and being licensed for use when other drugs have failed, **amiodarone** is still widely used in the UK for the management of AF due to its excellent efficacy. It is administered orally and, due to its long half-life, requires loading, i.e. it is given TDS for a week, then BD for a week before being continued OD. This loading allows for better tissue uptake. **Dronedarone** similarly shows good efficacy in maintaining sinus rhythm in patients with atrial fibrillation or atrial flutter, and is likely to be better tolerated, particularly long term, due to the absence of iodine in its structure. However, unlike amiodarone, it is contraindicated in heart failure, which has limited its use an alternative to amiodarone.

Sotalol tends to be better tolerated and can be administered orally OD without the need for loading.

Unwanted effects

Unwanted effects with **amiodarone** are common and extensive, affecting all organ systems in the body and although reversible, this may take some time to resolve due to its prolonged half-life. It distributes widely throughout the body, accumulating in fat, skeletal muscle, and well-perfused organs, such as the liver, lung, and spleen, leading to tissue fibrosis. Pulmonary fibrosis, for example, is relatively common and can be fatal. Liver function tests (LFTs) should be monitored while undergoing treatment as transaminases commonly increase shortly after initiation.

Thyroid function tests (TFTs) should also be carried out routinely as amiodarone inhibits the peripheral conversion of T4 to T3, leading to hypo- or hyperthyroidism. Furthermore, it has a high iodine content, which inhibits the production and release of T4 and T3. Within the eye, prolonged use can lead to the accumulation of micro-deposits, usually around the pupil, resulting in coloured halos or blurred vision. Prolonged use may also lead to deposits within the skin, causing hyperpigmentation. Hypersensitivity to the sun is also common and patients should be advised to avoid exposure. In addition, treatment with amiodarone is associated with the same cardiac effects (e.g. bradycardia and arrhythmias), as well as central and GI effects.

In general, **dronedarone** is better tolerated, although it has been linked to an increased risk of mortality in patients with heart failure, and it is therefore contraindicated in heart failure and left ventricular systolic dysfunction. It is also contraindicated in heart block or bradycardia. Aside from this, side effects tend to be GI in nature—in particular, diarrhoea.

Amiodarone toxicity

- Amiodarone therapy is associated with high levels of toxicity and should only be considered for use when other options have failed.
- While undergoing treatment, patients should be monitored for changes in thyroid, liver, and lung function.
- Patients should be counselled on the risks of treatment, advised to avoid exposure to sun, and report any signs of toxicity, such as altered vision.
- Where treatment is discontinued, side effects may persist for up to a month or more due to its long half-life.

Drug interactions

Both **amiodarone** and **dronedarone** are moderate inhibitors of CYP 3A4. As a result, they have the potential to increase the risk of toxicity of drugs such as **simvastatin** and, to a lesser extent, **atorvastatin**. Dronedarone is also a substrate for CYP 3A4 so may be affected by potent inhibitors and inducers of the CYP 3A4 enzyme, e.g. macrolides, **rifampicin,** respectively.

Class IV: Ca²⁺ channel antagonists

Class IV drugs selectively block the L-type Ca^{2+} channel, stabilizing phase 4 of the action potential and slowing the rate of spontaneous depolarization. For example, verapamil and diltiazem.

In the areas of the heart around the sino-atrial and atrioventricular nodes, conduction depends not on the fast inward Na^+ current, but on a slow inward Ca^{2+} current. This current is present throughout the myocardium (acting on its contraction), but has no role in conduction elsewhere. As a result, drugs capable of blocking these channels could prevent re-entrant arrhythmias dependent on this Ca^{2+} current.

Mechanism of action

Class IV drugs stabilize phase 4 of the action potential, particularly in the AV node, without significantly affecting the depolarization rates in the SA node, since this is largely dependent on T-type Ca^{2+} channels and the funny current. Given the specificity of its pharmacological action, they are only effective in the treatment of supraventricular arrhythmias.

Verapamil is the prototype for this class of drug, and acts by blocking the slow conducting (AV-nodal) limb of the re-entrant circuit. **Diltiazem** is also used for its rate controlling properties. The dihydropyridine Ca^{2+} antagonists (e.g. **nifedipine**) have no useful anti-arrhythmic properties.

Prescribing

Verapamil is available for oral and intravenous administration in the management of supraventricular arrhythmias; the latter should be used in acute disease administered over 2–3 minutes. Oral treatment can be used for either treatment or prophylaxis, and once stabilized on a dose, patients can be converted to a long-acting preparation to avoid dosing TDS.

Diltiazem, although advocated for use by numerous professional bodies, including NICE, for use in managing supraventricular arrhythmias, is not licensed for this indication.

Unwanted effects

For more information see Topic 2.1, 'Hypertension'.

Class IV in Wolff–Parkinson–White syndrome

In patients with atrial fibrillation or flutter associated with an accessory pathway (e.g. Wolff–Parkinson–White), the use of verapamil can promote conduction across this pathway, increasing the risk of ventricular fibrillation and should not, therefore, be used.

Cardiac glycosides

Digoxin reversibly inhibits Na^+/K^+ ATPase, increasing intracellular Ca^{2+} in myocardial tissue.

Mechanism of action

Digitalis glycosides (such as **digoxin**) increase the force and velocity of myocardial systolic contraction (positive inotropy), and decrease conduction velocity through the AV node, prolonging its refractory period. Although not an anti-arrhythmic drug in the strict sense of the term, they are used in the control of ventricular rate in atrial flutter and atrial fibrillation.

For more information on digoxin see Heart Failure Topic 2.6, 'Heart failure'.

Adenosine

Activation of the A1 G-coupled adenosine receptors activates inward rectifier K⁺ channel and enhances the flow of potassium out of myocardial cells, producing hyperpolarization of the cell membrane.

Mechanism of action

Adenosine belongs to the molecular group of nucleosides, composed of an adenine-group attached to a ribose sugar. In the heart, adenosine receptors are located in coronary arteries, SA node, atrial cells, AV node, and ventricular myocytes. Adenosine binds to receptors in the endothelium and smooth muscle cells of coronary arteries, causing vasodilation. In the SA node, adenosine produces a negative chronotropic effect and in very high doses can cause progressive sinus bradycardia and sinus arrest. As the SA nodal cells hyperpolarize in response to adenosine, their level of excitability is decreased. In addition, adenosine also antagonizes the stimulatory effects of the β-adrenergic component on Ca^{2+} currents. Although it slows impulse conduction through the AV node, it has no effect on conduction in the ventricles. The only effect adenosine has on the ventricle is indirect, as it acts to depress contractility when cyclic AMP levels are elevated. As most of the supraventricular tachycardias with a ventricular rate greater than 150 involve re-entry in the AV node, adenosine is well suited for treatment of this arrhythmia.

Prescribing

Adenosine is administered as a rapid IV bolus in the management of paroxysmal supraventricular tachycardias, with a short half-life and rapid onset of action, of about 10 seconds. Where ineffective, escalating doses can be administered at 1–2-minute intervals until sinus rhythm is achieved. Manufacturers recommend that treatment be given in a hospital setting with monitoring and resuscitation facilities available, due to the risk of significant cardiovascular toxicity, although due to its rapid elimination, cumulative effects are unlikely. BP should be monitored in the arm opposite to the adenosine infusion.

PRACTICAL PRESCRIBING

Adenosine and ATP are both effective in the management of supraventricular arrhythmias, although the phosphate salt is not available as a medicine.

Unwanted effects

Adenosine receptors are located throughout the body, particularly within the heart and brain. As adenosine acts non-selectively on these receptors, toxicity is therefore common and diverse. With its short half-life, effects tend to be short-lived and where intolerable, will resolve on cessation of treatment.

Stimulation of adenosine receptors within the brain, for example, causes sedation, dizziness, and more infrequently, convulsions and loss of consciousness. Meanwhile stimulation of adenosine receptors within the heart can cause heart block, arrhythmias (in particular AF) and, less commonly, bradycardia. Treatment is contraindicated in patients with pre-existing heart block or decompensated heart failure, due to the risk of deterioration in their condition. On the rare occasion where adenosine is given as an infusion, the vasodilatory effects may, in part, be overcome by slowing the rate of administration.

Respiratory effects also occur frequently with treatment such as dyspnoea and bronchospasm, and therefore should be avoided in asthmatics.

Drug interactions

Adenosine antagonists such as the xanthines (**aminophylline**, **theophylline**, **caffeine**) should be avoided for 24 hours before **adenosine** is administered, although this is less relevant in an emergency situation. Consideration should also be given to avoiding food containing xanthines within 12 hours of administration, such as coffee, tea, chocolate, and cola, particularly where patients are being admitted for planned testing within the catheter lab.

Dipyridamole can increase the effects of adenosine by up to four times as it inhibits cellular uptake and metabolism, and should therefore not be taken concurrently.

Atropine

Atropine is a competitive inhibitor of the muscarinic acetylcholine receptor, which reduces the inhibitory effect of the vagus nerve on the heart.

Mechanism of action

The blockade by **atropine** of the M_2 muscarinic acetylcholine receptors increases the firing rate of the SA node and conduction through the AV node.

Acetylcholine is the main neurotransmitter used by the parasympathetic nervous system, with ACh binding to muscarinic receptors found principally in the SA and AV nodes of the heart. This leads to the decrease in cAMP and activation of K-ACh channels, increasing K^+ efflux and hyperpolarizing the cells. By blocking muscarinic receptors in the heart, atropine inhibits the activation of inward rectifying K-ACh channels and prevents the hyperpolarization of the cell membrane. In doing so, it increases the firing rate of the SA node and conduction through the AV node.

Prescribing

Atropine is indicated for the acute management of bradyarrhythmias, administered either IV or by intramuscular injection. In the case of cardiac resuscitation, doses can be administered as small doses every 5 minutes until adequate sinus rhythm is achieved or, in the case of asystole, as a single large dose.

Unwanted effects

As an anti-muscarinic, predictable toxicity seen with **atropine** therapy includes dry mouth, blurred vision, glaucoma, drowsiness, constipation, and urinary retention. These effects are dose related and reverse on cessation of treatment.

Contraindications and drug interactions with atropine become irrelevant in the case of life-threatening emergencies, where the benefits of treating are likely to outweigh the risks.

PRACTICAL PRESCRIBING

Atropine administration

During resuscitation in patients with no IV access, doses of atropine can be administered via an endotracheal tube at 2–3 times the dose.

Magnesium sulfate

Magnesium sulfate has a negative chronotropic effect on cardiac and intra-atrial conduction.

Mechanism of action

Magnesium is the second most abundant cation in extracellular fluid, being important for the activity of many enzymes, neurochemical transmission and muscular excitability. It has the capacity to reduce striatal muscle contractions and block peripheral neuromuscular

transmission by diminishing the release of ACh at the neuromuscular junction. The multiple roles of magnesium in cardiac muscle has confounded interpretation of available data on hypo-magnesaemia as a cause or precipitant of arrhythmia.

Magnesium inhibits Ca^{2+} influx via voltage-operated Ca^{2+} channels, of the dihydropyridine sensitive type. Accordingly, in the treatment of arrhythmias the properties of magnesium sulfate resemble those of CCBs, significantly prolonging conduction time and refractory period at the AV nodal level, without significantly affecting sinus cycle length or infranodal conduction. The inhibition of the sinus node by magnesium is probably offset by inhibition of acetylcholine release at the vagal nerve terminals.

Prescribing

Magnesium sulfate is used in the treatment of Torsades de Pointes and VT, even where serum magnesium is within normal limits. In particular, it can be used to treat arrhythmias induced by drugs known to prolong the QT interval or with **digoxin** toxicity. Treatment is administered initially as a bolus over 1–2 minutes, followed by an IV infusion.

Unwanted effects

Predictably, the most likely side effect of treatment with magnesium sulphate is hypermagnesaemia. This can present as nausea, vomiting, diarrhoea, thirst, confusion, slurred speech, muscle weakness, and respiratory depression. While on treatment, patients should have serum electrolytes monitored, especially those with renal impairment where the risk of hypermagnesaemia is increased. It is contraindicated in severe renal impairment and in heart block.

PRESCRIBING WARNING

Magnesium sulfate in ventricular tachycardias

Although widely used in the management of ventricular tachycardias, magnesium sulfate remains unlicensed for this indication.

Further reading

Edhouse J, Morris F (2002) ABC of clinical electrocardiography: broad complex tachycardia—Part II. *British Medical Journal* 30(324), 776–9.

Edhouse J, Morris F (2002) Broad complex tachycardia—Part I. *British Medical Journal* 23(324), 719–22.

Haegeli LM, Calkins H (2014) Catheter ablation of atrial fibrillation: an update. *European Heart Journal* 35(36), 2454–9.

Hall MC, Todd DM (2006) Modern management of arrhythmias. *Postgraduate Medical Journal*, 82, 117–25.

Lilly LS (Ed.) (2003) *Pathophysiology of Heart Disease*, 3rd edn. Philadelphia, PA: Lippincott, Williams and Wilkins.

Lip GY, Boos CJ (2006) Antithrombotic treatment in atrial fibrillation. *Heart*, 92, 155–61.

Patel C, Yan GX, Kowey PR, et al. (2009) New drugs and technologies: dronedarone. *Circulation* 1(20), 636–44.

Roden DM (2000) Antiarrhythmic drugs: from mechanisms to clinical practice. *Heart*, 84, 339–46.

Guidelines

ACC/AHA/HRS (2015) ACC/AHA/HRS Guideline for the management of adult patients with supraventricular tachycardia: a report of the American College of Cardiology/American Heart Association Task Force on Clinical Practice Guideline and the Heart Rhythm Society. *Circulation* 132, e506–74. https://circ.ahajournals.org/content/early/2015/09/22/CIR.0000000000000311.full.pdf+html [accessed 21 March 2019].

EHRA/HRS/APHRS (2014) Expert Consensus on Ventricular Arrhythmias. http://www.hrsonline.org/Practice-Guidance/Clinical-Guidelines-Documents/2014-Expert-Consensus-on-Ventricular-Arrhythmias#axzz3eqwmpVXB [accessed 21 March 2019].

NICE (2014) Atrial fibrillation: the management of atrial fibrillation. NICE guidelines [CG180]Published date: June 2014. https://www.nice.org.uk/guidance/cg180 [accessed 21 March 2019].

Resuscitation Council UK Guideline (2010) Adult Advanced Life Support. http://www.resus.org.uk/pages/als.pdf [accessed 21 March 2019].

2.8 Venous thromboembolism

Venous thromboembolism (VTE) encompasses both deep vein thrombosis (DVT) and pulmonary embolism (PE). A thrombus may arise spontaneously, or be predisposed from changes involving increased blood coagulopathy, patient immobility, or blood vessel abnormalities from known risk factors (see 'Pathophysiology'); around 70% of patients with DVT have identifiable risk factors.

Collectively, VTE has an incidence of approximately 1:1000, with many of these patients being asymptomatic. It accounts for 25 000 avoidable hospital deaths in the UK alone. The clinical probability of VTE may be assessed using scoring tools like those of Wells' (see NICE CG144 in 'Guidelines') to guide further investigation.

Pathophysiology

The role of platelets in early haemostasis is dealt with in acute coronary syndrome (Topic 2.5, 'Acute coronary syndrome'). Here, emphasis is on the mechanisms involved in the blood coagulation cascade, which are responsible for thrombus formation. This cascade is activated later than platelet aggregation and is composed of two main pathways (see Figure 2.20):

- *The extrinsic pathway:* following tissue damage, normally circulating factor VII (FVII) binds to tissue factor (TF), which is expressed on fibroblasts and leukocytes. The resultant complex, TF–FVII, activates factors IX and X. The latter is activated to Xa, which with its co-factor FVa, forms the prothrombin complex that converts prothrombin to thrombin (in the *final common pathway*; see end of list). Thrombin itself can activate other procoagulant factors, such as V and VIII; releasing the latter from von Willebrand's factor (vWF). Activated

factor VIII is a co-factor for IX and collectively they activate factor X, potentiating thrombin formation.

- *The intrinsic pathway:* has less of an overall 'clotting effect'. It is a contact-activated pathway that is initiated when subendothelial collagen comes into contact with blood-borne factors like prekallikrein and factor XII (Hageman factor). The former is converted to kallikrein, while factor XII becomes activated (factor XIIa). In true cascade fashion, XIIa activates XI, XIa activates IX, and IXa with factor VIIIa as a co-factor, activates X. In common with the extrinsic pathway, Xa with co-factor Va drives thrombin formation.

The latter stage in both pathways is the early phase of the '*final common pathway*'. Here, thrombin converts fibrinogen to insoluble fibrin strands; these are cross-linked by factor XIII to form a clot. Thrombin also activates factors V and VIII, and their inhibitory (anticoagulant) modulator protein C.

Ca^{2+} and platelet phospholipids are required cofactors in the formation of activated factor X and prothrombin complex. The former is required at a number of other stages in coagulation.

Vitamin K is a key pro-coagulant co-factor for γ-glutamyl carboxylase, which carboxylates the glutamic acid residues of factors II, VII, IX, X, protein S, and protein C. The enzyme vitamin K epoxide reductase, reduces vitamin K to its active form, and can be inhibited by **warfarin** and other coumarins thus causing anticoagulant effects. The *extrinsic and common pathways* are affected by regulation of vitamin K levels and are clinically measured by assessment of prothrombin time (PT). PT measures factors I, II, V, VII, and X, and for most people is around 10–14 seconds when extracted or recombinant tissue factor is added to a patient test tube. Variations in source, batch,

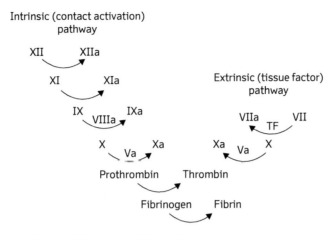

Figure 2.20 Overview of extrinsic and intrinsic coagulation pathway.
Reproduced with permission from Murphy, JG, & Lloyd, MA, *Mayo Clinic Cardiology: Concise Textbook*. Figure 48.3, page 447. Oxford, UK: Oxford University Press ©2012. Reproduced with permission of the Licensor through PLSclear.

and equipment used to calculate PT, means a standardized assay is required to accurately establish clotting. For this reason, the international normalized ratio (INR) is used.

For any tissue factor product, an international sensitivity index is established and the INR may be calculated as:

$$INR = \left(PT_{test} / PT_{control}\right)^{ISI}$$

A number of mechanisms regulate the clotting pathway by having anticoagulant actions. Protein C, which is vitamin K–dependent, and thrombin bind to cellular thrombomodulin, which acting with protein S and phospholipid degrades factors Va and VIIIa. This, in turn, holds back pro-thrombotic action. Dysfunction of protein C/S or insensitivity to them, as with factor V (Leiden), can have profound prothrombotic tendencies and increase the risk of DVT/PE. Factor VIII, on the other hand, is a cofactor for factor X, so its absence, as in haemophilia A, leads to a bleeding tendency.

Another key regulation in anticoagulant action is through antithrombin III (ATIII). Present in serum, this serine protease inhibitor inactivates thrombin, factors IXa, Xa, XIa, XIIa, kallikrein, and plasmin, thus having its predominant effects on the *intrinsic pathway*. Between around 1:2000–1:5000 of the normal population are thought to have antithrombin deficiency and are, therefore, predisposed to prothrombotic tendencies.

The heparins, as explained in Topic 2.5 ('Acute coronary syndrome'), are mucopolysaccarides that have widely varying molecular weights, from 3000 to 30 000 Da. Their action potentiates the activity of antithrombin,

which normally inhibits thrombin formation and factor Xa. Interestingly, certain heparins like **fondaparinux**, have a greater activity directed against factor Xa over thrombin. The LMWHs are commonly used clinically for prophylaxis and treatment, with the advantage over unfractionated heparins that they don't require continuous infusion or ongoing APTT monitoring.

Although VTE has the potential to affect anyone at any time, it most commonly occurs in at risk groups (e.g. heart failure, malignancy) in the presence of additional risk factors (e.g. immobility; see Table 2.21). A venous thrombosis is typically asymptomatic, but may lead to unilateral pain and calf swelling. Thrombi may break free and travel to the lung causing a PE, presenting as dyspnoea, chest pain ± haemoptysis. In PE, clinical clues may be seen on ECG (sinus tachycardia or S1Q3T3) or CXR, but diagnosis usually requires imaging, e.g. with computed tomography pulmonary angiogram (CTPA). In the case of DVT, diagnosis is usually obtained by ultrasound. Certain at-risk groups (e.g. protein C/S deficiency, factor V Leiden deficiency) require careful anticoagulation planning should they need hospitalization or a procedure, as these are associated with a high risk of morbidity and mortality.

For a full summary of the relevant pathways and drug targets, see Figure 2.21.

Management

The management of VTE focuses largely on prevention, as routine prophylaxis has been shown to significantly

Table 2.21 Risk factors for VTE

Risk factors for venous thromboembolism	
Age	Obesity
Family history of VTE	Thrombophilia
Varicose veins	Combined oral contraceptives/hormone replacement therapy
Pregnancy	Hospitalization
Immobility	Thrombotic states (cancer, HIV, severe acute infection)
Central venous catheter	Previous VTE
Surgery (hip or knee)	Prolonged surgery duration

reduce VTE incidence, and its associated morbidity and mortality. Hospitalized patients are routinely assessed on admission and at regular intervals during their stay, based on the presence of risk factors for VTE (Table 2.21). Non-pharmacological prophylactic measures, such as avoiding dehydration, mobilization plus or minus the use of anti-embolism stockings are applied universally; however, many patients at increased risk will require pharmacological prophylaxis.

Prophylaxis

Typically, hospitalized patients requiring prophylaxis are managed on a heparin, either LMWH or unfractionated, depending on renal function, duration of treatment and, in the case of surgical patients, type of surgery being performed. Certain situations preclude pharmacological prophylaxis (Table 2.22). **Fondaparinux**, **apixaban**, **dabigatran**, and **rivaroxaban** may also be used as primary prophylaxis, although the license use of novel oral anti-coagulants (NOACs) is more restricted. **Edoxaban**, the newest NOAC onto the market has only recently been licensed for this indication.

Treatment

Warfarin remains the most commonly used drug for the treatment and secondary prevention of VTE (e.g. AF), due to its licensing, cost, reversibility, and the greatest experience with its use. In suspected PE and DVT, patients

should be commenced as soon as possible on interim treatment with **heparin** or **fondaparinux**, at least within 24 hours of clinical suspicion, until a diagnosis is confirmed. Once diagnosis is confirmed, patients may be loaded on warfarin with heparin or fondaparinux continued until a therapeutic INR is achieved (at least 5 days). Warfarin treatment should be continued for a minimum of 3 months, although in some instances longer durations may be necessary. In the case of a massive PE thrombolysis (fibrinolytics) may be considered; the basis of this is dealt with in Topic 2.5 'Acute coronary syndrome'. Patients with unprovoked VTE will require investigations to exclude any underlying malignancy or thrombophilia.

In pregnant patients or those with cancer, LMWHs remain the drugs of choice over warfarin throughout treatment, except in severe renal impairment where unfractionated heparin is used. Oncology patients require a minimum of 6 months treatment, at which point they are assessed for the need for further treatment. Pregnant women will require treatment throughout pregnancy and for a minimum of 6 weeks post-partum; decisions to continue treatment beyond this will be made, depending on when the VTE was diagnosed and the presence of further risk factors.

All NOACs now also hold licenses for the treatment of VTE and have been advocated by NICE as a treatment option for this indication, increasingly in preference to warfarin.

Drug classes used in management

Coumarins

Warfarin and other synthetic derivatives of 4-hydroxycoumarin decrease blood coagulation by inhibiting vitamin K epoxide reductase, preventing the formation of the active vitamin K hydroquinone from vitamin K epoxide (inactive form).

Mechanism of action

The enzyme vitamin K epoxide reductase, acts to recycle oxidized vitamin K to its reduced form, after its involvement in the carboxylation of various coagulation factors, including prothrombin and factor VII. This carboxylation of N-terminal glutamate residues in factors II, VII, IX, and X leads to structural changes that promote Ca^{2+} binding. These Ca^{2+} moieties facilitate the interaction of negatively

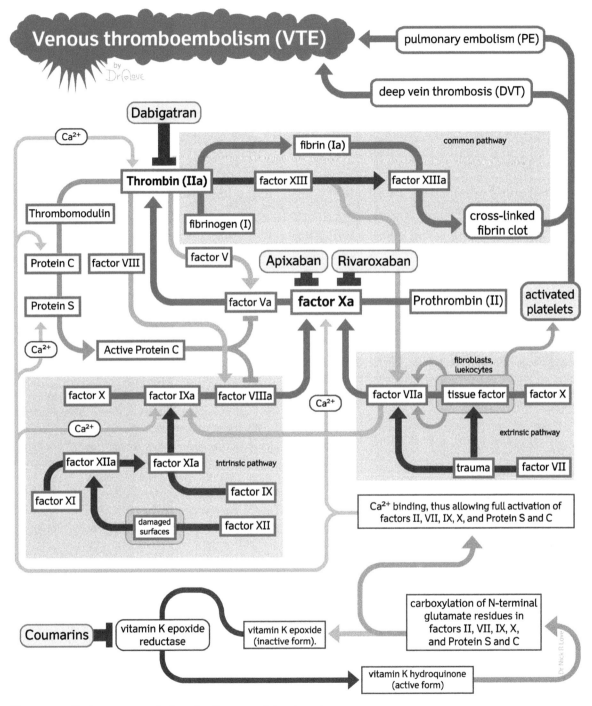

Figure 2.21 Topic: summary of relevant pathways and drug targets.

Table 2.22 Risk factors for bleeding

Risk factors for bleeding	
Active bleeding	Acute stroke
Acquired bleeding disorders (such as acute liver failure)	Thrombocytopenia (platelets less than 75 × 109/L)
Concurrent use of anticoagulants known to increase bleeding risk (e.g. warfarin with INR higher than 2)	Uncontrolled systolic hypertension (230/120 mmHg or higher)
Lumbar puncture/epidural/spinal anaesthesia expected within the next 12 hours	Untreated inherited bleeding disorders (such as haemophilia and von Willebrand's disease)
Lumbar puncture/epidural/spinal anaesthesia within the previous 4 hours	

charged phospholipids with clotting factors, for example, on platelets, thus stimulating the coagulation cascade and fibrin formation.

The protein carboxylation reaction is coupled to the oxidation of vitamin K, and the vitamin K epoxide must be reduced in order to be reactivated. Although it is sometimes defined as a vitamin K antagonist, **warfarin** only inhibits vitamin K recycling, causing a reduction in its active form. Administration of exogenous vitamin K reverses, albeit slowly, the effect of warfarin bypassing the blocked enzyme.

Prescribing

Warfarin is an orally administered drug with a long half-life, therefore requiring loading to facilitate a more rapid onset of action. In patients requiring urgent anticoagulation, i.e. VTE treatment, a heparin (usually a LMWH) is initiated concurrently and continued until a therapeutic INR is achieved.

As warfarin shows considerable inter-individual variation with regard to its effect on INR, and is easily affected by concomitant drugs, diet, and co-morbidities, patients require regular monitoring to ensure the INR remains within the desired therapeutic range. The frequency of monitoring can vary significantly between patients. Target ranges for INR vary with indication with higher levels required in the treatment of recurrent DVT or PE on anticoagulation (3.5), compared with that used as secondary prophylaxis, for example, in AF.

It is essential that newly initiated patients are adequately counselled on treatment to promote concordance with therapy, and reduce the risk and consequences of poor control (see 'Practical prescribing: warfarin counselling points').

PRACTICAL PRESCRIBING

Warfarin counselling points

- Doses should be taken daily at 18.00 hours.
- A missed dose should be taken as soon as remembered, but never doubled up.
- A regular blood test will be done to measure INR and therefore determine dose.
- The anti-coagulant clinic or GP will feedback the dose, depending on INR, this should be recorded in the yellow 'monitoring' book.
- Tablet colours are consistent between manufacturers, i.e. 0.5 mg tablets are white, 1 mg is brown, 3 mg is blue, and 5 mg is pink.
- Target range, i.e. 2–3 for prophylaxis or a primary clot, and 3–4 in recurrent VTE.
- Report any signs of excessive bleeding or bruising to GP or anti-coagulant clinic.
- Caution with interactions including alcohol, some foods with high vitamin K content, e.g. green vegetables and drugs, including non-prescribed and herbal medications.
- Advise to avoid 'binging' on things known to interact, and that they should speak to a pharmacist or doctor anytime a new medication (prescribed or otherwise) is initiated.

Unwanted effects

A raised INR resulting in excessive bleeding and bruising is the most common adverse effect reported with **warfarin** treatment, although this can, in part, be avoided by careful counselling and regular monitoring. Treatment

Table 2.23 Management of warfarin overdose

Indication	Action
Life-threatening haemorrhage	Stop warfarin. Discuss with haematologist Will probably require vitamin K and dried prothrombin complex
Non-life threatening haemorrhage	Stop warfarin, give phytomenadione IV if minor bleeding (if not bleeding give PO). Repeat at 24 hours if INR still raised. Restart warfarin when INR < 5
On long-term warfarin therapy without major haemorrhage • INR > 8 • INR 5–8 • INR < 6 and > 0.5 over target	• Stop warfarin, give phytomenadione IV if minor bleeding (if not bleeding withhold 1 or 2 doses). Restart warfarin when INR < 5 • Stop warfarin and restart when INR < 5 • Reduce dose or stop warfarin, restart when INR < 5
Not on long-term therapy without major haemorrhage	Give 10–20mg of vitamin K if INR > 4 or patient had ingested >0.25mg/kg. Monitor INR every 24–48 hours.

of overdose will depend on severity of bleed, INR, and whether or not the patient has a clinical need for warfarin treatment, see Table 2.23.

Due to the risk of bleeding, anticoagulant treatment should be withheld in high-risk patients, including those with haemorrhagic stroke, active bleeding or within 72 hours of surgery and 48 hours post-partum. Warfarin is contraindicated in pregnancy due to the risk of foetal malformations, although it may be used in breastfeeding.

On initiation warfarin has a paradoxical procoagulant action due to its inhibitory effect on protein C and protein S. It is therefore recommended that heparin be continued for at least 5 days after warfarin initiation, even if INR is within the therapeutic range. Other less common side effects include GI effects and hypersensitivity reactions, including rarely, warfarin-induced skin necrosis.

Drug interactions

Drug interactions with **warfarin** are common and complex, involving both drug therapy and many food types. These are, in part, due to the fact that warfarin is extensively metabolized through the cytochrome P450 pathway (primarily CYP1A2 and CYP3A4), although interactions are also likely with other drugs known to increase the risk of bleeding.

In particular, substances known to augment the effects of warfarin due to altered metabolism include azole antifungals, some statins (not **pravastatin**), **omeprazole**, some anti-depressants (including **St John's Wort**), quinolones, macrolide antibiotics, and cranberry juice. Concomitant use with drugs known to increase the risk of bleeding, such as antiplatelets, NSAIDs, thrombin inhibitors and other anticoagulants should be done with caution.

Conversely, items known to reduce the effects of warfarin include **carbamazepine**, **rifampicin**, and **vitamin K**; the latter present in some vitamin supplements, as well as foods including green leafy vegetables, liver, broccoli, and brussel sprouts.

Novel oral anti-coagulants/direct oral anti-coagulants

NOACs are relatively novel alternatives in anticoagulant therapy that are mainly divided into two classes, depending on the capacity to directly inhibit factor Xa or thrombin. Examples include apixaban, dabigatran, edoxaban, and rivaroxaban

Mechanism of action

Thrombin is a serine protease that functions as the final mediator in the coagulation cascade, which ultimately leads to fibrin production. In addition, thrombin is also a potent activator of platelets. The direct inhibition of thrombin offers advantages over more classical indirect inhibitors (heparins), as they can inactivate both free thrombin and also fibrin-bound thrombin, which generates thrombus expansion.

The inhibition of factor Xa is an especially attractive target for efficient anticoagulation, as factor Xa catalyses the conversion of prothrombin to thrombin, and is common to both the intrinsic and extrinsic pathway. As one molecule of factor Xa generates more than 1000 thrombin molecules, its inhibition significantly decreases the burst of thrombin and thrombin-mediated coagulation activities.

Rivaroxaban can inhibit factor Xa competitively, and has more than 10 000-fold selectivity when compared with relevant serine proteases (trypsin, thrombin, and activated protein C). It might also have the ability to inhibit clot-bound factor Xa. The maximum inhibition of factor Xa activity by rivaroxaban occurs 1–4 hours after administration, and it correlates with its plasma concentration.

Apixaban is a direct, competitive, reversible, and selective inhibitor of factor Xa that inhibits free factor Xa and prothrombinase activity, together with clot-bound factor Xa action. It has greater than 30 000-fold selectivity compared with other coagulation proteases.

Edoxaban is the most recent NOAC to come onto the market and, like apixaban, is a highly selective, reversible inhibitor of factor Xa. It has good oral bioavailability and is effective within 1–2 hours of the first dose being taken.

Dabigatran is a small-molecule direct thrombin inhibitor that needs ester cleavage to be converted to its active form. This reduces the number of drug–drug interactions and inter-individual differences, as esterases have low substrate specificity with high catalytic activity. In common with the other NOACs, because of its predictable pharmacokinetics and pharmacodynamics, dabigatran does not need routine coagulation monitoring.

Prescribing

The novel oral anti-coagulants (NOACs), **rivaroxaban**, **dabigatran**, **edoxaban,** and **apixaban**, are alternatives to **warfarin** for the treatment of VTE, and the prevention of recurrent VTE or VTE/stroke in non-valvular AF patients with a further risk factor (e.g. age ≥75 years, heart failure, hypertension, etc.). All but edoxaban are also indicated for prophylaxis following hip or knee surgery (see Table 2.24). Particular care should be taken when prescribing NOACs as doses and tablet strengths vary between indications,

and in the presence of other factors, such as impaired renal function or older age. Currently, NOACs are not indicated for use in patients with a prosthetic heart valve, with some evidence to suggest that dabigatran may be less effective than warfarin.

The main advantage of NOACs over warfarin is the superior relationship between dose and effect, thus enabling standardized dosing and negating the need for monitoring. Critics, however, express concerns about the inability to monitor their effects (INR is not a measure of activity) and only dabigatran currently has a licensed antidote in the case of overdose, **idarucizumab** (see ' Practical prescribing: switching between warfarin and NOACs').

PRACTICAL PRESCRIBING

Switching between warfarin and NOACs

- Warfarin to Rivaroxaban: Stop warfarin treatment and initiate rivaroxaban once INR ≤ 3.
- *Rivaroxaban to warfarin:* give the two concurrently until INR ≥2.5.
- *Warfarin to apixaban*: stop warfarin and start apixaban when INR <2.
- *Apixaban to warfarin:* give the two concurrently until INR >2, then stop apixaban.
- *Warfarin to dabigatran*: stop warfarin and start dabigatran once INR <2.
- *Dabigatran to warfarin:* for a CrCl ≥50 mL/min, run the two concurrently for 3 days; for INR 30–50 mL/min, run the two concurrently for 2 days.
- *Warfarin to edoxaban*: stop warfarin and start edoxaban once INR ≤2.5.
- *Edoxaban to warfarin*: give half usual edoxaban dose concurrently with warfarin until INR ≥2.

Table 2.24 Comparison of licensed indications for NOACs, note not all tablet strengths licensed for all indications

	Apixaban	Dabigatran	Edoxaban	Rivaroxaban
Treatment of DVT/PE	Yes	Yes	Yes	Yes
Prevention of recurrent DVT/PE	Yes	Yes	Yes	Yes
DVT/PE prophylaxis following elective hip or knee replacement surgery	Yes	Yes	No	Yes
Prevention of stroke and VTE in non-valvular AF with one or more risk factor	Yes	Yes	Yes	Yes

Unwanted effects

As with all anticoagulants excessive bleeding is the greatest risk associated with the NOACs, although this risk may be relatively less with **apixaban**. They are contraindicated in patients with clinically significant active bleeding or those at high risk of a major bleed, e.g. GI ulcers, arteriovenous malformations, recent neurosurgery, or intracranial haemorrhage. In patients undergoing surgery, NOACs should be discontinued prior depending on the type of surgery/bleeding risk, and reinstated post-operatively, based on bleeding risk. In patients with renal impairment the interval may need to be increased.

Until recently, there have been no antidotes available to reverse the effects of a NOAC, in part impacting on their widespread uptake as an alternative to warfarin. **Idarucizumab** is the first antidote to be made available. Effective against **dabigatran** only, it is indicated for rapid reversal in patients undergoing emergency surgery or in the case of a life-threatening or uncontrolled bleed. Doses are administered IV and dabigatran can be restarted after 24 hours. A further antidote (**andexanet alfa**) is currently under investigation, targeting the factor Xa inhibitors (apixaban, **edoxaban**, **rivaroxaban,** and **heparin**), whereas **ciraparantag** is being investigated as a possible reversal agent for all four licensed NOACs.

More generally, NOAC overdose is managed symptomatically with haemodynamic support, compression, and in severe cases, the use of agents such as prothrombin complex concentrate, under the advice of a haematologist.

Other more commonly reported side effects include GI toxicity, headaches, and confusion. Less commonly, treatment may lead to deranged LFTs; as this can increase bleeding risk by potentially impairing elimination, it is recommended LFTs are checked at baseline and monitored while on treatment.

Dose alterations and contraindications vary slightly between the NOACs based on their route of elimination (see Table 2.25). Rivaroxaban, edoxaban, and apixaban, for example, are extensively metabolized, albeit by different routes, before being partially cleared via the kidney, whereas dabigatran is predominantly cleared unchanged via the kidneys, with only small amounts metabolized in the liver. Limitations in dosing in some patient cohorts is based on lack of safety data where patients were excluded from original studies.

Drug interactions

As with **warfarin**, **rivaroxaban** is metabolized via the cytochrome P450 system and, therefore, has the potential to interact with drugs known to inhibit or induce these enzymes. Drugs known to inhibit clearance causing a significant rise in activity include the azole antifungals and protease inhibitors. Inhibition occurs to a lesser extent with **clarithromycin** and **erythromycin**, and is considered to be clinically insignificant. **Dabigatran**, although not metabolized through the cytochrome P450 enzyme system, is a substrate for the efflux transporter P-gp. Edoxaban is a substrate for both P-gp and to a lesser extent CYP3A4/5. Like dabigatran it has the potential to be affected by medication known to inhibit P-gp, such as **ciclosporin**, **amiodarone**, **dronedarone**, clarithromycin, erythromycin, **verapamil**, and **ketoconazole**, whereas **rifampicin** is an inducer.

Table 2.25 Dosing NOACs in renal and hepatic impairment

Drug	Dosing in renal impairment	Dosing in hepatic impairment
Apixaban	Contraindicated for CrCl <15mL/min In NVAF reduce dose if CrCl 15–29 mL/min OR CR ≥133 µmol/mL *and* 80 years old OR ≤60 kg	Contraindicated in severe hepatic disease or hepatic disease with associated coagulopathy and bleeding
Dabigatran	Contraindicated for CrCl <30 mL/min Reduce dose for CrCl 30–50 mL/min	Contraindicated where hepatic impairment is likely to impact on survival OR liver enzymes >2 ULN
Edoxaban	Contraindicated for CrCl <15mL/min Half dose for CrCl 15–50 mL/min	Contraindicated in severe hepatic disease and hepatic disease with associated coagulopathy and bleeding
Rivaroxaban	Contraindicated for CrCl <15mL/min Caution in CrCl 15–29 mL/min	Contraindicated in hepatic disease with associated coagulopathy and bleeding, incl. Child Pugh B and C

Predictably, there is an increased risk of bleeding when taken concurrently with other anticoagulants or antiplatelets, which requires caution.

Other reversal options

In many situations with ongoing life-threatening bleeding, prothrombin complex concentrate, activated prothrombin complex concentrate, and rFVIIa (**NovoSeven®**) should be considered; this will need discussion with a haematologist and is often driven by local hospital guidance, as NovoSeven® use is off-label in non-operable haemorrhage. NovoSeven® activates the extrinsic clotting cascade (via Factors IXa and Xa) generating an up-regulation in thrombin (Factor Xa complexes with Factor V to form the prothrombinase complex, which in turn, activates prothrombin, so thrombin then converts fibrinogen to fibrin so clot formation occurs).

Further reading

Bombeli T, Spahn DR (2004) Updates in perioperative coagulation: physiology and management of thromboembolism and haemorrhage. *British Journal of Anaesthesia* 93(2), 275–87.

Connors JM (2015) Antidote for factor Xa anticoagulants. *New England Journal of Medicine* 373, 2471–2.

Dahlbäck B (2008) Advances in understanding pathogenic mechanisms of thrombophilic disorders. *Blood* 112, 19–27.

Fareed J, Thethi I, Hoppensteadt D (2012) Old versus new oral anticoagulants: focus on pharmacology. *Annual Review Pharmacology and Toxicology* 52, 79–99.

López JA, Chen J (2009) Pathophysiology of venous thrombosis. *Thrombosis Research* 123(Suppl. 4), S30–4.

Martinelli I, Bucciarelli P, Mannucci PM (2010) Thrombotic risk factors: basic pathophysiology. *Critical Care Medicine* 38(Suppl. 2), S3–9.

Pallister CJ, Watson MS (2010) *Haematology*, 2nd edn. Banbury: Scion Publishing Ltd.

Sardar P, Chatterjee S, Mukherjee D (2013) Efficacy and safety of new oral anticoagulants for extended treatment of venous thromboembolism: systematic review and meta-analyses of randomized controlled trials. *Drugs* 73, 1171–82.

Guidelines

NICE CG92 (2015) Venous thromboembolism: reducing the risk for patients in hospital. https://www.nice.org.uk/Guidance/CG92 [accessed 21 March 2019].

NICE CG144 (2015) Venous thromboembolic diseases. http://guidance.nice.org.uk/CG144 [accessed 21 March 2019].

NICE Pathways (2019): venous thromboembolism. http://pathways.nice.org.uk/pathways/venous-thromboembolism [accessed 21 March 2019].

NICE QS29 (2016) Venous thromboembolism in adults: diagnosis and management. https://www.nice.org.uk/guidance/qs29 [accessed 21 March 2019].

NICE TA157 (2008) Dabigatran etexilate for the prevention of venous thromboembolism after hip or knee replacement surgery in adults. https://www.nice.org.uk/Guidance/TA157/ [accessed 21 March 2019].

NICE TA170 (2009) Rivaroxaban for the prevention of venous thromboembolism after total hip or total knee replacement in adults. https://www.nice.org.uk/Guidance/TA170/ [accessed 21 March 2019].

NICE TA245 (2012) Apixaban for the prevention of venous thromboembolism after total hip or knee replacement in adults. https://www.nice.org.uk/Guidance/ta245/ [accessed 21 March 2019].

NICE TA261 (2012) Rivaroxaban for the treatment of deep vein thrombosis and prevention of recurrent deep vein thrombosis and pulmonary embolism. https://www.nice.org.uk/Guidance/TA261 [accessed 21 March 2019].

NICE TA287 (2013) Rivaroxaban for treating pulmonary embolism and preventing recurrent venous thromboembolism. https://www.nice.org.uk/Guidance/TA287 [accessed 21 March 2019].

NICE TA327 (2014) Dabigatran etexilate for the treatment and secondary prevention of deep vein thrombosis and/or pulmonary embolism. https://www.nice.org.uk/Guidance/TA327 [accessed 21 March 2019].

NICE TA341 (2014) Apixaban for the treatment and secondary prevention of deep vein thrombosis and/or pulmonary embolism. https://www.nice.org.uk/Guidance/ta341 [accessed 21 March 2019].

NICE TA354 (2015) Edoxaban for treating and for preventing deep vein thrombosis and pulmonary embolism. https://www.nice.org.uk/Guidance/TA354 [accessed 21 March 2019].

3 Respiratory Medicine

3.1 Asthma

Asthma is a *reversible* chronic airways condition characterized by airway obstruction, bronchial hyperresponsiveness and chronic inflammation. Exposure to triggers causes an inflammatory cascade and symptoms, such as wheeze, dyspnoea, and cough. It is the most common medical condition in children, affecting 1 in 10 to varying degree. Peaks in prevalence occur at 10 and 59 years of age, with a tendency towards those of an atopic (hypersensitive allergic/genetic predisposition) nature.

Pathophysiology

In asthma, there is a swing in balance between two opposing T-helper (Th) cell populations towards persistent and excessive T-helper cell type 2 (Th2) dominated immune responses. Th1 cells are involved in response to infection, while Th2 cells are responsible for cytokine production (e.g. IL-4, IL-5, IL-6, IL-9, and IL-13) that are involved in allergic reaction, which may explain the overproduction of IgE, the presence of eosinophils and airway hyperresponsiveness. In the case of inhaled allergens, lung-based dendritic antigen-presenting cells ultimately stimulate Th2 cell production from naive Th0 cells (Figure 3.1). **Aspirin** and other NSAIDs can also initiate asthma symptoms, although this appears to be non-IgE dependant. Other dominant cells seen in asthma include mast cells and eosinophils.

Mast cells, when activated by inhaled antigen, release bronchoconstrictive factors like histamine, cysteinyl-leukotrienes, prostaglandin D_2, and eosinophil chemotactic factor. Mast cells in the airway may be sensitive to osmotic changes, thus account for exercise-induced asthma.

The production of IL-5 from activated Th2 and mast cells causes differentiation of eosinophils, which then migrate to the lung tissue, where they adhere to surface proteins like vascular-cell adhesion molecule 1 (VCAM-1) and intercellular adhesion molecule 1 (ICAM-1). Upon activation, these release pro-inflammatory cytokines like leukotrienes and granule proteins, which injure airway tissues. Additionally, eosinophil life is prolonged by the presence of IL-4 and granulocyte-macrophage colony-stimulating factor (GM-CSF). Collectively, the persistence and presence of eosinophils may potentiate chronic inflammatory changes and this correlates closely with the clinical severity of disease.

The overall cellular balance shift (Th2 dominance, mast cells, and eosinophils) and presence of an inflammatory stimulus results in bronchoconstriction (mainly via IgE-dependant release of mediators from mast cells constricting smooth muscle cells), airway oedema (through inflammation, mucus hypersecretion, and smooth muscle hypertrophy and hyperplasia), and airway hyperresponsiveness (through inflammation, dysfunctional neuroregulation, and structural changes).

Each clinical symptom therefore presents a potential target for therapy; be it acute or chronic treatment. β_2 adrenergic receptors (β_2 adrenoceptors) are located on airway epithelium and vascular smooth muscle; thus β_2-adrenoceptor agonists can relax bronchial smooth muscle, encourage mucocillary clearance, and inhibit release of mediators from mast cells. Steroids can improve overall lung function and reduce hyperresponsiveness by inhibiting transcription of cytokine genes within lymphocytes and macrophages that are responsible for the generation of inflammatory cytokines like IL-4, IL-5, IL-13, and GM-CSF. Methylxanthines are also beneficial in reducing bronchoconstriction and inflammation, although the mechanism is poorly understood. Other treatment options include leukotriene antagonists (**montelukast**) that inhibit leukotriene action, thereby reducing inflammation, by reduced synthesis through antagonism at leukotriene receptors or 5-lipoxygenase inhibition. New monoclonal therapies targeted specifically against IgE and IL-5 have recently been shown to be beneficial in asthma.

For a full summary of the relevant pathways and drug targets, see Figure 3.1.

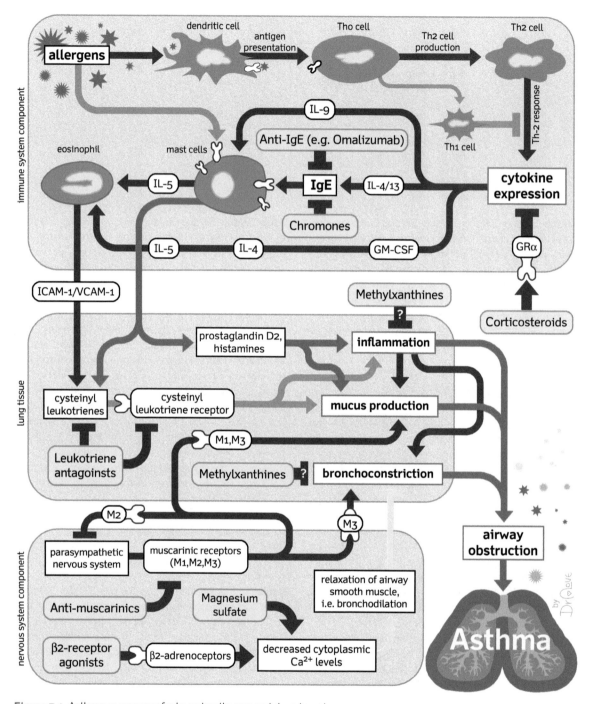

Figure 3.1 Asthma: summary of relevant pathways and drug targets.

Management

The primary aim of asthma management is to optimize disease control by preventing symptoms (day and night), and reducing the need for rescue medication and exacerbations. Patients should ideally attain a normal lung function so as to be able to participate in normal physical activity and exercise.

There is no single test that can be undertaken to diagnose asthma. Instead, the probability of respiratory symptoms being caused by asthma is made through a combination of structured clinical assessment,

diagnostic tests, and spirometry to assess for reversibility, and establish baseline measurements (see Figure 3.2). Where spirometry is not available peak expiratory flow (PEF) can be undertaken with the best of three efforts used.

Where the diagnosis of asthma is highly likely, a trial of treatment, usually with an inhaled corticosteroid for 6 weeks is recommended, with a follow-up appointment at the end of this period to assess response.

Where the probability of asthma is low/intermediate, or response to treatment is poor or equivocal, and inhaler technique/compliance has been assessed to be

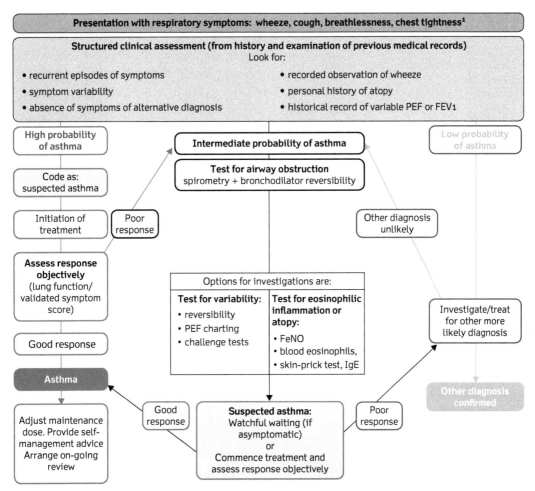

[1]In children under 5 years and others unable to undertake spirometry in whom there is a high or intermediate probability of asthma, the options are monitored initiation of treatment or watchful waiting according to the assessed probability of asthma.

Figure 3.2 Presentation with respiratory symptoms: wheeze, cough, breathlessness, chest tightness. This figure is reproduced from BTS/SIGN British Guideline on the management of asthma by kind permission of the British Thoracic Society. British Thoracic Society (BTS)/Scottish Intercollegiate Guidelines Network (SIGN). British Guideline on the management of asthma. Edinburgh: SIGN; 2016. (QRG 153). Available from URL: http://www.sign.ac.uk

reliable, further testing should be considered to establish an alternative diagnosis. The presence or absence of air-flow obstruction can be useful to differentiate from other diagnoses (see Table 3.1), although patients with asthma can produce normal results when they are asymptomatic. Where the diagnosis remains unclear, investigations such as CXR, serum IgE, and skin prick tests may be helpful to establish diagnosis.

Numerous risk factors have historically been attributed to asthma; however, supporting evidence is lacking with regards to allergen exposure (food or dust mite), weaning, or nutritional supplements, such as fish oils or probiotics. There is limited evidence to suggest that breastfeeding may offer a protective effect and exposure to smoking, unsurprisingly, is likely to be detrimental. Measures such as maintaining a healthy weight and avoiding smoking should be encouraged for better asthma control, especially as smoking in childhood doubles the risk of persisting asthma.

Management of chronic asthma

Once a diagnosis has been made, patients should be given advice on the importance of self-management to reduce the frequency of excerbations and ensure optimal control. This includes identifying signs/symptoms of deterioration and developing a personalized asthma action plan (PAAP), for use in the event of deterioration. The key is to generate an ethos of supported self-management.

In order to optimize control, while minimizing adverse effects, drug therapy for asthma is adjusted in a stepwise manner, starting at the level most appropriate for the patients' severity of symptoms (see Figure 3.3). Where inhalers are used, consideration should be given to the choice of device (see Table 3.2); ensuring patients are adequately counselled and able to demonstrate good inhaler technique.

Intermittent reliever therapy

All symptomatic patients require a short-acting bronchodilator to be used as a 'reliever'. Although short-acting β_2-adrenoceptor agonists (SABA) are preferred, other options include inhaled **ipratropium bromide**. Rarely, methylxanthines are used or, less favourably due to their high level of toxicity, oral β_2-adrenoceptor agonists. Patients requiring more than one short-acting bronchodilator inhaler device a month require an urgent review of their asthma control, as this is associated with an increased risk of fatal or near fatal asthma.

Table 3.1 Clinical clues to alternative diagnoses in adults

Clinical clue	Possible diagnosis
Without airflow obstruction	
Predominant cough without lung function abnormalities	Chronic cough syndromes; pertussis
Prominent dizziness, light-headedness, peripheral tingling	Dysfunctional breathing
Recurrent severe 'asthma attacks' without objective confirmatory evidence	Vocal cord dysfunction
Predominant nasal symptoms without lung function abnormalities	Rhinitis
Postural and food-related symptoms, predominant cough	Gastro-oesophageal reflux
Orthopnoea, paroxysmal nocturnal dyspnoea, peripheral oedema, preexisting cardiac disease	Cardiac failure
Crackles on auscultation	Pulmonary fibrosis
With airflow obstruction	
Significant smoking history (ie, >30 pack-years), age of onset >35 years	COPD
Chronic productive cough in the absence of wheeze or breathlessness	Bronchiectasis*; inhaled foreign body*; obliterative bronchiitis; large airway stenosis
New onset in smoker, systemic symptoms, weight loss, haemoptysis	Lung cancer*; sarcoidosis*

* may also be associated with non-obstructive spirometry

This table is reproduced from BTS/SIGN British Guideline on the management of asthma by kind permission of the British Thoracic Society. British Thoracic Society (BTS)/Scottish Intercollegiate Guidelines Network (SIGN). British Guideline on the management of asthma. Edinburgh: SIGN; 2016. (QRG 153). Available from URL: http://www.sign.ac.uk

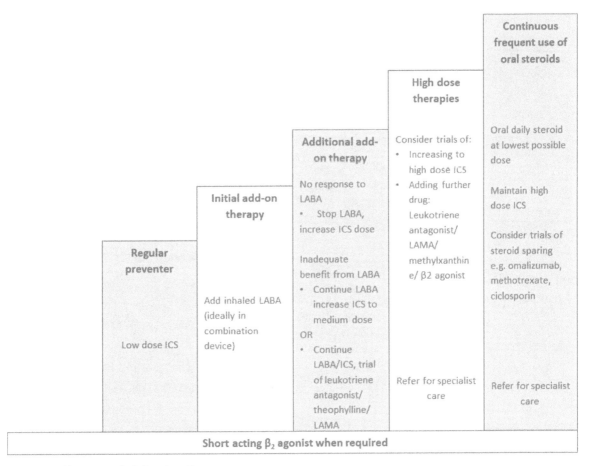

Figure 3.3 Management of chronic asthma.

This figure is reproduced from BTS/SIGN British Guideline on the management of asthma by kind permission of the British Thoracic Society. British Thoracic Society (BTS)/Scottish Intercollegiate Guidelines Network (SIGN). British Guideline on the management of asthma. Edinburgh: SIGN; 2016. (QRG 153). Available from URL: http://www.sign.ac.uk

Regular preventer therapy

First-line regular preventer therapy is with an inhaled corticosteroid, due to their superior efficacy in most patients and should be considered in any patient experiencing an asthma attack in the last 2 years, requiring a SABA three times a week or more or is waking one night a week. Clinically, there is little to choose between the corticosteroids or the type of available devices, so preference is determined by patient suitability (technique, age, dexterity, etc.) and resources (cost and availability). Initial doses should be based on severity of symptoms and titrated to achieve maximum response at minimum dose. Doses should be taken BD (except for **ciclesonide**), titrated so that the lowest effective dose to minimize the risk of long-term side effects with higher doses [in excess of 1000 µg of **beclometasone** (BDP) per day].

Alternative regular preventer therapy (e.g. leukotriene receptor antagonists, chromones, and methylxanthines), may be preferred in some patients, such as those unable to use an inhaler.

Initial add-on therapy

In adults who remain symptomatic on a first-line regular preventer (200–800 µg/day equivalent BDP), where poor adherence or inhaler technique has been excluded, add-on therapy may be necessary. For most patients long-acting β_2 agonists (LABAs) are the class of choice, as they demonstrate good efficacy in improving lung function and reducing exacerbations. These should always be used in combination with an inhaled corticosteroids (ICS), ideally in a combination device, of which **budesonide/ formoterol** is also licensed for reliever therapy.

Table 3.2 Choice of inhaler device

Inhaler type	Advantages	Disadvantages	Examples
Dry powder inhalers (DPI)	Numerous different devices Useful alternative especially in patients requiring combination therapy Unnecessary to coordinate actuation with inhalation Some devices 'click' to indicate dose has been taken correctly, e.g. NEXThaler®	Limited drug choice Dexterity to insert a capsule (e.g. HandiHaler®) Considerable respiratory effort to activate (e.g. Turbohaler®) Cost	Accuhaler® Turbohaler® HandiHaler® NEXThaler®
Metered dose inhalers (MDI)	Widely available Widely used Effective with adequate training Compatible with spacer devices	Requires coordination between actuation and inhalation Some patients find them difficult to use	
Breath-activated inhalers	Numerous devices Useful alternative in patients unable to manage MDI Unnecessary to coordinate actuation with inhalation Less respiratory effort than a DPI	Limited drug choice Cost	Autohaler® Easi-Breathe® Respimat®

Additional add-on therapies

In patients that fail to respond adequately to low-dose inhaled corticosteroid (ICS)/LABA, compliance and inhaler technique should be assessed, and an alternative diagnosis considered. If response is limited, doses of the ICS should be optimized or a leukotriene receptor antagonists/ long-acting muscarinic antagonist (LAMA)/methylxanthines added. Where there is no response to the LABA, this should be stopped and ICS optimized, a leukotriene antagonist added or a LAMA. **Tiotropium** Respimat® is a LAMA that has had its license extended for use in asthma.

High dose therapies

In adults who remain uncontrolled on a medium dose ICS plus a LABA (or alternative drug), should have treatment escalated by increasing ICS dose or adding in a further agent, i.e. a leukotriene receptor antagonist, LAMA, or methylxanthine), or the dose of ICS increased (equivalent of 800–2000 µg of BDP a day). There is little to choose between options, although a trial period for any agent is advisable and ineffective treatment withdrawn before trying further options.

Continuous/frequent use of oral corticosteroids

In very severe asthma long-term oral steroids may be required, with doses kept as low as possible. These patients will require monitoring to manage toxicity associated with long term corticosteroid use, including:

- Blood pressure.
- Glucose (blood and urine).
- Cholesterol.
- Bone mineral density.
- Growth (children).
- Cataracts.

Steroid-sparing therapies maybe considered under the supervision of a specialist. The anti-IgE monoclonal antibody, **omalizumab**, can play a role where symptoms are related to allergy. Immunosupressants, such as **methotrexate** or **ciclosporin**, are associated with significant toxicity, however, have been used in some patients following a successful 3-month trial. Steroid-sparing treatments should be managed in a specialist centre experienced with

Table 3.3 Levels of severity of acute asthma, adapted from BTS/SIGN guidelines 2016

Severity	Signs	
Moderate asthma	Increasing symptoms PEF > 50–75% best/predicted Absence of features of acute severe asthma	
Acute severe asthma	Any one of: • PEF 33–50% best/predicted • Respiratory rate ≥25/min • Heart rate ≥110/min • Unable to complete sentence in one breath	
Life-threatening asthma	Severe asthma + any one of the following: *Clinical signs*: • Altered conscious level • Exhaustion • Arrhythmia • Hypotension • Cyanosis • Silent chest • Poor respiratory effort	Measurements • PEF <33% best/predicted • SpO_2 <92% • PaO_2 <8 kPa • normal $PaCO_2$
Near fatal asthma	Raised $PaCO_2$ and/or requiring mechanical ventilation with raised inflation pressures	

This table is reproduced from BTS/SIGN British Guideline on the management of asthma by kind permission of the British Thoracic Society. British Thoracic Society (BTS)/Scottish Intercollegiate Guidelines Network (SIGN). British Guideline on the management of asthma. Edinburgh: SIGN; 2016. (QRG 153). Available from URL: http://www.sign.ac.uk

its use. Future treatment options include **mepolizumab**, an anti-IL5 that is currently being reviewed by NICE.

Management of acute asthma

Acute asthma is treated according to severity of the exacerbation (see Table 3.3), in a stepwise manner to achieve reversal of symptoms measured against predicted PEF and good oxygen saturation. Adults with any signs indicative of life-threatening/near fatal asthma or severe disease unresponsive to initial treatment will require rapid hospitalization for management.

Treatment of acute asthma includes:

• *β2 agonist bronchodilators* (**salbutamol** and **terbutaline**) are first-line treatment options for all episodes of acute asthma, regardless of severity. Salbutamol is the most widely used, administered either via an inhaler, with or without a spacer device; or in more severe cases, via a nebulizer (ideally oxygen driven). Doses can be repeated at frequent, regular intervals or, if necessary, administered continuously. In some cases of life-threatening asthma, salbutamol may be given IV, however, there is a greater risk of systemic side effects (e.g. cardiac arrhythmias). Where given IV monitor lactate levels to assess for toxicity.

• *Corticosteroids* are administered immediately in all patients on presentation with acute asthma and continued as necessary. Oral **prednisolone** is preferred, although where the oral route is not tolerated, **hydrocortisone** can be administered IV. Treatment should be continued for at least 5 days or until recovery, and ICS continued.

• *Oxygen* therapy is initiated in severe acute asthma (PEF <50% best or predicted) to maintain an SpO_2 of 94–98% (BTS). SpO_2 is measured with pulse oximetry except in patients with life-threatening asthma, where ABGs are taken.

• *Ipratropium* is used as additional nebulized therapy in severe or life-threatening acute asthma in patients failing to respond adequately to a SABA.

• *Magnesium sulfate* can be given as a single dose IV for its bronchodilator effects under guidance of senior medical staff where initial response to inhaled broncho-dilator therapy is poor.

- *Aminophylline* IV may be considered in life-threatening or near-fatal asthma at the discretion of senior clinicians. Where used, levels should be monitored and baseline levels taken in patients already on oral therapy to prevent toxicity.

Drug classes used in management

Bronchodilators: β2-adrenoceptor agonists

β$_2$-adrenoceptor agonists act on β$_2$-adrenoceptors that are widely distributed in the lung, resulting in relaxation of airway smooth muscle. Examples include short-acting salbutamol and terbutaline; and long-acting formeterol and salmeterol.

Mechanism of action

The β-adrenoceptors can be classified as β$_1$, β$_2$, and β$_3$ subtypes, with β$_2$ agonists being the most effective in the management of airway disease. A member of the superfamily of G protein receptors coupled to adenylate cyclase, activation increases production of cAMP and activation of cAMP-dependent protein kinase A (PKA). In airway smooth muscle, PKA activation leads to phosphorylation of key targets, such as myosin light chain kinase and Ca^{2+}-activated potassium channels. Simultaneous activation of Ca^{2+}–Mg^{2+}-ATPases in the endoplasmic reticulum and plasma membrane, reduces cytoplasmic Ca^{2+} levels. Together these actions lead to a decrease in Ca^{2+}-dependent actin–myosin interactions, which promotes the relaxation of airway smooth muscle.

It has also been suggested that some effects are cAMP independent and could be directly mediated by G proteins interaction with potassium channels in the smooth muscle or by non-Gs coupled pathways. Added to the bronchodilator effects of β$_2$-adrenoreceptor agonists, these drugs also protect against bronchoconstrictor stimuli actions.

The chemical structure of most of the β-adrenoceptors agonists commonly used is based on the endogenous catecholamine, **adrenaline**. SABAs, such as **salbutamol** are hydrophilic, thus rapidly metabolized and eliminated. They have a rapid onset of action (5 min) and last for up to 6 hours. LABAs, such as **salmeterol** and **formoterol** are more lipophilic, which allows for a more gradual release and sustained action. Formoterol has a more rapid onset of action than salmeterol (1–3 min versus 20 min) and so, more recently, has been advocated for use as both a reliever and preventer.

Prescribing

Short-acting β$_2$ adrenoceptor agonists

There are two commercially available SABAs, **salbutamol** and **terbutaline**, of which the former is more widely used, although both are indicated for the acute management or relief of breathlessness attributed to asthma. For mild to moderate symptoms, administration is via an inhaler device, selected according to patient preference, although greater choice is available for salbutamol.

For more severe symptoms, either drug may be nebulized, or in the case of life-threatening or unresponsive exacerbation, administered parenterally either as an IV infusion or intermittent injections (SC, IM, or slow IV). Patients requiring high doses require serum K^+ (as K^+ is driven into cells) and cardiac monitoring.

For chronic management, salbutamol may also be administered orally, although this is generally avoided due to unacceptable systemic toxicity.

Fenoterol, also a SABA, has been largely discontinued worldwide, as it has been linked with an increased risk of mortality. Although the risk is relevant to other SABAs, fenoterol was the most heavily implicated, possibly being the least selective of the agents available at the time. Although the association remains controversial; current practice dictates that SABAs should not be used regularly, but on an as-required basis.

Long-acting β$_2$ adrenoceptor agonists

Despite controversy over their safety, LABAs are a well-established step up in the management of asthma, as an add-on therapy in patients whose symptoms remain uncontrolled on inhaled corticosteroids. Administration is always by inhalation through a range of inhaler devices, either as a single or, preferably, combination product with a corticosteroid, i.e. **salmeterol** with **fluticasone** and **formoterol** with **beclometasone** or **budesonide**

Unwanted effects

At standard doses via an inhaler, the β_2-adrenoceptor agonists are well tolerated. However, at higher doses and with systemic therapy the risk of toxicity is increased. Common side effects include fine tremor, palpitations, headache, and muscle cramps, particularly with the SABAs. Frequent use of a SABA is associated with increased toxicity, increased risk of an exacerbation and, in some instances, tolerance to therapy; thus patients requiring more than one inhaler a month require a step-up in therapy.

Stimulation of β_2 adrenoceptors on smooth muscle within the heart, causes tachycardia and arrhythmias. Caution is, therefore, recommended in patients with pre-existing disease or at high risk of cardiac toxicity, e.g. hyperthyroidism, hypotension, or hypokalaemia. Furthermore, β_2 adrenoceptor stimulation of the Na^+/K^+ pump in skeletal muscle shifts potassium from the serum into cells causing hypokalaemia. Patients on high doses or on concurrent therapy known to cause hypokalaemia (e.g. loop or thiazide diuretics) require their serum K^+ levels closely monitored.

β_2 adrenoceptors stimulation also impairs glucose metabolism potentially affecting glycaemic control in diabetics. Other interactions of clinical significance are infrequent with inhaled used, generally being associated with high doses and systemic therapy.

Bronchodilators: antimuscarinics

Anticholinergic agents induce airway muscle relaxation by blocking muscarinic receptors, which mediate parasympathetic nervous system stimulation in the respiratory system responsible for bronchoconstriction. For example, ipratropium and tiotropium

Mechanism of action

The parasympathetic nerves mediate airway tone and hyperreactivity by releasing acetylcholine and activating muscarinic receptors. Three types of muscarinic receptors (M_1–M_3) can have physiological effects in the lungs, with airway smooth muscle, submucosal glands, and nerves having different expression profiles. Acetylcholine released from vagal nerve stimulation causes airway muscle contraction via activation of M_3 muscarinic receptors at the post-junctional level, as this leads to the generation of IP_3, diacyl glycerol, and intracellular Ca^{2+} increase. In addition, both M_1 and M_3 receptors mediate mucus secretion. The release of acetylcholine from the nerves can also be modulated by M_1 and M_2 receptors, with the presynaptic M_2 in particular acting as a negative feedback that can limit bronchoconstriction and be beneficial in asthma.

Ideally, treatment of asthma with an anticholinergic would reduce airway bronchoconstriction and mucus secretion via blockade of M_1 and M_3 muscarinic receptors, without inhibiting the M_2 subtype. **Atropine, ipratropium**, and **oxitropium** are non-selective antimuscarinics that bind M_2 and M_3 muscarinic receptors with equivalent affinity. See Topic 3.2, 'Chronic obstructive pulmonary disease' for information on **tiotropium**.

Prescribing

Of the inhaled short-acting muscarinic antagonists (SAMAs) only **ipratropium** is licensed in the UK for use in asthma, when a SABA is either unsuitable or inadequate, i.e. is a severe exacerbation. Ipratropium is administered either via an inhaler or nebulized, depending on severity of symptoms.

More recently, the LAMA, **tiotropium** Respimat® has been granted an extension to its license for use in the management of asthma. It can, therefore, be considered as an option in patients in step 4 as alternative add-on therapy in combination with an ICS and LABA.

Unwanted effects

Adverse effect reported with **ipratropium** are attributed to its antimuscarinic properties or local irritation, i.e. dry mouth, nausea, GI upset, cough, throat irritation, headache, and dizziness. Side effects are, therefore, primarily dose related and more pronounced with frequent, nebulized therapy. Although systemic toxicity is less common with inhaled therapy, cautions is still advised in patients where antimuscarinics are contraindicated, e.g. glaucoma, urinary retention, or prostatic hyperplasia. The risk of toxicity is increased when taken concurrently with other antimuscarinics and in combination with β_2 adrenoceptor agonist bronchodilators, as they, too, can increase the risk of glaucoma or raise intra-ocular pressure.

Bronchodilators: methylxanthines

Methylxanthines have anti-inflammatory and vaso-dilator actions, although the mechanisms of action are multiple and still not fully understood. For example, aminophylline and theophylline.

Mechanism of action

Despite their long history of use, the molecular mechanisms of action of methylxanthines remain unclear. **Theophylline** is a phosphodiesterase inhibitor at high concentrations, causing the increase of intracellular cAMP and cyclic guanosine monophosphate levels. Increased levels of cAMP in bronchial smooth muscle stimulates voltage-gated Ca^{2+}-activated K^+ channels in the cell membrane, leading to hyperpolarization and smooth muscle relaxation. Adenosine receptor antagonism may also be relevant to the clinical effect, through inhibition of adenosine-dependent mast cell release of histamine and leukotrienes, which promotes the constriction of hyper-responsive airways.

More recently, low doses of theophylline have been shown to have significant anti-inflammatory effects in the airways of asthmatic patients. At high doses, theophylline can inhibit eosinophil degranulation and the release of eosinophil basic proteins, block the release and expression of IL-1b and TNFα from blood monocytes, decrease IL-2 production by T cells and IL-2-dependent T cell proliferation and induce non-specific suppressor activity in human peripheral blood lymphocytes.

Prescribing

The methylxanthines have a narrow therapeutic index, increasing the risk of toxicity and making them a less favourable option in asthma management. Both **theophylline** and **amniophylline** are administered orally in chronic asthma management, usually as a slow-release preparation to improve tolerance and promote compliance. In severe exacerbations aminophylline can be given as an IV infusion, although serum monitoring is necessary during treatment and at baseline in patients already receiving oral therapy. Lower doses may be required in some patient groups (see next section, 'Unwanted effects').

Unwanted effects

Toxicity to methylxanthine treatment can be evident at levels as low as 15 μg/L, but more likely over 20 μg/L. For this reason, serum monitoring is recommended, particularly in patients where toxicity is suspected or clearance is likely to be impaired. Signs of toxicity include GI effects (nausea, vomiting) as well as anxiety, palpitations, headache, and restlessness. These effects occur more commonly in patients with underlying cardiovascular disease, hyperthyroidism, or hypertension. In some instance, severe toxicity or rapid administration can cause arrhythmias that may occasionally be fatal.

Clearance of methylxanthines may be reduced in hepatic impairment (this being the primary route of elimination), heart failure, acute febrile illness, and vulnerable patient groups, such as the elderly or infants under 6 months. Concomitant drugs known to affect clearance include macrolide antibiotics, **ciprofloxacin**, **furosemide**, and **diltiazem**. Conversely, **rifampicin**, **phenytoin**, St John's Wort, smoking, and alcohol can increase clearance, so that patients may require higher doses to achieve therapeutic levels.

Bronchodilators: magnesium sulphate

Magnesium sulfate promotes bronchodilation by blocking Ca^{2+} channels, reducing Ca^{2+} entry to the cell and overall muscle contractility.

Mechanism of action

The second most abundant cation of the intracellular domain, magnesium is essential for the activity of many enzymes, and has a fundamental role in neurochemical transmission and muscular excitability. In smooth muscle cell membranes, magnesium inhibits Ca^{2+} influx through dihydropiridine-sensitive voltage-dependent channels, which accounts for much of its relaxant effects in the respiratory system.

Prescribing

Magnesium sulfate is reserved for use in acute life-threatening episodes of asthma when other options have failed. Doses of 1.2–2 g are administered IV over 20 minutes; usually as a one-off dose, as there is little safety data regarding repeated use. This indication is unlicensed and reserved for use in patients under specialist/emergency care.

Unwanted effects

Single doses of magnesium are rarely associated with side effects, although with repeated doses and in at-risk patients (heart block, myocardial damage, myasthenia gravis, or in severe renal impairment) they have the potential to cause hypermagnesaemia, which in severe cases can present as flushing, thirst, hypotension, confusion, nausea, vomiting, slurred speech, muscle weakness, respiratory failure, electrolyte disturbances (hypocalcaemia), blurred vision, ECG changes, arrhythmias, coma, and cardiac arrest. In an acute situation, it is unnecessary to check levels pre-dose.

Hypermagnesamia, induced by magnesium sulphate treatment, can increase the risk of cardiac toxicity with cardiac glycosides (**digoxin**) and respiratory depression with drugs such as barbiturates, benzodiazepines, or opioids.

Anti-inflammatory agents: corticosteroids

> The anti-inflammatory activity of glucocorticoids occurs through activation of the cytoplasmic form of the glucocorticoid receptor (GR), which upon ligand binding translocates to the nucleus and inhibits the transcription of inflammatory cytokines. Examples include prednisolone, hydrocortisone, methylprednisolone, beclometasone, fludrocortisone, budesonide, ciclesonide, and mometasone.

Mechanism of action

The regulation of gene transcription by the GR complex occurs by direct binding with transcription factors activator protein (AP)-1 and nuclear factor (NF)-κB. These are up-regulated during inflammation and inhibit the pro-inflammatory effects of various cytokines. The complex can also promote the expression of the NF-κB inhibitor IkBa in specific cell types. Moreover, recruitment of deacetylases to the transcription complex of activated inflammatory genes, promotes deacetylation of core histones and gene silencing. Finally, glucocorticoids can augment the levels of cell ribonucleases and proteins capable of destabilizing mRNA, thus reducing mRNA levels of pro-inflammatory cytokines.

Glucocorticoids can have direct inhibitory effects on various cells involved in airway inflammation in asthma, a list that includes macrophages, T-lymphocytes, eosinophils, mast cells and airway smooth muscle, and epithelial cells. Glucocorticoids reduce mucosal oedema and macrophage eicosanoid (leukotrienes and thromboxane),

and cytokine synthesis. In the short-term, glucocorticoids can also up-regulate β-adrenoceptors, improving coupling to adenylyl cyclases, and have some effect on the relief of bronchoconstriction through the inhibition of ACh release via enhanced activity of M_2-muscarinic autoreceptors on acetylcholine nerve endings.

Prescribing

Corticosteroids form the mainstay of treatment in both acute exacerbations and chronic management of asthma, although the choice of agent and route of administration varies.

Inhaled corticosteroids

Of the inhaled corticosteroids licensed in the UK for the management of asthma; **beclometasone**, **budesonide**, and **fluticasone** are the most widely used. Budesonide and beclometasone are considered to have equal clinical effect at the same dose, whereas fluticasone and mometasone are as effective at half the dose. Although there is some suggestion that there are fewer side effects with the half-dose of fluticasone, this is not well established and the relative safety of mometasone remains unknown. **Ciclesonide**, the newest of the inhaled corticosteroids, has the least safety data, although studies to date suggest it may cause fewer systemic or local oropharyngeal side effects; furthermore, its long half-life enables OD administration. Despite this, choice of steroid is invariably dictated by inhaler device, patient preference, or the availability of combined preparations, where an inhaled corticosteroid alone is insufficient to control symptoms. More recently, fluticasone furoate in combination with **vilanterol** (Relvar®) has been launched, with the advantage of being more than five times as potent as fluticasone proprionate.

Treatment doses are generally described in beclometasone equivalents, for which the usual starting dose is 200 µg BD, increased to 600–800 µg/day in 2–4 divided doses. Higher doses of up to 2000 µg daily are associated with significant systemic toxicity and, therefore, reserved for patients who have failed other add-on options. As part of a PAAP, patients on lower doses (200 µg BD) may be advised to increase their own dose to a maximum of 1200 µg per day in order to optimize control.

Systemic corticosteroids

Prednisolone (40–50 mg/day) is the oral corticosteroid of choice in the management of acute exacerbations of asthma, or as add-on therapy for severe chronic asthma unresponsive to other treatment. In acute asthma it is given daily for at least 5 days in adults, or until symptoms resolve. For short courses, weaning is considered unnecessary;

however, those needing extended (over 3 weeks) or repeated courses require a more gradual withdrawal. In patients requiring chronic oral treatment, doses are adjusted to response enabling optimum control at minimum dose. Doses are best taken in the morning with food, to minimize the risk of adrenal suppression and GI toxicity, respectively.

In some cases, **hydrocortisone** may be administered IV or IM **methylprednisolone** where oral therapy is not possible. Patients should be converted to oral prednisolone as soon as practicable.

Unwanted effects

Although systemic toxicity is reduced when corticosteroids are inhaled, the risk is increased with higher doses and prolonged use. Patients may also experience local toxicity, such as dysphonia and oral candida, which may be avoided by promoting good inhaler technique, encouraging patients to rinse their mouth after use or by means of a spacer device.

See corticosteroids (Topic 6.6, 'Inflammatory bowel disease') for more information.

Anti-inflammatory agents: chromones

> Chromones inhibits IgE release from inflammatory cells, indirectly preventing vasoconstriction secondary to allergens or exercise. For example, sodium cromoglicate and nedocromil sodium.

Mechanism of action

Chromones can have a variety of actions that contribute to their clinical effect, including the inhibition of IgE-dependent release of mediators from human lung mast cells. This might be beneficial against bronchoconstriction induced by allergens or exercise. They also suppress the activation of and release from other inflammatory cells, including monocytes, eosinophils, and macrophages.

Antagonism on the effects of tachykinins, substance P, and neurokinin B, which are involved in the generation of sensory stimuli, might be responsible for the protection against irritant-induced bronchoconstriction.

Prolonged treatment with chromones inhibits eosinophil accumulation in the lungs, and the activation of eosinophils, neutrophils, and macrophages in inflamed lung tissue. This suggests a direct anti-inflammatory effect in human asthmatic airways. Together with reduced IgE production, these actions could help prevent

the late-phase response to allergens and bronchial hyper-reactivity.

Prescribing

In clinical practice the role of chromones in asthma management has been largely superseded by more effective therapy, although both **sodium cromoglicate** and **nedocromil sodium** inhalers remain licensed for asthma prevention. As they act indirectly in the inhibition of bronchoconstriction, they are of no value in acute management.

Unwanted effects

Side effects to chromones tend to be mild, but common, affecting more than 10% of patients; they include nausea, vomiting, headache, cough, and bronchospasm. Where treatment is discontinued, it should not be stopped abruptly, but gradually withdrawn over a week to reduce the risk of a rebound in symptoms

Anti-inflammatory agents: leukotriene receptor antagonists/leukotriene synthesis inhibitors

> Cysteinyl leukotriene receptor antagonists, which bind to cysteinyl leukotriene receptors, and leukotriene synthesis inhibitors can prevent leukotriene-mediated effects, including bronchoconstriction and mucus production. For example, montelukast and zafirlukast.

Mechanism of action

The function of cysteinyl leukotrienes in the origins of the pathology of asthma is well characterized. Both leukotrienes and histamine are released after contact with allergens from mast cells, eosinophils, and basophils. The cysteinyl leukotrienes play a role in sustaining the chronic airway inflammation response, in neurogenic inflammation and in the remodelling of airways.

Leukotrienes are synthesized in the cell from arachidonic acid by 5-lipoxygenase and induce biological effects by stimulating specific receptors that are localized on the plasma membrane of target cells. Cysteinyl leukotrienes, LTC4, LTD4, and LTE4 act via at least two distinct types of G protein–coupled receptors (CysLt1 and CysLt2). Expression of CysLT1 receptor is restricted to smooth muscle cells and tissue macrophages, while CysLT2 is localized to lung macrophages, airway smooth muscle and peripheral blood leukocytes. Stimulation of these receptors activates a guanosine triphosphate binding protein that transduces the intracellular signals.

Montelukast and **zafirlukast** are leukotriene receptor antagonists (sometimes referred to as *leukasts*), that are available in the UK for use in asthma, while **pranlukast** is available in other countries. **Zileuton** is a 5-lipoxygenase inhibitor, although its use has been associated with severe hepatic toxicity, probably linked to a toxic metabolite (2-actylbenzothiophene), so is not available for use.

Prescribing

The leukotriene receptor antagonists can be used chronically as add-on therapy in patients not adequately controlled with inhaled corticosteroids, being particularly beneficial in patients with exercise-induced asthma or associated seasonal rhinitis. Practically, they have the advantage of being taken orally, so provide an option in those unable to use an inhaler device. **Montelukast**, in particular, is widely used in paediatrics, being available in child-friendly chewable tablets and soluble sachet formulations. **Zafirlukast** is only licensed for use in patients over 12 years and is less frequently prescribed.

Unwanted effects

Side effects to the leukotriene antagonists, tend to be mild and of comparable frequency to that seen in patients receiving placebo. They include infection, headache, nausea, vomiting, diarrhoea, rash, and deranged LFTs. Rarely, leukotriene antagonists have been associated with systemic eosinophilia. This can present with symptoms such as a vasculitic rash, worsening pulmonary symptoms, cardiac symptoms, or neuropathy consistent with Churg–Strauss syndrome; where this is suspected, treatment should be discontinued.

Due to lack of safety data, manufacturers recommend avoiding **zafirlukast** in hepatic impairment and caution in renal impairment.

> **PRESCRIBING WARNING**
>
> **Risk of Churg–Strauss syndrome with leukotriene antagonists**
>
> Prescribers should be aware that leukotriene antagonists can occasionally induce a systemic eosinophilia and symptoms consistent with Churg–Strauss syndrome.

Monoclonal antibodies

> Monoclonal recombinant anti-IgE antibodies bind free, but not receptor-bound IgE, preventing IgE from binding to receptors and thus inhibiting the initiation of the allergic cascade. For example, omalizumab. Humanized monoclonal antibodies have also been developed against IL-5 that act to reduce circulating eosinophils. For example, mepolizumab and reslizumab

Mechanism of action

IgE is the effector antibody in atopic asthma and has a key function in the pathogenesis of allergic asthma. The antigen specific IgE is made by B cells that have undertaken isotype switching from IgM to IgE production, after the actions of IL-4 and IL-13. Circulating IgE binds to high affinity receptors that are expressed by mast cells and basophils in circulation. Two cell-surface receptors have been identified for IgE. A high affinity receptor (FcεRI) is mostly expressed on mast cells, basophils, and dendritic cells. A second receptor, FcεRII, binds with lower affinity to the carboxylic fragment of IgE and is present in various inflammatory cells, such as eosinophils, lymphocytes, mononuclear phagocytes, etc. IgE plays a key part in the early and late allergic responses via interaction with these two receptors. Because most asthma is allergic and initiated by IgE antibodies, factors that target this response are a novel strategy for developing new therapies.

Omalizumab is a monoclonal humanized recombinant anti-IgE antibody with a human IgG1 structure, and a complementary-determining region from an anti-IgE antibody of murine origin. It has a low potential for immunogenicity due to its low content of murine residues (less than 5%). Omalizumab recognizes an epitope on the fragment of IgE (Cε3) that binds to the α-chain of the IgE receptor, inhibiting IgE from binding to it. As a result, it blocks the IgE-mediated release of inflammatory mediators from mast cells and other inflammatory cells. Treatment with omalizumab appears to have two actions that potentially diminish allergic reactions—it reduces free plasma IgE levels and the density of high affinity receptors on inflammatory cells.

More recently, **mepolizumab** and **reslizumab** have been developed as humanized monoclonal antibodies effective against IL-5, a key interleukin for the growth, differentiation and activation of eosinophils, thereby reducing circulating levels.

Prescribing

Omalizumab is licensed and NICE approved for use in severe unstable IgE-mediated asthma, in patients that have required hospitalization at least twice in the previous 12 months for a severe exacerbation. It is administered subcutaneously every 2 or 4 weeks, with doses adjusted according to serum IgE levels and body weight. Doses are unaffected by renal or hepatic impairment as omalizumab is cleared via the reticular endothelial system (RES). It can take 12–16 weeks to achieve an effective response, so patients are reviewed at 16 weeks to assess for a marked improvement in overall asthma control, before continuing long-term.

Mepolizumab is administered by SC injection every 4 weeks for long-term management of severe eosinophilic asthma in adults, with efficacy assessed annually. **Reslizumab** is also administered every 4 weeks, but as an IV infusion for the same indication. Both agents are NICE approved.

Unwanted effects

Like all monoclonal antibodies these agents have the potential to cause serious immune-mediated reactions, in particular, hypersensitivity reactions (type I and type III). Type I reactions range from local skin reactions to, albeit rarely, anaphylaxis, which typically occur within hours of a dose (first or subsequent) or up to 24 hours later. Type III delayed allergic reactions to **omalizumab**, include serum sickness presenting as joint pain, rashes, fever, and lymphadenopathy, which may be prevented and treated with anti-histamines and corticosteroids. Churg–Strauss syndrome and hypereosinophilia have been reported with omalizumab therapy, although this may be a sign of severe asthma as a result of a decrease in oral corticosteroid therapy. More common side effects include pyrexia, headache, and upper abdominal pain.

As IgE and eosinophils are thought to be involved in the immune response to helminth infections, treatment may increase the risk of parasitic infection in some patients and reduce the efficacy of anti-helminth treatments.

> ### PRESCRIBING WARNING
>
> **Allergic reactions to monoclonal antibodies**
> Allergic reactions including anaphylaxis can occur more than 2 hours after administration and, in some cases, up to 24 hours following the dose. Patients should be advised accordingly to seek urgent medical help in the event of allergic symptoms. Further use should be avoided.

Further reading

Buhl R (2005) Anti-IgE antibodies for the treatment of asthma. *Current Opinions in Pulmonary Medicine* 11(1), 27–34.
Caramori G, Adcock I (2003) Pharmacology of airway inflammation in asthma and COPD. *Pulmonary Pharmacology and Therapy* 16(5), 247–77.

Guidance

BTS/SIGN British Guideline on the Management of Asthma, October 2016. https://www.brit-thoracic.org.uk/document-library/clinical-information/asthma/btssign-asthma-guideline-2016/ [accessed 22 March 2019].
Global Initiative for Asthma (2018) GINA Global Strategy for Asthma Management. https://ginasthma.org/gina-reports/ [accessed 29 March 2019].
NICE NG80 (2017) Asthma: diagnosis, monitoring and chronic asthma management. https://www.nice.org.uk/guidance/ng80 [accessed 22 March 2019].
NICE Pathway: Asthma http://pathways.nice.org.uk/pathways/asthma [accessed 22 March 2019].
NICE QS25 (2013) Asthma. https://www.nice.org.uk/guidance/qs25 [accessed 22 March 2019].
NICE TA278 (2013) Omalizumab for treating severe persistent allergic asthma (review of technology appraisal guidance 133 and 201). https://www.nice.org.uk/guidance/ta278 [accessed 22 March 2019].
NICE TA431 (2017) Mepolizumab for treating severe refractory eosinophilic asthma https://www.nice.org.uk/guidance/ta431 [accessed 22 March 2019].
NICE TA479 (2017) Reslizumab for treating severe eosinophilic asthma https://www.nice.org.uk/guidance/ta479 [accessed 22 March 2019].

3.2 Chronic obstructive pulmonary disease

COPD is an irreversible, or minimally reversible obstructive airway disease that responds partially, or not at all, to bronchodilators. It is a common progressive multifactorial disease that affects both the airway and lung parenchyma. It primarily affects smokers and has an element of genetic predisposition. Around 3 million people in the UK are thought to be affected, but only around a third possess a formal diagnosis, most not receiving this until their fifth decade. The prevalence increases with age and is thus growing worldwide.

Pathophysiology

COPD broadly affects the airways, from the large airways to bronchioles and down to the lung parenchyma itself. In the majority of cases, the effects are secondary to exposure of these areas to toxic stimuli (e.g. cigarette smoke, dusts, chemicals, or air pollution). In the large airways, mucus gland hyperplasia occurs with squamous metaplasia and loss of ciliary function (and the mucociliary escalator). In the medium and small airways, chronic inflammation and fibrosis occurs, and is primarily characterized by infiltration of CD8 lymphocytes, macrophages and neutrophils. In the lung parenchyma itself, emphysema occurs, which is characterized by alveolar wall destruction causing irreversible damage of end airspaces, and leading to loss in tissue elasticity and hyperinflation.

The key mechanisms involved in each of these lung damaging effects are thought to result from oxidative stress mechanisms, chronic inflammation, and protease–anti-protease enzyme imbalance, e.g. α1-antitrypsin deficiency, an autosomal recessive genetic risk factor that leads to accumulation in neutrophil elastase, responsible for the degradation of elastin, an essential protein in the connective tissue of lung parenchyma.

The three cell types that are predominant in COPD (neutrophils, macrophages, and lymphocytes) release numerous cytokines that perpetuate inflammation; neutrophils release IL-8 and leukotriene B4, recruiting more neutrophils to the area. Collectively, these neutrophils release proteolytic enzymes like elastase, proteinase 3, cathepsins, and matrix metalloproteinases (MMPs), which directly cause damage to the lung parenchyma. The macrophages release a number of cytokines, chemokines, and oxygen reactive species that activate MMPs, which are highly proteolytic. Furthermore, the lymphocytes, especially CD8+, release perforin and granzyme, which induce alveolar apoptosis.

Collectively, these processes result in mucus hypersecretion and ciliary dysfunction, airflow obstruction and hyperinflation, gas exchange abnormalities, pulmonary hypertension, and systemic effects. Each of these can thus pose as targets for pharmacological and non-pharmacological interventions in attempts to improve satisfactory gas exchange. In the case of antimucolytics, like **carbocisteine**, reduction in mucus viscosity can help reduce mucus plug formation and ease expectorating. Similarly, the use of bronchodilators, like β-adrenoceptor agonists, anticholinergics, and methylxanthines (phosphodiesterase inhibitors), can promote airway smooth muscle relaxation and thus ease expiration during tidal breathing, reducing airflow obstruction and easing hyperinflation.

For a full summary of the relevant pathways and drug targets, see Figure 3.4.

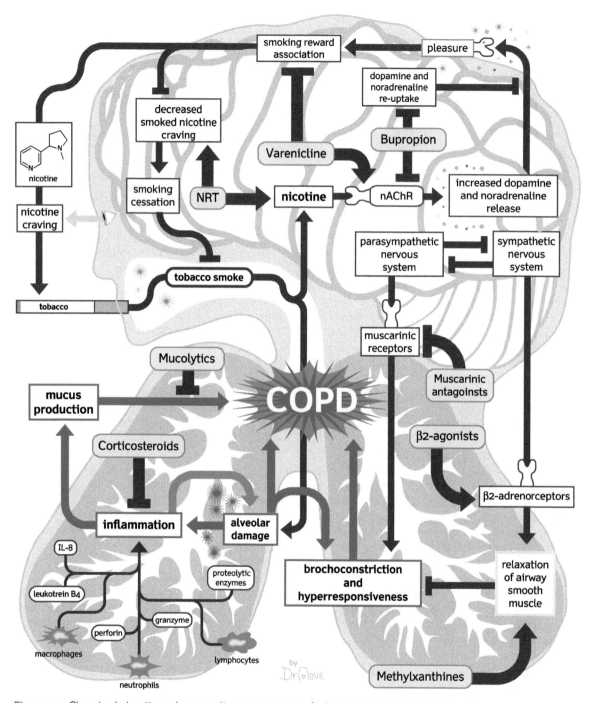

Figure 3.4 Chronic obstructive pulmonary disease: summary of relevant pathways and drug targets.

Management

COPD is a diagnosis based on clinical symptoms (dyspnoea, chronic cough/sputum production) confirmed with spirometry, and should be suspected in all smokers over 35. Diagnosis is confirmed by spirometry when FEV_1 (forced expiratory volume in 1 second)/FVC (forced vital capacity) <0.7, post-bronchodilator. Aside from a comprehensive history, additional investigations, such as reversibility testing with a short-acting bronchodilator or ECG, can exclude differentials such as asthma or cardiac causes of breathlessness (see Table 3.4).

Smoking is the primary cause of COPD, leading to irreversible structural damage, thereby accelerating the natural rate of decline in lung function. On stopping smoking, the rate of decline returns to that of a non-smoker, making smoking cessation a key factor in disease management, particularly in early disease. For more information on smoking cessation see Topic 10.4, 'Drug abuse, addiction, and dependency'.

Management of stable disease

Pharmacological management is advocated in patients experiencing breathlessness or exercise intolerance, and is based on severity of symptoms and the percentage of FEV_1 compared with predicted values, based on age, sex, and height (Table 3.5). Available treatment options are similar to those used in asthma; however, there are differences in choice hierarchy, as well as anticipated response (see Table 3.6). SABAs, or SAMAs are tried as a first line, on an 'as-required' basis in any patient with breathlessness or exercise intolerance; as unlike with asthma, the two show equal, albeit limited efficacy.

Patients that remain breathless or present with an $FEV_1 > 50\%$ of their predicted value, should be initiated on regular long-acting bronchodilator therapy, preferably a LAMA, or alternatively, a LABA, with additional inhaled corticosteroids (ICS) only in exacerbation. Patients escalated from a SAMA to a LAMA should have the former discontinued. At each stage, consideration should be

Table 3.4 Clinical features distinguishing asthma from COPD

Clinical feature	Asthma	COPD
Age of onset	Usually childhood, but can occur at any age	Usually >40 years of age
Pattern of respiratory symptoms	Symptoms vary over time, often limits activity. Usually triggered by exercise, emotions, dust/allergens	Chronic, often continuous symptoms, particularly during exercise. Have better/worse days
Lung function	Current and/or historical variable airflow limitation, e.g. BD reversibility	FEV_1 may improve with therapy, but post-BD FEV_1/FVC <0.7 persists
Lung function between symptoms	Can be normal between symptoms	Persistent air flow limitation
Past/family history	Commonly suffer allergies, personal/family history of asthma	History of exposure to noxious particles/gas (usually tobacco)
Time course	Often resolves spontaneously/with treatment. May result in fixed airflow limitation	Usually progresses slowly over years despite treatment
Chest X-ray	Usually normal	Severe hyperinflation and other changes of COPD
Exacerbations	Exacerbations occur, but risk significantly reduced with regular treatment	Exacerbations can be reduced by treatment. Co-morbidities where present can contribute to impairment
Typical airway inflammation	Eosinophils and/or neutrophils	Neutrophils in sputum, lymphocytes in airways, may have systemic inflammation

Adapted with permission from Global Initiative for Asthma: Diagnosis if Diseases of Chronic Airflow Limitation: Asthma, COPD and Asthma-COPD Overlap Syndrome (2015).

Table 3.5 Calculations for predicted FEV_1 and FVC

	Predicted FEV1	Predicted FVC
Male	$(0.043 \times height^*) - (0.029 \times age†) - 2.49$ (SD: ± 0.51 L)	$(0.0576 \times height^*) - (0.026 \times age†) - 4.34$ (SD: ± 0.61 L)
Female	$(0.0395 \times height^*) - (0.025 \times age†) - 2.60$ (SD: ± 0.38 L)	$(0.0443 \times height^*) - (0.026 \times age†) - 2.89$ (SD: ± 0.43 L)

*In cm; †in years.

given to choice of device and product license, with compliance assessed (both intentional and non-intentional) before escalation in the presence of persisting symptoms. Prescribers should be aware of the large and growing number of inhalers on the market, providing single and combination therapy treatment options in a wide range of inhaler devices with variations in licensed indications. As with all good prescribing practice a licensed product should always be selected in favour of a device used off-label. Furthermore, some devices may be unsuitable in certain patient groups, e.g. metered dose inhalers (MDIs) in patients unable to coordinate actuation with inhalation, or Turbohalers® in those with inadequate inspiratory flow.

Where patients remain symptomatic despite optimal inhaled therapy, add-on oral therapy may be of benefit with methylxanthines. Oral corticosteroids are generally reserved for use in acute exacerbations and, where possible, chronic use should be avoided due to

unacceptable toxicity. This may be unavoidable in end-stage disease where treatment cannot be withdrawn following an exacerbation. In this case, the lowest possible dose should be used and osteoporosis prophylaxis offered. In severe disease, long-term oxygen therapy (LTOT) may be considered in patients with severe resting hypoxaemia to improve survival.

Phosphodiesterase-4 inhibitors, like **roflumilast**, could also be used to reduce exacerbations for patients with chronic bronchitis, severe and very severe airflow limitation, and frequent exacerbations that are not well controlled by long-acting bronchodilators. It has recently been approved by NICE under the supervision of a specialist.

Management of acute exacerbations

In an acute exacerbation, bronchodilators in combination with corticosteroids form the mainstay of treatment. In less severe cases, patients may be treated at

Table 3.6 Management of COPD adapted from GOLD 2017

Group	Definition	Recommendation
Group A	≤1 exacerbation not leading to hospitalization mMRC* 0–1 and CAT <10†	Use of a bronchodilator (short- or long-acting based on symptoms)
Group B	≤1 exacerbation not leading to hospitalization mMRC ≥2 and CAT ≥10	LAMA (preferred) or LABA Escalate to LAMA + LABA
Group C	≥2 exacerbations or ≥1 leading to hospitalization mMRC 0–and CAT <10	LAMA Escalate to LAMA + LABA (preferred) or LABA + ICS
Group D	≥ 2 exacerbations or ≥ 1 leading to hospitalization mMRC ≥2 and CAT ≥10	LAMA Escalate to LAMA + LABA (preferred) or LABA + ICS Escalate to LAMA+ LABA + ICS Consider roflumilast

* mMRC, modified medical research council dyspnoea scale; † CAT, COPD assessment test.

Adapted with permission from the Global Strategy for the Diagnosis, Management and Prevention of COPD, Global Initiative for Chronic Obstructive Lung Disease (GOLD) 2017. Available from: https://goldcopd.org.

home, with some in possession of self-management plans and supplies of corticosteroids and antibiotics, to enable rapid response to symptoms. More severe cases or those unable to cope at home, will require hospitalization for management. Treatment options of acute exacerbations include:

- *Bronchodilators* are used at higher doses, administered via a hand-held inhaler or nebulizer, depending on severity of symptoms. Acutely unwell patients at risk of hypercapnic respiratory failure (see 'Prescribing warning: hypercapnic respiratory failure and oxygen-induced hypercapnia') should have air-driven nebulizer therapy (rather than oxygen-driven) with concurrent oxygen saturation monitoring. Patients failing to respond to inhaled bronchodilators may be managed with IV methylxanthines.

- *Corticosteroids* are recommended in all hospitalized patients and should be considered for those in the community in the event of an exacerbation. Treatment of choice is with oral prednisolone (30 mg) for 7–14 days. Courses beyond 14 days are unlikely to be of benefit, and are therefore not recommended. Patients requiring frequent courses of corticosteroids should be considered for osteoporosis prophylaxis.

- *Oxygen* therapy should be administered with care in patients with COPD, due to the increased risk of hypercapnia (see 'Prescribing warning: hypercapnic respiratory failure and oxygen-induced hypercapnia'). Acutely unwell patients require arterial blood gases prior to starting treatment and should be monitored using pulse oximetry. Treatment should be tailored to achieve an individualized target range.

- *Antibiotics* are recommended where the exacerbation is triggered by infection, i.e. an exacerbation with increased sputum volume or purulence. Empirical treatment should be initiated based on local guidelines, with either **amoxicillin**, macrolide, or **doxycycline** (see Topic 11.1, 'Bacterial infection').

Other treatment measures include non-invasive ventilation (NIV) or, in more severe cases, invasive ventilation. The respiratory stimulant **doxapram** is also an option on the rare occasion where NIV is unavailable or unsuitable.

PRESCRIBING WARNING

Hypercapnic respiratory failure and oxygen-induced hypercapnia

- Hypercapnia (elevated $PaCO_2$) is caused by increased CO_2 production and/or reduced elimination.

- Administration of uncontrolled oxygen in an acute exacerbation of severe COPD can induce hypercapnia, the mechanism of which is likely to be multifactorial:
  - Following oxygen administration there is an initial increase in minute ventilation, although this recovers and is only a small contributor to hypercapnia (reduced hypoxic drive was once thought to be the main cause).
  - Patients with COPD have an increased dead space due to a lower tidal volume/increased respiratory rate, leading to a ventilation/perfusion mismatch. This leads to reduced oxygen tension, normally compensated for by the release of local mediators, which act to induce pulmonary vasoconstriction. Administration of supplemental oxygen, however, increases oxygen tension, thus inhibiting pulmonary vasoconstriction. Ultimately, this leads to an increase in perfusion mismatch and dead space ventilation.
  - CO_2 is normally removed by deoxygenated haemoglobin. Administration of oxygen decreases the proportion of deoxygenated haemoglobin, thus reducing CO_2 clearance. Normally, this is accommodated for by an increase in minute ventilation, although patients with severe COPD are unable to achieve this.

Drug classes used in management

β_2-adrenoceptor agonists work via the direct relaxation of airway smooth muscle cells, thus acting as bronchodilators. They can be divided into short- or long-acting types, depending on the lipophilicity of each agent. Examples include salbutamol, terbutaline, salmeterol, formoterol, indacaterol, olodaterol, and vilanterol.

β₂-adrenoceptor agonists

Mechanism of action

For more details see Topic 3.1, 'Asthma'.

Prescribing

Short-acting β2-adrenoceptor agonists

SABAs have a rapid onset of action and are effective for acute symptom management in COPD. In addition to bronchodilation, they can increase mucociliary clearance and, with regular use, improve lung function and dyspnoea.

The preferred route of administration for **salbutamol** and **terbutaline** is via inhalation, at the same licensed doses as that used in asthma, although licensed devices may vary. In severe disease, nebulized therapy may be required for chronic treatment in patients that demonstrate an improvement in symptoms with its use, although consideration should be given to the provision of equipment and adequate support to ensure the nebulizer remains in good working order.

Long-acting β2-adrenoceptor agonists

LABAs (**salmeterol** and **formoterol**) have been shown to significantly improve lung function and overall health status. In addition, due to formoterol's fast onset of action, it can be used for both the relief of symptoms and maintenance medication in COPD.

Salmeterol and formoterol are available in a number of inhaler devices either alone or in combination with a corticosteroid (formoterol with **beclometasone**—Fostair®) or LAMA (e.g. formoterol with **aclidinium**—Duaklir®) for use in COPD. Care should be taken when prescribing combination products in COPD, as not all are licensed for this indication, e.g. Seretide®—where most strengths and devices are licensed for asthma only.

Indacaterol, **olodaterol**, and **vilanterol** the newer LABAs, are only indicated in the management of COPD either in single agent devices (except vilanterol), or in combination inhalers with corticosteroids or LAMAs. The long half-life of all three agents, enable OD dosing taken at the same time each day, and missed doses should be withheld until the following day.

Unwanted effects

See Topic 3.1, 'Asthma'.

Muscarinic antagonists

Anti-cholinergic agents decrease airway tone and improve expiratory flow limitation, hyperinflation, and exercise capacity in COPD patients. Examples include aclidinium, glycopyrronium bromide, ipratropium, tiotropium, and umeclidinium

Mechanism of action

In addition to the SAMA **ipratropium** (see Topic 3.1, 'Asthma'), the long-acting agents, **tiotropium**, **glycopyrronium bromide**, **aclidinium**, and **umeclidinium** also have a role to play in the management of COPD.

Like ipratropium, tiotropium, binds to all three receptor subtypes, but it has rapid dissociation constants from M2 receptors. The dissociation half-life from M3 receptors approaches 35 hours and has a terminal elimination half-life of 5–6 days, thus exerting a prolonged bronchodilatory effect.

Glycopyrronium bromide shows higher affinity for M3 than M2 receptors, and has a rapid onset of action. When delivered by inhalation, the device also promotes an extended duration of action by prolonging the half-life, thus retaining the active drug within the lung.

Umeclidinium is a further long-acting agent that like tiotropium, binds preferentially to M3 receptors. Its effects peak after about 3 hours and last for 24 hours enabling OD administration.

Aclidinium is selective for the M3 receptors, again with a long duration of action, albeit shorter than tiotropium and, therefore, best taken BD to ensure a sustained effect.

Prescribing

Short-acting muscarinic antagonists

Ipratropium is available in an inhaler or, in more severe symptoms, for nebulization in the management of COPD at the same doses as those used in the management of asthma.

Long-acting muscarinic antagonists

Tiotropium, **glycopyrronium bromide**, **aclidinium**, and **umeclidinium** are long-acting agents used solely in COPD, with little to distinguish between them clinically. All four agents are available in single agent devices or in combination with a LABA, in a variety of inhaler devices. Choice is determined by patient preference (based primarily on ability to use) and local availability. Patients started on a LAMA should have any SAMA therapy discontinued.

PRACTICAL PRESCRIBING

Tiotropium devices

- *HandiHaler®*: delivers a dose of 18 µg from a hard capsule, prescribed as a single dose OD as a dry powder device.
- *Respimat® device*: delivers a dose of 2.5 µg prescribed as two puffs (5 µg) OD in an inhaler device activated by pressing a button.

Unwanted effects

See Topic 3.1, 'Asthma'.

Corticosteroids

Glucocorticoids are the most potent of the anti-inflammatory agents used in the pharmacological control of airway disease. Examples inhaled include beclometasone, budesonide, fluticasone. Systemic examples include hydrocortisone and prednisolone.

Mechanism of action

See Topic 3.1, 'Asthma'.

Prescribing

Inhaled corticosteroids

Clinical trials investigating long-term treatment with high doses of inhaled glucocorticoids suggest that they do not arrest the progressive decline in lung function, even when treatment precedes symptomatic disease. There is, however, evidence to suggest that when used regularly in COPD patients with a $FEV_1 < 60$ predicted, they can improve symptoms, quality of life, and reduce the number of exacerbations. With long-term use, inhaled corticosteroids are associated with high prevalence of toxicity (oral candidiasis, hoarse voice, and skin bruising) so that use is increasingly reserved in those who have failed treatment with a LABA and LAMA.

Unlike with asthma, inhaled corticosteroids are only indicated in combination with a LABA, reflected in the availability of combination formulations only for use in COPD. Care should be taken when prescribing, as there are numerous combinations on the market with licensed indications that vary with inhaler strength and device.

Systemic corticosteroids

About 10% of patients with stable COPD have some symptomatic and objective improvement after oral glucocorticoids, although it is possible that they can have concomitant asthma, both being common diseases. There is also evidence to suggest that use in an acute exacerbation can reduce the rate of recurrent exacerbations in the following 30 days.

Systemic corticosteroids in COPD should be reserved for severe exacerbations, with courses restricted to 7–14 days, as longer courses are unlikely to be of benefit. Some patients, however, with end-stage disease, will require maintenance treatment to prevent relapse, bringing with it an increased risk of myopathy and respiratory failure.

Chronic users of oral therapy and high-dose inhaled therapy should be considered for osteoporosis prophylaxis. As with acute asthma management, **prednisolone** is preferred unless the oral route cannot be used, in which case **hydrocortisone** may be administered IV.

Unwanted effects

See Topic 3.1, 'Asthma'.

Methylxanthines/phosphodiesterase inhibitors

Theophylline is a non-selective phosphodiesterase inhibitor, acting as both a weak bronchodilator and respiratory stimulant. Examples include theophylline, aminophylline (non-selective), and roflumilast (phosphodiesterase-4 inhibitor)

Mechanism of action

See Topic 3.1, 'Asthma'.

Prescribing

Theophylline and **aminophylline** provide a useful oral option in patients where inhaled treatment is inadequate or unsuitable; however, as with asthma, use is restricted by the narrow therapeutic index and potential for toxicity. Doses are consistent with those used in asthma, adjusted according to response or to achieve a serum theophylline level of 10–20 µg/mL.

IV therapy is not commonly used in COPD, but may be of value in hospitalized patients who fail to respond adequately to nebulized bronchodilators. It is advisable to measure serum levels within 24 hours of initiation due to the high risk of toxic levels, particularly in patients on multiple drug therapy or those admitted on oral theophylline therapy.

Specific phosphodiesterase-4 inhibitors like **roflumilast** may also be an option in stable, but unresponsive COPD and has recently been advocated by NICE under specialist supervision.

Unwanted effects

See Topic 3.1, 'Asthma'.

Mucolytics

Mucolytics are classified as compounds with free sulphydryl groups that dissociate disulphide bonds and reduce the viscosity of mucus. Examples include carbocisteine, erdosteine, and mecysteine.

Mechanism of action

Although the facilitation of mucus clearance could provide some short-term relief, the effective long-term therapy of airway mucus hypersecretion in COPD is likely to demand more than just 'thinning' of mucus. Long-term benefit requires the reversal of the hypersecretory phenotype, which entails reducing the number of goblet cells and the size of the submucosal glands. This is not achieved with current anti-mucolytics.

Carbocisteine is a muco-active drug that has free radical scavenging and anti-inflammatory properties. Its mucolytic efficacy is related to its capacity to replace fucomucins by sialomucins, which reduces mucus viscosity.

Erdosteine is a thiol agent that has mucolytic activity due to a free sulphydryl group able to interact with the disulphide bridges of bronchial mucus. It also has antioxidant and anti-inflammatory activities.

Prescribing

Mucolytic therapy should be reserved for use in patients with chronic productive cough to reduce the viscosity of the sputum, and only continued where a trial of its use has demonstrated a symptomatic improvement. Of the available drugs **carbocisteine** tends to be most widely used, and is available in both capsule and liquid formulation. Doses are started higher and reduced as symptoms improve. Alternative agents include **mecysteine**, which is currently only marketed in the UK and, more recently, **erdosteine**. This latest addition to the class is only licensed for use in acute exacerbations, rather than for long-term use as the other agents are. Evidence of efficacy for this indication is inconclusive and it is therefore not generally advocated for use.

Unwanted effects

The mucolytics are well-tolerated and side effects rare. Some patients report GI effects and **erdosteine** has also been reported to cause headaches.

Further reading

Barnes PJ (2000) Chronic obstructive pulmonary disease. *New England Journal of Medicine* 343(4), 269–80.

Decramer M, Janssens W, Miravitlles M (2012) Chronic obstructive pulmonary disease *Lancet* 379(9823), 1341–51.

Hanania NA, Donohue JF (2007) Pharmacologic interventions in COPD: bronchodilators. *Proceedings of the American Thoracic Society* 4(7), 526–34.

MacNee W (2006) ABC of chronic obstructive pulmonary disease: pathology, pathogenesis, and pathophysiology. *British Medical Journal* 332(7551), 1202–4.

Yang IA, Ko FW, Lim TK, Hancox RJ (2013) Year in review 2012: asthma and chronic obstructive pulmonary disease. *Respirology* 18(3), 565–72.

Guidelines

Global Initiative for Asthma (2018) 2018 GINA Report, Global Strategy for Asthma Management and Prevention. https://ginasthma.org/gina-reports/ [accessed 29 March 2019].

Global Initiative for Chronic Obstructive Lung Disease (GOLD) Global strategy for the diagnosis, management and prevention of chronic obstructive pulmonary disease (2017). https://goldcopd.org/ [accessed 29 March 2019].

NHS Evidence (2012) Chronic obstructive pulmonary disease: Evidence Update. https://www.nice.org.uk/guidance/cg101/evidence

NICE CG115 (June 2010) Alcohol-use disorders: diagnosis, assessment and management of harmful drinking and alcohol dependence. https://www.nice.org.uk/guidance/cg115 [accessed 29 March 2019].

NICE Pathway Chronic obstructive pulmonary disease. https://pathways.nice.org.uk/pathways/chronic-obstructive-pulmonary-disease [accessed 29 March 2019].

NICE QS10 (July 2011) Chronic obstructive pulmonary disease in adults. https://www.nice.org.uk/guidance/qs10

NICE TA461 (2017) Roflumilast for treating chronic obstructive pulmonary disease https://www.nice.org.uk/guidance/ta461

Papi A, Rabe KF, Rigau D, et al. (2017) Management of COPD Exacerbations: An official ERS/ART Clinical practice guideline 2017. *European Respiratory Journal* 49, 1600791. https://www.thoracic.org/statements/resources/copd/mgmt-of-COPD-exacerbations.pdf [accessed 29 March 2019].

4 Endocrinology

4.1 The pituitary gland

The pituitary gland (hypophysis) is an endocrine organ located at the base of the skull in a bony recess, called the sella turcica, consisting primarily of an anterior (adenohypophysis) and posterior (neurohypophysis) lobe. Collectively, under the influence of the hypothalamus, these lobes control the hormone secretions responsible for growth, reproduction, behaviour/emotion, metabolism, and homeostasis, via a complex interplay of feedback loops. Dysfunction through failed synthesis of hormones, 'breaks' in the feedback pathways, or receptor malfunction can have diverse effects on plasma hormone levels and, hence, end organ function.

Pathophysiology

The *hypothalamus* is located within the base of the third ventricle in the diencephalon and is responsible for maintaining homeostasis, as well as influencing emotion and behaviour. It is linked to the pituitary gland, which sits outside the dura, via the pituitary stalk and the hypothalamic–hypophyseal portal system.

The *anterior pituitary lobe* makes up about 80% of the pituitary gland and is linked indirectly to the hypothalamus. It receives hormones released from neurosecretory cells in the paraventricular region of the hypothalamus, via a dense network of capillaries that make up the hypothalamic–hypophyseal portal system. These hormones subsequently bind to specific receptors on the pituitary cells to regulate a number of physiological processes including stress, growth, metabolism, reproduction, and lactation. There are six hormones released by the anterior pituitary—adrenocorticotropic hormone (ACTH), growth hormone (GH), thyroid-stimulating hormone (TSH), follicle-stimulating hormone (FSH)/luteinizing hormone (LH), and prolactin (PRH) (see Table 4.1).

The *posterior pituitary lobe* is controlled via axons and nerve terminals that extend down from the hypothalamus through the pituitary stalk and into the lobe, which subsequently releases neurohormones (oxytocin and vasopressin) into the blood stream (see Table 4.2). Vasopressin (also called antidiuretic hormone, ADH), is essential in maintaining fluid homeostasis to ensure adequate blood volume and salt concentration. Its release is modulated by osmoreceptors (rising osmolality) in the hypothalamus and baroreceptors (falling BP) in the cardiovascular system, and acts directly on the distal nephron to ensure water is conserved. Dysregulation of ADH may lead to conditions such as diabetes insipidus (DI) or SIADH (syndrome of inappropriate ADH).

Within the posterior pituitary lobe, oxytocin is stored packaged in vesicles bound to neurophysin I and is released under neural control from the hypothalamus. Oxytocin receptors are highly expressed in uterine and breast myometrial cells where, secondary to suckling response in feeding mothers, the hormone causes the 'let down' of milk to the sinuses, while also maintaining milk production. Cervical dilation also stimulates oxytocin release to cause uterine contraction in the latter stages of labour (hence, its historical use in the induction of labour).

Pituitary dysfunction results in disrupted downstream hormone levels, in either excess (hyperpituitarism) or deficiency (hypopituitarism), and can be the result of a number of causes including tumours, trauma, surgery, and inflammatory or vascular disorders. These endocrine disorders are generally classified according to the site of dysfunction, so that *primary disorders* occur as a result of abnormalities in the secreting target organ, e.g. thyroid (Topic 4.3, 'Thyroid disease'), adrenal gland (Topic 4.2, 'The adrenal gland'), *secondary disorders* refer to abnormalities of the pituitary per se and *tertiary disorders* defined as abnormalities of the hypothalamus (see Table 4.3).

Table 4.1 Hormones secreted by the anterior pituitary gland

Hormone	Release pattern	Upstream hormone/ neural	Target	Effect	Reference
Adrenocorticotropic hormone (ACTH)	Circadian rhythm. Peaks prior to waking	Corticotrophin-releasing hormone (CRH)	Adrenal gland	Glucocorticoid secretion (Cushing's disease)	Below and Topic 4.2, 'The adrenal gland'
Growth hormone (GH)	Short low-level pulses greater at night	GH-releasing hormone (GHRH) or GH inhibiting hormone (*somatostatin*)	Liver, adipose tissue, bone	On liver to release IGF-1 Muscle mass, bone mass, anabolic effects (lipolysis, gluconeogenesis, acromegaly)	Below
Thyroid-stimulating hormone (TSH)	10 pulses/ 24 hours night time peak	Thyrotropin-releasing hormone (TRH)	Thyroid gland	Thyroxine secretion	Topic 4.3, 'Thyroid disease'
Follicle-stimulating hormone (FSH)	Pulsatile	Gonadotropin-releasing hormone (GnRH)	Gonads	Germ cell maturation Initiate follicular growth	Topic 4.6, 'Female reproduction'
Luteinizing hormone (LH)	Pulsatile	Gonadotropin-releasing hormone (GnRH)	Gonads	Supports thecal cell hence androgens and oestradiol Supports Leydig cells hence testosterone	Topic 4.6, 'Female reproduction'
Prolactin hormone (PRH)	Bimodal Pulsatile-nocturnal peak		Ovaries Mammary glands	Lactation Weak gonadotroph (hyperprolactinaemia)	Below

'Hypo' pituitary function

Pituitary failure leading to a reduction in function typically occurs secondary to pituitary adenomas, which compress the normal tissues or obstruct blood flow to the gland itself. Less commonly, infection (e.g. meningitis), inflammation (e.g. haemochromatosis), vascular causes (e.g. Sheehan' syndrome), radiation, traumatic brain injury, or congenital gene mutation (e.g. transcription factor defects including Pit-1, PROP1, HESX1, LHX3, and LHX4) can affect pituitary function.

Hypopituitarism

Hypopituitarism is a condition where the gland fails to produce hormone or has insufficient upstream signalling, so that one or more hormones are deficient. Decreased secretion is generally a consequence of disrupted function, due to the presence of a tumour (non-functioning adenoma) or local trauma, e.g. following neurosurgery, infarction, radiation, infection, or brain injury. Congenital and genetic (e.g. PIT1, PROP1) causes of gland failure also occur.

Table 4.2 Posterior pituitary hormones and their actions

| Posterior pituitary gland | | | | | |
Hormone	Release pattern	Upstream hormone	Target	Effect	Reference
Vasopressin (ADH)	Circadian rhythm-highest at night	Neural synthesis and transport to PPG	Kidney collecting ducts Peripheral vasoconstriction Central	Conserve water Raise BP Drive thirst	Below
Oxytocin	Pulsatile	Neural synthesis and transport to PPG	Breast and uterine myometrial cells	Milk let down reflex, uterine contraction	Topic 4.6, 'Female reproduction'

Typically, it is the anterior pituitary cells that are affected and the hormones tend to fail in order of GH>FSH/LH>PRH>TSH>ACTH. This failure pattern is a gross simplification, but stems from the cellular lineage and structural organization within the anterior gland. Most patients are asymptomatic initially, but they may have progressive symptoms associated with specific or multiple hormone loss (e.g. GH-decreased muscle mass and fatigue, or TSH-hypothyroidism; see Topic 4.3, 'Thyroid disease'). As the pituitary adenoma expands, headaches, visual field defects, and nerve palsies may result. Sudden onset of ACTH deficiency and, hence, cortisol deficiency results in hypotension, hyponatraemia, and hypoglycaemia that can be life-threatening. Basal hormone levels may be diagnostic, but given the diurnal and pulsatile nature of some hormone release, dynamic tests may be required for particular hormone system identification (e.g. short Synacthen® test for adrenal insufficiency, insulin tolerance test for assessment of GH, and ACTH/cortisol reserve).

Table 4.3 Examples of primary, secondary, and tertiary causes of endocrine disease

	Examples
Primary	Grave's disease, Hashimoto's thyrotoxicosis
Secondary	Panhypopituitarism, acromegaly, Cushing disease, prolactinoma
Tertiary	Kallman's syndrome, hypothalamic failure (sarcoid/trauma)

Diabetes insipidus

There are two main types of DI:

- *cranial DI*: where there is failure of ADH release;
- *nephrogenic DI*: where kidneys are insensitive to ADH.

Central DI can be primary (idiopathic) disease or secondary to tumours, neurosurgery, or other causes of brain trauma. ADH is synthesized in the hypothalamus, transported to the posterior pituitary gland where its release is influenced by rising plasma osmolality, hypotension, and stress. Osmoreceptors are located in the hypothalamus and baroreceptors of the carotid sinus and aortic arch. Rising osmolality (higher concentrations) and/or falling BP leads to release of ADH so water is conserved and not lost through the collecting ducts of the kidney. This action via the kidney is mediated via V2 receptors where rising cAMP causes aquaporin-2 insertion to the apical membrane so water moves into the cells and is thus retained. Failure to secrete ADH results in an inability to concentrate urine so that large volumes of dilute urine can be lost (up to 20 L/day). This polyuria is commonly associated with polydipsia (chronic thirst), nocturia, and failure to thrive in children. Because of this symptom profile; diabetes mellitus, renal failure, and hypercalcaemia should be excluded prior to carrying out a 'water deprivation test' to investigate DI (see 'Management').

'Hyper' pituitary function

In general, excessive hormone production occurs in the presence of a 'functioning/secreting' adenoma.

These benign tumours secrete excessive levels of the same hormone produced by the cell from which they originate, independent of regulation by the hypothalamus. Adenomas occur most commonly in the anterior pituitary and can affect GH-producing cells (e.g. acromegaly), ACTH-producing cells (e.g. Cushing's syndrome), TSH-producing cells (hyperthyroidism), PRH-producing cells (causing galactorrhoea, infertility) and, less commonly, FSH/LH-producing cells (causing infertility).

Cushing's disease

Cushing's syndrome is a condition that may be caused by cortisol-like medications (called glucocorticoids) or by tumours, while Cushing's disease results from the excessive secretion of pituitary ACTH. These raised levels are produced by a pituitary ACTH-secreting adenoma and accounts for almost 70% of patients with Cushing's syndrome. The gene, ubiquitin-specific protease 8, has recently been found to be frequently mutated in Cushing's disease. For more information see Cushing's syndrome (Topic 4.2, 'The adrenal gland').

Hyperprolactinaemia

PRH is a 199 amino-acid polypeptide whose release, unlike the other anterior pituitary hormones, is under tonic inhibition from hypothalamic dopaminergic projections. PRH production can be stimulated by various factors: dopamine receptor antagonists, thyrotropin-releasing hormone (TRH), vasoactive intestinal peptide (VIP), and by suckling.

Oestrogens enhance release of PRH, so that during pregnancy the breasts are prepared for milk production, although the high levels of oestrogen and progesterone prevent lactation. The sudden drop in these two hormones during delivery allows PRH to initiate lactation (production), which is maintained with continued suckling via feedback from the nipple to hypothalamus. Abnormalities of PRH production is rare, but over secretion in the form of hyperprolactinaemia is relatively common with a prevalence of almost 0.4% in females. Hyperprolactinaemia is diagnosed when symptoms of amenorrhoea, oligomenorrhoea or galactorrhoea are seen in the presence of two raised serum PRH levels of >500 U/L (females) or >325 U/L (males). Physiological hyperprolactinaemia and symptoms/signs may be seen during pregnancy, but the most common abnormal cause is a secreting anterior pituitary adenoma that occurs in 20–50-year-old females. Other causes include drug-induced stimulation, such as with dopamine antagonists (e.g. phenothiazines,

butyrophenones, **metoclopramide**) or catecholamine depleting agents (e.g. **reserpine**), which can promote PRH release.

Symptoms can be accompanied by hypogonadism, as the high levels of PRH alter the pulsatile release of Gonadotropin-releasing hormone (GnRH), thus inhibiting LH and FSH release and impairing steroid production. Because of the effects that TRH has on the hypothalamus, around 40% of patients with hypothyroidism can have mildly elevated PRH levels, and, as such, TFTs should be performed given the subtleness of symptoms in hypothyroidism.

Acromegaly

Like many other pituitary abnormalities of hypersecretion, acromegaly is most often the result of an adenoma, but can rarely be seen in hypersecretion of hypothalamic GnRH or ectopic-releasing tumours (e.g. lung cancer and carcinoid). Numerous gene mutations have been linked to somatotroph (GH-secreting) adenomas, in particular a mutation in the guanine nucleotide stimulatory protein gene. Specific gene mutations can influence both tumour invasiveness and age of onset of acromegaly.

GH stimulates insulin-like growth factor (IGF-1, which acts at end-organ tissues to induce cell proliferation or to inhibit apoptosis. Clinical signs of acromegaly are therefore associated with IGF-1 production, giving rise to somatic (i.e. growth stimulation of tissue, skin, bone, enlarged jaw, osteoarthritis, etc.) and metabolic (increased gluconeogenesis, protein synthesis, and lipolysis) effects. Onset is insidious and affects multiple systems (see Table 4.4). Some patients present with local effects caused directly from tumour mass compression, giving rise to symptoms such as headache, visual field changes, or cranial nerve palsies.

Syndrome of inappropriate ADH

As outlined in diabetes insipidus, ADH is secreted from the hypothalamus via the posterior pituitary gland linked to osmoreceptors, where the sodium concentration per se and baroreceptors in the left atrium and aorta, where atrial pressure is detected have effects. In malignancy [e.g. lung (small cell), GI, lymphoma], pulmonary infections, CNS conditions (e.g. infection, trauma, haemorrhage, multiple sclerosis), and drugs [e.g. selective serotonin reuptake inhibitors (SSRIs), **amiodarone**, **carbamazepine**, **amitriptyline**, NSAIDs] inappropriate release of ADP can occur. This elevated level of ADH stimulates adenylate cyclase, and leads to increased intracellular cAMP and increased activity of aquaporin-2 channels in principal cells of the

Table 4.4 Characteristic signs/symptoms of acromegaly

	Organ/system	Symptoms/signs
Somatic	Skin	Hyperhidrosis, skin thickening
	Acral	Increased hand/foot size, frontal bossing, prominent nasolabial fold, enlarged jaw, coarsened facial features
	Soft tissue	Macroglossia, sleep apnoea (due to enlarged pharynx/larynx), carpal tunnel syndrome
	Bone/joints	Excessive growth/long bones in children. Arthropathy/joint pain in adults. Increased bone density
	Cardiovascular	Hypertension, congestive heart failure, cardiomyopathy
Metabolic/endocrine	Metabolic	Insulin resistance/DM
	Reproductive	Erectile dysfunction, amenorrhoea, infertility
	Thyroid	Goitre

apical membrane in the kidneys collecting ducts (Topic 5.1, 'The kidney, drugs, and chronic kidney disease'); this facilitates free water absorption, and subsequent concentration of urine, excess water intake resulting in hyponatraemia. Symptoms are very non-specific in mild SIADH, but may include nausea, vomiting, irritability, loss of appetite, and headache. Diagnosis is made by serum and urinary assessment of sodium and osmolality, and the identification of hypotonic (serum <280 mOsmol/kg, urine >100 mOsmol/kg) hyponatraemia (serum <135 mmol/L, urine >40 mmol/L). In asymptomatic patients with sodium ≥125 mmol/L fluid restriction and treatment of the underlying cause may be all that is required. However, in those with severe symptoms or sodium <125 mmol/L, hypertonic saline may be required acutely (in the emergency department) as this raises serum sodium by 8–10 mmol/L, lessening the possibility of acute neurological danger from hyponatraemia; central pontine myelinolysis (osmotic demyelination syndrome) may occur. In the chronic presentation, the mainstay of treatment is fluid restriction and hypertonic saline is rarely required, but this must be given under expert supervision, followed by the use of vasopressin receptor antagonists, such as non-selective **conivaptan**, for V1 and V2 receptors or **tolvaptan**, selective for V2. Serum sodium monitoring is required and the latter should not be used for greater than 30 days due to the risk of fatal liver injury.

For a full summary of the relevant pathways and drug targets, see Figure 4.1.

Management

'Hypo' pituitary function

In 'hypo' state, the general principles of management are in the identification and management of any underlying cause and, where necessary, the replacement of deficient pituitary or target organ hormones.

Hypopituitarism

Hypopituitarism is diagnosed through a combination of clinical history, MRI, and a series of hormone tests (see Table 4.5) to eliminate differentials and determine the underlying cause. The aim of treatment is to replace target hormones to normal endogenous levels (see Table 4.5), rather than the deficient pituitary hormone (except for GH). Doses of the replacement hormones require careful tailoring to patients needs with regular monitoring to assess whether target levels are being achieved.

Diabetes insipidus

DI should be considered in all patients presenting with polydipsia and polyuria (in excess of 3 L in 24 hours) who show signs of dehydration and an extended bladder. Primary investigations for DI should include serum biochemistry (U&Es, glucose) and measurement of plasma and urine osmolality, as well as a 24-hour urine collection (see 'Practical prescribing: water deprivation test/DDAVP

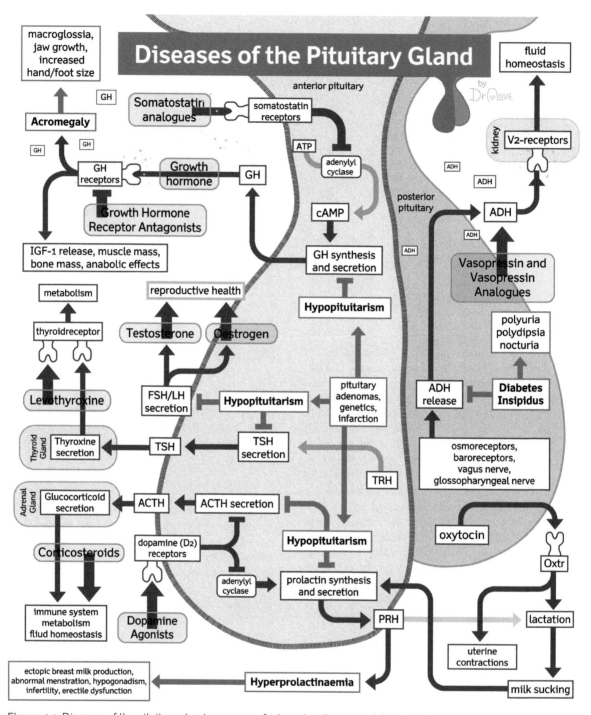

Figure 4.1 Diseases of the pituitary gland: summary of relevant pathways and drug targets.

Table 4.5 Deficient hormones, tests, and hormone replacement in hypopituitarism

Deficient pituitary hormone	Test	Replacement
Growth hormone	Insulin tolerance test (ITT)	Growth hormone
	Insulin-like growth factor (IGF1)	
Adrenocorticotrophic hormone (ACTH)	Short Synacthen® test	Hydrocortisone
	Basal cortisol level (09.00 hours)	
	ITT	
Thyroid-stimulating hormone	Thyroxine level	Levothyroxine
	TSH level	
Gonadotrophin	Luteinizing hormone (LH) level	Testosterone (men)
	Follicle-stimulating hormone (FSH) level	Oestrogen (women)
	Testosterone (men) level	
	Oestradiol (women) level	
Anti-diuretic hormone (ADH)	Water deprivation test	Desmopressin
Prolactin	Prolactin level	None

test'). Due to the risk of severe dehydration, the water deprivation test should only be carried out within a specialist service and patients closely monitored.

A full drug history can help to identify any drug-related causes of DI and, where possible, the causative agent discontinued (see Box 4.1).

Primary management of DI is to ensure adequate fluid intake and avoid dehydration, which in mild cases may be sufficient alone. In more severe cases of cranial DI however, replacement of **desmopressin** is necessary, taking care to avoid excessive use as this may lead to hyponatraemia. Patients will require U&Es repeated 1–3-monthly and some clinicians recommend omitting a dose

Box 4.1 Drugs known to cause diabetes insipidus

- Lithium
- Demeclocycline
- Amphotericin
- Gentamicin
- Colchicine
- Loop diuretics
- Foscarnet
- Ifosfamide
- Tenofavir

1 day a week to avoid hyponatraemia. Other less effective options for cranial DI include **carbamazepine** and thiazide diuretics.

In nephrogenic DI, the use of desmopressin is unlikely to be beneficial, except possibly at higher doses. Therefore, adequate hydration is the mainstay of treatment with regular follow-up to monitor for electrolyte disturbances. Some patients may benefit from treatment with thiazide diuretics or NSAIDs to reduce urine volume.

'Hyper' pituitary function

Management of hypersecretion of pituitary hormones requires hormone suppression either through surgery, radiation, or medication that inhibits hormonal activity.

Cushing's disease

Patients presenting with Cushingoid characteristics [i.e. mnemonic: cataracts, ulcers, skin (striae, thinning, bruising), Hypertension/ hirsutism/ hyperglycaemia, infections, necrosis, glycosuria, osteoporosis/obesity, immunosuppression, diabetes] require investigation to distinguish pituitary-related disease from other causes. This is achieved through a series of blood tests looking at baseline ACTH levels and serum potassium, in conjunction with a high-dose **dexamethasone** suppression test. An MRI can help confirm the presence of an adenoma, in combination with biochemical investigation. Primary management of Cushing's disease is trans-sphenoidal surgery to remove the adenoma, although with unresectable/residual disease radiotherapy or medical management may be appropriate (see Topic 4.2, 'The adrenal gland').

Hyperprolactinaemia

Hyperprolactinaemia can be diagnosed from a single serum prolactin level above the normal range, with additional investigations to identify any underlying cause, including drug history and an MRI (to identify any mass in the hypothalamic–pituitary region). In general, drug-induced hyperprolactinaemia in symptomatic patients is best managed by discontinuing or substituting the drug most likely to be the cause (see Table 4.6), although in the case of anti-psychotics, management decisions should be made in consultation with their psychiatrist. Repeat prolactin levels should be done 3 days after discontinuation. **Oestrogen** or **testosterone** therapy may be necessary in patients with a resultant hypogonadism and when hyperprolactinaemia persists, a dopamine agonist considered.

If the adenoma is small, symptoms are not troublesome, and there are no central mass effects, the pathology can be managed by judicious monitoring. Dopamine agonists form the mainstay treatment in symptomatic patients with prolactinomas, ideally with **cabergoline** to promote tumour shrinkage and a fall in prolactin levels. Doses may need to be escalated in non-responders and, very rarely, surgery may be considered for last-line management. Pharmacological treatment is continued long-term, but may be gradually withdrawn once patients demonstrate a resolution of prolactin levels and tumour shrinkage on MRI.

Acromegaly

Due to the pulsatile nature of GH release, random levels are not diagnostic and a dynamic evaluation, such as the glucose tolerance test should be performed. In normal circumstances, glucose suppresses GH levels, although failure to do so and the presence of a raised IGF-1 is diagnostic of acromegaly. An MRI scan is used to identify the presence of an adenoma.

Management of acromegaly aims to reduce GH levels (ideally, to less than 2.5 µg/L) either by pituitary surgery, medical treatment, or radiotherapy, as well as management of any complications (cardiovascular, endocrine, respiratory, and metabolic) associated with an increased risk of mortality (including screening for bowel cancer). A cure is defined as an IGF-1 within the normal age-adjusted limits and a random GH level of less than 1 µg/L. Trans-sphenoidal surgery to remove the adenoma is considered

Table 4.6 Examples of drugs known to cause hyperprolactinaemia (Torre, 2007)

Class	Likely stimuli	Examples
Benzodiazepines	GABA	Alprazolam
SSRI anti-depressants	Serotonin	Most likely with paroxetine
MAOIs	Unknown	Tranylcypromine
Tricyclic antidepressants	Serotonin, (mild)	Amitriptyline, clomipramine, desipramine
H2 receptor antagonists	Serotonin/dopamine	Cimetidine, rarely rantidine
Prokinetics	Dopamine (potent)	Domperidone, metoclopramide
Anti-hypertensives	Mixed	Methyldopa, labetalol (IV not PO), verapamil
Oral contraceptives	Dopamine	Oestrogen and progestogen
Opiates	Dopamine/unknown	Morphine
Atypical anti-psychotics	Dopamine	Risperidone, amisulpride
Typical anti-psychotics	Dopamine (common)	Haloperidol, chlorpromazine, thioridazine

Data from Torre, D. L., Falorni, A. Pharmacological causes of hyperprolactinaemia. *Ther Clinl Risk Manag* 3 (5) 929–951.

first-line treatment and should only be carried out by a suitably experienced surgeon.

Medical management is generally reserved for patients unsuitable for surgery or post-operatively in the presence of residual disease. Treatment options include somato-statin analogues (SSAs), e.g. **lanreotide/octreotide**, dopamine agonists or GH antagonists, of which SSAs are preferred, having demonstrated efficacy in reducing IGF-1/GH and to a lesser extent tumour size. Long-term treatment (10 years) can result in GH levels less than 2.5 ng/mL and a normal IGF-1 level in 70% of patients.

GH receptor analogues (**pegvisomant**) provide a second-line option in patients failing to respond to max-imum SSA therapy, either alone or in combination with an SSA. Due to their limited efficacy, dopamine agonists are reserved as a last-line option, possibly in combination with an SSA. As the only oral treatment option, they may be used infrequently in patients unwilling to have parenteral therapy, either for primary treatment or post-operatively.

Drug classes used in management

Growth hormone

The growth hormone is a single-chain polypeptide synthesized and secreted by somatotropic cells in the anterior pituitary gland that can stimulate growth and other metabolic processes in the body. Examples include recombinant human GH (somatotropin)

Mechanism of action

GH secretion is stimulated by GH-releasing hormone and inhibited by somatostatin. The receptor for the GH (GHR) is a type I cytokine receptor that uses the JAK (Janus kinase)/STAT (signal transducers and activators of tran-scription) signalling pathway.

The GHR is expressed as a monomer that forms a ligand-receptor complex made up of one GH molecule and two GHRs. The traditional model for GHR activation indicates that GH binding induces receptor dimerization leading to JAK/STAT signalling by transactivation. A more recent model suggests that GH binds to a constitutively homodimerized GHR, causing repositioning of the intracellular domain and activation of associated transduction pathways.

GHRs are present in many biological tissues and cell types, including bone, kidney, adipose, muscle, eye, brain, heart, hepatic, and immune tissue. A significant effect of GHR activation is the promotion of postnatal longitudinal growth, but it has also been associated with alterations in lipids, carbohydrate, nitrogen, and mineral metabolism. Other effects include adipocyte differentiation, immune system development, and various activities on the func-tion of the brain and cardiac system.

Prescribing

The synthetic GH, **somatotropin**, is identical to the en-dogenous GH excreted into the blood by somatotrope cells in the anterior pituitary gland. It is advocated by NICE for use in patients with GH deficiency (peak less than 9 mU/L, following an insulin tolerance test), already receiving treatment for other pituitary hormone deficien-cies, where quality of life is impaired. It is available in numerous injectable devices, designed to promote ease of administration, with selection based on patient pref-erences. Doses are started low and slowly titrated up to establish the lowest effective dose, to a maximum of 1 mg daily. Doses should be reviewed regularly as dose re-ductions may be necessary with increasing age. Patients failing to show an improved quality of life after 9 months should have treatment discontinued. In paediatrics, growth hormone is also used to achieve peak bone mass.

Unwanted effects

Toxicity to GH treatment more commonly includes local re-actions at the site of injection, as well as muscle pain/stiff-ness and the formation of antibodies. Other side effects related to its endocrine action include hypothyroidism, as GH increases conversion of T_4 to T_3. It is therefore advis-able to monitor thyroid function while on treatment, par-ticularly in those with a predisposition for hypothyroidism, such as in hypopituitarism. GH may also impair insulin sensitivity, thereby increasing the risk of DM or hypergly-caemia, and this again requires close monitoring.

The use of GH can promote tumour growth and is therefore contraindicated in the presence of a malignancy while being treated. Somatotropin should also be discontinued in acute critical illness, such as following major surgery or in acute re-spiratory failure, as there is an increased risk of mortality.

Aside from the effects on **levothyroxine** and **insulin**, clinically significant interactions with **somatotropin** are unlikely, despite reports that it may enhance clearance of drugs excreted via the CYP 3A4 enzyme.

Corticosteroids

> Corticosteroids produce their effect by activating corticosteroid receptors that are able to regulate the expression of key target genes. For example, hydrocortisone and prednisolone.

Mechanism of action

See Topic 6.6, 'Inflammatory bowel disease'.

Levothyroxine

> L-thyroxine (LT_4) is a synthetic form of the primary secretory product of the thyroid gland, 3,5,3',5'-tetraiodothyronine (T_4). Its administration can closely mimic glandular secretion and its conversion to T_3 can be appropriately regulated by tissue.

Mechanism of action

The peripheral deiodination of **levothyroxine**, either synthetic or endogenous forms, produces triiodothyronine (T_3), which can exert a broad spectrum of stimulatory effects on cell function and metabolism through its binding to thyroid hormone receptors. By acting as a replacement for the endogenous thyroxine, it relieves the symptoms of thyroxine deficiency, which include lack of energy, weight gain, hair loss, higher sensitivity to cold, and dry thick skin.

See Topic 4.3, 'Thyroid and Disease'.

Prescribing

See Topic 4.3, 'Thyroid and Disease'.

Unwanted effects

See Topic 4.3, 'Thyroid and Disease'.

Testosterone

> Testosterone is a steroid hormone from the androgen group, primarily secreted by the testes, ovaries, and adrenal glands. Used as hormone replacement therapy, it interacts with the endogenous androgen receptor stimulating metabolism and growth.

Mechanism of action

Testosterone, a member of the steroid hormone receptor family of molecules, is an endogenous ligand that is released in response to LH/FSH gonadotropic hormones stimulation on the testis. Low testosterone levels stimulate the hypothalamus to secrete gonadotrophin-releasing hormone, which in turn stimulates the release of FH/LSH from the anterior pituitary.

Testosterone binds to the ligand-binding domain on androgen receptors (AR), one of four main functional domains, which in turn induces a conformational change in the receptor. This leads to dimerization of two ARs, which subsequently translocate to the nucleus. In the nucleus, the ligand–receptor complex binds to promoter regions regulating the transcription of hormone-responsive genes that mediate the androgen effects. The molecular effects are dependent on a DNA binding domain, which is highly conserved among steroid hormone receptors.

For more information see Topic 4.7, 'Androgens and Steroids'.

Prescribing

Testosterone replacement in deficient males can be achieved through various methods of administration most often depot injection or gels (other routes include implants, capsules, injections, buccal tablets and patches). See Topic 4.7, 'Androgens and Steroids'.

Unwanted effects

See Topic 4.7, 'Androgens and Steroids'.

Oestrogen

> The oestrogen steroid hormones act on the oestrogen receptors, which are ligand-activated transcription factors that can regulate the activity of specific genes.

Mechanism of action

Conventionally associated with female reproduction, oestrogens are mostly produced in the ovary and testis in response to FSH stimulation, released from the anterior pituitary. Significant roles have also been observed for oestrogens in the male reproductive tissue, bone tissue, and the cardiovascular, immune, and central nervous system.

The oestrogen receptor (OR) has a highly conserved DNA-binding domain containing two zinc fingers, which is also involved in receptor dimerization. The ligand-binding domain is less conserved and also contains regions for receptor dimerization, nuclear localization, and interactions with co-activators and co-repressors of transcription. There are two functionally distinct oestrogen receptors, identified as ORα and ORβ, which have different tissue distributions and ligand activation properties.

See Topic 4.6, 'Female Reproduction', for further information

Prescribing

Hypogonadism in women is managed with oestrogen replacement, in combination with progesterone if the woman/girl has an intact uterus. The aim of treatment is to reduce symptoms (flushing, vaginal dryness, reduced libido, mood changes, etc.) and morbidity associated with oestrogen deficiency, e.g. loss of bone mass, increased risk of cardiovascular mortality/morbidity, and impaired cognition. Treatment strategy will depend on age of onset and symptoms, and can be delivered in numerous ways according to patient preference, i.e. tablets, patches, injections, implants, and gels.

In women over 50 in particular, oestrogen therapy is associated with an increased risk of breast, and to a lesser extent, endometrial and ovarian cancer. There is also a marginal increase in the risk of a VTE, DVT, stroke, or coronary heart disease, compared with the untreated population. The decision to replace in these women will therefore require an assessment of any underlying risk factors weighed up against the benefits of treatment (see Topic 4.6, 'Female reproduction').

Unwanted effects

Common side effects associated with oestrogen therapy aside from GI toxicity (nausea, vomiting, bloating, cramps), include breast enlargement/tenderness, altered libido, mood changes, depression, and headache. Sodium and water retention is also common, as is glucose intolerance and an altered lipid profile. For further information see Topic 4.6, 'Female reproduction'.

Vasopressin and vasopressin analogues

The neurohypophysial hormone arginine vasopressin (AVP) can regulate various physiological processes through binding to three distinct AVP receptors, all of which are part of a family of heptahelical transmembrane guanine nucleotide-binding protein coupled receptors. For example, desmopressin and vasopressin.

Mechanism of action

The regulatory roles of AVP include a wide range of physiological processes, such as renal water absorption, cardiovascular homeostasis, hormone secretion from the anterior pituitary, and regulation of emotional status.

The receptors V_{1a} and V_{1b} interact with the Gq protein to enhance the exchange of guanine nucleotides from GDP to GTP and couple to the phospholipase C (PLC) pathway, while V_2 receptors couple to the Gs and adenylate cyclase-signalling molecules. These, in turn, cause changes in several intracellular messengers, including cAMP, Ca^{2+}, inositol triphosphate, and diacylglycerol, depending on the type of cells and tissue targeted.

AVP and related peptides are strong vasoconstrictors in many vascular tissues. Feedback signals from the periphery on blood osmolarity and vascular tone are integrated in the AVP neurons to regulate hormone secretion from the posterior pituitary. Beyond its actions on the periphery, AVP also regulates cardiovascular homeostasis by acting on the baroreflex centre. In the kidney, AVP mainly contributes to the maintenance of body fluid homeostasis via the regulation of water, urea and ion transport, glomerular filtration rate, and renal blood flow.

Prescribing

Although both **vasopressin** and its analogue **desmopressin** are licensed for use in the management of diabetes insipidus, desmopressin is generally favoured, due to its longer duration of action and greater choice with regards to route of administration (sublingual, oral, intranasal, IM, and SC). Desmopressin is also used in the 'water deprivation test' to differentiate the underlying cause of diabetes insipidus i.e. cranial from nephrogenic (see 'Practical prescribing: water deprivation test/desmopressin test'). Where used for treatment, doses are started low and gradually increased to enable adequate diuresis at the minimum dose.

PRACTICAL PRESCRIBING

Water Deprivation Test/desmopressin Test

A water deprivation test is used to distinguish DI from other causes of polydipsia:

- From 08:30 hours only dry food is allowed, no fluids.
- At hourly intervals patients are weighed and a urine sample collected and tested for volume and osmolality. Bloods are also taken to check serum osmolality.
- In diabetes insipidus serum osmolality will increase and urine osmolality will remain low <300 mOsm/L as there is insufficient ADH to concentrate urine.

Desmopressin test will distinguish cranial from nephro-genic DI:

- desmopressin administered followed by further hourly urine collections and blood tests.
- In cranial DI patients serum and urine osmolality will normalize (293 and >750 mOsm/kg, respectively).

Unwanted effects

Desmopressin treatment requires careful monitoring to prevent hyponatraemia and fluid retention. In some instances, patients are advised to omit doses on a weekly basis to prevent this and, in all cases, patients require U&Es checked at regular intervals. Patients should be advised to seek help if they demonstrate symptoms of hyponatraemia, i.e. headaches, vomiting, weight gain, and, in severe cases, convulsions.

Treatment should be used with caution in patients with renal impairment, cardiovascular disease or other patients in whom the risk of fluid retention is high or the consequences severe, e.g. raised intracranial pressure. Where treatment is deemed necessary, care should be taken to restrict fluid intake and patients monitored closely.

Somatostatin analogues

Somatostatin analogues acting on the anterior pituitary gland mimic the physiological inhibitory action of somatostatin on GH secretion. For example, lanreotide and octreotide.

Mechanism of action

There are two biologically active forms of somatostatin that exist in the circulation and can act via seven subtypes of transmembrane G protein–coupled somatostatin receptor. The human pituitary gland expresses mostly SST1, SST2, SST3, and SST5 receptors. The patterns of activation of cellular pathways arising from these receptors can overlap, and include inhibition of adenylyl cyclase and activation of phosphotyrosine phosphatase (PTP) activity. Activation of somatostatin receptors can also couple to inward rectifying K^+ channels, voltage-dependent Ca^{2+} channels, and phospholipase C and A_2. The inhibition of secretion is normally linked to the inhibitory effects on adenylate cyclase activity and Ca^{2+}

influx, while the activation of PTP has a role in the regulatory actions that somatostatin has on the proliferation of cells.

The SST2 and SST5 somatostatin receptors are the most relevant in the inhibition of GH secretion by somatostatin. The somatostatin analogue **octreotide** is a long-acting octapeptide that binds to somatostatin receptors and mimics the effects of the endogenous hormone. **Lanreotide**, another synthetic analogue, has a longer half-life compared with endogenous somatostatin.

Prescribing

Octreotide, and the less frequently used **lanreotide**, are licensed for use in the management of acromegaly in patients unsuitable for surgery or in those where surgery alone has been insufficient to manage their symptoms. Doses are started low and gradually titrated until patients demonstrate a response without unacceptable side effects. Those that fail to respond within 3 months should have treatment discontinued. Once an effective treatment dose has been established, patients may be switched from standard preparations to depot injections, enabling less frequent injections (2–4-weekly as opposed to daily). Doses can be administered by IM, SC, or deep SC injection.

Where a depot preparation is being used presurgery, the last dose should be administered 3–4 weeks beforehand. There is some evidence to suggest that pre-operative use of octreotide may improve surgical outcome.

Unwanted effects

The most common side effects reported with the SSAs are GI and include abdominal discomfort, nausea, vomiting, diarrhoea, steatorrhoea, and constipation. These effects may be partly reduced by not taking short-acting preparations at mealtimes.

Like somatostatin, SSAs have an inhibitory effect on gallbladder motility, bile acid secretion, and bile flow, so that long-term use can cause gallstones. It is therefore recommended that an ultrasound scan be carried out prior to starting treatment and repeated every 6–12 months.

Somatostatin and its analogues also have an inhibitory effect on glucagon, GH, and to a lesser extent insulin, leading to impaired glucose control, particularly post-prandial. As a result, diabetic control may be affected leading to reduced insulin or oral hypoglycaemic requirements.

Other common adverse effects include impaired thyroid function and local reactions at the site of injection, although any redness and swelling generally resolves within 15 minutes.

Drug interactions

Aside from the effects of somatostatin analogues on insulin and oral hypoglycaemics, there are few known clinically significant drug interactions. Caution is advised with concomitant administration of **ciclosporin**, as both **lanreotide** and **octreotide** can increase ciclosporin levels.

Dopamine agonists

Dopaminergic agonists act on D_2 receptors located in the anterior pituitary gland and promote the inhibition of prolactin secretion. Examples include cabergoline, bromocriptine, and quinagolide.

Mechanism of action

Dopamine receptors are part of the family of seven transmembrane domain G protein–coupled receptors that, beyond their CNS functions, play numerous roles in the periphery, including the modulation of the endocrine system. Structural and functional analysis separates dopamine receptors into D_1-like, including D_1 and D_5 receptors, which usually mediate stimulatory functions, and D_2-like, including D_2–D_4 receptors, normally linked with inhibitory roles.

D_2 dopamine receptors are located in the anterior lobe of the pituitary gland, expressed mainly in lactotrope cells, but also in non-lactotrope cell populations. D_2 receptors in particular have also been found in the intermediate zone of the pituitary gland. Although D_4 dopamine receptors are present in the pituitary gland, too, their physiological role is unknown. The major role of D_2 dopaminergic receptors in the pituitary gland is the inhibitory control of prolactin synthesis and secretion, together with the growth of lactotrope cells. They do this by inhibition of adenylyl cyclase activity, reduction in intracellular cAMP concentrations and blockade of IP_3-dependent release of Ca^{2+} from intracellular stores. Reductions in intracellular Ca^{2+} may also occur after inhibition of Ca^{2+} influx through voltage-operated Ca^{2+} channels.

Cabergoline and **bromocriptine** are ergot alkaloid derivatives with potent dopaminergic activity, capable of activating D_2 receptors. They can inhibit prolactin secretion and are used to treat dysfunctions associated with hyperprolactinemia. **Quinagolide** is a non-ergot-derived dopamine agonist, structurally similar to **apomorphine**.

It has also been established that dopamine receptors, mainly of the D_2 type, are present in the majority of corticotrope pituitary tumours. In this case, dopaminergic agents can inhibit the secretion of ACTH, suggesting a physiological role in the capacity to regulate the release of ACTH. Like somatostatin analogues, the dopamine agonists can also inhibit GH secretion in pituitary tumours via the binding to D_2 receptors, albeit with inferior efficacy.

Prescribing

Dopamine agonists are indicated for use in prolactinomas and to a lesser extent in the management of acromegaly. All three drugs (**cabergoline**, **bromocriptine**, and **quinagolide**) are licensed for use in supressing lactation and hyperprolactinaemia, although cabergoline has the advantage of being administered once weekly compared with bromocriptine, which may be administered up to four times a day.

The role of dopamine agonists in acromegaly is less convincing and, although only bromocriptine is licensed for this indication, evidence suggests that cabergoline is the only dopamine agonist to be effective.

Unwanted effects

The side effect profile to the ergot alkaloids, **cabergoline** and **bromocriptine** are similar, although patients intolerant of one may get on better with the other. As doses used in hyperprolactinaemia are considerably lower than that used in Parkinson's disease, the risk of side effects are also reduced. The use of either, however, should be avoided in patients hypersensitive to ergot alkaloids or with an underlying valvulopathy. The ergot alkaloids can cause fibrotic reactions affecting the lungs, pericardium, and retroperitoneal. Patients should be advised of the risks and counselled to report symptoms such as dyspnoea, persistent cough, chest pain, and loin/ flank pain. Any evidence of valvulopathy may warrant investigation of cardiac by echocardiography and repeated at 6-monthly intervals.

Although more common with the ergot alkaloids, nausea, and vomiting can occur with all dopamine agonists (i.e. the non-ergot **quinagolide**), as can other GI effects such as pain, constipation, diarrhoea, and dyspepsia. Central effects also occur frequently, leading to confusion, dizziness, headaches, and insomnia. Hypotension is most likely on initiation.

Drug interactions

Predictably, the use of dopamine antagonist such as **metoclopramide** or **domperidone** will antagonize the effects of dopamine agonists and should be avoided. Concurrent use with other drugs known to cause hypotension, may aggravate the hypotensive effects of dopamine agonists.

Growth hormone receptor antagonists

GHR antagonists were developed by specific modifications of GH structure and are currently used for the treatment of clinical conditions resulting from elevated GH, such as acromegaly. For example, pegvisomant.

Mechanism of action

The drug **pegvisomant** was developed as a GH analogue with various amino acid substitutions to prevent agonist activity. The further addition of polyethylene glycol, a reagent that selectively conjugates to primary amino groups, significantly increased the half-life.

The GH antagonists do not prevent dimer formation and internalization, but it is presumed that they inhibit the 'correct' or functional activation of the GHR by sterically inhibiting conformational changes within the complex.

Prescribing

Pegvisomant provides an alternative treatment to somatostatin analogues in the medical management of acromegaly, i.e. in patients where response to surgery and radiotherapy is inadequate. Although available for use as monotherapy, it is safe and more effective in combination with an SSA, particularly in reducing tumour size. Pegvisomant is administered SC, OD with doses gradually increased according to response.

Unwanted effects

On the whole, **pegvisomant** is well tolerated, the most commonly reported adverse effect being deranged LFTs, which tend to be transient, although LFTs should be monitored 4–6-weekly for the first 6 months. Other common side effects include GI (nausea, diarrhoea, constipation),

weight gain, and neurological effects, such as headaches and dizziness.

As pegvisomant monotherapy has no effect on reducing tumour size, patients should be closely monitored for evidence of tumour growth requiring further treatment.

> **PRESCRIBING WARNING**
>
> **Effect of pegvisomant on female fertility**
> - The inhibitory effect of pegvisomant on IGF-1 may help to restore fertility in female patients previously unable to conceive.
> - Patients should there be advised of the possibility and the need for contraception where appropriate.

Drug interactions

As a GH receptor antagonist, **pegvisomant** increases insulin sensitivity so that patients with DM may require dose reductions in their insulin or oral hypoglycaemic therapy.

Further reading

Bhasin S, Cunningham GR, Hayes FJ, et al. (2010) Testosterone therapy in men with androgen deficiency syndromes: an Endocrine Society Clinical Practice Guideline. *Journal of Clinical Endocrinology and Metabolism* 95(6), 2536–59.

Cozzi R, Montini M, Attanasio R, et al. (2006) Primary treatment of acromegaly with octreotide LAR: a long-term (up to nine years) prospective study of its efficacy in the control of disease activity and tumor shrinkage. *Journal of Clinical Endocrinology and Metabolism* 91(4), 1397–140.

Giagulli VA, Triggiani V, Corona G, et al. (2011) Evidence-based Medicine update on testosterone replacement therapy (TRT) in male hypogonadism; focus on new formulations. *Current Pharmaceutical Design* 17(15), 1500–11.

Manjila S, Osmond C, Wu BA, et al. (2010) Pharmacological management of acromegaly: a current perspective. *Neurosurgery Focus* 29(4), E14.

Madsen M, Poulseb PL, Orskov H, et al. (2011) Cotreatment with pegvisomant and a somatostatin analogue in SA-responsive acromegalic patients. *Journal of Clinical Endocrinology and Metabolism* 96(8), 2405–13.

Makaryus AN, McFarlane SI (2006) Diabetes insipidus: diagnosis and treatment of a complex disease. *Cleveland Clinical Journal of Medicine* 73(1), 65–71.

Melmed S (2006) Acromegaly. *New England Journal of Medicine*, **355**, 2558–73.

Melmed S, Casanueva FF, Hoffman AR, et al. (2011) Diagnosis and treatment of hyperprolactinaemia: an Endocrine Society Clinical Practice Guideline. *Journal of Clinical Endocrinology and Metabolism*, 96(2), 273–88.

Neggers SJ, Van der Lely AJ (2011) Combination treatment with somatostatin analogues and pegvisomant in acromegaly. *Growth Hormone and IGF Research* 21(3), 129–33.

Prabhakar VKB, Shalet SM (2006) Aetiology, diagnosis and management of hypopituitarism in adult life. *Postgraduate Medicine* 82, 259–66.

Torre DL, Falorni A (2007) Pharmacological causes of hyperprolactinaemia. *Therapy and Clinical Risk Management* 3(5), 929–51.

Warrell DA, Cox TM, Firth JD (Eds) (2012) Endocrine disorders. In: *Oxford Textbook of Medicine*, Section 13, 5th edn. Oxford: Oxford University Press.

Wass JA, Karavitaki N (2009). Nonfunctioning pituitary adenomas: the Oxford experience. *Nature Review: Endocrinology* 5, 519–22.

Guidelines

Katznelson L, Atkinson JLD, Cook DM, et al. (2011) American Association of Clinical Endocrinologists medical guidelines for clinical practice for the diagnosis and treatment of acromegaly 2011 Update. *Endocrine Practice* 17(Suppl. 4), 1–44. https://www.aace.com/files/acromegaly-guidelines.pdf [accessed 25 March 2019].

Melmed S, Colao A, Barkan A et al. (2009) Guidelines for acromegaly management; an update (consensus statement). *Journal of Clinical Endocrinology and Metabolism* 94, 1509–17. http://www.seen.es/docs/apartados/815/Guidelines%20for%20acromegaly%20management%20JCEM%202009.pdf [accessed 25 March 2019].

Melmed S, Casanueva FF, Hoffman AR, et al. (2011) Diagnosis & treatment of hyperprolactinemia: an Endocrine Society Clinical Practice Guideline. *Journal of Clinical Endocrinology and Metabolism* 96(2), 273–88. https://academic.oup.com/jcem/article/96/2/273/2709487 [accessed 29 March 2019].

4.2 The adrenal gland

The adrenal glands are endocrine organs situated at the superior pole of the kidneys, composed of two parts—the inner medulla and an outer cortex. The *medulla* is made up of chromaffin cells that store adrenaline and noradrenaline, which are released in response to stress to act on adrenergic receptors. The *cortex* is composed of three zones, each of which secretes a different steroid hormone, i.e. the outer zona glomerulosa produces aldosterone, the middle zona fasciculata produces cortisol, and the inner zona reticularis produces androgens.

Adrenal gland dysfunction can result in excessive hormone production (e.g. Cushing's syndrome, phaeochromocytoma, or hyperaldosteronism) or hormone deficiency (e.g. Addison's disease or congenital adrenal hyperplasia), either as primary disease of the adrenal gland itself or secondary to impaired stimulation, e.g. from pituitary/hypothalamus dysfunction. The most common cause of adrenal insufficiency is adrenal atrophy following long-term corticosteroid therapy.

Pathophysiology

The *adrenal cortex* plays a fundamental role in regulating metabolism, BP and response to stress, through the secretion of three key steroid hormones:

- *Cortisol*: the hypothalamus releases corticotrophin-releasing hormone (CRH) in response to stress (both physical and psychological), which acts on the anterior pituitary, stimulating the release of corticotrophin (ACTH) into the general circulation. This, in turn, stimulates the adrenal cortex to produce cortisol. Activation is switched off through a negative feedback loop, as cortisol being lipophilic crosses the blood–brain barrier to interact with receptors and inhibit CRH release. Cortisol is a glucocorticoid with metabolic and immunomodulatory roles (see Table 4.7).

- *Aldosterone release*: regulated predominantly by the renin–angiotensin system within the kidneys, although ACTH also plays a role in its regulation. Aldosterone controls Na^+ and K^+ balance so that increased levels promote Na^+ and water reabsorption, and K^+ excretion by the kidneys, thus regulating BP and maintaining homeostasis. To a lesser extent, it also influences the metabolism of fat, carbohydrates, and protein. Interestingly, the chemical structures of cortisol and aldosterone are similar, so that a number of synthetic corticosteroids have both glucocorticoid and mineralocorticoids activity (e.g. **hydrocortisone**).

- *Androgen release*: like cortisol, is regulated via the hypothalamus (which releases CRH) and anterior pituitary (which releases ACTH), and is responsible for the development and maintenance of reproductive organs, and secondary sexual characteristics (e.g. hair growth, muscle mass, deepening of voice, etc.). See Topic 4.7 'Androgens, steroids', for more details.

Within the *adrenal medulla* chromaffin cells control the conversion of tyrosine into its downstream products like adrenaline, noradrenaline, and dopamine. The synaptic system has primary control over this region and thus modulates 'fight or flight responses' by releasing catecholamines into the circulating volume; these act directly on adrenergic receptors to increase heart rate, BP, reduce blood flow in the gut, and increase metabolism.

Dysregulation of adrenal hormones can therefore impact on metabolism, homeostasis, BP, and response to stress, so that response is either exaggerated 'hyper' or insufficient 'hypo'.

Table 4.7 Effects of increased glucocorticoid levels.

Immuno-modulatory roles	Metabolic effects
Inhibition of iNOS	Increased gluconeogenesis (increased storage of glucogen)
Inhibition of cytokines (e.g. IL-1,2,3,4,6,8,9,12, TNF; esp. reduced T-cell proliferation via IL-2)	Fat redistribution (secondary to catecholamines)
Inhibition of chemokines (e.g. IL-8)	Protein breakdown to synthesize glucose
Inhibition of COX-2	

'Hyper' adrenal function

Cushing's syndrome

Cushing's syndrome is the excessive production of cortisol, which can result from a number of mechanisms. Patients typically have symptoms of weight gain, lethargy, depression, proximal weakness, and irregular menses or erectile dysfunction. Signs of fat redistribution are characteristically seen with central obesity, buffalo hump, and a moon face, in addition to hypertension, hyperglycaemia, and an increased tendency for infection. Causes of Cushing's syndrome can be classified as ACTH-dependent or, less commonly, ACTH-independent.

ACTH-dependent: Cushing's disease is the most common cause of Cushing's syndrome (see Topic 4.1, 'The pituitary gland'). Excess ACTH production, however, can also arise from an ectopic source, e.g. bronchial carcinoma; or secondary to excess CRH production, which again can be from an ectopic source, e.g. medullary thyroid cancer, prostate carcinoma.

ACTH-independent: causes include adrenal adenoma and carcinoma. In general, adenomas secrete excess glucocorticoid, whereas carcinomas tend to secrete a mix of glucocorticoid and androgen, leading to virilisation, breast atrophy, voice changes and acne. ACTH-independent disease can also occur as part of a spectrum of disorders due to genetic mutations, e.g. McCune–Albright syndrome.

Investigations to distinguish between the causes include measurement of ACTH (in urine and saliva) to identify raised (ACTH-dependent) or suppressed levels (ACTH-independent), as well as identify diurnal variation; in conjunction with a **dexamethasone** suppression test.

Hyperaldosteronism

Mineralocorticoids, like aldosterone, may be affected with other corticosteroids or, less commonly, alone (e.g. Conn's syndrome). In Conn's syndrome primary hyperaldosteronism due to an adrenal adenoma results in Na^+ retention, via the Na^+–K^+-ATPase of renal tubules; and hypertension, with significant loss of urinary K^+. Idiopathic changes in bilateral adrenal cortex are responsible for most causes of hyperaldosteronism. Secondary causes arise from changes in renin levels, where renal artery stenosis or juxtoglomerular cell tumours increase aldosterone levels through the normal feedback system.

Phaeochromocytoma

A rare type of tumour that occurs in the adrenal medulla is a phaeochromocytoma, which is seen in approximately 1:1000 hypertensive patients. Most of these tumours are benign, with only 10% being malignant, although all increase catecholamine release into the circulation causing the classic triadic symptoms of headache, sweating, palpitation, and signs of hypertension, postural hypotension, and tremor. Pharmacological intervention has its place, but cure requires surgical resection.

'Hypo' adrenal function

Adrenal insufficiency and Addison's disease

As with glucocorticoid excess, adrenal deficiency is associated with primary (i.e. primary hypoadrenalism, Addison's disease), or secondary causes (i.e. ACTH deficiency). Globally, tuberculosis is another common cause making up 20% of cases in developed countries. Addison's results mainly from autoimmune adrenalitis (70%). Here, adrenal cortex antibodies cause gland atrophy and loss of cortical cells, thus decreasing production of cortisol and mineralocorticoids (aldosterone). Secondary adrenal deficiency arises from damage/disease of the hypothalamus or pituitary, e.g. pituitary tumours, although it is more commonly caused by chronic administration of glucocorticoids (see

Topic 4.1, 'The pituitary gland'). Primary iatrogenic causes of adrenal insufficiency can include adrenal surgery and drugs such as azoles, **rifampicin**, and **phenytoin**.

Symptoms of adrenal insufficiency include fatigue, weakness, joint pain, weight loss, and nausea and, in the case of Addison's disease, tend to be insidious in onset. Skin hyperpigmentation (affecting mainly skin creases and other areas of friction) is associated with chronic deficiency in primary disease, as both ACTH and melanocyte stimulating hormone are made from the same precursor molecule (pro-opiomelanocortin). Hyperpigmentation is not seen in secondary and tertiary hypoadrenalism.

Congenital adrenal hyperplasia

Congenital adrenal hyperplasia (CAH) refers to a family of inherited autosomal recessive conditions, where one of the enzymes essential for cortisol and/or aldosterone synthesis is deficient, most commonly 21 α-hydroxylase. Mutations in the gene coding for this enzyme (CYP21A) can be of varying severity and correlates with the severity of disease. Diagnosis is usually made in infants, often in the presence of ambiguous genitalia (in females) and signs of virilization (e.g. hirsutism). Males with severe disease will typically have normal genitalia, but can present with significant salt wasting (aldosterone deficiency).

For a full summary of the relevant pathways and drug targets, see Figure 4.2.

Management

'Hyper' adrenal function

Cushing's syndrome

Where Cushing's syndrome is suspected, diagnosis is made primarily with biochemical testing, by means of a 24-hour urinary-free cortisol, a late-night salivary cortisol, or a **dexamethasone** suppression test. The suppression test may be carried out as a low dose (1 mg) overnight or repeated doses (2 mg) over a 48-hour period, the latter being preferred as it is more accurate and can distinguish between different causes of Cushing's syndrome. Patients that have a negative test result are unlikely to have Cushing's syndrome, whereas those with a positive test will require further biochemical testing to improve the accuracy of diagnosis. The low dose test will be abnormal in Cushing's disease, but may be normal in ectopic

or adrenal causes of Cushing's syndrome. With an ectopic or adrenal cause the high dose test will detect if an abnormality exists.

> **PRACTICAL PRESCRIBING**
>
> ### Dexamethasone Suppression Test (Low Dose-Overnight)
>
> - In a healthy patient, dexamethasone suppresses ACTH and, therefore, cortisol secretion. In Cushing's syndrome, there is incomplete suppression.
> - Give 1 mg dexamethasone PO at 23.00 hours and the following morning, at around 09.00 hours, a blood sample (3 mL plain blood) is taken for plasma cortisol, where a level of <50 nmol/L excludes Cushing's syndrome.
> - If the patient is collecting a 24-hour urine sample for urinary-free cortisol, this should be done before taking the dexamethasone.
> - A normal response is shown by suppression of 09.00 hours cortisol to <50 nmol/L.
> - The low dose test is very sensitive, but if the blood sample is not taken at 09.00 hours this would yield a raised cortisol (a false positive test).

Once Cushing's syndrome has been confirmed, plasma ACTH is measured to differentiate between ACTH-dependent and ACTH-independent causes. Imaging in conjunction with biochemical testing can help establish a cause, e.g. evidence of tumour (ectopic source) or adrenal hyperplasia. As adrenal hyperplasia is seen in both ACTH-dependent and ACTH-independent causes of Cushing's syndrome, adrenal imaging cannot be used in isolation to distinguish between the two.

Management of Cushing's syndrome is complex and determined by the underlying cause, with the aim of normalizing serum cortisol levels. In general, surgery is the treatment of choice, removing any adrenal or pituitary adenoma or carcinoma, such as in Cushing's disease (see Topic 4.1, 'The pituitary gland'), or tumour responsible for ectopic secretion (e.g. bronchial carcinoma). Where surgery is unsuitable, other options include radiotherapy or medical management. Medical management may also be of value in patients with severe symptoms prior to surgery to reduce anaesthetic risks, in those waiting to see a benefit from radiotherapy or in the presence of residual disease following surgery. Treatment options available for Cushing's

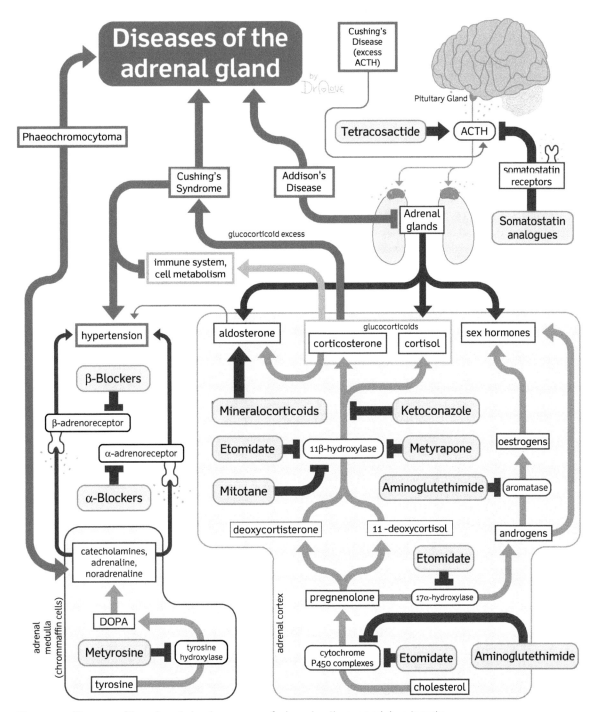

Figure 4.2 Diseases of the adrenal gland: summary of relevant pathways and drug targets.

syndrome can be broadly divided into three groups, i.e. drugs that:

- inhibit adrenal enzymes from converting cholesterol to cortisol (steroidogenesis inhibitors), e.g. **ketoconazole**, **metyrapone**, **mitotane**, and **aminoglutethimide**;
- act as neuromodulators, e.g. **pasireotide** and **cabergoline**;
- act as antagonists at glucocorticoid receptors, e.g. **mifepristone**.

Of these, the adrenal enzyme inhibitors are the preferred option; in particular, ketoconazole has historically been the most widely used due to its reasonable efficacy, rapid onset of action, and relatively acceptable tolerability. In comparison, mitotane, although demonstrating similar efficacy, is associated with a higher incidence of side effects, a slower onset of action and is more commonly used in adrenocortical carcinoma. As a rare disease, many of the enzyme inhibitors used in Cushing's were primarily developed for use in different indications and are, therefore, with the exception of metyrapone and ketoconazole, not approved for use in Cushing's syndrome.

More recently, pasireotide, a somatostatin analogue licensed for use in Cushing's disease, was developed to act specifically on excess ACTH secretion from a pituitary adenoma, thereby having less effect on other hormones. Dopamine agonists have also been investigated for their neuromodulator effects, although only cabergoline is currently used off-label in Cushing's syndrome. In patients unable to take oral therapy, **etomidate** may be administered IV, particularly in an acute situation.

Consideration will also need to be given to managing associated complications of Cushing's syndrome, such as hypertension and impaired glucose metabolism, although long-term these are best managed by inhibiting cortisol production.

Phaeochromocytoma

Phaeochromocytoma should be suspected in all patients presenting with malignant hypertension (sustained or paroxysmal) that shows poor response to conventional anti-hypertensive treatment. Patients are often asymptomatic, but may complain of headaches, palpitations, sweating, and a 'feeling of impending doom'. Tumours are often picked up incidentally on CT scan or with severe hypertension during surgery/general anaesthetic.

Where suspected, a diagnosis is made with two 24-hour urine collections to, ideally, metanephrines, rather than unmetabolized catecholamines, as they have greater

specificity. Failing that, serum levels or metanephrines may be carried out. Imaging by MRI or CT helps to confirm location and size, or alternatively MIBG or FDG-PET scans. Definitive treatment is by surgical removal, although drug therapy has a role to play in the initial stabilization of patients and peri-operatively to reduce the high and unpredictable anaesthetic risks associated with excessive catecholamine production.

The primary aim of drug therapy in phaeochromocytoma is to normalize BP and heart rate, prior to surgery. This is achieved through the use of an α-adrenoceptor antagonist, typically **phenoxybenzamine**, started up to 2 weeks prior to surgery. Although potent and effective, phenoxybenzamine is associated with high levels of toxicity due to its lack of selectivity. This includes a high risk of circulatory collapse and syncope related to postural hypotension; doses should be started low, ensuring first that patients are well hydrated. **Phentolamine** is a shorter-acting alternative that is administered IV and often used in anaesthesia to manage hypertension.

Prazosin and **doxazosin** are selective α₁-adrenoceptor antagonists and as such are preferred by some clinicians due to their lack of effect on pre-synaptic α₂-adrenoceptors, which causes tachycardia. As competitive inhibitors, however, they tend to be less effective in controlling surges in BP caused by sudden catecholamine release when the tumour is manipulated during surgery. Of the two, doxazosin is favoured due to its longer duration of action, which ensures it remains effective throughout surgery in patients who have taken it pre-operatively.

Once patients have been stabilized on an α-adrenoceptor antagonist, a β-blocker may be required to reverse symptoms of tachycardia. Although tachycardia could be a result of predominantly adrenaline secreting tumours, most phaeochromocytomas secrete noradrenaline and, therefore, β-blockers are generally used to antagonize the effects of non-selective α-blockers on α₂-adrenoceptors. Treatment should not be initiated until adequate α-blockade has been achieved, as this may aggravate hypertension or heart failure in patients with underlying myocardial dysfunction. Where a β-blocker is required, cardioselective β-blockers that act selectively on β₁-receptors, such as **propranolol** or **atenolol** can be used. While **labetalol** causes competitive α₁-adrenergic blockade and nonselective competitive β-adrenergic blockade.

Metirosine is an inhibitor of tyrosine hydroxylase that has been used in inoperable or malignant tumours. As it is not licensed in the UK, it can be obtained through specialist importing companies or as an unlicensed special.

'Hypo' adrenal function

Addison's disease

About half of patients with Addison's will present with an adrenal crisis, although the underlying principle of replacing deficient cortisol applies to all patients. Depending on severity at presentation, patients may require resuscitation to ensure cardiovascular stability and the correction of electrolyte imbalance (typically, hyponatraemia and hyperkalaemia). Diagnosis can be made through measurements of serum cortisol and ACTH levels, ideally simultaneously at about 09.00 hours, where ACTH levels are raised relative to cortisol levels. Preferably a 'Synacthen®' (**tetracosactide**) test (see 'Practical prescribing: Synacthen® (tetracosactide)/ACTH stimulation test') is required to confirm diagnosis, although priority should be given to urgent cortisol replacement in the case of a suspected adrenal crisis. Once diagnosis has been confirmed, further testing is required to establish the underlying cause, e.g. autoimmune disease or tuberculosis. In some cases, such as with tuberculosis, it may be necessary to treat the underlying cause.

PRACTICAL PRESCRIBING

Synacthen® (tetracosactide)/ACTH stimulation test

- Used to investigate adrenal insufficiency.
- Baseline cortisol taken immediately prior to administration of ACTH.
- 250 µg of ACTH administered IM or IV.
- Further cortisol level taken at 30 minutes.
- A 30-minute level of <450–550 nmol/L or a rise of <200 nmol/L, is considered abnormal.

Addison's disease requires lifelong glucocorticoid and mineralocorticoid replacement:

- **Hydrocortisone** is the favoured glucocorticoid due to its short duration of action, enabling more accurate diurnal variations in cortisol levels, compared with longer-acting agents, such as **prednisolone** or **dexamethasone**. The usual dose is 20–30 mg/day orally in two to three divided doses for chronic management, or IV in the case of an adrenal crisis, with doses titrated to requirements. On initiation, patients should be counselled on the signs and symptoms of an adrenal crisis, to facilitate urgent treatment, and educated on principles of self-management to prevent hospitalization.

For example, provision of dose escalations of their hydrocortisone for dealing with periods of 'stress' (e.g. viral illness, infection, surgery) and IM hydrocortisone in the case of an emergency. If patients are unable to tolerate oral administration due to nausea and vomiting it is important they attend hospitals for IV administration.

- **Fludrocortisone** is the only mineralocorticoid available for replacement therapy and, as with hydrocortisone, usually started at a low dose (100 µg daily) and titrated to response. Patients should be advised to monitor for signs suggestive of fluid or electrolyte disturbances, such as oedema, hypertension, and salt cravings. Unlike hydrocortisone, however, dose alterations are not necessary during 'stress'.

Congenital adrenal hyperplasia

Management of CAH involves replacement of deficient hormones (**hydrocortisone**, **fludrocortisone**), and correction of electrolyte imbalance (sodium). Treatment is tailored to severity of symptoms.

Drug classes used in management

Steroidogenesis inhibitors: ketoconazole

Ketoconazole is an imidazole derivative with antifungal properties that can reduce adrenal steroid production via inhibition of multiple steroidogenic enzymes.

Mechanism of action

Ketoconazole has to be used in high doses (400–1200 mg/day) in order to reduce cortisol production in patients with Cushing's syndrome of various aetiology. It acts on various mitochondrial cytochrome P450-dependent enzymes to inhibit several steps in adrenal steroidogenesis, which includes cholesterol side-chain cleavage enzyme, 17-α hydroxylase, and 17,20-lyase enzymatic activities. With long-term treatment, adrenal insufficiency is avoided by adjusting the dose to achieve physiological cortisol levels. Early reports have suggested that patients with ACTH-independent Cushing's have a more sustained suppression, but not all disease types respond in a similar manner.

Although it has been found that ketoconazole can bind competitively to the adrenal receptor (AdR), the dose required for 50% occupancy of the receptor is unlikely to be achieved in the plasma. In addition, it has also been suggested that ketoconazole may have pituitary effects in Cushing's syndrome, by inhibiting ACTH secretion.

Prescribing

Originally developed as an anti-fungal, **ketoconazole** has recently been approved for use in Cushing's syndrome, at considerably higher doses of 400–1200 mg/day in two or three divided doses. Furthermore, it has been withdrawn in the EU for use as an anti-fungal. Doses are started low and gradually titrated up according to response, with larger doses divided into four equal doses in the day. Of the steroidogenesis inhibitors available for use in Cushing's syndrome, ketoconazole tends to be the best tolerated, even with extended use and, therefore, the drug of choice.

Unwanted effects

Ketoconazole is associated with significant hepatic toxicity, particularly with higher doses and extended use. It is, therefore, essential to monitor patients closely for both efficacy (plasma cortisol) and toxicity (LFTs) to ensure that treatment is adjusted to the lowest effective dose. As a potent inhibitor of CYP 3A4, ketoconazole has a high potential for drug interactions. Furthermore, absorption is affected by drugs that alter gastric acidity (e.g. proton pump inhibitors) and, therefore, these are best avoided. For more information on unwanted effects and drug interactions (see Topic 11.2, 'Fungal infections').

Steroidogenesis inhibitors: metyrapone

> Metyrapone blocks the last step of cortisol synthesis through the inhibition of 11β-hydroxylase, and can diminish the production of cortisol in patients with ectopic ACTH production, adrenal tumours and Cushing's syndrome.

Mechanism of action

The inhibition of 11β-hydroxylase by **metyrapone** can generate a compensatory increase in ACTH production, as a result of the reduction in cortisol-mediated negative feedback on the corticotropic adenoma. This may not only lead to an increase in adrenal production of cortisol, but also of androgens and mineralocorticoid precursors. The increase in androgens may be beneficial in patients with significant catabolic effects from hypercortisolaemia, although less desirable in women.

Prescribing

Like **ketoconazole**, **metyrapone** has been used for several decades in the management of Cushing's syndrome with good results and, until recently, was the only drug approved for this use. Usual doses range from 750–6000 mg a day in three or four divided doses, due to its short duration of action, and adjusted to achieve normal cortisol levels. It is best taken with milk or food to reduce the risk of nausea and vomiting. Metyrapone is also licensed for the diagnosis of Cushing's syndrome, although rarely used for this indication.

Unwanted effects

On the whole, **metyrapone** is well tolerated, even with extended courses, the most common side effects being nausea and vomiting, hypotension, dizziness, and headache. With extended courses, treatment may result in hirsutism or hypoadrenalism, particularly with inadequate monitoring. Patients with deranged LFTs may show a delayed response to treatment due to impaired cortisol metabolism by the liver, with the effects also impaired in the presence of hypothyroidism.

Steroidogenesis inhibitors: mitotane

> Mitotane is an adrenolytic agent used in the treatment of adrenal carcinoma. It can supress cell growth, but also inhibit cholesterol side-chain cleavage and 11β-hydroxylase, which decreases cortisol production.

Mechanism of action

Mitotane has a cytotoxic effect on adrenocortical tissue, as well as having extra-adrenal effects that includes steroidogenesis inhibition. The precise mode of action, however, is not completely understood. The adrenolytic effects of mitotane require its transformation to an acyl chloride via cytochrome P450-mediated hydroxylation, this subsequently binds covalently to bionucleophiles within the mitochondria of adrenocortical cells, causing mitochondrial destruction and cell necrosis. In addition, it causes oxidative damage through the formation of free radicals, such as superoxide, which generates hydroxylated radicals and induces lipid peroxidation. Inhibition of steroidogenesis by mitotane alters metabolism so that cortisol is metabolized to 6-β-hydroxycortisol, reducing the production of 17-hxydroxycorticosteroid.

The non-specific action of mitotane on other enzyme pathways leads to toxicity including hypercholesterolaemia (through inhibition of cholesterol oxidase) and an increase in hormone-binding globulins. It also acts to accelerate the metabolism of synthetic glucocorticoids (e.g. **dexamethasone** and **fludrocortisone**), thereby potentially increasing requirements.

Prescribing

Mitotane is licensed for use in adrenocortical carcinoma to relieve symptoms in patients with inoperable tumours, although off-label it provides an alternative drug therapy in Cushing's syndrome. It is highly lipophilic and, as such, distributes into adipose tissue, where it accumulates. As a result, onset of action and elimination is slow (half-life of 18–159 days) due to delayed clearance from fat storage sites. Dose titrations typically involve an initial loading to achieve optimum effect and then titration to response, usually 3–6 g/day in divided doses. Once treatment is established, glucocorticoid replacement therapy should be initiated as needed. With its slow onset of action and significant toxicity, it is a less favourable treatment option.

Unwanted effects

Side effects to **mitotane** are very common and a significant limiting factor to its use. In particular, patients complain of GI (nausea, vomiting) and neurological toxicity (vertigo, drowsiness, headaches, confusion), the latter having a marked effect on the ability to drive or operate heavy machinery. Treatment also adversely affects liver enzymes, and plasma cholesterol and triglyceride levels; patients therefore require baseline measurements and monitoring throughout therapy.

Adrenal insufficiency occurs in about 75% of patients receiving mitotane, so that patients require glucocorticoid replacement. Furthermore, as an inducer of the CYP 3A4 enzyme; metabolism of **dexamethasone**, among other drugs (e.g. **warfarin**, anticonvulsants, **rifampicin**, and St John's Wort), is increased. **Hydrocortisone** is unaffected.

Other side effects to be aware of include rashes and blood dyscrasias, such as leucopenia and thrombocytopenia.

Steroidogenesis inhibitors: aminoglutethimide

Aminoglutethimide binds and inhibits aromatase, which is essential for the generation of oestrogens from androstenedione and testosterone. It also blocks the conversion of cholesterol to pregnenolone, through inhibition of cytochrome P450 complexes.

Mechanism of action

The pharmacological effects of **aminoglutethimide** result in a reduction in the adrenal mineralocorticoids, glucocorticoids, oestrogens, and androgens production. The decrease in cortisol secretion leads to an augmented production of pituitary ACTH, which can overcome the steroid synthesis blockade. This can be supressed by the concomitant administration of **hydrocortisone**.

Prescribing

Aminoglutethimide, once used in Cushing's syndrome and metastatic breast cancer, has been widely withdrawn from the market worldwide due to unacceptable toxicity.

Steroidogenesis inhibitors: etomidate

The anesthetic etomidate is an imidazole derivative that inhibits cholesterol side-chain cleavage and the 17α-hydroxylase, 11β-hydroxylase and C17-20 enzymes, leading to the suppression of steroidogenesis.

Mechanism of action

Etomidate reduces levels of serum cortisol and aldosterone, but increases ACTH, 11-deoxycortisol, and deoxicorticosterone, probably through the inhibition of the cytochrome P450 complex. It has a rapid onset of action and is useful in patients with acute complications of Cushing's, typically with ectopic generation of ACTH and overwhelming cortisol production.

Prescribing

Etomidate is the only steroidogenesis inhibitor available for IV use in Cushing's syndrome and therefore of value in patients unable to tolerate oral therapy, particularly in acute management in an intensive care or high-dependency setting. It is licensed as an anaesthetic induction agent due to its rapid onset and short duration of action.

In Cushing's syndrome, it is administered by continuous infusion at a dose of 0.04–0.05 mg/kg/hour, titrated to achieve a serum cortisol of around 500 nmol/ L. Throughout treatment, serum cortisol levels should be closely monitored and normalization should occur within 12–24 hours of initiation. In the case of adrenal insufficiency, doses may need to be reduced or failing that, replacement with IV **hydrocortisone** may be necessary.

Unwanted effects

Within the terms of its license as an anaesthetic agent, **etomidate** is restricted for use in induction, rather than maintenance of anaesthesia, due to the risk of adrenal suppression associated with continuous infusions. Although clearly not a contraindication in managing patients with acute hypercortisolaemia, patients should be closely monitored so that adequate replacement can be initiated in those affected. Patients will require management by experienced staff in a high dependency setting with resuscitation facilities available. Close monitoring of BP and respiratory rate is necessary to detect signs of hypotension and apnoeas, respectively.

Neuromodulators: somatostatin analogues

> Somatostatin analogues bind to somatostatin receptors, which inhibit ACTH secretion and reduce cortisol levels, and is thus of value in Cushing's disease. Secondary benefits include the inhibition of tumour cell proliferation. For example, pasireotide.

Mechanism of action

Somatostatin was primarily described as a hypothalamic peptide that strongly inhibits growth hormone secretion by the pituitary gland. It has since been shown that the peptide has extensive activity on several neuro-endocrine systems, such as the GI tract and pancreas. There are two biologically active forms of somatostatin (SS-14 and SS-28), which act via high affinity G protein–coupled membrane receptors. They link to various second messenger systems, including inhibition of adenylyl cyclase activity

and Ca^{2+} channels linked to inhibition of secretory processes, as well as stimulation of phosphotyrosine phosphatase or MAP kinase activity, which could have a part in the regulation of cell proliferation.

Pasireotide is a synthetic cyclic hexapeptide with a broad spectrum affinity for somatostatin receptors.

Prescribing

Pasireotide is the only somatostatin analogue approved for use in Cushing's disease, due to its specific mechanism of action. It is administered SC at a dose of 600 μg BD, increased to 900 μg BD if tolerated. Response to treatment, defined by normalization of urinary-free cortisol levels, is demonstrated within 2 months, although in phase 3 studies only about 13/25% of patients achieved this at 600 and 900 μg, respectively. In those who fail to respond at 2 months, consideration should be given to discontinuing therapy.

Unwanted effects

In general, side effects to **pasireotide** are similar to other somatostatin analogues (see Topic 4.1, 'The pituitary gland'), although the risk of hyperglycaemia is greater (see 'Prescribing warning: hyperglycaemia with pasireotide').

PRESCRIBING WARNING

Hyperglycaemia with pasireotide

- Patients on pasireotide are at increased risk of hyperglycaemia.
- The risk is increased in patients with pre-diabetic conditions.
- Fasting glucose levels and HbA1c should be measured at baseline and weekly for 2–3 months after initiation or following a dose change. Monitoring thereafter should be repeated intermittently.
- Affected patients may be managed with oral hypoglycaemics or have treatment discontinued.

Glucocorticoid receptor antagonists: mifepristone

> Mifepristone exerts its anti-glucocorticoid effects though binding to glucocorticoid receptors.

Mechanism of action

Mifepristone binds to glucocorticoid receptors with 18 times the affinity of cortisol, thus blocking its activity. Peripherally, there is an increase in cortisol levels as the negative feedback that would normally control secretion of CRH/ACTH is lost. Consequently, treatment is associated with a potential increase in mineralocorticoid effects, as action at these receptors is not lost. This leads to hypokalaemia and an increase in BP.

Prescribing

Mifepristone is reserved for use in patients with hyperglycaemia secondary to Cushing's syndrome, for which it has been approved in the USA. In the UK it is only licensed for medical termination in early pregnancy. Doses are administered orally at a usual starting dose of 300 mg/day and titrated to clinical response (weight, glucose, and BP). As treatment can lead to an increase in serum cortisol levels, these cannot be used to monitor therapy.

Unwanted effects

Aside from nausea and vomiting, the most common side effect with prolonged use occur as a result of increased mineralocorticoid activity, i.e. hypokalaemia and hypertension, which can be managed with **spironolactone** and potassium supplements. Antiprogestin effects include endometrial hyperplasia with long-term use and, therefore, vaginal ultrasounds are recommended.

Corticotrophins (tetracosactide)

Tetracosactide is a synthetic analogue of ACTH, which acts on the adrenal gland to stimulate the production of steroid hormones.

Mechanism of action

Tetracosactide can be used as a diagnostic agent to assess adrenal reserve, thus distinguishing the cause of apparent adrenal gland malfunction as either adrenal damage or lack of pituitary ACTH.

Prescribing

Doses are administered by IM or IV injection, followed by serial sampling of serum cortisol levels at predefined intervals to assess response. If the response to **tetracosactide** is inadequate, a serum ACTH should be carried out. In the case of Addison's disease the level should be raised.

Unwanted effects

As an analogue of ACTH, side effects to **tetracosactide** are as for corticosteroids, although as it is only used diagnostically, the risk of toxicity is minimal. For this reason, it may be used for diagnosis in pregnant or breastfeeding women, and in those with renal or hepatic impairment where use is deemed essential.

Synthetic corticosteroids: glucocorticoids

Loss of cortisol in adrenal insufficiency requires exogenous replacement with synthetic corticosteroids that possess glucocorticoid and mineralocorticoid activity, administered to mimic diurnal variations seen endogenously (see Table 4.8).

Glucocorticoids are a class of steroid hormones released by the adrenal gland. They bind to the glucocorticoid receptor and regulate the expression of various target genes. For example, hydrocortisone.

Table 4.8 Activity of exogenous corticosteroids

	Glucocorticoid activity	Mineralocorticoid activity	Replacement dose
Cortisone	++	++	–
Dexamethasone	++++	–	–
Hydrocortisone	++	++	20–30 mg
Methylprednisolone	+++	+	–
Prednisolone	+++	+	2.5–15 mg
Fludrocortisone	+	++++	50–300 µg

Mechanism of action

Loss of glucocorticoid function in adrenal insufficiency results in an impaired response to 'stress', affecting carbohydrate, glucose, and protein metabolism, as well as immune response. Exogenous replacement with synthetic corticosteroids helps to maintain function.

Prescribing

Hydrocortisone is the corticosteroid of choice for glucocorticoid replacement, due to its short duration of action. Administration is typically split into TDS timed doses adjusted to individual response, with the larger dose given in the morning to best reflect normal diurnal variation (e.g. 10 mg on waking, 5 mg at noon, and 5 mg at 17.00 hours). In case of 'stress', e.g. sepsis/surgery, doses are doubled, again to mimic normal cortisol response.

Unwanted effects

As replacement therapy, doses are tailored to mimic physiological levels so that the risk of chronic toxicity from corticosteroid use is reduced. See Topic 6.6, 'Inflammatory bowel disease' for more information.

Synthetic corticosteroids: mineralocorticoids

Mineralocorticoids, such as aldosterone, are steroids produced by the adrenal cortex. Angiotensin II stimulates aldosterone secretion, which circulates in the plasma and regulates target tissues by interacting with the mineralocorticoid receptor. For example, fludrocortisone.

Mechanism of action

The synthetic mineralocorticoid **fludrocortisone** acts by binding to intracellular mineralocorticoid receptors (MRs) belonging to the steroid nuclear receptor superfamily. These are ligand-dependent transcription factors, interacting with hormone responsive elements in the promoter regions of regulated genes. MRs are found in epithelial (renal distal nephron, colon, sweat ducts, and salivary glands) and non-epithelial (heart, brain, vascular muscle, liver, and leucocytes) tissues.

Activation of the MRs increases Na^+ reabsorption in the kidney and at other secretory epithelial sites, at the expense of H^+ and K^+ ions. In vascular smooth muscle, MR activation results in changes in pressor responsiveness to stimulation of adrenergic receptors and may regulate collagen formation. In the CNS, MRs regulate sympathetic outflow, together with thirst and salt intake. In brief, excessive aldosterone can elevate blood pressure through various MR-dependent mechanisms.

Prescribing

Fludrocortisone is the only corticosteroid with sufficient mineralocorticoid properties (100 times more potent than **hydrocortisone**) for use in adrenocortical deficiency. Although it has a short plasma half-life of 3.5 hours, it biological half-life is prolonged (18–36 hours) enabling once daily dosing.

Unwanted effects

See Topic 4.6, 'Female reproduction'.

Alpha-blockers

Alpha-blockers are antagonists of α-adrenergic receptors, used in the treatment of hypertension. Examples include phenoxybenzamine, phentolamine, doxazosin, and prazosin.

Mechanism of action

Alpha-blockade in phaeochromocytoma minimizes hypertension secondary to vasoconstriction, mediated through excessive stimulation of $α_1$-adrenoceptors.

Prescribing

Alpha-blockade with **phenoxybenzamine** is the preferred agent pre-operatively, started 10–14 days before surgery. Due to its profound effect on BP and tachycardia, doses are started low and gradually increased to achieve a BP of 130/80 mmHg or less.

Phentolamine, can be administered IV as a bolus injection or infusion, and is the preferred option in a hypertensive crisis. Patients will require an initial test dose of 1 mg.

In patients requiring chronic therapy, the longer-acting agents, **prazosin** or **doxazosin** are more commonly used, as they tend to be better tolerated. Again, doses are tailored to achieve optimal BP.

Unwanted effects

See Topic 2.1, 'Hypertension'.

Beta-blockers

> Beta-blockers are antagonists of β-adrenoceptors, blocking the actions of endogenous catecholamines, adrenaline, and noradrenaline in particular. For example, propranolol, atenolol, and labetolol.

Mechanism of action

Beta-blockade is used to overcome the effects of excess cateocholamines that act on cardiac β-adrenoceptors to cause tachycardia. As β-blockers also cause peripheral vasoconstriction, they should not be initiated until α blockade has been established (a postural BP drop of 15–20 mmHg), as they may otherwise act to further aggravate hypertension.

Prescribing

The cardioselective β-blockers (e.g. **propranolol**) are used preferentially in the management of phaeochromocytoma to manage tachycardia. Doses are administered orally, starting at a low dose (e.g. 10–20 mg TDS) and titrated to achieve a pulse of about 70 bpm.

Unwanted effects

See Topic 2.1, 'Hypertension'.

Metyrosine

> Metyrosine inhibits tyrosine hydroxylase, the enzyme that catalyses the conversion of tyrosine to dihydroxyphenylalanine (DOPA).

Mechanism of action

Inhibition of this rate-limiting step in the production of catecholamines leads to depletion of dopamine, adrenaline, and noradrenaline levels, which are excessively produced in patients with phaeochromocytoma.

Prescribing

Although infrequently employed, **metyrosine** has been used orally pre-operatively in phaeochromocytoma in combination with **phenoxybenzamine** to establish better BP control during surgery. Treatment is started 1–3 weeks prior to surgery at a dose of 250–500 mg every 2–3 days then increased as needed to between 1.5 and 2 g/day. The drug is not licensed in the UK and can only be obtained through specialist importing companies.

Unwanted effects

Adverse effects to **metyrosine** are predominantly neurological, commonly causing sedation and, less frequently, extrapyramidal side effects, confusion, and hallucinations. Treatment is also associated with crystalluria, which may be overcome by ensuring adequate fluid intake of at least 2 L/day.

Further reading

Baudry C, Coste J, Bou Khalil R (2012) Efficiency and tolerance of mitotane in Cushing's disease in 76 patients from a single center. *European Journal of Endocrinology* 17(4), 473–81.

Chakera AJ, Vaidya B (2010) Addison disease in adults: diagnosis and management. *American Journal of Medicine* 123, 409–13.

Colao A, Petersenn S, Newell-Price J (2012) A 12-month phase 3 study of pasireotide in Cushing's disease. *New England Journal of Medicine* 366, 912–24.

Feelders RA, Hofland LJ, de Herder WW (2010) Medical treatment of Cushing's syndrome: adrenal-blocking and ketaconazole. *Neuroendocrinology* 92(1), 111–15.

Findling JW, Raff H (2006) Cushing's syndrome: important issues in the diagnosis and management. *Journal of Clinical Endocrinology and Metabolism* 91(10), 3746–53.

Gross BA, Mindea SA, Pick AJ (2007) Medical management of Cushing Disease. *Neurosurgery Focus* 23(3), E10.

Pacek K (2007) Preoperative management of the phaeochromocytoma patient. *Journal of Clinical Endocrinology and Metabolism* 92(11), 4069–79.

Preda VA, Sen J, Karavitaki N, et al. (2012) Etomidate in the management of hypercortisolaemia in Cushing's syndrome; a review. *European Journal of Endocrinology* 167, 137–43.

Prys-Roberts C (2000) Phaeochromocytoma—recent progress in its management. *British Journal of Anaesthesia* 85, 44–57.

Rizk A, Honegger J, Milian M (2012) Treatment options in Cushing's disease. *Clinical Medicine Insights: Oncology* 6, 75–84.

Schteingart DE (2009) Drugs in the medical treatment of Cushing's syndrome. *Expert Opinions in Emergency Drugs* 14(4), 661–71.

Guidelines

Nieman LK, Biller BMK, Findling JW, et al. (2008) The diagnosis of Cushing's syndrome: an Endocrine Society Clinical Practice Guideline. *Journal of Clinical Endocrinology and Metabolism* 93(5), 1526–40.://www http.endocrhttps://academic.oup.com/jcem/article/93/5/1526/2598096 [accessed 29 March 2019].

Nieman LK, Biller BMK, Findling JW, et al. (2015) Treatment of Cushing's syndrome: an Endocrine Society Practice Guideline. *Journal of Clinical Endocrinology and Metabolism* 100(8), 2807–31. http://press.endocrine.org/doi/pdf/10.1210/jc.2015-1818 [accessed 25 March 2019].

4.3 Thyroid disease

The thyroid is a gland located anteriorly in the lower neck and contains the two biologically active thyroid hormones—thyroxine (T_4) and, to a lesser extent, 3,5,3'-triiodothyronine (T_3). Collectively, these hormones play a role in numerous metabolic processes, regulated by TSH released from the anterior pituitary. In dysfunction patients may present thyrotoxic (e.g. Grave's disease), hypothyroid (e.g. autoimmune thyroiditis) or euthyroid often as a result of autoimmune disease, but also a consequence of adenomas and changes in iodine supply. Treatment aims to restore normal function and may involve pharmacological or surgical management.

Pathophysiology

The thyroid gland is comprised of two elongated lobes that are connected by a median isthmus. It is divided up by fibrous septa into lobules, each containing follicles that are surrounded by a network of capillaries and contain thyroglobulin, the precursor to the two biologically active thyroid hormones—T_4 and T_3.

Thyroid hormone regulation is through the hypothalamic–pituitary axis, which fundamentally controls the basal metabolic status of an individual through a negative feedback loop. Low serum levels of T_3/T_4 stimulate the release of TRH from the hypothalamus, which in turn acts on the anterior pituitary to produce TSH. TSH acts to stimulate the production and release of thyroid hormones, both within the thyroid and, in the case of T_3, in peripheral tissues. Conversely, raised thyroid hormone levels inhibit the synthesis and release of both TSH and TRH.

Thyroid hormones are iodine-containing molecules that are synthesized within the thyroid, following active transport of sodium iodide into the follicles. Here iodide binds to the tyrosyl residue of thyroglobulin to produce monoiodotyrosine (MIT) and diiodotyrosine (DIT). Subsequently, two DIT molecules are bound together by thyroid peroxidase (TPO) to form T_4, which is produced by the thyroid gland only and stored in thyroglobulin. The same enzyme within the thyroid also acts to bind a DIT and MIT molecule to make T_3. T_3, however, is predominantly synthesized in other tissues (liver, kidney) through deiodination of circulating T_4. Collectively, these are abundant hormones, both within the thyroid gland and in the circulation bound to thyroxine-binding globulin (TBG), ensuring they are rapidly available. It is, however, in their free form that T_4 and T_3 are biologically active. T_3 has a short half-life of 1.5 days, while that of T_4 is 7 days.

The main actions of T_3 are as a regulator of gene transcription acting through four classes of thyroid hormone receptors located on different tissues:

- α_1 (cardiac and skeletal).
- α_2 (widely distributed, but does not bind hormone).
- β_1 (brain, liver, and kidney).
- β_2 (hypothalamus and pituitary).

Activated receptor forms bind to DNA, and through a number of co-factors can activate or suppress gene function; thus, in addition to metabolic influences, actions are also essential for nervous system development and puberty.

Hypothyroidism

Predictably, thyroid hormone production may be altered by iodine deficiency or gland dysfunction (thyroid, hypothalamus, or pituitary).

Primary hypothyroidism

Primary hypothyroidism occurs when the gland is devoid of chemical precursors (e.g. through altered iodine supply, iodine contrast media, **amiodarone**, or **lithium**) or undergoes autoimmune modulation, e.g. autoimmune thyroiditis.

- *Change in iodine supply*: hypothyroidism can be seen with endemic goitre when iodine intake is <30 µg/day. This can result in severe mental, physical, and profound neurological delay in the new born, or altered development in the infant. In a sporadic goitre or multinodular goitre, most patients will be euthyroid, while others may be hypothyroid secondary to deficits in hormone synthesis.

- *Drug-induced*: **Amiodarone** has high iodine content and, as such, can act to alter thyroid function, affecting around 30% of patients on treatment; in 5–10% of patients this can cause hyperthyroidism. This can be through direct inhibition of T_3 and T_4 entry to peripheral tissues and cytotoxicity to follicular cells, or indirectly by affecting iodine signalling/synthesis. Two clinical effects have been described:

  - The Wolff–Chaikoff effect, where there is *hypo*thyroidism caused by ingestion of a large amount of iodine; and

  - The Jod–Basedow effect, where *hyper*thyroidism occurs following administration of iodine.

  Amiodarone has the potential to cause both effects. In most cases of drug-induced hypothyroidism replacement with **levothyroxine** will suffice, although alternative treatments to amiodarone should be considered.

- *Autoimmune mediated*: (e.g. Hashimoto's disease). Autoimmune thyroiditis (AIT) occurs in the presence of antibodies to TPO, thyroglobulin, and TSH receptors, leading ultimately to thyroid gland failure. Patients may present with a goitre due to infiltration of lymphocytes (especially B-cells) and macrophages; or thyroid atrophy due to loss of follicular cells, caused by antibody action against TPO and thyroglobulin. These antibodies, especially anti-TSH receptor 'blockers', break the negative feedback system so there is insufficient thyroxine production, causing symptoms of fatigue, weight gain, cold intolerance, and depression. Patients with autoimmune thyroiditis may also present with normal thyroid function or, rarely, with thyrotoxicosis. The risk of AIT is higher in women than men and is probably the result of a combination of environmental (e.g. radiation, pregnancy, and stress) and genetic risk factors, as demonstrated with familial clustering and an increased risk with certain HLA genotypes, such as HLA-DR5.

Secondary hypothyroidism

Secondary hypothyroidism results from upstream changes in the negative feedback system that may be pituitary or hypothalamic in origin (see Topic 4.1, 'The pituitary gland'). TSH levels are key to the diagnosis of hypothyroidism (Table 4.9). If upstream changes are suspected, TSH levels would normally be low, although in the presence of raised TSH, free-T_4 should also be measured.

Hyperthyroidism and thyrotoxicosis

Thyrotoxicosis is a condition that results from excessive production of thyroid hormones from any source, whereas in hyperthyroidism excess secretion is originated specifically from the thyroid gland. Hyperthyroidism is thus a form of thyrotoxicosis.

The most common cause of primary thyrotoxicosis is Grave's disease (60–80%), an autoimmune condition where autoantibodies stimulate TSH receptors causing raised levels of thyroxine. High-circulating thyroxine levels can cause symptoms of weight loss, diarrhoea, tachycardia, agitation/anxiety, heat intolerance, and palpitations (e.g.

Table 4.9 Summary of laboratory findings in common thyroid disorders

Thyroid disorder	T_4	T_3	Free T_4	TSH	TR Ab
Hypothyroidism					
Primary	L	L	L	H	–
AIT	L*	L*	L*	H*	+
Secondary	L	L	L	N/L	–
Hyperthyroidism					
Grave's disease	H	H	H	L	+
Secondary	H	H	H	H/N	–

Key: (TSH) thyroid-stimulating hormone, (TR Ab) thyrotropin receptor antibody, (AIT) autoimmune thyroiditis, (N) normal, (L) low, (H) high, (+) positive, (–) negative.
*Levels can vary with type of AIT.

atrial fibrillation). More specific signs may be seen in Grave's, such as exophthalmos, pretibial myxedema, and thyroid acropachy. Eye signs (exophthalmos) are due to infiltration of immune responses (T-cells and macrophages) to tissues, so oedema, inflammation, and latterly fibrosis occurs, increasing the volume of extra-ocular tissues. As with autoimmune hypothyroidism there is a genetic element and this has strongest associations with HLA-DR and CTLA4. Environmental factors have also been identified, including stress, high iodine intake, or infection.

The T-cell mediated autoimmune response (again type IV) means that cells and antibodies, to the TSH receptors, flood the thyroid, and cause smooth glandular hypertrophy and hyperplasia. The strategy to modulate the effects of these antibodies and the subsequent high thyroxine levels (see Table 4.9) is to initially manage symptoms (tachycardia, diarrhoea, anxiety) and, subsequently, antithyroid therapy.

The second most common cause of primary thyrotoxicosis is a toxic multinodular goitre; here the gland has undergone localized changes, such that focal adenomatous regions secrete thyroxine. Other secreting lesions of the thyroid, such as a benign solitary nodule or follicular carcinoma, should also be considered and investigated. It should also be noted that some drugs (e.g. **amiodarone**, **lithium**; see previously) can rarely lead to hyperthyroid status.

Secondary hyperthyroidism is rare and may be due to a TSH-secreting pituitary tumour or chorionic gonadotrophin-secreting tumour. Typically, TSH, T_3 and T_4 are all raised.

For a full summary of the relevant pathways and drug targets, see Figure 4.3.

Management

Hypothyroidism

Diagnosis of hypothyroidism is made through clinical observations in combination with assessment of end organ damage, i.e. skin, eyes, heart, etc. Symptoms tend to be non-specific (lethargy, apathy, hair loss, weight gain), so that measurement of serum thyroid hormones, i.e. TSH, T_4, and T_3, is required for a definitive diagnosis. Further blood tests are needed to exclude anaemia, liver dysfunction, raised cholesterol levels, and altered calcium levels, all of which may be caused by hypothyroidism. A thorough drug history will help identify iatrogenic causes and ensure that, where possible, treatment is discontinued. Management is through

replacement with **levothyroxine**, with doses adjusted to render patients asymptomatic.

Hyperthyroidism

Hyperthyroidism management will depend on the underlying cause, with initial investigations carried out to distinguish primary from secondary causes. As with hypothyroidism, initial investigations include clinical examinations to **assess** for raised pulse, BP and respiratory rate, and weight loss, in combination with assessment of end-organ damage, e.g. eye or cardiac symptoms. Serum measurements of TSH, free T_4 and T_3 are necessary to confirm the diagnosis, assess severity, and distinguish between causes. For example, with overt disease TSH is barely detectable, whereas T_4 and T_3 are significantly raised.

In patients with symptomatic thyrotoxicosis, the primary aim of treatment is to manage end-organ symptoms. β-blockers (e.g. **atenolol**, **propranolol**) are used first-line to manage symptoms of increased adrenergic stimulation, i.e. tachycardia, hypertension, and anxiety. However, where contraindicated, a Ca^{2+} channel blocker, such as **diltiazem** or **verapamil** may be used.

A thyrotoxic crisis or 'thyroid storm', the most severe presentation of thyrotoxicosis, is considered a medical emergency, which if left untreated may be fatal. Patients typically present with hyperpyrexia (as high as 40–41°C), tachycardia, agitation, seizures, delirium, vomiting, diarrhoea, and even coma. Management will often require invasive monitoring and inotropic support, so is often carried out in an intensive care setting (see Table 4.10).

In patients with overt Grave's disease, antithyroid strategies may be required; either through surgery (thyroidectomy), radioiodine ablation or the use of a thionamide (antithyroid drug), e.g. **carbimazole** or **propylthiouracil**. Choice will be determined by factors such as age and severity. Pharmacological treatment is continued for 12–18 months with the intention of rendering the patient euthyroid, although as precise inhibition may be difficult, a 'block and replace' technique may be necessary. Following treatment cessation, more than half of patients will relapse within 3–6 months or even years later.

In patients that are hypersensitive to thionamides or iodine, **lithium** may be used off-label in hyperthyroidism, to reduce the secretion of thyroid hormones by the thyroid. Doses of 600–1000 mg daily are given in divided doses, although not without potentially serious side effects and drug interactions, in part, due to its narrow therapeutic index.

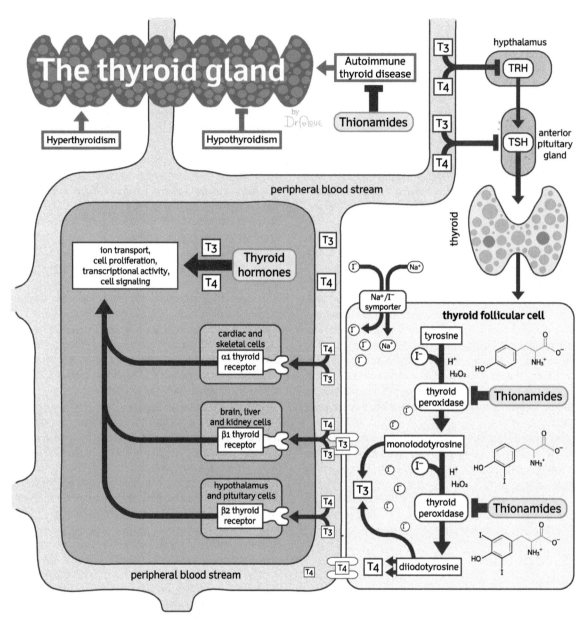

Figure 4.3 The thyroid gland: summary of relevant pathways and drug targets.

Drug classes uses in management

Thionamides

The anti-thyroid drugs or thionamides inhibit thyroid peroxidase and reduce the synthesis of T_3 and T_4 hormones. Additionally, they can also be immunosuppressive in individuals with auto-immune thyroid disease. For example, carbimazole, propylthiouracil, and methimazole.

Mechanism of action

First introduced in the 1940s, the thionamides are grouped into two classes—thiouracils and imidazoles. **Methimazole** and **carbimazole** are part of the imidazole group, while

Table 4.10 Management of thyrotoxic storm

Symptom/ sign	Management
Thyrotoxicosis	• β-blockers (e.g. propranolol, esmolol) or if contraindicated calcium channel blockers (e.g. diltiazem) to overcome adrenergic effects • Thionamide (e.g. propylthiouracil)—high dose to inhibit thyroid hormone production • Radioiodine to reduce the activity of the thyroxine producing cells • Oral iodine to invoke Wolff–Chaikoff effect (see previously) • Glucocorticoids to reduce conversion of T_4 to T_3 • Bile acid sequestrants to reduce enterohepatic recycling of thyroid hormones
Hypovolaemia	Fluids +/– inotropes
Hyperthermia	Cooling, anti-pyretics (paracetamol)
Electrolyte disturbances	Appropriate correction
Arrhythmias	Defibrillation, anti-arrhythmics
Agitation	Benzodiazepines, anti-psychotics

propylthiouracil is the only thiouracil. Carbimazole is rapidly metabolized to methimazole once ingested.

The thionamides main action is to halt the synthesis of thyroid hormone by interfering with TPO-mediated oxidation of iodide, iodide organification, and iodotyrosine coupling. In addition, thionamides inhibit the TPO-catalysed coupling process, by which iodotyrosine residues (DIT and MIT) are combined for the formation of T_4 and T_3. Propylthiouracil also inhibits type 1 deiodinase in peripheral tissue, thus blocking the conversion of T_4 to T_3. This extrathyroidal action is useful in cases of thyroid storm or severe thyrotoxicosis.

In addition to the inhibition of thyroid hormone production, in vitro and in vivo studies have shown that thionamides have an inhibitory effect on the immune system. Here, they act to decrease immune-related molecules, such as intracellular adhesion molecule 1 and soluble interleukin-2, as well as lower the levels of TSH-receptor antibodies over time. Antithyroid drugs also decrease human leukocyte antigen class II expression and induce apoptosis of intrathyroidal lymphocytes.

Prescribing

Antithyroid drugs are associated with a high incidence of unwanted effects, although **carbimazole** (or **methimazole** available in the USA) is better tolerated than **propylthiouracil** and preferred for long-term treatment. In thyrotoxicosis treatment is continued for 12–18 months, at which point it may be tapered or discontinued if TSH levels have returned to normal. Patients on

carbimazole who have failed to respond at this point may opt to continue treatment, although treatment failure is likely to require surgery or radioactive iodine therapy.

Both drugs are administered orally, usually in divided doses, although carbimazole can be given OD, with doses started high, then subsequently reduced to a maintenance dose once the patient becomes euthyroid; this usually takes 1–2 months. In some cases, higher doses are continued in combination with **levothyroxine** in a 'block and replace' regimen, although this is associated with more adverse effects and generally considered less favourable.

In thyrotoxic crisis, propylthiouracil tends to be the preferred agent as, unlike carbimazole, it blocks the extrathyroidal conversion of T_4 to T_3. Here, high doses of 200–300 mg are given 4–6-hourly until thyroid function has stabilized, at which point treatment is generally switched to carbimazole.

Unwanted effects

The thionamides, in particular **propylthiouracil**, are known to cause serious hypersensitivity reactions, including agranulocytosis (see 'Prescribing warning: agranulocytosis with propylthiouracil and carbimazole'), hepatitis, and cutaneous vasculitis, all of which require urgent management. Patients with a history of hypersensitivity should not be re-exposed and other drugs in the class should be used with caution, as there is a risk of cross-sensitivity.

Prior to initiating antithyroid therapy, it is recommended that baseline bloods are carried out, i.e. full blood counts (white cell count) and LFTs (bilirubin and transaminases), repeated at regular intervals to assess for toxicity.

PRESCRIBING WARNING

Agranulocytosis with propylthiouracil and carbimazole

- Agranulocytosis is a severe hypersensitivity reaction associated with thionamides.
- Reactions occur more commonly with propylthiouracil, regardless of dose, whereas with carbimazole the risk is dose dependent.
- Affects approximately 1:200 prescribed.
- All patients should be counselled on the risks prior to starting treatment, and advised to stop taking it and seek help immediately should they experience symptoms such as sore throat, mouth ulcers, fever, malaise, bruising, or bleeding.
- A full blood count should be carried out in case of suspected agranulocytosis.

Other non-specific adverse effects include nausea, vomiting, and headache. Although both propylthiouracil and **carbimazole** cross the placenta and can cause foetal goitre, propylthiouracil is preferred in the first trimester as it has rarely been associated with congenital malformations. Propylthiouracil is also favoured in breastfeeding mothers, despite both being present in breastmilk.

Thyroid hormones

The actions of thyroid hormones at the cellular level can originate in the nucleus, at the plasma membrane, in the cytoplasm, and at the mitochondrion. It can lead to local membrane actions on ion transport, control of cell proliferation, or regulation of transcriptional activity. For example, levothyroxine and liothyronine.

Mechanism of action

The thyroid hormone nuclear receptors (TR), are DNA-binding proteins that regulate transcription by interacting with thyroid hormone response elements in the promoter region of T_3 target genes. There are four receptor isoforms (α_1, β_1, β_2, β_3), which are tissue dependent and mediate subtype-specific functions. Activity is also regulated by a host of nuclear co-regulator proteins, so that diverse protein complexes of TR can achieve the variously different effects of thyroid hormones.

The non-genomic actions of thyroid hormones are those not mediated by the nuclear receptors, and may begin at the plasma membrane or the cytoplasm. The plasma membrane protein, integrin $\alpha v \beta 3$, has been shown to contain a binding domain for iodothyronines, which acts as an initiation site for hormone-directed cellular events, such as cell proliferation and angiogenesis. Proteins in the cytoplasm can also bind thyroid hormones, which could be either translocated nuclear receptors or native cytoplasmic proteins. These receptors can activate intracellular signalling cascades, such as PI3K and ERK, leading downstream to specific gene transcription.

Prescribing

Levothyroxine (T_4) is the thyroid hormone of choice in the management of hypothyroidism, although it has been used in combination with **liothyronine** (triiodothyronine, T_3). Doses of levothyroxine for replacement therapy are based on age, weight and sex; which in the presence of a non-functioning thyroid, equates to about 1.6 µg/kg/day based on lean body weight. Doses are administered orally, ideally in the morning with water, 30–60 minutes before breakfast.

Compared with levothyroxine, liothyronine has a more rapid onset and shorter duration of action, with greater potency making it valuable in treating severe or acute hypothyroid states such as myxoedema coma. Doses may be administered IV (unlike with levothyroxine) and patients switched to oral therapy once they are stabilized; availability can, however, be a problem.

PRACTICAL PRESCRIBING

Absorption of levothyroxine

- Levothyroxine demonstrates significantly superior bioavailability if taken with water on an empty stomach either 60 minutes before breakfast or 4 hours after an evening meal.
- For compliance, however, it is better to advise patients to take it with water 30–60 minutes before breakfast.
- Iron and calcium supplementation can cause malabsorption of levothyroxine/liothyronine, so should be taken at least 4 hours apart.

Unwanted effects

Side effects to **levothyroxine** are more commonly seen in overdose, in particular GI (diarrhoea, vomiting) and cardiac (palpitations and arrhythmias) toxicity. In order to distinguish levothyroxine-induced cardiac toxicity from any underlying cardiovascular disease, manufacturers advocate the use of a baseline ECG before starting treatment. Careful titration to establish the lowest effective dose helps minimize the effects of excessive use or subclinical hyperthyroidism, such as osteoporosis, weight loss, restlessness, insomnia, and headaches.

The side effects profile to **liothyronine** is similar, although with its rapid onset and short duration of action they are likely to be more pronounced (e.g. tachycardia, anxiety), especially with higher doses.

Drug interactions

Although numerous drugs have the potential to interact with **levothyroxine** and **liothyronine**, interactions of clinical significance are rare. Drugs that can reduce absorption, such a calcium salts, antacids, and iron are best spaced by a few hours. As the anti-coagulant effects of **warfarin** may be enhanced by levothyroxine/liothyronine, caution is recommended on initiation or following a dose change.

Further reading

Cheng S-Y, Leonard JL, Davis PJ (2010) Molecular aspects of thyroid hormone actions. *Endocrine Review* 31(2), 139–70.

Narayana SK, Woods DR, Boos CJ (2011) Management of amiodarone-related thyroid problems. *Therapeutic Advances in Endocrinology and Metabolism* 2(3), 115–26.

Nayak B, Hodak SP (2007) Hyperthyroidism. *Endocrinology and Metabolism Clinics* 36(3), 617–56.

Wass JA, Stewart PM, Amiel SA, Davies MC (2011) The thyroid. In: Wass JAH, Stewart P (Eds) *Oxford Textbook of Endocrinology and Diabetes* (2nd Ed) Part 3, pp. 301–631. Oxford: Oxford University Press.

Guidelines

Bahn RS, Burch HB, Cooper DS, et al. (2011) Hyperthyroidism and the other causes of thyrotoxicosis: management guidelines of the American Thyroid Association and American Association of Clinical Endocrinologists. *Endocrine Practice* 17(3), e3.

Garber JR, Cobin RH, Gharib H, et al. (2012) Clinical practice guidelines for hypothyroidism in adults: cosponsored by the American Association of Clinical Endocrinologists and the American Thyroid Association; *Endocrine Practice* 18(6), e2.

4.4 Parathyroid disease

The parathyroid glands are a number of, usually four, small glands located posterior to the thyroid gland, and are responsible for the production of parathyroid hormone (PTH), which regulates Ca^{2+} and phosphate metabolism. Dysfunction therefore leads to hyper/hypocalcaemia, which can affect neurotransmitter release, bone metabolism, and muscle contraction. Abnormal Ca^{2+} levels can occur as a result of primary disease of the parathyroid (e.g. autoimmune disease) or secondary to iatrogenic causes, vitamin D deficiency, renal failure, or malignant tumours. Severe Ca^{2+} deficiency (<1.9 mmol/L) requires urgent correction.

Pathophysiology

PTH is an 84 amino acid polypeptide, secreted from chief cells in a circadian rhythm fashion that is influenced by 'free' ionized Ca^{2+}. Ca^{2+}-sensing receptors either promote preproPTH mRNA in the case of low Ca^{2+}, or for high Ca^{2+}, induce intraglandular metabolism of the PTH. Almost 50% of circulating Ca^{2+} is protein bound, mainly to albumin, although only the 'free' ionized form is active. Clinically, therefore, it is crucial to use corrected Ca^{2+} measurement on blood results, as altered proteins levels (e.g. in dehydration, myeloma, renal failure, liver disease) can affect the amount of total Ca^{2+}, even if the 'free' Ca^{2+} is normal.

PTH tightly maintains circulating Ca^{2+} levels through a negative feedback system, acting directly on the kidney, bone, and GI tract. PTH, rapidly activates receptors on the kidney and stimulates 1α-hydroxylase to convert 25-hydroxyvitamin D to the active 1,25-(OH)2D (calcitriol), which increases circulating Ca^{2+}. Calcitriol acts in the gut to increase absorption and in the bone to induce skeletal resorption of Ca^{2+}. Vitamin D also acts in the kidney to promote phosphate retention and in the gut to increase its absorption.

A separate Ca^{2+}-regulating hormone **calcitonin** is released from the C cells of the thyroid gland. This hormone, although less potent on overall Ca^{2+} control, has the reverse effects to PTH, i.e. lowers Ca^{2+} by:

- Inhibiting gut Ca^{2+} absorption.
- Inhibiting bone resorption.
- Inhibiting renal tubular cell reabsorption of Ca^{2+}, but like PTH also inhibits kidney phosphate reabsorption.

As such, exogenous **calcitonin** can be used to treat hypercalcaemia, osteoporosis, and Paget's disease.

As PTH regulates Ca^{2+}, dysfunctional changes in PTH levels will therefore affect Ca^{2+} levels.

Hyperparathyroidism

Primary hyperparathyroidism is the most common cause of hypercalcaemia, affecting 3/1000 adults in the UK. It is usually caused by a parathyroid adenoma and is associated with gene abnormalities such as retinoblastoma, MEN (multiple endocrine neoplasia) type 1 (*MEN1*), and MEN type 2 (*MEN2*). Most patients are asymptomatic, but in severe/chronic disease inadequately managed it can lead to end-organ damage, i.e.:

- *Bones*: osteoporosis, osteopenia.
- *Kidney*: renal calculi, renal impairment.
- Pancreatitis.
- *Joints*: pseudogout.
- *Cardiovascular*: hypertension, ECG changes (shortened QT interval).
- Muscle weakness.

In general severe complications are rare, mainly due to earlier detection and management.

Secondary hyperparathyroidism most commonly occurs as a result of chronic renal failure, where there is phosphate retention and decreased production of 1,25-(OH)2D. This leads to hypocalcaemia, which increases secretion of PTH in a normal physiological response. Similarly, other causes of hypocalcaemia can precipitate secondary hypoparathyroidism, e.g. vitamin D deficiency, rickets, drugs, such as bisphosphonates (reduced bone resorption), and **phenytoin** (increased vitamin D metabolism).

Tertiary hyperparathyroidism occurs when long-standing hypocalcaemia (i.e. in chronic renal failure) and chronic parathyroid stimulation results in parathyroid glands that become hyperplastic and autonomous, thus producing excessive amounts of PTH and leading to hypercalcaemia. Consequently, tertiary disease patients are hypercalcaemic, hyperphosphataemic, and hyperparathyroid.

Hypoparathyroidism

Hypoparathyroidism is relatively uncommon, but typically occurs post-surgery (i.e. following thyroidectomy), due to the inadvertent removal of parathyroid glands. Subsequent loss of PTH input to the negative feedback system causes hypocalcaemia. Since acute hypocalcaemia can be life-threatening, it must be recognized though symptoms (e.g. paraesthesia of fingers/lips, muscle cramps) and signs (e.g. Chvostek's, Trousseau's, and lengthening QT on ECG). Severe hypocalcaemia (corrected Ca^{2+} less than 1.9 mmol/L) will require acute replacement IV. In chronic or resistant hypocalcaemia long-term supplementation is necessary.

For a full summary of the relevant pathways and drug targets, see Figure 4.4.

Management

Hyperparathyroidism

Primary hyperparathyroidism is diagnosed in the presence of a raised serum Ca^{2+} and parathyroid hormone and cured by a parathyroidectomy, removing the affected gland(s). Post-operatively, patients will routinely require calcium replacement, which in more severe cases is administered IV with **calcium gluconate**.

Asymptomatic patients may be managed without surgery, through close monitoring of serum Ca^{2+}, serum creatinine, and bone density. Where necessary, pharmacological treatment may be used to reduce serum Ca^{2+} or improve bone mineral density, i.e. bisphosphonates, selective oestrogen receptor modulators, and calcimimetics.

In secondary or tertiary hyperparathyroidism, primary management is through the identification and treatment of any underlying cause, e.g. drug therapy, vitamin D deficiency, etc. The calcimimetic, **cinacalcet** may be used to reduce PTH in primary hyperphosphataemia where parathyroidectomy is inappropriate, or in secondary disease in patients with end stage renal disease on renal dialysis, i.e. not in patients with hypocalcaemia.

Hypoparathyroidism

Hypoparathyroidism is diagnosed in the presence of a low serum Ca^{2+} and PTH. In the case of pseudohypoparathyroidism, PTH levels remain normal despite low Ca^{2+} levels, although there is an end-organ resistance to PTH effects. In either case the aim of treatment is to achieve normal serum Ca^{2+} levels through calcium supplementation usually in combination with vitamin D (**calcitriol** or **alfacalcidol**). Treatment will also include correction of low magnesium levels or raised phosphate levels.

Drug classes used in management

Bisphosphonates

> Bisphosphonates are stable analogues of naturally occurring pyrophosphate-containing compounds that are adsorbed to bone mineral and inhibit bone resorption. They decrease bone breakdown and are used for the treatment of complications related to bone metastasis in thyroid cancer. For example, pamidronate, alendronate, and risedronate.

For more information see Topic 7.4, 'Metabolic bone disease'.

Phosphate binders

> These agents work by binding to phosphate in the GI tract, reducing their absorption. The serum phosphate and Ca^{2+} levels are both regulated by the PTH. In patients with chronic renal failure, serum phosphate control is important due to its association with bone pathology. Examples include aluminium hydroxide, calcium acetate, lanthanum, sevelamer carbonate, and sevelamer hydrochloride.

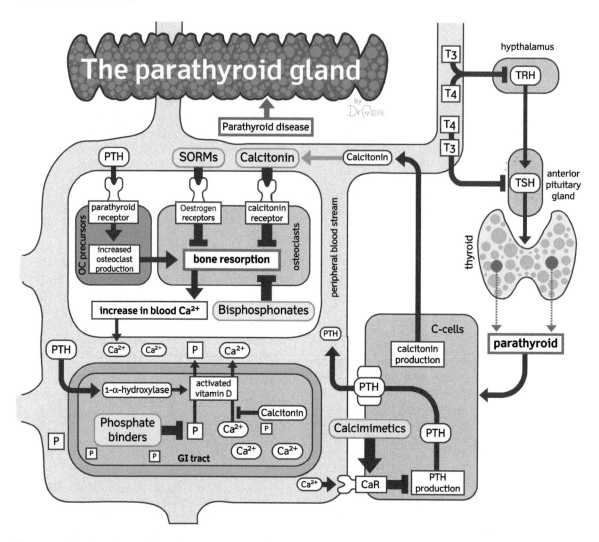

Figure 4.4 The Parathyroid gland: Summary of relevant pathways and drug targets

For more information see Topic 5.2, 'Acute kidney injury'.

Calcimimetics

Calcimimetics modulate the Ca²⁺ receptor (CaR) by increasing their sensitivity to activation by extracellular Ca²⁺, leading to the inhibition of PTH secretion. In turn, the decrease in PTH levels is associated with a concurrent reduction in serum Ca²⁺. For example, cinacalcet.

Mechanism of action

Extracellular ionized Ca²⁺ levels are tightly controlled and largely regulated by PTH, which increases serum Ca²⁺

levels to maintain homeostasis. The CaR responds to Ca²⁺ with high affinity and is a member of the G protein–coupled superfamily of receptors; expressed in cells controlling systemic Ca²⁺ homeostasis, mainly in the parathyroid gland, kidney, thyroid C-cell, bone, and intestines.

Activation of CaR on the parathyroid gland cells leads to the stimulation of intracellular signalling pathways, coupling to PLC via G protein, and then indirectly to phospholipase A2. This leads to the release of arachidonic acid, conversion to leukotriene metabolites, and inhibition of PTH secretion.

Prescribing

Cinacalcet is an oral therapy licensed for use in primary hyperparathyroidism (where a parathyroidectomy is inappropriate) and secondary hyperparathyroidism in patients with end-stage kidney disease on dialysis. It is not indicated in CKD for patients not on dialysis, where serum Ca²⁺ levels are likely to be low.

Tablets are administered OD at escalating doses to achieve optimal PTH levels, or increasingly, according to serum Ca²⁺ levels as this is considered to be more cost effective. Where corrected Ca²⁺ levels fall below normal limits, treatment should be withheld or discontinued.

Unwanted effects

As calcimimetics act to increase PTH levels and Ca²⁺ loss, treatment is contraindicated in hypocalcaemia, as its use can cause profound and even fatally low levels. Patients should be advised to report symptoms or signs of hypocalcaemia such as tetany, paraesthesia, myalgia, and convulsions. In case of severe hypocalcaemia, patients will require urgent correction with **calcium gluconate** 10%. The risk of toxicity is increased in hepatic dysfunction, where clearance is impaired.

Other common side effects to **cinacalcet** include GI effects, in particular nausea and vomiting, as well as dyspepsia and diarrhoea, and hypersensitivity reactions.

Drug interactions

Cinacalcet is a substrate for CYP 3A4 and, to a lesser extent, CYP 1A2. Potent inhibitors (e.g. azole anti-fungals, **telithromycin**, **ritonavir**) or inducers (e.g. **rifampicin**) of CYP 3A4 can alter cinacalcet levels and dose adjustments may be necessary. Cinacalcet itself is a potent inhibitor of CYP 2D6. This is of greatest clinical significance with **tamoxifen** where it inhibits conversion of tamoxifen to its active metabolite.

Calcitonin

Calcitonin is a 32 amino acid linear polypeptide hormone, produced by the C cells of the thyroid gland that has a potent inhibitory effect on osteoclasts through the calcitonin receptor. It acts to reduce blood Ca²⁺, in opposition to the parathyroid hormone.

Mechanism of action

The calcitonin receptor in bone remodelling osteoclasts, and also in the kidney and the brain, is a G protein–coupled receptor linked to adenylate cyclase and cAMP production, as well as the phosphatidyl–inositol–Ca²⁺

pathway. Receptor activation increases the generation of vitamin D producing enzymes (25-hydroxyvitamin D-24 hydroxylase) and leads to greater retention of Ca²⁺ and enhanced bone density. The reduction in blood Ca²⁺ levels is also achieved by inhibition of renal tubular cell Ca²⁺ reabsorption, which allows for increased urine excretion.

Prescribing

Following an MHRA alert on the long-term safety of **calcitonin**, it is no longer advocated for use in osteoporosis (see Topic 7.4, 'Metabolic bone disease'). It may, however, be used where the benefits are thought to outweigh the risks, such as treating hypercalcaemia of malignancy. Calcitonin is not currently licensed for use in hypercalcaemia due to other causes.

Unwanted effects

See Topic 7.4, 'Metabolic bone disease'.

Selective oestrogen receptor modulators

Selective oestrogen receptor modulators (SORMs) are a class of compounds that lack the steroid structure of oestrogens, but possess a tertiary structure that allows binding to the oestrogen receptors. Unlike pure receptor agonists or antagonists, SORMs exert selective agonist or antagonist actions depending on the target tissue. Examples: raloxifene

For more information see Topic 7.4, 'Metabolic bone disease'.

Further reading

Bilezikian JP, Khan AA, Potts JT, et al. (2011) Hypoparathyroidism in the adult: epidemiology, diagnosis, pathophysiology, target-organ involvement, treatment and challenges for future research. *Journal of Bone and Mineral Research* 26(10), 2317–37.

Cooper MS, Gittoes NJ (2008) Diagnosis and management of hypocalcaemia. *British Medical Journal* 336(7656), 1298–302.

Drueke TB (2004) Modulation and action of the Ca²⁺-sensing receptor. *Nephrology, Dialysis and Transplantation* 19(5), v20–6.

Hendy GN (2005) Calcium regulating hormones. Vitamin D and parathyroid hormone. In: Melmed S, Conn PM (Eds)

Endocrinology. Basic and Clinical Principles, 2nd edn, pp. 283–99. New York City, NY: Humana Press.

Marx SJ (2000) Hyperparathyroid and hypoparathyroid disorders. New England Journal of Medicine 343, 1803–75.

Thakker RV (2000). Parathyroid disorders. Molecular genetics and physiology. In: Kirollos R, Helmy A, Thomson S, Hutchinson P. (Eds) Oxford Textbook of Surgery, pp. 1121–9. Oxford: Oxford University Press.

Guidelines

Bilezikian JP, Brand ML, Eastell R, et al. (2014) Guidelines for the management of asymptomatic primary hyperparathyroidism: summary statement from the Fourth International Workshop. Journal of Clinical Endocrinology and Metabolism 10, 3561–9.

Eastell R, Brandi M, Costa A, et al. (2014) Diagnosis of asymptomatic primary hyperparathyroidism: Proceedings of the Fourth International Workshop. Journal of Clinical Endocrinology and Metabolism 10, 3570–9.

NICE TA117 (Jan 2007) Cinacalcet for the treatment of secondary hyperparathyroidism in patients with end-stage renal disease on maintenance dialysis therapy. https://www.nice.org.uk/Guidance/ta117 [accessed 26 March 2019].

4.5 Diabetes mellitus

DM is a metabolic disorder with acute and chronic implications, due to deficiency or reduced effectiveness of endogenous insulin. There are two main types; type 1 diabetes mellitus (DM1)—which is a *failure* in the production of insulin, and type 2 diabetes mellitus (DM2)—which is *resistance* to insulin. Around 5% of DM is due to other causes (e.g. endocrine, drug-induced, maturity onset diabetes of the young (MODY)) or, in the case of secondary diabetes, occurs in the presence of a syndrome or condition (e.g. pancreatic disorder or endocrinopathies). The hormone insulin normally acts on muscle cells, adipocytes, and hepatocytes to stimulate glucose uptake and suppress glucose production, respectively. When this fails, high-circulating plasma glucose levels may cause diabetic ketoacidosis in the short term, and long term lead to serious microvascular (e.g. ocular, diabetic neuropathy/foot disease/nephropathy) and macrovascular complications (e.g. coronary heart disease, acute MI, peripheral vascular disease, hypertension, and dyslipidaemias).

Overall, DM is exceptionally common with around 3 million sufferers in the UK and a prevalence of ~4.5%. Of these 83% have DM2, which typically presents in those >30 years old, with associated risk factors (see Box 4.2). DM1 (12%), on the other hand, is more commonly seen as juvenile onset.

Pathophysiology

Insulin and the control of blood glucose

Insulin is a potent anabolic hormone that is synthesized and secreted from the β-cells within the islets of Langerhans in the pancreas. It is coded by the *INS* gene (chromosome 11) and transcription/translation produces pre-proinsulin, which is cleaved to proinsulin within the Golgi apparatus. Proinsulin then undergoes further cleavage to reveal insulin and C-peptide, which are stored in β-cell granules ready for secretion. C-peptide, previously considered inert, is now known to have vasoactive properties.

Circulating blood glucose levels are tightly controlled by β-cells, through a direct glucose positive feedback mechanism (via GLUT-2 receptors) and other factors (e.g. glucagon, the autonomic nervous system—parasympathetic/sympathetic; see Table 4.11). Basal release of insulin is pulsatile, with low-amplitude peaks every 10 min, although average basal levels remain more or less constant throughout the 24-hour period. However, upon eating levels rise significantly in response to glucose and gut neuroendocrine release of incretin. The early response to glucose consists of two phases influenced by circulating levels and rate of change. During phase 1, response is rapid, peaks at 5 minutes and lasts 10 minutes with insulin available from a stored pool. Phase 2 is a slow rising increase that peaks at approximately 60 minutes, and comes from a stored and newly synthesized pool.

The insulin response to glucose is controlled through the GLUT-2 transporter receptor, located on β-cells. Here, circulating glucose is transported into cells and undergoes metabolism by glucokinase, to glucose-6-phosphate. It then enters glycolysis and the tricarboxylic acid cycle, with the proportional liberation of ATP. Intracellular ATP acts to close ATP-sensitive K^+ channels, so that depolarization occurs with consequential influx of Ca^{2+} (voltage-gated) to cause granule translocation, fusion with the cell membrane and release of insulin (Figure 4.5). When there is insulin insensitivity or failing release of insulin, the K_{ATP} channel can be augmented through binding of sulphonylureas. This inhibits the hyperpolarizing actions of K^+, so that membranes are more likely to depolarize and release insulin. Furthermore, these compounds can sensitize β-cells to glucose, limit hepatic glucose production and decrease lipolysis, all of benefit in DM.

During overnight fast, circulating insulin levels are 20–50 pmol/L. However, they can be markedly lower in patients with DM1, secondary diabetes or in insulin

Box 4.2 Risk factors for DM2

- Obesity, especially central (truncal) obesity
- Lack of physical activity
- *Ethnicity*: South Asian, African, African-Caribbean, Polynesian, Middle-Eastern and American-Indian
- History of gestational diabetes
- Impaired glucose tolerance
- Impaired fasting glucose
- *Drug therapy*: e.g. combined use of a thiazide diuretic with a β-blocker
- Low-fibre, high-glycaemic index diet
- Metabolic syndrome
- Polycystic ovarian syndrome
- *Family history*: 2.4-fold increased risk for type 2 diabetes

Table 4.11 Factors affecting insulin release from pancreatic β-cells

Stimulation of insulin release	Inhibitors of insulin release
Glucose	Low glucose
Parasympathetic (ACh via muscarinic receptors)	Sympathetic (adrenaline via α2 receptors)
Glucagon-like peptide (α-cells)	Somatostatin (δ-cells)
Amino acids	
Fatty acids	
Gastrin	
Secretin	
Cholecystokinin	

sensitivity. Conversely, in patients with an insulinoma (a rare secreting tumour of pancreatic β-cells), levels are significantly raised. Insulin acts on almost every cell in the body, to control intermediate metabolism and favour a fuel storage state. Hepatocytes, skeletal muscle cells, and adipocytes show profound responses to insulin, mediated via transmembrane insulin receptors to cause:

- *Carbohydrate metabolism*: in the liver insulin *stimulates* glycogen storage from glucose and non-glucose sources (gluconeogenesis), and *inhibits* breakdown of glycogen (glycogenolysis). While in muscle it promotes the recruitment of glucose transport into cells via GLUT-4, stimulating glycolysis and glycogen synthesis (Figure 4.5).
- *Fat metabolism*: in the liver there is increased triglyceride synthesis (lipogenesis) and subsequent reduced circulating free fatty acid levels through lipase inhibition. Lipolysis is also decreased, by opposing the actions of adrenaline and growth hormone on adenylate cyclase.
- *Protein metabolism*: in muscle cells amino acid uptake is increased promoting protein synthesis, while in the liver there is decreased proteolysis (protein breakdown).

Insulin is also important in the transport of K^+, Ca^{2+}, and phosphate into cells. The ability of insulin to drive circulating K^+ into cells is important clinically as it can, like **salbutamol**, help to treat hyperkalaemia (see Topic 5.1, 'The Kidney, drugs, and chronic kidney disease'). There

are also longer-term actions of insulin on DNA and RNA via the RAS complex (Raf, MEK, MAPK) to regulate growth and gene expression.

DM1

DM1 is a T cell-mediated autoimmune disease that destroys the β-cells of the pancreas and accounts for about 15% of DM. It has a genetic predisposition, but also a strong environmental element, with patients typically presenting younger. Genetically, it is associated with HLA DR3, DR4, insulin gene promoter region, >20 other genetic loci, and islet autoantibodies. Of this patient group it is predicted that around 30–40% show immunogenetic and familial concordance.

Many environmental triggers have been proposed, including viruses, toxins, dietary factors, and stress. These factors may initiate damage to β-cells and reveal specific antigens, like GAD65 and IGRP (islet-specific glucose-6-phosphatase catalytic subunit-related protein). In DM1 patients, 90% have autoantibodies against the former. Over 25% of individuals without one of these or islet cytoplasmic autoantibodies will have positive antibodies to ZnT8, a pancreatic beta-cell-specific zinc transporter. T-cell (cytotoxic CD8+) action and β-cell proliferation can lead to patchy insulitis, which may lead to insidious

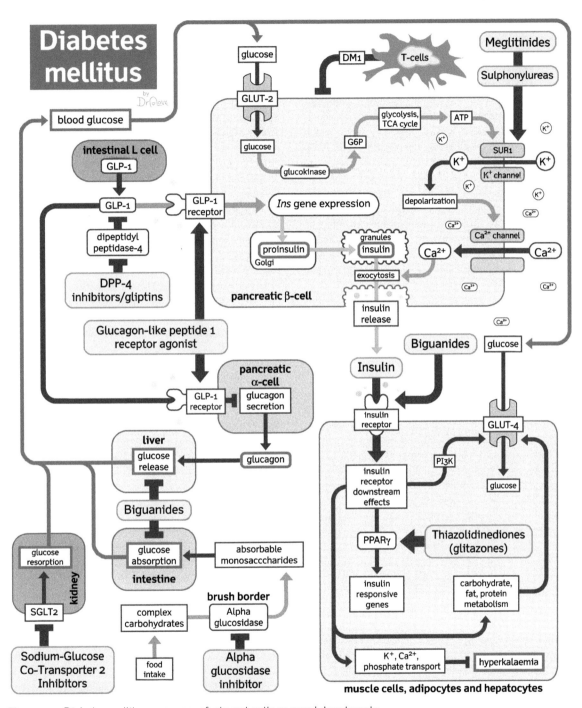

Figure 4.5 Diabetes mellitus: summary of relevant pathways and drug targets.

onset and a prediabetic phase that is not clinically an insulin-dependent state.

The increasing loss of β-cells and, hence, insulin production, means the body's anabolic (storage) potential is lost and metabolism of carbohydrate, fat, and protein is increased. This results in a hyperglycaemic state with excess free fatty acid production. The disinhibited lipolysis generates free fatty acids that, in turn, lead to ketone body formation and the characteristic signs seen in diabetic ketoacidosis (DKA); weight loss, acetone breath, nausea and acidotic breathing.

DM1 can present as DKA, but most features develop over a week or so, and are related to catabolism and hyperglycaemia; only when 80–90% of beta cells have been destroyed does hyperglycaemia develop. The osmotic effects of glucose in the kidney results in urinary loss of water with ketones and electrolytes, giving rise to polyuria/polydipsia, characteristic symptoms. Osmotic shift can also cause changes in vision, which includes acute and reversible effects due to changes in the refraction of the lens. Metabolic changes lead to weight loss, malaise, and weakness with an increased predisposition to infection due to persistent hyperglycaemia. The only real effective therapies are replacement of insulin and long-term management of any complication (see 'Management DM1').

DM2

DM2 is a complex multifactorial disease, where a combination of insulin resistance and β-cell failure results in a net hyperglycaemic state, as insulin release is unable to overcome resistance. Typically, the early response to glucose is *impaired*, so that the initial phase is lost and phase 2 becomes more prominent, therefore, supplying constant, relatively high doses of insulin and inhibiting lipolysis. This leads to weight gain and increased body fat, further driving insulin resistance.

DM2 is the most common form of DM and accounts for 85% of the disease with a rising prevalence. It is associated with environmental and genetic factors (see Box 4.2). A number of genetic loci have been identified that affect insulin resistance (PPAR-γ), insulin secretion (TCF7L2), and obesity (FTO), although their strength in predicting disease is poor. Nonetheless, having a first-order relative with DM still confers a lifetime risk of ~40%. The largest single risk factors remain obesity and a sedentary lifestyle (Box 4.2).

A heterogeneity of DM2 pathophysiology exists around the world, with some patients suffering as a result of insulin resistance progressing to failed release (e.g. USA and European obesity), whereas with others (e.g. Asian) hyposecretion is predominant. For most with DM2, background insulin levels are sufficient to prevent lipolysis and ketogenesis, so insulin replacement per se is not required. For others, however, disease progression and failure of control through diet and anti-diabetic medications means replacement is fundamental to survival. The overall 'long game' in DM2 management is to prevent

acute hyperglycaemia and the complications of chronic poor control.

The mechanism of insulin resistance in DM2 is complex and a number of models have been proposed. It is suggested that insulin activity is reduced in the presence of obesity, due to the increased metabolic activity of visceral adipocytes, as these tend to be more resistant to insulin than subcutaneous deposits. Furthermore, the increased sensitivity of visceral fat to catecholamines, means more lipolysis occurs so that more free fatty acids are delivered to the liver. A second possible mechanism suggests that free-circulating fatty acids (due to impaired suppression of lipolysis) impair insulin-mediated glucose deposition, accelerate hepatic glucose production, and directly suppress endogenous insulin secretion. This fatty acid load may impede insulin action through mitochondrial dysfunction and (through TNFα, which inhibits tyrosine kinase activity) affect GLUT-4 translocation. Finally, persistently high glucose levels can reduce insulin-mediated tyrosine kinase activity, so that failure of GLUT-4 translocation occurs and insulin receptor substrates become altered. This leads to decreased glucose utilization and decreased uptake of glycogen, fat, and protein formation.

The normal response to insulin resistance is to increase the amount of insulin released from β-cells so that normoglycaemia can be maintained. Unregulated circulating levels of insulin may prevent DM symptoms, although high levels may cause non-specific receptor activation of IGF-1. This, in turn, activates keratinocytes and melanocytes, leading to clinical signs of acanthosis nigrans tattooing and skin thickening; as well as androgenization. The resistant phase of DM2 can also lead to, by definition, *metabolic syndrome* (syndrome X). Here, there is insulin resistance, glucose intolerance, obesity, dyslipidaemia, and hypertension. This syndrome is a strong indicator of impending DM2, atheroma formation, and cardiovascular complications.

Early signs of β-cell failure are the loss of phase one responses to a glucose challenge. This glucose intolerance and insulin resistance drives the β-cells to produce more insulin, but at a certain point the system 'breaks' and no further insulin can be secreted. There is a therapeutic window in which, if resistance and β-cell failure are addressed, function can return to physiological-like levels, avoiding the requirement for insulin replacement. As outlined previously, use of sulphonylureas, weight loss, diet control, and other insulin-sensitizing drugs may ameliorate this progression. The meglitinides may act at β-cells via closure of the K_{ATP} channel to enhance insulin release especially in the phase one release. Other approaches include insulin sensitizers, like glitazones (see 'Management

Thiazolidinediones'), where activity is in the peripheral tissues via PPAR-Y changing gene expression. Adipocytes are therefore more sensitive to insulin, increasing GLUT-1 and GLUT-4 expression, and improving dyslipidaemias. Another commonly used drug, **metformin**, acts peripherally to inhibit fat and muscle cell mitochondrial respiration, so increases GLUT-1 and GLUT-4 translocation.

For a full summary of the relevant pathways and drug targets, see Figure 4.5.

Management

Diagnosis of diabetes is made through the identification of hyperglycaemia, either by measuring plasma glucose (fasting plasma glucose or an oral glucose tolerance test) or, as endorsed more recently by WHO, through the measurement of HbA1c (see Table 4.12). HbA1c reflects plasma glucose levels over a period of 8–12 weeks and can be taken at any time of the day without the need for fasting; however, due to expense and availability, fasting plasma glucose remains the test of choice for some.

In symptomatic patients, a single abnormal reading can be used to confirm diagnosis; however, in patients that are asymptomatic, confirmation requires a second abnormal result, ideally using the same test. Subsequent investigations aim to distinguish the type of DM, i.e. DM1, DM2, or secondary DM (see Table 4.13)

Following diagnosis, patients will require extensive education. Lifestyle advice should be offered to all patients with confirmed diabetes and those with an impaired glucose tolerance (defined as 7.8–11 mmol/L), in order to reduce the risk of cardiovascular disease and premature death. This will include dietary, as well as general healthy living advice, i.e. stopping smoking, weight loss in obesity, regular exercise, and moderate alcohol consumption. Patients will require 3–6-monthly reviews to reassess their diabetes control, considering both pharmacological and non-pharmacological factors, as well as their ability to deal with a diabetic crisis.

The primary aim of medical management of diabetes mellitus is to achieve optimal glycaemic control (an HbA1c less than 48 mmol/mol), thus reducing the risk of microvascular and macrovascular complications. Consideration should also be given to managing other cardiovascular risks, i.e. hypertension and dyslipidaemias, in order to reduce these complications.

DM1

Management of DM1 is with **insulin** therapy to achieve a target plasma glucose of 4–7 mmol/L pre-meals, and an HbA1c of 48 mmol/mol or less. Insulin is formulated to achieve short, intermediate, or long durations of action. Increasingly, the insulin analogues (e.g. insulin glargine—long acting, insulin aspart, short-acting) are being used in preference to the soluble human or animal insulins. Patients are managed with a regimen (see Table 4.14) based on patient preference and trends in insulin

Table 4.12 Diagnostic tests for DM

Test	Diagnostic level	Advantages	Disadvantages
Fasting plasma glucose	≥ 7 mmol/L	Widely available / Inexpensive / Unaffected by presence of haemoglobinopathies	Inconvenient (sample storage, timing requirements) / Affected by daily variations in glucose levels
OGTT	≥ 11.1 mmol/L	Widely available / Inexpensive / Unaffected by presence of haemoglobinopathies	Inconvenient (sample storage, time-consuming) / Affected by daily variations in glucose levels
HbA1c	≥ 48 mmol/ mol (6.5%)	Convenient / Avoids daily variations in plasma glucose levels	Cost / Worldwide issues with availability and standardization of assay technique

Table 4.13 Investigations to distinguish type of DM

	DM1	DM2
Common presenting signs/symptoms	Polydipsia, polyuria, weight loss, lethargy, DKA (30%), repeated candidiasis (thrush)	Polyuria/polydipsia, asymptomatic (40%), rarely DKA (~10%), repeated candidiasis (thrush)
Age at presentation	Usually in childhood	Usually in adulthood
Body size	Rarely obese, recent history of weight loss	Typically obese/overweight
Family history	About 10% have affected close relative	75–90% have affected close relative
Antibodies	Can have pancreatic autoantibodies	Lower incidence of autoantibodies
Other signs, co-morbidities		Acanthosis nigricans, hypertension, polycystic ovarian syndrome

requirements, e.g. avoiding basal insulin in patients with severe nocturnal hypoglycaemia, or the use of an insulin pump.

To optimize control, patients will require education on monitoring blood sugars and adjusting insulin requirements, as well as advice on recognizing signs of hypoglycaemia. They should also be advised to rotate injection sites to prevent the formation of hard fatty lumps. In practice, few succeed in achieving good glycaemic control, so it is recommended that HbA1c levels are checked every 3–6 months, or more often in case of poor control.

DM2

As with DM1, management strategies include a combination of non-pharmacological (e.g. lifestyle, education, diet, weight management) and pharmacological interventions. Blood glucose control is managed primarily with oral hyperglycaemics, to achieve an HbA1c of 48 mmol/mol or less (unless drug therapy is associated with a risk of hypoglycaemia then aim for 53 mmol/mol. This should be measured every 3–6 months until stable and then 6-monthly. First-line treatment in the UK is with **metformin**, although where contraindicated or poorly tolerated, NICE advocates the use of a sulfonylurea or a newer agent, e.g. DPP-4 inhibitors or **pioglitazone** is recommended. In general, choice of agent should be based on patient factors such as pre-existing co-morbidities (e.g. cardiovascular disease, renal impairment), ease of administration and tolerance (see Table 4.15). In all cases, doses should be titrated to achieve target HbA1c levels. Where monotherapy is insufficient, a second agent should be added

Table 4.14 Insulin regimens

Regimen	Description
Multiple daily injections (basal-bolus)	Short-acting insulin administered before meals and longer-acting insulin administered OD or BD. This is the preferred regimen
One, two, or three daily injections	Injections of short and intermediate insulin mixed by the patient prior to use or pre-mixed biphasic insulin
Continuous SC insulin pump	Continuous or regular administration of usually a short-acting insulin via a pump.

Table 4.15 Comparison of oral hypoglycaemics

	Examples	Weight change	Hypoglycaemia	Frequency of admin	Effect on reducing HbA1c (%)
Biguanides	Metformin	↓	0	2–3/day	1–1.5%
Sulfonylureas	Gliclazide, glimepiride, glibenclamide, glipizide	↑	+++	Varies	1–1.5% but wears off
Thiazolidinediones 'glitazones'	Pioglitazone	↑↑	+	1/day	0.5%
GLP 1 agonists	Exenatide, liraglutide, dulaglutide, lixisenatide	↓↓	0*	Weekly/daily	Exentaide 0.5–1% liraglutide 0.8–1.5%
DPP-4 inhibitors 'gliptins'	Alogliptin, linagliptin, saxagliptin, sitagliptin, vidagliptin	0	0*	1/day	0.6–0.9%
SGLT	Dapagliflozin, canagliflozin, empagliflozin	↓	0*	1/day	
Meglitinides	Repaglinide, nateglinide	↑	+	3/day	Repaglinide 1–1.5%, nateglinide 0.6–1%
Alpha-glucosidase inhibitors	Acarbose	0	Unlikely	3/day	0.5–0.8%

*Commonly used in combination therapy where risk of hypoglycaemia may be increased.

in and, failing that, a third may be considered or **insulin** therapy initiated.

Drug classes used in management

Insulin

Insulin is the major regulator of energy functions in the body, acting as an anabolic hormone that favours the uptake, utilization, and storage of glucose, the storage of lipids and the prevention of protein breakdown. It binds and activates the insulin receptor tyrosine kinase, which mediates the activation of intracellular signalling cascades in the target cells.

Mechanism of action

The insulin receptor is a heterotetramer composed of two α and two β glycoproteins subunits, connected by disulphide bridges. Insulin binds to a site in the extracellular α subunits, which triggers activation of the tyrosine kinase domain on the intracellular portion of the β subunits. This intracytoplasmic domain attaches phosphate groups to tyrosine residues elsewhere on the receptor and on additional intracellular proteins. The phosphorylation and recruitment of insulin receptor substrate (IRS) proteins, which vary in their tissue distribution and subcellular localization, initiates the intracellular transduction pathways within the target cell. Tyrosine-phosphorylated IRS then displays binding sites for numerous signalling partners, all possessing specific sarcoma homology region SH2 domains, and leads to the effects of insulin on glucose, lipid, and protein metabolism.

The phosphatidylinositol 3-kinase (PI3-K) signal transduction pathway, mainly via the activation of the protein kinase Akt/PKB and the protein kinase C-δ (PKC δ) cascades, is a crucial transduction step that appears to mediate virtually all of insulin's effects on glucose transport, lipogenesis, and glycogenesis. By contrast, the mitogen-activated protein kinase (MAPK) pathway has more relevance to the actions of insulin on cell growth.

Beyond the actions on glucose, lipid, and protein metabolism, insulin also has effects on nitric oxide-mediated vasodilation, growth, and differentiation of the foetal nervous system, and increased Na^+ absorption by the kidneys.

Prescribing

Insulin is predominantly used in patients with DM1, although it may also be beneficial in patients with DM2 who remain poorly controlled, despite mono or combined therapy with oral hypoglycaemics. As a polypeptide hormone, it is inactivated in the gut and therefore must be administered by injection, preferably SC. The short-acting or soluble insulins are administered 15–30 minutes before a meal, as they have an onset of action of 30–60 minutes when administered SC and faster when given IV. For this reason, many patients prefer the more rapidly acting insulin, e.g. **aspart** or **lispro**, as these are taken immediately before a meal (see Table 4.16).

The onset and duration of action of insulin is increased by preparing the insulin as a suspension, either by forming a complex with protamine (**isophane** insulin) or protamine zinc; or modifying the particle size, such as with insulin zinc suspensions. This provides background (basal insulin) cover administered once (at night) or BD. In patients experiencing nocturnal hypoglycaemia with BD intermediate acting or for those using a rapid-acting agent with meals, a longer-acting agent (**glargine**) should be considered as the basal insulin.

Biphasic insulins are pre-mixed combinations of short- and intermediate-acting insulin analogues, available in different ratios (e.g. 40:60 or 30:70 of soluble:isophane insulin). Where used, they are usually administered SC two to three times a day, 15 minutes before a meal, although they have been largely superseded by basal-bolus regimens, which offers more flexible control.

Unwanted effects

Hypoglycaemia, local reactions, and allergy account for the main adverse effects reported with insulin therapy, the latter being very rare. Care should be taken when transferring between different insulin analogues as requirements may vary, particularly between human, porcine, and bovine analogues.

As with endogenous insulin, the effects of insulin analogues can be altered by some drugs, to either reduce (corticosteroids, growth hormone, **salbutamol**, etc.) or increase (hypoglycaemics, salicylates, and some ACE inhibitors) their effects.

Biguanides

Biguanides are anti-hyperglycemic drugs that can decrease glucose absorption by the intestines and glucose production in the liver, while also improving insulin sensitivity. They can lower blood glucose concentrations without causing overt hypoglycaemia. For example, metformin.

Mechanism of action

The activation of AMP-activated protein kinase (AMPK) is closely linked to the multiple actions of **metformin**.

Table 4.16 Onset and duration of action of insulins

	Onset of action	Duration of action	Examples
Rapid-acting	15 minutes	2-5 hours	Aspart, lispro
Short-acting	30–60 minutes	Up to 8 hours	Soluble
Intermediate-acting	1–2 hours	16–35 hours (maximal effect 4-12 hours)	Isophane (NPH)
Long-acting	2–3 hours	Up to 36 hours (maximal effect at 10-20 hrs). Takes 2-4 days to reach steady state	Glargine

AMPK is a serine/threonine protein kinase that acts as a sensor for cellular energy status. In normal conditions, AMPK is activated by an increase in the AMP/ATP ratio, which results from an imbalance between the production and consumption of ATP. When activated, AMPK switches cells from an anabolic to a catabolic state, inhibiting ATP-consuming synthetic pathways through phosphorylation of key metabolic enzymes and transcription factors. This leads to an inhibition of glucose, lipid, and protein synthesis, while the oxidation of fatty acids and glucose uptake are stimulated.

Most of the evidence suggests that metformin does not directly activate AMPK, but that this is a secondary effect, resulting from a transient decrease in cellular energy status, prompted by the specific but weak inhibition of the mitochondrial respiratory chain complex I. The added improvement in insulin sensitivity is due to the positive effects on insulin receptor expression and tyrosine kinase activity.

Prescribing

Metformin is the only biguanide widely available worldwide and the most frequently used oral hypoglycaemic in the management of DM2. Like the sulfonylureas, it can result in a ~1.5% decrease in HbA1c percentage point, although unlike sulphonylureas, these effects tend to be more sustainable, with some evidence to suggest it may confer an additional benefit in reducing cardiovascular risk. Metformin should not be given in any disorder that reduces oxygen, i.e. severe COPD, heart failure, and must be used with caution in renal failure (avoid initiation if the eGFR is <45 mL/minute/1.73 m² and monitor U&E). Doses are preferably taken orally with food, to improve tolerance, two to three times a day, either as monotherapy or in combination with further hypoglycaemic agents or insulin.

Unwanted effects

Metformin is generally well tolerated, being associated with neither hypoglycaemic episodes nor weight gain (some patients may achieve some weight loss). It is, however, contraindicated in patients with severe renal impairment or an underlying condition that predisposes them to renal impairment, due to the risk of lactic acidosis (see 'Prescribing warning: lactic acidosis with metformin'). More common side effects include GI toxicity (nausea, vomiting) particularly on initiation, and taste disturbances.

PRESCRIBING WARNING

Lactic acidosis with metformin

- Lactic acidosis is a rare but severe or even fatal metabolic complication of metformin therapy caused by accumulation secondary to renal impairment. This can be prevented by:
  - Avoiding in severe renal impairment (CrCl < 30 mL/min), reducing in moderate impairment (<60 mL/min).
  - Avoiding in conditions predisposing to renal impairment, e.g. shock, dehydration.
  - Avoiding in periods of tissue hypoxia, e.g. myocardial infarction, respiratory failure.
  - Annual monitoring of renal function in patients with normal renal function, two to four times a year in patients at risk of renal impairment, e.g. elderly.
  - Discontinuing treatment 48 hours prior to and at least 48 hours after surgery once normal renal function confirmed.
  - Discontinuing prior to administration of contrast media and for 48 hours after.
  - Avoiding alcohol intoxication.

Sulfonylureas

The anti-hyperglycaemic sulfonylureas are a class of insulin secretagogues that act by stimulating insulin release from pancreatic β cells, while also increasing the number and sensitivity of insulin receptors. They can also reduce hepatic gluconeogenesis and augment peripheral glucose utilization. Examples include gliclazide, glibenclamide, glipizide, and glimepiride.

Mechanism of action

Insulin release is stimulated by binding to the sulphonylurea receptor, a subunit of the octameric inward-rectifier K_{ATP} ion channel complex in the β-cell membrane. This leads to channel closure and membrane depolarization, which in turn causes influx of Ca^{2+} and exocytosis of insulin granules.

The various types of sulfonylureas have diverse cross-reactivity with cardiovascular K_{ATP} channels. As such, the agents closing these channels can oppose ischaemic preconditioning. This effect has generated concern due to a possible deleterious effect of sulfonylureas in cardiovascular disease.

Prescribing

The sulfonylureas can be subdivided into first (**glibenclamide** and **chlorpropamide**, which has been widely discontinued) and second generation (**gliclazide**, **glipizide**, **glimepiride**) agents, with second generation more widely used due to the reduced risk of hypoglycaemia. As a class they are effective in reducing HbA1c by about 1.5 percentage points with a relatively fast onset of action, although effects when used as monotherapy tend to wear off with time.

Unwanted effects

In practice sulfonylureas, with the exception of **gliclazide**, are infrequently used due to the risk of hypoglycaemia and weight gain. Hypoglycaemia is particularly problematic in elderly patients, with high doses, in patients with erratic eating habits, i.e. a tendency to miss meals, or in the presence of a declining renal or hepatic function.

Thiazolidinediones (glitazones)

Thiazolidinediones activate the intracellular receptor of the peroxisome proliferator-activated class, specifically the PPAR-Y, which regulates the transcription of insulin-responsive genes involved in the regulation of glucose production, transport, and use. For example, pioglitazone and rosiglitazone.

Mechanism of action

Thiazolidinediones, through the activation of PPAR-Y, act by selectively enhancing or partially mimicking some of the actions of insulin, thus producing a slow antihyperglycaemic effect in DM2. The PPAR-Y is expressed principally in white and brown adipocytes, and since thiazolidinediones are lipophilic, they can enter the cells and bind to receptors with high affinity. This produces a conformational change in the receptor complex, which displaces a co-repressor and allows the activation of DNA regulatory sequences. Because some of these genes are also controlled by insulin, thiazolidinediones can increase expression of genes that encode lipoprotein lipase, the fatty acid transporter protein, the adipocyte fatty acid-binding protein, fatty acyl-CoA synthase, malic enzyme, and glucokinase. Overall, this leads to an increase in fatty acid uptake and lipogenesis in adipocytes. Thiazolidinediones also promote the differentiation of pre-adipocytes into adipocytes.

Prescribing

In 2010, **rosiglitazone** was withdrawn from the market as it was shown to increase cardiovascular mortality and MI.

Although the risk is likely to be lower with **pioglitazone** and despite being advocated for use by NICE as an option where metformin is not suitable, the potential for cardiovascular morbidity has seen it generally fall out of favour. Where used, pioglitazone may be initiated as monotherapy or in combination with additional oral therapy or **insulin**. Doses are administered orally OD, starting low and titrated up slowly according to response. Patients should be reviewed every 3–6 months to assess for response, ideally aiming to achieve >0.5% reduction in HbA1c.

Unwanted effects

The increased risk of cardiac mortality, MI, and heart failure remains the main concern associated with glitazone treatment, thus **pioglitazone** is contraindicated in all patients with heart failure or a history of (see 'Prescribing warning: cardiovascular toxicity with pioglitazone'). Weight gain is also commonly reported which may, in part, be due to fluid retention and a possible indicator of a deteriorating heart. Diabetic macular oedema may be aggravated in diabetic patients receiving pioglitazone, which is likely to be secondary to increased fluid retention. Patients should be advised to report any deterioration in eyesight and, where appropriate, a referral made to ophthalmology.

More recent data has linked glitazone therapy to an increased risk of osteoporosis and bladder cancer, patients therefore require initial screening to identify any underlying predisposition and routine monitoring while on treatment.

Pioglitazone is extensively metabolized in the liver by CYP 2C8; consequently, it is contraindicated in hepatic impairment and has the potential to interact with drugs known to induce (**rifampicin**) or inhibit (**gemfibrozil**) this enzyme. Furthermore, it is hepatotoxic so patients will require baseline and periodic measurements of transaminases.

PRESCRIBING WARNING

Cardiovascular toxicity with pioglitazone

- Pioglitazone is associated with an increased risk/worsening of heart failure, secondary to fluid retention.
- These effects are increased when used in combination with insulin.
- Patients with any single given risk factor (e.g. previous MI) should be initiated on the lowest possible dose, with the dose increased gradually.
- While on treatment, patients should be monitored and pioglitazone discontinued in the case of worsening cardiac disease.

Glucagon-like peptide 1 (GLP-1) receptor agonist

Glucagon-like peptide receptor agonists are degradation-resistant peptides similar in sequence to the incretin hormone GLP-1, but with better pharmacokinetic properties that permit their use in antidiabetic therapy. Examples include exenatide, liraglutide, dulaglutide, and lixisenatide.

Mechanism of action

Glucagon-like peptide 1 (GLP-1) is an incretin hormone derived from the gut that can stimulate insulin and suppress glucagon secretion, inhibit gastric emptying, and decrease appetite and food intake. Most GLP-1 is generated in enteroendocrine L cells, located in the ileum and colon, with a mixture of endocrine and neural signals mediating the fast stimulation of GLP-1, before the food that is being digested transits through the gut.

GLP-1 activates a G protein–coupled receptor (GLP-1R) expressed in islet α and β cells, and in peripheral tissues, including the CNS and PNS, heart, kidney, lung, and GI tract. Activation of GLP-1R produces a fast increase in cAMP levels and intracellular Ca^{2+}, with subsequent insulin exocytosis in a glucose-dependent manner.

Exenatide (synthetic exendin-4) is a biologically active peptide from lizard venom that shares ~ 50% of its amino acid sequence with mammalian GLP-1, and is a potent degradation-resistant agonist at the mammalian GLP-1R. It has a half-life of 60–90 minutes, and reaches peak plasma concentrations 4–6 hours after a single SC injection. **Liraglutide** is a partially DPP-4 resistant GLP-1 analogue, which has an Arg34Lys substitution, and a glutamic acid and 16-C free fatty acid addition to Lys26. The acyl moiety helps non-covalent binding to albumin. It has a half-life of 10–14 hours after SC administration.

Prescribing

There are currently four GLP-1 agonists on the market, each with specific licensed indications. **Exenatide**, the first to be licensed, is administered as a weekly SC injection in combination with **metformin** and/or a sulfonylurea/thiazolidinedione as dual or triple therapy. In studies it has been shown to reduce HbA1c by about 1.3 percentage points, as well as promote marked weight loss.

In comparison, **liraglutide** is administered SC OD, and can be given as mono or combination therapy with oral agents or **insulin**. Head to head studies with exenatide have demonstrated its superior efficacy both in its ability to reduce HbA1c (about 1.5 percentage points) and promote weight loss. Of the two, exenatide tends to be better tolerated. **Lixisenatide** and **dulaglutide** the most recent to appear on the market, appear to date to be comparable with other agents in terms of administration and efficacy. Despite differences in licensing all agents are generally used in combination therapy when other treatment options have failed. More recently, evidence suggests that the use of liraglutide is associated with a reduced risk of cardiovascular-related mortality.

Unwanted effects

GI toxicity is commonly reported on initiating treatment with GLP-1 agonists, particularly with **liraglutide** (nausea, vomiting, and diarrhoea). Effects tend to be mild to moderate in nature and settle with time, although the manufacturer advises caution in patients with inflammatory bowel disease. This toxicity may in part explain the weight loss of 2–3 kg seen in the first 6 months of treatment and which is more pronounced with liraglutide. Other less common, but potentially more serious effects associated with treatment include pancreatitis and thyroid disease. Although relatively rare, patients should be advised to look out for signs of acute pancreatitis (severe, persistent abdominal pain) and seek help. There are also anecdotal reports of pancreatic cancer linked to GLP-1 agonists.

Dipeptidyl peptidase-4 inhibitors (DPP-4 inhibitors/ gliptins)

DPP-4 inhibitors increase levels of GLP-1 in circulating plasma by inhibiting its rapid degradation by the dipeptidyl peptidase-4. Examples include alogliptin, linagliptin, saxagliptin, sitagliptin, and vidagliptin.

Mechanism of action

DPP-4 is a ubiquitous cell-surface aminopeptidase that spans across the membrane and is expressed in several tissues, including the liver, kidney, lung, intestinal membranes, endothelial cells, and lymphocytes. Once cleaved from its membrane-anchored form, the extracellular domain can circulate in the plasma with full enzymatic activity.

Inhibitors of DPP-4 mimic several of the effects associated with GLP-1R agonists, including stimulation of insulin and inhibition of glucagon secretion, and stimulation of β-cell proliferation. However, unlike the GLP-1 receptor agonists they are not generally linked with weight loss, probably due to the fact that they increase the levels of other incretins, as well as GLP-1, which have adipogenic effects. There are many small-molecule DPP-4 inhibitors developed for oral administration, reducing DPP-4 activity by more than 80%.

Prescribing

The first of the DPP-4 inhibitors, **sitagliptin** was licensed for use in 2006 and has been shown to reduce HbA1c by between 0.6 and 0.9 percentage points. As a class they are indicated for use second-line, either as monotherapy or in combination with one or two further agents including **insulin**, with slight differences in specific licenses between agents. They are all available in combination tablets with **metformin**. Of the drugs in the class, **linagliptin** has the advantage of being licensed for use in renal impairment, as unlike the other agents is not renally excreted.

Compared with the GLP-1 agonists they have the advantage of being administered orally, although they are less effective in improving glycaemic control and tend to be weight neutral.

Unwanted effects

In general, the DPP-4 inhibitors are well tolerated, the most commonly reported side effect being nasopharyngitis and upper respiratory tract infection, possibly secondary to interference with immune function. Hypoglycaemia can occur, particularly when taken in combination with sulfonylureas and **metformin**. There have also been reports of pancreatitis with treatment, which although rare is potentially serious so that patients should be advised to report any severe, persistent abdominal pain.

Drug interactions

Of the gliptins, **linagliptin**, **sitagliptin** and **saxagliptin** are metabolized through the liver via cytochrome P450 or p-glycoprotein, although this rarely leads to interactions of clinical significance.

Linagliptin is a weak to moderate inhibitor of CYP 3A4 and a substrate for p-glycoprotein, with the potential to increase **simvastatin** levels and have its own levels altered in combination with potent inhibitors, e.g. **ritonavir** (increased levels) and potent inducers **rifampicin** (decreased levels).

Saxagliptin is a substrate for CYP 3A4 and when used in combination with **diltiazem** or **ketoconazole** (moderate and potent inhibitors, respectively) shows significant increases in serum levels, where as potent inducers (e.g. rifampicin) may impair glucose control.

Interactions with sitagliptin and **alogliptin** are unlikely as they are primarily really cleared with minimal CYP450 metabolism.

Sodium-glucose co-transporter 2 inhibitors

The sodium-glucose co-transporter (SGLT) couple the transport of glucose against a concentration gradient with the concurrent transport of Na^+ down a concentration gradient. Inhibition of SGLTs decreases the transport of glucose across the proximal tube epithelium in the kidneys, thus reducing its reabsorption. Examples include dapagliflozin, canagliflozin, and empagliflozin

Mechanism of action

During fasting state, plasma glucose levels are mainly maintained through the production of endogenous glucose by the liver via glycogenolysis and gluconeogenesis. In turn, the kidney contributes to glucose homeostasis by gluconeogenesis and the added reabsorption of filtered glucose. In physiological conditions about 180 g of glucose is filtered a day, and the kidney can prevent this loss by active reabsorption (importantly, glucosuria results when the reabsorptive capacity is overwhelmed by filtered load).

Glucose can enter eukaryotic cells via two types of membrane-located carriers: the facilitative glucose transporters (GLUTs) and the SGLTs, which are responsible for glucose reabsorption from glomerular filtrate. SGLTs can be grouped into two types, SGLT1, located primarily in small intestinal cells, plus kidney and heart, and SGLT2, which are present exclusively at the apical domain of the epithelial cells in the early proximal convoluted tubule (S1 segment). SGLT2 is a low-affinity, high capacity SGLT responsible for almost 90% of reabsorbed filtered glucose. Thus, SGLT2 inhibition leads to a reduction in filtered glucose reabsorption, a decrease in the renal threshold for glucose and subsequent increase in glucose excretion.

Prescribing

Dapaglaflozin, **canagliflozin**, and **empagliflozin**, are the first in the newest class to be launched for use in DM2. As well as effectively optimizing glycaemic control, they have been shown to be beneficial in reducing weight and lowering BP. As with many of the newer agents,

NICE only advocate its use in combination therapy with **metformin** and/or **insulin**, regardless of licensed indications. Empagliflozin like **liraglutide** has been shown to reduce the risk of cardiovascular-related mortality.

Unwanted effects

The sodium-glucose-co-transporter 2 is expressed selectively in the kidney where it promotes glucose reabsorption; thus, in order to be effective, renal function must be adequate. Treatment is therefore not recommended in patients with moderate to severe renal impairment (CrCl <60 mL/min) and treatment is associated with a small risk of an increase in serum creatinine and dysuria. As glucose is excreted in the urine, patients are at increased risk of urinary tract infections (UTIs; particularly in women) and genital mycotic infections, e.g. vulvovaginal candidiasis, especially in those with a previous history.

Furthermore, these drugs act to promote diuresis and, as such, should be avoided in patients at risk of volume depletion, hypotension, or electrolyte disturbances, particularly if they are already taking diuretics. Of greatest concern with treatment is the risk of atypically presenting DKA, which can be severe and even life-threatening (see 'Prescribing warning: risk of DKA with SGLT-2 inhibitors').

Despite this, treatment is generally well tolerated, hypoglycaemia, the most common adverse effect, usually occurs in combination with **insulin** or a sulphonylurea. For this reason, NICE does advocate its use as triple therapy with **metformin** and a sulfonylurea. Other side effects tend to be non-specific (nausea, dizziness, and rash) with incidence comparable with placebo.

PRESCRIBING WARNING

Risk Of Dka With SGLT2 Inhibitors

- In June 2015 the MHRA/EMA published advice warning of the risk of severe DKA associated with SGLT2 inhibitors.
- Patients on treatment can present with atypical symptoms of DKA, where serum glucose levels are only moderately increased.
- Where DKA is suspected, treatment should be discontinued and ketones measured even if plasma glucose levels are near normal.
- Patients should be advised on how to recognize signs of DKA.

Meglitinides

Meglitinides are short-acting insulin secretagogues, which bind to β-cells in the pancreas and stimulate insulin release. In contrast to the sulfonylureas class they have no effect on insulin release in the absence of glucose. For example, nateglinide and repaglinide.

Mechanism of action

In normal conditions, glucose enters the cells where it is metabolized to produce ATP. Inside the cell, high concentrations of ATP inhibit the ATP-sensitive K^+ channels, leading to membrane depolarization and opening of L-type Ca^{2+} channels. This leads to Ca^{2+}-dependent exocytosis of insulin granules. Inversely, low ATP production causes K^+ channels to open to restore membrane potential. **Nateglinide** and **repaglinide** inhibit the ATP-sensitive K^+ channels in a glucose-dependent manner, and do not appear to affect skeletal, cardiac, or thyroid tissue. Meglitinides have a distinct binding site at β cell membranes, which is different to sulphonylureas, although like sulphonylureas they will only be effective where there is some level of β cell function.

Prescribing

The meglitinides **nateglinide** and **repaglinide** may be taken orally as monotherapy or in combination with **metformin** to optimize reductions in HbA1c. Due to their short half-life, they have a rapid onset and short duration of action, so are taken TDS, ideally 30 minutes before a main meal to optimize efficacy. Evidence suggests that repaglinide may be more effective in reducing HbA1c, and both drugs are of equal or lesser efficacy than metformin monotherapy.

Unwanted effects

The meglitinides are generally well tolerated, although they can cause symptomatic hypoglycaemia, with the risk increased at higher doses, in case of strenuous exercise, or with excessive alcohol intake. As with all secretagogues, treatment is associated with an increased risk of weight gain, which is possibly more pronounced with **repaglinide** compared with **nateglinide**. Other mild side effects tend to be GI in particular diarrhoea. Both drugs are hepatically metabolized and thus contraindicated in severe hepatic impairment.

Drug interactions

The meglitinides are substrates for the cytochrome P450 enzyme and, as such, are prone to interactions with drugs known to induce or inhibit these enzymes. **Repaglinide** is metabolized predominantly via CYP 2C8 and to a lesser extent CYP3A4. Potent inhibitors of these enzymes such as **gemfibrozil**, **clarithromycin**, azole anti-fungals, some anti-depressants, ACE inhibitors, NSAIDS, mono-amine oxidase inhibitors (MAOIs), and alcohol can therefore increase serum levels, increasing the risk of toxicity. Conversely, the effects of repaglinide may be reduced in combination with potent inducers, such as **rifampicin**, **phenytoin**, and **St John's Wort**.

Nateglinide is predominantly metabolized via CYP2C9 and to a lesser extent CYP3A4. Of note, significant reactions include reduced efficacy with rifampicin, St John's wort, and phenytoin, and increased toxicity with ACE inhibitors, NSAIDs, and MAOIs.

Alpha glucosidase inhibitor

The inhibition of intestinal alpha-glucosidase enzyme reduces the rate of digestion of starch and sucrose, flattens post-prandial blood glucose excursions and mimics the effects of dieting on hyperglycaemia, hyperinsulinaemia, and hypertriglyceridaemia. For example, acarbose.

Mechanism of action

The alpha-glucosidases in the brush border of the small intestine are responsible for the metabolism of complex carbohydrates into absorbable monosaccharide units. The alpha-glucosidase inhibitors bind competitively to the carbohydrate-binding region of the enzyme, thus competing with the binding of oligosaccharides leading to a decrease in glucose absorption due to the diminished amount of glucose molecules.

Acarbose is a nitrogen-containing pseudotetrasaccharide that reversibly inhibits the alpha-glucosidases and is efficacious in improving glycaemic control in type 2 diabetic patients, particularly with regard to post-prandial hyperglycaemia. It acts primarily in the gut because is not significantly absorbed.

Prescribing

Acarbose is rarely used due to its inferior efficacy compared to **metformin** and many of the newer agents (reduces HbA1c by about 0.5–0.8 percentage points). It is generally reserved for patients where other therapy is not tolerated or contraindicated. Doses are started low and can be increased at intervals of 6–8 weeks if treatment is ineffective. Tablets should be chewed with the first mouthful of food or immediately before with water.

Unwanted effects

GI side effects are common with **acarbose**, in particular flatulence, diarrhoea, and abdominal pain secondary to altered digestion of carbohydrates. These symptoms may be reduced by slow dose titrations and by strict adherence to a diabetic diet. Acarbose may also cause hepatic dysfunction and therefore liver transaminases should be monitored for the first 6–12 months. Due to its mechanism of action, hypoglycaemia is unlikely to occur with acarbose, unless used in combination with other drugs known to cause hypoglycaemia.

Further reading

Alberti K, Zimmet P, Shaw J (2005) The metabolic syndrome—a new worldwide definition. *Lancet* 366, 1059–62.

Andujar-Plata P, Pi-Sunyer X, Laferrere B (2012) Metformin effects revisited. *Diabetes Research and Clinical Practice* 95(1), 1–9.

Bazelier MT, Vestergaard P, Gallagher AM, et al. (2012) Risk of fracture with thiazolidinediones: disease or drugs? *Calcified Tissue International* 90, 450–7.

Black C, Donnelly P, McIntyre L, et al. (2009) Meglitinide analogues for type 2 diabetes mellitus. *Cochrane Database of Systematic Reviews* 18(2), 1–52.

Buse JB, Naruck M, Forst T, et al. (2012) Exentaide once weekly versus liraglutide once daily in patients with type 2 diabetes (DURATION-6): a randomised open-label study. *Lancet* 381, 117–24.

Chan HW, Ashan B, Jayasekera P, et al. (2012) A new class of drug for the management of type 2 diabetes: sodium-glucose co-transporter inhibitors, glucuretics. *Diabetes Metabolic Syndrome* 6(4), 224–8.

Drucker DJ, Nauck MA (2006) The incretin system: glucagon-like peptide-1 receptor agonists and dipeptidyl peptidase-4 inhibitors in type 2 diabetes. *Lancet* 368(9548), 1696–705.

Gallagher AM, Smeeth L, Seabroke S, et al. (2011) Risk of death and cardiovascular outcomes with thiazolidinediones: a study with the general practice research database and secondary care data. *PLoS ONE*, 6(12), e21857.

Kuzuya T, Matsuda A (1997) Classification of diabetes on the basis of etiologies versus degree of insulin deficiency. *Diabetes Care*, 20, 219–20.

Lind M (2012) Incretin therapy and its effects on body weight in patients with diabetes. *Primary Care Diabetes* 6(3), 187–91.

Marso SP, Daniels GH, Brown-Frandshen K, et al. (2016) Liraglutide and cardiovascular outcomes in type 2 diabetes. *New England Journal of Medicine* 375, 311–22.

Peters A (2010) Incretin-based therapies: review of current clinical trial data. *American Journal of Medicine* 123(3a), S28–37.

Pickup JC, Williams G (2002) *Textbook of diabetes*, 3rd edn. Oxford: Blackwell Science.

Scott L (2012) Repaglinide: a review of its use in type 2 diabetes mellitus. *Drugs* 72(2), 249–72.

Warrell DA, Cox TM, and Firth JD (2012) Endocrine disorders. In: Warrell DA, Cox TM, Firth JD (Eds) *Oxford Textbook of Medicine*, 5 edn, Section 13, 1787–2074. Oxford: Oxford University Press.

Zinman B, Wanner C, Lachin JM, et al. (2015) Empagliflozin, cardiovascular outcomes, and mortality in type 2 diabetes. *New England Journal of Medicine* 373, 2117–28.

Guidelines

International Diabetes Federation (2012) Clinical Guidelines task force global guideline for type 2 diabetes. https://www.iapb.org/wp-content/uploads/Global-Guideline-for-Type-2-Diabetes-IDF-2012.pdf [accessed 3 April 2019].

Nathan DM, Buse JB, Davidson MB, et al. (2009) Medical management of hyperglycaemia in type 2 diabetes mellitus: a consensus algorithm for the initiation and adjustment of therapy. A consensus statement from the American Diabetes Association and the European Association for the Study of Diabetes. *Diabetologia* 52, 17–30. http://care.diabetesjournals.org/content/35/6/1364.full.pdf+html [accessed 27 March 2019].

NICE NG17 (2016) Type 1 diabetes in adults: diagnosis and management. https://www.nice.org.uk/guidance/ng17 [accessed 27 March 2019].

NICE NG28 (2015) Type 2 diabetes in adults: management. https://www.nice.org.uk/guidance/ng28 [accessed 27 March 2019].

NICE TA288 (2013) Dapagliflozin in combination therapy for treating type 2 diabetes https://www.nice.org.uk/guidance/ta288 [accessed 27 March 2019]. NICE TA315 (2014) Canagliflozin in combination therapy for treating type 2 diabetes https://www.nice.org.uk/guidance/ta315 [accessed 27 March 2019].

NICE TA336 (2015) Empagliflozin in combination therapy for treating type 2 diabetes https://www.nice.org.uk/guidance/ta336 [accessed 27 March 2019].

SIGN 116 (2010) Management of diabetes: a national clinical guideline https://www.sign.ac.uk/sign-116-and-154-diabetes.html [accessed 3 April 2019].

WHO (2011) Use of glycated haemoglobin (HbA1c) in the diagnosis of diabetes mellitus: abbreviated report of a WHO consultation. https://www.who.int/diabetes/publications/report-hba1c_2011. [accessed 27 March 2019].

WHO/IDF (2006) Definition and diagnosis of diabetes mellitus and intermediate hyperglycaemia; Report of a WHO/ IDF consultation. https://www.who.int/diabetes/publications/diagnosis_diabetes2006/en/ [accessed 27 March 2019].

4.6 Female reproduction (abnormal menstruation, contraception, assisted reproduction)

The menstrual cycle and ovulation is driven under the tight control of gonadotrophic hormones—FSH and LH, which are released via the hypothalamic-pituitary axis to act on the ovaries. GnRH secreted from the hypothalamus stimulates the pituitary to produce gonadotrophic hormones, which in turn act on the ovaries to alter circulating levels of ovarian hormones (e.g. oestrogen, progesterone, and inhibin), and regulate follicular growth and ovulation.

During the lifetime of a female around 400–500 oocytes will be ovulated, while the remaining 99% will never complete meiosis. Dysregulation of the hypothalamus–pituitary–ovarian axis can predictably lead to impaired menstruation and infertility.

Pathophysiology

The menstrual cycle

In general terms, the menstrual cycle is split into two phases (see Figure 4.6);

- *follicular phase*, when 'adult' follicular development occurs to the point of ovulation;
- *luteal phase* when the corpus luteum forms, leading to either pregnancy of luteolysis.

The luteal phase is generally fixed at 14 days length, while the follicular phase varies, explaining the variation in length of menstrual cycle observed in the population (21–35 days; average of 28 days). During the follicular phase, sustained low levels of FSH and LH select out and promote a single follicle (Graafian follicle) to become dominant within the ovary. Under the influence of FSH and LH, granulosa cells secrete oestrogen (converted from androgens produced by thecal cells in the follicle), which encourages endometrial proliferation, thereby optimizing the environment for implantation. The rising oestrogen levels have a negative feedback on the hypothalamus (via inhibin), ceasing further release of FSH. This continued rise in oestrogen concentrations peaks, and the negative feedback flips to become positive feedback via the hypothalamus (involving GnRH and kisspeptin), which initiates a massive LH surge lasting 24–48 hours. This LH surge, in conjunction with a minor FSH rise, initiates the final stages of oocyte maturation and activates a cascade of inflammatory responses [associated with prostaglandins (PG) and cytokines] before ovulation at the thinning ovarian cortex and follicular rupture. In the early stages of the LH surge, the granulosa cells start to express LH receptors and under hormonal influence begin to secrete progesterone independent of PGs.

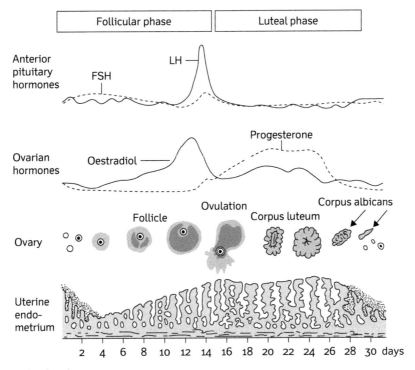

Figure 4.6 The menstrual cycle.

Reproduced with permission from Sanders, S, Dawson, J, Datta, S, et al. (Eds), *Oxford Handbook for the Foundation Programme*, Oxford, UK: Oxford University Press ©2005. Reproduced with permission of the Licensor through PLSclear.

As the follicle collapses it becomes the corpus luteum, producing progesterone from the thecal cells and oestrogen; with both hormones acting to increase endometrial thickening and vascularity should implantation occur. Progesterone levels start low, but as these rise from the corpus luteum, the cervical mucus becomes thicker and fallopian tube motility decreases, increasing the likelihood that sperm and egg will meet. Progesterone production is dependent on LH, but over time the corpus luteum diminishes, leading to a rapid decline in progesterone if fertilization fails to occur. Over this period, the corpus luteum has also been secreting oestrogen and inhibin, which represses FSH secretion, with the failing corpus luteal secretions triggering menstruation

Pregnancy

Should fertilization of the oocyte occur, β-human chorionic gonadotrophin (βhCG) is secreted by the trophoblast, and acts on the LH receptors of the thecal cells within the corpus luteum, so that progesterone release continues.

Ongoing progesterone secretion by the corpus luteum maintains the endometrium and trophoblast implantation until foetal autonomy ensues. By week 8 of pregnancy, the placenta is sufficiently developed to provide the pregnant woman with the necessary progesterone, thus the corpus luteum is no longer required. As progesterone is the only circulating steroid required to maintain pregnancy, the use of the anti-progesterone drug **mifepristone** leads to endometrial loss and may be used in the termination of early pregnancy or as an emergency contraceptive.

Menopause

Menopause is the permanent loss of menses, amenorrhoea, for 12 consecutive months and occurs at a mean age of 52 years. It is associated with a variety of symptoms linked with the loss of hormone cycles. In the perimenopausal period (first symptoms of menopause), oestrogen levels are highly variable, and may decline or rise, with a consequent increase in FSH. During normal menses, failing oestrogen alone causes a rise in FSH, although in the peri-menopause period there is a failing numbers of follicles, with a corresponding drop in the release of inhibin and the associated anti-mullarian hormone (see Topic 4.7, 'Androgens, steroids'). Progesterone levels also decline in anovulation as the corpus luteum does not form and produce the hormone. This occurs more frequently as menopause approaches (full anovulation) and, as oestrogen and progesterone levels drop across the whole cycle, FSH and LH concentrations rise dramatically to stimulate (FSH) and maintain (LH) any remaining follicles. As the ovaries fail, with a consequential rise in gonadotrophins, the main source for sex hormones becomes the adrenal gland.

Abnormal menstruation and contraception

Dysmenorrhoea

Within the first 6–12 months following menarche, around 40% of females present with dysmenorrhoea, i.e. symptoms of 'unacceptable' pain associated with menstruation. Typically, this cramp-like pain starts within the first 1–2 days of menstruation, lasts for 48–72 hours, is localized to the suprapubic region and can be associated with nausea/vomiting, fatigue, and headache. *Primary* dysmenorrhoea is diagnosed when no organic cause can be found, whereas *secondary* dysmenorrhoea may result from pelvic inflammatory disease, endometriosis, adenomyosis, or pelvic adhesions, requiring additional investigations and intervention (see 'Management'). *Primary* dysmenorrhoea only occurs in ovulatory cycles and is due to higher, or abnormal, release of prostaglandins, which may cause abnormal uterine contraction, hypoxia, and ultimately ischaemia. Exogenous prostaglandins given to enhance uterine contraction of labour can emulate these symptoms, so intervention in this signalling pathway can be of benefit. However, despite the knowledge of this 'end-stage' mechanism, the underlying aetiology is poorly understood.

The declining progesterone levels of premenstruation (due to loss of the corpus luteum) means lysosomal instability occurs, with increasing levels of phospholipase A2 and subsequent arachidonic acid. The latter undergoes oxidation via the COX pathway (see Figure 4.7) to produce prostaglandins (e.g. prostaglandin E_2 and cyclic endoperoxides), which can hypersensitize pain fibres within the pelvis, resulting in disproportionate pain. Intervention within the COX pathway, by NSAIDs (e.g.

mefenamic acid, see Topic 7.1, 'Osteoarthritis') is of benefit for many females, although around 30% have unresponsive symptoms. An alternative pathway in resistant females may involve signalling via 5-lipoxygenase, where arachidonic acid is converted to leukotrienes that may directly stimulate uterine contraction.

Menorrhagia

Menorrhagia is defined as menstrual blood loss that interferes with a female's physical, psychological, social, and day-to-day quality of life; it affects some 6.5% of women aged between 15 and 51 years of age. For the purposes of research studies, it is defined as menstrual loss of >80 mL. Menorrhagia with regular and heavy menstrual bleeding tends to occur during the extremes of age and may be associated with ovulation and abnormal PG ratios. If cycles are irregular, with periods of amenorrhoea, lack of cyclic progesterone can lead to a fragile endometrium that easily bleeds. Causes may be local [e.g. fibroids, sexually transmitted disease (STI)] or systemic (e.g. thyroid dysfunction, coagulopathy); however, in the majority of cases no organic cause is identified, making it a primary endometrial disorder. If no pathology is found, dysfunctional uterine bleeding as a diagnosis of exclusion can be made, but the aetiology remains elusive. Studies have shown there to be increased levels of circulating PG, which result in vasodilatation and failed aggregation of platelets, leading to increased bleeding tendency. Excessive fibrinolysis has also been reported, so the use of antifibrinolytics, such as **tranexamic acid**, as a non-hormonal treatment, have been shown to reduce bleeding by about 40%. NSAIDS also have a significant role in the PG pathway. For patients where pregnancy is not currently intended, hormonal interventions can be more appropriate and effective. The Mirena® intrauterine device (coil) releases **levonorgestrel** into the endometrium so atrophy occurs, and reduces blood loss by up to 90%. It acts as a contraceptive by thickening the cervical mucus, which inhibits sperm entry. It also reduces sperm mobility within the uterus, making it more difficult for sperm to reach the egg. Oral contraceptives also have a role and, should these fail, upstream intervention with GnRH analogues can be used to down-regulate the hypothalamic–pituitary–ovarian axis and induce ovarian suppression, resulting in amenorrhoea.

Amenorrhoea/oligomenorrhoea

The absence of menses, amenorrhoea, can be divided into *primary* or *secondary* conditions. *Primary amenorrhoea* is

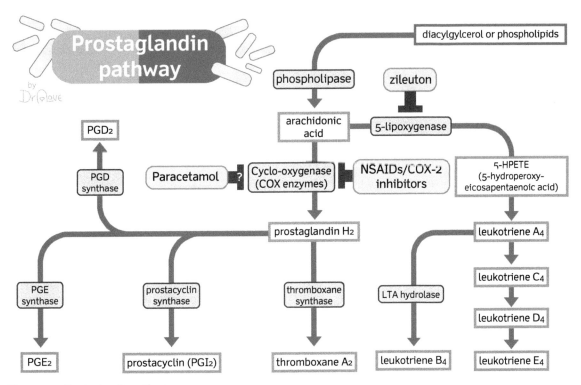

Figure 4.7 Prostaglandin pathway.

defined by a failure to start menstruating by the age of 15 years, whereas *secondary amenorrhoea* refers to the cessation of menstruation (>6 months) in a woman who previously had a menstrual cycle. Aside from pregnancy, causes include failure of the hypothalamic–pituitary–ovarian axis, thereby affecting stimulation and feedback of gonadotrophic hormones, e.g. Turner's syndrome, trauma, excessive weight loss, cancer, drug therapy, etc. In most cases of primary amenorrhoea, however, women will start spontaneously by the age of 18.

By examining a patient's hormone profile a diagnosis, as per the WHO system (Insler, 1988), can be made (Table 4.17) and appropriate treatment of the underlying cause made.

Raised prolactin (hyperprolactinaemia; Topic 4.1, 'The pituitary gland') levels, idiopathic or resulting from a pituitary adenoma, will lead to hypogonadotrophic hypogonadism and amenorrhoea. Hypothyroidism (Topic 4.3, 'Thyroid disease') can also cause oligomenorrhoea or amenorrhoea, so it is important to assess thyroid-stimulating hormone levels since raised thyrotrophin-releasing hormone will stimulate prolactin and suppress FSH production.

With oligomenorrhoea, menses occurs infrequently, i.e. a cycle of more than 35 days, secondary to numerous causes including, most commonly, low body weight and polycystic ovary syndrome (PCOS; this may also cause either primary or secondary amenorrhoea—see Topic 4.7, Androgens, steroids). Hormonal contraception can also affect the menstrual cycle leading to a reduced frequency.

Table 4.17 Diagnosis of amenorrhoea

Group	Hormone profile
Group I	Low oestrogen, low FSH, and no hypothalamic-pituitary pathology = hypogonadotrophic hypogonadism
Group II	Normal oestrogen, normal FSH, and normal prolactin = polycystic ovary syndrome
Group III	Low oestrogen and high FSH = gonadal failure

Endometriosis

During the reproductive years, it is estimated that around 10–12% of females may possess ectopic (outside the uterine) endometrial tissue that is oestrogen dependant, and capable of giving symptoms of pain or infertility. The true cause is unknown, but the likely source of this tissue is via retrograde menstrual flow, since many women have blood in the pelvis at the time of menstruation. Symptoms of pain may be constant or, more commonly, cyclical and chronic in nature, although some may be completely asymptomatic and present with infertility. Because this tissue is maintained by the presence of oestrogen, pharmacological therapy to manage symptoms include local oestrogen suppression (e.g. aromatase inhibitors—Topic 13.1, 'Haemato-oncology and malignancy') or ovarian suppression (e.g. combined oral contraceptive, GnRH analogues, or **danazol**). Medically, little can be done to restore fertility, so surgical treatment and IVF may be required. The GnRH analogues (e.g. **goserelin**) act like the endogenous decapeptide of the hypothalamus to stimulate FSH and LH from the anterior pituitary gland, which with continued stimulation, leads to a drop in FSH/LH levels and a subsequent downstream suppression of oestrogen.

Contraception

Exogenous oestrogen and progestogens are used as contraceptives and act to interfere with normal feedback on FSH and LH. High levels of oestrogen lead to suppression of FSH release and LH surge, thereby suppressing ovulation, thickening cervical mucosa, and endometrial thinning. The use of progestogen alone again causes endometrial thinning, decreased fallopian motility, and thickening of the cervical mucus.

Menopausal symptoms and hormone replacement therapy

During the perimenopausal period, symptoms may be complex due to varied oestrogen levels (high = breast tenderness, short cycle; low = hot flush), but as gonadotrophin levels rise and oestrogen declines, stable symptoms of menopause occur. These tend to fall into three categories and are mainly the result of falling oestrogen:

- *Vasomotor*: hot flushes, night sweats.
- *Genitourinary*: vaginal dryness, dysuria.
- *Psychological*: anxiety, depression.

Since symptoms can be severe and associated long-term with an increased risks of osteoporosis and fractures from falls, a risk-balanced approach to hormone replacement

is prudent. Local and/or systemic use can be considered, with oestrogen replacement alone in women who have undergone hysterectomy or oestrogen with progestogen (if systemic) in women with a uterus. **Tibolone** is a synthetic steroidal compound with oestrogenic, progestogenic, and androgenic activity that may be used as an alternative to combined hormone replacement therapy (HRT).

For a full summary of the relevant pathways and drug targets, see Figure 4.8.

Management

Abnormal menstruation and contraception

Primary dysmenorrhoea

Primary dysmenorrhoea is managed first-line with an NSAID and, failing that, with hormonal contraceptives in patients that remain symptomatic. NSAIDs are significantly more effective than **paracetamol** in symptom control of dysmenorrhea, although paracetamol may be considered where NSAIDs are contraindicated. As the efficacy of NSAIDs is likely to be a class effect, choice is determined by licensed indications and toxicity profile; consequently, **mefenamic** acid, **ibuprofen**, and **naproxen** are the preferred options.

Hormonal contraceptives (progestogen only and combined) provide an effective second-line option in patients that remain symptomatic on NSAIDs or paracetamol. Choice should be made in consultation with the patient, taking into consideration route and choice of hormones, as well as any co-morbidities that may preclude the use of hormonal therapy. In some patients, NSAIDs and contraceptives may be required together. In addition, patients should be advised of non-pharmacological options, such as heat application with a hot water bottle or bath, or the use of a TENS machine.

Menorrhagia

Pharmacological management of menorrhagia may be initiated once any underlying causes such as fibroids, endometriosis, carcinoma, or pelvic inflammatory disease have been excluded. Treatment of choice is NSAIDs and **tranexamic acid**, which may be enough to control the symptoms. If this fails, an intrauterine progestogen only device (e.g. Mirena®) may be used, although the patient should be made aware that, ideally, it would remain in place for a year. Alternatively, a combined oral contraceptive may be used in combination with NSAIDs and tranexamic acid. The third line option is with a

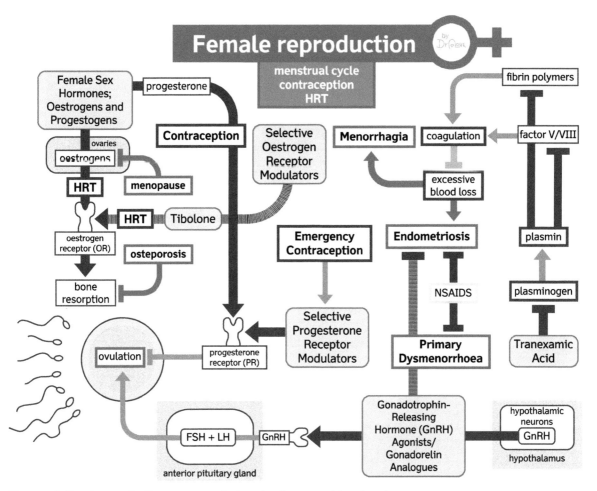

Figure 4.8 Female reproduction: summary of relevant pathways and drug targets.

progestogen, such as **norethisterone** or a longer-acting depot injection, e.g. **medroxyprogesterone**.

Endometriosis

Women with symptoms of endometriosis should be referred to a gynaecologist for investigation, particularly if symptoms are severe or if there is a possibility of impaired fertility. Following referral, treatment options (surgical or medical) can be discussed with the patient, with consideration given to preferences, severity of symptoms, and any desire to retain fertility. Surgical options range from the conservative use of laparoscopic techniques to remove any endometriosis (e.g. diathermy ablation) and breakdown adhesions, to more radical hysterectomies and/or salpingo-oophorectomies.

NSAIDs and contraceptives (combined oral contraceptive pill or progestogen only contraceptives) can be used to manage any pain associated with endometriosis; however, they will not restore fertility. Other treatment options initiated in secondary care include androgens (although rarely used now) or GnRH agonists to provide pain relief and reduce the number of lesions.

Contraception

There are numerous hormonal contraceptives available on the market, either as a combination of an oestrogen and progestogen, or as a progestogen only (see Table 4.18). When considering options, patients should be made aware of the relative risks and benefits, in particular any contraindications, such as oestrogens in patients with a history of DVT or at high risk of developing one, e.g. smokers. Where compliance is an issue, longer-acting devices such as implant or intrauterine devices (IUDs) may be an advantage.

Table 4.18 Comparison of hormonal contraceptive treatments

Contraceptive hormone	Route/ administration	Active ingredient	Advantages/ disadvantages	Efficacy*
Combined hormonal contraceptives	Oral (COC) OD either continuously (7-inactive pills) or for 21 days with a week break	Oestrogen (ethinylestradiol, estradiol) plus progestogen (norethisterone, levonorgestrel, drospirenone, desogestrel, gestodene)	A: Ease of administration, readily reversible. D: Dose must be taken at same time each day. Breakthrough bleeding	92%
	Transdermal Applied weekly for 3 weeks then 7 days patch-free	Ethinylestradiol and norelgestromin	A: Improved compliance in some D: Loss of adhesion	92%
	Vaginal ring Inserted and left in for 21 days, repeat after 7-day interval	Ethinylestradiol and etonogestrel	A: Improved compliance in some D: Risk of expulsion or breaking	92%
Progestogen-only	Oral (POP) OD taken continuously	Desogestrel, norethisterone, levonorgestrel, ethynodiol	A: Fewer contraindications compared with COC and maybe better tolerated D: Less effective than COC, smaller administration 'window' than COC.	92%
	Parenteral Long-acting depo injections administered IM every 8–12 weeks	Medroxyprogesterone acetate, norethisterone enantate	A: Compliance D: Not easily reversible, troublesome bleeding, clinic attendance	97%
	Implant Remove after 3 years	Etonogestrel	A: Compliance, efficacy, effects reversed on removal D: Clinic attendance	99.9%
	Intra-uterine device Remove after up to 5 years	Levonorgestrel	A: Compliance, efficacy, effects reversed on removal D: Clinic attendance	99.9%

*Percentage of women not pregnant after first year of use.

Emergency contraception can be administered following unprotected intercourse with oral **ulipristal** or **levonorgestrel**, or by using a copper IUD. Choice will, in part, be dictated by patient preference/circumstance and the time elapsed since intercourse, i.e. ulipristal can be used up to 5 days post-intercourse, whereas oral levonorgestrel only 3 days after. A copper IUD as emergency contraception can be used for up to 5 days post-intercourse, with the added benefit of providing future protection against pregnancy. In all cases, efficacy is increased by administering as early as possible. Both ulipristal and oral levonorgestrel are available to purchase over the counter from a pharmacy, to facilitate more rapid access.

Hormone replacement therapy

Before commencing HRT, the relative risks and benefits should be discussed with the woman to enable her to make an informed decision (see Table 4.19), with treatment tailored to address individual symptoms. In general, topical preparations are associated with a lower risk of serious morbidity and, for this reason, is often preferred. Advice on non-pharmacological strategies to help with symptoms such as flushing, night sweats, sleep disturbances, and mood disturbances may be helpful, and can include weight loss, regular exercises, wearing light clothing, and avoiding triggers such as spicy food or caffeine. For those that opt to take HRT, choice will partly depend on whether or not the woman has a uterus, i.e. the use of systemic oestrogen-only HRT is suitable for women without

a uterus, or combination HRT for those with. **Tibolone** is a useful alternative in women intolerant of standard HRT treatment and **raloxifene** in those at high risk of post-menopausal osteoporosis.

Drug classes used in management

Tranexamic acid

Synthetic derivative of the amino acid lysine, tranexamic acid is an antifibrinolytic used to reduce or prevent excessive blood loss during surgery and various conditions, including menstruation or trauma.

Mechanism of action

Tranexamic acid competitively inhibits activation of plasminogen, and reduces its conversion to plasmin, the enzyme that degrades fibrin clots, procoagulant factors V and VIII, fibrinogen, and other plasma proteins. At higher concentrations, it can directly inhibit plasmin activity in a non-competitive manner.

Prescribing

Tranexamic acid is administered orally for short-term management of bleeding, including menorrhagia, starting on the day of menstruation and continued for up to 4 days.

Table 4.19 Summary of risks with HRT

Risk	HRT	Relative risk
Breast cancer	All	Increases with duration of use
Endometrial cancer	Oestrogen-only	Risk increases with dose and duration
		Risk reduced with addition of progestogen in women with a uterus
Ovarian cancer	All	Risk is small
Venous thromboembolism	All	Risk higher in first year and in those with predisposing risk factors, e.g. smokers, personal or family history, obesity, varicose veins, etc.
Stroke	All	Only small increase in risk
		Tibolone increases risk by 2.2 times in the first year
Coronary heart disease	Combined	Risk greater in women starting HRT more than 10 years after menopause

Unwanted effects

As **tranexamic acid** inhibits the breakdown of fibrin clots, its use is contraindicated in patients with active or a history of VTE, and caution should be exercised in high risk patients such as those on hormonal contraceptives. In general, treatment is well tolerated, although it can accumulate in renal impairment and dose reductions are recommended.

Female sex hormones: oestrogens and progestogens

Synthetic progestins are functionally similar to progesterone, but structurally distinct and with longer biological half-lives. Ethinylestradiol is the synthetic oestrogen used in combination with progestins. They activate specific subtypes of steroid receptors, which are members of the ligand-binding transcription factors superfamily with both transcription dependent and independent effects. Examples include progestogens (norethisterone, levonorgestrel, etonogestrel, medroxyprogesterone, drospirenone, desogestrel, gestodene) and oestrogens (ethinylestradiol, estradiol).

Mechanism of action

Progestogens

The biological effects of progesterone and synthetic progestins are mediated by the progesterone receptor (PR), a member of the nuclear/intracellular receptor superfamily of ligand-dependent transcription factors. Progesterone binding induces a conformational change in the PR, which leads to its dissociation from multiprotein chaperone complexes, homodimerization and binding to specific progesterone response elements within the promoter of target genes. There is also increasing evidence that PG can mediate rapid, membrane-initiated cytoplasmic effects, independent of gene transcription, mediated by various second messengers and signal transduction pathways. These effects seem to be mediated by the same PR that regulates gene transcription.

The progesterone receptors are expressed in the female reproductive tract, mammary gland, brain, and pituitary gland. They play a crucial role in the establishment and maintenance of pregnancy, mammary gland development, and sexual behaviour. Their contraceptive value is based on the inhibitory effect of progesterone on ovulation and changes in cervical mucus that inhibit sperm penetration.

Progesterone can also bind with low relative affinity to the glucocorticoid receptor and displays weak partial agonist activity. Like natural progesterone, synthetic progestins have been reported to have no binding or transactivation activity via the oestrogen receptor (OR), which is expressed in the female reproductive system, brain, lung, and heart.

Oestrogens

Oestrogens are primarily produced in the ovary and testis, and play a role in reproduction, bone metabolism, and cardiovascular function. Synthetic oestrogens include, amongst others, **ethinylestradiol**, a synthetic derivative of the natural oestrogen estradiol, and **mestranol**, which is activated through conversion to ethinylestradiol. As with endogenous oestrogens, these derivatives act on ORs, of which two functionally distinct types have been identified; ORα and ORβ. These receptors differ in terms of tissue distribution and ligand activation properties. The ORs regulate cell function by targeting specific genes through oestrogen response elements, or by interacting with other transcription factors. They also have ligand-independent activity via a variety of signalling pathways. Post-translational modifications, such as phosphorylation by the MAPK, protein kinase A (PKA) or PKC pathways can regulate its interaction with other co-factors and affect ligand binding, receptor dimerization, or DNA binding.

Activation of oestrogen receptors in target tissues increases the hepatic synthesis of sex hormone-binding globulin, thyroid-binding globulin, and other serum proteins, and suppress follicle-stimulating hormone from the anterior pituitary. In combination with progestin, they suppress the hypothalamic–pituitary system, decreasing GnRH secretion.

Prescribing

Contraception

Hormonal contraception with an implant or intrauterine device provides the most effective method of birth control, and is reversible. Consideration should be given to risks and patient preferences in order to minimize adverse effects or ineffective control.

The combined contraceptives (oestrogen- and progestogen-containing) are usually administered orally, and are available in low or standard strength preparations determined by the **ethinylestradiol** content (20 versus 30-40 µg). Lower-strength preparations provide an option for women at increased risk of VTE, such as those who are obese or have a family history of VTE. Combined contraception may also be administered as a patch (standard strength) or as a vaginal ring (low strength), particularly in patients where compliance with daily oral therapy is in question.

Progestogen-only oral contraception, although less likely to cause VTE than a combined pill, is of inferior efficacy. Furthermore, a patient who misses a dose by as little as 3 hours (up to 12 hours with desogestrel) is considered to be unprotected (compared with up to 24 hours with a combined pill). The progestogen-only intra-uterine device, however, is a highly effective method of contraception, with the added benefit of reducing symptoms of primary menorrhagia within 3–6 months. Progestogens can also be administered parenterally or as an implant, and like the IUD may be preferred in patients struggling to comply with oral therapy.

HRT

Hormone replacement therapy is the administration of oestrogens (ideally natural; **estradiol** or **estrone**) to overcome symptoms of oestrogen deficiency, with the intention of improving quality of life.

Women with urogenital symptoms alone, such as vaginal dryness or increased urinary frequency, may be best managed with topical low-dose oestrogen treatment (i.e. cream, pessary, ring, or tablet). However, patients with vasomotor symptoms (flushing, night sweats) will require systemic therapy either with oestrogen alone in women without a uterus, or in combination with a progestogen in women with a uterus, to protect against endometrial cancer. Combined preparations are available with progestogens administered cyclically or continuously.

Systemic therapy may be administered orally or preferably transdermally as either a patch or less commonly a gel, to reduce the risk of toxicity in particular thrombosis compared with oral administration. In either case, the lowest possible dose should be prescribed and treatment continued for the shortest possible time.

PRACTICAL PRESCRIBING
Hormone replacement therapy

- HRT should be prescribed at the lowest possible dose for the shortest possible time.
- Neither continuous combined preparations (progestogen and oestrogen) nor tibolone are suitable for use in the peri-menopausal period, due to the risk of irregular menstruation.
- Initiation is not recommended until at least 12 months since last menstrual bleed.
- Women without a uterus may receive oestrogen alone, although those with endometriosis may benefit from additional progestogen depending on the site of endometrial tiissue.

Unwanted effects

Toxicity associated with hormonal therapy depends on the relative content of oestrogen and progestogen. Progestogen-related side effects include fluid retention, mood swings, depression, and acne, whereas oestrogen is more commonly associated with nausea and leg cramps. Breast tenderness and headaches/migraines are linked to both hormones. When considering the use of HRT and contraception, it is important to be aware of the risks associated with therapy and make sure that the woman is fully informed of these. As the absolute risks, although small, are associated with a high level of morbidity and mortality, this may outweigh the benefits for some and a less risky alternative may be more appropriate.

Myocardial infarction and stroke

Hormonal therapy for both contraception and HRT leads to a slight increase in cardiovascular risk, which is most pronounced with HRT in women more than 10 years after the menopause. Use of HRT and hormonal contraception is contraindicated following a recent MI, stroke, or active angina, and should be used cautiously in high-risk patients.

Venous thromboembolism

Although there is an increase in the relative risk of a VTE, the absolute risk remains low and can be further minimized by avoiding in patients with a history of VTE. Caution should be taken with high-risk patients, such as those who are obese. Risk can be reduced by the use of lower strength oestrogen preparations and avoiding the progestogens **desogestrel** or **gestodene**.

Breast cancer

The risk of breast cancer is slightly increased with the combined oral contraceptives, although this is largely age-related and returns to baseline 10 years after stopping therapy. Combined HRT increases the risk by 1.6 times after 5 years and 2.3 times after 10 years, whereas the increased risk associated with oestrogen-only therapy is likely to be less. Breast cancer, either active or historical, is a contraindication to use and consideration should be given to avoid in patients with a family history.

Cervical cancer

The risk of cervical cancer is associated with a small increase with long-term use of combined contraceptives. Use of oral contraceptives, however, is not recommended in patients with a history of cervical cancers or in the presence of undiagnosed vaginal bleeding.

Ovarian cancer

The risk of ovarian cancer may be slightly increased with HRT, but is reduced with the use of combined contraceptives.

Endometrial cancer

The risk of endometrial cancer is reduced by the addition of progestogen to HRT in women with a uterus. Both combined and progestogen-only contraceptives reduce the risk of endometrial cancer.

Drug interactions

Oestradiol is metabolized in the liver via the cytochrome P450 enzyme system and, as such, its metabolism may be affected by drugs known to induce or inhibit this pathway. Of note are the enzyme inducers—**phenytoin**, **carbamazepine**, and **rifampicin**, and enzyme inhibitor **erythromycin**.

Tibolone

Tibolone is a synthetic steroid hormone with weak agonist activity at all five of the steroid hormone receptors, thus having combined oestrogenic, progestrogenic, and androgenic properties.

Mechanism of action

The global effects of **tibolone** are predominantly oestrogenic, but in the endometrium the activation of both progesterone and androgen receptors produce mostly progestogenic actions. Although tibolone displays a full range of oestrogenic effects on the development of vaginal epithelia, the endometrium differs in response, with clinical studies showing that it remains atrophied in the majority of women. The action of tibolone on bone is mediated via the oestrogen receptor, acting as a bone resorption inhibitor.

Prescribing

Tibolone can be used in post-menopausal women (more than a year) or immediately following a hysterectomy as an alternative to oestrogen therapy; for example, in women who prefer amenorrhoea or report a reduced libido. Despite its rapid onset and short duration of action,

it is administered OD (orally), providing relief of menopause symptoms within a few weeks. It is also effective in preventing osteoporosis, as it increases bone mineral density in 75–85% of women after 2 years of treatment.

Unwanted effects

As with other HRT, treatment is not without risks and the benefit of treating should be carefully weighed up against risks before starting treatment. See 'Hormone replacement therapy'.

Selective progesterone receptor modulators

The selective progesterone receptor modulators have mixed agonist–antagonist properties on the progesterone receptor, occupying an intermediate position in the spectrum of progesterone receptor ligands. For example, ulipristal.

Mechanism of action

The main difference between selective progesterone receptor modulators (SPRMs) and progesterone receptor full agonists (progesterone) or antagonists (**mifepristone**) is that their agonist/antagonist effect can vary depending on the target tissue. Unlike progesterone, which upon binding with the progesterone receptor shifts the conformational balance towards a state that favours upregulation of gene expression, SPRMs binding to the receptor leads to a more finely balanced equilibrium between activator and repressor conformations. Hence, the presence or absence of co-activators and co-repressors can regulate the effect of SPRM in the different target tissues. Interactions with other signalling pathways, cAMP in particular, as well as the ratio of progesterone receptor isoforms in the cell, may also be important.

Prescribing

Ulipristal was first licensed for use as an emergency contraceptive and, subsequently, in the management of uterine fibroids. As an emergency contraceptive, it is taken as a single dose as soon as possible after unprotected intercourse, although it can be taken up to 5 days later. In comparison, **levonorgestrel** (the first hormonal emergency contraceptive) is only effective for up to 3 days post-intercourse.

Unwanted effects

Nausea and vomiting are common with **ulipristal** and when vomiting occurs within 3 hours of taking a dose, a further dose should be taken. Ulipristal may impair the efficacy of hormonal contraception, so combination management with a barrier method is recommended until the next menstrual cycle. Furthermore, it is suggested that a second dose of ulipristal should not be used within the same menstrual cycle and only occasional use considered. Other side effects include headaches, dizziness, breast tenderness, and fatigue. Women should also be advised that irregular bleeding may occur and the timing of the next menstrual period may be early or late. An MHRA alert was issued in February 2018 regarding the use of ulipristal for the treatment of uterine fibroids due to the risk of serious liver injury. Patients on treatment will now require routine monitoring of liver function prior to starting and whilst on treatment.

Gonadotrophin-releasing hormone agonists/gonadorelin analogues

These synthetic peptides interact with the GnRH receptor leading to the secretion of the pituitary hormones FSH and LH. Their structure is based on the natural GnRH decapeptide, with specific amino acid substitutions. Examples include buserelin, goserelin, leuprorelin, nafarelin, and triptorelin.

Mechanism of action

The endogenous GnRH is processed in hypothalamic neurons and acts as a key regulator of the reproductive hormonal cascade. Released in a pulsatile fashion, it acts on the pituitary GnRH type I transmembrane receptor, leading to the activation of Gq protein transduction cascades, although other G proteins or G protein–independent processes can also occur.

The role of GnRH in the reproductive system has prompted the development of various peptide analogues. These synthetic agonists are modelled after the endogenous GnRH, with a double or single substitution at glycine 6 and 10, which inhibits rapid degradation and affects receptor interactions. Initial stimulating action on the receptor is followed by receptor down-regulation and a sustained drop in gonadotropin secretion, preventing their use for prolonged periods.

Prescribing

The gonadotrophin-releasing hormone agonists can be used for endometriosis, administered by injection on either a monthly or 3-monthly basis (**goserelin**, **leuprorelin**, **nafarelin**, and **triptorelin**), or intranasally daily (**buserelin**). For all agents oral bioavailability is poor. Treatment is limited to 6 months as there is the risk of osteoporosis with continued use. In cases where there is a wish to continue, it should be combined with HRT to reduce this risk.

Unwanted effects

Breakthrough bleeding occurs commonly with the GnRH agonists, particularly in the first month secondary to oestrogen withdrawal. Although intensity and duration can vary between patients, extended periods should be investigated. Other common side effects include hot flushes, nausea, vomiting, impaired memory, and concentration.

Long-term use of GnRH agonists is restricted due to its effect on bone mineral density, losing on average 1% a month over the 6-month period. This may be more pronounced in the presence of other predisposing risk, such as smoking, corticosteroid use, malnutrition, etc. In some cases, treatment to counteract the effects may be considered.

Further reading

Brynhildsen J. (2014) Combined hormonal contraceptives: prescribing patterns, compliance, and benefits versus risks. *Therapy and Advances in Drug Safety* 5(5), 201–13.

Insler V. (1988) Gonadotropin therapy: new trends and insights. *International Journal of Fertility* 33, 85–6, 89–97.

Jensen DV, Andersen KB, Wagner G. (1987) Prostaglandins in the menstrual cycle of women. A review. *Danish Medical Bulletin* 34(3), 178–82.

Pitkin J (2007) Dysfunctional uterine bleeding. *British Medical Journal* 334(7603), 1110–1.

Prentice A (1999). Medical management of menorrhagia. *British Medical Journal* 319, 1343–5.

Sarris I, Bewley S, Agnihotri S, et al. (2009) Menstrual disorders In: Sarris I, Bewley S, Agnihotri S (Eds) Training in Obstetrics and Gynaecology, pp. 320–43. Oxford, Oxford University Press.

Smith RP and Kaunitz AM (2013). Treatment of primary dysmenorrhea in adult women. http://www.uptodate.com/contents/treatment-of-primary-dysmenorrhea-in-adult-women [accessed 27 March 2019].

Guidelines

Marjorbanks J, Proctor M, Faruhar C, et al. (2015) Nonsteroidal anti-inflammatory drugs for dysmenorrhoea (Review), Cochrane Collaboration Jan 2010. *Cochrane Database Systems Review* (7):CD001751. https://www.cochranelibrary.com/cdsr/doi/10.1002/14651858.CD001751.pub3/full [accessed 3 April 2019].

Lethaby AE, Cooke I, Rees M (2007) Progesterone or progestogen-releasing intrauterine systems for heavy menstrual bleeding. *Cochrane Database of Systematic Reviews*. Issue 2, 1–73.

NICE (2008) Inducing Labour NICE Clinical guideline CG70. https://www.nice.org.uk/guidance/cg70 [accessed 27 March 2019].

4.7 Androgens, anti-androgens, and anabolic steroids

Androgens are a group of hormones that are synthesized naturally in the adrenal cortex and gonads (e.g. testosterone), or synthetically produced (e.g. anabolic steroids). They influence reproductive tract development and initiation/maintenance of secondary sexual characteristics. Before puberty, androgens are released in low levels, but once through puberty, men have plasma concentrations approximately 10 times that of females. Androgens are under the control of the hypothalamic–pituitary axis, and in females are precursors in oestrogen synthesis. Excess androgens in the female may result in hirsutism, amenorrhoea, acne, and increased muscle mass; secondary to polycystic ovarian syndrome or congenital adrenal hyperplasia, among other causes.

Pathophysiology

Androgens are produced by the steroid-producing cells of the testes, ovaries, and adrenals. The major circulating androgen in men is testosterone, which is produced in the Leydig cells of the testis under the control of LH released by the anterior pituitary gland. Most testosterone travels in the bloodstream bound to sex-hormone-binding globulin (SHBG) and is converted to dihydrotestosterone (DHT) by 5α-reductase.

The 5α-reductases are a class of three enzymes that have function in bile acid synthesis, androgen metabolism, prostate cancer, and benign prostatic hyperplasia (BPH). The three enzymes are expressed differentially in a number of tissues including testes, ovaries, and epididymis; with distribution also varying with age. In addition to reducing testosterone to DHT, other substrates include progesterone, androstenedione, epi-testosterone, cortisol, aldosterone, and deoxycorticosterone.

Both testosterone and DHT act on androgen receptors to stimulate the differentiation and maintenance of external genitalia and secondary sexual characteristics, although DHT binds preferentially and has two or three times the potency of testosterone. Testosterone also acts during sexual differentiation in the foetus, and is pivotal in the development of male sexual organs (i.e. Wolffian duct system). Beyond this, androgens act as agonists to stimulate bone marrow production of red blood cells, especially in aplastic anaemia of hereditary cause (e.g. Fanconi's syndrome or dyskaryosis) or acquired disease. Androgens are responsible for the higher basal RBC noted in men.

Hypogonadism

Reduced gonad function, or hypogonadism, may reduce sex-hormone synthesis, or impair gamete regulation. In males diminished prepubertal testosterone levels leads to delayed puberty, while diminished post-pubertal levels can impair spermatogenesis, reduce sex drive, and cause muscle wasting. Hypogonadism occurs as a result of primary or secondary dysfunction:

- *Primary hypogonadism* is dysfunction of the gonads themselves, leading to reduced production of testosterone and/or spermatozoa. In most cases, primary hypogonadism is acquired (e.g. mumps, trauma, chemotherapy), but can also result from congenital causes such as in Klinefelter's (XXY) or Turner's (XXO) syndrome. Alcohol can directly lower testosterone levels and alter androgen metabolism, resulting in testicular atrophy and gynaecomastia.

- *Secondary hypogonadism* results from dysfunction of the hypothalamic–pituitary axis, thereby impairing the release of LH and its subsequent stimulation of the testis to produce testosterone. Secondary causes of hypogonadism include congenital conditions (e.g. Kallmann's syndrome), structural abnormalities within the hypothalamus/pituitary (e.g. trauma, tumours, radiotherapy) or as a consequence of functional anomalies (e.g. stress, obesity, medication/illicit drugs). Drugs known to affect the normal pituitary–testicular axis include **cimetidine**, **spironolactone**, and anabolic steroids.

Androgen insensitivity syndrome

Androgen insensitivity syndrome (AIS) is a rare condition where mutations in the androgen receptor gene on the X chromosome leads to alterations in the receptor, making them partially (PAIS) or completely (CAIS) resistant to the action of androgens. In PAIS patients are phenotypically male, with varying degrees of under-virilization, whereas in CAIS, patients are phenotypically female at birth with an inguinal hernia that contains testis.

Benign prostatic hyperplasia

In BPH, hyperplasia of stromal and epithelial cell within the prostate leads to nodules forming in the transitional zone, ultimately obstructing urinary outflow. Androgens are important in the development and maintenance of stromal and epithelial cells; however, DHT is potent and causes growth factor expression, which is mitogenic and causes nodular hyperplasia; hence, the benefit of 5α-reductase inhibitors.

Hyper-androgenization/polycystic ovary syndrome

Excessive androgen production, hyperandrogenism, is most commonly associated with polycystic ovary syndrome (PCOS). Affected women present with signs and symptoms of over-virilization, e.g. hirsutism, menstrual disturbances (e.g. amenorrhoea), impaired fertility, and obesity. PCOS is associated with significantly increased cardiovascular risk. Risk factors such as metabolic syndrome, DM, dyslipidaemia, and obesity and hypertension are significant associations. Lifestyle changes and **metformin** are the mainstay of treatment. Although men can also be affected by hyper-androgenization, the clinical effects are generally less significant.

For a full summary of the relevant pathways and drug targets, see Figure 4.9.

Management

The androgens and anabolic steroids have a broad range of therapeutic uses in both men and women.

Hypogonadism

Patients with symptoms suggestive of hypogonadism should be worked up to distinguish between primary (testicular) and secondary (hypothalamic-pituitary axis) causes. In symptomatic patients, and in the absence of contraindications (prostate cancer, raised PSA or breast cancer); replacement with **testosterone** is recommended to maintain secondary sexual characteristics, improve muscle mass and bone mineral density, and improve general well-being. Choice of agent is based on patient preference and serum testosterone should be monitored every 3–6 months to assess response.

Benign prostatic hyperplasia

The 5α-reductase inhibitors (**finasteride**, **dutasteride**) are indicated for androgen inhibition in benign prostatic hypertrophy (BPH) to reverse prostatic enlargement, thus providing symptomatic relief. This reduction in prostate volume also leads to a reduction in the serum biomarker prostate specific antigen (PSA), used in the diagnosis of prostate cancer; as such finasteride use may be falsely reassuring to patients with early or undiagnosed prostate cancer. The 5α-reductase inhibitors are usually used in combination with α-adrenoceptor blockers (e.g. **tamsulosin**), which is considered to be a first-line treatment and acts to relax smooth muscle within the bladder and prostatic urethra in order to overcome urinary obstruction. Patients intolerant of α-adrenoceptor blockers may be managed with 5α-reductase inhibitors as monotherapy.

Hyper-androgenization/polycystic ovary syndrome

Anti-androgens act to reduce libido and spermatogenesis, and as such have been used for 'chemical castration' in male sex offenders. In women, treatment with **cyproterone** (in combination with **ethinylestradiol**; co-cyprindiol) can reduce the unwanted effects of hyper-androgenization associated with PCOS, such as acne and hirsutism.

Aplastic anaemia

Androgens may be used to promote erythropoiesis in aplastic anaemia (**danazol**, **testosterone**), although anabolic steroids are more commonly used for this indication.

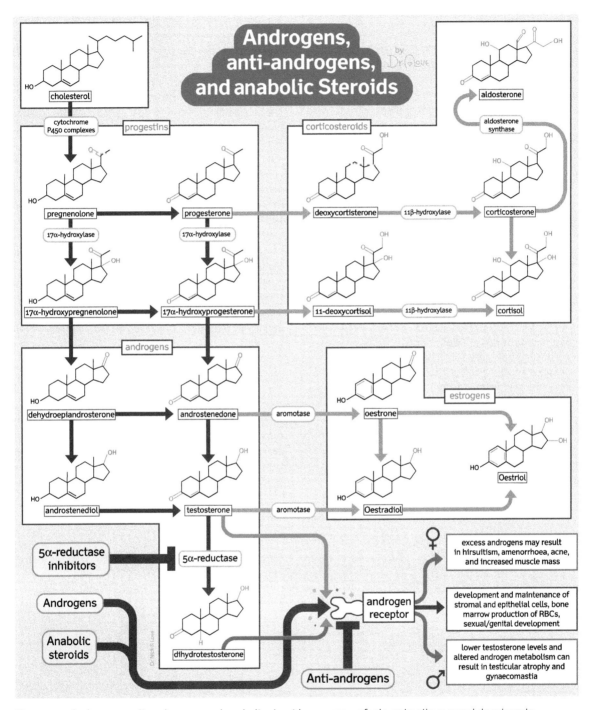

Figure 4.9 Androgens, anti-androgens, and anabolic steroids: summary of relevant pathways and drug targets.

Prostate cancer

In patients with locally advanced prostate cancer the anti-androgens (**bicalutamide**, **flutamide**, **cyproterone**, **abiraterone**) may be used either alone, or in combination with radical prostatectomy or radiotherapy to control disease. While on treatment, patients should have PSA levels monitored and treatment may be intermittently interrupted when PSA levels are low. Cyproterone or **megestrol acetate** may be offered to men who experience hot flushes secondary to androgen deprivation treatment.

Drug classes used in management

Androgens

> Androgens are responsible for the development and maintenance of male reproductive organs, skeletal muscle, and hair cycle, mostly through activation of the androgen receptor, a member of the steroid/thyroid hormone nuclear receptor superfamily. Examples: testosterone, methyltestosterone, danazol.

Mechanism of action

The two endogenous ligands, **testosterone** and its more potent metabolite, 5α-dihydrotestosterone (DHT), act as paracrine hormones and bind to the nuclear androgen receptor. This acts as a transcription factor, activating gene expression via specific binding to the androgen responsive elements. At the cellular level, steroid-converting enzymes modulate the effects of androgens. In reproductive tissues in particular, 5α-reductase converts testosterone to DHT. In other tissues, testosterone can be converted to oestradiol by aromatase.

In the target tissues, modulation also occurs via a variety of co-regulators and co-regulator complexes that can support ligand-dependent control of transcriptional activity. Androgens can also affect cellular processes in a non-genomic fashion; for example, by activation of intracellular signalling pathways, such as ERK1/2, tyrosine kinase c-Src, cAMP and PKA, or increasing intracellular Ca^{2+} concentrations. These effects can occur independently or in tandem with the genomic effects.

Danazol is a modified testosterone, a derivative of the synthetic ethisterone. A gonadotrophin inhibitor that supresses the pituitary–ovarian axis, it can also bind to androgen receptors, progesterone, and glucocorticoid receptor.

Prescribing

Testosterone is available for use in a variety of formulations (see Table 4.20) to promote bioavailability, as due to extensive first-pass metabolism in the liver, its oral bioavailability is poor. The more efficacious routes of administration are parenteral, implants, or transdermal (either as a patch or gel). Choice of formulation is dictated by

Table 4.20 Usual doses of various testosterone formulations

Form	Salt	Dose	Frequency	Notes
IM (oily)	Testosterone enanthate/various	250 mg	2–4-weekly	Fluctuations in mood/libido, cough after injection
	Testosterone undeconate (Nebido®)	1000 mg	10–14-weekly	
Gel	Testosterone (e.g. Testim®)	50–100 mg	Nightly	Cover site with clothing, wash before skin to skin contact
Buccal tablet	Testosterone	30 mg	12-hourly	Taste alterations, risk of gum/mucosa irritation
Implant	Testosterone	100–200 mg	3–6-monthly	
Oral	Testosterone undeconate	120–160 mg	Daily	

licensed indication, availability, and patient preference, although the gel preparations and implants are more likely to maintain serum testosterone levels within the desired physiological range.

Regardless of preparation choice, testosterone levels should be measured at baseline and initially repeated 3–6-monthly. Once stabilized, levels should be checked annually, together with assessments of response, including bone mass density and screening for prostate cancer.

Danazol, with its weak androgenic effects, is only available in an oral formulation (capsule), licensed for use in endometriosis and benign fibrocystic breast disease. Off-label however, it has been used to treat gynaecomastia, hereditary angioedema, and aplastic anaemia.

Unwanted effects

The predominant side effects of androgen therapy predictably include acne, hirsutism, oily skin, weight gain, fluid retention, increased libido, and deepening of voice, the significance of which depends on the desired effects and the patient group they are being used in. The risk of fluid retention is increased in patients with pre-existing heart or renal failure, and can aggravate hypertension. As testosterone can stimulate the bone marrow to cause overproduction of red blood cells, patients will need full blood count monitoring while on treatment.

Patients should be advised to report signs of intolerance as these are invariably dose related; in particular, the fluctuations seen with the ester salts administered IM may be resolved by dose modifications or switching between products.

As **danazol** also acts to inhibit the pituitary–ovarian axis, this gives rise to menstrual disturbances, hot flushes, sweating, vaginal dryness, and altered mood.

There is some controversy as to whether extended use of androgens can increase the risk of prostate cancer, which is known to be androgen-dependent (see 'Prescribing warning: the controversial relationship between testosterone and prostate cancer'). Before starting and while on treatment, routine monitoring should include a digital rectal examination and PSA to exclude benign prostatic hypertrophy or preclinical prostatic cancer, as well as a haematocrit and LFTs. Other malignancies such as breast (men) and primary liver cancer are also associated with androgen use.

PRESCRIBING WARNING

The controversial relationship between testosterone and prostate cancer

- In 1941 Huggins and Hodges demonstrated that reducing endogenous testosterone through castration led to the regression of prostate cancer, whereas testosterone supplementation promoted its growth.

- More recently, a meta-analysis of 18 prospective studies demonstrated that there was no association between prostate cancer and prediagnostic androgen levels.

- Other studies have demonstrated a potential for worse prognosis with low testosterone levels (<2.5 ng/mL).

- On initiation, testosterone causes a slight increase in PSA, although this does not seem to be associated with an increased risk of prostate cancer.

Testosterone is metabolized through the liver and has the potential to interact with drugs that alter enzyme activity, as well as alter LFTs.

Anti-androgens

Anti-androgens compete with endogenous androgens for the ligand-binding pocket in the androgen receptor. In this way, they induce conformational changes that prevent efficient transcriptional activity. Examples include abiraterone, bicalutamide, cyproterone, and flutamide.

Mechanism of action

Incorrect activation of the androgen receptor (AR) axis is a significant factor in the progression of prostate cancer, leading to the development of drugs that directly target the AR.

The anti-androgens currently available still promote translocation of the androgen receptor to the nucleus and binding to DNA, but the inability to recruit co-activators prevents its normal transcriptional role. Anti-androgens can be divided in two general classes, steroidal and non-steroidal. The latter were developed to circumvent the off-target effects of general steroid stimulation. As such, they do not interact with other nuclear receptors, apart from the androgen type.

Prescribing

The non-steroidal anti-androgens **bicalutamide** and **flutamide** are oral anti-androgens licensed for the suppression of testosterone in the treatment of prostate cancer. Of the two, bicalutamide is advocated by NICE due to its superior efficacy and favourable dosing frequency (OD versus TDS). The decision to use is based on extent of disease, prognosis, and patient preferences.

Other drugs with anti-androgen properties **abiraterone** and **cyproterone** may also be used in the management of prostate cancer, although usually in palliative disease where surgery or radiotherapy are deemed unsuitable. Cyproterone in alternative oral formulations is licensed for treating hypersexuality in males, or combined with oestradiol as an oral contraceptive in women for the treatment of hyperandrogenization symptoms, i.e. severe acne and hirsutism.

Unwanted effects

Inhibition of androgens results in flushing, gynaecomastia or breast tenderness with or without galactorrhoea, reduced libido and sperm count, and weight gain. In patients receiving **bicalutamide** monotherapy for metastatic prostate cancer, NICE recommends either pretreatment with radiotherapy to both breast buds, or weekly **tamoxifen** while on treatment to prevent gynaecomastia.

As treatment with anti-androgens can cause fluid retention, it should be used with caution in patients with pre-existing cardiovascular disease, such as heart failure or hypertension. Treatment is also associated with hepatic toxicity, again requiring caution and monitoring.

Drug interactions

Biculatmide is a relatively potent inhibitor of CYP 3A4 so has the potential to affect the levels of drugs known to be cleared via this pathway, particularly those with a narrow therapeutic index. The drug manufacturers recommend avoiding co-administration with **terfenadine**, **astemizole**, and **cimetidine**. Although **flutamide** is activated by CYP 1A2, the only drug interaction of any likely significance is an increase in **warfarin** efficacy.

5α-reductase inhibitors

> α-reductase inhibitors decrease the activity of 5α-reductase, preventing the conversion of testosterone into its more active metabolite DHT. For example, dutasteride and finasteride.

Mechanism of action

Finasteride is a synthetic 4-azasteroid drug, which acts as a competitive and specific inhibitor of type II and III 5α-reductase, forming a stable complex with the enzyme. Inhibition results in a decrease in the concentrations of serum and tissue DHT, moderate increase in serum testosterone, and a significant increase in prostatic testosterone. **Dutasteride** is another 4-azasteroid, which inhibits all three isoforms of 5α-reductase. Type I is predominant in the sebaceous glands, skin, and liver, with Type II 5α-reductase found in prostate, seminal vesicles, and epididymis, plus liver and hair follicles.

Although the AR antagonists show significant benefit in blocking AR activity, the affinity of these inhibitors for the receptor is lower than that of DHT. As a result, when intratumoral androgen synthesis increases, DHT outcompetes the inhibitors, leading to re-activation of the AR pathway. The use of 5α-reductase inhibitors that block conversion of testosterone to DHT is thus under investigation in hormone refractory prostate cancer.

Prescribing

Finasteride and, more recently, **dutasteride**, have been licensed to reduce prostate size in benign prostatic hyperplasia (BPH). Treatment is oral and OD, requiring review every 3–6 months to assess for efficacy. Although not licensed for use in prostate cancer, dutasteride has demonstrated a benefit in hormone refractory disease.

Unwanted effects

Unsurprisingly, the adverse effects of the 5α-reductase inhibitors are comparable with the anti-androgens with specific caution recommended in pregnancy. Exposure to **finasteride** or **dutasteride** during pregnancy can affect the development of male foetal genitalia, so it is recommended that pregnant women avoid handling broken finasteride tablets or dutasteride capsules that are leaking.

Anabolic steroids

> Anabolic steroids are synthetic derivatives of testosterone, modified in order to maximize anabolic and minimize androgenic actions. They activate the androgen receptor and increase protein levels within skeletal muscle and bone mineral density. For example, oxymetholone and nandrolone.

Mechanism of action

Anabolic steroids have both androgenic (associated with masculinization) and anabolic (linked to protein building in muscle and bone) effects. Since synthesis of anabolic steroids cannot completely eliminate the androgenic effects, anabolic steroids are more accurately termed anabolic-androgenic steroids (AAS). The anabolic effects of AAS are mediated mainly by ARs in skeletal muscle, but collagen and bone are also target tissues. AAS also exert other anabolic effects, including glucocorticoid antagonism, stimulation of insulin-like growth factor axis and psychoactive effects in the brain.

The dissociation of anabolic versus androgenic properties can happen at cellular level, depending on the metabolism of anabolic steroids in the target tissues, and the activity of 5α-reductase. It can also occur as a consequence of anabolic steroids inducing conformational changes in the receptor complex, which can modify the interaction with specific co-regulators in different tissues. To date, several structural modifications have been introduced into testosterone in order to increase the anabolic effect, without significant androgenic actions.

Nandrolone is a naturally occurring steroid in the human body, which is only produced in low amounts and acts as an androgen receptor agonist. **Oxymetholone** is a synthetic anabolic steroid, primarily used in the treatment of osteoporosis and anaemia.

Prescribing

Due to their lack of specificity and high abuse potential, anabolic steroids have largely been replaced by other agents. **Oxymetholone** is no longer licensed for use in many countries, although is occasionally used off-label in aplastic anaemia for patients failing other therapy. Similarly, **nandrolone**, although licensed for use in women for osteoporosis, is no longer advocated for this, but instead occasionally used off-label for aplastic anaemia and HIV-associated muscle wasting to increase lean body mass.

Unwanted effects

Characteristic findings of anabolic steroid use include low testosterone and low FSH/LH with normal or increased muscle bulk. Testicular atrophy or softening may also be present. Continuous treatment with high-dose anabolic steroids leads to virilization and increased lean body mass, thereby making them susceptible to abuse. In women, these effects lead to hirsutism, increased libido, amenorrhoea, and acne, as well as hoarseness, which may be irreversible. In men symptoms include impaired spermatogenesis. As both drugs also possess androgenic properties, side effects will also include those seen with testosterone and other androgens. Prolonged use is associated with liver tumours and should be used cautiously in hepatic impairment, if at all. Like the androgens, anabolic steroids are contraindicated in prostate and male breast cancer.

Further reading

Brinkmann AO (2011) Molecular mechanisms of androgen action: a historical perspective. *Methods in Molicular Biology* 776, 3–24.

Foradori CD, Weiser MJ, Handa RJ (2008) Non-genomic actions of androgens. *Frontiers in Neuroendocrinology* 29(2), 169–81.

Kicman AT (2008) Pharmacology of anabolic steroids. *British Journal of Pharmacology* 154(3), 502–21.

Matsumoto T, Shiina H, Kawano H, et al. (2008) Androgen receptor functions in male and female physiology. *Journal of Steroid Biochemistry and Molecular Biology* 109(305), 236–41.

Ramasamy R, Fisher ES and Schlegel PN (2012) Testosterone replacement and prostate cancer. *Indian Journal of Urology* 28(2), 123–8.

Guidelines

Bhasin S, Cunningham GR, Hayes FJ, Matsumoto AM, Snyder PJ, Swerdloff RS, Montori VM. (2010) Testosterone therapy in adult men with androgen deficiency syndromes: Endocrine society clinical practice guidelines. *Journal of Clinical Endocrine Metabolism* 95(6), 2536–59. https://academic.oup.com/jcem/article/95/6/2536/2597900 [accessed 28 March 2019].

Curtis Nickel J, Méndez-Probst CE, Whelan TF, et al. (2010) CUA Guideline 2010 Update: guidelines for the management of benign prostatic hyperplasia *Canadian Urology Association Journal* 4(5), 310–16. http://www.ncbi.nlm.nih.gov/pmc/articles/PMC2950766/ [accessed 28 March 2019].

NICE CG175 (2014) Prostate cancer; diagnosis and management. https://www.nice.org.uk/guidance/cg175 [accessed 28 March 2019].

NICE TA259 (2012) Abiraterone for castration resistant metastatic prostate cancer previously treated with a docetaxel-containing regimen. https://www.nice.org.uk/guidance/ta259 [accessed 28 March 2019].

5 Renal medicine

5.1 The kidney, drugs, and chronic kidney disease

The kidneys are of fundamental importance in the regulation of fluid and electrolytes, maintaining permissive extracellular fluid composition (salts and water), pH, and volume, while also mediating the removal of waste products. Based on the anatomy of the nephron, three main processes occur in order to deliver this balance: *glomerular filtration, tubular secretion*, and *tubular resorption*. Drugs can act at different sites within this system, so that functional equilibrium can be restored in various disease states (e.g. hypertension, heart failure, liver failure, nephrotic syndrome).

CKD is a long-term condition that lasts more than 3 months and affects the function of both kidneys. It results from any pathology that reduces renal functional capacity and produces a decrease in GFR to less than 60 mL/min/1.73 m². Prevalence within the UK is high, particularly in the elderly and affects 6–8% of the population. The most common cause of CKD is idiopathic (unknown, usually with small kidneys), then diabetes mellitus. In both, glomerular damage and mesangial injury (causing metabolic and haemodynamic effects) occur. Mild-moderate essential hypertension does not cause CKD.

The kidney and drugs

Knowledge of the functional anatomy of the proximal tubule and loop of Henle is essential in understanding therapeutic targets and treatment of pathologies, as each region and transporter system has a key role. In brief, the journey of solutes from the blood to the production of urine occurs at five main anatomical sites—the glomerulus, the proximal tubule, the loop of Henle, the distal tubule (proximal part and distal part), and the collecting ducts (Figures 5.1 and 5.2).

Glomerulus

The glomerulus is a network of capillaries (like a ball of string), which merge with the nephron via Bowman's capsule. It is the first site of filtration and the place where solutes, toxins, and small proteins are removed from the wider circulatory system, after delivery by the renal arteries (via an afferent arteriole).

Blood and larger proteins remain in the arteriole and leave via an efferent branch, while the filtrate enters the proximal convoluted tubule. The *afferent:efferent* system ensures that a constant filtration pressure is maintained irrespective of variations in arterial pressure.

The capillary bed is very large, so that permeability and filtration rates are high. A normal glomerular filtration rate (GFR) i.e. 90–120 mL/min/1.73 m², depends on hydrostatic pressure, the colloid osmotic pressure and hydraulic permeability. Vascular filtration pressure at the Bowman's capsule is high and constant in order to favour filtration, which is achieved by:

- *Myogenic autoregulation*: stretch then contraction of afferent arteriole.
- *Osmotic autoregulation* (Na^+–Cl^--sensing): where local macular densa cells release prostaglandins to control afferent arterial flow.
- *Autonomic innervation* of afferent arteriole smooth muscle, which constricts or dilates vessels.

In the event of a drop in BP, renin is released from the kidney into the circulation in response to a reduction in Na^+, Cl^- reaching the macular densa cells or through direct stimulation of β1-adrenoreceptors in the juxtaglomerular apparatus. This, in turn, converts angiotensinogen (from the liver) to angiotensin I, which is then converted by

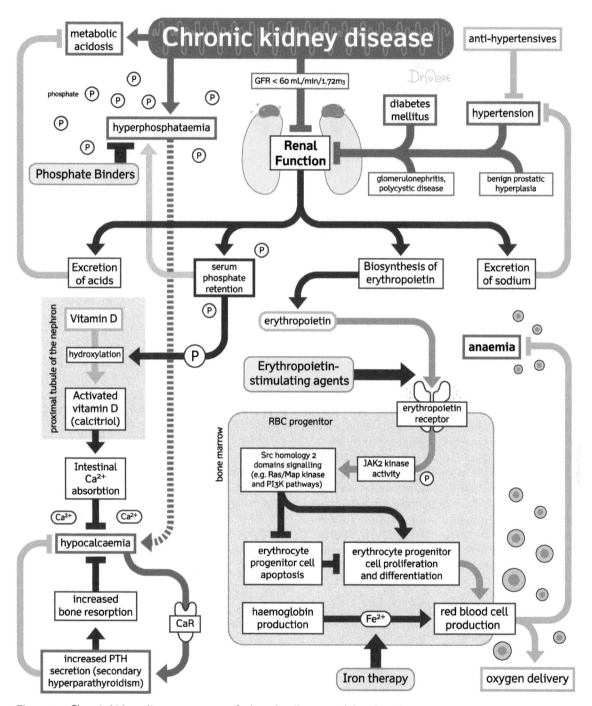

Figure 5.1 Chronic kidney disease: summary of relevant pathways and drug target.

ACE to angiotensin II (see Renin-angiotensin system, in Topic 2.1, 'Hypertension, Pathophysiology'). Angiotensin II causes:

- at low levels, constriction of efferent arterioles, raising glomerular filtration;
- at higher levels, constriction of both efferent and afferent arterioles, reducing glomerular filtration;
- increased reabsorption of Na^+ (and water) in distal tubule;
- release of aldosterone (adrenal cortex) and vasopressin (pituitary), which increases reabsorption of Na^+ and water in the distal tubule.

Glomerular filtration rate is a good overall index of kidney function, although there is more than one eGFR equation, which can make the issue confusing for a student or junior doctor. For all equations, adjustments have to be made for age, sex, and body size, and black ethnicity. So a serum creatinine of 200 μmol/L could mean an eGFR of 15 mL/min and CKD5 (and imminent need for dialysis) for an 80-year-old White or Asian female; or eGFR of 45 mL/min and CKD3, in a 30-year-old Black male. Values decline with age and in CKD. The CKD-EPI creatinine equation (2009), among others, can be used to estimate GFR.

$$eGFR = 141 \times min(S_{Cr} / \kappa, 1)^{\alpha} \times max(S_{Cr} / \kappa, 1)^{-1.209}$$
$$\times 0.993^{Age} \times 1.018 \text{ [if female]} \times 1.159 \text{ [if Black]}$$

Where, eGFR (estimated glomerular filtration rate) = mL/min/1.73 m², S_{Cr} (standardized serum creatinine) = mg/dL, κ = 0.7 (females) or 0.9 (males), α = −0.329 (females) or −0.411 (males), min = indicates the minimum of S_{Cr}/κ or 1, max = indicates the maximum of S_{Cr}/κ or 1.

It is important to note that eGFR should not be used in AKI, AKI on CKD, childhood, pregnancy, or advanced CKD (GFR <15 mL/min), where its validity is not certain. Remember GFR goes up (and serum creatinine down) in the first trimester of pregnancy. If it is important to measure GFR accurately, then an isotope GFR or creatinine clearance needs to be requested. This is often done, for example, with a Black male and a creatinine of 130 μmol/L (70–120 μmol/L is the normal range).

In perspective, GFR only tells you about one function (clearance), it is no direct reflection of the six other primary functions; i.e. two excretory—water balance, acid-base, and four endocrine/paracrine: BP (renin), EPO, activation of Vit D, and PG production. So CKD is a chronic disease, where all seven functions are affected, and usually slowly deteriorate.

Proximal tubular

The proximal convoluted tubule (PCT) of the nephron is where around 70% of salts that have been filtered by the glomerulus are reabsorbed back into the blood stream. Approximately two-thirds of water and Na^+ are reabsorbed at this site, with sodium passively entering renal tubular cells along an electrochemical gradient. This gradient is established via the K^+/Na^+ pump; a P-type ATPase, which acts on the basolateral membrane of the tubular cells, exchanging $3Na^+$ out, for $2K^+$ in. Cl^- ions are co-transported along the same gradient with Na^+, to create an increase in intercellular osmolality so that water is reabsorbed by osmosis. Similarly, almost 100% of glucose and amino acids are reabsorbed at the proximal tubule, via passive co-transport with Na^+ (see Figure 5.2). The proximal tubule also regulates filtrate pH by exchanging hydrogen ions in the interstitium for bicarbonate ions in the filtrate, in a process dependent on the enzyme carbonic anhydrase.

Osmotic diuretics

See also Topic 5.2 'Acute kidney injury'. Osmotic diuretics (e.g. **mannitol**) act at the proximal convoluted tubule (PCT) and elsewhere in the kidney (i.e. descending limb of loop of Henle). Mannitol induces diuresis by elevating the osmotic pressure of the glomerular filtrate, thereby reducing reabsorption of water and promoting the excretion of Na^+. The osmotic effect of these agents causes water to be drawn from cells, increasing circulating systemic volume, which limits its clinical use; however, these fluid shifts *are* particularly useful in conditions like cerebral oedema; where they reduce brain mass and cerebrospinal fluid (CSF) pressure. Osmotic diuretics are also of use in raised intraocular pressure or as an add-on therapy in cystic fibrosis. Unfortunately, these agents do cause a rise in serum Na^+, but reduction in K^+ and urea, so that fluid and electrolyte balance, serum osmolality, and renal function should be monitored.

Carbonic anhydrase inhibitors

See also 'Drug classes used in management'. Carbonic anhydrase inhibitors (e.g. **acetazolamide**) also act at the proximal tubule, leading to an increase in HCO_3^-, Na^+ and K^+ secretion, causing urine to become more alkaline. These inhibitors have limited use as a diuretic as they lead to the retention of H^+ ions, causing a mild acidosis, which up-regulates carbonic anhydrase rapidly leading to drug tolerance. In practice, carbonic anhydrase inhibitors are used topically in the short-term (e.g. **dorzolamide**

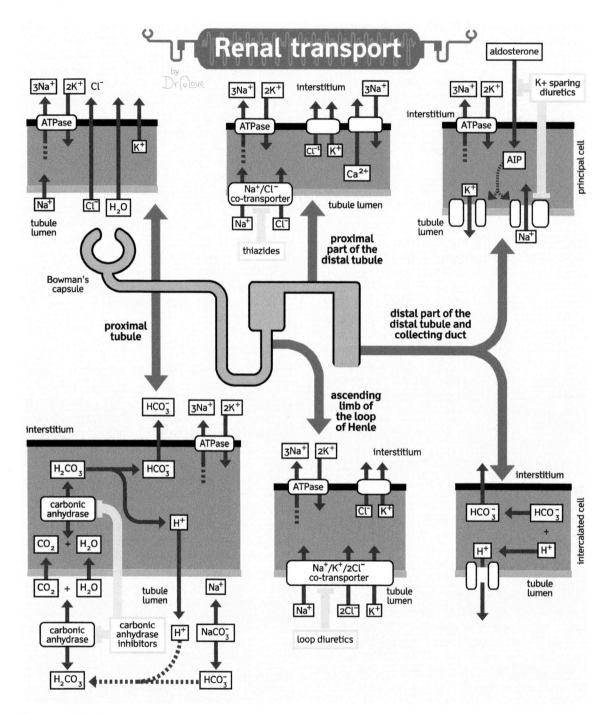

Figure 5.2 Renal transport.

and **brinzolamide**) to reduce the raised intraocular pressure of glaucoma in patients with β-blocker resistant glaucoma.

Loop of Henle

The loop of Henle can be divided into several parts that contribute to its overall function:

- *The descending limb of loop of Henle* receives isotonic filtrate (300 mOsmol) from the PCT, which increases to approximately 1400 mOsmol (hypertonic) as it descends down the loop, due to water loss being highly permeable to water, but not Na^+ or other solutes.

- *The ascending limb of loop of Henle* membranes are impermeable to water, but contain luminal active co-transporter of $Na^+/K^+/2Cl^-$. These are driven by the gradient produced by the Na^+/K^+ ATPase pump, which actively transports Na^+ out of the tubular cells in exchange for K^+ ($3Na^+/2K^+$) ions. K^+ that is co-transported from the tubular lumen into the cells, is recycled back into the lumen so there is sufficient to assist in Na^+ removal along its gradient. Up to 30% of Na^+ is reabsorbed along the ascending limb, so that the filtrate becomes increasingly hypotonic (100 mOsmol). Because two sides of the loop of Henle perform opposing functions, it acts as a counter-current multiplier diluting solutes.

- *Cortical thick ascending limb*: at the end of the ascending limb, the lumen is thick and the reabsorption of Na^+ is greatest in the intersitium, creating an osmotic gradient that permits the formation of hypertonic urine in the collecting ducts.

Loop diuretics

See also Topic 2.6, 'Heart failure'. The loop diuretics (e.g. **furosemide**, **bumetanide**) act at the intraluminal co-transporter of $Na^+/K^+/2Cl^-$ in the ascending limb. By binding to the co-transporter, Cl^- and Na^+ reabsorption is reduced, thus decreasing the medullary concentration gradient and preventing urine concentrating at the collecting ducts (i.e. more water is lost as urine). The increased retention of Na^+ in the filtrate at the distal tubule results in a negative luminal gradient, so more K^+ is lost in urine which can result in dose-dependent hypokalaemia. The increased luminal Na^+ concentration will also, via renin release, stimulate aldosterone release, which acts at the distal tubule to increase Na^+ resorption and K^+ loss (in urine) via the Na^+/K^+ channels of principle cells.

Loop diuretics are highly potent, can in most cases be given IV or orally, and are licenced in a number of therapeutic areas where fluid unloading is of clinical benefit such as the management of oedema in heart failure (Topic 2.6, 'Heart failure') or nephrotic syndrome (see 'Nephrotic syndrome'), or in hepatic cirrhosis (Topic 6.7, 'Liver disease'). Bumetanide is more potent than furosemide and more completely absorbed, although both have relatively short half-lives and can result in volume depletion (hypotension), hyponatraemia (commonly seen), and hypomagnesemia. Hypokalaemia can be dangerous in severe cardiovascular disease and in patients receiving cardiac glycosides. In hepatic failure, hypokalaemia caused by diuretics can precipitate encephalopathy, particularly in alcoholic cirrhosis.

Distal convoluted tubule (proximal)

Filtrate leaves the thick limb of the loop of Henle in a hypotonic state and enters the proximal region of the distal convoluted tubule (DCT). This region is again impermeable to water, but possesses a luminal Na^+/Cl^- co-transporter that is driven by a Na^+ gradient established by a basolateral membrane ATPase ($3Na^+$ out, $2K^+$ in; Figure 5.2). The blood supply to this region is extensive so that many solutes (Na^+, Cl^-, Ca^{2+}) can be reabsorbed to plasma. It is located close to the glomerulus so the macular densa cells detect luminal Na^+ and Cl^- to limit Na^+ losses. This is achieved through constriction of afferent arterioles and secretion of renin (see Topic 2.1, 'hypertension'), with subsequent aldosterone release.

The proximal DCT is also the site of Ca^{2+} reabsorption via the transient receptor potential cation channel subfamily V member 5 (TRPV5), located on the luminal surface of epithelial cells. This channel passes Ca^{2+} intracellularly for subsequent extrusion into the circulation via the $Ca^{2+}/3Na^+$ basolateral antiporter. The rate of Ca^{2+} uptake at this site is influenced by parathyroid hormone (see Topic 4.4, 'Parathyroid disease'), but is limited and inversely proportional to Na^+ transport, as it inhibits the TRPV5 channel or decreases antiporter ($Ca^{2+}/3Na^+$) activity.

Thiazides

See also Topic 2.1, 'Hypertension'. The thiazide diuretics act at the proximal DCT to inhibit reabsorption of Na^+ and Cl^- via the luminal membrane co-transporter, thus more water is lost in urine. They are less potent than the loop diuretics, achieving around 8% diuresis from the Na^+ load and include **bendroflumethiazide**, **hydrochlorothiazide**, chlortalidone, metolazone, and indapamide, which are structurally related to the sulphonamides. The drugs generally have a slower onset of action, but act for longer, so are useful in adult hypertension (see Topic 2.1, 'Hypertension'); they are often used in combination with ACEi or ARBs. Potassium excretion is increased with thiazide diuretics as more Na^+ reaches the distal tubular site; where Na^+/K^+ exchange occurs. As such, long-term thiazide therapy can cause metabolic alkalosis associated with hypokalaemia and hypochloraemia, with most clinical presentations of hypokalaemia occuring within 2 weeks of initiating therapy. Glucose intolerance can also be seen with thiazides, which is associated with hypokalaemia via dampened-down cellular responses to insulin. Thiazides increase bicarbonate excretion, but this does not affect acid-base balance. In general, thiazides are less effective with reduced GFR, with the exception of metolazone, which remains effective in advanced renal failure. In the elderly, doses should be initiated lower as they are particularly susceptible to the side effects; monitoring of electrolytes is prudent.

Distal convoluted tubules (distal) and collecting ducts

Hypotonic filtrate that leaves the proximal DCT enters the distal DCT before draining into the collecting ducts. Within the distal DCT a further 3–5% of Na^+ is reabsorbed via an 'amiloride' sensitive Na^+ channel, located on the luminal surface of principal cells. This channel is linked to an ATP sensitive K^+ channel that, following depolarization, pumps K^+ back into the luminal filtrate. The distal DCT is the primary site responsible for maintaining circulating K^+. The Na^+ flux is again driven by a basolateral membrane $3Na^+/2K^+$ ATPase, whose activity is enhanced by the actions of aldosterone. Circulating aldosterone also induces a number of proteins in the principal cell to activate and increase the expression of Na^+ channels.

This region, and the principal cell, is also the main site of action for antidiuretic hormone (vasopressin; ADH), which increases water absorption and the concentrating of urine along the collecting ducts. ADH, from the posterior pituitary gland (see Topic 4.1, 'The pituitary gland'), acts at vasopressin 2 receptors on the basolateral membrane to up-regulate aquaporin channels, so cells are more permeable to water that is drawn into the systemic circulation.

Another cell type in this region, the intercalated cell, (especially the collecting duct) is important for acid-base homeostasis. These cells actively secrete H^+ into urine and conserve HCO_3^- (Figure 5.2). They are up-regulated during systemic acidosis and driven by a recently discovered system, which relies on an H^+ ATPase.

Aldosterone antagonists/K^+ sparing diuretics

See also Topic 2.6, 'Heart failure'. The K^+ sparing diuretics (e.g. spironolactone, eplerenone, amiloride, triamterene) act at diverse, but specific sites within distal DCT and collecting ducts. Although weak diuretics, they enhance Na^+ and water loss whilst preserving serum K^+ due to the reduction in Na^+/K^+ change at the luminal surface. Maintenance of K^+ is particularly important when loop or thiazide diuretic have led to clinical hypokalaemia.

Aldosterone is a steroid hormone and part of the renin–angiotensin system. It acts on mineralocorticoid receptors at DCT and collecting ducts to cause transcription of proteins such as SGK1, which phosphorylates and activates Na^+ channels. This activation causes Na^+ reabsorption and water retention. Spironolactone and eplerenone, respectively, are non-selective and selective aldosterone receptor antagonists used to treat oedema and ascites of liver disease, heart failure, malignancy, resistant hypertension, and nephrotic syndrome. Antagonizing aldosterone activity phosphorylation of Na^+ channels decreases Na^+ uptake from the tubular lumen channels. Basolateral membrane Na^+ extrusion by the ATPase is also decreased, thereby reducing water uptake. Because most Na^+ is reabsorbed in the proximal renal tubules, spironolactone is relatively ineffective when administered alone. For that reason, concomitant administration of a diuretic, which blocks reabsorption of Na^+ proximal to the distal portion of the nephron, such as a thiazide or loop diuretic, is required for maximum diuretic effects.

Amiloride and triamterene are K^+ sparing diuretics not usually used alone in the treatment of oedema (as monotherapy; see Topic 2.6, 'Heart failure'). They are used as an adjunct when K^+ conservation is required following treatment with thiazides or loop diuretics in hypertension (see Topic 2.1, 'Hypertension') or the ascites of hepatic cirrhosis. These two drugs act directly on the distal renal tubule of the nephron to inhibit Na^+–K^+ ion exchange at the luminal Na^+ channel; their actions being independent of the aldosterone pathway. Because of the mechanism of action of K^+ sparing diuretics, hyperkalaemia is possible in those with CKD or receiving ACEi. Hyponatraemia is also possible but only seen in those patients receiving diuretic combination therapy.

Box 5.1 Primary causes of nephrotic syndrome

- *Primary causes of nephrotic syndrome in adults*: focal and segmental glomerulosclerosis (FSGS). Focal sclerotic lesions affecting the glomeruli. Less responsive to corticosteroids
- *Membranous nephropathy*: thickening of the glomerular basement membrane
- *Minimal change nephropathy*: lesions on the podocytes and glomerular epithelial cells. Tends to be steroid sensitive
- *Mesangiocapillary (membranoproliferative) glomerulonephritis*: proliferation of mesangial cells and thickening of glomerular walls. Pathologically, it is like a combination of membranous and IgA nephropathy.

Nephrotic syndrome

Nephrotic syndrome is characterized by a collection of symptoms indicative of kidney damage, such as *oedema, proteinuria*, and *hypoalbuminaemia*, with or without *hyperlipidaemia*. It has an overall incidence of ~3/100,000 in adults and it affects slightly more men than women (as does AKI and CKD), presenting with signs of oedema, salt retention, and lethargy. It can result from many causes that directly (primary disease) or indirectly (secondary disease) affect the glomerular matrix (see Boxes 5.1 and 5.2)

Pathophysiology

The exact pathophysiology of each primary or secondary causative condition of nephrotic syndrome is subtly

Box 5.2 Secondary causes of nephrotic syndrome

- *Drugs*: NSAIDs, penicillamine, gold, lithium, tamoxifen, anti-TNF drugs
- *Infections*: HIV, hepatitis B/C, malaria, toxoplamosis
- *Systemic disease*: DM (commonest cause), amyloidosis, systemic lupus erythematosus (SLE)
- *Cancer*: myeloma, lymphoma
- *Congenital*: Denys–Drash, Pierson's syndrome, Alport's syndrome

different, but each essentially leads to the breakdown of the glomerular filtration system, causing albumin to leak through. The changes in membrane matrix proteins and persistence of hyperglycaemia leads to three major histological changes—mesangial expansion; thickening of the glomerular basement membrane; and glomerular sclerosis (see Figure 5.2). Clinical diagnosis is based on the presence of:

- raised proteinuria (>3.5 g in 24 hours, see Topic 5.2, 'Acute kidney injury', protein:creatinine ratio of >300 mg/mmol);
- hypoalbuminaemia (<30 g/L);
- peripheral oedema;
- severe hyperlipidaemia (in some cases).

Proteinuria

Proteinuria is the presence of excess levels of serum proteins in the urine and indicates insufficiency of absorption or impaired filtration. Proteins loss leads to a decrease in plasma oncotic pressure, preventing fluid being drawn out of the tissues. As such, the kidneys tend to retain salt and water further exacerbating fluid retention.

Hypoalbuminaemia

Albumin loss occurs predominantly as a result of increased urinary excretion, although there are likely to be other factors involved as serum levels appear lower than apparent loss. Although hepatic synthesis of albumin increases, this is not sufficient to maintain plasma levels so that oncotic pressure falls. So, with a failing liver and albumin synthesis, the extent of hypoalbuminaemia may be dramatic.

Peripheral oedema

Peripheral oedema is caused by Na^+ retention and exacerbated by a fall in oncotic pressure. Pulmonary oedema is unusual, unless CKD is present and worsening. If the patient is short of breath, pleural effusion and/or pulmonary embolism should be excluded.

Hyperlipidaemia

The declining oncotic pressure and subsequent liver expansion associated with rising protein synthesis, means augmented serum lipoproteins causing hypercholesterolaemia and lipiuria.

Complications

Many small anti-coagulant proteins are lost in urine, while large *pro*coagulant proteins remain or increase (possibly in an attempt to balance plasma oncotic pressure); this swing, plus changes in liver expression of factors V, VII, and X, and fibrinogen means a pro-coagulant state predominates. As such, around 30% of patients with nephrotic syndrome develop a deep vein thrombosis (~10%) or renal venous thrombosis (5–50%). If bilateral, this may present as AKI, or AKI on CKD. Further complications of nephrotic syndrome include infection (e.g. *Streptococcus pneumoniae)*, through the loss of urinary immunoglobulins. Some patients may also present with AKI and require treatment (see Topic 5.2, 'Acute kidney injury'), although management is complex and requires specialist advice (see Figure 5.3).

Management

A diagnosis of nephrotic syndrome is made clinically in the presence of proteinuria (>3.5 g in 24 hours or, more recently, protein:creatinine ratio of >300 mg/mmol), hypoalbuminaemia (<30 g/L) and peripheral oedema, with further tests to identify underlying causes, e.g.

- Glucose and HbA1c (diabetes).
- C-reactive protein (CRP).
- Renal immunology.
- Viral serology (Hep B, Hep C, HIV).
- *Renal biopsy:* if the cause of nephrotic syndrome is not obvious from history, examination, and these blood tests, most (adult) patients will need a renal biopsy.

With regards to treatment, primary measures involve treatment of the underlying cause—e.g. stop offending

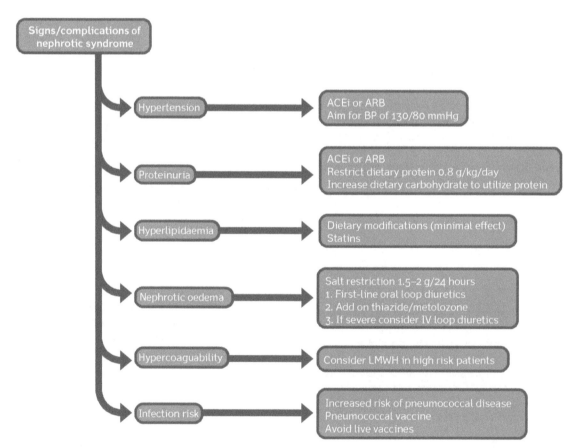

Figure 5.3 Complications of nephrotic syndrome.

drug, antiviral therapy for hepatitis B, treat malignancy, etc. Primary disease may require additional treatment with corticosteroids or immunosuppressants, e.g. glucocorticoids plus **cyclophosphamide** in severe idiopathic membranous nephropathy. Patients will, in addition, require supportive measures to manage symptoms.

Proteinuria

Management of proteinuria is through lowering of intraglomerular pressure to reduce protein loss, by means of an ACE inhibitor or ARB. ACEi and ARBs reduce intraglomerular pressure by inhibiting angiotensin II–mediated efferent arteriolar vasoconstriction. Moreover, they possess renoprotective properties due to the other haemodynamic and non-haemodynamic effects by reducing the breakdown of bradykinin (an efferent arteriolar vasodilator), restoring glomerular cell walls, and reducing cytokines production (e.g. TGF-beta, which contributes to glomerulosclerosis and fibrosis). A number of studies have shown ACEi and ARBs can reduce protein secretion by 40% and, as such, this can slow the progression of CKD, although they have not been shown to prevent dialysis.

Peripheral oedema

Salt restriction is recommended, in combination with lifestyle modifications (weight loss, exercise, and smoking cessation, particularly in the presence of hypertension or hyperlipidaemia). Diuretics are almost always required to reduce intravascular circulating volume, in particular loop diuretics, usually **furosemide**, with titrated doses according to response. With resistant oedema, thiazides diuretics, or aldosterone antagonists, or **amiloride** may be considered.

Hyperlipidaemia

Patients with evidence of hyperlipidaemia with chronic disease should be provided with advice on lifestyle modifications and, where necessary, statin therapy considered.

Complications

All adults with nephrotic syndrome will be considered for anticoagulation; especially those at high risk where albumin is <20 g/L. Patients at high risk of infection with *Streptococcus pneumoniae* may be considered for prophylactic **phenoxymethylpenicillin** plus vaccination.

Chronic kidney disease

Early stage CKD can present without signs or symptoms; however, as a risk factor for cardiovascular disease, early identification and implementation of preventative measures is crucial. As the pathologies of CKD progress this may lead to end-stage renal disease (ESRD) and the requirement for renal replacement therapy.

Pathophysiology

Failure of kidney function, acutely or chronically, has several important implications for the removal of waste products, conservation of essential nutrients and regulation of acid-base balance and electrolyte concentrations (see Table 5.1). In severe AKI or CKD (see Table 5.2), dysfunction of the latter two systems can result in systemic metabolic acidosis and/or hyperkalaemia, which can be life threatening. See Figure 5.1.

Decreased excretion

Sodium, as the predominant ion in extracellular fluid, accounts primarily for serum osmolality and BP. The kidney is the main regulator of Na^+ levels and homeostasis, although even in dysfunction, it manages to maintain control; so that even in severe failure, the incidence of hypo/hypernatraemia is low. That said, the incidence of hypertension is high, in part due to impaired excretion of

Table 5.1 Summary of consequences of altered kidney function

Mechanism of failure	Product	Pathological effect
Decreased excretion of	Urea	Uraemic syndrome
	Sodium	Hypertension
	Phosphate	Hyperparathyroidism
	Potassium	Hyperkalaemia
	Acid	Metabolic acidosis
Decreased biosynthesis of	Erythropoietin	Anaemia
	Vitamin D activation	Hyperparathroidism
Altered metabolism	Dyslipidaemia	Athersclerosis

Table 5.2 Stage of kidney disease based on the NKF-KDOQI classification

GFR categories (mL/min/1.73 m²) Description and range			A1 Normal to mildly increased <30 mg/g <3 mg/mmol	A2 Moderately increased 30–300 mg/g 3–30 mg/mmol	A3 Severely increased >300 mg/g >30 mg/mmol
G1	Normal or high	≥90	Low risk	Moderately increased risk	High risk
G2	Mildly decreased	60–89	Low risk	Moderately increased risk	High risk
G3a	Mild to moderately decreased	45–59	Moderately increased risk	High risk	Very high risk
G3b	Moderately to severely decreased	30–44	High risk	Very high risk	Very high risk
G4	Severely decreased	15–29	Very high risk	Very high risk	Very high risk
G5	Kidney failure	<15	Very high risk	Very high risk	Very high risk

NB: CKD1-2 cannot be diagnosed unless the patient has evidence of structural renal disease, e.g. significant proteinuria/albuminuria (A2 or A3), or abnormal ultrasound. CKD5 or ESRD implies the need for dialysis, transplantation or supportive care.
*Low risk if no other markers of kidney disease, no CKD.

Reprinted from Inker, L. A. et al., KDOQI US Commentary on the 2012 KDIGO Clinical Practice Guideline for the Evaluation and Management of CKD. *American Journal of Kidney Diseases*, 63(5), 713-735. https://doi.org/10.1053/j.ajkd.2014.01.416. Copyright © 2014 Published by Elsevier Inc.

sodium, but also due to increased activation of the renin–angiotensin pathway.

The decreased function of the H^+/K^+ luminal antiporter in the PCT means H^+ is resorbed by an alternative pathway in conjunction with Cl^- resulting in a compensatory hyperchloraemic metabolic acidosis. Generally, if the renal damage affects glomeruli and tubules, the acidosis is a high-anion gap acidosis. This mechanism relies on carbonic anhydrase, where CO_2 is converted to bicarbonate. Carbonic anhydrase inhibitors like **acetazolamide** (used in respiratory/metabolic alkalosis) can, therefore, decrease resorption of bicarbonate. At Stage 4 CKD, around 20% of patients have a metabolic acidosis.

In renal failure, the electrochemical gradient responsible for secretion of K^+ in the distal tubule and collecting duct may be lost, leading to retention of K^+ and hyperkalaemia. Interestingly, loop diuretics (see 'Loop diuretics') may be of benefit in fluid overloaded or oedematous patients, as more Na^+ reaches the collecting ducts so is resorbed with a counter-current loss of K^+ aiding return to normokalaemia.

Decreased biosynthesis

As renal function deteriorates and GFR falls, serum phosphate is retained and the hydroxylation activation of vitamin D is impaired. This initially leads to decreased circulating levels of Ca^{2+} and, with time, secondary hyperparathyroidism (see Topic 4.4, 'Parathyroid disease') develops with symptomatic itching. Increased bone resorption of both Ca^{2+} and phosphate can lead to metabolic bone disease.

The kidney is also the site of erythropoietin production. Erythropoietin acts on pluripotent stem cells in the marrow leading to their differentiation and multiplication, ultimately producing red blood cells. In CKD, erythropoietin production is impaired, reducing RBC production, causing anaemia.

Altered metabolism

With declining renal function, dyslipidaemias are common due to alterations in lipid enzymes. In general, reductions in lipoprotein lipase and hepatic lipase, in combination with increased activity of HMG-CoA reductase, gives rise to—increased triglycerides, increased intermediate density lipoproteins (IDL) and a reduction in HDL. LDL cholesterol associated with increased cardiovascular risk, generally remain unaffected.

The most common causes of CKD are hypertension and diabetes, leading to vascular disease and diabetic nephropathy. In addition, chronic atherosclerosis in the renal artery can cause ischaemic nephropathy contributing to glomerulosclerosis. Renal failure secondary to DM is due to intraglomerular hypertension. This is a result of mesangial expansion induced by persistent hyperglycaemia, which causes increased matrix production, glomerular basement membrane thickening, and hyaline thickening of afferent and efferent arterioles.

Patients with CKD typically present with non-specific symptoms, related to the kidneys key regulatory roles, i.e. fatigue and weakness due to failure in the production of erythropoietin (EPO), polyuria from filtration failure, hypertension from Na$^+$ retention, and disequilibrium in the renin–angiotensin system and pruritus secondary to hyperphosphataemia/hyperuraemia. As these signs and symptoms present late, it is important to have a high index of suspicion in those at risk, i.e. diabetics (e.g. diabetic nephropathy), hypertensive or hyperlipidaemic patients (e.g. renovascular disease), those with a family history (e.g. glomerulonephritis or polycystic disease), and the elderly (e.g. benign prostatic hyperplasia). Prolonged AKI, failure to recover from the insult or extended exposure to nephrotoxins (e.g. **gentamicin**, contrast-dyes) may also lead to CKD.

Management

The aim of management in CKD is to delay progression through modification of risk factors (see Box 5.3), and where relevant, the identification and subsequent treatment of any reversible causes. This may include the discontinuation of nephrotoxic drugs (see Table 5.3), in particular chronic NSAID use, ACEi/ARBs, or other factors such as urinary obstruction or volume depletion. Reversible causes are usually associated with a more rapid decline in renal function.

In addition to establishing GFR to assess renal function, other investigational clues of dysfunction may exist in the form of persistent microalbuminuria, proteinuria, and haematuria from urine analysis. Urinary dipstick is not sufficient. Urine samples should be sent for midstream specimen of urine (MSU) (M,C&S), and urinary

Box 5.3 Risk factors for progression of CKD

- Cardiovascular disease
- Smoking
- Race/ethnicity
- Level of GFR/albuminuria
- Serum calcium
- CVD
- Diabetes
- Proteinuria
- Obesity
- Haemoglobin
- Serum phosphate
- Diabetes
- Hypertension
- Chronic NSAID use
- Sex
- Age
- Serum bicarbonate
- Hypertension

albumin and protein. Ultrasound may demonstrate structural abnormalities like polycystic kidney disease and obstructive nephropathy, while biopsy may identify chronic glomerulonephritis.

Patients with CKD should be offered advice on lifestyle modifications, such as weight loss, smoking cessation, restricted salt intake, and restricted dietary protein (0.8 g/kg day); patients with hyperphosphataemia should also have their phosphate intake restricted. Advice on restrictions should be carried out under the direction of a suitably trained professional. Other modifiable risk factors should be addressed, such as optimizing BP control in hypertension and glycaemic control in diabetics. With progressive disease, complications of CKD will require additional pharmacological management, i.e. anaemia, renal bone disease/osteodystrophy (now called CKD-MBD).

Hypertension

ACE inhibitors or angiotensin receptor II antagonists are the treatments of choice for managing hypertension in both diabetic and non-diabetic patients with CKD. Treatment should be modified to achieve a BP of less than 130 mmHg systolic and 80 mmHg diastolic. If such patients develop AKI or rapidly progressive CKD, these drugs should be stopped.

Table 5.3 Common example of nephrotoxic drugs.

Class	Examples	Toxicity
Aminoglycosides	Gentamicin, amikacin	Acute tubular necrosis
Thiazides	Bendroflumethiazide, indapamide	Acute interstitial nephritis, pre-renal
Loop diuretics	Furosemide	Acute interstitial nephritis, pre-renal
NSAIDs	Indometacin, diclofenac, ibuprofen, naproxen	Acute interstitial nephritis, chronic renal failure, nephrotic syndrome
ACE inhibitors + ARBs	Enalapril, ramipril, losartan, irbesartan	Prerenal (renal artery stenosis)
Penicillins	Amoxicillin, phenoxymethylpenicillin, flucloxacillin	Acute interstitial nephritis
Amphotericin	N/A	Prerenal, acute tubular necrosis
Lithium	N/A	Acute tubular necrosis, acute interstitial nephritis
Ciclosporin	N/A	Prerenal

Glycaemic control

In diabetic patients, glycaemic control should be optimized to achieve an HbA1c of <48 mmol/mol, although slightly higher levels are acceptable in patients at risk of hypoglycaemia or in those with multiple co-morbidities. Consideration should also be given to managing other cardiovascular risk factors, with the addition of **aspirin** or statins as appropriate. In advanced CKD (CKD4 or above), the doses of insulin or oral hypoglycaemic agents often need to reduced (or the drugs even stopped), as insulin is renally excreted, otherwise hypoglycaemic attacks will occur.

Hyperkalaemia

Hyperkalaemia is a real risk in patients with CKD, particularly in those not treated with ACEi or ARB therapies. The management of hyperkalaemia is outlined in chapter 5.2 AKI.

Anaemia

Anaemia is a common complication of CKD associated with poor outcomes. Routine monitoring of haemoglobin is therefore essential, with treatment offered to symptomatic patients or those with a haemoglobin of <100 g/L.

The target haemoglobin is 110–120 g/L for a patient with ESRD. Further blood tests should be carried out to determine the nature and severity of any anaemia, including full blood count (FBC), serum ferritin, serum vitamin B12, and folate. Although oral iron supplementation may suffice in non-dialysed patients, more severe cases and those on dialysis will probably require IV therapy. Erythropoietin-stimulating agents (ESAs) may be required to maintain haemoglobin levels.

Bone metabolism and osteoporosis

Hyperphosphataemia, secondary to CKD leads to altered bone mineral metabolism, as well as increased cardiovascular risk. This is called renal bone disease or renal osteodystrophy (and now CKD-MBD). Patients with CKD Stage 3 or 4 and above, therefore require routine monitoring of serum calcium, phosphate, and alkaline phosphatase every 3–6 months, and PTH every 6–12 months. In addition, levels of 25-hydroxycholecalciferol (25(OH)D) should be measured at baseline and repeated according to baseline levels, i.e. more frequently in those with altered levels.

Phosphate, calcium, and vitamin D levels should be maintained within the normal range, through treatment with phosphate binders, calcium supplements, and vitamin D supplements as appropriate. Where PTH remains elevated despite these measures, calcimimetics may be added. In early stage 3 or less, **colecalciferol** and **ergocalciferol** are the vitamin D supplements of choice, whereas in stage 4 or 5 disease, supplementation with **alfacalcidol** or **calcitriol** is preferred, as renal insufficiency prevents the conversion of 25(OH)D to its active form.

Patients with osteoporosis or at risk of fracture secondary to CKD should be managed as for those without CKD [see Topic 7.4, 'Metabolic bone disease (Paget's, osteoporosis')], i.e. with bisphosphonates, etc. Consideration, however, should be given to any dose modifications due to impaired renal function, and in patients with stage 4 or 5 disease, bisphosphonates should be avoided.

Bicarbonate

Patients with low serum bicarbonate (less than 22 mmol/L) may require supplementation with oral sodium bicarbonate to help reduce disease progression.

Drug classes used in management

Carbonic anhydrase inhibitors

Inhibition of the carbonic anhydrase enzyme reduces the reabsorption of Na^+ in the proximal tubule, promoting the excretion of Na_+, HCO_3^- and K. For example, acetazolamide.

Mechanism of action

Within the proximal tubule carbonic anhydrase catalyses the conversion of H_2CO_3 to CO_2 and H_2O following movement of H^+ ions into the lumen in exchange for Na^+ ions, where it interacts with HCO_3^- to promote its reabsorption. CO_2 and H_2O then diffuse intracellularly, where again under the influence of carbonic anhydrase the reaction is reversed to produce H^+ and HCO_3^-. HCO_3^- subsequently leaves the cell in exchange for Na^+ ions, enabling the reabsorption of Na^+ against an electrochemical gradient.

As the proximal tubule is a minor site for Na^+ reabsorption the effects of carbonic anhydrase inhibition on diuresis is minimal, although they do prevent the initial reabsorption of HCO_3^-, thereby promoting loss, which may be utilized in metabolic alkalosis. Increased secretion of HCO_3^- also leads to urinary alkalinization, which can

promote the excretion of some drugs thus reducing their toxicity, e.g. **methotrexate**.

Prescribing

In practice the carbonic anhydrase inhibitors are rarely used for their diuretic properties. They are, however, of value in promoting urinary alkalinization and in the management of metabolic and respiratory alkalosis. They are also used acutely in the management of glaucoma to reduce intraocular pressure and in the management of altitude sickness.

Unwanted effects

Unwanted effects with **acetazolamide** tend to be mild, in-line with its mild diuretic effects, furthermore, with continued use tolerance develops to its diuretic effects. Side effects can include tingling sensations and altered appetite. Due to their effects on bicarbonate, acetazolamide will also affect the taste of carbonated drinks.

Erythropoietin-stimulating agents

The glycoprotein erythropoietin, produced primarily in the kidney in response to decreased oxygen in circulation, is the key regulator in the homeostatic system that controls cell blood mass and oxygen delivery to tissues: Examples include erthyropoetin alfa/beta and darbepoetin.

Mechanism of action

Erythropoietin and **darbepoetin** are indicated for the symptomatic treatment of anaemia secondary to CKD or ESRD, once any folate or iron deficiency has been corrected. Erythropoietin binds to the erythropoietin receptor, a transmembrane protein with an extracellular and intracellular domain. One erythropoietin molecule interacts with two erythropoietin receptors leading to a conformational change that brings constitutively associated JAK2 kinases in close proximity and stimulates their activation by transphosphorylation. In turn, JAK2 molecules phosphorylate tyrosine residues in the intracellular domain of the erythropoietin receptor, serving as a dock for various signalling processes that contain Src homology 2 domains, the Ras/Map kinase, and Pi3K pathways. Erythropoietin stimulation results in the activation of anti-apoptotic cascades, preventing the death of erythrocyte progenitor cells, stimulating proliferation and terminal differentiation. Although mainly expressed in cells of the erythroid lineage, the erythropoietin receptors have also been found in brain, retina, heart, muscle kidney, and endothelial cells, suggesting paracrine extra-erythropoietic actions.

The three main erythropoietic agents for the treatment of anaemia are the recombinant human erythropoietins (rHuEpo), **erythropoietin** α and **erythropoietin** β, and **darbepoetin**-α, a hyperglycosylated derivative.

Prescribing

The recombinant human erythropoietins (rHuEpo), α and β tend to be used more frequently, and are administered either SC or as a slow IV injection depending on brand, and whether or not the patient is on haemodialysis. Doses are usually given one to two times a week (or when target haemoglobin is achieved, a dosage every 2 weeks may be adequate).

Darbepoetin has the advantage of a longer duration of action, enabling less frequent administration (weekly), again with doses adjusted according to response. For all ESAs, treatment is initiated and managed in specialist renal centres, and stopped in those resistant to its effects.

PRACTICAL PRESCRIBING

Prescribing erythropoietin

Erythropoetin should be prescribed by brand due to lack of bioequivalence between products.

Unwanted effects

Common side effects to ESAs include GI toxicity and hypertension (dose-dependent). BP should therefore be monitored, particularly in those with poorly controlled hypertension. The sudden onset of a 'stabbing' migraine-like pain could indicate a hypertensive crisis.

Haematological toxicity associated with ESA treatment, includes thrombosis and, less frequently, thrombocythaemia and pure red cell aplasia. Patients should have platelets monitored in the first 8 weeks of treatment and haemoglobin monitored throughout. Levels beyond target Hb levels increases the risk of thrombosis, particularly in patients with cardiovascular disease. In patients with a recent history of a stroke or MI, treatment is best avoided. Also, if the haemoglobin level achieved by an ESA is too high (e.g. >120 g/L), the fistula (or graft) of a patient on chronic haemodialysis can clot.

Neurological effects such as headaches and generalized tonic-clonic seizures are also commonly reported, which may or may not be associated with a hypertensive crisis. Patients with a history of seizures should use with caution.

Iron therapy

Essential for a wide variety of metabolic processes, iron is required for erythropoietin to effectively stimulate red blood cell production, and is used to treat iron deficiency anaemia. Examples include ferrous sulfate, ferrous gluconate, ferrous fumarate, iron sucrose, iron dextran, ferric carboxymaltose, and iron isomaltoside 1000.

Mechanism of action

Reduced secretion of erythropoietin by the kidney or decreased response to it in the bone marrow can lead to anaemia; defined by a shortage in new erythrocyte production relative to the removal rate of aged erythrocytes. The production of red blood cells (erythropoiesis) requires 30–40 mg of iron per day to produce sufficient haemoglobin, which accounts for about 95% of the dry weight of red blood cells.

Since iron is potentially highly toxic to various cell structures in solution, various mechanisms have evolved to minimize free iron. Approximately two-thirds of iron is utilized in the bone marrow and circulating red blood cells, while the remaining one-third is stored mostly in liver tissue and macrophages of the reticuloendothelial system. Active transport of iron from tissue stores to the bone marrow is essential for haematopoiesis to occur. Almost all iron not taken up by haem- proteins, is bound to transferrin for transport in the circulation or ferritin for tissue storage. Serum ferritin and transferrin saturation are relatively good markers for assessing iron stores and the circulating iron pool, respectively.

PRACTICAL PRESCRIBING

Factors affecting oral absorption of iron

Oral absorption of iron is enhanced when the body's iron stores are low, including during pregnancy, whereas food, certain drugs, and caffeinated drinks may impair absorption. Despite this, it is often recommended that it is taken with food to reduce GI toxicity.

The percentage of iron absorbed decreases with dose, thus taking smaller doses BD or TDS is more effective than taking a single larger daily dose.

Prescribing

The treatment of iron deficiency anaemia with iron replacement therapy is usually with oral therapy, available in a number of different salts, e.g. fumarate, sulfate, and gluconate. Although the salts contain varying amounts of elemental iron per mg, they demonstrate comparable efficacy at therapeutic doses. Absorption of oral iron, however, can be affected by a number of factors (see 'Practical prescribing: oral and parenteral iron interaction').

PRACTICAL PRESCRIBING

Oral and parenteral iron interaction

- Administration of parenteral iron impairs absorption of oral iron.
- Any oral therapy should not be resumed until 5 days after an iron injection.

Parenteral iron therapy provides an option when oral supplementation is inadequate due either to severe deficiency, in renal dialysis, or in those unable to tolerate oral supplements. There are a number of available options—**iron dextrose**, **iron sucrose**, **ferric carboxymaltose**, **ferumoxytol**, and **iron isomaltoside 1000**. In all cases, doses are calculated on haemoglobin levels (current and desired) and patient's body weight, although they vary in their method, duration, and frequency of administration. Ferric carboxymaltose and iron isomaltoside have the advantage of being administered as a single dose (for doses less than 1000 mg) over 15–30 minutes, compared with 6 hours required with some alternative preparations.

Unwanted effects

GI effects are common, particularly with oral iron, giving rise to constipation and nausea, as well as darkened stools. Although switching between salts may help improve toxicity, there is no evidence to suggest which salt is less likely to cause GI effects.

Hypersensitivity reactions are a well-documented risk to all parenteral iron therapy, with the risk increased in patients that have an underlying immune or inflammatory condition. For all agents except ferric carboxymaltose, treatment is contraindicated in patients with a history of allergic disorders including asthma and eczema.

PRESCRIBING WARNING

Risk of severe hypersensitivity reactions to intravenous iron

- Hypersensitivity reactions are widely reported and potentially severe with IV iron product.
- They may occur with any dose, so test doses are no longer recommended.
- Practitioners are advised to closely monitor all doses and to continue to monitor for a further 30 minutes after completion.
- Doses should be given by appropriately trained staff with resuscitation facilities on hand.

Phosphate binders

Phosphate binders act by binding to phosphate in the gut, forming an insoluble compound and thus preventing its absorption. Examples include sevelamer, lanthanum, aluminium hydroxide, calcium salts, magnesium carbonate, and colestilan.

Mechanism of action

With progressive CKD, phosphate binders prevent phosphate absorption from the gut, providing an effective way of reducing serum levels when restricted diets become insufficient. Traditionally, this was achieved with the use of **aluminium**, **magnesium**, and **calcium** salts, but the realization of the toxic effect of long-term aluminium, made calcium salts the preferred option.

Sevelamer is a non-metal, non-calcium polymer that lacks strong binding action, but may have added advantages with its ability to bind cholesterol in the gut. More recently, the rare earth metal **lanthanum carbonate** has been introduced, which is minimally absorbed in the gut and does not rely on the kidney for its elimination. **Colestilan** is a bile acid sequestrant that also acts to bind phosphate in the duodenum, and like sevelamar it has the advantage of being non-calcium and non-metal. However, it is more likely to adversely affect absorption of fat soluble vitamins.

Prescribing

Calcium acetate is the treatment of choice in the management of hyperphosphataemia of CKD. As well as having the benefit of providing additional calcium supplementation, it tends to be better tolerated than some binders, such as the **aluminium** and **magnesium** salts, and is less costly than **sevelamer** or **lanthanum**. Where patients have calcium levels on the upper limit of normal, treatment is poorly tolerated or phosphate levels remain raised, then a non-calcium based binder such as sevelamer may be added or used in its place.

All phosphate binders are taken orally, invariably involving large amounts of unpalatable tablets. Lanthanum should be chewed, some swallowed whole (sevelamer hydrochloride, aluminium hydroxide), and calcium acetate may be broken, but not chewed due to its bitter taste. Sevelamer carbonate is also available as a powder for suspension.

Unwanted effects

GI side effects are those most widely reported to phosphate binders, including nausea, vomiting, constipation, and bloating. Absorption of fat soluble vitamins is likely to be impaired in the presence of phosphate binders, particularly **colestilan**. Long-term unsupervised treatment runs the risk of causing hypophosphataemia, hypercalcaemia, or hypermagnesaemia depending on the agent used. **Calcium** salts are also associated with an increased risk of vascular calcification, thus increasingly, the newer non-calcium-based binders are being introduced earlier. Long-term treatment with **aluminium**-containing salts is associated with aluminium toxicity and dementia, and is now not often used.

Further reading: chronic kidney disease

Arora P (2012) Chronic kidney disease. *Medscape.* https:// emedicine.medscape.com/article/238798-overview [accessed 28 March 2019].

El Nahas AM, Bello AK (2005) Chronic kidney disease: the global challenge. *Lancet* 365(9456), 331–40.

Levey AS, Coresh J (2012) Chronic kidney disease. *Lancet.* 379(9811), 165–80.

Ritz E, Drüeke TB, Firth JD (2013) Chronic kidney disease. In: Wilkinson IB, Raine T (Eds) *Oxford Textbook of Medicine*, Ch 21.6. Oxford: Oxford University Press.

Guidelines: chronic kidney disease

KDIGO (2012) Clinical Practice Guideline for Anaemia in Chronic Kidney Disease. *Kidney International* (Suppl. 2;4), 279–335. https://kdigo.org/guidelines/ anemia-in-ckd/ [accessed 24 April 2019].

KDIGO (2017) Clinical practice guidelines for the diagnosis, evaluation, prevention and treatment of chronic kidney disease—Mineral and bone disorders (CKD-MBD). *Kidney International Supplements* 7, 1–59. https://kdigo. org/wp-content/uploads/2017/02/2017-KDIGO-CKD-MBD-GL-Update.pdf [accessed 10 April 2019].

NICE CG157 (2013) Hyperphosphataemia in chronic kidney disease: Management of hyperphosphataemia in patients with stage 4 or 5 chronic kidney disease. NICE guideline CG157. https://www.nice.org.uk/guidance/ cg157 [accessed 10 April 2019].

NICE NG8 (2015) Chronic kidney disease: managing anaemia. NICE guideline NG8. https://www.nice.org.uk/ guidance/ng8 [accessed 28 March 2019].

SIGN 103 (2008) Diagnosis and management of chronic kidney disease. http://www.seqc.es/download/gpc/62/ 3729/1043258133/1073968/cms/sign-diagnosis-and-management-of-chronic-kidney-disease_guideline.pdf/ [accessed 10 April 2019].

Further reading: Nephrotic syndrome

Crew RJ, Radhakrishnan J, Appel G (2004) Complications of the nephrotic syndrome and their treatment. *Clinical Nephrology* 62, 245–59.

Haraldsson B, Nyström J, Deen WM (2008) Properties of the glomerular barrier and mechanisms of proteinuria. *Physiology Review* 88(2), 451–87.

Hogan J, Radhakrishnan J (2013) The treatment of minimal change disease in adults. *Journal of the American Society for Nephrology* 24(5), 702–11.

Hull RP, Goldsmith DJA (2008) Nephrotic syndrome in adults. *British Medical Journal* 336, 1185–9.

Kerlin BA, Ayoob R, Smoyer WE (2012) Epidemiology and pathophysiology of nephrotic syndrome-associated thromboembolic disease. *Clinical Journal of the American Society for Nephrology* 7(3), 513–20.

Kodner C (2009) Nephrotic syndrome in adults: diagnosis and management. *American Family Physician* 80(10), 1129–34.

Guidelines: nephrotic syndrome

KDIGO (2012) Clinical practice guidelines for glomerularnephritis. *Kidney* 2 (Suppl. 2). https://kdigo.org/guidelines/anemia-in-ckd/.

5.2 Acute kidney injury

AKI is a rapid loss of kidney function. It takes into consideration a spectrum of disease (see 'Pathophysiology') and has replaced the term acute renal failure (ARF). It is surprisingly common in primary and secondary care, in the presence or absence of acute illness, and exists in nearly 20% of hospital admissions. A national confidential enquiry into patient outcome and death in 2009 revealed that AKI was poorly managed throughout the UK, so guidance now exists on the importance of early intervention/recognition, risk assessment, and treatment.

Pathophysiology

The glomerulus is the functional unit for the filtration of blood and relies on a regulated renal blood flow from afferent and efferent arterioles. Reduction of renal blood flow directly decreases glomerular filtration rate (GFR). To this end, AKI can result from three potential mechanisms:

- *Pre-renal failure* (and acute tubular necrosis): the most common form of AKI, resulting from decreased intravascular circulating volume, secondary to multiple causes, e.g. hypovolaemia or haemorrhage, oedematous states (e.g. heart failure), sepsis, or anaphylaxis. Iatrogenic causes of prerenal failure include NSAIDs, ACEi, ARBs, aminoglycosides (like **gentamicin**), or radiocontrast dyes, all of which can reduce renal perfusion.

- The term *acute tubular necrosis* (ATN), describes a pathological condition, which may follow AKI (especially pre-renal) if the cause is not corrected. It usually encompasses AKI in a specific clinical context that results in oliguria/anuria and recovers to normal renal function in days to weeks (most in 10–14 days). In ATN, the injured kidney fails to maintain a high medullary solute concentration so that urine osmolality is affected (in prerenal it is >500 mOsm/kg, whereas in intrarenal it is typically <300 mOsm/kg). The key to management

is early restoration of renal blood flow. Although the condition normally reverses itself, once blood flow to the kidneys has been restored, inadequate treatment, such as nephrotoxic drugs in the volume depleted or an elderly patient, can make pathology advance from pre-renal to ATN, resulting in toxin accumulation and hyperkalaemia. Dialysis may be required if AKI (pre-renal leading to ATN) cannot be reversed for the duration of the ATN.

- *Intrinsic (intra) renal failure*: occurs when direct damage or injury to the kidney produces a rapid loss of kidney function. It can typically be divided into two categories: patients with glomerular aetiologies (e.g. glomerulonephritis, thrombosis, haemolytic uraemic syndrome) and those with tubular dysfunction (i.e. from ATN following prolonged ischaemia after nephrotoxin exposure; or acute tubule-interstitial nephritis, often caused by penicillins, cephalosporins, and NSAIDs). ATN secondary to prerenal AKI rarely leads to long-term ESRF due to intrinsic renal failure, i.e. when AKI does not recover. Vasculitic disease may also cause intrinsic renal failure. In the case of glomerular disease, patients will often present with nephrotic syndrome as well; i.e. a urinary protein:creatinine ratio (UPCR) of >300 mg/mmol Cr. Previously, this was defined as proteinuria (>3.5 g/24 hours*), hypoalbuminaemia (<30 g/L), and oedema (see Topic 5.1, 'The kidney, drugs, and chronic kidney disease').

- *Obstructive (post)-renal failure*: mechanical obstruction of the urinary collecting system can occur anywhere along the tract (i.e. renal pelvis, ureters, bladder, or urethra) and may result in post-renal AKI. Causes include tumours (benign or malignant), haematomas, or strictures. Stone disease is a rare cause, as both kidneys have to be affected. Unilateral obstruction may have little impact on serum creatinine. However, a bilateral obstruction from BPH and prostate (or bladder),

Box 5.4 Criteria for AKI

- A rise in serum creatinine of 26 μmol/L or greater within 48 hours
- A >50% rise in serum creatinine (presumed) within the past 7 days
- A fall in urine output to < 0.5 mL/kg/hour for more than 6 hours in adults

tumours in men, or pelvic malignancy (including gynaecological and bladder tumours) in women may present as AKI.

The detection and criteria for AKI is defined in Box 5.4. The staging is outlined in guidance set out in RIFLE (2004), AKIN (2007), and KDIGO (2012) all of which use specific criteria for GFR decline.

As with CKD, AKI has implications on the excretion, biosynthesis, and metabolic functions of the kidney, leading to a broad spectrum of pathologies. In addition, some patients who present with AKI, may be suffering an acute-on-chronic renal failure (or AKI on CKD) secondary to decompensation of a previously undiagnosed chronic condition; this emphasizes the importance of a systematic approach to clinical investigation. AKI can be diagnosed in the presence of a rise in serum creatinine of >26 μmol/L over 48 hours, a fall in urine output of <0.5 mL/kg/hours for 6 hours or a >25% fall in eGFR over the last 7 days. As a 'rule of thumb', that is a >25% rise in serum creatinine over the last 48 hours is AKI until otherwise proven.

For a full summary of the relevant pathways and drug targets, see Figure 5.4.

Management

AKI is common in primary and secondary care, but often remains undetected and affects an increasing number of patients with no underlying acute illness. Optimal management is facilitated by improved detection and through identification of at-risk groups for subsequent monitoring of serum creatinine relative to baseline levels (see Box 5.5). Early detection helps to enable the reversal of any precipitating causes, e.g. drug therapy (like ACEi) or dehydration, and to avoid the use of further nephrotoxic drugs (such as aminoglycoside antibiotics) or contrast media.

Where AKI is detected, urinalysis (blood, protein, leucocytes, and nitrites) should be carried out to identify an underlying cause. An ultrasound scan of the urinary tract

should be carried out in most cases, particularly where the cause remains unknown or pyonephrosis is suspected. Any potentially nephrotoxic drugs, prescribed or otherwise, should be discontinued (e.g. herbal remedies, OTC medication, illicit drugs). In addition, consideration should be given to any necessary dose modifications for renally cleared drugs, such as **digoxin** and **allopurinol**.

Although some causes of AKI may be managed in primary care, patients with established severe AKI or AKI of unknown cause benefit from early referral to a nephrologist. Some patients, such as those failing to respond to medical interventions for hyperkalaemia, metabolic acidosis, pulmonary oedema, or complications of uraemia, *will* require immediate and specialist treatment in the form of renal replacement therapy (RRT). The indications for RRT are outlined in Box 5.6.

Pharmacological therapy has a limited role in the management of AKI, as to date there is little evidence to suggest that any drug can effectively treat or prevent AKI. Drug therapy is therefore limited to managing complications, often with limited success. However, an important first step in the management is to discontinue precipitating/causative agents, and initiate a fluid challenge to encourage renal perfusion.

Haemodynamic instability

Where haemodynamic instability secondary to septic shock or dehydration precipitates AKI, patients will require urgent fluid correction to restore fluid volume and BP, thus improving renal perfusion. Fluids should be carefully titrated to reverse AKI without causing fluid overload, as this is associated with an increase in mortality, in part linked to pulmonary oedema. Choice of fluids remains controversial, with recent studies suggesting no difference in outcome between isotonic crystalloids (e.g. sodium chloride 0.9%) and colloids (e.g. albumin), although the former have the advantage of a reduced cost (see 'Fluids'). The use of Hartmann's solution with 5 mmol/L of K^+, is best avoided in those with hyperkalaemia secondary to AKI.

To date, optimum fluid targets have not been established in AKI, but proactive administration of fluids before and after a timed insult, such as in radiological contrast dyes, can reduce contrast-induced nephropathy. Fluid overload, however, should be avoided, especially in those with sepsis, AKI, and oliguria and/or anuria, as it significantly worsens outcome. It can increase intra-abdominal pressure causing venous congestion resulting in reduced GFR and worsening urine output. Diuretics may be required to encourage offload of fluids.

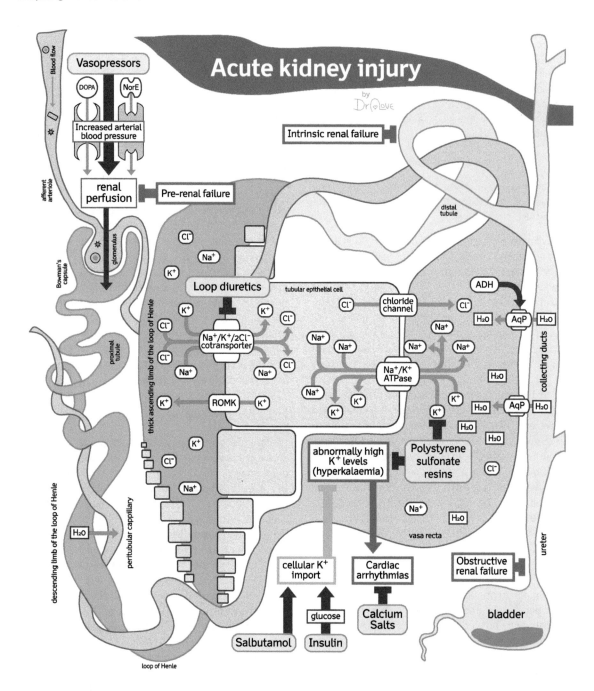

Figure 5.4 Topic: summary of relevant pathways and drug targets.

Vasopressors are widely used in the treatment and prevention of AKI. Historically, low dose **dopamine** was frequently used to reduce renal vascular resistance, this practice in AKI is no longer advocated. Evidence to support the use of other vasopressors (**noradrenaline**, **vasopressin** and **terlipressin**), although more convincing in terms of improving urine output and creatinine clearance, still fails to demonstrate a reduced

Box 5.5 Risk factors for AKI

- Chronic kidney disease
- Diabetes
- Hypovolaemia
- Sepsis
- Urological obstruction
- History of AKI
- Liver failure
- Nephrotoxic drugs
- Deteriorating physiological (modified) early warning score
- Oliguria
- Heart failure
- Impaired fluid intake
- Recent iodine contrast
- Over 65 years of age
- Malignancy

need for renal replacement therapy or improvement in overall survival. The mortality of dialysis-dependent AKI remains high at 50%. That said, they remain widely used in the treatment of septic shock and are included in international guidelines to prevent AKI. Ultimately, maintaining optimal BP is paramount so that renal perfusion is preserved.

Box 5.6 Indications for renal replacement therapy in AKI

- Clinical features of uraemia (e.g. pericarditis, gastritis, hypothermia, fits, or encephalopathy)
- *Pulmonary oedema*: unresponsive to diuretics with urine volume < 200 mL over 12 hours
- Severe hyperkalaemia (>6.5 mmol/L) unresponsive to medical management
- Serum sodium above 155 mmol/L or below 120 mmol/L
- Severe acid-base disturbance (pH <7.0) unresponsive to sodium bicarbonate
- Severe renal failure (urea >30 mmol/L, creatinine >500 μmol/L)
- Drug-induced toxicity with drugs that can be cleared by dialysis

Oedema

Loop diuretics should only be offered to patients with pulmonary oedema, taking care not to over-diurese. Excessive diuresis and routine use of loop diuretics to prevent AKI can be detrimental and may increase mortality.

Hyperkalaemia

ACEi are a common cause of hyperkalaemia in AKI since intrinsic autoregulation of renal blood flow, and GFR is tightly controlled by angiotensin II and the sympathetic system. When perfusion pressures drop, as in hypovolaemia or CKD, renin release occurs from afferent arterioles, with a resulting rise in angiotensin II causing efferent arterioles vasoconstriction, which then maintains renal perfusion pressure. ACEi act to reduce levels of angiotensin II thereby reducing GFR leading to hypoperfusion and impaired Na^+ resorption. As such they cause inadequate constriction of the efferent arteriole resulting in decreased hydrostatic pressure across the glomerulus decreasing GFR. ACEis also lower plasma aldosterone levels so urinary K^+ excretion from the collecting duct is reduced (c.f. potassium sparing diuretics). The frequency of AKI induced by ACE inhibitors varies between 5% and 20%.

Hyperkalaemia secondary to AKI should be monitored for and managed according to severity. Mild-moderate hyperkalaemia will respond to diuretic treatment in patients who are fluid overloaded, or with polystyrene sulfonate resins (e.g. Calcium Resonium®), whose onset of action is slow. However, with higher levels (e.g. greater than 6.5 mmol/L), urgent correction is usually necessary, ideally with **insulin** therapy (after initial cardiac stabilization with **calcium salts**) or, less commonly, **salbutamol**. Prescribers should be aware Calcium Resonium® may cause GI disturbance while high doses of salbutamol can cause fine tremor and malignant tachycardia. In all instances, drugs known to cause hyperkalaemia should be discontinued, e.g. ARBs, β-blockers, **spironolactone**, potassium sparing diuretics, potassium supplements, **trimethoprim**. Hyperkalaemia, in AKI, is commonly due to a combination of these drugs. When the patient is discharged, it should be made clear in the discharge summary, which drugs have been stopped and why. The GP may want to reintroduce them (perhaps at lower dosage) when the patient is stable.

Anuric patients will not clear circulating K^+, and will require specialist intervention and renal replacement therapy.

Metabolic acidosis

In severe AKI, metabolic acidosis is common, requiring urgent correction with a **sodium bicarbonate** infusion. In some instances, patients may require dialysis, particularly those who are fluid overloaded or have uraemia.

Drug classes used in management

Fluids

Fluid replacement in the form of crystalloids, colloids, and blood can minimize hypovolaemic causes of AKI and reduce the risk of further AKI in those at risk groups exposed to nephrotoxins. Examples include crystalloids—sodium chloride 0.9%, sodium lactate solution (Hartmann's); colloids—albumins, gelatins, starches.

Mechanism of action

The body is composed of approximately 60% water by weight, with almost two-thirds of this being intracellular. Around 20% of the extracellular fluid, some 3.5 L in a 70 kg individual, is made up of plasma and is regulated by hydrostatic pressure due to the proteins and cells contained within it. This oncotic and osmotic pressure dictates, in conjunction with fluid intake and output, where water and electrolytes are distributed around the body (i.e. fluid shifts).

Fluid replacement is generally achieved with volume expanders, which have the property of delivering volume to the circulatory system. There are two principal varieties of volume expanders—crystalloids and colloids.

Crystalloids are aqueous solutions composed by mineral salts or other water-soluble molecules, with **sodium chloride 0.9%** (often referred to as 'normal saline') being the most commonly used.

Colloids, such as starches, **Gelofusine®**, or **albumin**, contain larger insoluble molecules that tend to stay in the intravascular circulatory space, and should theoretically increase the intravascular volume. However, since colloids are not linked to better survival and are considerably more expensive than crystalloids, their use is difficult to justify.

Prescribing

To date, the exact type of fluid to be used in AKI remains controversial, as it is unclear which is best to encourage end-organ renal function. As in fluid resuscitation, crystalloids are a good starting point to correct water and electrolyte deficiencies in hypovolaemia and AKI, although research indicates hyperchloraemia is a risk from normal saline infusions and may, itself, affect renal function. In severe hypovolaemia, however, colloids and blood do have their place, and may be more beneficial in maintaining organ microcirculation in AKI. Patients will need to be monitored, as hyperoncotic renal failure may occur if insufficient crystalloid is not maintained. As such, balanced salt solutions or Hartmann's may be best used in those at risk of AKI, but may run the theoretical risk of contributing to hyperkalaemia.

Loop diuretics

Loop diuretics act by blocking the luminal Na^+–K^+–$2Cl^-$ transporter in the thick ascending limb of the loop of Henle, inhibiting Na^+ and Cl^- reabsorption. For example, bumetanide, furosemide, and torasemide.

Mechanism of action

See Topic 2.6, 'Heart failure'.

Prescribing

Loop diuretics have historically been used at high doses to treat AKI, in particular **furosemide** at doses greater than 1 g/day. More recently, however, evidence suggests that these doses are associated with high levels of toxicity, in particular ototoxicity, and evidence of efficacy is lacking. Usage should therefore be reserved for managing fluid overload and doses titrated to achieve the desired effect. They may be useful, in higher than normal doses, for a short period to treat pulmonary oedema (and reduce serum K^+) until a definitive decision on dialysis can be made. They do not reduce the need for dialysis or mortality. For more information see Topic 2.6, 'Heart failure'.

Vasopressors

Potent systemic vasopressor agents, like noradrenaline or high dose dopamine, can be employed to restore arterial pressure in order to sustain organ perfusion in the kidney. However, noradrenaline provokes vasoconstriction in various vascular beds, and can reduce renal and visceral blood flow, a concern that has stopped a more extended use. For example, noradrenaline, vasopressin, and terlipressin

Mechanism of action

In all regional circulations, including renal, the blood flow is autoregulated to maintain BP above the autoregulatory threshold, thus maintaining organ blood flow. A decrease in BP below this threshold produces an almost linear decrease in organ blood flow, leading to organ ischaemia and failure. Restoration of BP is therefore logical for renal protection. The main concern with the use of noradrenaline comes from the observation that it can induce AKI when infused into the renal artery. However, intensive renal vasoconstriction has only been seen to occur with direct infusion into the renal artery and not via clinically relevant systemic routes. Based on current evidence, in hypotensive vasodilated patients with AKI, the restoration of BP towards auto-regulatory values should be attempted with noradrenaline, and continued until vasodilation disappears. In most hospitals, this can only be done in a critical care setting (e.g. GCC, HDU, CCU etc.). In other words, in a patient with AKI with low BP, who you think is (or was) hypovolaemic, and whose BP is not coming up after 2 hours of rehydration (and other measures), you need a senior review, and probable transfer to a critical care setting.

Noradrenaline is very effective in augmenting arterial BP, inducing vasoconstriction by increasing vascular tension of the vascular smooth muscle via α-adrenergic receptor stimulation (see Table 5.4).

Vasopressin is an antidiuretic hormone secreted from the posterior pituitary that promotes peripheral vascular resistance by acting on V1a receptor, increasing arterial BP. The V1a is a G protein receptor that couples to GTP binding proteins and activates phospholipase C activity, increasing IP_3 levels and cytosolic Ca^{2+} concentrations. **Terlipressin** is an analogue of vasopressin used as vasoactive drug mainly in the management of low BP.

Prescribing

Noradrenaline is the only vasopressor licensed to restore BP in severe hypotension. It is administered as an IV infusion via a central venous catheter, due to the risk of necrosis with extravasation. Doses are based on weight, with the rate carefully titrated to achieve an optimal mean arterial pressure (MAP). **Terlipressin** and **vasopressin**, although not licensed for this indication, have also been used in the management of shock, with some evidence to suggest vasopressin is effective in patients refractory to treatment with noradrenaline.

Unwanted effects

Patients receiving vasopressors require careful, regular haemodynamic monitoring to prevent serious complications such as profound hypertension, plasma volume depletion, and peripheral vasoconstriction, which in severe cases, can lead to a reduced cardiac output or peripheral ischaemia. Treatment should be given in combination with appropriate fluids to maintain plasma volume and prevent rebound hypotension when the vasopressor is discontinued.

Table 5.4 Summary of action of vasoactive compounds useful in AKI. Dopamine's haemodynamic effects are highly dose dependent

Drug	Mean arterial pressure	Cardiac output	Systemic vascular resistance	Receptors	Mechanism
Noradrenaline	⇧	⇧	⇧	α1, β1	Vasoconstriction and increased cardiac contractility
Dobutamine	⇔	⇧	⇩	β1, mild β2	Increases cardiac contractility with mild vasodilation
Adrenaline	⇧	⇧	⇧	α1, β1, β2	Increases cardiac contractility, causes peripheral vasoconstriction and smooth muscle relaxation
Vasopressin	⇧	⇩	⇧	V1, V2, V3	Vasoconstriction of vascular smooth muscle

Other unwanted effects include headaches, anxiety, dyspnoea, and local skin reactions, as vasopressors are vesicant.

Calcium salts

> IV calcium salts antagonize the effects of hyperkalaemia in inducing arrhythmias. For example, calcium chloride and calcium gluconate.

Mechanism of action

Calcium salts act to reduce the excitability of myocardial cells by decreasing the depolarization effects of raised intracellular K^+ levels, which may otherwise lead to altered membrane excitability and arrhythmias. There is a tendency for tachyarrhythmias to occur if the serum K^+ is >6.5 μmol/L, and brady arrhythmias, if K^+ is <2.5 μmol/L. However, this distinction is not a clear one, i.e. any serious arrhythmias can occur with either state. Calcium salts, however, do not affect serum levels of K^+.

Prescribing

Calcium salts (gluconate or chloride) are administered slowly IV (over 5–10 minutes) in patients with severe hyperkalaemia or in those who are symptomatic. The onset of action is 3 minutes, so patients who remain symptomatic may receive a further dose after 5–10 minutes.

Insulin

> Insulin promotes the intracellular uptake of K^+ by regulating the Na^+/K^+ ATPase pump, thus correcting hyperkalaemia.

Mechanism of action

The activity of kidney tubule Na^+/K^+ ATPase is under tight multi-hormonal control, which can regulate its surface expression or modify the function of single-pump units. **Insulin** stimulates the Na^+/K^+ ATP pump by regulating its phosphorylation on the α-subunit, promoting the intracellular uptake of K^+. In order to prevent hypoglycaemia it is given in combination with glucose.

Prescribing

In the management of hyperkalaemia, **insulin** can be administered as a bolus or continuous IV infusion (see local guidelines) made up in glucose. The effects can occur within 10 minutes of starting treatment, peaking within the hour and lasting for 4–6 hours. Patients will need to have their blood glucose levels monitored throughout treatment to prevent hypoglycaemia. For more information on insulin see Topic 4.5, 'Diabetes mellitus'.

Salbutamol

> The short acting β₂-adrenoceptor agonist salbutamol is used in hyperkalaemia due to its ability to increase the intracellular uptake of K^+.

Mechanism of action

Salbutamol acts by binding to β₂-adrenoceptors in the liver and muscle, activating the conversion of ATP to AMP. This, in turn, stimulates the ATP Na^+/K^+ pump, again promoting the intracellular uptake of K^+.

Prescribing

Salbutamol may be a useful add-on in the management of severe hyperkalaemia where **insulin** treatment is inadequate. Treatment can be administered IV or nebulized, although the former has a more profound effect and faster onset of action. For more information on salbutamol see Topic 3.1, 'Asthma'.

Salbutamol is commonly used in initial medical therapy (e.g. in ED), but given the risks of malignant tachycardia and fine tremor, it tends to be avoided by many nephrologists, in particular where there is access to RRT to ameliorate hyperkalaemia. It may be useful in a hospital environment where dialysis is not available, to 'buy you time' to transfer the patient to a renal centre.

Polystyrene sulfonate resins

> Polystyrene polymers with a sulfonate functional group are cross-linked to form a resin and as ion exchange K^+ binding complexes can be used for the treatment of abnormally high K^+ levels (hyperkalaemia).

Mechanism of action

The polystyrene sulfonates are indigestible resins that bind to excess K^+ forming a complex that is excreted with the stools, thus preventing systemic absorption. Ion exchange resin function depends on the ion selectivity, contact time with the solution, relative concentration of the ions, and the resin capacity.

Prescribing

The polystyrene sulfonate resins (calcium and sodium) can be used in the treatment of mild to moderate hyperkalaemia, although of little value in acute severe hyperkalaemia. There is little to choose between them, both administered as powders orally QDS, made up with small amounts of water or syrup to improve palatability. Doses should not be prepared in fruit juice due to the high potassium content. The powder can also be administered rectally as an enema that is retained for 9 hours before being removed by irrigation.

Unwanted effects

GI effects are common with the polystyrene sulfonate resins, especially nausea, gastric irritation, faecal impaction, constipation, and diarrhoea. Treatment is therefore contraindicated in obstruction or in patients at high risk of developing it, e.g. metastatic carcinoma. Treatment may also lead to hypomagnesaemia, and hypercalcaemia or hypernatraemia, depending on the salt used. Concurrent use with sorbitol should be avoided as this can lead to intestinal necrosis.

Further reading

Briguori C, Visconti G, Focaccio A, et al. (2011). Renal insufficiency after contrast media administration trial II (REMEDIAL II): RenalGuard system in high-risk patients for contrast-induced acute kidney injury. *Circulation* 124, 1260–9.

Koshimizu T, Nakamura K, Egashira N, et al. (2012) Vasopressin V1a and V1b receptors: from molecules to physiological systems. *Physiological Review* 92, 1813–64.

Kyung Jo S, Rosner MH, Okusa MD (2007) Pharmacological treatment of acute kidney injury: why drugs haven't worked and what is on the horizon. *Clinical Journal of the American Society for Nephrology* 2, 356–65.

Rottembourg J, Kpade F, Dansaert A (2010) Hyperkalemia and ion exchange resins—limitations. *Dialysis and Transplantation*, 39(6), 260–3.

Shankar S, Brater DC (2002) Loop diuretics: from the Na-K-2Cl transporter to clinical use. *American Journal of Physiology* 284(1), F11–21.

Guidelines

KDIGO (2012) Clinical Practice Guideline for Acute Kidney Injury. *Kidney International* (Suppl. 2(1)). https://kdigo.org/wp-content/uploads/2016/10/KDIGO-2012-AKI-Guideline-English.pdf [accessed 10 April 2019].

NICE (2013) Acute kidney injury; prevention, detection and management of acute kidney injury up to the point of renal replacement therapy. NICE guideline CG169. https://www.nice.org.uk/guidance/cg169?unlid=9291282542016214516o [accessed 29 March 2019].

UK Renal Association (2011) Clinical practice guidelines: acute kidney injury, 5th edn. https://renal.org/wp-content/uploads/2017/06/acute-kidney-injury-5th-edition9e74a231181561659443ff000014d4d8-1.pdf [accessed 10 April 2019].

5.3 Disorders of micturition

Urinary incontinence is the complaint of any involuntary leakage of urine. Around 3.5 million people are affected in the UK and it is almost twice as common in females. Urinary incontinence can be broadly classified into two types:

- *Urge incontinence*: occurs when there is sudden, strong desire to void before, or during, involuntary leakage of urine. This can be due to detrusor (bladder wall smooth muscle) overactivity or low bladder compliance.

- *Stress incontinence*: where involuntary urinary leakage occurs as a result of exertion, sneezing or coughing. This is due to weakness of the pelvic floor or urethral sphincter that normally supports the bladder and regulates the release of urine. Risk factors are associated with physicomechanical (e.g. being female, childbirth) or neurological changes that disrupt the complex synergy responsible for continence (e.g. spinal cord injury and diabetes).

Urinary retention is the failure to empty the bladder, presenting as difficulty voiding. This is often preceded by symptoms of hesitancy (difficulty in starting urination), poor stream, with increased frequency and urgency of urination. It occurs more commonly in men, and is most often caused by bladder outlet obstruction secondary to benign BPH. In fewer cases, urinary retention is as a result of neurological disease affecting the bladder or urethral sphincter (e.g. multiple sclerosis, cauda equina, spinal cord trauma).

Pathophysiology

The control of urinary continence results from a balance of factors under the control of both the central and peripheral nervous systems. Maintenance of continence relies on the bladder (detrusor muscle) being able to maintain a low pressure as bladder volume increases on filling, and a dynamic resting urethral sphincter tone that contains urine within the bladder. There are two normal functional states for the bladder—a storage phase (filling) and an emptying phase (voiding) (see Table 5.5).

Understanding the nervous anatomy is pertinent to bladder control, as micturition is coordinated by the nervous system and involves many different pathways. The peripheral nervous system has sensory (afferent) inputs and motor (efferent) outputs, each of which may be somatic (under conscious control) or autonomic (e.g. visceral or endocrine). Autonomic pathways may be sympathetic (cranio-sacral) or parasympathetic (thoracolumbar) as defined by their emergence from the spinal cord. Parietal lobes and the thalamus receive and coordinate detrusor afferent stimuli, with frontal lobes and basal ganglia providing signals to inhibit voiding. The pontine micturition centre integrates these inputs into socially appropriate voiding, with coordinated urethral relaxation and detrusor contraction until the bladder is empty.

At low bladder volumes, and during the storage phase, inhibition of sacral parasympathetic preganglionic neurons occurs as the main mechanism of bladder relaxation. Bladder filling activates the sensory afferent fibres of the bladder wall stretch receptors, which stimulate the sympathetic (hypogastric nerve) pathway so that bladder neck and internal urethral sphincter muscle contraction occurs via α1-adrenoceptors. This closure of the bladder outlet occurs with concomitant bladder wall relaxation via inhibition of the detrusor parasympathetic neurones. Activation of detrusor sympathetic β3-adrenoceptors during the storage phase also contributes to bladder wall relaxation. Efferent somatic activity (pudendal nerve) maintains the tone of the striated muscle of the external urethral sphincter during bladder filling, thereby augmenting continence.

Normal voiding is a voluntary event initiated in the cerebral cortex leading to inhibition of both sympathetic neurones to the bladder wall and somatic efferents to the external urethral sphincter, so that parasympathetic outflow predominates to allow bladder wall contraction. Bladder contraction is mediated via muscarinic receptors (mainly M3), and urethral smooth muscle relaxation via nitric oxide (NO), so as to overcome the parasympathetic

Table 5.5 Summary of the processes involved with bladder filling and voiding

Bladder filling (storage phase)	Bladder emptying (voiding phase)
Contraction of the (striated) external urethral sphincter (somatic innervation)	Relaxation of the (striated) external urethral sphincter (somatic innervation)
Contraction of (smooth muscle) internal urethral sphincter (sympathetic innervation)	Relaxation of the (smooth muscle) internal urethral sphincter and opening of the bladder neck (sympathetic innervation)
Inhibition of detrusor activity (sympathetic innervation)	Detrusor contraction (parasympathetic innervation)

cholinergic contractile activity of ACh to the bladder neck and urethral smooth muscle, which normally maintains continence during bladder filling.

Urinary incontinence

Urge incontinence is associated with involuntary detrusor overactivity during the filling phase and can be due to an underlying neurological cause, such as multiple sclerosis or Parkinson's disease, but can be idiopathic where there is no defined cause. The basis is usually multifactorial and involves intrinsic over-activity between muscle cells, disruption of neural control, and abnormal or exaggerated peripheral autonomic activity within the myovesical plexus.

Within the smooth muscle of the bladder wall, ACh, and muscarinic M3 receptors control contraction via a G protein–mediated process. This causes Ca^{2+} release from the sarcoplasmic reticulum, which binds calmodulin to activate myosin-light chain kinase. Hence, during filling, muscarinic antagonists (e.g. **oxybutynin**) are of benefit in maintaining continence, while centrally acting compounds like **desmopressin** (see 'Desmopressin' in 'Drug classes used in management') have the ability to reduce urinary volume. The potency of ACh innervation to the detrusor can also be ameliorated by **botulinum toxin**, which acts by inhibiting ACh release from presynaptic cholinergic nerve terminals; it is particularly useful in neurogenic (NDO) or idiopathic detrusor overactivity (IDO) and detrusor-sphincter dyssynergia (where there is an over-active external urethral sphincter that does not relax during voiding due to underlying neurological disease).

Stress incontinence results from a failure of the sphincter mechanisms to maintain urethral closure during bladder filling. Any leak is typically due to impaired pelvic support (from pelvic floor weakness) or weakness of the urethral sphincters (due to previous surgery such as prostatectomy or intrinsic sphincter deficiency). Two theories of stress incontinence pathogenesis may involve laxity of the anterior vaginal wall and pubo-urethral ligaments, causing bladder neck hyper-mobility, or failure of support of urethra by the endopelvic fascia and vaginal wall. Somatic motor neurons in the sacral spinal cord (Onuf nucleus) control urethral function and are densely populated with noradrenergic (NA) and serotonergic (5-HT) presynaptic terminals, so up-regulation of this tone can potentially maintain continence. **Duloxetine** is a selective NA/5-HT uptake blocker so can maintain normal physiological innervation, but augment the resting tone and, hence, be of benefit in stress incontinence.

Urinary retention

Outlet obstruction is the second most common cause of urinary incontinence in older men; most obstructed men, however, are not incontinent. Causes include BPH, prostate cancer and urethral stricture. Bladder outlet obstruction as a result of BPH has both a static component due to the obstructing size of the enlarged prostate, as well as a dynamic component due to α1-adrenoceptor mediated prostatic smooth muscle contraction. Those with lower urinary tract symptoms (e.g. reduced flow, urgency, post-micturition dribble) may benefit from pharmacological intervention in the form of α1-adrenoceptor blockers (e.g. **doxazosin**), which can reduce the resting tone of prostate smooth muscle cells. Alternatively, 5α-reductase inhibitors (e.g. **finasteride**) can induce apoptosis of prostate epithelial cells, thereby reducing prostate bulk by 25% at 12 months treatment. Combination of these two approaches may also be of clinical benefit.

For a full summary of the relevant pathways and drug targets, see Figure 5.5.

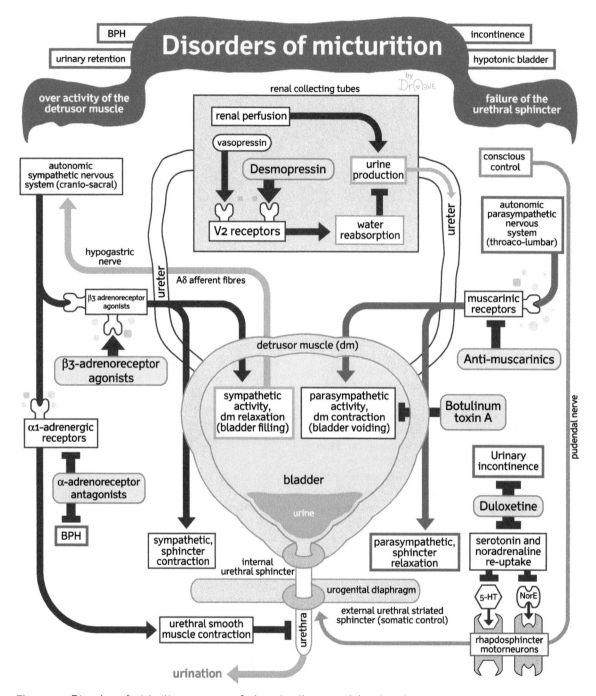

Figure 5.5 Disorders of micturition: summary of relevant pathways and drug targets.

Management

Urinary incontinence

On presentation, a clinical history is carried out to determine the type of incontinence (stress, urge, or a mixture of both) and identify any triggers or risk factors, such as childbirth, medication, weight, or any underlying neurological or gynaecological pathologies. Investigations should also eliminate the possibility of UTI.

In the absence of any underlying pathology, conservative management forms the mainstay of treatment, aimed at addressing potential precipitating factors (weight, caffeine, fluid restriction, smoking, and constipation) and offer bladder training (where the goal is to increase the amount of time between needing to urinate and the amount of volume the bladder can hold). With stress or mixed incontinence, strengthening the pelvic floor muscle either through physical training or electrical stimulations may be beneficial; whereas with urge or mixed incontinence behavioural training is preferred.

Where these measures fail, pharmacological therapy is recommended, primarily with antimuscarinics. Patients should be advised prior to initiation that side effects are common. However, this can be minimized by starting with low doses and titrating slowly to establish the lowest effective dose. **Oxybutynin** immediate release should be avoided in frail and older women (as it may cause acute confusional states in the elderly and contribute to falls). Second-line options include **desmopressin** (off-licence) for nocturia or **duloxetine** in patients unsuitable for surgery. More recently, the β3-adrenoreceptor agonist, **mirabegron** has been approved by NICE and the European Association of Urology to improve sympathetically mediated detrusor relaxation and, thereby, increases bladder capacity in over-active bladder syndrome.

In patients with detrusor overactivity, injections of **botulinum toxin A** may be administered directly into the detrusor muscle, but can lead to side effects of urinary retention and UTI.

In some instances, patients may require referral for surgical management, such as those who are intolerant of, or have failed to respond to pharmacological or conservative therapy. Surgical techniques aim to improve the strength of the bladder outlet and urethral sphincter, and include synthetic mid-urethral tape, intramural bulking, and the use of an artificial urinary sphincter. In patients unwilling or unable to have treatment, pads or catheterization provide alternative options.

Urinary retention

Investigations to identify common causes of urinary retention include urinalysis, prostate examination, and a complete drug history to identify any likely causative drugs (see Table 5.6), which will need to be discontinued.

Acute management of retention requires catheterization, followed by management of the underlying cause, i.e. treatment of infection/constipation or referral for management of chronic underlying obstruction of neurogenic cause.

In most cases, however, urinary retention occurs secondary to BPH, thus occurring in older men. In these patients, treatment with α1-adrenoceptor blockers is recommended before a trial without catheter (TWOC) to increase the success rate of voiding without the catheter.

Drug classes used in management

Antimuscarinics

> Antimuscarinic drugs are considered to work in the syndrome of overactive bladder by blocking muscarinic receptors on the detrusor muscle, which are stimulated by cholinergic parasympathetic nerves. Examples include oxybutynin, tolterodine, darifenacin, festerodine, propiverine, solifenacin, trospium, and flavoxate.

Mechanism of action

In the simplest interpretation, blocking detrusor muscle activity is understood to decrease the contraction capacity of the bladder. However, antimuscarinic

Table 5.6 Drugs known to cause urinary retention

Class	Drugs
Antimuscarinics	Oxybutynin, tolterodine, solifenacin, darifenacin, trospium
Antihistamines	Chlorphenamine, cetirizine
Tricyclic antidepressants	Amitriptyline, imipramine

action of decreasing urge and increasing capacity is mainly achieved during the storage phase, when there is normally no activity in parasympathetic nerves. It is thus believed that the mechanism behind the effect of antimuscarinic drugs is more complex than initially anticipated.

There are five subtypes of muscarinic receptors coupled to various signal transduction systems. M_1, M_3, and M_5 couple mainly to G_q proteins and activate phospho-inositide hydrolysis and Ca^{2+} mobilization. M_2 and M_4 receptors couple to G_i protein, resulting in the inhibition of adenylyl cyclase activity. The M_2 and M_3 receptor subtypes are the ones found in the human detrusor muscle, and while M_2 predominates, the M_3 receptors are the ones mainly responsible for normal micturition contraction. The M_2 receptors may oppose the detrusor relaxation mediated by β-adrenoceptors.

Muscarinic receptors are also found on presynaptic nerve terminals where they regulate neurotransmitter release, both in inhibitory (M_4) or excitatory (M_1) fashion. There is some indirect clinical evidence to suggest that the release of acetylcholine during bladder filling and storage phase, both from neuronal and non-neuronal sources (the urothelium) can, directly or indirectly, excite afferent nerves in the sub-urothelium and within the detrusor muscle, thus making it a mechanistic target for antimuscarinic drugs.

Antimuscarinic drugs, which are defined by the purity of their anti-muscarinic effects, include **propantheline** and **trospium**, which have no subtype selectivity, and **tolterodine**, which although it has no subtype selectivity, is claimed to have functional selectivity for the bladder over the salivary gland. Other antimuscarinic drugs, such as **oxybutynin** and **propiverine**, are defined as having 'mixed' actions, due to the fact that in addition to their pronounced antimuscarinic effect, they can have a 'poorly' defined action on bladder muscle, which might involve blockade of voltage-gated Ca^{2+} channels.

Prescribing

As well as showing variations in their purity and selectivity, the antimuscarinics available to treat urinary urgency and incontinence vary in their route of administration and tolerability. **Oxybutynin**, one of the more widely used antimuscarinics, is standardly administered orally either BD or TDS, although the use of an OD slow-release preparation or patch may be better tolerated and promote compliance. Oral alternatives to oxybutynin include

tolterodine, **festerodine**, **propiverine**, and **trospium**, of which the latter is less likely to demonstrate neurological toxicity, being less lipophilic.

Solifenacin and **darifenacin**, more selective antimuscarinics, are administered orally OD. Due to their selectivity, they tend to be better tolerated and demonstrate good efficacy compared with the older antimuscarinics. NICE advocates the use of **darifenacin** as a first line in women with overactive bladder syndrome (OAB), based on cost.

Unwanted effects

Side effects to antimuscarinics are common and constitute the main limitation to their use. They include dry mouth, constipation, blurred vision, drowsiness, and confusion. Elderly patients are particularly susceptible to toxicity and the risk of anticholinergic burden (see 'Prescribing warning: anticholinergic burden'). Use should be avoided in patients with glaucoma, myasthenia gravis, or urinary or intestinal obstruction. Antimuscarinics are also associated with increased cardiovascular risk and mortality, particularly in combination and in patients with underlying co-morbidities.

Patients travelling to hot climates should be advised that the use of antimuscarinics can reduce their ability to sweat thus leading to overheating or fainting.

PRESCRIBING WARNING

Anticholinergic burden (ACB)
- Antimuscarinics act on receptors on the brain to affect cognition.
- Risks are augmented with increasing anticholinergic burden, i.e. the use of multiple drugs with anticholinergic properties, and with increasing age.
- Drugs that readily cross the blood–brain barrier are more likely to cause neurological effects.

Drug interactions

Drugs with antimuscarinic properties that have the potential to increase ACB include antihistamines or tricyclic antidepressants. There is also an increased risk of ventricular arrhythmias when antimuscarinics are used concurrently with anti-arrhythmics, such as **flecainide**, **amiodarone**, or **sotalol**.

Desmopressin

> Desmopressin is a synthetic structural analogue of the endogenous antidiuretic hormone vasopressin, which regulates extracellular fluid volume in the body. It binds to V2 receptors in the renal collecting tubes, augmenting water reabsorption.

Mechanism of action

Vasopressin is produced by the hypothalamus and stored in the posterior pituitary gland. In physiological conditions, its secretion is determined by the effective osmotic pressure of plasma, mediated by specialized osmoreceptor cells in the hypothalamus. When vasopressin activates the V2 receptors, preformed water channels increase the permeability of the apical membrane of cells in the distal nephron tubules, allowing reabsorption of water without solute. By increasing osmotic reabsorption of water in the distal and collecting tubes of the kidney, vasopressin increases urine osmolality, and decreases urine volume.

Desmopressin is a nonapeptide, more potent, stable, and longer-acting than vasopressin. Unlike vasopressin, it is V2-receptor specific so can reduce urine production without inducing pressor activity.

Prescribing

Desmopressin helps reduce symptoms of nocturia in patients (particularly women) with OAB. Following oral administration much of the dose is destroyed in the stomach, resulting in poor oral bioavailability; thus oral doses are 10 times greater than those required for intranasal administration, where it is well absorbed through the oral mucosa. Doses slightly smaller than oral doses may be administered sublingually. Desmopressin is licensed in a tablet formulation for use in primary nocturia to be taken at night, and may also be administered intranasally off-label.

Unwanted effects

Due to its anti-diuretic properties, treatment is contraindicated in patients with underlying medical conditions managed with diuretics, such as heart failure; or with disturbed fluid balance such as with profound diarrhoea and vomiting. Steps should be taken to reduce the risk of water intoxication by avoiding excess fluid consumption 1 hour before the dose and 8 hours after.

While on treatment, patients commonly complain of headaches and nausea, which may be indicative of water intoxication or hyponatraemia, and in severe cases can lead to convulsions. With larger doses administered IV, **desmopressin** can have a profound vasodilator effect causing a drop in BP, tachycardia, and flushing. In patients with CKD, the diuretic effects of desmopressin are reduced and dose alterations may be necessary.

Duloxetine

> Duloxetine is a potent and selective inhibitor of serotonin and noradrenaline re-uptake. Its efficacy is due to an increase in the synaptic levels of both of these neurotransmitters that control rhabdosphincter motorneurons.

Mechanism of action

Serotonin and noradrenaline are important monoamine neurotransmitters distributed throughout the peripheral and central nervous system, and responsible for the coordination of a variety of somatic and visceral responses. Both the serotoninergic and noradrenergic terminals that project from the brain stem, are dense in spinal areas associated with lower urinary tract functioning.

The normal micturition cycle of alternating urinary storage and voiding phases, is controlled by the communication between the bladder reservoir and bladder outlet structures in the lower urinary tract. These are controlled by a complex interchange between the CNS, and the afferent sensory and efferent somatic and autonomic branches of the peripheral nervous system. Glutamate is the primary excitatory neurotransmitter for the spinal somatic storage reflex, activating somatic pudendal motor neurons to contract the striated rhabdosphincter muscle fibres as part of the external urethral sphincter. The serotoninergic and noradrenergic neurons from the brain stem, are two important modulatory systems that control motor neurons responsiveness to glutamate. Increases in noradrenergic and sertotoninergic response has been shown to inhibit detrusor contractility and increase capacity.

Prescribing

Duloxetine is the only SNRI licensed for use in moderate to severe stress urinary incontinence (SUI) in women. Due to its unfavourable side effect profile however, it is reserved for use second-line in women unsuitable for surgery. In SUI it is administered orally BD, at doses considerably lower than those used in depression.

Unwanted effects

Side effects to **duloxetine** are common and despite using lower doses in SUI, patients are still likely to complain of GI effects, headache, and fatigue. Treatment is contraindicated in severe renal and hepatic impairment. For more details see Topic 10.2, 'Depression'.

β3-adrenoceptor agonists

β$_3$ adrenoceptor agonists contribute to the relaxation of the detrusor smooth muscle and are used for the treatment of overactive bladder, as they allow larger bladder capacity. For example, mirabegron.

Mechanism of action

Although first identified in adipose tissue, the β$_3$-adrenoceptor can also be found in smooth muscle tissue, particularly in the GI tract and urinary bladder. In humans, the β$_3$-adrenoceptor is the predominant subtype in sympathetically mediated detrusor muscle relaxation. Activation of the receptor couples, via G proteins, to adenylyl cyclase, leading to an increase in cAMP and subsequent activation of protein kinase A (PKA). The PKA-dependent phosphorylation of myosin light chain kinase supresses Ca^{2+}-calmodulin-dependent interaction of myosin with actin. The increase in cAMP also results in the decrease of cytoplasmic Ca^{2+} concentrations, which contributes to the β$_3$-adrenoceptor-mediated relaxation of smooth muscle. It has been suggested that cAMP-independent pathways also exist, involving direct interaction of G proteins with K$^+$ channels. **Mirabegron** is a potent and selective agonist of β$_3$-adrenoceptor, with a recommended daily dose of 50 mg. At this dose, the effect on other β-adrenoceptors are rare, but can cause tachycardia as a side effect and is contraindicated in those with severe uncontrolled hypertension.

Prescribing

Mirabegron is the first β$_3$-adrenoceptor agonist to be launched for the treatment of urinary frequency and urgency in over-active bladder. It has been approved by NICE in patients failing treatment with antimuscarinics.

Unwanted effects

Although the incidence of adverse effects to **mirabegron** is comparable with antimuscarinics, the nature of these adverse effects differs, notably with a reduced incidence of dry mouth. The most frequently reported side effects to treatment include UTIs and tachycardia. Less commonly, patients may present with atrial fibrillation, dyspepsia, or hypersensitivity reactions, e.g. rashes.

Mirabegron is metabolized through multiple pathways including the cytochrome P450 enzyme system, before being excreted through the kidneys. Consequently, in severe renal and hepatic impairment, a 50% dose reduction is recommended or treatment avoided altogether if patients also take enzyme-inhibiting drugs. Dose reductions are also recommended in mild to moderate renal or hepatic impairment in patents on concurrent enzyme inhibitors (see 'Drug interactions').

Drug interactions

Although a substrate for multiple enzyme pathways, including CYP3A4 and, to a lesser extent, CYP2D6, altered clearance of **mirabegron** is only likely to reach any significance in combination with potent CYP 3A4 inhibitors, e.g. **ketoconazole**, **itraconazole**, where there is co-existing renal or hepatic impairment. Mirabegron is itself a moderate inhibitor of CYP 2D6 and should be used cautiously in combination with drugs that have a narrow therapeutic index metabolized through the same pathway, e.g. type 1c anti-arrhythmics (**flecainide**, **propafenone**) and tricyclic antidepressants (**imipramine**, **desipramine**).

Botulinum toxin A

Botulinum toxin A is a presynaptic neuromuscular blocking agent that induces selective and reversible muscle weakness when injected intramuscularly. It is mainly used to treat muscular hypercontraction.

Mechanism of action

The botulinum toxin is produced by the bacteria *Clostridium botulinum*, and consists of a heavy (H) and light (L) chain bound together by heat labile disulphide bonds. The H chain is bound to the nerve terminals at the neuromuscular junction, and the L chain is internalized by endocytosis and acts as the neurotoxic component. Neither chain can exert neurotoxicity independently. After being internalized, the L chain compromises the intracellular protein SNAP-25, producing a lesion in the secretory pathway, without affecting synthesis or storage of neurotransmitters. Different types of botulinum toxin cleave different parts of the protein complex, which is necessary for the docking of ACh vesicles and subsequent neurotransmitter release. This results in a temporary chemodenervation, and the loss or reduction of neuronal activity at the target organ. The recovery of the denervation after 3–6 months is due to a turnover of presynaptic molecules and the growth of new nerve sproutings leading to the formation of a new functional synapse.

The injection of **botulinum toxin A** transurethrally or transperineally, effectively treats detrusor-sphincter dyssynergia. This leads to a decrease in external urethral sphincter pressure, voiding pressure and post-void residual volume. The effects lasts between 2 and 9 months, depending on the number of injections.

Prescribing

The different brands of **botulinum toxin A** are produced through different techniques, so that dosing units between brands are not equivalent and doses non-interchangeable. Currently Botox® is the only brand licensed for injection into the detrusor muscle in the treatment of over-active bladder or neurogenic detrusor activity, when patients fail treatment with antimuscarinics. Treatment is administered on a day-case basis, at a dose of 200 units every 6 months or sooner if the effects have worn off. Some patients may opt for a lower, less effective dose of 100 units to reduce the risk of catheterization.

Unwanted effects

Short-term side effects of **botulinum toxin A** for this indication, include increased risk of UTIs and urinary retention requiring the patient to perform intermittent self-catheterization; however, less is known of the long-term effects on bladder function beyond two doses. In general, extensive use leads to an exaggerated muscle weakness, toxin spread to other parts of the body and production of neutralizing antibodies; the risk of muscle weakness is increased in patients with underlying neurological conditions.

α1-adrenoceptor antagonists

α_1-adrenoceptor antagonist block the α_1-adrenoceptors present in the urethra and bladder smooth detrusor muscle tissue, facilitating urine flow and decreasing lower urinary tract symptoms. Examples include alfuzosin, doxazosin, indoramin, prazosin, tamsulosin, and terazosin.

Mechanism of action

Adrenoceptors can be divided into α and β categories, with several subtypes distinguished by their pharmacology, structure, and activation of second messenger systems. α_1-adrenoceptors exist in various organs and tissues, but in terms of the urinary tract system, their expression in the smooth muscle of the prostate, urethra, spinal cord, and bladder is most relevant. These receptors generally activate the Gq type of G proteins leading to the stimulation of inositol phosphate hydrolysis. Molecular and contraction studies demonstrate the predominance of α_{1a}-adrenoceptor subtype in the prostate stroma, with blockade resulting in relaxation of prostate smooth muscle. The bladder neck and intraprostatic urethra also contain α_{1a}-adrenoceptors, while bladder smooth muscle expresses mainly α_{1d}-adrenoceptors. It is suggested that α_{1a}-adrenoceptor selective antagonists relieve obstructive outflow symptoms and improve flow through relaxation of prostate smooth muscle, which accounts for approximately 40% of the area density of the hyperplastic prostate in BPH, while α_{1d}-adrenoceptor specific antagonists act on the bladder and/or spinal cord to relieve bladder symptoms.

Terazosin, **doxazosin**, and **alfuzosin** are non-subtype selective and block all three subtypes of α_1-adrenoceptor. In contrast, **tamsulosin** is a subtype-selective antagonist, with 10 times greater affinity for α_{1d} over α_{1b}. All α_1-adrenoceptor antagonists have similar efficacy in terms of symptom relief, but differ in their side effect profile.

Prescribing

Although all α_1-adrenoceptor antagonists are licensed for use in BPH and of comparable efficacy; **tamsulosin** is the most widely prescribed due to its favourable dosing regimen and reduced hypotensive effects, particularly in the elderly, due to its greater selectivity. It is only available as a slow release preparation, enabling OD dosing and optimizing tolerance; this negates the need for gradual dose titrations on initiation compared with other drugs in the class. As **tamsulosin** capsules are slow release, they should be swallowed whole and ideally taken at the same time of day.

Unwanted effects

Hypotension, drowsiness, dizziness, and fainting are the most common side effects reported with **tamsulosin** treatment, which may affect ability to drive and patients should be made aware of this. Patients should also be informed of the side effect of retrograde ejaculation, where semen is redirected into the bladder rather than down the urethra during ejaculation. This is due to failure of closure of the bladder neck and internal urethral sphincter as a result of taking tamsulosin.

For more details see Topic 2.1, 'Hypertension'.

Further reading

Andersson A, Arner A (2004) Urinary bladder contraction and relaxation: physiology and pathophysiology. *Physiological Review* 84, 935–86.

Andersson K-E (2004) Antimuscarinics for treatment of overactive bladder. *Lancet Neurology* 3(1), 46–53.

Clemens JQ (2010) Basic bladder neurophysiology. *Urology Clinics of North America* 37, 487–94.

Leippold T, Reitz A, Schurch B (2003) Botulinum toxin as a new therapy option for voiding disorders: current state of the art. *European Urology* 44(2), 165–74.

Norgaard JP, Hashim H, Malmberg L, et al. (2007) Antidiuresis therapy: mechanism of action and clinical implications. *Neurourology and Urodynamics* 26(7), 1008–13.

Yeo EKS, Hashim H, Abrams P (2013) New therapies in the treatment of overactive bladder. *Expert Opinions in Emerging Drugs* 18(3), 319–37.

Guidelines

EAU (2011) Guidelines on neurogenic lower urinary tract dysfunction. www.uroweb.org/guidelines/online-guidelines [accessed 10 April 2019].

European Association of Urology (2014) Guidelines on urinary incontinence. https://uroweb.org/wp-content/uploads/EAU-Guidelines-Urinary-Incontinence-2015.pdf [accessed 10 April 2019].

NICE CG97 (2015) Lower urinary tract symptoms: The management of lower urinary tract symptoms in men. https://www.nice.org.uk/guidance/cg97 [accessed 29 March 2019].

NICE CG171 (2015). Urinary incontinence in women: management. https://www.nice.org.uk/guidance/cg171 [accessed 29 March 2019].

NICE CG148 (2012) Urinary incontinence in neurological disease. https://www.nice.org.uk/guidance/cg148 [accessed 29 March 2019].

NICE TA290 (2013) Mirabegron for treating symptoms of overactive bladder. https://www.nice.org.uk/guidance/ta290 [accessed 29 March 2019].

NICE Pathway: urinary incontinence in neurological disease https://pathways.nice.org.uk/pathways/urinary-incontinence-in-neurological-disease [accessed 29 March 2019].

NICE Pathway: urinary incontinence in women. https://pathways.nice.org.uk/pathways/urinary-incontinence-in-women [accessed 29 March 2019].

5.4 Erectile dysfunction

Erectile dysfunction (ED) is the inability to consistently achieve or sustain an erection, sufficient for satisfactory sexual performance. ED has a high worldwide incidence and prevalence affecting approximately 50% of men aged 40–70 years old and can have significant psychosocial impact on patients, their partners, and families. The causes of ED are usually multifactorial, and can be broadly classified as organic or psychogenic. Organic causes are conditions that are associated with reduced nerve and endothelium function, which cause arterial insufficiency and defective smooth muscle relaxation in the penile tissues. Diabetes is therefore an important cause. Around 50% of cases in men over the age of 50 result from vascular disease, including atherosclerosis, hypertension, and peripheral vascular disease. Approximately 10% of total cases are primary psychogenic, but almost all patients latterly will have an element of psychogenic contribution.

Pathophysiology

Anatomy

The penis is constructed of three muscular beds, two corpora cavernosae and the corpus spongiosum, which surrounds the urethra. For erection, both cavernosae and the sinuses (also called lacunae) that lie within them, fill with blood delivered by the cavernosal arteries. The lacunae are lined with trabecular tissue and are involved in contraction. Arterial relaxation leads to increased blood flow and engorgement of the lacunar spaces such that erection ensues. The vascular pattern of erection is split into five phases:

- Increased arterial, but unchanged cavernosal pressure.
- Venous outflow reduction and increased cavernosal pressure.
- Attainment of intracavernosal pressure of ~100 mmHg.
- Contraction of pelvic floor muscles and maintenance of a rigid erection before ejaculation.
- Reduction of arterial flow and veno-occlusive influences so that flaccidity ensues (detumescence) after removal of sexual stimulation.

Sexual stimulation

This is a complex process that involves psychological and emotional factors, direct neurological pathways, and hormonal influences. Psycho-emotional sexual stimulation appears to be regulated via the limbic system causing excitatory and inhibitory modulation via the spinal cord. This leads to a functional antagonism mediated by the release of neurotransmitters (norepinephrine, endothelin and contractile prostanoids) and relaxing factors (e.g. nitric oxide) from cavernosal nerves.

Erection and ejaculation

The development and maintenance of an erection and subsequent ejaculation is a complex interplay involving central neural pathways in combination with the parasympathetic and sympathetic systems. The dominant neural pathways for erection initiation and maintenance (*P*oint) is via parasympathetic innervation (S2–S4), while the dominance in ejaculation is sympathetic (*S*hoot). Erection itself is mediated through thoracolumbar (T12–L2) sympathetic inhibition, parasympathetic (S2–S4) stimulation and non-adrenergic-non-cholinergic (NANC) pathways. Sexual stimulation activates the parasympathetic pathway via the cavernosal nerve supplying the corpora cavernosa. This causes arterial blood to flow into the sinusoidal spaces with relaxation of the cavernosal smooth muscle. The expansion of the sinusoidal spaces with blood is limited by the rigid tunica albuginea covering each corpus cavernosus muscle. During erection, the subtunical venous plexuses are compressed against the tunica albuginea and, therefore, contributes to maintenance of erection through decreasing venous outflow. Post-ganglionic NANC fibres are ultimately responsible for local control of erection, by releasing nitric oxide (NO) from terminals and local endothelial cells. The fibres themselves are inhibited by sympathetic innervation (NA), and activated by ACh and testosterone (via nitric oxide synthase; NOS). NOS is an enzyme that manufactures nitric oxide from the precursor L-arginine and is located in neural (nNOS) or epithelial tissues (eNOS). NO itself crosses smooth muscle membranes where it activates guanylate cyclase to convert GTP into cGMP. The cGMP activates protein kinase G, which hyperpolarizes the cell causing a decrease in Ca^{2+} influx and increased deposition to the endoplasmic reticulum, so that smooth muscle relaxation occurs and erection ensues. Any surplus cGMP is broken down by type 5 phosphodiesterase (PDE5) activity and detumescence occurs.

ED may occur as a result of psychogenic (anxiety–sympathetic driven), vascular (atherosclerosis), hormonal (hypogonadism- decreased testosterone), metabolic (diabetes), neuronal (pelvic trauma), or iatrogenic (drugs—Table 5.7) influences. By far the commonest risk factor is vascular disease, with atherosclerosis the prime culprit, through the reduced arterial inflow causing relative hypoxia and resulting in endothelial dysfunction. In such instances, as with hypertension, it is possible that NO signalling cannot overcome sympathetic and proflaccidity mediators (e.g. NA, ET-1, neuropeptide Y) thereby decreasing smooth muscle response.

Nitric oxide as a therapeutic target

Beyond primary prevention (including diet and exercise), the single most important pharmacological target to treat ED is through the improvement in local NO levels. As a neurotransmitter, NO is incredibly short-lived; *inhibiting* cGMP hydrolysis by the enzyme PDE5 is the most effective mechanism in promoting erection, while cGMP persists. PDE5 is highly expressed in penile smooth muscle and at other sites throughout the body, thus inhibition is not without adverse effects, due to action at other capillary smooth muscle sites (e.g. facial flushing, headache). The PDE5 inhibitors have good specificity for this subtype of enzyme, although off-target effects occur with other PDE subtypes (e.g. PDE6-retina, PDE11-heart, liver). Prostaglandin E1 (PGE1) is an alternative treatment, as this drug ligand (**alprostadil**) binds to G protein–coupled

Table 5.7 Potential drug causes of erectile dysfunction

Drug type	Drug class
Antihypertensive drugs	• Diuretics • β-blockers • Centrally-acting anti-hypertensive agents, e.g. clonidine, methyldopa
Centrally-acting agents	• Phenothiazines • Serotonin reuptake inhibitors • Tricyclic antidepressants, e.g. phenytoin
Endocrine drugs	• LHRH analogues anti-androgens • Oestrogens
Recreational drugs	• Alcohol • Cocaine • Opiates • Amphetamines • Anabolic steroids
Other drugs	• Cimetidine • Metoclopramide • Digoxin

Adapted from Eardley, I. Sexual dysfunction. In *Oxford Textbook of Medicine, Fifth Edition*, Table 13.8.5.1, page 1942. Oxford, UK: Oxford University Press © 2010. Reproduced with permission of the Licensor through PLSclear.

receptors and activates adenylate cyclase to catalyse the conversion of AMP to cAMP. This, in turn, activates protein kinase A, decreasing intracellular Ca^{2+} concentrations as NO does.

For a full summary of the relevant pathways and drug targets, see Figure 5.6.

Management

As ED shares many of the risk factors with CVD, clinical examination should include BP, peripheral pulses, carotid bruit and any other atherosclerotic signs. Examination of the genitourinary system is also important in order to identify any anatomical abnormalities (e.g. Peyronie's disease, micropenis) or endocrine signs (e.g. hypogonadism, secondary sexual characteristics). Before referral, work-up should include investigation of likely risk factors, e.g.

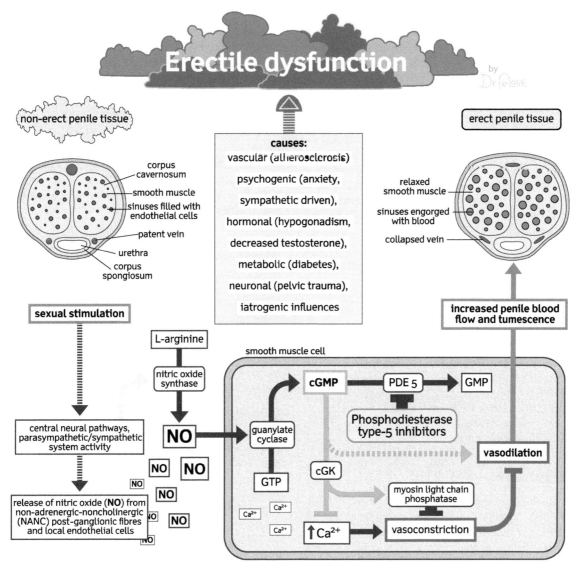

Figure 5.6 Erectile dysfunction: summary of relevant pathways and drug targets.

diabetes mellitus (HbA1c), hyperlipidaemia (lipid profiles), and free testosterone. Evidence of endocrine abnormalities, anatomical abnormalities, or underlying organic disease are likely to require hospital referral for further investigation (e.g. vascular studies, such as duplex ultrasound of cavernous arteries, nerve conduction studies in neuropathies). A complete drug history should be carried out to identify possible iatrogenic causes e.g. β-blockers, diuretics, and antidepressants.

Where possible any underlying causes of ED should be managed, in many cases through reduction of risk factors (i.e. lifestyle changes including diet, exercise, and prevention of smoking) or where possible modification of current precipitating drug therapies. There is a strong likelihood that these simple modifications will fail, but this approach combined with psychosexual therapy can improve outcomes. For those with treatable causes like testicular failure or traumatic injury, outcomes are normally better. In others, there is a high chance of failure and pharmacotherapy is required.

Oral phosphodiesterase inhibitors are first line treatment in ED, but contraindicated in those taking nitrates, those who suffer from hypotension, or in patients who have had a recent stroke or myocardial infarction. Most classes of oral therapy have similar efficacy, but the onset and duration of action varies depending on the exact PDE inhibitor prescribed (see 'Prescribing'). 75% of men have improved erections, but those who have trialled eight doses at the maximum tablet strength, may be non-responders and require referral to urology.

Second-line therapies include intra-urethral pellet insertions of **alprostadil** (prostaglandin E1), which produces an erection in 30–66% of men, but is less effective than the same drug given by corpora caveronsa injection where success rates of 70% are reported. Vacuum devices, topical vasoactive drugs, and penile prosthesis also have a place in treatment.

Drug classes used in management

Phosphodiesterase type-5 inhibitors

PDE5 is the predominant phosphodiesterase in the corpus cavernosum and is responsible for the breakdown of cGMP. Inhibition of PDE5 can thus promote vasodilation and penile erection by locally increasing cGMP levels and PKG activity. Examples include avanafil, sildenafil, tadalafil, and vardenafil.

Mechanism of action

In physiological conditions, the degradation of cGMP by PDE5 counteracts penile erection, by removing the positive effect of a NO-dependent increase in cGMP in the relaxation of arterial and trabecular smooth muscle. Crucially, inhibition of PDE5 is ineffective in the absence of a stimulatory action on the NO pathway, which is specifically stimulated in the penis following sexual arousal. As a result, PDE5 inhibitors can promote penile erection, while having a relatively small effect on other tissues.

PDE5 competitive inhibitors employ a common mechanism of action and have similar chemical formulae. However, they have significant clinical differences in terms of onset, duration of action, and side effect profile. All of the available PDE5 inhibitors have strong selectivity for PDE5, compared with the other known PDE enzymes, although **avanafil** demonstrates less inhibition of PDE1, PDE6, and PDE11, which are located in the heart, retina, and testicles, respectively. As a result of this high

selectivity and low cross-reactivity, avanafil could exhibit reduced incidence of side effects, such as visual disturbances, haemodynamic changes and musculoskeletal effects. Its faster onset and short half-life also allows for quicker functional erections.

Prescribing

There are currently four PDE5 inhibitors on the market in the UK for use in erectile dysfunction, of which **sildenafil** and **tadalafil** are also licensed for use in pulmonary hypertension. Doses are taken orally, on an as-required basis prior to sexual intercourse, although the specific timing varies between agents according to onset of action, from 15 minutes to 1 hour (sildenafil is the slowest to take effect). Tadalafil also has a license for repeated daily dosing in patients who anticipate intercourse at least twice a week.

Unwanted effects

As PDE5 inhibitors cause peripheral vasodilation, common side effects predictably include headache, flushing, and dizziness. There have also been reports of priapism, although this has only been reported on post-marketing surveillance.

Drug interactions

Patients taking α-adrenoceptor antagonists run the risk of experiencing increased side effects of PDE5 inhibitors, in particular hypotension, and thus manufacturers of **vardenafil** and **avanafil** recommend using lower doses initially.

Tadalafil, **sildenafil**, vardenafil, and avanafil are all substrates predominantly for CYP 3A4 and, as such, have a high tendency to be affected by drugs that potently inhibit (e.g. **erythromycin**, protease inhibitors) or induce (e.g. **rifampicin**) this enzyme. Although partly metabolized via other enzyme, CYP450 interactions with other isoenzymes are unlikely to be of clinical significance.

Prostaglandins

Prostaglandin E1 has diverse pharmacological actions, but in the case of ED acts as a potent vasodilator. It produces corporal smooth muscle relaxation through its action at PGE receptors activating adenylate cyclase and causing a rise in cAMP and decrease intracellular Ca^{2+}. For example, alprostadil.

Mechanism of action

Alprostadil (prostaglandin E_1) is one of a family of naturally occurring acidic lipids with various pharmacological effects. In terms of ED, this compound acts via prostaglandin E (PGE) receptors to activate adenylate cyclase, resulting in elevated concentrations of cAMP. This in turn decreases intracellular Ca^{2+} concentrations, which leads to relaxation of trabecular smooth muscle and dilation of cavernosal arteries. Erection is achieved through subsequent expansion of lacunar spaces and entrapment of blood by compressing the venules against the tunica albuginea.

Prescribing

Alprostadil can be used for ED (and neurogenic ED specifically) in a number of pharmaceutical forms, i.e. intraurethral pellet insertion, direct topical application, or intracavernosal injection. Prescribing of these products is generally via a specialist. Typically, the onset of action of alprostadil is 10 minutes with average erection maintenance for ~15 minutes.

Unwanted effects

Side effects include hypotension and, as such, should be prescribed with caution in those taking anti-hypertensives (e.g. ACEi, β-blockers) or nitrates. For topical preparations urethral burning and pain are possible, while for other direct routes penile pain and haematoma are common. Abnormal penile anatomy is an absolute contraindication (e.g. hypospadias).

Further reading

Costa P, Potempa AJ (2012) Intraurethral alprostadil for erectile dysfunction: a review of the literature. *Drugs* 72(17), 2243–54.

Lasker GP, Maley JH, Kadowitz PJ (2010) A review of the pathophysiology and novel treatments for erectile dysfunction. *Advances in Pharmacological Sciences* Article ID 730861.

Matsui H, Sopko NA, Hannan JL, et al. (2015) Pathophysiology of erectile dysfunction. *Current Drug Targets* 16(5), 411–19.

Wright PJ (2006) Comparison of phosphodiesterase type 5 (PDE5) inhibitors. *International Journal of Clinical Practice* 60(8) 967–75.

Guidelines

EAU Guidelines on Erectile Dysfunction (2016) Premature ejaculation, penile curvature and priapism. European Association of Urology. https://uroweb.org/wp-content/uploads/EAU-Guidelines-Male-Sexual-Dysfunction-2016.pdf [accessed 10 April 2019].

European Association of Urology (2013) Guidelines on Male Sexual Dysfunction: erectile dysfunction and premature ejaculation. https://uroweb.org/wp-content/uploads/14-Male-Sexual-Dysfunction_LR.pdf [accessed 29 March 2019].

Hackett G, Kell P, Ralph D, et al. (2008) British Society for Sexual Medicine guidelines on the management of erectile dysfunction. *Journal of Sexual Medicine* 5(8), 1841–65.

6 Gastroenterology

6.1 Nausea and vomiting

Nausea and vomiting can be defined, respectively, as the urge to or the actual act of expelling undigested food from the stomach. It is thought to be an evolutionary defence mechanism to protect against toxic insult (drugs or microbes) and over-eating, while it can also be triggered during pregnancy, or by unpleasant sights or smells. In some instances, it may be the symptom of a more severe underlying pathology. Severity of nausea and vomiting varies considerably between individuals exposed to the same stimulus and symptoms can be highly detrimental to patient quality of life affecting not only their nutritional intake, but also mood and well-being.

Pathophysiology

Although nausea itself is a subjective term, vomiting is a pathophysiological reflex triggered by the vomiting centre located in the medulla. The vomiting centre receives signals from a number of afferent inputs, i.e. the chemoreceptor trigger zone (CTZ), vestibular nucleus, abdominal and cardiac vagal afferents, and cerebral cortex (Table 6.1). It may also be activated by hormonal triggers, which accounts for hyperemesis in pregnancy, and the increased incidence of nausea and vomiting associated with the female gender. As the vomiting centre is located close to centres responsible for salivation and breathing, vomiting is often associated with hypersalivation and hyperventilation. The CTZ is highly vascularized and located at the floor of the fourth ventricle, just outside the blood–brain barrier and, therefore, is itself directly sensitive to chemical stimuli.

Afferent inputs activate the vomiting centre through several known neurotransmitter pathways; dopamine (D_2), serotonin (5-HT$_3$, 5-HT$_4$), acetylcholine (ACh), and substance P (neurokinin 1; NK$_1$). Each of which provides a potential pharmacological target in the management of nausea and vomiting, once the cause has been established.

Efferent pathways from the vomiting centre induce autonomic changes, including vasoconstriction, pallor, tachycardia, salivation, sweating, and relaxation of the lower oesophagus and fundus of the stomach. In vomiting, oesophageal relaxation leads to contraction of the pyloric sphincter, thereby emptying the contents of the jejunum, duodenum, and pyloric stomach into the relaxed fundus. Coordination of muscle contraction occurs within the diaphragm and abdomen, and retrograde contractions from the intestine then expel the contents of the fundus.

In all instances, the underlying cause of the nausea and vomiting must be established first, to prevent the masking of a more serious pathology. A careful clinical history is paramount before initiating treatment, taking into consideration the nature and timing of the vomit, and any accompanying symptoms (see Table 6.2). In general terms, symptoms fall into three categories; GI (e.g. gastritis, inflammatory bowel disease), non-GI (e.g. pregnancy, infection), or neurological (e.g. vestibular).

For a full summary of the relevant pathways and drug targets, see Figure 6.1.

Management

Left untreated, nausea and vomiting can have a profound effect on both the physical and psychological well-being of a patient. Optimizing management can help reduce complications such as dehydration, electrolyte imbalance, malnutrition, impaired wound healing, and delays in essential treatment. Furthermore, patients find nausea and vomiting extremely distressing, particularly where symptoms are persistent, thus impacting on quality of life. Poor management increases the risk of psychogenic symptoms, particularly with chemotherapy where patients require multiple cycles of emetogenic chemotherapy.

Baseline investigations including blood tests (FBC, U&Es and LFTs) or urinalysis, may be useful in establishing

Table 6.1 The afferent inputs modulating the vomiting centre of the medulla

Afferent input	Stimulus	Transmitter/receptor
Abdominal vagal afferents	Infection, drugs, obstruction, alcohol, post-operative eating	D_2, 5-HT_3, NK_1
Chemoreceptor trigger zone (CTZ)	Drugs either inhaled or blood-borne, toxins, alcohol, hepatic impairment, renal impairment, hypercalcaemia, and other biochemical abnormalities	D_2, 5-HT_3, opioid, NK_1, ACh, H_1
Vestibular nuclei	Motion sickness, vertigo, middle ear surgery, post-operative movement	ACh, H_1
Cortical afferent nerves (higher centres)	Sights, smells, anxiety, fear, raised ICP, hypoxia	

a cause (see Table 6.3). Where an underlying GI pathology is suspected, such as gastric ulceration, endoscopy may be considered.

Once the underlying cause has been identified and appropriately managed, patients who remain symptomatic may require pharmacological management with anti-emetics. The choice of drug in the treatment of nausea and vomiting is determined by the underlying cause. Drugs are routinely used for both the treatment and prevention of symptoms, often in combination so as to target the various implicated receptor sites. It is generally

accepted that nausea and vomiting is easier to manage through regular effective prophylaxis, than by treating already established symptoms. By the same principle, treatment prescribed on an as-required basis is often less effective than regular treatment.

Gastrointestinal

Common GI causes of nausea and vomiting include obstruction and infection (gastritis, pancreatitis, appendicitis), but chronic diseases such as liver failure or inflammatory bowel disease (IBD) may also induce symptoms. First-line treatment is usually with a dopamine antagonist, with or without a 5HT3 antagonist depending on symptom severity. Although substance P is also implicated in this pathway, **aprepitant** or **fosaprepitant** are the only products currently on the market that influence this neurotransmitter, and neither is licensed for this indication.

Non-gastrointestinal

Pregnancy-induced

Pharmacological therapy in pregnancy is only used where the benefits of treating are believed to outweigh any potential risk to the foetus. Patients are advised to use medication only when lifestyle measures, such as avoiding precipitating foods, and eating little and often have proved unsuccessful. Alternative therapies such as ginger and acupressure wristbands may be of benefit in some patients. Where pharmacological therapy is

Table 6.2 Clinical history in nausea and vomiting.

Signs and symptoms	Possible causes
Appearance of vomit	Blood stained, coffee-ground, faecal smell (e.g. GI obstruction)
Timing and onset	In relation to ingestion of possible toxin (e.g. infection, drug, etc.), raised ICP associated with morning symptoms, sudden onset
Accompanying symptoms	Diarrhoea (infection), constipation (obstruction), pain (ulcers, pancreatitis, appendicitis), headache (migraines, raised ICP), double vision (raised ICP, intracranial tumour), dizziness (labyrinthitis), appetite (possibly unaffected in psychogenic disease)

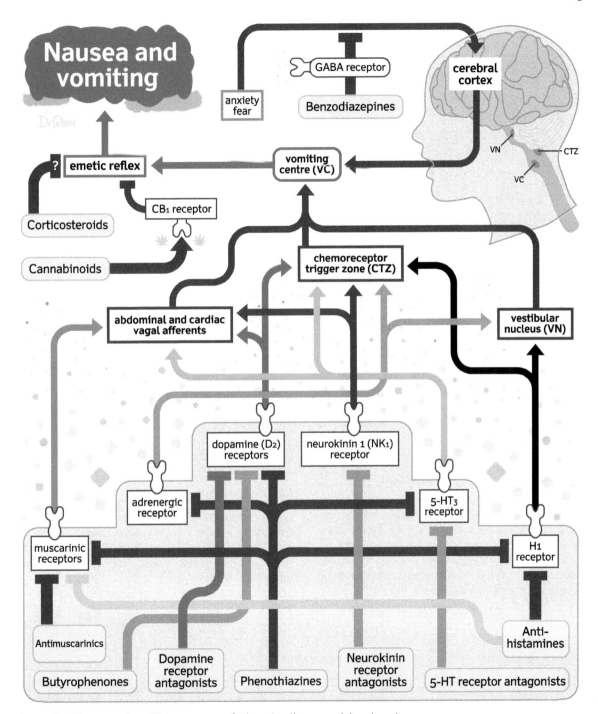

Figure 6.1 Nausea and vomiting: summary of relevant pathways and drug targets.

deemed necessary, antihistamines are the drug of choice, followed by **prochlorperazine** or 5HT$_3$ antagonists; **metoclopramide**, once widely used is now used less frequently due to associated risk of neurological toxicity. In severe hyperemesis gravidium requiring hospitalization, corticosteroids such as **dexamethasone** and **prednisolone** have been used, although they are not without risk, so are reserved as last-line usage.

Table 6.3 Baseline investigations in nausea and vomiting

Test	Cause
FBC	Anaemia, bleeding
U&Es	Hypercalcaemia, renal dysfunction, derangement secondary to vomiting, acidosis
LFT	Excess alcohol, hepatic disease
Amylase	Pancreatitis
Urine dip	UTI

Systemic toxicity

The chemoreceptor trigger zone responds to toxic stimulus within the blood, such as drug therapy (e.g. chemotherapy), alcohol, or biochemical abnormalities. As so many receptors are involved in the pathway, treatment is effective with a wide range of anti-emetics. Where symptoms are mild, first line treatment will invariably be with a dopamine antagonist or anti-muscarinic, with the option to add on a 5-HT$_3$ antagonist in more severe cases.

Treatment of drug-induced nausea and vomiting is rarely necessary, as invariably symptoms tend to be mild and self-limiting, and if not, drug treatment is discontinued. The exception to this is nausea and vomiting induced by chemotherapy or opioids, where treatment is likely to be essential. Effective prophylaxis is paramount in the management of chemotherapy-induced nausea and vomiting (CINV), tailored to the emetogenicity of the chemotherapy agents used. In the case of highly emetogenic chemotherapy, combination therapy with a 5-HT$_3$ antagonist and **dexamethasone** forms the gold standard, with addition of agents such as **levomepromazine**, neurokinin inhibitors, dopamine antagonists, and anti-muscarinics where

necessary. **Aprepitant** and **fosaprepitant** are generally reserved for use in highly emetogenic **cisplatin**-based chemotherapy regimens or equivalent, again given as part of combination therapy. As all patients are unique in the way they are affected by chemotherapy, consideration should be given to experience from previous cycles and effective anti-emetics.

Post-operative nausea and vomiting

The choice of anti-emetics in the prevention of post-operative nausea and vomiting (PONV) is determined by the relative risk of symptoms. Risk can be calculated through consideration of risk factors (see Table 6.4) and used to direct therapy (Table 6.5).

Neurological
Vestibular disorders

Nausea and vomiting is also common in vestibular disorders, such as Meniere's disease, motion sickness, vertigo and labyrinthitis. Pharmacological management with antimuscarinics and anithistamines will not only control the sickness, but also ameliorates symptoms of any related dizziness. These classes should also be considered for post-operative prophylaxis following middle ear surgery, or in treating nausea induced by post-operative movement.

Psychogenic causes

Where the cause of nausea and vomiting is thought to be non-organic in nature, i.e. induced by feelings of anxiety or fear, or in some cases from memories of previous episodes; pharmacological management is most effective with benzodiazepines. In this instance, **lorazepam** is the benzodiazepine of choice, e.g. in patients prior to chemotherapy or surgery.

Table 6.4 Risk factors for post-operative nausea and vomiting

Patient risk factors	Surgical risk factors	Anaesthetic risk factors
Female post-puberty	Duration of surgery	General anaesthesia
Young adults and children	Type of surgery (ENT, neurosurgery, breast, laparotomy, plastic, cholecystectomy)	High dose neostigmine
Non-smoker		Nitrous oxide
Previous history	Dehydration	Duration of anaesthesia
History of motion sickness		Intra- and post-operative opioid

Table 6.5 Management of PONV

Risk	Definition	Treatment strategy
Low risk	1 risk factor or no previous history	Prescribe PRN anti-emetics in case they are required
Moderate risk	2 risk factors or previous history	Single agent prophylaxis with $5HT_3$ antagonist, droperidol, dexamethasone, hyoscine, cyclizine, or promethazine.
High risk	3 or more risk factors	Combination of 2 drugs, e.g. a $5HT_3$ antagonist plus dexamethasone or droperidol

Drug classes used in management

Antihistamines

The antihistamines used in the management of nausea and vomiting are first generation non-selective H_1 receptor antagonists with significant antimuscarinic and central H_1 effects. Examples include cyclizine, promethazine, and cinnarizine.

Mechanism of action

The anti-emetic actions of histamine receptor antagonists are through the blockade of H_1 receptors located in the vestibular nuclei and vomiting centre. In addition, the majority of antihistamines are potent muscarinic receptor antagonists, and this can make a significant contribution to their therapeutic effects against emesis. Indeed, the H_1 receptor antagonist **chlorphenamine**, which does not inhibit motion sickness, also lacks centrally mediated cholinergic effects. In addition to its antihistamine action, **promethazine** can also block some 5-HT receptors.

Prescribing

Not all antihistamines are used as anti-emetics, however those that are include; **cyclizine**, **promethazine**, and **cinnarizine**. Cyclizine tends to be the most widely used showing good efficacy in managing sickness post-operatively, drug-induced, or that associated with vestibular disorders. Although used less frequently, promethazine is useful in the management of pregnancy-induced nausea and vomiting, where extensive experience suggests it to be non-teratogenic. Both agents are available in oral and parenteral formulations, the latter potentially of value in patients unable to manage oral therapy due to sickness.

Cinnarizine, although marketed for use in vestibular disorders, is generally only used for the prevention of motion sickness and in acute Meniere's attacks. There is no parenteral preparation available.

More recently **doxylamine** in combination with **pyridoxine** has been licensed for use in pregnancy induced nausea and vomiting.

Unwanted effects

All four agents used in the treatment of nausea and vomiting are first generation antihistamines, so by definition are less selective in nature, showing activity against muscarinic and H_1 receptors (central and peripheral). Consequently, sedation is the most widely reported side effect, followed by common antimuscarinic effects, i.e. dry mouth, blurred vision, and urinary retention. Glaucoma is more likely to be precipitated in patients receiving antimuscarinic therapy.

The increased risk of central toxicity with parenteral administration can be reduced by slow administration (over 3–5 minutes). Antihistamines are eliminated hepatically and therefore best avoided in severe hepatic impairment, where there is a risk of accumulation and more severe central toxicity.

PRESCRIBING WARNING

Cyclizine

There have been reports of cyclizine being abused for its hallucinogenic and euphoric potential, and is believed to work synergistically with opiates.

Cyclizine should be avoided in acute alcohol intoxication; it may increase the toxicity of alcohol.

Drug interactions

Unsurprisingly, there is an additive effect when these agents are used with other drugs that possess sedating or antimuscarinic properties. This is of particular concern in patients who are driving or operating heavy machinery, and they should therefore be advised appropriately.

Antimuscarinics

> Antimuscarinic agents block muscarinic receptors controlling the visceral afferent input from the gut. For example, hyoscine (scopolamine).

Mechanism of action

Muscarinic receptor antagonists inhibit cholinergic transmission in receptors located within the vomiting centre, which are stimulated by afferent pathways from the CTZ and vestibular nucleus. **Hyoscine** also potently inhibits GI movements through antimuscarinic effects on bowel smooth muscle, which might further contribute to its antiemetic action.

Prescribing

Hyoscine is licensed for use in the prevention of motion sickness as oral (hyoscine hydrobromide) or transdermal formulations. Choice of formulation will depend on the intended journey time. Oral tablets may be administered half an hour before the journey commences, but the duration of action is short and requires repeated doses to be administered every 6 hours. In contrast, the transdermal patch only requires changing every 3 days, but needs to be applied for 5–6 hours before it takes effect.

Although beyond the scope of the licence, hyoscine treatment may be a useful add on in the prevention of chemotherapy induced nausea and vomiting, particularly in longer cycles where effects are sustained and a patch allows for non-invasive administration.

Unwanted effects

Predictably given the antimuscarinic properties, the most commonly reported side effects to **hyoscine** are dry mouth, sedation, and blurred vision. Hyoscine is best avoided in patients with a history of glaucoma. Transdermal patches may also cause a local irritation.

PRESCRIBING WARNING

Transdermal Hyoscine

- Once a hyoscine patch is removed, hyoscine will continue to enter the blood from the skin, so that after 24 hours, levels will only have reduced by one-third.

- After handling a patch, ensure your hands are washed thoroughly; any remaining traces can cause a transient cyclopegia and papillary dilatation on direct contact with the eye.

Drug interactions

Concomitant use of **hyoscine** with other drugs known to have anticholinergic effects will increase the risk of toxicity, particularly in elderly patients who are susceptible to falls, delirium, and cognitive impairment. Anticholinergic risk scores (ARS) provide a useful tool for elderly or polypharmacy patients to assess the relative risk of unacceptable toxicity, and provide guidance on the choice of drug therapy.

PRACTICAL PRESCRIBING
Anticholinergic risk scores

- Anticholinergic risk scores were devised to assess the risk of toxicity (falls, delirium and cognitive impairment) in elderly patients (over 65 years).
- Drugs are categorized according to their predicted risk of adverse effects (1, 2 or 3 points), with a total score calculated for all the medication a patient is taking.
- A total score of 3 or higher is associated with increased risk.
- Antimuscarinic drugs such as hyoscine are attributed 3 points.

Rudolph JL, Salow MJ, Angelini MC, McGlinchey RE. (2008) Archives of Internal Medicine *168(5), 512.*

Phenothiazines

> The antipsychotic phenothiazines act as antagonists on numerous receptors implicated in nausea and vomiting. Examples include prochlorperazine, levomepromazine, perphenazine, chlorpromazine, and trifluoperazine.

Mechanism of action

Phenothiazines are antagonists at more than one receptor site, i.e. muscarinic, histaminergic, dopaminergic, adrenergic, and 5-HT receptors, all of which are potential targets within the CTZ. This makes them particularly valuable in treating nausea and vomiting associated with drug therapy or metabolic toxicities, although their primary class effect is as an anti-psychotic.

Prescribing

The phenothiazines are best known for their role in palliative care and chemotherapy- or radiotherapy-induced nausea and vomiting. Within the class, **prochlorperazine** is the most widely prescribed, not only for the indications above, but also in vestibular disorders such as vertigo and labyrinthitis. There is also a good body of evidence to support its use in PONV where it is routinely prescribed for prophylaxis. Doses can be administered orally or parenterally and, unlike other anti-emetics, is available as a buccal preparation, which undoubtedly plays a large part in its popularity. Of the remaining drugs, **levomepromazine** tends to be preferred, used at doses considerably smaller than those in schizophrenia, i.e. 6–50 mg daily compared with 200–1000 mg.

Unwanted effects

Cautions and side effects

The non-selectivity of the phenothiazines, although valuable in the management of nausea and vomiting, also accounts for its broad side effect profile, in particular those affecting the nervous system. As a class, they are profoundly lipophilic and protein bound, so accumulate readily in the brain, lung, and other highly vascular tissues.

In general, toxicity is associated with higher doses and long-term use, and is thus unlikely when used acutely as an anti-emetic; but more common with the higher, extended doses used in palliation. **Chlorpromazine** tends to be the most poorly tolerated, which explains why it is rarely used.

The prominent adverse class effect is sedation, although in some instances this may be considered a benefit, with effects wearing off after a few days of treatment.

Antagonistic action on dopamine receptors and their ability to cross the blood–brain barrier accounts for the relatively high frequency of extrapyramidal side effects, such as dystonia, akathisia, and tardive dyskinesia. They are therefore best avoided in Parkinson's disease. Patients are also potentially at risk of neuroleptic malignant syndrome, particularly with chlorpromazine.

PRESCRIBING WARNING

QT interval prolongation with phenothiazines
- Phenothiazines are associated with QT prolongation.
- Although this is unlikely at anti-emetic doses (with the exception of chlorpromazine), consider alternatives in patients with risk factors for QT prolongation, e.g. elderly, family history, hypokalaemia, severe renal or hepatic failure, or those taking other drugs known to cause it.

Drug interactions

Interactions of clinical significance associated with short-term use of phenothiazines as anti-emetics are negligible. In palliation, where sustained higher doses are being used, interactions with other drugs known to prolong the QT interval such as some anti-arrhythmics or other anti-psychotics are best avoided where possible. Unsurprisingly sedation will be augmented when phenothiazines are taken with other sedating drugs.

Butyrophenones

The antipsychotic butyrophenones are structurally related to phenothiazines and used in anti-emetic therapy for their antagonism of dopaminergic receptors. For example, haloperidol and droperidol.

Mechanism of action

Butyrophenones are weak antihistamines with dopamine receptor antagonist activity. They are structurally related to phenothiazines and possess many similarities. **Haloperidol** and **droperidol** act centrally by binding to dopamine D_2 receptors located in the vomiting centre and the CTZ.

Prescribing

Droperidol was originally developed for use as an antipsychotic back in 1961, although in March 2001 all oral preparations were withdrawn worldwide due to the risk of QT interval prolongation and torsades de pointes associated with chronic use. It is now only available in an injectable form for use in PONV, or nausea and vomiting secondary to post-operative opioid patient-controlled analgesia (PCA). However, outside of the license, there is evidence to suggest it is effective in managing CINV.

Haloperidol is licensed for use in managing nausea and vomiting in palliative care, particularly secondary to metabolic causes, such as renal failure or hypercalcaemia, with some evidence to suggest it may be useful for preventing PONV. Unlike droperidol it is available in oral and IV formulations.

With both drugs, anti-emetic doses are lower than those used in psychoses.

Unwanted effects

Due to structural similarities, the unwanted effects associated with butyrephenones mirror those seen with phenothiazines. However, due to the previous withdrawal of **droperidol**, manufacturers are considerably more cautious with its use, highlighting numerous contraindications related to the risk of QT interval prolongation.

Dopamine receptor antagonists

Dopamine receptor antagonists block dopamine D_2 receptors and inhibit dopaminergic neurotransmission in the CTZ. For example, metoclopramide and domperidone.

Mechanism of action

The observation that most dopamine agonists used in the treatment of Parkinson's disease could induce nausea and vomiting through stimulation of dopaminergic receptors in the CTZ, led to the use of highly potent antagonists of the dopamine receptors as anti-emetics. In high doses **metoclopramide** is also known to have anti-5-HT_3 activity; however, high dose treatment has been largely replaced by the significantly better tolerated selective 5-HT_3 antagonists.

Prescribing

Both **domperidone** and **metoclopramide** are well absorbed orally, and while domperidone is also formulated for rectal administration, metoclopramide is available in parenteral formulations.

Unwanted effects

Aside from the possible methods of administration, the main difference between the **domperidone** and **metoclopramide** is in the ability of the latter to cross the blood–brain barrier and thus affect the striatal areas of the basal ganglia, increasing the central toxicity of metoclopramide.

Extrapyramidal side effects to metoclopramide (see 'Prescribing warning: metoclopramide neurological toxicity') can occur after a single dose, and are more likely to affect children and young adults, particularly when doses higher than 500 µg/kg are administered. Acute dystonic reactions, such as oculogyric crisis, are best treated with dopamine agonists, such as **bromocriptine** or **procyclidine**.

Rare side effects commonly include GI toxicity and hyperprolactinaemia. The production of prolactin is normally suppressed by the presence of dopamine, therefore continued use of domperidone and metoclopramide can raise prolactin levels leading to galactorrhoea, gynaecomastia, and amenorrhoea.

PRESCRIBING WARNING

Sudden Cardiac Death with Domperidone

Epidemiological studies have suggested an association between domperidone and sudden cardiac death, possibly attributed to QT prolongation. To minimize the risk:

- Use only in the treatment of nausea and vomiting.
- Use the smallest possible dose for the shortest duration (max daily dose of 30 mg).
- Avoid use with other drugs known to cause QT prolongation, especially ketoconazole.
- Contraindicated in patients with a history of cardiac disease.

PRESCRIBING WARNING

Metoclopramide Neurological Toxicity

Due to the increased risk of neurological toxicity with metoclopramide, the MHRA and EMA recommend:

- Maximum of 30 mg a day for 5 days in adults.
- Consider as second-line option in patients 1–18 years.
- Children under 1 should not receive metoclopramide.
- It should no longer be used for the management of chronic conditions.

Drug interactions

Ketoconazole possibly increases the risk of arrhythmias when prescribed concurrently with **domperidone**.

5-HT receptor antagonists

> The 5-HT antagonists used in emesis block 5-HT3 receptors in the CTZ and gut. Examples include ondanestron, granisetron, and palonosetron.

Mechanism of action

The development of serotonin receptor antagonists that are selective for the $5HT_3$ subtype, produced a significant improvement in the treatment of nausea and vomiting. They act by preventing serotonin from binding to $5\text{-}HT_3$ receptors present in high density in the CTZ and on the gut vagal afferent nerve endings. The $5\text{-}HT_3$ antagonists inhibit various relevant functions that are induced by serotonin release, such as the splanchnic afferent nerve responses to painful distension and the vagal reactions to chemotherapy. In addition, they also inhibit the discharge of secreto-motor nerves. Although it is understood that $5\text{-}HT_3$ receptor antagonists prevent nausea and vomiting at the nucleus tractus solitarius and CTZ sites, it is not completely clear whether the main location of receptor blockade is situated within the central or the peripheral nervous system or if, indeed, blockade at both sites is equally important.

Prescribing

The $5HT_3$ antagonists are effective in both prevention and treatment of established emesis, particularly involving afferent inputs from the CTZ or gut, e.g. nausea and vomiting induced by chemotherapy, radiotherapy, or surgery. This is due to the fact that chemotherapeutic drugs evoke a significant release of serotonin from small enterochromaffin cells stimulating $5\text{-}HT_3$ receptors on vagal afferent fibres. The $5HT_3$ receptor antagonists have no effect on motion sickness or in other vestibular disorders.

Of the three available for therapy, **ondansetron** and **granisetron** tend to be the most widely used. They are both rapidly absorbed orally and can also be administered by IV or IM injection. Both drugs have relatively short half-lives requiring multiple daily dosing; compared with the 40-hour half-life of **palonosetron**, which is only licensed to be used prophylactically as a single dose administered 30 minutes before chemotherapy. Two further drugs in this

class **tropisetron** and **dolasetron** were discontinued in the UK in 2008 and 2009, respectively.

Unwanted effects

Constipation and headache are the most commonly reported side effects to the $5\text{-}HT_3$ antagonists, the former due to the effect they have on increasing bowel transit time.

All drugs are hepatically metabolized, but only **ondansetron** requires caution in severe hepatic impairment.

Drug interactions

The $5\text{-}HT_3$ antagonists are all, to varying degree, substrates for different cytochrome P450 enzyme subgroups, however, are themselves neither inducers nor inhibitors. Interactions of clinical significance are unlikely, but in patients taking potent enzyme inducers that fail to achieve adequate control of their emesis, higher doses, or alternative therapy may need to be considered.

Corticosteroids

> Corticosteroids are only used in emesis at low doses and for short periods, when they are unlikely to cause significant immunosuppression. Examples include dexamethasone, methylprednisolone, and prednisolone.

Mechanism of action

Dexamethasone and, to a lesser extent, **methylprednisolone** and **prednisolone** are routinely used for their anti-emetic effects. Although the precise mechanism of action is unknown, evidence suggests that the effect might be due to activation of glucocorticoid receptors in the nucleus tractus solitarius in the medulla, and it may involve the inhibition of prostaglandin synthesis.

Prescribing

Dexamethasone is a corticosteroid widely used in the management of nausea and vomiting post-operatively and in patients receiving chemotherapy. In the latter, dexamethasone is used in combination with a $5\text{-}HT_3$ antagonists as the gold standard for the prevention of sickness associated with highly emetogenic chemotherapy. Loading doses are often necessary when dexamethasone is used as an anti-emetic either before chemotherapy or with PONV at the induction of anaesthesia. Less commonly, **methylprednisolone** is used for the same indication.

All three agents have a role to play in severe hyperemesis gravidarum where all other measures have failed, and the impaired nutritional status of the mother poses a risk to her and the unborn baby.

Unwanted effects

Used in low doses and for short durations, as they are as anti-emetics, there are few reported side effects to corticosteroids. The main exceptions include sleep disturbances and neuropsychiatric reactions such as altered mood, anxiety and irritability (particularly in patients with predisposing risk factors) or mild GI toxicity. In short courses, they are unlikely to cause significant adrenal or immunosuppression effects, attributed to much of the toxicity associated with corticosteroid therapy. Slow withdrawal is therefore unnecessary and they can invariably be used without problem in patients with severe systemic infection.

Drug interactions

Dexamethasone, **methylprednisolone**, and **prednisolone** are all substrates for CYP 3A4, and are therefore affected by inhibitors and inducers of this subgroup.

Interactions with potent inhibitors such as **clarithromycin**, **erythromycin**, and **ritonavir** can lead to increased serum corticosteroid levels. Of particular note is the interaction seen with the potent inhibitor **aprepitant**. Where used concomitantly with aprepitant, doses of dexamethasone and oral doses of methylprednisolone should be reduced by 50% and IV doses of methylprednisolone by 25%.

Potent enzyme inducers such as **carbamazepine**, **phenytoin**, and **rifampicin** can reduce levels, thereby impairing anti-emetic effects.

Neurokinin receptor antagonist

> Neurokinin receptor antagonists act at the substance P NK_1 receptor subtype in the CNS. For example, aprepitant and fosaprepitant.

Mechanism of action

The capacity that substance P has to induce neural excitation in the area postrema of the dorsal brainstem, raises the possibility that it can act together with other tachykinins as important mediators of the emetic reflex.

Antagonists of the NK_1 substance P receptor subtype appear to have broad-spectrum anti-emetic activities, inhibiting the emesis that is evoked by different drugs and also motion sickness. This broad extent of anti-emetic properties might indicate an inhibitory action on the final pathways of the emetic reflex.

Prescribing

Aprepitant, the first of the neurokinin 1 inhibitors, was licensed in 2003 making it the newest class of anti-emetics. More recently, **fosaprepitant**, a pro-drug of aprepitant, has been developed as an IV formulation. Studies comparing aprepitant to **ondansetron** in controlling emesis secondary to **cisplatin**, demonstrated equal efficacy in acute emesis, but aprepitant to be more effective in controlling delayed emesis. Aprepitant is well absorbed in the gut and has a long half-life, allowing for OD administration.

Unwanted effects

Both **aprepitant** and **fosaprepitant** are highly selective for the neurokinin receptors and therefore possess a side effect profile distinct from other classes of anti-emetics. Commonly reported side effects include hiccups, constipation, headache, decreased appetite, dyspepsia, and fatigue.

Aprepitant is extensively metabolized by the liver so is best used cautiously in severe hepatic impairment.

Drug interactions

Aprepitant is a substrate, inhibitor, and inducer of the CYP3A4, as well as an inducer for CYP2C9 and therefore has a high potential for drug interactions. Co-administration with **pimozide**, **terfenadine**, and **astemizole** are contraindicated as aprepitant can increase serum levels, giving rise to unacceptable toxicity in particular QT interval prolongation.

Clear advice is provided by the manufacturers on the concomitant use of aprepitant with corticosteroids (see 'Corticosteroids'). This is, in part, down to the fact that the licensed use is as add-on therapy to a 5-HT_3 and dexamethasone combination, so the two have been extensively investigated together.

Cannabinoids

> Cannabinoid receptors agonists act on CB_1 receptors making them effective anti-emetics, but generally poorly tolerated. For example, nabilone.

Mechanism of action

Nabilone acts on CB_1 receptors, which are present in larger quantities than most other G protein–coupled neurotransmitter receptors throughout the brain, particularly in areas implicated in chemotherapy-induced nausea and vomiting. Unlike other receptors, where anti-emetics act as antagonists at receptor sites, nabilone acts as an agonist on CB_1 receptors to induce its anti-emetic actions. The effect may be mediated by indirect activation of somatodendritic $5-HT_{1A}$ receptors in the dorsal raphe nucleus, which can reduce the release of serotonin in terminal forebrain regions.

Naloxone, an opioid receptor competitive antagonist, can antagonize the anti-emetic properties of cannabinoid agents, which implies that opioid receptors may also have a role in the action of these drugs.

Prescribing

Nabilone is licensed solely for use in chemotherapy-induced nausea and vomiting in patients who have failed first-line or conventional treatment. Administered orally, it is well absorbed in the GI tract and is hepatically metabolized. Nabilone itself has a short half-life of 2 hours, although the longer half-life of some of its active metabolites allow for BD dosing.

Unwanted effects

CB_1 receptors are present in large numbers throughout the CNS, and their stimulation leads to both excitatory and inhibitory unwanted effects, e.g. sedation, dizziness, euphoria, and sleep disturbances. Although effects tend to be mild and resolve with continued use, **nabilone** should be used cautiously in patients with a history of psychiatric illness or substance abuse, and generally restricted to use in hospitalized patients for the minimum effective duration.

Drug interactions

The CNS toxicity of **nabilone** is likely to be increased when used in combination with hypnotics, narcotic analgesics, alcohol, or other psychoactive drugs.

Benzodiazepines

Benzodiazepines act by binding to GABA receptors in the CNS and increasing their affinity for the endogenous neurotransmitter. Examples include chlordiazepoxide, diazepam, lorazepam, and midazolam.

Mechanism of action

Benzodiazepines act on GABA receptors within the cerebral cortex, inducing anxiolytic and amnesic effects. They therefore do not act as anti-emetics per se, but have a role to play in emesis associated with anxiety or memory, and are of particular value in anticipatory nausea and vomiting associated with chemotherapy.

Prescribing

Lorazepam, the benzodiazepine of choice, is usually prescribed as a stat dose prior to chemotherapy, although in some instances doses may be repeated BD. It has a relatively short half-life (12 hours), allowing for sustained action without the risk of rapid withdrawal or 'hangover' effects. Doses may be administered orally or IV and it is not treated as a controlled drug as other agents in the class are.

Unwanted effects

Sedation is the most widely reported side effect to benzodiazepines, although in this instance it is a desired effect. Treatment is also likely to cause confusion, dizziness, and muscle weakness, particularly in elderly patients and those with hepatic impairment where levels can accumulate. Anti-emetic courses should be kept short to avoid the risk of dependence or symptoms on withdrawal. Benzodiazepines are contraindicated in myasthenia gravis.

PRESCRIBING WARNING

Paradoxical reactions with benzodiazepines

Some patients, in particular children or the elderly, may experience a paradoxical excitatory effect with benzodiazepines presenting as anxiety, excitation, aggression, or sleep.

Drug interactions

The effects of benzodiazepines will be augmented in the presence of other CNS depressants, such as anxiolytics, barbiturates, sedatives, and anticonvulsants. At low doses further potential interactions are unlikely to cause problems.

Further reading

Horn CC, Wallisch WJ, Hormanics GE (2014) Pathophysiological and neurochemical mechanisms of postoperative nausea and vomiting. *European Journal of Pharmacology* 722, 55–66.

Hornby PJ (2001) Central neurocircuitry associated with emesis. *American Journal of Medicine* 111(8a), 1065–125.

Quigley EM, Hasler WL, Parkman HP (2001) AGA technical review on nausea and vomiting. *Gastroenterology* 120(1), 263–86.

Smith HS, Cox LR, Smith EJ (2012) 5-HT$_3$ receptor antagonists for the treatment of nausea/vomiting. *Annals of Palliative Medicine* 1(2), 115–20.

Guidelines

Gan TJ, Diemunsch P, Habib AS (2014) Consensus guidelines for managing postoperative nausea and vomiting. *Anaesthesia and Analgesics* 118(1), 85–113.

MacKinnon CJ, Arsenault MY, Bartellas E, et al. (2002) SOGC Clinical Practice Guidelines 120: The Management of Nausea & Vomiting of Pregnancy. https://www.sciencedirect.com/science/article/pii/S1701216316304753?via%3Dihub [accessed 5 April 2019].

NICE (2013) Antenatal care, NICE guideline CG62. https://www.nice.org.uk/guidance/cg62 [accessed 31 March 2019].

Roila F, Herrstedt J, Aapro M, et al. (2010) Guideline update for MASCC and ESMO in the prevention of chemotherapy- and radiotherapy-induced nausea and vomiting: results of the Perugia consensus conference *Annals of Oncology* 21(Suppl. 5), v232–43.

Scottish Palliative Care Guidelines. Symptom Control—Nausea and Vomiting. http://www.palliativecareguidelines.scot.nhs.uk/guidelines/symptom-control/Nausea-and-Vomiting.aspx [accessed 31 March 2019].

6.2 Dyspepsia (peptic ulceration and gastro-oesophageal reflux disease)

Dyspepsia is a disturbed digestion that is associated with symptoms of epigastric pain, nausea, heartburn, or vomiting. Around 40% of the adult population suffer these symptoms and approximately 10% seek medical advice. The majority of cases are functional and non-ulcer related, while around 25% are due to peptic ulcer disease and 25% to gastro-oesophageal reflux disease (GORD). Collectively, the proton pump inhibitors **lansoprazole** and **omeprazole**, account for more than 30 million prescriptions in the UK alone, making them some of the most widely used drug therapies.

Pathophysiology

The mammalian stomach contains a 0.1 M solution of hydrochloric acid (H^+Cl^-). Gastric acid secretion from gastric parietal cells, which line the stomach, occurs by activation of a membrane-bound proton-pump (an exchange of K^+ and H^+ ions; the H^+/K^+-ATPase). The hydrogen ions are obtained from hydrolysed carbonic acid (H_2CO_3), so HCO_3^- enters plasma in exchange for chloride ions (Cl^-). The Cl^- thus imported into the cell exits, via Cl^- channels in the apical membrane before reaching the stomach lumen (Figure 6.2). In order to maintain electroneutrality, each Cl^- that moves into the stomach lumen is accompanied by a K^+ that moves outward through a separate channel. Thus, the excess K^+ ions pumped inside the cell by the H^+/K^+-ATPase are returned to the lumen, helping maintain intracellular K^+ concentration. The end result is an accumulation of both H^+ and Cl^- ions in the gastric lumen, while the pH of the cytosol remains neutral and the excess OH^- and HCO_3^- transported into the blood.

The activity of this proton pump is controlled by histamine, gastrin, and acetylcholine, the latter two work through a Ca^{2+}-dependent pathway (adenylate cyclase) and the former via cAMP-dependent pathway; modification of these receptor pathways are some of the pharmacological targets used to treat dyspepsia, peptic ulcer disease, and GORD.

The acid secreted is normally protected from causing mucosal damage via several mechanisms; production of viscoelastic mucus, secretion of HCO_3^-, tight intracellular junctions and mucosal blood flow (delivering buffering HCO_3^-). Most of these processes are mediated by prostaglandin E_2 and PGI_2 and, in addition, these inhibit acid secretion and reduce endogenous histamine.

Dyspepsia

Dyspepsia symptoms are primarily a result of alterations in gastric motility (e.g. impaired fundus relaxation, antral dilation, and/or hypomotility, gastroparesis) and visceral sensation. In the latter it is thought that hypersensitivity to gastric distension results in bloating, pain, and nausea; the exact site is unknown, but may be mechanoreceptor, spinal, or brain in origin. The role of *Helicobacter pylori* in functional dyspepsia remains controversial, but there is

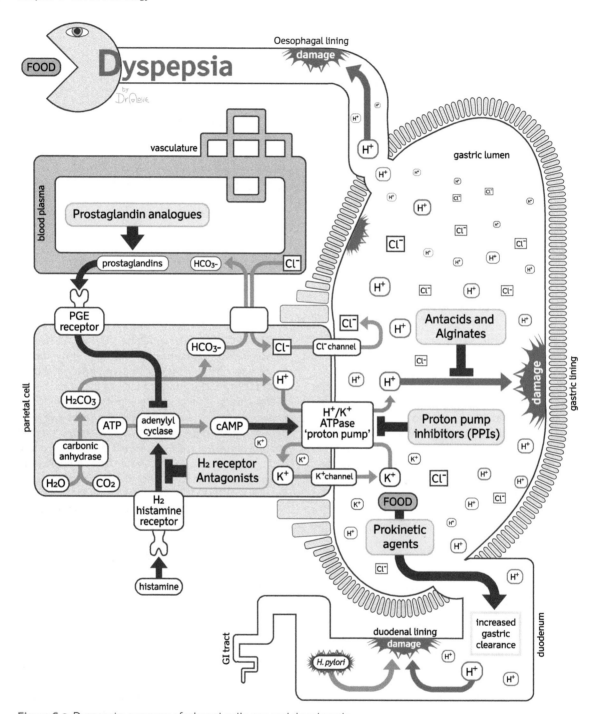

Figure 6.2 Dyspepsia: summary of relevant pathways and drug targets.

Table 6.6 Risk factors contributing to damaged mucosa

Proximal (type I) gastric ulcers	Distal ulcers (type II)—duodenum (80%), distal gastric portion (20%)
H. pylori infection in 70% of cases	Virtually all duodenal ulcers are associated with *H. pylori*
Drugs: NSAIDS, bisphosphonates, K+, corticosteroids	*Drugs*: NSAIDS, bisphosphonates, K+, corticosteroids
Smoking, alcohol	Smoking (strong), alcohol
Low or normal acid production	High acid production (including Zollinger–Ellison syndrome)
Age (peaks 30–55 years)	Age (peak incidence 20–35 years)
Male sex (M:F 3:1)	Male sex (M:F 4:1)

a known association in peptic ulceration (especially duodenal ulcer).

Peptic ulcer disease

Peptic ulcer disease is complete damage to the columnar mucosa of the GI wall caused by abnormal exposure to peptide juices; it encompasses gastric (proximal-type I) and duodenal (type II) ulcers primarily. The precise mechanism of mucosal erosion is unknown, but a number of risk factors are known to contribute (Table 6.6), damaging muscular mucosa, submucosa and beyond.

Where *H. pylori* is involved (e.g. duodenal ulcers) the gram-negative spiral micro-aerophilic bacillus is found in the gastric mucosal layer. It is abundant with urease and breaks down stomach urea to carbon dioxide and ammonia. Ammonia is converted to ammonium by accepting a proton that neutralizes gastric acid; *H. pylori* thus lives in an 'alkaline cloud' with its bi-products, ammonia, proteases, vacuolating cytotoxin A, and phospholipases being toxic to epithelial cells. Bacterial colonization leads to inflammation and gastritis, which overcomes the prostaglandin-mediated mucosa protective mechanisms.

NSAIDs can cause gastric erosion, primarily by inhibiting cycloxygenase-1 (COX-1), reducing levels of PGE_2 and PGI_2, and thus decreasing mucosal protective defence. This causes reduced gastric blood flow, which in turn reduces mucus and bicarbonate secretion and produces mucosal breakdown resulting in H^+ leaking and cytotoxicity through the uncoupling of cellular oxidative phosphorylation. Furthermore, the acidic nature of NSAIDs means they reduce the hydrophobicity of the mucoviscous layer.

Clinical presentation of peptic ulcer disease tends to fall into three categories: asymptomatic, typical symptoms, or complications. Typically, patients with gastric ulcers have epigastric pain on eating—weight loss, nausea, and vomiting may also occur. The duodenal ulcer (type II) may reveal itself as epigastric pain, worse at night (awaking the patient) or when fasting, that is relieved by foods/antacids and presents as relapsing/remitting 2-week cycles. While in GORD, symptoms are a mixture of heartburn, water-brash, nausea, nocturnal cough/exacerbation of asthma. Some patients present with ALARM flag symptoms (Box 6.1) and require urgent endoscopy.

For a full summary of the relevant pathways and drug targets, see Figure 6.2.

Management

In patients who present with dyspepsia, clinicians will need to exclude the presence of ALARM symptoms (see Box 6.1) and therefore the need for urgent referral (see Figure 6.3). In patients without these symptoms, primary management is through lifestyle advice, medication review, removal of precipitating factors (see Box 6.2) and

Box 6.1 ALARM flag symptoms in dyspepsia

ALARM Symptoms
- Persistent dyspepsia in patient aged over 55 years
- Unintentional weight loss (≥3 kg)
- Unexplained iron-deficiency anaemia
- GI bleeding
- Dysphagia and odynophagia
- Epigastric mass
- Previous gastric surgery or gastric ulcer

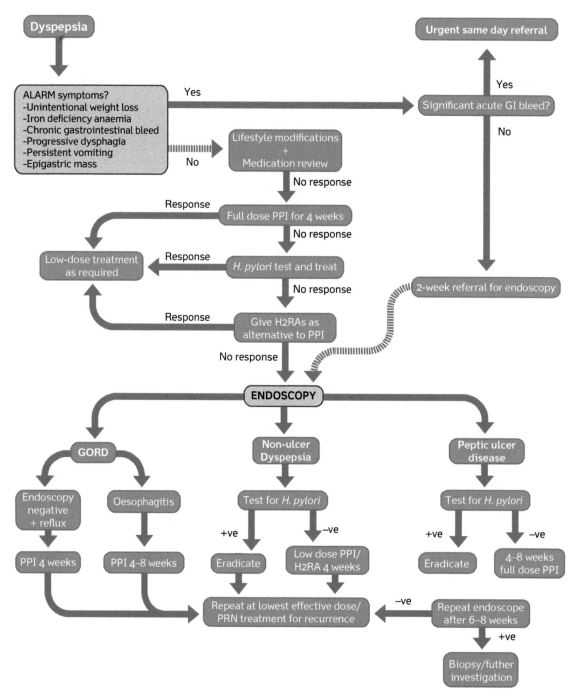

Figure 6.3 Management of dyspepsia.

Box 6.2 Lifestyle modifications to relieve symptoms of GORD

- Avoid dietary factors that precipitate symptoms, e.g. alcohol, coffee, spicy food, fatty food, chocolate
- Smaller meals
- Eat evening meal 3–4 hours before going to bed
- Weight loss in overweight/obese patients
- Stop smoking
- Raise the head of the bed
- Manage stress and anxiety, e.g. relaxation techniques
- Avoid drugs that may precipitate or aggravate symptoms (NSAIDs, steroids, calcium antagonists, nitrates, theophyllines, and bisphosphonates)

treatment. Antacids can benefit many, but in those where symptoms persist or return consider:

- *Empirical acid suppression [with proton pump inhibitor (PPI)]*: full dose for 1 month.
- *H. pylori* testing (e.g. stool antigen or laboratory serology) and eradicate if positive (see 'Helicobacter pylori').

GORD

GORD can be diagnosed by the presence of oesophagitis on endoscopy, or where there are predominant signs of reflux with a negative endoscope. First-line treatment is with a proton pump inhibitor used for a month. In patients who remain symptomatic, courses can be repeated and doses doubled where symptoms are severe. Failing this, H_2 receptor antagonists maybe considered as adjunctor alternative therapy. Where treatment remains unsuccessful prokinetics may be of value, although current advice only advocates their use in the short term. Patients should be encouraged to manage their symptoms through lifestyle measures and repeated courses of PPIs, stepping treatment up or down to find the lowest effective dose.

Dyspepsia

Patients with uninvestigated dyspepsia should be offered testing and treatment for *H. pylori*, allowing for a 2 weeks washout period if they are taking PPIs. In the absence of *H. pylori* or where not tested, patients can be offered 4 weeks of full-dose PPI. Where symptoms recur, patients

should be managed on the lowest possible dose of a PPI or H2RA, ideally on a when-required basis.

Helicobacter pylori

H. pylori is most commonly tested for by means of a stool antigen test or blood test (laboratory-based). Where a patient tests positive for *H. pylori* at any stage, an eradication programme should be initiated. This comprises a 7-day course of BD doses of a proton pump inhibitor in combination with two antibiotics from **amoxicillin**, **clarithromycin**, and **metronidazole**. Choice is determined from previous (failed) therapy and penicillin allergy (see Table 6.7), with an eradication rate of around 80%. Resistance to antibacterials used for the eradication of *H. pylori* is a growing problem that can lead to treatment failure and the need for subsequent courses of alternative agents. This may include the use of quadruple therapy.

Peptic ulcer disease

As with dyspepsia, patients with proven peptic ulcer disease should have any NSAID therapy stopped and be tested for *H. pylori*. The recommended treatment is 4–8 weeks (8 weeks if induced by an NSAID) with full dose proton pump inhibitors or, less commonly, a histamine antagonist and *H. pylori* eradication where tests are positive. A follow-up endoscopy after 6–8 weeks is necessary to ensure the gastric ulcer has healed, and where they remain unhealed a biopsy performed to exclude malignancy or other possible underlying causes. In patients who continue to require a NSAID, the risks should be discussed with the patient and consideration given to the use of low-dose ibuprofen or COX-2. A PPI should be prescribed concurrently in all cases.

Table 6.7 Eradication program for *H. pylori*

	Drug combination
First-line treatment	PPI + amoxicillin + clarithromycin/metronidazole
Treatment in penicillin allergy	PPI + clarithromycin + metronidazole
Penicillin allergy with previous clarithromycin use	PPI + bismuth + metronidazole + tetracycline

Drug classes used in management

Antacids and alginates

Antacids act mainly by neutralizing hydrochloric acid in the gastric secretions thus raising the gastric pH. Examples include aluminium hydroxide, calcium carbonate, magnesium carbonate, magnesium trisilicate, alginic acid, and sodium alginate.

Mechanism of action

The increase in gastric pH has the effect of inhibiting peptic activity, but beyond their ability to buffer gastric acid secretion, antacids can also modulate some of the processes that are part of the pathogenesis of peptic ulcer. The antacids that have **aluminium hydroxide** in particular have been shown to chelate bile salts, stimulate mucoprotein secretion, and decrease pepsin concentration. Since antacids produce similar results in the treatment of duodenal ulcer patients with hypersecretion and normal secretion; this might indicate a cytoprotective effect that is dependent on the augmented production of substances that are capable of protecting the mucosa, i.e. endogenous prostaglandins.

Alginates are natural polysaccharide polymers isolated from brown seaweed, which are widely used in the pharmaceutical industry. Alginate preparations react with gastric acid to create a strong viscous gel, or alginate 'raft', of a near-neutral pH that floats on the gastric contents and protects the oesophageal mucosa during reflux. Preparations are normally combined with an antacid, which might be responsible for much of the clinical effect.

Prescribing

Antacids and alginates for the symptomatic relief of dyspepsia are available over the counter (without prescription) enabling self-medication, but should not be used frequently or long-term. Preparations contain either single agents or more commonly a combination of salts intended to neutralize acidity and/or prevent reflux. There is little to choose between them, although many favour the alginate preparations, which tend to be better tolerated. Choice is otherwise dictated by taste, formulation, cost, and familiarity.

Unwanted effects

Although generally well tolerated, antacids in particular can cause side effects depending on the salts used. Adverse effects are invariably GI such as diarrhoea with **magnesium**, or constipation with **aluminium hydroxide** or **calcium carbonate**-containing preparations. Preparations containing calcium carbonate, magnesium trisilicate, and magnesium carbonate form carbon dioxide within the acidic pH of the stomach leading to flatulence. This may be partly overcome by the presence of **simeticone** within the formulation.

Due to the presence of electrolytes in many of the preparations, serum levels may be deranged with frequent or long-term use. The prolonged use of silica-based products may also cause renal stones, while calcium carbonate can cause a rebound in acid secretion when used long term.

PRACTICAL PRESCRIBING
Sodium content
It is worth checking the sodium content of antacids before recommending to a patient on a low sodium diet, as levels in some combination products are high.

Drug interactions

As antacids affect the gastric pH and gastric emptying time, there is a theoretical risk of interacting with other drugs that are reliant on an acidic pH for absorption. Manufacturers of some drugs therefore recommend that they should not be taken at the same time of day as some oral therapies, e.g. **ciprofloxacin** (and other quinolones), tetracyclines, **azithromycin**, and **itraconazole** (capsules only). Manufacturers of **ulipristal** advise avoiding concomitant use.

Proton pump inhibitors

Proton pump inhibitors reduce gastric secretions by inhibiting H^+/K^+-ATPase of parietal cells, affecting the final common step in acid production. Examples include esomeprazole, lansoprazole, omeprazole, pantoprazole, and rabeprazole.

Mechanism of action

Omeprazole is a weak base that is inactive at neutral pH in the cell cytoplasm, but gains a proton when it passes to the acidic environment of parietal canaliculi, being converted to a sulphonamide. As such, omeprazole couples irreversibly to the cysteine in the α-subunit of the H^+/K^+-ATPase, so that the expulsion of H^+ and intrusion of K^+ ions is halted. Inhibition of the pump lasts for 16–18 hours and returns to normal within 4 days. It is eliminated via the liver and has a short plasma half-life, although the effects are considerably prolonged (up to a day) due to the irreversible inhibition of the ATPase.

Although PPIs were first synthesized as racemic mixtures of two optical isomers, it has now been established that S-omeprazole (**esomeprazole**) has greater efficacy, albeit with similar pharmacology. This is due to the fact that the S-form is metabolized less efficiently, which results in more sustained serum concentrations. While the clinical significance of optical pure isoforms has been questioned, various delayed-delivery systems are being tested, including multilayer coatings that allow the interval release of agents.

Prescribing

Despite data to suggest that **esomeprazole** is more effective than other PPIs in controlling stomach acid, this is not reflected in prescribing trends, largely due to cost and the good results achieved with other agents in the class. All agents are inactivated by the acidic pH of the stomach and so are presented in gastro-resistant formulations to ensure they reach the small intestine where they are absorbed. Consequently, neither tablets nor the contents of the capsule should be crushed to aid with administration. All agents are available as either a capsule and/or a tablet to be taken OD; with **omeprazole**, esomeprazole, and **pantoprazole** also available in IV formulations. Oral doses are best taken in the morning to optimize their effects.

> ### PRESCRIBING WARNING
>
> **Proton pump inhibitors**
> If empirical acid suppression is given, patients should be monitored after 1–2 months of treatment to ensure there are no emergent ALARM symptoms. Do not continue repeat prescriptions in perpetuity.

Unwanted effects

As proton pump inhibitors can mask the symptoms of a gastric malignancy, any patients presenting with ALARM symptoms should be investigated before starting treatment. Elimination is primarily via the liver, thus lower doses are recommended in severe hepatic impairment.

In general, the PPIs are well tolerated, the most commonly reported side effect being GI (abdominal pain,

nausea, constipation, diarrhoea, and flatulence) and headaches. More severe side effects are rare, but may include hypersensitivity reactions such as anaphylaxis or Stevens–Johnson syndrome.

As treatment has a profound effect on gastric pH, there is the potential for an increased risk of infections, such as *Clostridium difficile*.

Drug interactions

Drug interactions are surprisingly frequent with PPIs, in particular with **esomeprazole** and **omeprazole**, due to their inhibitory effects on the CYP2C19; an enzyme implicated in the metabolism of numerous drugs. Interactions to be particularly aware of include the increased effects of **warfarin**, **phenytoin**, **cilostazol**, and **diazepam**. Alternative PPIs may be worth considering in patients requiring these drugs.

As a class, their effect on gastric pH can disrupt the absorption of some drugs, causing either a reduction in the plasma levels, e.g. **nelfinavir**, **atazanavir**, and **clopidogrel**, or an increase, e.g. **digoxin** levels. As with other antacids, manufacturers of **ulipristal** recommend avoiding concurrent use.

> ### PRESCRIBING WARNING
>
> **Clopidogrel and PPIs**
> Concomitant use of clopidogrel with PPIs has been associated with reduced efficacy of clopidogrel and an increased risk of MI and death. Prescribing of PPIs in patients on clopidogrel should therefore be done with caution

H$_2$ receptor antagonists

Histamine H$_2$ antagonists act at surface histamine receptors on gastric parietal cells, inhibiting a cAMP-dependent pathway and reducing the activity of the H$^+$/K$^+$-ATPase, hence decreasing acid extrusion. For example, famotidine, nizatidine, and ranitidine.

Mechanism of action

The discovery that there was more than one type of histamine receptor led to the development of novel agents targeting the H$_2$ subtype. **Cimetidine** was introduced in the 1970s, and became the mainstay of acid suppression before the development of PPIs. The competitive antagonism on H_2 receptors reduces direct acid secretion by 60% and pepsin production. It also inhibits the increased production of secretin following stimulation in the acidic pH of the duodenum. Above pH 4 secretin production is halted. Hence, H_2 receptor antagonists are not as effective as PPIs at reducing acid levels.

With prolonged usage, there is a change in the response to the histamine antagonists and a surge in basal acid secretion after cessation of treatment. Potential reasons for these observations are the 'up-regulation' of the H_2 receptors (rise in number and/or sensitivity) or the growth in parietal cell mass, thereby increasing the response to stimuli, both endogenous and/or exogenous.

Prescribing

Of the H_2 receptor antagonists, **ranitidine** is the most widely used, being available in the widest range of formulations (tablets, effervescent tablets, liquids, injection) for the greatest range of indications and at low cost. At lower doses, it may also be purchased over the counter.

Cimetidine, although the first in the class to be licensed, is no longer available in the UK as it causes QT prolongation leading to ventricular arrhythmias, responsible for over 100 patient deaths worldwide. It is also prone to drug interactions, (see 'Drug interactions'). **Nizatidine** is the only other H_2 receptor antagonist available in an IV formulation, but as with **famotidine** it is rarely prescribed.

Unwanted effects

As with PPIs, H_2 receptor antagonists can mask symptoms of gastric ulceration and so should be withheld in patients with ALARM symptoms until they have been investigated. As a class they are well tolerated, the incidence of side effects similar to placebo. The most commonly reported effects include diarrhoea, headache, dizziness, rash, and fatigue. **Cimetidine** is also reported to possess anti-androgen properties, which can rarely cause gynaecomastia. Side effects are dose-related and tend to resolve with continued use.

In agents available as injections, IV administration should be slow (over at least 2 minutes) to reduce the risk of bradycardia.

Drug interactions

Cimetidine is an inhibitor of numerous subgroups of the cytochrome P450 enzyme, increasing the effects of many drugs metabolized though this pathway. Of particular significance is its effect on **warfarin** (and other anticoagulants), **carbamazepine**, **phenytoin**, **theophylline**, **amiodarone**, CCBs, and IV **lidocaine**.

As with the PPIs, H_2 receptor antagonists can alter the absorption of some drugs reliant on the acidic pH of the stomach, thereby decreasing absorption, e.g. **itraconazole**, **posaconazole**, **atazanavir**, and **ulipristal**.

Prokinetic agents

> Prokinetic agents are used to stimulate, either directly or indirectly, smooth muscle contractions leading to enhancement of gastric emptying and acceleration of bowel transit. For example, domperidone and metoclopramide.

Mechanism of action

Dopamine receptor antagonists, serotonergic agents acting as agonists at the 5-HT_4 receptor and motilin receptor agonists are the drugs presently used for stimulation of gastric movements. Newer drugs are also being developed, targeting dopaminergic and serotonergic receptors, as well as cholecystokinin receptor antagonists.

Among the existing prokinetic compounds **metoclopramide** and **domperidone** are the most commonly used. Domperidone is a butyrophenone derivative that exerts anti-dopaminergic properties at peripheral D_2 receptors without crossing the blood–brain barrier.

Metoclopramide, a substituted benzamide, is a major dopamine receptor antagonist that has been used as a prokinetic for at least 35 years. In addition to its action on D_2 receptors, metoclopromide binds to serotonergic receptors at high doses, having moderate partial 5-HT_4 receptor agonism and weak 5-HT_3 receptor antagonism. It has been indicated that 5-HT_4 receptor activation by metoclopramide provides its GI prokinetic action by increasing the release of acetylcholine (ACh) from intrinsic cholinergic motor neurons.

Opioid receptor antagonists have also been developed as prokinetic agents, given that opioids can inhibit propulsive motility and cause constipation in healthy subjects. **Alvimopan** is an orally active opioid antagonist that is peripherally restricted and has promising prokinetic properties

Prescribing

The use of prokinetics as an add-on in dyspepsia has fallen out of favour due to unacceptable toxicity. More recently, warnings have been issued by the MHRA for both **domperidone** (cardiac toxicity) and **metoclopramide** (neurological toxicity) with regards to their usage. Where used, they are only recommended as anti-emetics and should be used for the shortest possible duration (see 'Prescribing warning: metoclopramide-induced neurotoxicity' and 'Prescribing warning: domperidone induced cardiac toxicity').

> ### PRESCRIBING WARNING
>
> **Metoclopramide-induced neurotoxicity**
> - Metoclopramide can cause neurological effects, including extrapyramidal disorders and tardive dyskinesia.
> - To reduce the risk it should only be prescribed for up to 5 days and no longer used for chronic conditions, including dyspepsia and GORD.

> ### PRESCRIBING WARNING
>
> **Domperidone induced cardiac toxicity**
> - Domperidone has been associated with an increased risk of cardiac toxicity, particularly in patients over 60 years of age, or taking QT-prolonging drugs or CYP 3A4 inhibitors concomitantly.
> - To reduce the risk domperidone should be prescribed at the lowest possible dose for the shortest possible duration (<1 week).
> - Use is contraindicated in patients with severe hepatic impairment, cardiac conduction disorders, heart failure, or with concomitant CYP3A4 inhibitors/QT-prolonging drugs.

Unwanted effects

For more information on **domperidone** and **metoclopramide** see Topic 6.1, 'Nausea and vomiting'.

Prostaglandin analogues

> Prostaglandin analogues, like misoprostol, are used to reduce NSAID-induced gastric damage. For example, misoprostol.

Mechanism of action

Dyspepsia, gastric irritation, and gastric ulceration are some of the GI problems derived from inhibition of mucosal production of prostaglandins associated with NSAID treatment.

Misoprostol is a prostaglandin E_1 analogue used for the prevention and treatment of gastric ulcers associated with the use of NSAIDs. In addition to its gastric acid antisecretory effects, misoprostol increases the thickness of the mucosa layers, diluting the concentrations and increasing the distance that NSAIDs must go through to reach susceptible cells. As an analogue of prostaglandins, misoprostol can prevent the release of various tissue-damaging cytokines and inflammatory mediators from the intestinal mucosa.

Prescribing

Although **misoprostol** is indicated for the treatment or prevention of gastric ulcers specifically associated with the use of NSAIDs, it is rarely used in clinical practice and where used, is done so as prophylaxis in combination preparations with NSAIDs such as **diclofenac** or **naproxen**. Changes in practice have seen its use replaced with PPIs in combination with a NSAID, when a NSAID is indicated in at risk patients, as this is supported by a greater body of evidence.

Misoprostol is now generally used more often off-label in the medical management of miscarriage or as a treatment option in post-partum haemorrhage (see Topic 4.6, 'Female reproduction (abnormal menstruation, contraception, assisted reproduction)').

Unwanted effects

As a prostaglandin analogue, **misoprostol** increases uterine tone and contraction, which can lead to the premature expulsion of the foetus. When not used specifically for this purpose, it is therefore contraindicated in pregnancy and should be avoided in women of childbearing age unless they are taking effective contraceptive measures and have been counselled on the risks.

The most common adverse effect to misoprostol is diarrhoea, affecting over 8% of users and although dose-related, is usually mild and self-limiting; in some patients it can be severe enough to necessitate withdrawal. Manufacturers caution its use in patients who are predisposed to diarrhoea, e.g. IBD. Other common effects include abdominal pain, nausea, dyspepsia, headache, dizziness, and rash.

Drug interactions

Care should be taken when co-prescribing with other drugs known to cause diarrhoea, in particular magnesium-containing antacids or laxatives.

Further reading

Devault KR and Talley NJ (2009) Insights into the future of gastric acid suppression. *Nature Review: Gastroenterology and Hepatology* 6(9), 524–32.

Leontiadis GI, Sharma VK, Howden CW (2006) Proton pump inhibitor treatment for acute peptic ulcer bleeding (Cochrane Review). *The Cochrane Library*, Issue 1. Harlow: John Wiley & Sons, Ltd.

Malfertheiner P, Megraud F, O'Morain C et al. (2007) Current concepts in the management of Helicobacter pylori infection: the Maastricht III Consensus Report. *Gut* 56(6), 772–81.

Neale G (2003) Symptomatology of gastrointestinal disease. In: Warrell DA, Cox TM, Firth JD and Benz EJ (Eds) *Oxford textbook of medicine: volume 2*, 4th edn, pp. 486–9. Oxford: Oxford University Press.

Thumshirn M (2002) Pathophysiology of functional dyspepsia. *Gut* 51(Suppl. I), i63–6.

Wang X, Fang JY, Lu R, Sun DF (2006) A meta-analysis: comparison of esomeprazole and other proton pump inhibitors in eradicating *Helicobacter pylori*. *Digestion* 73(2–3), 178–86.

Guidelines

NICE CG184 (Sept 2014) Gastro-oesphageal reflux disease and dyspepsia in adults: investigation and management. NICE guideline CG184. https://www.nice.org.uk/guidance/cg184 [accessed 31 March 2019].

NICE Pathway Dyspepsia and gastro-oesophageal reflux disease overview http://pathways.nice.org.uk/pathways/dyspepsia-and-gastro-oesophageal-reflux-disease [accessed 31 March 2019].

NICE QS96 (July 2015) Dyspepsia and gastro-oesophageal reflux disease in adults. NICE guideline QS96. https://www.nice.org.uk/guidance/qs96 [accessed 31 March 2019].

6.3 Diarrhoea

Diarrhoea is an increase in stool water and volume, leading to unformed or liquid stool that is increased in frequency or quantity (typically >200 mL/day). This can be due to:

- Increased intestinal secretion that occurs in the absence of macroscopic or microscopic injury, following exposure to secretory enterotoxins.
- Decreased intestinal absorption as a consequence of intestinal damage or inflammation.

In reality, the pathogenesis involves a combination of both. Diarrhoea is either acute (<4 weeks) or chronic (>4 weeks) in nature.

Pathophysiology

The pathophysiological basis of diarrhoea is due to four mechanisms, which can act alone or in combination:

- Increased osmotic load in the gut lumen occurring when a soluble compound cannot be absorbed and draws fluid into the intestinal lumen (Figure 6.4). It stops with fasting.
- Uncontrolled secretion of water into the bowel lumen that results from prolonged opening of Cl⁻ channels. Infections (e.g. *Vibrio cholera*), drugs (e.g. diuretics, **theophylline**), and gut allergies cause secretory diarrhoea; it persists with fasting. In colonization, bacterial enterotoxins have a variety of effects on gut mucosa epithelial ion transport; they stimulate adenylate cyclase causing intracellular rise in cyclic adenosine monophosphate, which leads to Cl⁻ channel opening and augmented Cl⁻ secretion into the bowel (Figure 6.4).
- Inflammation of the intestinal lining and breakdown of the GI barrier leads to exudation of serum and blood into gut lumen, with water absorption being substantially affected. Activation of leucocytes causes production of inflammatory mediators, cytokines (TNF-α, interferon-γ and IL-1), and reactive oxygen species, which further stimulates secretion and damages intestinal epithelial cells.

- Increased intestinal motility and accelerated transport time decreases absorption of fluid and nutrient; hypermotility can be seen in all causes of diarrhoea (see Topic 6.5, 'Irritable bowel syndrome' and Topic 6.6, 'Inflammatory bowel disease').

Acute episodes in adults typically occur once per year and are self-limiting, lasting for 2–5 days. Most causes are infective, so it is important to establish the characteristics of the stool, presence of fever, and any contact they may have had with others who have diarrhoea (viral gastroenteritis); have they eaten the same food or in the same restaurant (*Salmonella*), or travelled with others who have symptoms. Bacterial causes tend to include infections from *Campylobacter jejuni*, *Shigella* spp., and *Escherichia coli*, the former being most common in primary care. The presence of blood in the diarrhoea may also be related to bacteria (e.g. *C. jejuni*, *E. coli* O157:H7, *Shigella*, *Yersinia*, *Aeromonas*, *Cl. difficile*), viruses (cytomegalovirus), or parasites (*Entamoeba histolytica*, schistosomiasis).

Patients starting on new drugs (e.g. **allopurinol**, angiotensin-II receptor blockers, magnesium-containing antacids, NSAIDs, proton pump inhibitors, SSRIs, statins, **levothyroxine**, or antibiotics) may report diarrhoea. Recent antibiotic use should prompt consideration of *Cl. difficile*, which causes pseudomembranous colitis. Viral gastroenteritis is more common than a bacterial cause in children.

In chronic diarrhoea, the causes may not only be related to infection, but also to ongoing systemic pathology and, as such, they can present clinically in subtly different ways (see Table 6.8).

If the history indicates a public health risk or community risk, then Public Health England (PHE) can be

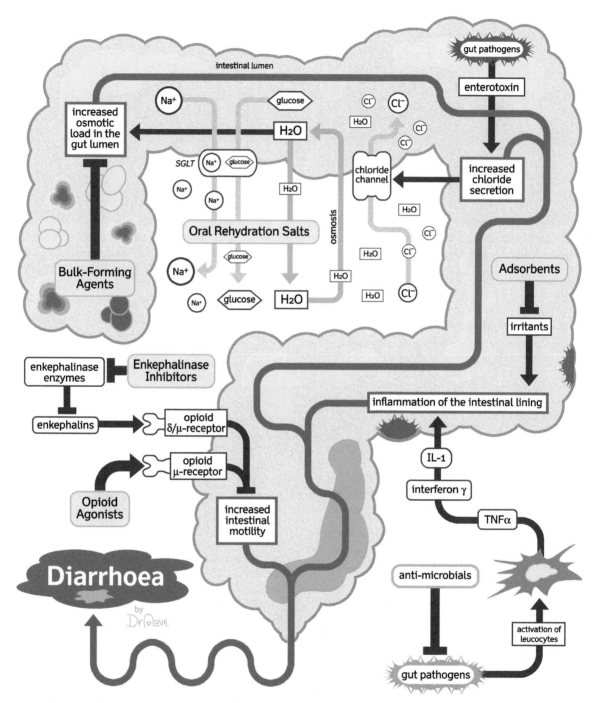

Figure 6.4 Diarrhoea: summary of relevant pathways and drug targets.

Table 6.8 Causes and clinical presentation of chronic diarrhoea

Causes of chronic diarrhoea	Clinical presentation
Infection with *Giardia*	Chronic diarrhoea, malabsorption, weight loss, abdominal pain, flatulence, bloating; fever is uncommon
Infection with *Cryptosporidium*	Sudden onset of watery diarrhoea (often green and offensive ± blood) with abdominal cramps
Infection with *Entamoeba histolytica*	Lower abdominal pain and diarrhoea with latterly blood and mucus in stool
Inflammatory bowel disease	Relapsing/remitting GI symptoms (diarrhoea ± blood and mucus). Abdominal pain, fever, weight loss, and extra-abdominal manifestations (see Topic 6.6)
Irritable bowel syndrome	low-volume diarrhoea, often in mornings and following meals, and may involve faecal urgency (see Topic 6.5)
Coeliac disease	Folate or iron deficient anaemia, abdominal discomfort, arthralgia, and malaise. Diarrhoea, steatorrhoea and malabsorption are common
Bile acid malabsorption (e.g. Crohn's disease, after ileal resection, cholecystectomy)	Levels of bile acids to increase, which stimulates electrolyte and water secretion, resulting in diarrhoea
Colorectal cancer	Altered bowel habit, blood may be mixed in the stool, weight loss, and abdominal pain

contacted for advice. In all patients with acute or chronic presentation, it is important to assess for signs of clinical dehydration or shock (Table 6.9) and treat effectively (see 'Management').

For a full summary of the relevant pathways and drug targets, see Figure 6.4.

Management

Acute diarrhoea is invariably self-limiting, with further investigation often unnecessary. Patients should be asked about current medication or treatment, including chemotherapy, radiotherapy, or even chronic laxative abuse. Patients who are systemically unwell, have blood or pus in their stool, have recently received antibiotics, or have travelled, should have stools sent for culture and sensitivities. In the case of severe dehydration or shock, patients should be referred to secondary care for fluid management. Referral should also be considered with symptoms such as bloody stools, fever, or abdominal pain, particularly in the elderly or those with chronic co-morbidities. Patients with chronic diarrhoea lasting more than 14 days and where infection has been excluded, should undergo further investigations (see Table 6.10).

Management of diarrhoea will be determined by the underlying cause, such as the introduction of a gluten-free diet in coeliac disease or the use of antibiotics with some bacterial infections. Where drug therapy is implicated as the cause, consideration should be given to stopping, switching, or reducing doses where possible to manage symptoms.

Primary management of acute diarrhoea is with oral rehydration therapy (ORT) to replace losses, although in severe cases, or in patients unable to tolerate oral input, IV therapy may be necessary. Patients may eat as they are able, but should ideally avoid dairy products (due to the risk of dairy intolerance), carbonated drinks, and caffeine. Additional symptomatic management with anti-motility agents, such as **loperamide** or **racecadotril**, may be used cautiously in acute mild or moderate diarrhoea, but avoided in the case of infection or colitis due to the risk of toxic megacolon (acute toxic colitis with dilatation of the colon).

Antibiotics are rarely indicated for the acute management of diarrhoea (including traveller's diarrhoea), unless symptoms persist or they are caused by certain organisms, e.g. *Cl. difficile*, *Shigella* and *Salmonella*. Quinolones, such as **ciprofloxacin**, are effective in the management of most infectious causes of diarrhoea, with the exception of *Cl. difficile*

Table 6.9 Signs of clinical dehydration

Symptom	Minimal or no dehydration (<3% loss of body weight)	Mild to moderate dehydration (3%–9% loss of body weight)	Severe dehydration (>9% loss of body weight)
Mental status	Well; alert	Normal, fatigued or restless, irritable	Apathetic, lethargic, unconscious
Thirst	Drinks normally; might refuse liquids	Thirsty; eager to drink	Drinks poorly; unable to drink
Heart rate	Normal	Normal to increased	Tachycardia, with bradycardia in most severe cases
Quality of pulses	Normal	Normal to decreased	Weak, thread, or impalpable
Breathing	Normal	Normal: fast	Deep
Eyes	Normal	Slightly sunken	Deeply sunken
Tears	Present	Deceased	Absent
Mouth and tongue	Moist	Dry	Parched
Skin fold	Instant recoil	Recoil in <2 seconds	Recoil in >2 seconds
Capillary refill	Normal	Prolonged	Prolonged; minimal
Extremities	Warm	Cool	Cold; mottled; cyanotic
Urine output	Normal to decreased	Decreased	Minimal

Sources: Adapted from Duggan C, Santosham M, Glass RI. (1992) The management of acute diarrhea in children: oral rehydration, maintenance, and nutritional therapy. *Mortality and Morbidity Weekly Report* 41(No. RR-16), 1–20; and World Health Organization (1995) The treatment of diarrhoea: a manual for physicians and other senior health workers. Geneva: World Health Organization. https://apps.who.int/iris/bitstream/handle/10665/43209/9241593180.pdf;sequence=1 [accessed 1 April 2019]. Data from King, C.K. et al. Centers for Disease Control and Prevention. Managing acute gastroenteritis among children: oral rehydration, maintenance, and nutritional therapy. *MMWR Recomm Rep.* 2003 Nov 21;52(RR-16):1–16.

Table 6.10 Investigations and systemic causes of chronic diarrhoea

Investigation	Possible cause
Full blood count	Anaemia, inflammation
LFTs including albumin	Alcoholic liver cirrhosis
Calcium, vitamin B_{12}, ferritin, folate	Malabsorption
Thyroid function tests	Hyperthyroidism
ESR, CRP, FBC	IBD
Antibody testing	Coeliac disease
Sigmoidoscopy, colonoscopy	IBD, cancer

where oral **vancomycin** or **metronidazole** can be used. More recently the role of faecal transplantation has gained popularity in managing resistant cases of *Cl. difficile*. Some causes of diarrhoea, such as *E. coli* and food poisoning, are notifiable diseases, for which PHE should be informed.

Drug classes used in management

Oral rehydration salts

Polymeric solutions for oral rehydration therapy allow the treatment of diarrhoea with a sharp reduction of nausea and vomiting, decrease of fluid loss, and illness duration.

Mechanism of action

The discovery that the intestinal mucosa requires the translocation of a Na^+ for each molecule of glucose, led to the development of the oral rehydration salts (ORS) formula for the treatment of diarrhoea. Although early ORS formulations did not shorten illness or reduce the amount of purging or vomiting, it was later found that when food polymers (starches and proteins) are substituted for glucose or sucrose, the duration of diarrhoea can be reduced. This is due to the increase in co-transporting molecules that are made available at the intestinal epithelium. As a result, more Na^+ and with it water, can be moved from the lumen of the gut into the blood stream and lymphatics, without any increase in the osmolality of the solutions used.

Prescribing

Commercially available formulations of ORSs are based on the ORS formula (see Table 6.11), with an osmolarity of 245 mmol/L to prevent it from causing osmotic diarrhoea.

Solutions available in the UK tend to have lower sodium content, as sodium loss in the UK secondary to diarrhoea is often less severe. Sachets are made up with cool water and 200–400 mL taken following each loose motion. In an adult, the fluid requirement is equivalent to about 20–40 mL/Kg/day.

Unwanted effects

When oral rehydration solutions are used in primary care, patients should be advised to seek help if symptoms persist for longer than 48 hours. Care should be taken in patients that are fluid restricted, e.g. in renal impairment, and glucose content taken into consideration when administered to diabetic patients.

Overdose, although rare, is possible in patients with renal impairment, potentially causing hyperkalaemia or hypernatraemia, particularly with prolonged or excessive use.

Bulk-forming agents

Bulking agents absorb water in the intestinal tract and can be used in some cases of non-acute diarrhoea. For example, sterculia, ispaghula husk, and methylcellulose.

Mechanism of action

Bulk-forming agents are better known for their role in constipation, but the ability of some organic polymers to hold extra water in the stool means that they are also indicated in the management of diarrhoea. By absorbing water, bulking agents can increase faecal mass and adjust faecal consistency.

Prescribing

The bulking agents **methylcellulose**, **ispaghula husk**, and **sterculia**, although rarely used in the management of diarrhoea, may be of benefit in reducing symptoms associated with diverticular or IBD as part of a 'high residue' or high fibre diet.

Unwanted effects

Bulk-forming agents are not recommended for acute diarrhoea and should be avoided in diarrhoea of infectious causes, and in the case of severe dehydration. Neither should they be used in faecal impaction. Flatulence and abdominal discomfort are the most widely reported side effects.

Table 6.11 ORS formula (WHO/UNICEF)

Ingredient	g/L	Electrolyte	mmol/L
Sodium chloride	2.6	Sodium	75
Glucose, anhydrous	13.5	Chloride	65
Potassium chloride	1.5	Glucose, anhydrous	75
Trisodium citrate, dehydrate	2.9	Potassium	20
		Citrate	10

Reprinted from WHO/ UNICEF (2006). Oral Rehydration Salts: Production of the new ORS. © World Health Organization 2006. http://apps.who.int/iris/bitstream/10665/69227/1/WHO_FCH_CAH_06.1.pdf?ua=1&ua=1

Opioid agonists

Opioid agonists decrease gut motility and are useful first line drugs for the treatment of diarrhoea. For example, loperamide, diphenoxylate, and codeine.

Mechanism of action

Opioid receptor agonists, such as **loperamide**, are the main pharmacological agents used to decrease gut motility. Their anti-motility action is a result of binding to opioid μ-receptors on neurons in the submucosal neural plexus of the intestinal wall. They increase the tone and segmental contractions in the colon and diminish propulsive activity, as well as increasing luminal water absorption and decreasing secretion, mostly due to the prolonged transit time of intestinal contents.

Loperamide has a relatively selective action on the GI tract and in addition to its effect on opioid receptors, it has additional antimuscarinic activity that inhibits peristalsis and may also increase rectal tone. Its high first-pass metabolism limits systemic absorption and, in contrast to other opiates, **morphine**-like dependence is not a problem. Both loperamide and **codeine** have antisecretory actions in addition to their effects on gut motility, but the latter should generally be avoided due to the high risk of opioid dependence. Although large doses of **diphenoxylate** can also produce dependence, therapeutic doses suitable for the treatment of diarrhoea should be safe from opioid effects in the CNS.

Prescribing

Where an anti-motility agent is deemed appropriate **loperamide** is invariably the drug of choice, available as capsules, orodispersible tablets, and liquid. Although **codeine** is also used for this indication, it has the potential for abuse and is associated with a greater side effect profile. Remedies available over the counter include co-phenotrope, which contains a combination of **diphenoxylate** with **atropine**.

PRACTICAL PRESCRIBING

Formulation choice

Formulations that are more rapidly absorbed, such as liquids or orodispersible tablets, may be more beneficial than capsules in patients where absorption is impaired, such as stomas or short bowel syndrome.

Unwanted effects

Anti-motility agents should not be used in patients where inhibition of peristalsis could lead to toxic megacolon or paralytic ileus. For this reason they are best avoided in acute ulcerative colitis, intestinal obstruction, and antibiotic associated colitis.

Common side effects to anti-motility agents include constipation and abdominal discomfort. As **codeine** is less selective than **loperamide** for the GI tract, it is less well tolerated and associated with significantly greater neurological toxicity such as dizziness and drowsiness.

Adsorbents

Adsorbents such as kaolin and pectin are relatively ineffective in the treatment of diarrhoea and are no longer recommended for therapy.

Mechanism of action

In theory, adsorbents are capable of interacting with irritants and other harmful substances that are present in the intestine (e.g. micro-organisms). In the process that leads adsorbents to be moved through the intestine and excreted, irritants would be carried with them. Their real efficacy, however, has never been proven and no effect on either the severity or duration of diarrhoea has been demonstrated.

Prescribing

Despite the fact that **light kaolin** is no longer recommended for use, it remains available either on its own (for use in children), or in combination with **morphine** in some preparations available over the counter to relieve 'occasional' diarrhoea.

Unwanted effects

Although **light kaolin** itself is relatively well tolerated, it can mask the presence of a more severe underlying aetiology; therefore, patients self-medicating with adsorbents should be advised to avoid long-term use. Many of the common side effects are associated with the presence of **morphine**.

Drug interactions

Adsorbents have the potential to impair the absorption of medication from the GI tract and should not be taken at the same time as other medication, in particular, **chloroquine**, **aspirin**, and **tetracyclines**.

Enkephalinase inhibitors

These agents inhibit the action of endogenous peptides, including enkephalin thereby reducing hypersecretion of water and electrolytes. For example, racecadotril.

Mechanism of action

Racecadotril, the first in its class, is a pro-drug of the enkephalinase inhibitor, thiorphan. Enkephalinase enzymes are membrane bound and responsible for the degradation of the endogenous opioids, enkephalins. By inhibiting enzyme degradation, there is a subsequent increase in opioid availability and therefore greater activation of δ opioid receptors. This leads to a reduction in cAMP levels in the mucosa and, therefore, reduced secretion of water and electrolytes into the intestinal lumen.

Prescribing

Racecadotril is indicated for use in adults, children, and infants for the symptomatic relief of uncomplicated acute diarrhoea in combination with rehydration. It is administered orally TDS until diarrhoea stops, for a maximum of 7 days. Doses are available as capsules or granules, the latter to aid with dosing and administration in young children and infants.

Unwanted effects

Racecadotril is generally well tolerated, although it has been known to cause rashes. The granules for suspension contain a high concentration of sucrose, which may be an issue in diabetics.

Further reading

Baldi F, Bianco, MA, Nardone G, et al. (2009) Focus on acute diarrhoeal disease. *World Journal of Gastroenterology* 15(27), 3341–8.

Kroser JA, Metz DC (1996) Evaluation of the adult patient with diarrhoea. *Primary Care* 23(3), 629–47.

Matheson AJ, Noble S (2000) Racecadotril. *Drugs* 59(4), 829–35.

Schiller LR (2007) Management of diarrhoea in clinical practice: strategies for primary care physicians. *Reviews in Gastroenterological Disorders* **7**(Suppl. 3), S27–8.

Thomas PD, Forbes A, Green J, et al. (2003) Guidelines for the investigation of chronic diarrhoea, 2nd edition. *Gut* 52(Suppl. 5) v1–15.

Guidelines

NICE CG61 (2008) Irritable bowel syndrome in adults: diagnosis and management of irritable bowel syndrome in primary care. NICE guideline CG61. https://www.nice.org.uk/guidance/cg61 [accessed 1 April 2019].

NICE ESNM11 (2013) Acute diarrhoea in adults: racecadotril. NICE guideline ESNM11. https://www.nice.org.uk/advice/esnm11/chapter/Relevance-to-NICE-guidance-programmes [accessed 1 April 2019].

World Gastroenterology Organisation (2008) World Gastroenterology Practice Guideline Acute diarrhea. http://www.worldgastroenterology.org/guidelines/global-guidelines/acute-diarrhea [accessed 1 April 2019].

WHO/ UNICEF (2006). Oral rehydration salts: production of the new ORS http://apps.who.int/iris/bitstream/10665/69227/1/WHO_FCH_CAH_06.1.pdf?ua=1&ua=1 [accessed 1 April 2019].

6.4 Constipation

The basic definitions identifying constipation include two or more of the following symptoms for a period greater than 3 months (Rome Criteria):

- Straining at defaecation >25% of time.
- Sensation of incomplete evacuation > 25% of time.
- Hard lumpy stools >25% of time.
- Less than two bowel motions per week.

  Data from Drossman, D. The functional gastrointestinal disorders and the Rome II process. *Gut.* 1999 Sep; 45(Suppl 2): II1–II5.

It is important to establish that the 'normal' bowel can have motions from two to three times per day to three times per week. Thus, individual *change* in bowel habit, especially with regards to frequency, is more descriptive of an underlying pathology.

Pathophysiology

The colon is responsible for the absorption of water, energy, and electrolytes, and the excretion of non-absorbable GI products. The intrinsic muscular tone of the colon varies throughout the day, with an increased tone following food and a decreased one during sleep. Random, low amplitude contractions bring gut contents together, while those of high amplitude coordinate peristaltic contractions to move contents along the colon; this happens approximately twice per day.

There are a number of pathophysiological mechanisms that account for constipation, and can be loosely divided into:

- *General lifestyle*: low levels of dietary fibre lead to stools of low volume and high density. Fibre, like wheat bran, makes the stools bulkier with increased solid weight and water content, thus lessening constipation.
- *Prolonged colonic transit time*: transit time can be affected by many factors, including autonomic or enteric nerve dysfunction, neuroendocrine dysfunction, or colonic myopathy. Levels of acetylcholine and serotonin (5-HT) are reduced in constipated individuals. Some drugs can impair colonic transit time.
- *Impairment of defecation*: intra- or extraluminal masses (colorectal or anal cancers) may directly obstruct the passage of stool. Distortion in shape of the anorectum and pelvic floor or sphincter dysfunction (e.g. from damage at childbirth) can also lead to outlet obstruction.

Primary constipation (functional constipation) is idiopathic and chronic constipation, while secondary constipation results from an identifiable pathology or iatrogenic causes (see Table 6.12). The retention of stool in the rectum or faecal impaction can occur as part of constipation. This can result in overflow incontinence, where loose stool bypasses as diarrhoea without sensation.

Constipation is a symptom of multiple pathologies and, hence, requires proficient questioning to make a diagnosis and avoid missing potentially life-threatening diseases. Age and duration of symptoms are crucial to rule out 'ALARM' symptoms of organic disease, such as colorectal cancer (see Box 6.3). If patients have been constipated for many months a functional cause is most likely.

It is important to enquire about frequency of defaecation and what form the stool takes (Figure 6.5). Specifically, ask about blood mixed in or on the stool, and the presence of further bleeding post-defaecation to differentiate between sinister or benign pathology (e.g. colorectal cancer or haemorrhoids, which may have resulted from excessive straining). Pain on performing a motion should be clarified as this may suggest anal fissure or anal cancer.

Associated abdominal pain or bloating could suggest irritable bowel syndrome (IBS) [see Topic 6.5, Irritable Bowel Syndrome] or, in the presence of acute complete constipation, a pseudo- or true bowel obstruction. Psychological stress and depression can affect bowel

Table 6.12 Causes for secondary constipation

Predisposing factors	GI causes	Metabolic causes	Drug causes	Neurological
Low fibre diet	Colorectal carcinoma	Hypercalcaemia	Opiates	Multiple sclerosis
Accessibility to toileting	IBD (strictures)	Hyperparathyroidism	Antipsychotics	Parkinson's disease
Reduced mobility	Pelvic mass	Hypothyroidism	Antidepressants	Cauda equina
Reduced exercise	Pseudo-obstruction	Hypokalaemia	Antiepileptics	Neurofibromatosis
Anxiety or depression	Anal fissure	Porphyria	Diuretics	Hirschsprung's
Abnormal eating patterns	Rectal prolapse	Diabetes (as autonomic myopathy)	Iron supplements	
Pyrexia	Proctalgia fugax		Antispasmodics	
Dehydration			Antihistamines (sedating)	

function directly or indirectly through poor sleep, diet and exercise.

Abdominal examination should check for abdominal distension, hyper-resonance, high pitch bowel sounds, or vacuous rectum, which may indicate pseudo-obstruction or megacolon. Digital rectal (DRE) examination will identify anal fissure (skin tags, painful ++), rectal mass (hard craggy mass, fresh blood on glove), or impaction (hard stool). A diagnosis of idiopathic constipation can be made when systemic or GI causes have been excluded.

For a full summary of the relevant pathways and drug targets, see Figure 6.5.

Management

In the majority of cases, constipation can be managed in primary care (see Figure 6.6). However, if the history,

Box 6.3 Alarm symptoms of constipation

ALARM symptoms/signs
- **A**naemia (lethargy, pale conjunctivae, etc.)
- **L**oss of weight
- **A**norexia
- **R**ecent change in bowel habit or '**R**elatives' (family history of colonic cancer)
- **M**elaena (dark = proximal GI, fresh = distal GI) or haematemesis

examination, or investigations leaves any suspicion of cancer, then an urgent referral for colonoscopy should be made. If a non-cancerous pathology or pseudo-/true obstruction is suspected then refer to a surgeon. Where relevant, any secondary causes of constipation should be addressed, such as discontinuing any constipating medication (e.g. **codeine**, **amitriptyline**, iron tablets) or correcting any metabolic disturbances.

In healthy individuals, an increase in dietary fibre to 20–30 g/day (e.g. five large carrots, five slices wholegrain bread) can increase stool bulk, frequency, and rate, but in the constipated individual it may be ineffective. However, fibre is contraindicated in the megacolon, those bedbound, and those with neurological causes. In the absence of medical contraindications (e.g. heart failure), an increase in fluid intake should also be encouraged.

The approach to pharmacological management of constipation can be considered in a stepwise manner.

First line

Bulk-forming agents, such as **isphagula husk,** can produce results within 2–3 days, with good levels of hydration required.

Second line

Osmotic laxatives (in particular **macrogols**) or stimulant laxatives such as **senna** or **bisacodyl** are licensed for

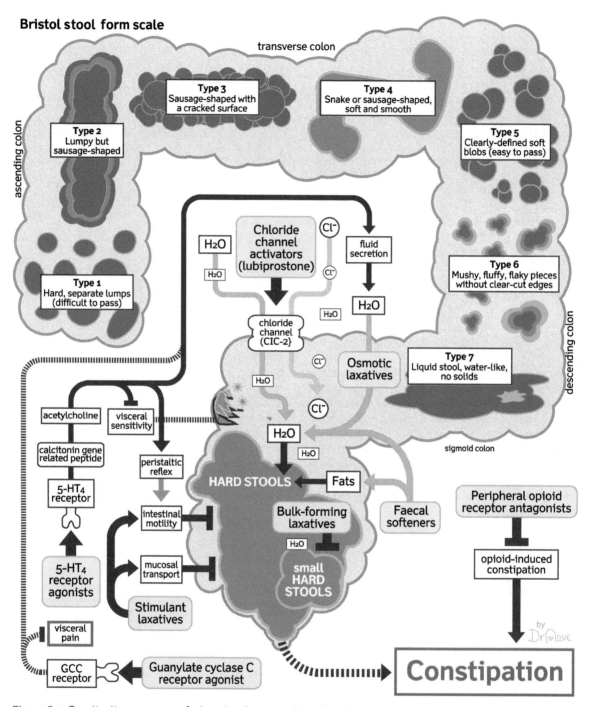

Figure 6.5 Constipation: summary of relevant pathways and drug targets.

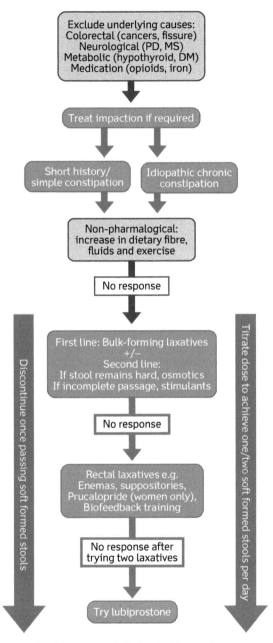

Figure 6.6 Management of chronic idiopathic constipation.

short-term use, and they must not be used in suspected bowel obstruction.

Third-line therapy

Difficult constipation should prompt re-evaluation of causes and consideration of impaction (see 'Faecal impaction treatment'). If not consider trying:

- **Magnesium sulfate** orally in water daily (avoid in pregnancy and renal impairment).
- A stimulant agent, e.g. **senna** 30 mg or **bisacodyl** 20 mg orally daily at night.
- **Glycerin** suppository PR.
- **Phosphate** enema PR.

Fourth-line therapy

In a minority of patients, resistant constipation can occur, which might require repeated enemas (e.g. **macrogols**, **sodium phosphates**, or **sodium picosulfate** bowel preparations) and/or manual evacuation.

Faecal impaction treatment

To disimpact the bowel the following is a practical approach:

- High dose oral **macrogol** laxative.
- After 3–4 days add in oral stimulant laxative.
- If oral laxatives are insufficient consider:
  - *Suppository*—for soft stool use **bisacodyl**, if hard stool **glycerol**.
  - *Mini-enema*—**sodium docusate** or **sodium citrate**.
- If treatment still insufficient, and stool still hard and compact, try **phosphate enema**.

Drug classes used in management

Pharmacologic treatment of constipation includes the use of traditional laxatives, together with agents that aim to correct apparent defects in the function of the neuromuscular control.

Bulk-forming laxatives

Bulk laxatives are particularly useful in those patients with small hard stools, but have a delayed onset and might exacerbate bloating and cramping. For example, bran, ispaghula husk, methylcellulose, and sterculia.

Mechanism of action

Bulk-forming laxatives tend to be the mildest class of laxatives. They include many organic polymers, usually of plant origin, which have a hydrophilic action and are capable of holding extra water in the gut lumen, thus expanding and softening the faeces. The concomitant increase in intraluminal volume owing to the occurrence of increased solids and obligated water, can also stimulate colonic mucosal receptors, promoting peristalsis and accelerating the transit of luminal contents past the colon. The effect on stool consistency can also make defecation easier, contributing to the overall clinical outcome.

The capacity of bulking agents to increase stool water content depends on their ability to escape small intestine digestion and absorption, while avoiding bacterial metabolism in the colon. Therefore, the dose taken, capacity to hold water, and extent of destruction by fermentation, together with the potential contribution of fermentation products, are crucial for determining the laxative effect.

Prescribing

The bulk-forming laxatives, **ispaghula husk** and **sterculia**, are formulated as granules that must be taken with plenty of fluids, causing them to swell. **Methylcellulose** is available in a tablet formulation, but as this also swells on contact with water it should be crushed before it is taken. Many consider these agents unpalatable, which may affect compliance.

PRACTICAL PRESCRIBING

Bulk-forming laxatives

Bulk-forming laxatives swell on contact with liquid so should be swallowed carefully with water and not taken immediately before bedtime.

Unwanted effects

Fermentation of fibre in the colon produces gas, responsible for the side effects of bloating and flatulence; which can be minimized by optimizing fluid intake. Bulk-forming laxatives are best avoided in patients who are severely dehydrated or in the case of obstruction, faecal impaction or colonic atony. As they remain within the gastrointestinal tract, they can be safely used in pregnancy and breast-feeding, and are otherwise well tolerated.

Osmotic laxatives

Osmotic laxatives are poorly absorbed by the intestine and force retention of water within the lumen, due to the need to maintain isotonicity with the plasma. Examples include lactulose, macrogols, magnesium salts, and sodium acid phosphate.

Mechanism of action

The small intestine and colon do not keep an osmotic gradient between luminal contents and plasma, a process that it is attained in the stomach. As a result, even hypertonic solutions are rapidly equilibrated and cause water to be retained intraluminally. The osmotic laxatives include incompletely absorbed salts (**phosphate** salts, **sulphate**, and **magnesium**), disaccharides that are poorly absorbed (such as **lactulose**), sugar alcohols (such as sorbitol or **mannitol**) and polyethylene glycol (**macrogol**).

The success of osmotic agents is dependent on the capacity to be kept within the lumen. As such, the ability of the intestinal mucosa to absorb them, together with the precipitation by other chemicals and the metabolism by luminal bacteria, will have a negative impact on their effectiveness.

Magnesium, which is used in many laxative preparations, may also stimulate cholecystokinin release from the intestinal mucosa, increasing intestinal secretions and colonic motility. Sulphate, another ion used as an osmotic laxative, is more easily absorbed than magnesium, which means the dose and timing of administration are crucial. Phosphate salts are also important as osmotic laxatives that can be absorbed by the small intestine.

Lactulose is a synthetic disaccharide of fructose and galactose, linked by a bond that cannot be hydrolysed by lactase in the small intestine. In the colon, bacterial action releases fructose and galactose, which are then fermented to lactic and acetic acids with release of gas. This acidifies the stool and forces the excretion of stool water to the extent that the colon does not absorb these fermentation products.

Prescribing

Of the osmotic laxatives, **lactulose** is one of the most widely used and has been shown to be more effective than the bulk-forming laxative **ispaghula husk** in the management of constipation in terms of both frequency and consistency. In more severe constipation, **macrogol 3350** is both superior and better tolerated than lactulose, and is useful for the management of faecal impaction. Treatment is formulated as a powder that is taken in water, with up to eight sachets taken in the case of faecal impaction.

Magnesium hydroxide is a mild laxative that is recommended for a maximum duration of 3 days. The effects of **magnesium sulfate** (or Epsom salts) tend to be less mild and associated with more abdominal cramps.

Sodium citrate and **sodium phosphate** are available in rectal formulations and are generally reserved for the management of faecal impaction, or for bowel evacuation prior to a colonoscopy or bowel surgery, due to their high potency and rapid onset of action.

PRACTICAL PRESCRIBING
Osmotic laxatives

Patients taking osmotic laxatives should be advised to ensure adequate fluid intake in order to optimize efficacy and minimize side effects, i.e. flatulence, abdominal discomfort, and cramping.

Unwanted effects

Although osmotic laxatives have a similar mechanism of action, their distinct structure gives rise to variations in unwanted effects. As a class, they largely remain within the GI tract and are therefore contraindicated in obstruction or paralytic ileus. **Macrogols** are also best avoided in severe inflammatory conditions of the GI tract, such as Crohn's and ulcerative colitis.

PRESCRIBING WARNING
Macrogol

Macrogol preparations tend to have high sodium content so should be used cautiously in patients on low sodium diets.

In addition to fructose and galactose, **lactulose** contains lactose so should be used cautiously in patients with lactose intolerance or galactosaemia. Furthermore, the excessive production of gas secondary to fermentation within the gut can lead to abdominal distention, bloating, cramping, and excess flatus. Patients should be advised to optimize fluid intake to reduce side effects.

Magnesium salts should be used cautiously in patients with renal impairment due to the risk of hypermagnesaemia, particularly with prolonged use. Prolonged use of **magnesium hydroxide** can alter gastric pH, leading to impaired absorption of tetracyclines and **digoxin**.

Stimulant laxatives

Although these agents were mainly believed to act by stimulating intestinal motility, it has been now determined that they can also affect mucosal transport. Examples include bisacodyl, dantron, senna, and sodium picosulfate.

Mechanism of action

The stimulant laxatives include a variety of drugs and herbal preparations that can induce defaecation by a variety of mechanisms, including the stimulation of local reflexes through myenteric nerve plexuses in the gut. This enhances gut motility and increases water transfer into the lower intestine. Long-term use has been associated with atonic bowel and should generally be avoided.

Diphenylmethane derivatives include phenolphthalein, the now more commonly used diacetic ester **bisacodyl**, and the disulphuric acid semi-ester **sodium picosulfate**. Bisacodyl can inhibit water absorption through effects on prostaglandins and other eicosanoids, kinins, and possibly the Na^+/K^+-ATPase that exists in enterocytes. Sodium picosulphate is just activated in the colon, where considerable bacterial flora is normally present. It is biotransformed to the same active moiety as bisacodyl.

Anthraquinones, such as **senna** and **dantron**, are a group of chemicals based upon the tricyclic anthracene nucleus. They are bulky molecules that are poorly absorbed and are mostly unaffected by passage via the small intestine. Bacterial metabolism converts them to active forms in the colon. Rhein and other anthraquinone metabolites produce net fluid secretion in the human jejunum and colon. Nevertheless, the actions on the motility of the colon are probably more relevant than those on fluid transport.

Prescribing

Senna is available in liquid and tablet formulation usually administered at bedtime to enable a motion in the morning, as onset of action tends to be 6–12 hours. The same is true of **bisacodyl** when taken orally (tablets only), although rectal administration can work within 20–45 minutes.

Glycerol suppositories have both stimulant and osmotic activity. Suppositories should be wetted before use and are generally prescribed on an as needed basis.

The use of **dantron** is limited to patients that are terminally ill, as although highly effective, it is a potential carcinogen. **Sodium picosulfate** is a potent oral stimulant generally used for bowel evacuation prior to bowel surgery or colonoscopy.

PRACTICAL PRESCRIBING
Timing of stimulants

Doses of oral stimulant laxatives are best taken at night, as onset of action tends to be about 12 hours. Rectal formulations are considerably faster and are, therefore, best taken in the morning.

Unwanted side effects

As stimulant laxatives induce peristalsis, abdominal cramping is the most common side effect associated with their use. Long-term use can lead to diarrhoea or rebound constipation secondary to an atonic bowel. In common with other laxatives, they are contraindicated in GI obstruction, perforation, and ileus.

> ### PRESCRIBING WARNING
>
> **Sodium picosulfate**
>
> Sodium picosulfate is branded under the name Dulcolax® Pico and bisacodyl as Dulcolax®, to avoid confusion prescribe generically, rather than by trade name.

   Dantron use has been reported to cause liver and intestinal tumours in rats and mice, which is why it is only licensed for use in terminally ill patients. It can also stain urine and the peri-anal area a red/pink colour, which patients should be made aware of.

Faecal softeners

> Faecal softeners increase fluid and fat penetration into hard stool, but with the exception of of docusate sodium are relatively ineffective laxatives. Examples include docusate sodium, liquid paraffin, and arachis oil.

Mechanism of action

Surface-active agents such as **docusate sodium** are mainly detergents believed to exert fairly modest effects on mucosal transport of ions. They were originally devised to permit water to interact in a more effective way with stood solids, thus promoting their softening.

Prescribing

Docusate sodium is the most frequently used and effective of the faecal softeners, administered orally as a capsule, with the dose decreased as constipation improves. In addition to its effects as a softener, it also acts as a stimulant. **Liquid paraffin** once widely used as a faecal softener in the past, is now infrequently prescribed due to the unacceptable level of toxicity (anal seepage and irritation, granulomatous reactions).

   Arachis oil may be administered as an enema in the case of faecal obstruction. As it contains peanut oil and soya, however, it is contraindicated in patients with a peanut allergy and caution advised in soya hypersensitivity.

Unwanted effects

See 'Stimulant laxatives' for unwanted effects of docusate sodium. Use of liquid paraffin is also known to cause lipoid pneumonia in patients with impaired swallow.

> ### PRESCRIBING WARNING
>
> **Liquid paraffin**
>
> Use of liquid paraffin as a faecal softener has largely been superseded due to toxicity, where used the duration should be minimized.

Peripheral opioid receptor antagonists

> Antagonists of opioid receptors are useful in the treatment of opioid-induced constipation, but more studies in non-opioid-dependent patients are needed before its use can be extended to more general functional constipation. For example, methylnaltrexone, alvimopan, and naloxegol.

Mechanism of action

The peripheral opioid receptor antagonists have a specific role in the management of opiate-induced constipation and post-surgical ileus, where constipation is specifically induced through stimulation of peripheral μ-opioid receptors. Until recently, **naloxone** was the only available opioid antagonist, however, as it crosses into the CNS, it can also reverse the therapeutic effects of opioids. Unlike naloxone, the newer drugs **methylnaltrexone** and **alvimopan**, act selectively on μ-receptors and do not cross the blood–brain barrier.

   More recently, naloxone has been reformulated as a pegylated derivative, **naloxegol**, which reduces its passive permeability and makes it a substrate for the P-glycoprotein transporter, this promotes increased efflux from the CNS across the blood–brain barrier. As a result, CNS levels are minimized.

Prescribing

Methylnaltrexone bromide is licensed in the UK for the treatment of opioid-induced constipation, in palliative patients that show an inadequate response to other therapy. It is administered IV on alternate days, with a rapid onset of action (30–60 minutes).

   Alvimopan is licensed in the USA only for oral administration to treat post-operative ileus following bowel resection. Lack of efficacy of alvimopan in the treatment of chronic idiopathic constipation and negative results for naltrexone in combination with tegaserod in constipation-type IBS, has restricted their use to opioid-dependent constipation only.

Naloxogel is taken orally OD in opioid-induced constipation where other agents have failed. It is advocated by NICE for this indication, although is not widely used.

Naloxone has rarely been used off-licence to reverse GI side effects of opioids. Licensed compound preparations containing **oxycodone** and naloxone may help improve opioid tolerance; however, use is restricted by cost and evidence suggests it to be no better than oxycodone prescribed with regular laxatives.

Unwanted effects

The most common side effects associated with **methylnaltrexone bromide** include nausea, abdominal pain, diarrhea, and flatulence, although these effects tend to be mild. Also in line with other laxatives it is contraindicated in patients with GI obstruction or acute surgical abdomen. Approximately half of the dose is excreted in the urine, so that patients with severe renal impairment (i.e. eGFR <30 mL/min/1.73 m²) require dose reductions of about 50%. As a relatively new drug, experience is limited and, consequently, use in certain patient groups is cautioned, e.g. patients with colostomy, faecal impaction, and those at higher risk of perforation.

5-HT$_4$ receptor agonists

5-HT4 receptor agonists target the serotoninergic presynaptic receptors in the enteric nervous system, facilitating the release of acetylcholine and calcitonin gene-related peptide. For example, prucalopride and tegaserod.

Mechanism of action

Activation of presynaptic 5-HT$_4$ receptors starts the peristaltic reflex, promoting fluid secretion in the intestine, and inhibiting visceral sensitivity. This leads to a decrease in colonic transit time and improves the quantity of bowel movements, ameliorating abdominal discomfort, and promoting bowel satisfaction.

The benzofurancarboxamide **prucalopride** is a highly selective, high affinity 5-HT$_4$ agonist. Unlike other 5-HT$_4$ receptor agonists (**cisapride**, **tegaserod**, **mosapride**, and **renzapride**), it does not act on 5-HT$_3$ and 5-HT$_{1B}$

receptors, and certain K$^+$ channels (hERG), which give it a more favourable risk–benefit profile. Recent reports have indicated that prucalopride improves GI transit, stool frequency, and consistency, significantly reducing the symptoms of severe chronic constipation.

Prescribing

The licensed use of **prucalopride** is restricted to chronic constipation as an OD oral preparation where other laxatives have failed. The license of prucalopride has only more recently been extended to men, although NICE still only advocate its use in women. It is well absorbed orally, regardless of food intake and can be taken at any time of the day.

> **PRACTICAL PRESCRIBING**
>
> **Prucalopride**
>
> NICE recommend the use of prucalopride in women with chronic constipation that have tried and failed at least two laxatives from different classes at full dose, for a period of at least 6 months. Efficacy should be reviewed after 4 weeks. (NICE, Dec 2010)
> https://www.nice.org.uk/guidance/ta211/resources/prucalopride-for-the-treatment-of-chronic-constipation-in-women-82600244622277.

Unwanted effects

In common with other laxatives, **prucalopride** can cause abdominal pain, nausea, diarrhea, and flatulence in about 20% of patients; it also commonly causes headaches. As with other drugs in the class, there is an increased risk of QT interval prolongation (through the K$^+$ hERG channel) with prucalopride, although being more selective for the 5-HT$_4$ receptor, this risk is reduced. The risk of palpitations is increased with doses exceeding 2 mg, and it is cautioned in patients with a history of arrhythmias. Prucalopride is contraindicated in intestinal obstruction and in patients at risk of perforation, i.e. with severe inflammatory conditions such as Crohn's and toxic megacolon.

Doses should be halved in severe renal and hepatic impairment as, although it is primarily excreted via the kidney, hepatic metabolism does occur and is very slow.

Chloride channel activators

These drugs target the Cl$^-$ channels in the apical membrane of the GI epithelium. For example, lubiprostone.

Mechanism of action

Lubiprostone is a bicyclic functional fatty acid (prostaglandin E1 derivative), which acts as a selective Cl⁻ channel (CIC-2) activator in the epithelium of the GI tract to raise intestinal chloride secretion into the lumen. In order to maintain isoelectric neutrality, there is an efflux of Na^+ through a paracellular pathway, which is followed by water to preserve isotonic equilibrium. Overall, this process increases intraluminal fluid collection in the intestine, augmenting intestine motility and facilitating the passage of stools.

Prescribing

Lubiprostone is the first in its class to be licensed for use in chronic idiopathic constipation and in the USA for opioid-induced constipation in patients with chronic non-cancer pain. More recently, it has been advocated for use by NICE, in patients who have previously failed treatment with at least two different types of laxatives at optimal doses over a 6-month period. Prescribing should be restricted to clinicians with specialist experience of managing chronic idiopathic constipation. Doses are administered orally BD for 2–4 weeks.

Unwanted effects

Trial data suggests that **lubiprostone** is well tolerated, the most frequently seen adverse effects being diarrhoea and nausea, with the latter in part relieved by taking it with food. As with other laxatives it is not to be used in patients with GI obstruction. On rare occasions, lubiprostone has been reported to cause chest pain or dyspnoea, which resolves within a few hours. Affected patients should avoid future use.

Lubiprostone is hepatically metabolized and as such should be used with caution in moderate to severe hepatic impairment. Patients should be started on a half dose that may be increased if ineffective and tolerated.

Guanylate cyclase C receptor agonist

Linaclotide binds to the GCC receptor located on the luminal surface of the intestinal epithelium, where it increases colonic transit and reduces visceral pain. For example, linaclotide.

Mechanism of action

The guanylate cyclase C receptors are normally activated by endogenous ligands following a meal to promote intestinal secretions, through an increase in cGMP levels. Increased cGMP levels activates cGMP protein kinase, which leads to the activation of the cystic fibrosis transmembrane conductance regulator (CFTR) ion channel. This is turn promotes secretion of Cl⁻ and HCO_3^- ions into the intestinal lumen, thereby promoting fluid secretion and GI transit. **Linaclotide** acts as an agonist on these receptors directly within the GI tract and is minimally absorbed.

Prescribing

Linaclotide is an orally administered treatment for constipation in IBS. It is taken OD for up to 4 weeks, at which point it should only be continued if patients have shown a response.

Unwanted effects

Due to its effect on promoting GI secretions and transit, potential side effects to **linaclotide** include electrolyte disturbances, dehydration, abdominal cramping, and diarrhoea, particularly in overdose. Patients should be advised to hold treatment if they are affected.

Further reading

BMJ Best Practice (2019) Constipation. http://bestpractice.bmj.com/best-practice/monograph/154.html [accessed 1 April 2019].

BMJ Best Practice (2019) Evidence at the point of care. http://clinicalevidence.bmj.com/ceweb/conditions/spc/2407/2407_I16.jsp [accessed 1 April 2019].

Crowell MD, Harris LA, Lunsford TN, et al. (2009) Emerging drugs for chronic constipation. *Expert Opinions in Emergency Drugs* 14(3), 493–504.

NICE (2017) Constipation. Clinical knowledge summaries. http://cks.nice.org.uk/constipation#!management [accessed 1 April 2019].

Pohl D, Tutuian R, Fried M (2008) Pharmacologic treatment of constipation: what is new? *Current Opinions in Pharmacology* 8(6), 724–8.

Tadataka Y (2008) *Textbook of Gastroenterology*. Philadelphia, PA: Lippincott Williams and Wilkins.

Guidelines

NICE TA211 (2010) Prucalopride for the treatment of chronic constipation in women. https://www.nice.org.uk/guidance/TA211 [accessed 1 April 2019].

NICE TA318 (July 2014) Lubiprostone for treating chronic idiopathic constipation. https://www.nice.org.uk/guidance/TA318 [accessed 1 April 2019].

NICE TA435 (July 2015) Naloxogel for treating opioid-induced constipation. https://www.nice.org.uk/guidance/TA345 [accessed 1 April 2019].

NICE Pathway (July 2015) Constipation overview. http://pathways.nice.org.uk/pathways/constipation [accessed 1 April 2019].

6.5 Irritable bowel syndrome

IBS is a chronic disease of relapsing-remitting course characterized by abdominal pain/discomfort, bloating, and altered bowel habit (constipation and/or diarrhoea). It has a prevalence of 10–20%, affecting women more commonly than men (2:1) and is biphasic in distribution, peaking at 20–30 years and also in the elderly.

Pathophysiology

The aetiology and pathophysiology of IBS is poorly understood. Causal theories include infection (e.g. following gastroenteritis), inflammation, diet, antibiotics, surgery, and hereditary and psychological disturbances; in reality, the aetiology is likely to be multifactorial and includes:

- *Abnormal autonomic activity*: about a quarter of patients have abnormalities in the extrinsic autonomic innervation of GI viscera. Cardiovagal dysfunction has a particular role in IBS constipation-predominant (IBS-C), while sympathetic adrenergic dysfunction is important in IBS diarrhoea-predominant (IBS-D). Extrinsic lumbosacral parasympathetic outflow over-activity via M_2 and M_3 muscarinic acetylcholine receptors on smooth muscle causes symptomatic hyper-contraction and hypermobility.

- *Abnormal CNS modulation of the gastrointestinal tract*: the brain–gut axis is a two-way communication system, functioning at the unconscious level. The limbic and paralimbic systems (e.g. medial prefrontal cortex, amygdala, and hypothalamus), functioning through the autonomic system, convey emotional changes, and modulate GI motility, secretion, and blood flow. Peripheral afferents send signals to the thalamus and brain stem, which are then modulated centrally by higher centres affecting central efferent outflow to the gut.

- Serotonin (5-HT) is a neurotransmitter and a local hormone in the GI peripheral vascular system that modulates GI motility, sensation, blood flow, and secretion. About 90% is stored in enterochromaffin cells and 10% in enteric neurons, with release triggered by luminal distension and chemical signals. Serotonin acts at GI-located 5-HT_{1-4} and 5-HT_7 G protein–coupled receptors; with 5-HT_3 and 5-HT_4 being the most important in IBS. 5-HT_3 modulates visceral pain, aids peristalsis, and influences the emotional component of visceral stimulation within the CNS. 5-HT_4 is important in gastric emptying, colonic secretions, facilitation of the peristaltic reflex, and the contraction or relaxation of the smooth muscle. The variation in central response/gate-keeping to visceral stimuli is based on prior experiences, so cognitive manipulation with agents like tricyclic antidepressants or corticotropin-releasing factor receptor antagonists may be of benefit.

- *Visceral hypersensitivity*: IBS patients are likely to have enhanced perception of visceral events, and notice events like bowel contraction and gas. It is postulated that acute inflammation sensitizes the peripheral, spinal, and central system, while chronic inflammation may down-regulate.

- *Abnormal GI immune function*: in IBS, increased numbers of mast cells, lymphocytic infiltrates, and increased inducible NOS levels have been noted, suggestive of augmented GI immune function.

Clinically, a large proportion of IBS sufferers report motility abnormalities. Patients show augmented responses to stimuli like meals, distension, and stress. In those

with IBS-D there are increased frequency of high amplitude propagating contractions, which are more likely to
be associated with abdominal pain. As such, the changes
in motility may be attenuated with antispasmodics like
antimuscarinics and smooth muscle relaxants.

For a full summary of the relevant pathways and drug
targets, see Figure 6.7.

Management

Irritable bowel syndrome should be considered in any
patient presenting with **A**bdominal pain or discomfort,
Bloating, or a **C**hange in bowel habit. A diagnosis is made
based on the Rome II criteria as set out in Box 6.4, once
other causes have been excluded. As IBS is often associated with emotional stress, a link between the onset of
symptoms and life events can help confirm diagnosis.

A careful history, rectal examination, and routine bloods
[FBC, erythrocyte sedimentation rate (ESR), C-reactive
protein (CRP), coeliac disease (endomysial antibodies or
tissue transglutaminase)] should be carried out to establish any organic disease, and identify any 'red flag' indicators (see Box 6.5), requiring urgent referral.

Patients with raised inflammatory markers suggestive
of IBD (e.g. ESR, CRP) also require referral to secondary
care for specialist management. In females at risk of
ovarian cancer, measurement of CA-125 is prudent.

Once an IBS diagnosis is made patients should be
offered lifestyle advice (see Box 6.6) to help manage
symptoms, although if symptoms persist pharmacological
treatment may be necessary.

The choice of pharmacological management will depend on symptoms, with doses titrated to response in
order to produce a soft, formed stool (Figure 6.8).

First-line

- *Antispasmodics*: can be broadly divided into two
classes, antimuscarinics (**hyoscine**, **dicycloverine**,
propantheline) and smooth muscle relaxants
(**alverine**, **mebeverine**, and **peppermint oil**). There is
a lack of evidence to suggest superiority of one agent
over another; therefore, choice is determined by tolerance and the dominant IBS symptoms. Patients should
be treated with one antispasmodic at a time and a substitution made should the first not work. Prolonged use
can lead to a loss of efficacy so patients should be advised to use on a when-required basis.

- *Laxatives*: (but not **lactulose**) in patients with
constipation-predominant symptoms. They are
best taken in small, regular amounts (see Topic 6.4,
'Constipation').
- *Anti-diarrhoeals*: in patients with diarrhoea predominant symptoms, first choice being **loperamide** (see
Topic 6.3, 'Diarrhoea').

Second-line

- *Anti-depressants*: there is greater evidence available
for tricyclic anti-depressants than selective serotonin
re-uptake inhibitors in the management of IBS, with
amitriptyline the drug of choice starting at 5–10 mg
at night, titrating to 30 mg if necessary. Where a TCA is
not effective, however, an SSRI may be considered.

- *Linaclotide*: a first in class drug, licensed for use in
IBS-C, may be a useful option in some patients that fail
to respond to other treatment options. NICE highlight
it as an option in patients that have failed to respond to
conventional laxatives at optimal doses and have had
constipation for 12 months. **Lubiprostone**, an alternative agent is licensed in some countries (not the UK) for
use in IBS-C, where it has been shown to be effective in
managing constipation. In the UK it is only licensed for
use in chronic idiopathic constipation (see Topic 6.4,
'Constipation').

Drug classes used in management

Antispasmodics: antimuscarinics

Antimuscarinics are believed to have an effect on IBS
treatment through the decrease in intestinal smooth
muscle activity. Substantial side effects and inconclusive clinical trials make these agents a suboptimal
choice for therapy. Examples include hyoscine butyl
bromide, dicycloverine, and propantheline.

Mechanism of action

Muscarinic receptors can stimulate the turnover of phosphatidyl inositol in intestinal smooth muscle, which
leads to the mobilization of Ca^{2+} and muscle contraction. The signalling mechanism is somewhat unclear, because the source of Ca^{2+} for the tonic phase of

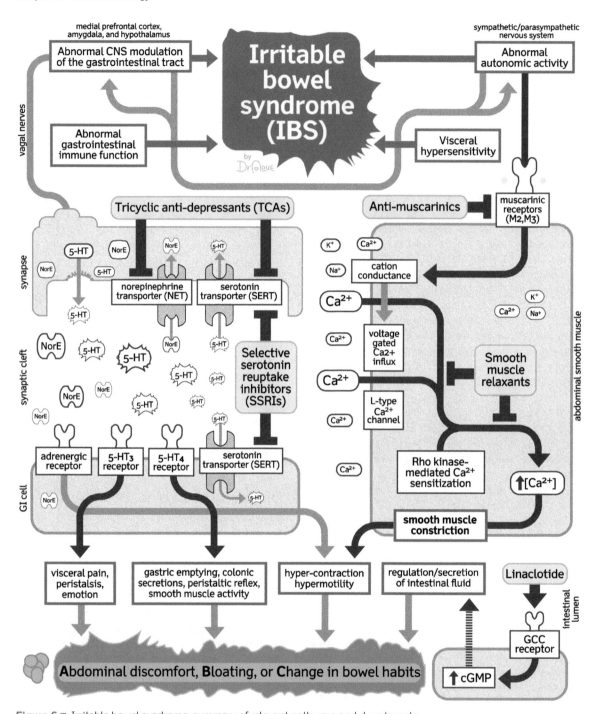

Figure 6.7 Irritable bowel syndrome: summary of relevant pathways and drug targets.

contraction is normally extracellular and not through the IP_3-mediated release of Ca^{2+} from the endoplasmic reticulum. It is thought that muscarinic receptors elicit a non-selective cation conductance, which provides the necessary depolarization for an influx of Ca^{2+} through voltage-dependent Ca^{2+} channels.

Based on the idea that disrupted intestinal motility may contribute to many of the symptoms of IBS, muscarinic

Box 6.4 Rome II criteria for IBS

At least 12 weeks (which need not be consecutive) in the preceding 12 months of abdominal discomfort or pain with two or more of the following features:
- Relief with defaecation
- Onset associated with a change in stool frequency
- Onset associated with a change in stool form

Symptoms that cumulatively support the diagnosis of IBS:

- Abnormal stool frequency
- Abnormal stool form (lumpy/hard or loose/ watery stool)
- Abnormal stool passage (straining, urgency, or feeling of incomplete evacuation)
- Passage of mucus
- Bloating or feeling of abdominal distension

Reproduced from Drossman, D. The functional gastrointestinal disorders and the Rome II process. *Gut*. 1999 Sep; 45(Suppl 2): II1–II5. Copyright © 1999, BMJ Publishing Group Ltd and the British Society of Gastroenterology. http://dx.doi.org/10.1136/gut.45.2008.ii1

receptor antagonists are used for treatment, mostly for the relief of abdominal pain and discomfort.

Non-selective muscarinic antagonists, such as **dicycloverine** and **hyoscine butylbromide** have shown some limited value in relieving symptoms. M₃-selective muscarinic antagonists have a more favourable side effect profile than non-selective antagonists, as they preferentially target M_3 muscarinic receptors located in the gut, i.e. **zamifenacin** and **darifenacin**.

Prescribing

Of the available antimuscarinics used for their antispasmodic properties, **hyoscine butylbromide** is the most widely prescribed and the only drug in the class specifically licensed for use in IBS. Furthermore, unlike **dicycloverine** and **propantheline**, hyoscine butylbromide is available to

Box 6.5 Red flag indicators requiring urgent referral

Unintentional weight loss
- Rectal bleeding
- Family history of bowel or ovarian cancer
- Increased frequency and looser stools for more than 6 weeks in patients over 60 years
- Anaemia
- Abdominal/rectal mass

Box 6.6 Lifestyle advice in IBS

- Small frequent meals
- Review of fibre intake, to use soluble fibres (e.g. oats not bran)
- Limit fruit to three portions a day
- Avoid resistant starch (often present in reheated food)
- Avoid sorbitol/artificial sweeteners with diarrhoea
- Four-week trial of probiotics at optimal dose
- Avoid trigger foods one at a time for 1 month under dietician guidance, e.g. chocolate, caffeine
- Encourage good fluid intake, avoiding caffeine, fizzy drinks, and alcohol
- Increase physical activity
- Optimize leisure and relaxation time

buy over the counter, enabling patients to self-medicate. Patients should be advised that chronic use should be avoided unless the cause of symptoms has been established. **Atropine** is not recommended for use in IBS. In general, antimuscarinics are of greater value in patients where diarrhoea is the dominant symptom.

Unwanted effects

As with all antimuscarinics, the antispasmodics are contraindicated in patients with myasthenia gravis, pyloric stenosis, paralytic ileus, and enlarged prostate. As doses for IBS are relatively low, the risk of complications is reduced, although care is still required in conditions characterized by tachycardia or urinary retention, and in those susceptible to narrow angle glaucoma.

On the whole, the antimuscarinic, antispasmodics are reasonably well tolerated, with the most commonly reported side effects being predictably dry mouth, blurred vision, dizziness, and constipation. Their use is discouraged in the elderly due to the increased risk of confusion and falls.

Drug interactions

Adverse effects are potentiated when used with other drugs known to have antimuscarinic effects, including tricyclic anti-depressants.

Antispasmodics: smooth muscle relaxants

Antispasmodics of the smooth muscle relaxant type inhibit GI contractions, but unlike the muscarinic antagonists, they do so by directly affecting the Ca^{2+} dynamics in smooth muscle. Examples include peppermint oil, mebeverine, and alverine citrate.

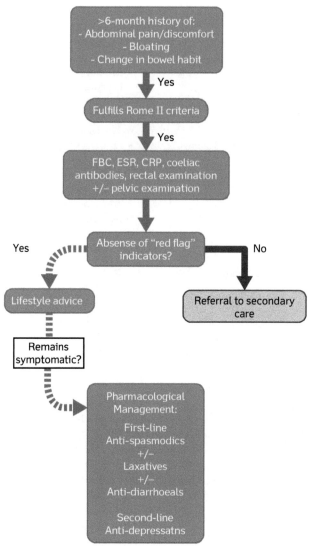

Figure 6.8 Management of IBS.

Mechanism of action

The mechanism by which **peppermint oil** might improve IBS symptoms is not completely understood. The muscle contraction induced by acetylcholine is only marginally modified with peppermint extract, indicating that its effects are not due to cholinergic antagonism. However, it has been suggested that it directly acts by relaxing the intestinal smooth muscle, possibly due to the menthol's interference with the passage of Ca^{2+} across the cell membrane. Although only a limited number of clinical trials have been carried out, all have shown a clear superiority against placebo.

Ca^{2+} channel blockers, such as **pinaverium bromide**, are smooth muscle relaxants that may also be useful in IBS. They can be effective through decreasing post-prandial and distension-induced rectal hypermotility, increasing colonic transit time and improving rectal sensory thresholds.

The spasmolytic drug **alverine** has shown the capacity to decrease the duration of spontaneous contractions in the gut and uterus. Some of the effects are a consequence of complex mechanisms, including inhibition on both K^+ channel-mediated negative feedback to L-type Ca^{2+} channels and Rho kinase-mediated Ca^{2+} sensitization.

The antimuscarinic **mebeverine**, a derivative of phenylethylamine, is a musculotropic agent with antispasmodic activity and regulatory actions on the function of the bowel. At doses used for oral administration it shows no typical anticholinergic side effects, such as dry mouth, blurred vision, and impaired micturition.

Prescribing

The smooth muscle relaxants **alverine**, **mebeverine**, and **peppermint oil** are increasingly popular in the management of IBS and are widely available for purchase over the counter. As they are not known to cause constipation, they should be considered in patients with constipation dominant IBS in preference to antimuscarinic agents. Doses are best taken before meals (20 minutes in the case of mebeverine).

Unwanted effects

The smooth muscle relaxants have a better side effect profile than the antimuscarinics, rarely causing non-specific reactions such as headache, nausea, or rash. However, peppermint oil is known to cause heartburn. As with the antimuscarinics they are contraindicated in paralytic ileus.

Tricyclic antidepressants

> The mechanism of action of tricyclic antidepressants (TCAs) relates to their ability to regulate central and peripheral pain perception, and may take at least 4 weeks to become efficacious. For example, amitriptyline, trimipramine, and doxepin.

Mechanism of action

Most TCAs act as serotonin-norepinephrine reuptake inhibitors, blocking the serotonin, and norepinephrine transporters, leading to an increase in the extracellular levels of these neurotransmitters, thus enhancing neurotransmission (see Topic 10.2 'Depression'). Serotonin release is triggered by luminal distension and chemical signals. With the exception of 5-HT_3, which is a ligand-gated ion channel, most serotonin receptors are G protein–coupled. Those 5-HT receptor subtypes known to act on the GI tract are 5-HT_{1-4} and 5-HT_7. The 5-HT_3 and 5-HT_4 subtypes appear to be the most important in IBS, with 5-HT_3 modulating visceral pain, aiding peristalsis and influencing the emotional constituent of visceral stimulation within the CNS. Although their mode of action is not fully elucidated, it has been suggested that it links to the capacity to regulate central and peripheral pain perception, and the neurotransmitter activity that controls gut motility.

Most TCAs also have typically high affinity for antagonizing histamine and muscarinic receptors, thus acting as potent antihistamines and anticholinergics. Most also potently inhibit sodium channels and L-type Ca^{2+} channels, which can contribute to cardiotoxicity in overdose.

Prescribing

The tricyclic anti-depressants **amitriptyline**, **trimipramine**, and **doxepin** may be useful in improving global symptoms, as well as more specific bloating and bowel habits, in patients who demonstrate an inadequate response to first-line treatment. Doses should be started low (5–10 mg equivalent of amitriptyline) and gradually increased to a maximum of 30 mg amitriptyline (30–50 mg trimipramine and 50–75 mg of doxepin) according to response. Doses above this are unlikely to confer any additional benefit. None of the TCAs are licensed for this indication.

Unwanted effects

It is the potential cardiotoxicity of the TCAs that largely limits their use, particularly as the risk with SSRIs is lower. Therefore, in patients with underlying cardiac disease such as arrhythmias, recent myocardial infarction and heart block, TCAs are best avoided. The link to sudden cardiac death is generally associated with doses over 100 mg (**amitriptyline**) and, therefore, unlikely to be a problem in IBS.

TCAs also possess antimuscarinic and antihistamine activity, which accounts for most of their unwanted effects, such as dry mouth, blurred vision, and drowsiness. Although these side effects tend to wear off with continued use and by slow introduction of treatment, they are best administered at night.

As with other antimuscarinics, they should be avoided in paralytic ileus and used cautiously in urinary retention, prostatic hypertrophy, or glaucoma.

Drug interactions

See Topic 10.2, 'Depression'.

PRESCRIBING WARNING

Potentially fatal interactions between MAOIs and TCAs or SSRIs

There have been reports of severe and sometimes fatal cases of neuroleptic malignant syndrome when an MAOI has been taken in combination with an SSRI or TCA. Concurrent use is therefore contraindicated and a 2-week wash-out period recommended for anyone switching between the two.

Selective serotonin reuptake inhibitors

Selective serotonin reuptake inhibitors (SSRIs) inhibit the re-uptake of serotonin, promoting neurotransmission. As they lack effects on other monoamine transporters, they have fewer contraindications compared with TCAs. For example, fluoxetine and paroxetine.

Mechanism of action

SSRIs act by inhibiting serotonin reuptake, thereby increasing levels of the neurotransmitter at the synaptic cleft (see Topic 10.2, 'Depression'). Their mechanism of action with regards to IBS therapy is similar to TCAs, although they only inhibit the re-uptake pumps responsible for serotonin. Compared with the TCAs, they have fewer and milder side effects, and a much higher toxic dose, although studies examining their use in IBS have had inconsistent results. It is unclear whether SSRIs would be most useful in constipation-predominant IBS, given that diarrhoea is often a side effect. Of the SSRIs, only **fluoxetine** and **paroxetine** have evidence to support their use in IBS management.

Prescribing

SSRIs are a useful alternative to TCAs in patients where the latter are either ineffective or unsuitable due to intolerance or contraindications. As with TCAs doses are started low and high doses unlikely to be beneficial (max 20mg **fluoxetine**). Their use in IBS falls outside the product licence. Although there is evidence to suggest they can give a global improvement in symptoms, they are less likely than TCAs to improve symptoms such as bloating, pain, or bowel movements; which is likely due to their lack of antimuscarinic activity.

Unwanted effects

SSRIs are generally better tolerated than TCAs, particularly as they are less likely to cause significant cardiotoxicity. They also lack the antimuscarinic and antihistamine properties seen with TCAs and, conversely, are more likely to cause insomnia or agitation than drowsiness. Doses are, therefore, better taken in the morning. Other common side effects tend to be GI (nausea and diarrhoea), fatigue, or headache.

Drug interactions

See Topic 10.2, 'Depression'.

PRACTICAL PRESCRIBING
TCAs versus SSRIs

- The decision to use a TCA or an SSRI in the management of IBS will depend on any co-morbidities the patient may have.
- In the absence of any contraindications or cautions, TCAs are more likely to be effective.
- Treatment should be reviewed every 4 weeks until considered effective and then in a 6–12-monthly period.

Linaclotide

A first in class, linaclotide is a 14 amino acid peptide of the guanylin peptide family. It can act as a selective agonist at the guanylate cyclase-C receptor that is located on the luminal side of intestinal enterocytes.

Mechanism of action

The guanylin peptide hormones promote intestinal secretions in response to a meal by binding to guanylate cyclase-C receptors. Activation of these receptors leads to increased levels of cGMP, which has a role in the regulation and secretion of intestinal fluid.

Prescribing

Linaclotide is administered orally in adults who suffer with constipation-predominant IBS, with doses taken in the morning, 30 minutes before breakfast. Clinically, it is infrequently used, largely due to its relatively high cost compared with conventional laxatives. NICE advocates its use in patients who have failed to respond to optimal doses of laxatives and who have suffered constipation for over 12 months. Patients should have treatment reviewed for efficacy after 3 months.

Unwanted effects

Predictably, diarrhoea is the most common side effect associated with **linaclotide**, which is usually mild–moderate in presentation. In severe, persistent cases patients are advised to withhold treatment and seek medical advice. Use is contraindicated in mechanical GI obstruction. The observation of infrequent adverse events suggestive of drug hypersensitivity has led the FDA to suspect the possible production of autoantibodies against the peptide; this has not as yet been substantiated.

Further reading

Ehlert FJ, Pak KJ, Griffin MT (2012) Muscarinic agonists and antagonists: effects on gastrointestinal function. *Handbook of Experimental Pharmacology* 208, 343–74.

Drossman DA, Camilleri M, Mayer EA, et al. (2002) AGA technical review on irritable bowel syndrome. *Gastroenterology* 123(6), 2108–31.

Ford AC, Talley NJ, Spiegel BM, et al. (2008) Effect of fibre, antispasmodics, and peppermint oil in the treatment of irritable bowel syndrome: systemic review and meta-analysis. *British Medical Journal* 337, a2313.

Hammerle CW, Surawicz CM (2008) Updates on treatment of irritable bowel syndrome. *World Journal of Gastroenterology* 14(17), 2639–49.

Talley NJ (2003) Pharmacologic therapy for the irritable bowel syndrome. *American Journal of Gastroenterology* 98(4), 750–8.

Guidelines

NICE CG61 (2015) Irritable bowel syndrome in adults: Diagnosis and management of irritable bowel syndrome in primary care. https://www.nice.org.uk/guidance/cg61 [accessed 1 April 2019].

NICE ESNM16 (2013) Irritable bowel syndrome with constipation in adults: linaclotide. https://www.nice.org.uk/guidance/esnm16 [accessed 1 April 2019].

NICE Pathway (2019) Irritable bowel syndrome in adults overview. http://pathways.nice.org.uk/pathways/irritable-bowel-syndrome-in-adults [accessed 1 April 2019].

NICE QS114 (2016) Irritable bowel syndrome in adults. https://www.nice.org.uk/guidance/qs114 [accessed 1 April 2019].

6.6 Inflammatory bowel disease (ulcerative colitis and Crohn's Disease)

IBD encompasses two distinct conditions; *ulcerative colitis* (UC) and *Crohn's disease* (CD). Both are idiopathic chronic relapsing-remitting diseases, with complex pathophysiology, presentation, and clinical sequelae. CD has an incidence of approximately 10/100 000, although this is increasing, with two peaks of incidence at 15–30 and 60–80 years old; it is increasingly more common in children. UC has a similar incidence with two peaks at slightly lower ages of 15–25 and 55–65 years old. In CD there is a stronger genetic concordance of disease than in UC, and while smoking is a known risk factor in the former, it is protective in UC.

Pathophysiology

Genome-wide association studies have identified around 100 genetic loci where the risks of developing IBD lie; currently 30% of loci are shared between CD and UC, despite their distinct clinical features. The dysfunction of pathways that control intestinal homeostasis, microbial defence, innate immune regulation, reactive oxygen species generation, autophagy, the regulation of adaptive immunity, and metabolic stress all have a role in IBD.

Crohn's disease

Given the genetic concordance in CD, research has highlighted that deficits in cellular and humoral immunity have the prominent role in mucosal inflammation. Altered innate immunity is central to pathogenesis of CD and causes may be multifactorial:

- Th1 cytokines, e.g. IL-12 and tumour necrosis factor (TNFα) stimulate the inflammatory response. Inflammatory cells (e.g. macrophages) are thus recruited and then release non-specific inflammatory products, including arachidonic acid metabolites, proteases, platelet activating factor, and free radicals. These products result in direct injury to the intestine.

- The macrophages may themselves fail to secrete cytokines in response to a bacterial challenge, so enhanced recruitment of neutrophils occurs.

- The Crohn's patient is less able to control autophagy and, hence, bacterial replication and antigen presentation.

- Abnormal regulation of antimicrobial peptides like defensins produced by Paneth cells (in small intestine crypts), may also reduce normal bacterial defensive mechanisms and cause mucosal changes.

- There is increasing evidence that the IL-12/IL-23—Th-1/Th-17 axis is important in modulation between the innate and acquired immune responses in Crohn's pathogenesis. IL-23 can stimulate formation of Th17 cells, which produces IL-17, a cytokine that then causes T cell priming and stimulates release of further molecules such as IL-1, IL-6, TNFα, NOS-2, and chemokines resulting in inflammation.

- TNFα modulates granuloma formation so numerous anti-TNFα drugs have been developed for use in CD.

Whatever the precise mechanism in CD, non-caseating granulomas result at multiple foci along the GI tract. Typically, these multifocal and discontinuous areas produce 'skip lesions', that occur anywhere from the mouth to the anus, and can extend across the bowel wall into mesentery and lymph nodes. Neutrophils infiltrate the crypts and form crypt abscesses, destroying crypt architecture. Typically, disease is confined to the terminal ileum and caecum, while 30% is in the small bowel, 20% in the large bowel, with the rectum often spared. Because of the transmural nature, advanced lesions can result in fissures, fistulae, large ulcers, sinus tracts, fibrosis, and perforations.

Clinically, patients tend to present with abdominal pain and weight loss, which with colonic disease may be associated with diarrhoea (± blood). Often systemic symptoms of malaise, anaemia, anorexia, and fever are seen. Signs of abdominal tenderness/distension, peri-anal skin tags, abscess, and fistulae are common. Extra-intestinal manifestations may also be present, such as finger clubbing or arthritis (see Table 6.13).

Ulcerative colitis

Unlike CD, UC is confined to the mucosa and submucosa of the colon, typically affecting the rectum (proctitis); it can extend proximally to involve other areas of large bowel; areas of inflammation are usually in continuity.

The aetiology of UC is less well understood than CD, but has a certain degree of overlap as demonstrated in genome-wide association studies, although the influence of non-genetic factors is much greater in UC. As with CD, it is thought that microbial antigen exposure plays a role in initiating and maintaining UC. Dysregulation in the innate immune system (e.g. toll-like receptors, dendritic cells, etc.) and in the adaptive immune system (e.g. effector T-cells, regulatory T-cells, eosinophils, neutrophils, etc.) contribute significantly to pathogenesis. Unlike CD, however, T-cell response to antigens is not Th1 dominant, but rather thought to be a Th2 disease (IL-4, IL-13) probably mediated by specialized natural killer T cells that secrete IL-13. This is evidenced by the fact that interferon-γ production, although raised in CD, is near normal levels in UC. In contrast, raised levels of IL-1, IL-6, and TNFα, is present in both CD and UC, thus anti-TNFα therapy is effective in the management of both diseases.

T cell accumulation in the lamina propria occurs in diseased segments, and these cells produce high levels of IL-13 that are ultimately cytotoxic to colonic epithelium and induce hypersecretion of mucin.

In addition to an increase in T cells, production of B cells and plasma cells is also increased, effecting an increase in immunoglobulin production, in particular IgG. Increased mucosal IgG1 antibodies have activity against colonic epithelial antigens, suggesting that autoimmunity plays a part in the disease. A concept strengthened by the presence of autoantibodies against perinuclear anti-neutrophil cytoplasmic antibodies (pANCA), which are not present in Crohn's disease. Furthermore, the epithelial antigen targeted by IgG1, is also present in other sites that are prone to extra-intestinal manifestation such as the skin, eyes, and joints.

Symptoms in UC are usually insidious in onset, although can be acute, and typically involve bloody diarrhoea and mucus with an increased urgency to defecate. Weight loss is common and abdominal discomfort may occur (left-hypochondrum). Anorexia, fever, and vomiting are systemic associations in severe attacks probably as a result of infectious colitis. Much like CD, UC may have extra-intestinal manifestations (Table 6.14).

The Truelove and Witts severity index, based on the number of stools passed, and systemic symptoms can be

Table 6.13 Extra-intestinal manifestations in Crohn's disease

Manifestation	Examples		
Arthritis	Large joint arthritis	Sacroileitis	Ankylosing spondylitis
Ocular manifestations	Scleritis	Episcleritis	Conjunctivitis
Metabolic bone disease	Osteopenia		
Mucocutaneous manifestation	Apthous ulcers	Pyoderma gangrenosum	Erythema nodosum
Renal stones	Oxalate stones		

Table 6.14 Extra-intestinal manifestations in Ulcerative colitis

Extra-intestinal manifestations in UC	Related to colitis activity	Unrelated to colitis activity
Arthritis	Peripheral arthropathy	Sacroiliitis
		Ankylosing spondylitis
Ocular manifestations	Episcleritis	
Mucocutaneous manifestation	Erythema nodosum	
	Apthous ulcers	
Other		Primary sclerosing cholangitis

used to establish if admission and/or urgent treatment is required.

Further considerations in IBD

The diagnosis of Crohn's or UC should be based on clinical suspicion and findings from sigmoidoscopy/colonoscopy and histology. Less frequently, serology can be performed to differentiate between the two. More recently, a faecal calprotectin test has been advocated by NICE as a tool to differentiate between IBD and non-IBD (including IBS).

The main aim in the treatment of IBD is to induce and preserve a state of remission so patients can maintain a good quality of life and avoid/delay the requirement for surgery; 75% of patients require surgery within 20 years. The two primary considerations in management are treatment of active disease and maintenance therapy.

For a full summary of the relevant pathways and drug targets, see Figure 6.9.

Management

Crohn's disease

Diagnosis is based on a combination of clinical history backed up by endoscopic, biochemical, histological, and radiographic findings. Preliminary investigations will include laboratory tests; FBC, U&Es, LFTs, and inflammatory markers (ESR and CRP), as well as stool samples taken to exclude infectious causes. Diagnosis, however, is confirmed by endoscopy, used to establish the extent of disease and to obtain a biopsy to identify pathological markers consistent with CD.

As neither medical nor surgical management of Crohn's provides a cure; the aim of treatment is to induce a

remission, or failing that optimize symptom management and quality of life, while minimizing toxicity and long-term complications. The disease is managed according to its site, severity, and pattern, determined through CRP and symptoms where possible, in order to minimize the excessive imaging required by IBD patients during their lifetime.

Some controversy exists over the medical treatment strategies used in Crohn's, such as adopting a step-up or step-down approach, or which drug therapies offer the better risk/benefit profile; however, there is universal acceptance that exposure to corticosteroid therapy should be minimized. Surgery plays a large role in the management of CD, particularly in those failing medical therapy, obstructive disease, and fistulas. Medical treatment aims to minimize/delay surgical resection, thereby reducing the risk of short bowel syndrome and its associated complications. In all cases, patients should be actively involved in treatment decisions, ensuring they are adequately informed on the relative risks and benefits of all available options.

Active disease

Ileocolonic disease accounts for the vast majority of cases of Crohn's; less commonly disease occurring in the peri-anal, oral, or gastroduodenal areas, requires greater tailoring of treatment. On first presentation of ileocolonic disease, or in patients that have not had an exacerbation for over 12 months, monotherapy with conventional glucocorticoids (**prednisolone**) is the preferred treatment option, supported by the greater body of evidence for superior efficacy. Treatment is generally continued for 1–4 weeks until resolution of symptoms, before being gradually tapered over an 8-week period according to patient's response. Oral **budesonide**, although less effective, can be used as an alternative where conventional glucocorticoids fail or where disease is more distal.

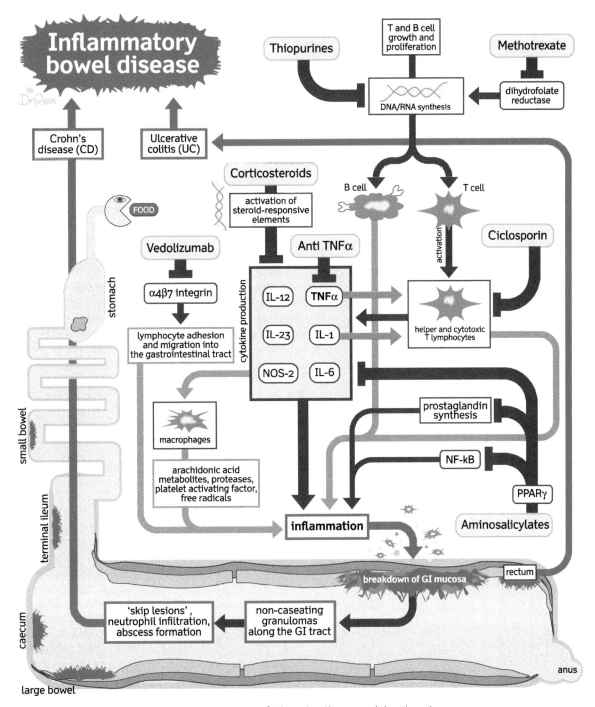

Figure 6.9 Inflammatory bowel disease: summary of relevant pathways and drug targets.

In mild to moderate disease an amino salicylate can be used if steroid treatment is not possible. Patients should be made aware, however, that although aminosalicylates are generally well tolerated the evidence behind their use is variable, with inferior efficacy. Neither budesonide nor aminosalicylates are recommended for use in severe disease. Where an aminosalicylate is used, choice of agent should be based on the site of disease, for example,

sulfasalazine relies on colonic bacteria to release the active moiety and is therefore unlikely to be effective in ilieitis. A response should be expected within 3–4 weeks, and in the case of treatment failure, prednisolone is necessary, unless contraindicated. Elemental enteral feeds are an option in acute disease in children and young adults for inducing remission, with the benefit of being steroid-sparing in the long term.

In patients with severe disease or recurrent flares, i.e. 2 or more exacerbations in the preceding 12 months, or where tapering of glucocorticoids leads to a relapse in remission, a thiopurine (ideally **mercaptopurine** or less favourably **azathioprine**) is recommended in addition to steroid treatment to induce a remission. Prior to initiating treatment, a viral screen should be carried out to assess CMV/EBV status and thiopurine methyltransferase (TMPT) status should be assessed. Patients in whom TMPT activity is lower than normal will likely require lower thiopurine doses; however, in TMPT deficiency, they should be avoided and methotrexate considered as an alternative. **Methotrexate** is frequently used, particularly where thiopurines are contraindicated or poorly tolerated.

In severe active Crohn's disease, unresponsive to conventional treatment, anti-TNFα therapy (**infliximab** or **adalimumab**), forms the mainstay of treatment. Patients on anti-TNFα therapy are reassessed annually and treatment discontinued in the event of treatment failure, or in the case of stable remission where this is deemed appropriate by the treating specialist. Patients that achieve remission and subsequently relapse, are offered the option of restarting.

More recently, the introduction of a further monoclonal antibody **vedolizumab**, offers a treatment option for those unsuitable for anti-TNFα therapy, either due to lack of efficacy, intolerance, or contraindications. As with the anti-TNFα's, it is reserved for use in moderate to severe disease, although an initial assessment is made at 14 weeks to determine whether the patient has responded before treatment continues. Reassessments are carried out annually and treatment continued where a benefit is sustained in the absence of stable remission. As with anti-TNFα treatment, those that do enter remission can restart treatment in the event of a relapse.

Additional supportive management such as replacement of electrolytes, total parenteral nutrition (TPN) or elemental diet may be required in some patients, as well as antibiotic therapy to treat any underlying sepsis.

Peri-anal or fistulizing disease is usually associated with disease elsewhere in the GI tract. However, additional treatment such as **metronidazole** and an earlier introduction of immunomodulating therapy or biologics may be necessary. Specifically, **infliximab** is licensed for active fistulizing Crohn's disease, with the same requirements for annual reassessment.

Maintenance

Maintenance treatment is recommended in patients that have required dual therapy to induce a remission, or in the presence of poor prognostic factors such as more than one previous resection or previous complicated disease. Some patients, however, choose not to have maintenance treatment.

Thiopurines are the preferred agents for maintenance, although this indication falls outside of the product license for both **azathioprine** and **mercaptopurine**. Where treatment is poorly tolerated, contraindicated (e.g. TMPT deficiency), or where **methotrexate** was required to induce a remission, maintenance with methotrexate is the preferred option.

There is limited evidence of benefit with aminosalicylate therapy in maintaining remission in CD, although **mesalazine** (but not **sulfasalazine**) has been used to maintain remission in preference to no therapy, in patients with mild disease who have responded successfully to therapy. Mesalazine is also used for maintenance where surgery has been carried out to induce remission.

The use of conventional glucocorticoids or **budesonide** is not recommended for maintenance therapy, due to the associated toxicity with long-term steroid use. Furthermore, although budesonide has been shown to maintain remission in some patients, any benefit appears to be lost after 6–12 months (Figure 6.10).

Ulcerative colitis

As with Crohn's disease, UC is diagnosed through a combination of clinical history and investigations including laboratory tests, stool samples, and more definitively, with colonoscopy or sigmoidoscopy. Similarly, disease management aims to induce and maintain a remission of symptoms, in order to optimize quality of life, while minimizing toxicity associated with therapy; in particular, long-term corticosteroid use. Medical treatment, especially in severe disease, can help reduce the need for a colectomy.

Treatment will be determined by severity and extent of disease, i.e. distal disease (up to the sigmoid descending junction and includes proctitis), left-sided disease (extending from the sigmoid descending junction to the splenic flexure) and extensive disease (extending proximal to the splenic flexure).

In general, the medical management of UC is better supported with consistent evidence of efficacy than CD,

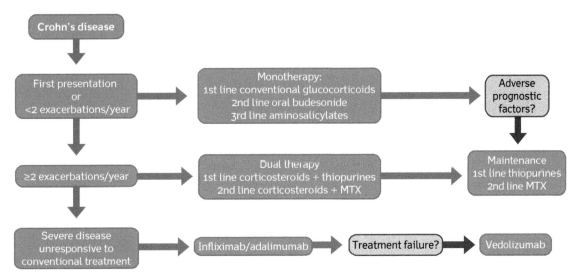

Figure 6.10 Medical management of ileocolonic CD.

reflected in the number of drugs licensed for its treatment and a greater consensus on the way it is managed.

Active disease

In most cases mild/moderate disease can be managed in an outpatient setting, avoiding the need for hospital admissions. Unlike Crohn's, there is good evidence to show successful treatment with aminosalicylates given topically and/or orally in the management of active mild to moderate UC, for which all four aminosalicylates are licensed. Choice and route of aminosalicylate will depend on site of disease, i.e. in proctitis and proctosigmoiditis topical treatment is preferred, whereas oral therapy is treatment of choice in left-sided or extensive disease. **Mesalazine** is invariably the drug of choice, as it shows good efficacy in treating UC at all sites, is well tolerated and competitively priced. **Balsalazide** is a useful alternative and **olsalazine** may be preferred in the management of left-sided disease or in patients intolerant of first line choices. **Sulfasalazine** is usually avoided due to its poor side effect profile, but may be of value in patients with co-existing reactive arthropathies.

Topical therapy with mesalazine is a viable treatment option, particularly in patients with distal disease and is most effective when used in combination with oral therapy. In patients unable to use topical mesalazine, topical steroids may be considered, although they are of inferior efficacy.

Where optimal treatment with an aminosalicylate fails, oral **prednisolone** is the drug of choice in inducing remission in active disease. Once patients are symptom free, doses should be tapered gradually over an 8-week period to reduce the risk of relapse.

In severe acute disease, patients will require hospitalization where the need for surgery is assessed. Ideally, first-line treatment is with IV corticosteroids (**methylprednisolone**, **hydrocortisone**), while any maintenance aminosalicylate therapy is continued.

In addition, patients will require parenteral fluids and electrolytes to replace any losses and may need nutritional support with either TPN or enteral feeds. Antibiotics are reserved for patients with infection or those requiring surgery. Topical therapy may be used adjunctively, particularly in distal disease. An intensive medical management approach can help reduce the risk of colectomy, although this remains unavoidable in some patients.

In patients with moderate to severe disease that fail to respond to conventional therapy, anti-TNFα therapy with **infliximab**, **adalimumab**, or **golimumab** is recommended. Once on treatment, patients may continue while they continue to demonstrate a benefit, with annual reviews to assess disease activity. **Vedolizumab** is another option in patients who fail to respond to anti-TNFα therapy. The use of immunosupressants such as **tacrolimus** and **ciclosporin** in refractory disease has largely been superseded with the introduction of anti-TNFα therapy.

Maintenance treatments

Lifelong maintenance is recommended in all patients with left-sided and extensive disease, as well as those with distal disease who relapses within 1 year of treatment. As with CD, the choice of drug for maintenance therapy will depend on what was used to successfully treat active disease. Oral aminosalicylates are effective in maintaining remission, with topical therapy preferred in distal disease. An escalation to thiopurine therapy is recommended in patients who relapse more than twice a year, or in those who are steroid dependent. Corticosteroids should not be used for maintenance treatment (Figure 6.11).

Drug classes used in management

Aminosalicylates

5-aminosalicylic acid (5-ASA) is the active anti-inflammatory component of all salicylates used in the treatment of IBD. Examples include balsalazide, mesalazine, olsalazine, and sulfasalazine.

Mechanism of action

Sulfasalazine is the prototype drug of this group, and was the first aminosalicylate shown to have efficacy in the treatment of IBD. It is a chemical compound of a salicylate; 5-ASA, and a sulfonamide, **sulfapyridine**, joined by a nitrogen bond. Hydrolysis to its two components is done by bacteria in the large bowel, and while the sulfapyridine is absorbed and excreted in the urine, the 5-ASA acts locally as an anti-inflammatory agent in the wall of the gut. Most of the adverse effects of sulfasalazine are due to its sulfapyridine component, which led to the development of formulations where 5-ASA is given on its own (**mesalazine**) or as two 5-ASA molecules joined by a diazo bond (**olsalazine**).

Mesalazine is rapidly absorbed and has to be protected in special formulations, in order to prevent absorption before reaching the large bowel. Olsalazine, in contrast, is poorly absorbed and is hydrolysed by gut bacteria to a single 5-ASA molecule. The mucosal concentration will determine the therapeutic efficacy of 5-ASA,

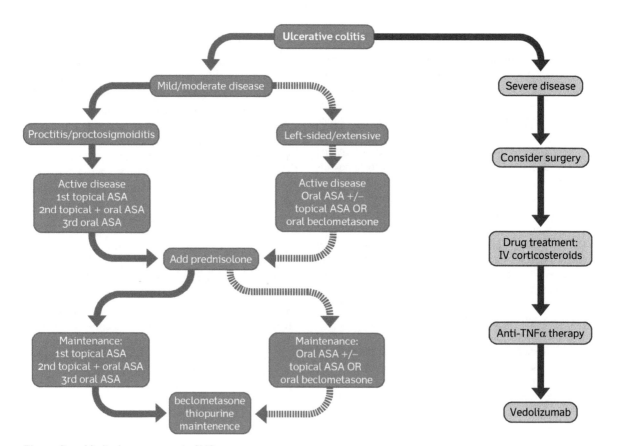

Figure 6.11 Medical management of UC.

with the combination of topical and oral therapy producing a 100-fold increase. Novel delivery systems control the colonic release of 5-ASA via a multi-matrix (MMX) of hydrophilic polymer and lipophilic excipients enfolded in a coated tablet, which might increase the mucosal delivery to the sigmoid colon. **Balsalazide** is a prodrug that is enzymatically cleaved by bacterial azoreduction in the colon to produce mesalazine, also releasing the inert 4-aminobenzoyl-β-alanine.

The 5-ASAs compounds have been suggested to have various mechanisms of action, such as inhibition of the NF-kB pro-inflammatory signal pathway, modulation of cytokine production and prostaglandin synthesis inhibition. These actions seems to be produced by induction of and binding to the peroxisome proliferator-activated receptor-Y (PPARY) expressed on epithelial cells, a nuclear receptor that is highly expressed in the colon, and has a crucial role in bacterial-induced inflammation.

Prescribing

Aminosalicylates are widely used in the management of IBD both in the induction and maintenance of remission, although evidence for their efficacy is considerably superior in UC. **Sulfasalazine** was the first in the class to be developed and, although potentially more effective, is largely limited by its poor tolerability. **Mesalazine**, the only other aminosalicylate licensed for use in Crohn's, is tolerated in 80% of patients intolerant of sulfasalazine, primarily due to the toxicity associated with the sulfapyridine moiety in sulfasalazine. **Olsalazine** and **balsalazide**, the newer of the aminosalicylates, are only licensed for use in UC.

PRACTICAL PRESCRIBING

Sulfasalazine monitoring

- *Baseline*: FBC (differential white cell, red cell and platelet counts), LFTs, and renal function.
- *Routine*: FBC should be checked fortnightly for the first 12 weeks, and then 12-weekly thereafter; LFTs (including ALT or AST) should be checked every 4 weeks for the first 12 weeks, and then 12-weekly. Regular renal function may be considered in some patients.

Choice of aminosalicylate will primarily depend on tolerance, cost, and dosing schedule; although consideration should also be given to the site of the disease as different drugs and formulations vary in their release profiles so that they act at different sites. Olsalazine and balsalazide, for example, may be preferred in distal disease as they are released by bacterial activity within the colon. Although mesalazine preparations are formulated to target different sites within the gut, in reality there is little to distinguish them in terms of efficacy. Mesalazine is also available as rectal formulations as enemas and suppositories that are useful in distal disease, although monotherapy is not recommended.

PRACTICAL PRESCRIBING

Topical mesalazine formulations

- Mesalazine suppositories are superior to enemas in delivering drug to the rectum and therefore indicated in disease up to the rectosigmoid junction.
- Foam enemas deliver drug up to the proximal sigmoid colon and liquid enemas can deliver drug to the splenic flexure.
- There is little difference in efficacy between foam and liquid enemas; however, foam enemas tend to be easier to use, more comfortable to retain, and thus preferred by patients

---

Unwanted effects

Side effects occur most commonly with **sulfasalazine**, affecting about 45% of patients; where the incidence with **mesalazine** and **olsalazine** are more comparable with placebo. The most common adverse effects to aminosalicylates are dose dependent and tend to occur within 3–6 months of starting treatment; they include nausea, headache, rash, and diarrhoea.

As a class, aminosalicylates are associated with renal toxicity and undergo renal excretion; they should therefore be avoided in severe renal impairment. All patients will require close monitoring pretreatment and at regular intervals thereafter.

The **sulfapyridine** moiety in sulfasalazine in particular is associated with hypersensitivity reactions including blood dyscrasias (leukopenia, thrombocytopenia), rashes (including rarely, severe reactions such as toxic epidermal necrolysis and Stevens–Johnson Syndrome), serum sickness, and anaphylaxis. Patients with a history of hypersensitivity to 'sulfa' drugs should avoid sulfasalazine. Treatment is also associated with DRESS (drug, rash, eosinophilia, systemic symptoms; see 'Prescribing warning: DRESS with sulfasalazine'.

Drug rash eosinophilia systemic symptoms with sulfasalazine

- Drug rash eosinophilia systemic symptoms (DRESS) is a rare, but potentially fatal systemic hypersensitivity reaction characterized by a maculopapular rash, fever, facial oedema, lymphadenopathy, eosinophilia, and internal organ involvement, e.g. heart, lung, liver, and kidneys.
- Onset is usually within 2–6 weeks of initiating drug therapy.
- Management is primarily with high dose corticosteroids.

Sulfasalazine, and rarely mesalazine therapy, can induce oligospermia and cause infertility, which usually resolves within 2–3 months of withdrawal

Drug interactions

As aminosaliclyates are poorly absorbed from the GI tract, drug interactions are infrequent and of minimal clinical significance.

Corticosteroids

Corticosteroids activate receptors present in immune cells and regulate the expression of various steroid-responsive target genes controlling the inflammatory process. Examples include prednisolone, budesonide, beclometasone, hydrocortisone, and methylprednisolone.

Mechanism of action

Corticosteroids have been very effective in the reduction of the inflammatory component and clinical induction of remission. They suppress active inflammation acutely, but are not effective as maintenance agents, having side effects that preclude their long-term use. Moreover, therapeutic response is lost in most patients over time. One year after corticosteroid treatment, only 48% of UC and 32% of Crohn's patients are corticosteroid-free without surgery, underscoring how maintenance therapy after steroid-induced remission is a crucial step in the management of the disease.

Although the specific mechanisms are not fully understood, corticosteroids affect immune cells by activating corticosteroid receptors. This could lead to the induction or suppression of several steroid-responsive target genes transcription, with many relevant in the inflammatory process. Corticosteroids can decrease the production of many pro-inflammatory proteins, such as interleukin 1-6, TNFα, Y-interferon, prostaglandins, adhesion molecules, and cytosolic phospholipase A2. This regulation of gene expression is not necessarily direct, as many of these genes do not present recognizable glucocorticoid response elements in their promoter regions, indicating the existence of inhibitory mechanisms. Indeed, corticosteroid receptors can also alter the stability of messenger RNA, or translation rates, thus affecting protein levels.

The interaction of corticosteroid receptors with other transcription factors has also been recognized as a crucial mechanism regulating the anti-inflammatory action. In particular, the transcription factor NF-κβ, known to control the transcription of key inflammatory molecules, can be inhibited via straight protein interaction and increased production of the NF-κβ inhibitor I-κβ. Given the key role of NF-κβ signalling in the regulation of the inflammatory process, the inhibition by corticosteroids might be a crucial anti-inflammatory effect.

The inhibition of the production of several pro-inflammatory cytokines, chemokines, and adhesion molecules, contributes towards the strong anti-inflammatory effects. At the cellular level, these molecular mechanisms are transduced into reduced intercellular interactions crucial to antigen presentation and inflammatory cell activation, decreased migration of immune cells, and reduced phagocytic and degranulation functions. Moreover, there is evidence that corticosteroids can prevent intestinal mucosal natural killer cell activity, and increase the GI tract water and sodium absorption, thus alleviating diarrhoea.

Prescribing

Corticosteroids are effective in managing relapses of both UC and Crohn's, showing greater efficacy than aminosalicylates in inducing remission. However, due to their toxic profile every effort is made to minimize patient exposure. This is partly addressed by minimizing doses to 40 mg/day of **prednisolone**, to allow optimal efficacy with minimal toxicity. Doses are tapered gradually over an 8-week period to reduce the risk of relapse.

IV therapies of **hydrocortisone** (the main glucocorticoid secreted by the adrenal cortex) or **methylprednisolone** are used in severe disease, where patients are unable to tolerate oral therapy or where absorption is thought to be compromised.

The other oral agents **beclometasone** (synthetic halogenated glucocorticoid licensed in UC) and **budesonide** (with high affinity to the glucocorticoid receptor and weak mineralocorticoid activity, which is licensed in Crohn's affecting the ileum or ascending colon), are poorly absorbed and formulated to promote a local action. They therefore have minimal effect on systemic or extensive disease.

Topical treatment with rectal formulations may be beneficial in combination with systemic therapy in patients with distal disease, although the aminosalicylate rectal formulations are preferred. Available rectal corticosteroid formulations include suppositories (prednisolone) or enemas (prednisolone, hydrocortisone, and budesonide), each formulated to promote release at distinct distal sites.

Unwanted effects

Side effects to corticosteroids are numerous and can be acute in onset, associated with prolonged use, or occur following withdrawal, all of which are relevant in the management of IBD. Side effects are dose-dependent and may be severe, so it is generally accepted that the lowest effective dose should be used for the shortest possible period, thus not used for maintenance treatment in IBD.

Corticosteroids possess varying combinations of mineralocorticoid and glucocorticoid activity, the proportion of which will determine their side effect profile. **Prednisolone**, **beclometasone**, and **methylprednsiolone** possess predominantly glucocorticoid activity, associated with metabolism of glucose and fats, as well as bone formation. They also act within the brain to affect mood and cognitive ability. Acutely, they can impair glucose metabolism, particularly in diabetic patients, increase appetite, and induce or exacerbate psychiatric reactions ranging from mood disturbances to psychosis. Prolonged use is associated with osteoporosis and muscle wasting. Patients, in particular post-menopausal women, receiving frequent courses (steroid dependent) should undergo regular DEXA scans to assess bone density and receive primary osteoporosis prophylaxis with a bisphosphonate. Long-term use also leaves the skin very fragile and easy to bruise.

Glucocorticoids have potent anti-inflammatory properties, adversely affecting immune response to infections by impairing white cells, such as neutrophils, lymphocytes, and macrophages, in terms of numbers and activity. As a result, prolonged use of corticosteroids increases susceptibility to infection and may mask symptoms due to an impaired response to infection. Frequent users of corticosteroids are therefore advised to avoid contact with chicken pox, measles, and tuberculosis. Live vaccines should be avoided and response to other vaccines is likely to be impaired.

Hydrocortisone possesses equal mineralocorticoid and glucocorticoid activity. Mineralocorticoid effects include sodium and water retention, which can lead to oedema and hypertension, and electrolyte disturbances. In some instances, prolonged use may result in congestive cardiac failure, particularly in high-risk patients.

As with many drugs, GI effects such as nausea, vomiting, dyspepsia, etc., are common, particularly with oral therapy. Prolonged use also carries a risk of peptic ulceration, so that a PPI may be considered prophylactically and use avoided in patients with active peptic ulceration.

Prolonged use of steroids (more than 3 weeks) at doses exceeding physiological levels (equivalent to 7.5 mg of prednisolone), leads to adrenal atrophy, so that abrupt withdrawal can lead to adrenal insufficiency. This can be avoided by administering doses in the morning, minimizing doses and duration of treatment, and ensuring that prolonged or frequently repeated courses are tapered slowly. Adrenal atrophy can persist for years after treatment is stopped, leaving patients at risk of an adrenal crisis if poorly managed.

Drug interactions

Aside from vaccines (see 'Unwanted effects') there are few interactions to be aware of with corticosteroids, with the exception of **methylprednisolone** as it is metabolized via the CYP 3A4 isoenzyme. Consequently, potent inhibitors, e.g. macrolides (**clarithromycin**, **erythromycin**), can significantly increase levels of methylprednisolone, whereas potent inducers, e.g. **rifampicin**, **phenytoin**, can reduce its effect. Methylprednisolone can increase **ciclosporin** levels, increasing the risk of convulsions.

Thiopurines

Thiopurines have immunosuppressive properties due to their capacity to be incorporated into DNA and RNA, impeding growth and proliferation of T and B cells. For example, azathioprine and mercaptopurine.

Mechanism of action

The development of **azathioprine** (AZA) as an innovative immunosupressive drug in the 1950s laid the basis for the current concept of steroid-sparing treatment strategies in IBD. As with **mercaptopurine**, azathioprine needs to undergo significant metabolic transformation before being active as an immunosuppressant. Bioavailability is highly variable (16–72 %) due to incomplete absorption, with significant inter- and intra-individual variation. A high proportion of absorbed AZA suffers a rapid non-enzymatic liver conversion to yield 6-mercaptopurine (6-MP) and 1-methyl-4-nitro-5-thioimidazole. 6-MP has a very short half-life (1–2 hr) and is metabolized by three competing enzymatic pathways—xanthine oxidase, thiopurine S-methyltransferase, and hypoxanthine phosphoribosyltransferase, producing the active nucleotide metabolites 6-thioguanine nucleotides (6-TGN) and 6-methylmercaptopurine.

6-TGNs are the pharmacologically active end-metabolites of thiopurines. The activation of cytotoxic pathways is normally used to explain their mechanism of action. Due to their structural similarity to endogenous purine bases, they can be integrated into DNA or RNA, and produce strand breakage, inhibition of replication, and DNA repair, plus disruption of *de novo* protein synthesis. This can affect the cellular growth and proliferation of T and B cells resulting in immunosupression. Moreover, 6-TGNs have been shown to inhibit the inflammatory mediator interferon α, while genome-wide expression studies have shown that AZA has the capacity to inhibit the stimulus-induced expression of various genes that can regulate the metabolism, signalling pathways and immune functions of T cells.

Elucidating the detailed molecular mechanism of AZA's immunosuppressive effects could help in the development of biochemical modifications that can overcome the delayed effect of action. In this respect, novel findings point towards an inhibition of T lymphocytes proliferative capacity, together with pro-apoptotic effects. The fact that the capacity of human T cells to produce effector cytokines, and therefore contribute to the pro-inflammatory environment, seems to be unaffected by AZA, and could partly explain the delayed onset of action.

Prescribing

Thiopurines are effective in treating active disease and for maintenance in IBD. They are generally used for their steroid-sparing effect, although onset of action is considerably faster with corticosteroids. Treatment is usually second-line to aminosalicylates, which are better tolerated.

Prior to initiating therapy, patients should have their TPMT status assessed (see 'Practical prescribing: thiopurine methyl transferase levels') to ensure they have the ability to metabolize and clear the drug. Doses are started low and titrated up slowly to achieve optimal effect,

thereby reducing the risk of a patient developing leucopenia. Monitoring is therefore essential, with FBCs carried out weekly for the first 8 weeks and then 3-monthly. A viral screen should also be carried out pretreatment to rule out the presence of CMV or EBV.

> ## PRACTICAL PRESCRIBING
> ### Thiopurine methyl transferase levels
> - About 1 in 300 patients lack the enzyme thiopurine methyl transferase (TPMT) required to metabolize thiopurines.
> - These patients are therefore more susceptible to toxicity, in particular leucopenia, which is a common dose-limiting side effect.
> - Current recommendations advocate baseline TPMT levels to reduce the risk of toxicity.
> - Patients with lower than normal levels will likely require a dose reduction.
> - Patients that are TPMT deficient should not receive thiopurines.

Unwanted effects

Bone marrow suppression (leucopenia and thrombocytopenia) is the most commonly reported side effect to thiopurines, affecting more than 10% of patients; who should thus be advised to report symptoms such as unexplained bruising or bleeding. Other common side effects, including GI effects (nausea, vomiting, diarrhoea, and pancreatitis) and flu-like symptoms (fever, muscle pain, and headache) are dose-dependent and resolve on drug withdrawal. Severe hypersensitivity reactions such as Stevens–Johnson syndrome can occur, but are rare.

Regular LFTs should be carried out with thiopurine therapy, as both drugs are hepatotoxic and extensively metabolized via the liver. Dose reductions may be necessary in hepatic impairment, particularly if patients show signs of toxicity.

As with other immunosuppressants, patients should be advised to avoid the use of live vaccines while on treatment and be aware of the increased risk of infection.

Drug interactions

The effects of thiopurines are increased with **allopurinol** and a dose reduction to 25% of the usual dose is recommended, unless being used therapeutically to boost levels. Drugs known to cause haematological toxicity should be used cautiously in combination with thiopurines, as the effect is likely to be augmented. Of particular concern are anticoagulants, **clozapine** (increased risk of agranulocytosis) and **trimethoprim**.

Methotrexate

Methotrexate is an inhibitor of the enzyme dihydrofolate reductase that is required for DNA synthesis. In addition, it can also have anti-inflammatory effects through increased adenosine receptor activation.

Mechanism of action

The folate antagonist **methotrexate** was developed for the treatment of malignancies, with later use in non-neoplastic diseases as an anti-inflammatory and/or immunosuppressive drug.

Methotrexate inhibition of AICAR transformylase results in augmented release of adenosine by fibroblasts and endothelial cells among others. Adenosine is an effective anti-inflammatory purine nucleotide that reduces superoxide anion generation in neutrophil-mediated injury to endothelial cells. This and other observations show that the anti-inflammatory effects of methotrexate are due to the action of adenosine and its A2-receptors.

The active promotion of effector T cell apoptosis is one of the main anti-inflammatory mechanisms that allows the control of inflammatory reactions in the intestinal mucosa of patients. The role of apoptosis in the cell death generated by methotrexate at high doses was first established in the 1990s and subsequently confirmed for human T lymphocytes, hepatoma cell lines, and keratinocytes. Further studies with low doses of methotrexate also demonstrated that it can induce apoptosis to activated T cells.

Methotrexate inhibits dihydrofolate reductase and produces a diminished thymidylate synthesis, which is required for DNA production. It acts during the synthesis of DNA and RNA, and is cytotoxic during the S-phase of the cell cycle. Thus, it has more toxicity on fast-dividing cells (i.e. GI and oral mucosa), which undergo more repeated DNA replication.

Prescribing

Methotrexate is administered orally, IM or SC in the management of Crohn's disease as a treatment option in patients failing conventional therapy. Higher doses (25 mg) are used to induce remission and then reduced for maintenance (15 mg IM, 10–15 mg PO). In all instances, doses are administered weekly, with weekly folic acid taken approximately 3 days later, to reduce adverse effects without impairing efficacy of methotrexate. Although used in UC off-label, there is a lack of high-quality evidence to support this indication.

PRACTICAL PRESCRIBING

Methotrexate monitoring

- *Baseline investigations*: renal function, ALT and/or AST, albumin, and FBC.
- *Frequency*: every 2 weeks until on stable dose for 6 weeks, then monthly for 3 months and thereafter at least every 12 weeks.

Reproduced from Ledingham, J. et al. BSR and BHPR guideline for the prescription and monitoring of non-biologic disease-modifying anti-rheumatic drugs. Rheumatology, 56(6), 865–868. https://doi.org/10.1093/rheumatology/kew479. Copyright © 2017, Oxford University Press.

PRESCRIBING WARNING

Methotrexate weekly—never event

- In IBD, methotrexate is always prescribed as a weekly dose and, as such, has been the victim of numerous prescribing and dispensing errors.
- To reduce the risk of errors, patients should be clearly counselled on the dosing frequency and advised to report any signs of toxicity, such as unexplained bruising, bleeding, mouth ulcers, or nausea.
- Clinicians prescribing methotrexate should always ensure the frequency is clearly indicated and never prescribed as directed. F1 doctors should not prescribe methotrexate.

Unwanted effects

Side effects commonly include GI intolerance such as nausea, vomiting, and mouth ulcers. Bone marrow suppression is also common and patients should be counselled on signs of toxicity. For more information see Topic 13.1, 'Haemato-oncology and Malignancy').

PRESCRIBING WARNING

Chronic methotrexate toxicity

Hepatotoxicity and pneumonitis associated with chronic use are side effects of particular concern in IBD patients who receive methotrexate at low doses for prolonged periods.

Anti-TNFα monoclonal antibodies

Anti-TNFα are monoclonal antibodies that bind TNFα on T cells to promote apoptosis and cell death. For example, infliximab, adalimumab, and golimumab.

Mechanism of action

Tumour necrosis factor α (TNFα) is a pro-inflammatory cytokine, which together with interferon-Y, interleukin-1 (IL-1), have a central role in IBD. Increased expression of IL-1 and TNFα has been recognized in IBD, with a role of TNFα also being established in the pathogenesis of the disease.

IL-1 and TNFα have various common pro-inflammatory properties and are critical in the amplification of mucosal inflammation. Principally secreted by monocytes and macrophages after activation, they are able to induce neutrophils, fibroblasts, intestinal macrophages, and muscle cells to generate other soluble mediators of inflammation and injury, together with other inflammatory cytokines. TNFα may affect mucosal inflammation by interfering with the epithelial barrier, promotion of villous epithelial cells apoptosis, and chemokine secretion from cells of the intestine epithelia.

The chimeric monoclonal antibody **infliximab** targets human TNFα, and binds soluble bioactive TNFα in the intestinal mucosa, neutralizing its effects. This probably reduces pro-inflammatory cytokine (IL-1, IL-6) production, leucocyte migration and infiltration, and neutrophil and eosinophil activation. In addition, infliximab binds membrane-bound TNFα, leading to the destruction of immune cells in vitro, via antibody-dependent cellular toxicity. The binding to membrane-bound TNFα on activated T cells can promote apoptotic T cell death.

Infliximab is made of a human constant region IgG1k light chain (approximately 75% of the antibody), connected to a mouse variable region (25%), which is associated with a risk of immunogenicity. With a very long half-life (9 days), its mechanism of elimination is still poorly understood.

The fully human **adalimumab** IgG1 monoclonal antibody to TNFα is given SC. Preliminary studies have shown that it could be well tolerated in patients with CD who lost response, or developed infliximab-induced infusion reactions or hypersensitivity. Adalimumab is given by subcutaneous injection once every 2 weeks, due to the very long half-life of about 12 days. Although not well defined, the mechanism of elimination is likely to be proteolysis.

Golimumab is a human IgG1k monoclonal antibody that binds to the soluble and transmembrane bioactive forms of TNFα. After SC administration, it can achieve maximum serum concentrations in 2–6 days, with a long half-life of about 2 weeks.

Prescribing

The anti-TNFα drugs **infliximab**, **adalimumab**, and **golimumab** are increasingly being used for their steroid sparing effects in IBD (see Table 6.15). They are reserved for patients with moderate to severe disease-failing treatment with conventional therapy, including corticosteroids and other established therapy. Infliximab, the first on the market, and adalimumab are licensed for use in both Crohn's and UC patients, whereas golimumab only holds a license for use in UC. All three agents are advocated by NICE for use in UC, and infliximab and adalimumab in CD, as treatment options in moderate to severe disease, where conventional therapy has been ineffective. Patients should receive treatment for 12 months or until treatment failure, with annual reviews carried out to ensure benefit in the presence of active disease. More recently, the launch of infliximab and adalimumab biosimilars onto the market has meant a potential reduction in the cost of anti-TNFα treatment. In general, these biosimilars are considered to be of comparable efficacy to the original brand.

Unwanted effects

Hypersensitivity and infection (secondary to bone marrow suppression) are the most commonly reported adverse effects to the monoclonal antibodies. Infusion-related reactions affect up to 18% of patients receiving **infliximab**, and it is therefore recommended that initial infusions are administered over 2 hours and the patient observed for a further 2 hours. In patients that tolerate this, subsequent infusions maybe administered over an hour. Local reactions to **adalimumab** include erythema and itching. Over time, patients are known to develop antibodies to infliximab, which can diminish its efficacy; furthermore there is a risk of delayed hypersensitivity where patients are retreated after a prolonged period off treatment.

The risk of infections, including opportunistic infections, is increased with long-term use of monoclonal antibodies and therefore, prior to treatment, tuberculosis should be excluded. Once on treatment, patients should be monitored and counselled to report symptoms of infection. Similarly, the risk of malignancy is also increased on treatment, in particular melanoma or malignancies

Table 6.15 Comparison of anti-TNFα agents

	Infliximab	Adalimumab	Golimumab
Moderate to severe UC	Yes	Yes	Yes
Moderate to severe CD	Yes	Yes	No
Fistulizing CD	Yes	No	No
Patients 6–17 years CD	Yes	Yes	No
Patients 6–17 years UC	Yes	No	No
Route of administration	IV infusion	SC injection	SC injection
Loading dose	0, 2, and 6 weeks	80 mg at week 0, 40 mg at week 2, **OR** 160 mg at week 0 +/– 80 mg at week 2 (CD only)	200 mg at week 0, 100 mg at week 2
Maintenance dose	8-weekly	2-weekly increased to weekly if necessary	100 mg 4-weekly
Expected response time	2 doses CD 3 doses fistulizing CD 3 doses UC	4–12 weeks CD 2–8 weeks UC	12–14 weeks of starting

of the head, and neck or lung. Patients at increased risk, e.g. those with previous PUVA therapy, COPD, or heavy smokers, require additional precautions.

Other commonly reported side effects include GI effects, headaches, muscle pain, chest pain, fatigue, and fever. The response to vaccination may be impaired in patients on monoclonal antibodies and live vaccines avoided.

Vedolizumab

The recombinant humanized IgG1 monoclonal antibody vedolizumab targets the α4β7 integrin, which is a crucial mediator of gastrointestinal inflammation. For example, vedolizumab.

Mechanism of action

The α4β7 integrin is involved in the recruitment of lymphocytes to the normal and inflamed gut mucosa, and the lymphoid tissue. The selective targeting of α4β7 integrin by **vedolizumab** inhibits the adhesion of lymphocytes to mucosal-addressing cell adhesion molecule 1 (MAdCAM-1). In this way, it prevents lymphocytic cells entering the gut lamina propria and gut-associated lymphoid tissue.

Prescribing

Vedolizumab is indicated for use in UC or CD, in patients who have failed conventional first-line therapy and anti-TNFα treatment. As with **infliximab**, vedolizumab is administered as an IV infusion at weeks 0, 2, and 6, and then 8-weekly, so patients will need to be admitted for day care treatment. Patients failing to respond after 10 weeks are unlikely to benefit and should have treatment discontinued. The dosing interval can be reduced to 4-weekly, where benefits are thought to have reduced over time.

Unwanted effects

As with other MABs, side effects tend to be infusion-related, hypersensitivity-type reactions. Again, patients are at increased risk of infection and malignancy, thus those at risk should be managed cautiously and tuberculosis excluded before treatment started.

Ciclosporin

Ciclosporin is a potent immunosuppressive agent with inhibitory effects on the activation of helper and cytotoxic T lymphocytes.

Mechanism of action

A cyclic undecapeptide from an extract of soil fungi, **ciclosporin** binds to cyclophilin and this complex regulates calcineurin-calmodulin activity, and inhibits the nuclear factor of activated T lymphocytes and cytokine gene expression. Studies have also shown that ciclosporin has negative effects on interferon-Y and TNFα mRNA expression, together with anti-CD3-induced cytotoxic activity, in mucosal T lymphocytes isolated from UC patients. *In vitro* experiments demonstrated that it also has suppressive effects on neutrophil activation, superoxide generation, and chemokine production.

Prescribing

Ciclosporin is a last-line option in UC for the management of severe disease where standard therapy with IV corticosteroids has failed, although with the introduction of biological therapy, its use is largely outdated. Its use in UC is unlicensed and reserved as last line in severe acute disease, as toxicity and long-term failure rates are high; however, in some patients it may provide a 'bridge' to surgery. It is of no value in Crohn's disease.

The dose is administered IV as a continuous infusion titrated up according to serum levels and response. Rarely, it may be converted to oral therapy to continue for up to 6 months thereby forming a 'bridge' to thiopurine therapy.

Unwanted effects

Up to half of patients will experience a mild adverse effect to **ciclosporin** therapy, and as many as 25% a more severe complication, such as renal impairment, opportunistic infections (secondary to immunosuppression), neurotoxicity (seizures) and less commonly hepatic toxicity.

Due to its narrow therapeutic index, and a high risk of severe complications associated with higher levels, blood level monitoring is essential with ciclosporin therapy. As it is extensively metabolized (via CYP 3A4) before being renally cleared, baseline serum creatinine levels and LFTs should be carried out and repeated regularly during treatment. Dose reductions are necessary in renal impairment and should be considered in severe hepatic impairment, based on bilirubin and liver enzymes. As an immunosuppressive, patients on continuous therapy may require antibiotic prophylaxis with **co-trimoxazole** against *Pneumocystis jiroveci*.

Other mild, commonly observed adverse effects include paraesthesia, hypertension, headache, hyperlipidaemia, hypomagnesaemia, and GI effects.

Drug interactions

As **ciclosporin** has a narrow therapeutic index and is metabolized via CYP 3A4, it has a high potential for toxicity, prescribers should be aware of clinically significant interactions with drugs known to affect its serum levels. Potent inhibitors known to increase levels include **methylprednisolone** (and, to a lesser extent, **prednisolone**), macrolides (**erythromycin**, **clarithromycin**), azole antifungals, anti-retrovirals (**atazanavir**, **ritnoavir**) **metoclopramide**, and **omeprazole**. Patients taking concomitant methylprednisolone and ciclosporin are at an increased risk of seizures and therefore ciclosporin monotherapy (not with corticosteroids) is advocated where possible to manage disease. Concomitant therapy with **rosuvastatin** and **tacrolimus** is contraindicated.

Potent enzyme inducers known to decrease ciclosporin levels include the anti-epileptics **phenytoin** and **carbamazepine**.

Other significant interactions occur with drugs possessing similar side effects such as renal toxicity with NSAIDs and hyperkalaemia with ACE inhibitors and potassium sparing diuretics.

In common with other immunosupressants, immune response to vaccination may be impaired.

Further reading

Bosani M, Ardizzone S, Bianchi Porro G (2009) Biologic targeting in the treatment of inflammatory bowel disease. *Biologics* 3, 77–97.

Chevaux JB, Peyrin-Biroulet L, Sparrow MP (2010) Optimizing thiopurine therapy in inflammatory bowel disease. *Inflammatory Bowel Disease* 17(6), 1428–35.

Clemett D, Markham A (2000) Prolonged-release mesalazine: a review of its therapeutic potential in ulcerative colitis and Crohn's disease. *Drugs* 59(4), 929–56.

Danese S, Fiocchi C (2011) Ulcerative colitis. *New England Journal of Medicine* 365, 1713–25.

de Boer NKH, van Bodegraven AA, Jharap B, et al. (2007) Drug insight: pharmacology and toxicity of thiopurine therapy in patients with IBD. *Nature Reviews: Gastroenterology and Hepatology* 4, 686–94.

Engel M, Neurath MF (2010) New pathophysiological insights and modern treatment of IBD. *Journal of Gastroenterology* 45(6), 571–83.

Kaser A, Zeissig S, Blumberg RS (2010) Inflammatory bowel disease. *Annual Reviews of Immunology* 28, 573–621.

Ledingham J, Gullick N, Irving K, et al. (2017) BSR and BHPR guideline for the prescription and monitoring of non-biologic disease-modifying anti-rheumatic drugs. *Rheumatology*, 56(6), 865–8.

Loftus CG, Loftus EV, Sandborn WJ (2003) Ciclosporin for refractory ulcerative colitis. *Gut* 52(2), 172–3.

Yang YX, Lichtenstein MD (2002) Corticosteroids in Crohn's disease. *American Journal of Gastroenterology* 97(4), 803–23.

Guidelines

Carter MJ, Lobo AJ, Travis SPL (2004) on behalf of the IBD Section of the British Society of Gastroenterology: guidelines for the management of inflammatory bowel disease in adults. *Gut* 53(Suppl. V); v1–6. https://gut.bmj.com/content/gutjnl/53/suppl_5/v1.full.pdf

Kornbluth A, Sachar DB (2010) Ulcerative colitis practice guidelines in adults: American College of Gastroenterology, Practice Parameters Committee. *American Journal of Gastroenterology* 105, 501–23

Lichtenstein GR, Hanauer SB, Sandborn WJ (2009) American College of Gastroenterology; Management of Crohn's Disease in Adults. *American Journal of Gastroenterology* 104(2), 465–83.

NICE NG129 (2019) Crohn's disease: management. https://www.nice.org.uk/guidance/ng129 [accessed 21 July 2019].

NICE CG166 (2013) Ulcerative colitis: management. https://www.nice.org.uk/guidance/CG166 [accessed 2 April 2019].

NICE DG11 (2013) Faecal calprotectin diagnostic tests for inflammatory diseases of the bowel. https://www.nice.org.uk/Guidance/DG11 [accessed 2 April 2019].

NICE Pathway—Crohn's disease http://pathways.nice.org.uk/pathways/crohns-disease [accessed 2 April 2019].

NICE Pathway—Ulcerative colitis. (2019) https://pathways.nice.org.uk/pathways/ulcerative-colitis [accessed 10 April 2019].

NICE TA163 (2008) Infliximab for acute exacerbations of ulcerative colitis. https://www.nice.org.uk/guidance/ta163 [accessed 2 April 2019].

NICE TA187 (2010) Infliximab (review) and adalimumab for the treatment of Crohn's disease. https://www.nice.org.uk/guidance/ta187 [accessed 2 April 2019].

NICE TA329 (2015) Infliximab, adalimumab and golimumab for treating moderately to severely active ulcerative colitis after the failure of conventional therapy. https://www.nice.org.uk/guidance/ta329 [accessed 2 April 2019].

NICE TA342 (2015) Vedolizumab for treating moderately to severely active ulcerative colitis. NICE Technology https://www.nice.org.uk/guidance/ta342 [accessed 2 April 2019].

NICE TA352 (2015) Vedolizumab for treating moderately to severely active Crohn's disease after prior therapy. NICE Technology https://www.nice.org.uk/guidance/ta352 [accessed 2 April 2019].

NICE TA456 (2017) Ustekinumab for moderately to severely acting Crohn's disease after previous treatment. NICE Technology https://www.nice.org.uk/guidance/ta456 [accessed 2 April 2019].

NPSA Patient safety alert 13 (2006) Improving compliance with oral methotrexate guidelines http://www.nrls.npsa.nhs.uk/resources/?entryid45=59800 [accessed 2 April 2019].

6.7 Liver disease

The liver is key in the maintenance of metabolic homeostasis. It processes dietary amino acids, carbohydrates, lipids, and vitamins; metabolizes cholesterol and toxins; produces clotting factors; and stores glycogen. In liver failure, toxic waste accumulates (acutely or chronically) affecting CNS function; termed hepatic encephalopathy (HE). Injury to the liver parenchyma in the presence of acute or chronic inflammatory cells is called hepatitis.

Failure of liver function can result from numerous causes, including viral infection, drug/alcohol toxicity, and autoimmune disease. Liver failure can be classified as:

- *Acute*: failure in a previously healthy liver
- *Acute on chronic*: acute failure in a chronically damaged liver (e.g. alcohol).
- *Chronic*: gradual failure in liver function due to progressive parenchyma destruction, from fibrosis and cirrhosis.

Acute liver failure

Pathophysiology

The precise definition of acute liver failure (ALF) is the development of HE and an INR >1.5 without previous liver disease, evidence of which can be defined as:

- *Hyperacute*: within 7 days of onset of jaundice.
- *Acute*: between 7 and 28 days.
- *Subacute*: 5–26 weeks.

Collectively, drug-induced failure and viral hepatitis are the most common causes of ALF; **paracetamol** overdose is, most common in the UK/US/Australia, whereas worldwide viral hepatitis affects more than a third of the population and is the leading cause in Asia and some parts of Europe. In most cases of ALF, liver dysfunction results from hepatocellular necrosis beginning in the central zone of the acinus (the functional unit of the liver) and migrating towards portal tracts.

Following ingestion, paracetamol undergoes hepatic sulfonation and glucuronidation, enabling normal urinary excretion. Normally, approximately 5%, is metabolized via P450 CYP2E1, to form a toxic metabolite N-acetyl-p-benzoquinoneimine, which is also excreted in urine. However, in overdose this metabolite is directly responsible for necrosis in centrilobular hepatocytes around the central vein (i.e. perivenular or zone 3). If significant hepatocyte death occurs, ALF will result. Nausea, vomiting, and abdominal pain are most common presentations in overdose, while jaundice, confusion, and changes in consciousness are rare.

The clinical consequences of acute failure are:

- *Cerebral oedema and HE*: build-up of ammonium products (see 'Hepatic encephalopathy').
- *Coagulopathy*: abnormal liver synthesis and reduced vitamin K.
- *Inflammation and infection*: impaired host-defence mechanisms (e.g. opsonization, chemotaxis, and action of NK) increasing risk of Gram-positive and fungal sepsis.
- *Metabolic dysfunction*: hypoglycaemia and metabolic acidosis following paracetamol overdose.
- *Renal failure*: toxin-related acute tubular necrosis, vasculitic injury in leptospirosis, hepatorenal syndrome.

For a full summary of the relevant pathways and drug targets, see Figure 6.12.

Management

When diagnosing ALF, a distinction between acute causes (e.g. toxic liver challenges or viral infections) and acute on

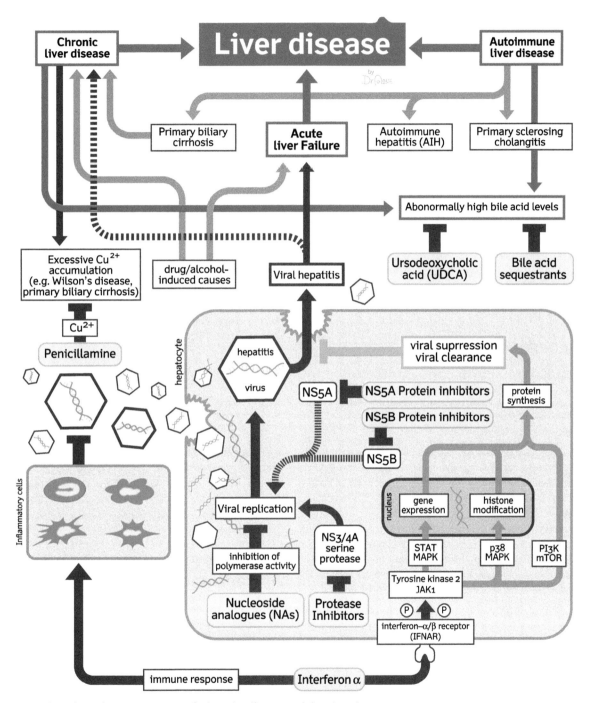

Figure 6.12 Liver disease: summary of relevant pathways and drug targets.

chronic causes is necessary Table 6.16). Once GI examination for signs of chronic disease, and LFTs (including clotting) have been assessed, more specific investigations can be carried out (Table 6.16). Treatment is initially supportive, then targeted to diagnosis.

Generally, ALF with hepatic encephalopathy is managed in the intensive treatment unit (ITU)/high dependency unit (HDU) until the underlying cause is identified. Hepatotoxic drugs (e.g. NSAIDs) and those that worsen complications of ALF (e.g. ACE-inhibitors, opiates) should be avoided.

Table 6.16 Causes of acute liver failure

Cause	Diagnosis in ALF	Comments
Hepatitis A	Anti-HAV IgM	Possible ↑ rate of ALF if also chronic hepatitis C
Hepatitis B	IgM Anti-HB core (HBsAg may be –ve in ALF)	ALF in 1% of acute infections, especially if co-infection with hepatitis D
Hepatitis C	HCV RNA (anti-HCV Ab often –ve)	Extremely rarely causes ALF
Paracetamol overdose	Plasma-paracetamol levels, history	Most common cause of ALF in UK
Drug reactions, e.g. NSAIDs, isoniazid, rifampicin, herbal remedies, 'ecstasy'	Drug history, eosinophils blood/urine analysis	See drug-induced hepatotoxicity
Toxins (e.g. *Amanita phalloides* mushrooms)	History of ingestion	
Wilson's disease	Urinary copper, caeruloplasmin	Usually presents with ALF <20 years of age
Budd–Chiari syndrome	Imaging, history for risk factors	May present with ascites
Autoimmune hepatitis	AutoAbs, Igs	ALF unusual

Reproduced from Stuart Bloom, George Webster, Daniel Marks, *Oxford Handbook of Gastroenterology and Hepatology, Second Edition*, Table 5.2, page 584. Oxford, UK: Oxford University Press © 2012. Reproduced with permission of the Licensor through PLSclear.

Treatment options for ALF may include **vitamin K** IV for 3 days, particularly where ALF is caused by biliary obstruction, and rarely proton pump inhibitors. In some cases, liver transplantation assessment may be indicated unless contraindicated (i.e. septic shock, infection, cardio-pulmonary disease). Targeted treatments may be required such as **penicillamine** in Wilson's disease and cortico-steroids (e.g. **methylprednisolone**) in autoimmune hepatitis (see chronic), with acute hepatitis B **entecavir** or **tenofovir** are the preferred agents ('Nucleoside and nucleotide analogues').

Paracetamol overdose

In **paracetamol** overdose, the major objective is to min-imize liver damage, with **acetylcysteine** considered in all patients to prevent progression to severe encephalopathy. Treatment is indicated where serum levels exceed specified thresholds, or liver biochemical tests (e.g. AST, ALT) and in symptomatic patients. If hepatotoxic doses are apparent (intake of >75 mg/kg) within 1 hour, then activated charcoal may be of benefit. All patients require a 4-hour, or at-presentation, paracetamol level which is typically plotted on a standardized graph to establish the requirement for initiating acetylcysteine treatment (Figure 6.13). The risk of ALF is considerably greater in pa-tients taking CYP-inducing drugs (e.g. **carbamazepine**, **rifampicin, phenobarbital, phenytoin**), following alcohol intake or in glutathione deficiency.

Drug classes used in management of acute liver failure

Acetylcysteine

Acetylcysteine enhances glutathione stores so the liver is protected from *N*-acetyl-p-benzoquinone imine tox-icity. For example, acetylcysteine.

Mechanism of action

Acetylcysteine is a derivative and a pro-drug of cysteine, with an acetyl group attached to the amino group of cyst-eine. Once activated, cysteine acts directly to replenish hepatic glutathione stores. Sufficient glutathione in the

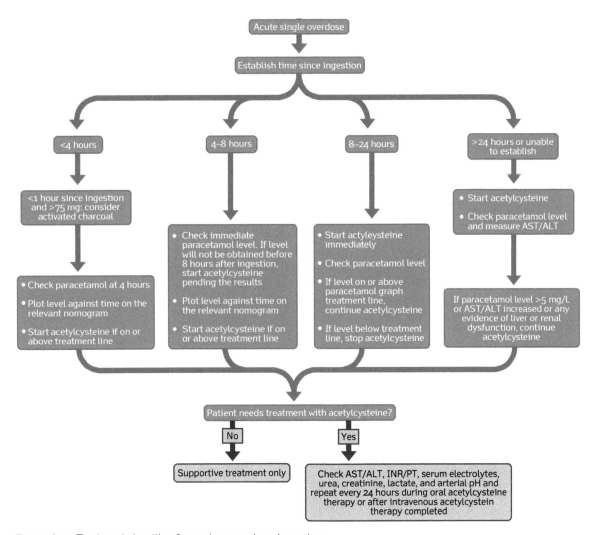

Figure 6.13 Treatment algorithm for acute paracetamol overdose.

liver protects it from injury by the toxic **paracetamol** metabolite N-acetyl-p-benzoquinone imine.

Prescribing

Acetylcysteine is licenced for use in **paracetamol** overdose. It is administered IV, in 5% glucose over a total period of 21 hours, initially as a high/loading dose over 1 hour, followed by a lower dose over 4 hours and then a moderate dose over 16 hours. In some cases, extended treatment may be required.

Unwanted effects

Generally, **acetylcysteine** is well tolerated, although hypersensitivity reactions are relatively common (18%).

Bronchospasm, angioedema, urticaria, and local injection site reaction are most common during the loading dose, requiring careful monitoring and extra caution in asthmatics; this is not, however, a contraindication. Nausea and vomiting are also frequently seen.

Cirrhosis and chronic liver disease

Pathophysiology

Chronic liver disease is a clinical and investigational diagnosis, based on the presence of unexplained jaundice and abnormal LFTs. Cirrhosis, however, is usually clinically

Box 6.7 Signs of chronic liver disease

- Gynaecomastia
- Clubbing
- Palmar erythema
- Leukonychia
- Peripheral oedema
- Spider naevi
- Portal hypertension
- Recurrent infection

silent until advanced stages, i.e. decompensated liver disease, although patients may present with fatigue, right upper quadrant pain, jaundice, arthralgia, and a number of clinical signs (Box 6.7). There are numerous causes, including chronic viral infection (e.g. hepatitis B/C), alcohol abuse, non-alcoholic steatohepatitis (associated with the metabolic syndrome), drugs (e.g. **nitrofurantoin**, **methyldopa**, **isoniazid**), primary biliary cirrhosis, autoimmune hepatitis, sarcoidosis, and Wilson's disease. Progressive disease results in liver cirrhosis, and latterly portal hypertension and/or ascites. Cirrhosis is a histological diagnosis with evidence of diffuse fibrosis and nodule formation.

Two clinical patterns emerge in chronic liver disease, neither mutually exclusive, but each with unique clinical problems.

Compensated cirrhosis

Patients generally have good LFTs despite cirrhosis with no HE or ascites (see 'Ascites'). The course of disease is still progressive fibrosis and liver dysfunction, but treatment/changes in lifestyle can slow down or even reverse clinical progression.

Decompensated cirrhosis

Commonly occurs as a result of acute deterioration in chronic liver function, resulting in jaundice, HE, and ascites. Triggers for deterioration include binge-drinking, infection, and new drugs, or the development of hepatocellular carcinoma (HCC).

Ascites

This is the accumulation of fluid within the peritoneal cavity, usually secondary to portal hypertension in the case of cirrhosis; it is associated with a poor prognosis. Fibrosis of the sinusoid system within the liver leads to increased resistance and congestion in the portal system.

Local vasodilation (splanchnic) reduces circulating blood volume, activating the renin–angiotensin system causing salt and water retention; transudation of fluid then occurs into the peritoneal cavity. Raised portal pressures lead to the generation of a portosystemic shunt, putting patients at risk of gastro-oesophageal variceal bleed. Therefore, treating the underlying disease and reducing portal pressure can lessen bleeds. Salt restriction and diuretics can help reduce ascites.

Hepatic encephalopathy

As the liver fails, nitrogenous toxic waste builds up and crosses the blood–brain barrier, where astrocytes attempt to remove it by converting glutamate to glutamine; the increased glutamine levels forces an intracellular fluid shift, causing cerebral oedema. The presence of ammonia and worsening oedema leads to altered mood, confusion, slurred speech, asterixis (flapping tremor), coma, and eventually death. In chronic disease, an acute insult (e.g. infection) may trigger HE, requiring prompt treatment with antibiotics and supportive measures. Other less common precipitating factors include GI bleed, diuretic overdose, electrolyte disorders, and constipation.

Autoimmune liver disease

Autoimmunity against the liver presents in three typical forms:

Primary biliary cirrhosis

Primary biliary cirrhosis (PBC) is the most common autoimmune hepatic condition affecting ~10/100 000, mainly females, with a peak presentation of 50 years old. The aetiology is unclear, but intrahepatic bile ducts are damaged by chronic granulomatous inflammation. Retention of toxic substances like bile acids and copper can further damage ducts and hepatocytes, leading to cholestasis, which may progress to cirrhosis and portal hypertension. Around half of patients are asymptomatic and identified from a random LFT. Symptomatic patients report pruritis and lethargy, with osteoporosis a common finding, as cholestasis impairs the absorption of fat soluble vitamins (A, D, E, K).

Primary sclerosing cholangitis

Primary sclerosing cholangitis (PSC) is another cholestatic liver disease, characterized by biliary stricture and dilatation. It has an overall prevalence of around 50/million, mainly affects men, and is associated with IBD. The aetiology is unknown, but immunogenic (HLA A1, B8, DR3) and environmental factors (bacteria) are thought to be important. Symptoms are of chronic biliary obstructive disease (i.e. fatigue, pruritus, intermittent jaundice, and right upper quadrant pain), which lead ultimately to liver failure. Signs of chronic liver disease and portal hypertension may be seen with initially raised alkaline phosphatase and latterly bilirubin; p-ANCA is raised in 65–85%.

Autoimmune hepatitis

Autoimmune hepatitis (AIH) is a liver disease of unknown cause. It is strongly associated with HLA DR3 (young onset, severe) and DR4 (older onset, benign), and may be triggered by exposure to environmental triggers (e.g. hepatitis A/B, Epstein–Barr virus infection, drugs/immunizations). Cell-mediated attack occurs against antigen expressing hepatocytes, which activates undifferentiated T helper cells (Th0). The activated Th0 cells then differentiate to Th1 (secreting IL-2 and interferon-Y), which in turn activates macrophages and attenuates the system; and Th2 cells (secreting IL-4, IL-5, and IL-10), which stimulate B cells to produce autoantibodies against hepatocytes.

Diagnosis is based on typical serological findings and liver histology, as well as by exclusion of other diseases. There may be an overlap with PBC or PSC. Three true clinical types of AIH have been identified, which express different autoantibodies (see Table 6.17).

Management

Treatment of cirrhosis targets the underlying cause to reduce clinical progression, i.e. viral ('Viral hepatitis'), alcohol abuse (see chapter 8.7 drug abuse, addiction, and dependency) or autoimmune ('Autoimmune liver disease'). The failing liver will also manifest as clotting abnormalities, vitamin/fat malabsorption/deficiency, accumulation of toxins and the subsequent pathology of these (e.g. osteoporosis, ascites, portal hypertension, and HE).

Antifibrotic therapies are currently under development, but to-date none are licensed. Drugs known to exacerbate HE must be avoided, e.g. opiates, diuretics, oral hypoglycaemics, and saline fluids; and hepatotoxic drugs such as **paracetamol**, **methotrexate**, **isoniazid**, salicylates, and tetracyclines.

Good nutrition and alcohol abstinence is vital. As cholestatis impairs absorption of fat and fat soluble vitamins (A, D, E, and K), supplementation of these is recommended with calcium to prevent osteoporosis secondary to cirrhosis. Triggers for decompensation should also be managed (e.g. potential sepsis).

Decompensated cirrhosis

Ascites

This is primarily managed by achieving a negative sodium balance, i.e. with salt restriction (80–120 mmol of Na^+/day) and diuretics to promote renal excretion. Renal sodium retention in ascites occurs secondary to hyperaldosteronism, which promotes reabsorption along the distal tubule. Therefore, aldosterone antagonists (e.g. **spironolactone**) are more effective than loop diuretics in ascites management. Response to diuretic treatment tends to be slow, so doses are increased every 7 days to response, adjusted to optimal weight loss. In patients who fail to respond adequately, a loop diuretic (e.g. **furosemide**) may be added in. Once ascites has resolved, patients are reduced to a maintenance dose. Fluid restriction is only recommended in the case of a dilutional hyponatraemia. In refractory ascites (10%) large volume paracentesis, surgical shunting, transjugular intrahepatic portosystemic shunt (TIPS) or liver transplantation may be required.

Portal hypertension

The risk of portal hypertension and associated variceal bleeds can be reduced by splanchnic vasoconstrictors,

Table 6.17 Clinical types of AIH

	Type 1	Type 2	Type 3
Symptoms	Acute hepatitis (jaundice, hepatic encephalopathy), fever, malaise, urticaria, polyarthritis		
Age affected	10 year to elderly (bimodal peaks)	2–15 years	30–50 years
Diagnostic autoantibodies	ASMA ANA Antiactin	Anti-LKM P-450 IID6 Synthetic core motif peptides 254–271	Soluble liver-kidney antigen Cytokeratins 8 and 18

i.e. non-selective β-blockers (e.g. **propranolol**). Acute bleeding can be managed with variceal banding, or TIPS in uncontrolled bleeding. Pharmacological options for acute bleeds include **terlipressin**; a synthetic vasopressin analogue that causes splanchnic vasoconstriction, or **octreotide/somatostatin**.

Hepatic encephalopathy

HE management is primarily through controlling any underlying precipitant, as this alone will resolve ~90% of episodes; however, some patients may require ITU admission and supportive measures, such as reducing toxic load through bowel cleansing and diet. The non-absorbable disaccharide **lactulose** is used at high doses for its perceived advantage as a prebiotic and to reduce the ammonia load from the gut, thereby helping in HE. That said, studies suggest its primary advantage is as a laxative. **Rifaximin**, a non-absorbable oral antibiotic, is supported by the most convincing evidence in HE, improving cognitive impairment and reducing ammonia load. It is used in combination with lactulose in recurrent HE. Other treatment strategies with less convincing evidence include **sodium benzoate** (again, in combination with lactulose) to improve ammonia clearance by increasing nitrogen excretion, and antibiotics (**neomycin** or **metronidazole**), active against urease-producing gut bacteria.

Autoimmune liver disease

The mainstay of treatment in autoimmune liver disease is symptomatic alleviation, specific replacement of deficits (e.g. vitamin deficiencies), the use of stents, and latterly liver transplantation.

Primary biliary cirrhosis

Symptomatic relief in PBC can include **colestyramine** for pruritus, and **ursodeoxycholic acid** to possibly slow disease progression and significantly reduce the need for transplantation. Immunosuppressants are ineffective in the disease process. Cirrhosis is associated with advanced disease and managed as outlined previously. Vitamin deficiency is managed through supplementation of affected vitamins i.e. A, D, E, and K, and calcium/vitamin D to prevent osteoporosis.

Primary sclerosing cholangitis

Drug therapy in PSC is much like that for PBC, except the use of **ursodeoxycholic acid** is controversial, i.e. improves LFTs, but has no effect on symptoms or survival. In proven cholangitis antibiotics such as **ciprofloxacin** are of benefit.

Autoimmune hepatitis

In AIH, the mechanism of autoimmunity can be reduced by immunosuppression, the mainstay of treatment being corticosteroids, with 80% remission at 2–4 yrs. Although corticosteroids are used long-term to maintain remission, adjunctive **azathioprine** has a steroid-sparing effect and can help maintain remission. Other immunosuppressants like **tacrolimus** and **ciclosporin** may be effective, although their role requires further investigation.

Drug classes used in management of cirrhosis and chronic liver disease

Bile acid sequestrants

> Bile acid sequestrants are big polymers with the capacity to bind negatively charged bile salts in the small intestine. For example, colestyramine.

Mechanism of action

The water-soluble bile acids are amphipathic end products of cholesterol metabolism that are produced in the liver and actively absorbed in the small intestine. After synthesis from cholesterol, they are conjugated to glycine- or taurine-forming bile salts. Conjugated bile acids are mainly in their deprotonated (A-) form in the duodenum, which increases their water solubility and makes them much more able to fulfil their physiological role of emulsifying fats to aid with digestion and absorption. High levels of bile acids are concentrated in bile and intestinal contents, with multiple enterohepatic circulations achieved before excretion. Importantly, bile acids are toxic to cells at abnormally high concentrations, both at intra- or extracellular level.

   Colestyramine is a resin that can exchange its chloride anions with anionic bile acids in the intestinal tract. The resin adsorbs and associates with the bile acids to produce an insoluble complex that is excreted with the faeces. The binding of bile salts in the intestine leads to the partial removal of bile acids that are present in the enterohepatic circulation.

Prescribing

Colestyramine is used to treat pruritus secondary to raised serum bile acids, associated with partial biliary obstruction and primary biliary cirrhosis, and can reduce bile acid levels by 30–40%, although it rarely achieves a complete resolution of pruritis. With complete biliary obstruction, bile is not secreted into the intestine so colestyramine is ineffective. It is taken mixed with liquid, e.g. water, juice, skimmed milk, pureed fruit, and thin soups, which may also help improve compliance. It may not be taken dry.

Unwanted effects

As it remains in the GI tract, adverse effects to **colestyramine** tend to be GI, i.e. nausea, vomiting, constipation, and abdominal discomfort.

As well as binding to bile, colestyramine binds to fat soluble vitamins and potentially other drugs (including **ursodeoxycholic acid**), inhibiting their absorption; administration should therefore be spaced by an hour. Manufacturers also suggest supplementing fat soluble vitamins in patients on long-term therapy.

Ursodeoxycholic acid

> UDCA stabilizes plasma membrane against cytolysis and also halts apoptosis caused by excessive accumulation of tension-active bile acids.

Mechanism of action

Ursodeoxycholic acid (UDCA) is a 3α, 7β-dihydroxy-5β-cholanoic acid, with far higher hydrophilicity than structural analogues, thus less able to interact with and disturb lipid membranes. Excessive levels of hydrophobic bile acids can damage cell membranes, especially in the biliary tree. The enrichment of UDCA in the bile renders it more hydrophilic and less cytotoxic. In normal individuals, UDCA comprises no more than 4% of the total endogenous bile acid pool, which increases to 40–60% at a conventional treatment dosage.

Evidence suggests that in addition to its protective actions against membrane damage by cytotoxic bile acids, UDCA's therapeutic properties also include stimulation of hepatobilliary secretion and protection of hepatocytes against apoptosis induced by bile acids. The anti-apoptotic effects of UDCA have been associated with a reduction in the mitochondrial membrane permeability transition and of cytochrome-c release.

Prescribing

UDCA is widely used at standard doses to slow disease progression in primary biliary cirrhosis. Its role in primary sclerosing cholangitis is more controversial; furthermore,

treatment with higher doses may be associated with an increased mortality.

Unwanted effects

Side effects and cautions

As **UDCA** relies on enterohepatic circulation for excretion, it should not be used in liver or intestinal disease where this is impaired, e.g. biliary tract inflammation or occlusion, non-functioning gall bladder, chronic liver disease, inflammatory disease of the intestine, and frequent biliary colic. Adverse effects tend to be GI, i.e. nausea, vomiting, diarrhoea, and pasty stools.

Interactions

UDCA increases **ciclosporin** absorption, thereby increasing the risk of toxicity. As a bile acid it will bind to bile acid sequestrants such as **colestyramine**, which may be avoided by spacing administration by at least 2 hours.

Penicillamine

> Penicillamine is a chelating agent mainly used for its hepatic copper decreasing and immunomodulatory properties.

Mechanism of action

Penicillamine is mainly used as a copper-chelating drug in the treatment of Wilson's disease, since primary biliary cirrhosis has been linked with augmented hepatic levels of copper. *In vitro* evidence has shown that one atom of copper combines with two molecules of penicillamine, while its use relies on the binding to accumulated copper and subsequent elimination through urine.

Prescribing

As **penicillamine** chelates heavy-metal ions, it is best taken on an empty stomach to avoid any interaction with food. It is used in autoimmune hepatitis once LFTs indicate that the disease has been controlled with corticosteroids. Doses of penicillamine are gradually increased as corticosteroid doses are decreased. In recent clinical trials, however, penicillamine showed no improvement in survival, but was linked with a four-time increase in adverse effects.

Unwanted effects

Penicillamine is poorly tolerated, with a high incidence of side effects that may be severe. As these are dose related, treatment is initiated at low doses and titrated up slowly. Proteinuria and thrombocytopenia are the most common side effects reported with therapy, the former affecting up to 30% of patients. Patients should be closely monitored and advised to report any unexplained bruising or bleeding.

There are numerous other potential side effects associated with penicillamine including GI (nausea, vomiting, diarrhoea, and stomatitis), neurological (headache, dizziness), haematological, rashes (including Stevens–Johnson syndrome), hepatic toxicity, renal toxicity, and inflammatory disorders (arthritis, pulmonary fibrosis). Being renally excreted, dose reductions are recommended in mild renal impairment and its' use contraindicated in moderate/severe impairment.

Interactions

Due to the high incidence of haematological toxicity associated with **penicillamine**, caution is recommended when taking with other drugs known for their haematological toxicity; in particular, **clozapine** due to the risk of agranulocytosis.

Viral hepatitis

Pathophysiology

There are three main hepatic viruses which cause liver disease:

Hepatitis A

A DNA virus spread via the faecal–oral route and responsible for 50% of acute viral hepatitis in the UK; it is vaccine preventable.

Hepatitis B

A DNA virus spread by perinatal transmission, blood, and sexual transmission resulting in chronic, or rarely, acute hepatitis. Clinically, hepatitis B (HBV) can vary from an inactive carrier state, to a chronic progressive disease leading to cirrhosis and even hepatic cell carcinoma (HCC). The course of disease can be affected by the presence of other chronic infections (e.g. HIV, HCV etc.) or patient factors such as obesity and alcohol abuse. Approximately 95% of patients will clear the virus without intervention and, subsequently, develop immunity through seroconversion (hepatitis B surface antigen (HBeAg) to anti-HBe); however, 5% go on to develop chronic disease, i.e. HBeAg persists for more than 6 months. Chronic disease is characterized by

four phases (see Table 6.18), although these do not necessarily occur sequentially and time course can vary significantly between patients. About 15–20% of patients with chronic disease will go on to develop serious complications, i.e. decompensated liver disease and HCC, thus disease management aims to promote seroconversion of HBeAg to anti-Hbe to achieve an inactive state.

Hepatitis C (HCV)

An RNA virus, spread via blood either directly or indirectly, although most commonly transmitted via IV drug use or blood transfusion. Like with HBV, disease course varies considerably, from minimal histological changes to chronic progressive disease and associated cirrhosis, extensive fibrosis or HCC; however, the incidence of chronic infection is significantly higher (60–85%). There are six different genotypes of HCV, of which genotye 1 and to a lesser extent 4, are associated with poorer treatment outcomes. The primary aim of treatment is to cure the infection and achieve a sustained viral response (SVR), as in the absence of cirrhosis this will usually resolve liver disease.

Essentially, the virus invades hepatocytes in the liver, replicates, and is recognized as foreign by the immune-system activated CD4+ and CD8+ lymphocytes. An inflammatory process in the parenchyma and portal ducts occurs, leading to hepatic cell necrosis, cellular collapse, and increase of necrotic tissue in the lobules and portal ducts, impairing bilirubin excretion. The final stage of disease is cirrhosis and liver decompensation. Antiviral drugs are the mainstay of treatment to either suppress replication or eradicate viral load.

Management

Hepatitis A

There is no specific treatment for hepatitis A (HAV), but vaccination is effective in at-risk groups (IV drug users, haemophilia, males with multiple sexual male partners, HBV/HCV co-infection). Management options of acute hepatitis secondary to HAV are limited (3–4 weeks after infection), although a small number have prolonged cholestasis for which 2–4 weeks of **prednisolone** can speed resolution.

Hepatitis B

In HBV chronic disease, antiviral therapy is used to suppress viral replication and ideally promote HBeAg loss and

Table 6.18 Phases of chronic HBV infection

Phase	HBV DNA levels	HBeAg	ALT	Anti-HBe	Liver pathology
Immune tolerant	↑↑↑	+ve	Normal	–ve	Minimal change
HBeAg +ve chronic HB	↑↑	+ve	Abnormal	–ve/↑	Active inflammation, fibrosis, progressive liver injury
Inactive carrier	↓↓	↓/-ve	Normal	+ve	Risk of cirrhosis low, absence of progressive disease
HBeAg –ve chronic HB	↑	-ve	Abnormal	+ve	Progressive damage, advanced fibrosis, cirrhosis, HCC

seroconversion to anti-HBe (see Figure 6.14). HBV infection cannot be completely eradicated, so treatment is used to induce and sustain a remission, thereby preventing progression to severe liver injury, i.e. advanced fibrosis, cirrhosis, and hepatocellular carcinoma. Treatment is indicated in active disease (HBeAg positive or negative chronic disease) based on HBV DNA levels, ALT levels, and presence of liver damage, although strategies differ between HBeAg positive and negative disease. In recent years, there have been considerable advances in the availability of anti-viral therapies to target HBV, leading to improved outcomes.

Peginterferon alfa remains the first-line treatment in both HBeAg positive and negative chronic disease, as 48 weeks of treatment induces seroconversion in 30% and 20% of adults at 1 year, respectively, compared with approximately 20% and 5% with a nucleotide/nucleoside analogue (NA). In patients who fail to achieve seroconversion, second-line treatment is with a nucleoside (**lamivudine**, **entecavir**, **telbivudine**, **emtricitabine**) or nucleotide (**adefovir**, **tenofovir**) analogue:

- Tenofovir and entecavir are most potent with optimal resistance profile and thus the preferred agents.
- Lamivudine induces HBeAg seroconversion in 25% after 1 year of use, although the risk of treatment resistance is high so it is currently avoided as monotherapy.
- Adefovir and telbivudine are not currently advocated in chronic HBV in the UK, although are approved for use in other countries.
- Emtricitabine is not licensed for use in chronic HBV.

Hepatitis C

In HCV alcohol can accelerate disease progression, as can co-infection with HAV or HBV; vaccination against these is therefore advisable. Patients should be advised to protect others by not donating blood, sharing razors, or needles.

Until recently, **peginterferon alfa** and **ribavirin** formed the mainstay of treatment in chronic HCV, achieving an SVR in 40–80% of patients depending on genotype. The more recent introduction of the direct-acting antivirals (DAAs) has led to marked improvements in outcome, particularly in the management of HCV genotype 1 and 4, albeit at a high financial cost. Antiviral treatment is considered in all patients with HCV and compensated or decompensated liver disease, particularly in those with co-existing infections (HIV, HBV) or where transmission is likely (e.g. women of child-bearing age, IV drug users, etc.). Treatment strategy depends in part on genotype, as some agents are only effective/licensed against specific genotypes, presence of cirrhosis, and whether it has been previously treated.

Drug classes used in management of viral hepatitis

Interferon alfa

Interferons are cytokines that have antiviral, antiproliferative, antitumour, and immunomodulatory properties. For example, peginterferon alfa.

Mechanism of action

The inflammatory reaction to intruding pathogens includes the secretion of cytokines and chemokines, which can activate or attract innate immune cells to coordinate a response at the infection site. Endogenous interferons are produced by dendritic cells, macrophages, fibroblasts,

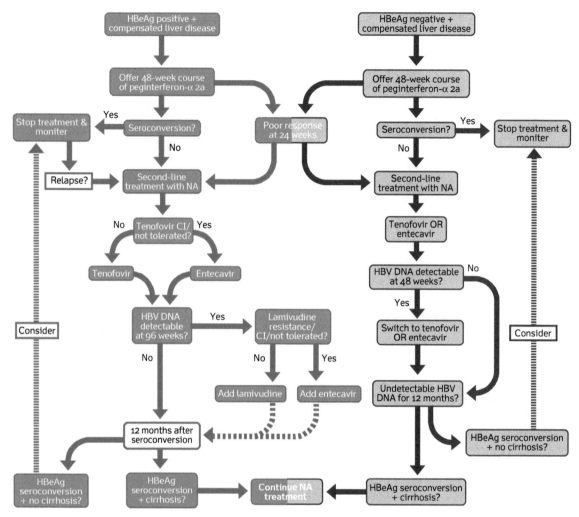

Figure 6.14 Management of viral hepatitis.

and endothelial cells, and are fundamental effectors of the innate immune response induced by viral infections.

The interferon-α/β receptor (IFNAR) is a heteromeric cell surface receptor with two subunits (the α-chain IFNAR1 and β-chain IFNAR2). Interferon binding to the receptor induces phosphorylation of the receptor-bound tyrosine kinases, tyrosine kinase 2 and JAK1, which leads to:

- control of protein synthesis by the PI_3k and mammalian target of rapamycin (mTOR) pathways;
- gene expression through the phosphorylation of STAT proteins and MAPk activation;
- histone modification via the p38 MAPk pathway.

Overall, activation of the IFNAR promotes the expression of interferon-stimulated genes encoding antiviral proteins that are able to supress viral replication, while helping viral clearance.

In addition to the regulation of gene expression and protein synthesis, interferons can promote neutrophil survival, and the activation of macrophages, dendritic cells, natural killer cells, and other cells that mediate the immune response. As a result, interferons can co-ordinate the immune system in response to virus infection. This crucial role has generated many pathogenic viruses that have generated mechanisms to disrupt and limit the interferon response (e.g. the NS3/4A HCV serine protease targets proteins required for the production of interferon). Determining the basis of these antagonistic processes constitutes a fundamental aspect for optimizing interferon treatment as a viable therapy for acute viral infections.

Addition of a polyethylene glycol to the interferon (pegylation), increases the half-life compared with the native form, i.e. **peginterferon**.

Prescribing

Chronic hepatitis B

Treatment is initiated early in order to minimize any inflammatory hepatic necrosis caused by the virus, and continued for 12 months where effective. Long-term use, however, is associated with unacceptable toxicity, although patients failing to achieve seroconversion at 12 months are converted to NA therapy. Response rates to both **peginterferon** and **interferon** in hepatitis B are only 30–40%, with a high level of relapse, so treatment should be discontinued after 6 months if patients fail to respond. Poor response is defined by insufficient reduction in HBV DNA or where HBeAg remains above 200 000 units/mL.

Chronic hepatitis C

Peginterferon in combination with **ribavirin** (unless contraindicated) is the therapy of choice in chronic hepatitis C, as this has been shown to be superior to either **interferon** plus ribavirin, peginterferon monotherapy, or treatment with a nucleoside/nucleotide analogue. Treatment is continued for 16, 24, or 48 weeks depending on genotype, with a sustained viral response achieved in 40–85% of patients.

There are two interferon α alfa products on the market, 2a and 2b, differentiated by their amino acid code, although practically there is little to distinguish between them. Both are administered SC three times a week at slightly differing doses, whereas peginterferon is administered SC once a week.

Unwanted effects

Flu-like symptoms (fever, chills, headaches, myalgia), nausea, anorexia, and diarrhoea are common with interferon therapy, although tend to be transient and rarely require discontinuation.

More serious, infrequent reactions include (among others); suicidal ideation (see prescribing warning), hypersensitivity reactions, cardiovascular toxicity (including arrhythmias), haematological toxicity (bone marrow suppression), ocular toxicity, and hepatic and renal toxicity. Treatment is therefore contraindicated in severe cardiac disease, renal impairment, and hepatic impairment, with long-term treatment not recommended. Interferon α should not be used in combination with **telbivudine** due to the increased risk of peripheral neuropathy.

> **PRESCRIBING WARNING**
>
> **Suicidal ideation with interferon and peginterferon alfa**
> - Suicidal ideation and suicide attempt have been reported in adults and particularly children whilst on interferon α treatment and for up to 6 months after.
> - Adults with a severe psychiatric history should be assessed and closely monitored.
> - Treatment is contraindicated in children and adolescents with severe psychiatric conditions.

Nucleoside and nucleotide analogues

> The nucleoside analogues work mainly by inhibiting DNA polymerase activity of the hepatitis B virus, supressing viral replication. Examples include lamivudine, adefovir, entecavir, ribavirin, and telbivudine tenofovir.

Mechanism of action

Nucleotide analogues (NAs) are one of the two major drug classes currently used as antiviral agents for the treatment of chronic hepatitis B. Unlike the immunomodulatory actions of interferon, NAs target HBV polymerase, which has RNA- and DNA-dependent DNA polymerase functions, vital for viral replication. NAs inhibit by competitively binding with endogenous substrates, or via integration into viral DNA, which leads to chain termination.

Lamivudine (first in class) is a cytidine nucleoside analogue, which is phosphorylated to its active metabolites and acts as a chain terminator following integration into viral DNA. It has a high rate of resistance to mutations, i.e. 10–25% of patients after 1 year.

Tenofovir disoproxil fumarate undergoes phosphorylation and can competitively inhibit the endogenous substrate deoxyadenosine 5'-triphosphate. After integration into HBV DNA polymerase it acts as a chain terminator. There are no cases of primary resistance so far described.

Entecavir is a guanosine carboxylic analogue, which is phosphorylated intracellularly to its active 5' triphosphate metabolite. It competes with the endogenous substrate deoxy guanosine triphosphate inhibiting HBV DNA polymerase. Resistance to entecavir is rare, <2% after 5 years.

Adefovir is a nucleotide analogue of adenosine monophosphate with relatively slow rates of viral suppression. Its main advantage is its efficacy against lamivudine-resistant mutants, although genotypic resistance rates are 28% after 5 years. It can also enhance immune responsiveness via the stimulation of TNFα production.

Ribavirin is a synthetic nucleoside analogue capable of inhibiting viral RNA synthesis through the blockade of uridine and cytidine incorporation. Although on its own it has little effect on viral replication, it enhances the efficacy of interferon α against HCV, and can increase the production of antiviral cytokines.

Telbivudine is a synthetic unsubstituted L-nucleoside analogue of thymidine. Cellular kinases convert it to its triphosphate form, which can lead to premature chain termination by competing with thymidine 5'-triphosphate. It has high antiviral potency, but a relatively high resistance rate of 10–25% after 2 years.

Prescribing

Chronic hepatitis B

Nucleotide analogues are now widely used for viral suppression in chronic hepatitis B as long-term therapy or until there is evidence of viral resistance. There are currently five drugs on the market for this indication (**adefovir**, **entecavir**, **lamivudine**, **telbivudine**, and **tenofovir**), of which lamivudine and tenofovir are also licensed for use in HIV. Agents vary in terms of potency and resistance rates, for which entecavir and tenofovir have shown to be superior, thus recommended for initial therapy. Other agents may be considered if there is an inadequate response after 6–9 months.

All agents are administered orally OD and indicated in decompensated liver disease, except for telbivudine, due to a lack of safety data and known risk of hepatotoxicity.

Chronic hepatitis C

Ribavirin is used in combination with **peginterferon** to treat chronic hepatitis C for 24 or 48 weeks depending on the presenting viral load, initial response and disease genotype (genotype 1 and 4 require longer treatment). There are currently two oral products (Copegus®, Rebetol®) on the market, both only licensed for use in combination with peginterferon produced by the same manufacturer. Doses are administered orally BD based on patient's weight and, in the case of Copegus®, genotype, and co-infection with HIV. Ribavirin is also used in conjunction with DAAs in a variety of interferon-free regimens.

Unwanted effects

Nucleoside analogues frequently cause exacerbations of hepatitis both on treatment and after discontinuation.

Patients require close monitoring of ALT, particularly with advanced disease or cirrhosis, due to the increased risk of decompensated disease. Severe hepatic toxicity is more common in decompensated disease, as is hepatorenal disease and lactic acidosis, and most commonly associated with **telbivudine**.

As all nucleoside analogues are renally cleared; dose modifications are required or treatment stopped with severe impairment. They are rarely known to induce renal impairment.

Other common side effects include headache, fatigue, dizziness, GI effects (nausea, diarrhoea, abdominal pain, flatulence), and rash. **Telbivudine** is associated with peripheral neuropathy and should not be used in combination with interferon α.

As **ribavirin** is primarily used with **peginterferon**, this affects side effects reported and contraindications listed by its manufacturer, e.g. both are contraindicated for use in children with a history of severe psychiatric conditions. Where peginterferon therapy is discontinued due to toxicity, ribavirin should also be stopped, as it has not shown to be effective as monotherapy.

For more details and drug interactions see Topic 11.3, 'Viral infection'.

Protease inhibitors

Specific protease inhibitors can prevent viral replication by inhibiting NS3 serine proteases and are a valuable treatment in patients where first line therapy failed. Examples include boceprevir, paritaprevir, simeprevir, and telaprevir.

Mechanism of action

Telaprevir is a highly selective and potent inhibitor of the HCV NS3/4A serine protease. This is part of the chymotrypsin serine protease family that produces some of the components of the RNA viral replication complex, via cleavage of the non-structural part of the viral polyprotein.

Boceprevir forms covalent reversible complexes with NS3 protease, acting as a peptidomimetic inhibitor it has strong antiviral activity in the HCV virus replicon system.

Simeprevir is another HCV NS3/4A serine protease inhibitor, which belongs to the class of organic compounds known as macrolactams.

Paritaprevir is an acylsulphonamide inhibitor of the HCV NS3/4A serine protease that is formulated with **ombitasvir** and **ritonavir**, the latter present to augment exposure to paritaprevir through inhibition of CYP3A.

Prescribing

The recent introduction of protease inhibitors in chronic HCV has provided valuable treatment options both *de novo,* and in those who have failed first-line treatment, particularly with unfavourable genotypes and compensated liver disease. Treatment is used in adjunct to standard therapy with **ribavirin** and **peginterferon** with the exception of **paritaprevir**. Paritaprevir, formulated with **ritonavir** and **ombitasvir**, in part to promote efficacy, is licensed for use in combination with **dasabuvir** and/or ribavirin. All agents are taken orally, with **simeprevir** having the advantage of being given OD and choice determined by genotype, patient factors, and availability.

Unwanted effects

Side effects are common with protease inhibitors (see Topic 11.3, 'Viral infection' for more details); of particular note with these agents is the high incidence of rash associated with **telaprevir** therapy (see 'Prescribing warning: rash with telaprevir').

Drug interactions

Clinically significant drug interactions with protease inhibitors are common, in particular **boceprevir** and **telaprevir** are potent inhibitors of CYP3A4, and **paritaprevir** is formulated with **ritonavir**, also a potent inhibitor of CYP3A. Prescribers should be aware of the high potential for drug interactions when prescribing any new medication and patients made aware of the importance of informing other clinicians that they are taking these drugs.

> **PRESCRIBING WARNING**
>
> **Rash with telaprevir**
> - Up to 5% of patients will develop a rash on telaprevir, which in severe cases may include Stevens–Johnson syndrome or DRESS.
> - Patients should be advised to report any new rash or worsening of an existing rash, and treatment discontinued in moderate to severe cases

NS5A protein inhibitors

> The non-structural NS5A protein has been identified as a target for viral inhibition due to its key role in viral replication. For example, daclatasvir, ledipasvir, and ombitasvir.

Mechanism of action

NS5A is a zinc-binding and proline-rich phosphoprotein with pleiotropic functions, including roles in viral replication and assembly. It exists in phosphorylated and hyperphosphorylated forms, and can influence cellular functions through inhibition of apoptosis and promotion of tumorigenesis, both implicated in triggering hepatocarcinogenic mechanisms.

Inhibition of NS5A in HCV replicon-containing cells results in redistribution of NS5A from the ER to lipid droplets, which coincides with the onset of inhibition of replication. They have pangenotypic activity, but the exact mechanism of antiviral action of NS5A inhibitors is unknown. Evidence suggests they have multiple effects contributing to their potency, one proposed mechanism being inhibition of NS5A hyperphosphorylation, likely vital for viral production.

Daclatasvir is a highly selective NS5A inhibitor with broad coverage of HCV genotypes in vitro. It has been shown to block hyperphosphorylation of NS5A, as well as altering its subcellular localization. **Ledipasvir** is a potent NS5A inhibitor against genotypes 1a, 1b, 4a and 5a in vitro, with lower activity against 2a and 3a genotypes. **Ombitasvir** is a potent pan-genotypic inhibitor of NS5A.

Prescribing

Of the NS5A protein inhibitors, only **daclatasvir** is available as a single agent, whereas **ledipasvir** is formulated with **sofosbuvir** (see 'NS5B Protein inhibitors'), and **ombitasvir** with the protease inhibitors—**paritaprevir** and **ritonavir**. All agents are taken orally OD in chronic hepatitis C, with dosing and combination therapy determined by genotype and extent of liver disease.

Unwanted effects

As a class, these agents are generally well-tolerated with side effects often mild and self-limiting, e.g. fatigue, headache, and nausea, although as they are all only taken as part of combination therapy, the risk of more frequent/severe adverse effects is high. For example, combination treatment with **ombitasvir/paritaprevir/ ritonavir** and **dasabuvir** is associated with significant hepatotoxicity, and should be discontinued in patients with hepatic decompensation, whereas **ledipasvir** and **sofosbuvir** is cautioned in patients with bradycardia or heart block.

Drug interactions

The risk of drug interactions with the NS5A protein inhibitors is high, due either to the drug itself or other drugs with which it is combined. **Daclatasvir** is both a substrate and weak inducer of CYP3A4, as well as being a substrate for P-gp. Drugs that are potent inhibitors or inducers of these pathways can therefore increase the risk of toxicity or treatment failure, respectively. Although drug interactions with **ombitasvir** are less likely, **ritonavir** and **paritaprevir** with which it is formulated, have a high tendency for drug interactions.

NS5B protein inhibitors

> The HCV non-structural NS5B protein is the RNA-dependent RNA polymerase that is responsible for the replication of the RNA viral genome, thus becoming a target of choice for the development of antiviral agents. For example, dasabuvir and sofosbuvir.

Mechanism of action

NS5B protein is needed for viral RNA replication and, although many small molecules are recognized as allosteric inhibitors of it, only a few are active in clinical applications. NS5B polymerase inhibitors have been broadly classified as nucleoside and non-nucleoside classes.

The prodrug **sofosbuvir** is a pangenotypic nucleotide analogue that after metabolism to its active form, can act as a defective substrate for HCV NS5B protein.

Dasabuvir is a non-nucleoside analogue inhibitor capable of binding outside of NS5B active site, this means it has reduced activity across genotypes. Its efficacy is limited to HCV 1a and 1b genotypes.

Prescribing

Sofosbuvir is used in chronic HCV in combination with **ribavirin** and **peginterferon alfa**, or ribavirin alone in patients intolerant of peginterferon. It is only advocated for use in genotypes 1, 4, 5, and 6 and as with other new DAAS is associated with high cost.

Dasabuvir is used in combination with **ombitasvir/ paritaprevir/ritonavir** against chronic HCV genotype 1a/ b. It is taken orally BD with food to optimize absorption.

Unwanted effects

As **sofosbuvir** and **dasabuvir** are always used as part of a combination therapy, drug specific side effects are less well defined. For example, dasabuvir in combination with **ombitasvir/paritaprevir/ritonavir** commonly causes nausea, fatigue, pruritis, and insomnia. Manufacturers report that sofosbuvir with **peginterferon alfa** and **ribavirin**, displays a toxicity profile similar to that of peginterferon alfa/ribavirin used alone, i.e. insomnia, headache, nausea, etc.

Drug interactions

Drug interactions are common with both **sofosbuvir** and **dasabuvir**, as part of a combination therapy. Dasabuvir, for example, potently inhibits UGT1A1 (responsible for glucoronidation) and to a lesser extent P-gp. Sofosbuvir, conversely, is a substrate for P-gp, but is not known to inhibit or induce this or other enzymes.

Further reading

de Boer NKH, van Bodegraven AA, Jharap B, et al. (2007) Drug insight: pharmacology and toxicity of thiopurine therapy in patients with IBD. *Nature Reviews: Gastroenterology and Hepatology* 4, 686–94.

Deutsch M, Hadziyannis SJ (2008) Old and emerging therapies in chronic hepatitis C: an update. *Journal of Viral Hepatology* 15, 2–11.

Dienstag JL (2009) Benefits and risks of nucleoside analog therapy for hepatitis B. *Hepatology* 49, S112–21.

Ferenci P (2012) Treatment of chronic hepatitis C—are interferons really necessary? *Liver International* 32(1), 108–12.

Fung J, Lai C-L, Seto W-K, et al. (2011) Nucleoside/nucleotide analogues in the treatment of chronic hepatitis B. *Journal of Antimicrobial Chemotherapy* 66(12), 2715–25.

Heidelbaugh JJ, Bruderly M (2006) Cirrhosis and chronic liver failure: Part I. Diagnosis and evaluation. *American Family Physician* 74(5), 756–62.

Out C, Groen AK, Brufau G (2012) Bile acid sequestrants: more than simple resins. *Current Opinions in Lipidology* 23(1), 43–55.

Roma MG, Toledo FD, Boaglio AC, et al. (2011) Ursodeoxycholic acid in cholestasis: linking action mechanisms to therapeutic applications. *Clinical Science* 121(12), 523–44.

Guidelines

EASL (2010) Clinical practice guidelines on the management of ascites, spontaneous bacterial peritonitis and hepatorenal syndrome in cirrhosis. *Journal of Hepatology* 53, 397–417.

EASL (2012) Clinical practice guidelines: management of chronic hepatitis B virus infection. *Journal of Hepatology* 57, 167–85.

EASL (2014) Clinical practice guidelines: hepatic encephalopathy in chronic liver disease: 2014 practice guidelines by the European association for the study of the liver and the American association for the study of liver diseases. *Journal of Hepatology* 61(3), 642–59.

EASL (2015) Clinical practice guidelines: vascular diseases of the liver. *Journal of Hepatology* 64(1), 179–202.

EASL (2015) Recommendations on treatment of hepatitis C. *Journal of Hepatology* 63, 199–236.

NICE Pathway (2019) Hepatitis B (chronic). http://pathways. nice.org.uk/pathways/hepatitis-b-chronic [accessed 3 April 2019].

NICE Pathway (2019) Liver conditions. http://pathways. nice.org.uk/pathways/liver-conditions [accessed 3 April 2019].

NICE TA96 (2006) Adefovir dipivoxil and peginterferon alfa-2a for the treatment of chronic hepatitis B. https://www.nice. org.uk/guidance/ta96 [accessed 3 April 2019].

NICE TA153 (2008) Entecavir for the treatment of chronic hepatitis B. https://www.nice.org.uk/guidance/TA153 [accessed 3 April 2019].

NICE TA154 (2008) Telbivudine for the treatment of chronic hepatitis B. https://www.nice.org.uk/guidance/TA154 [accessed 3 April 2019].

NICE CG165 (2013) Hepatitis B (chronic): diagnosis and management. https://www.nice.org.uk/guidance/cg165 [accessed 3 April 2019].

NICE TA173 (2009) Tenofovir disoproxil for the treatment of chronic hepatitis B. https://www.nice.org.uk/guidance/ TA173 [accessed 3 April 2019].

NICE TA200 (2010) Peginterferon alfa and ribavirin for the treatment of chronic hepatitis C. https://www.nice.org.uk/ guidance/TA200 [accessed 3 April 2019].

NICE TA253 (2012) Boceprevir for the treatment of genotype 1 chronic hepatitis C. https://www.nice.org.uk/guidance/ TA253 [accessed 3 April 2019].

NICE TA330 (2015) Sofosbuvir for treating chronic hepatitis C. https://www.nice.org.uk/guidance/TA330 [accessed 3 April 2019].

NICE TA331 (2015) Simeprevir in combination with peginterferon alfa and ribavirin for treating genotypes 1 and 4 chronic hepatitis C. https://www.nice.org.uk/guidance/ TA331 [accessed 3 April 2019].

NICE TA 363 (2015) Ledipasvir-sofosbuvir for treating chronic hepatitis C. https://www.nice.org.uk/guidance/TA363 [accessed 3 April 2019].

NICE TA364 (2015) Daclatasvir for treating chronic hepatitis C. https://www.nice.org.uk/guidance/TA364 [accessed 3 April 2019].

NICE TA365 (2015) Ombitasvir-paritaprevir-ritonavir with or without dasabuvir for treating chronic hepatitis C. https:// www.nice.org.uk/guidance/TA365 [accessed 3 April 2019].

7 Musculoskeletal medicine

7.1   Osteoarthritis

Osteoarthritis (OA) is best described as a chronic pain syndrome affecting one, or more frequently, multiple joints. It most commonly affects the knees, hips, hands, neck and lower back, although any joint can be affected. Defining OA by pathological changes is no longer considered best practice, as the correlation between pathology and symptoms is frequently discordant, i.e. patients with severe structural changes may present with minimum symptoms and vice versa. For this reason, patients should be assessed using a biopsychosocial model, which takes into consideration impact on social and psychological well-being, alongside pathological changes. OA can create substantial mobility problems and is the most common cause of disability in elderly people in the developed world. Prevalence rises with age such that approximately one-third of people in the UK over 45 have sought treatment for OA compared with 40–50% of people over the age of 75.

Pathophysiology

In the pathological conditions of OA, there are specific hallmarks of damage that affect load-bearing articular cartilage, the formation of new bone at the joint margins (osteophytosis), subchondral bone changes (sclerosis), thickening of the joint capsule, loss of cartilage, and joint space narrowing (Figure 7.1B). In general, structural changes seen on X-ray or CT do not correlate with the pain of OA, but an association does occur between the presence of synovitis, subchondral bone oedema and osteophytes. In OA the vasculature of the osteochondral junction also expresses higher levels of nerve growth factors (NGF) so pain sensitization associated with inflammation is likely to occur.

OA is considered by some to be the result of physiological processes originally targeted at joint repair that, over time, cause tissue damage resulting in symptomatic OA. In many cases, severe trauma or pathological repair processes may be contributory factors. Other risk factors for OA include genetic and patient factors, such as age and obesity (see Box 7.1).

Anti-NGF drugs may be of benefit, primarily via pain modulation, but OA is not considered to be a disease of inflammation and the mainstay of treatment relies on effective analgesia. The presence of synovitis in late disease is controversial and the presence of joint crystals may confound inflammation in OA. It is clear that wear, tear, and damage is associated with the breakdown of collagen and increased presence of proteolytic enzymes called matrix metalloproteinases (MMPs). Healthy collagen is normally 'protected' from breakdown by aggrecans, but some MMPs (e.g. aggrecanase 1) appear to degrade aggrecans, an early marker of OA, and latterly cause collagen cleavage (e.g. with MMP-13 (collagenase 3). These early processes progress to degenerate the osteochondral matrix resulting in the hallmarks of damage outlined above.

In most cases, patients present to a GP with pain and stiffness where the joint is increasingly inflexible and the pain aggravated by exercise, but calmed by rest; the stiffness can be worsened by inactivity. In advanced disease, rest and night pain can also occur with some degree of functional difficulties (e.g. knee giving way or locking). OA-related knee pain is usually bilateral, and experienced in and around the knee. Hip pain that is due to OA is sensed in the groin, and anterior or lateral thigh; it can also be felt as referred pain to the knee.

On examination, patients have a reduced range of joint movement with pain. There is often joint swelling, periarticular tenderness, and crepitus. Bony swelling and deformity due to osteophytes formation in the fingers is common at the distal interphalangeal joints (Heberden's nodes, Figure 7.1A), or at the proximal interphalangeal joints (Bouchard's nodes). For a full summary of the relevant pathways and drug targets, see Figure 7.2.

(a)

(b)

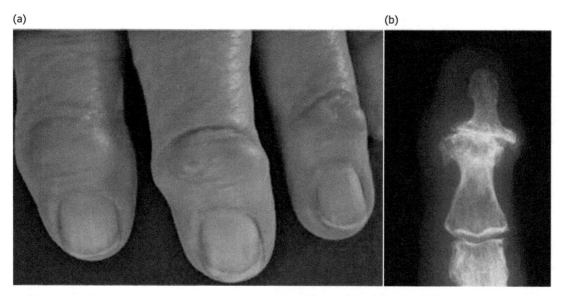

Figure 7.1 (a) Heberden's nodes. (b) Radiographic features of osteoarthritis (e.g. joint-space narrowing, sclerosis, osteophyte).

Reproduced with permission from Watts, RA, et al. (Eds). *Oxford Textbook of Rheumatology*. Oxford, UK: Oxford University Press ©2013. Reproduced with permission of the Licensor through PLSclear.

Management

As the correlation between pathological changes and symptoms is poor, a diagnosis of OA is often made clinically without the need for imaging. Pain that is relieved by activity or morning stiffness that persists beyond

Box 7.1 Risk factors for OA

- 40–60% of cases are heritable, gene unknown
- High bone density (risk for developing osteoarthritis)
- Low bone density (risk for progression of osteoarthritis)
- Occupational/recreational stresses on joints
- Obesity
- Age
- Females
- Joint laxity
- Acromegaly
- Joint injury
- Reduces muscle strength
- Joint malalignment

Data from National Collaborating Centre for Chronic Conditions at the Royal College of Physicians (2008). Osteoarthritis. London: Royal College of Physicians.

30 minutes is more likely to be associated with inflammatory arthritis. However, imaging is necessary in cases of diagnostic uncertainty, or where patients are being considered for arthroplasty, to ensure evidence of significant joint pathology.

To optimize the management of OA, a holistic approach is essential, taking into consideration the patient's health beliefs, quality of life, support network, mood, pain, and attitude towards exercise (see Figure 7.3). Chronic pain can be physically and emotionally debilitating so the whole range of treatments should be considered, including ultimately joint surgery if the patient is fit enough. By working with the patient to establish the impact of symptoms on quality of life, clinicians should actively encourage patients to self-manage their symptoms through advice and goal setting.

Treatment strategies primarily include patient education, strengthening exercises, and aerobic training (regardless of their age), and help with weight loss in cases of obesity. Involvement of allied health professionals can help with supportive measures such as physiotherapy, walking aids, and footwear advice. Where these measures fail to manage symptoms, drug therapy may be necessary, primarily with **paracetamol** and/ or topical NSAIDs for use in knee or hand OA. In practice, only one in seven patients are likely to derive a benefit from paracetamol treatment.

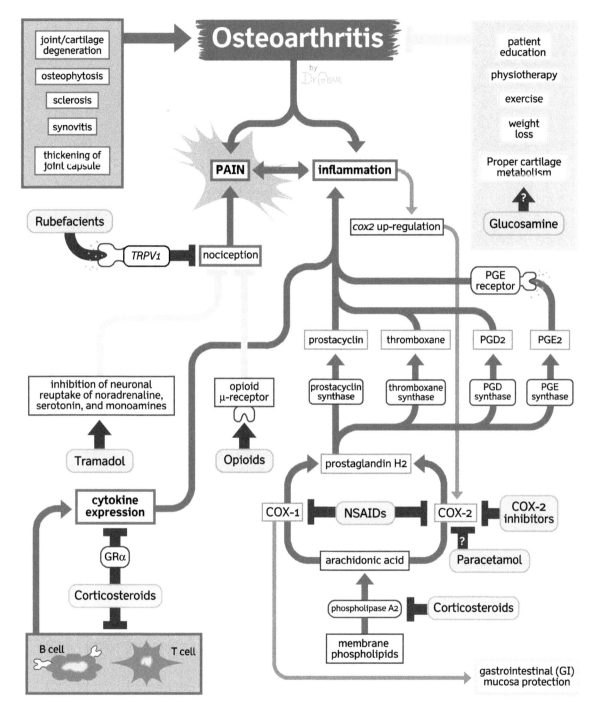

Figure 7.2 Osteoarthritis: summary of relevant pathways and drug targets.

Where patients remain symptomatic, adjunctive treatments with a low-dose oral NSAID or COX-2 inhibitor (with the exception of **etoricoxib** at 60 mg) may be considered, e.g. **naproxen** or low dose **ibuprofen**. The NSAID **diclofenac**, high-dose ibuprofen (to a lesser extent) and COX 2 inhibitors are associated with an increase in cardiovascular risk. In all cases, treatment should be with the lowest dose for the shortest period of time, with an

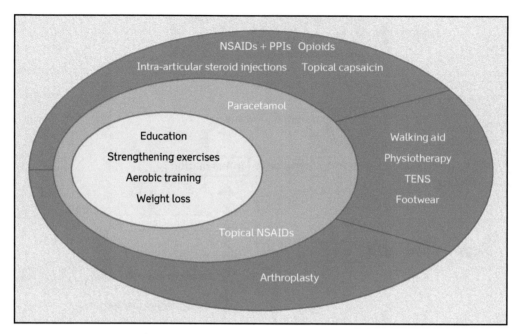

Figure 7.3 Management of osteoarthritis.
Adapted with permission from Conaghan PG, et al., Care and management of osteoarthritis in adults: summary of NICE guidance. *BMJ* 336(7642):502-3. Copyright © 2008, British Medical Journal Publishing Group. [doi: https://doi.org/10.1136/bmj.39490.608009.AD]

adjunct proton pump inhibitor to protect against GI toxicity. Any topical NSAIDS should be discontinued. Before starting treatment, the potential risks and benefits should be weighed up, taking into consideration factors such as age (over 65 years), pre-existing cardiovascular risk, renal impairment, and a history of gastric ulcers. Patients requiring low dose **aspirin** should consider alternative analgesic options to oral NSAIDs first.

In patients unsuitable for NSAIDs, or where NSAIDs and paracetamol are ineffective, opioids may be considered either as an alternative or add-on therapy. Patients may also benefit from add-on therapy administered locally, such as intra-articular corticosteroid injections for the relief of moderate-to-severe pain or topical **capsaicin**, in the case of hand or knee OA. Treatment with intra-articular **hyaluronic acid** is not widely advocated due to limited evidence on its efficacy, although it may be beneficial in the short term, as well as having the potential to reduce the long-term toxicity associated with recurrent corticosteroids.

Patients wishing to supplement their diet with **glucosamine** and/or **chondroitin** should be advised that they might do so, although effects may vary between patients and treatment is associated with only a small reduction in pain. On the converse, risks are likely to be

minimal. Where electing to self-medicate, patients should be recommended to trial treatment for 3–6 months to determine if it is of any benefit.

In patients who remain resistant to pharmacological and non-pharmacological management, arthroplasty may be considered to reduce pain and restore joint function.

Drug classes used in management

Paracetamol

Paracetamol works by decreasing cyclo-oxygenase products, but the precise pharmacological mechanism is still unknown.

Mechanism of action

See Topic 8.3, 'Local anaesthetics'.

Prescribing

Paracetamol is widely accepted as the first-line option for pain management in patients with OA, although this is largely influenced by its excellent safety record. In terms of efficacy, the best available evidence suggests it to be superior to placebo in reducing pain (at rest and on movement), but only by about 4 points on a scale of 0–100. More recent evidence, however, does suggest that chronic daily use exceeding 3 g/day, is associated with an increased risk of GI haemorrhage and perforation. Consequently, the use of lower doses with chronic therapy would appear to be prudent. For more information, see Topic 8.3, 'Local anaesthetics'.

NSAIDs (topical and oral)

> The anti-inflammatory and anti-nociceptive effects of NSAIDs have been linked to the inhibition of cyclo-oxygenase enzymes and a subsequent reduction in inflammatory prostaglandins. Examples include diclofenac, felbinac, ibuprofen, ketoprofen, naproxen, and piroxicam.

Mechanism of action

NSAIDs exert their anti-inflammatory effects through inhibition of cyclo-oxygenase-2 enzyme, reducing prostaglandins, thromboxanes, and prostacyclins. Topical formulations are absorbed by diffusion through the skin and via connective (blood) transport, although systemic exposure is incomplete.

In comparison, following oral administration, the absorption of NSAIDs is normally rapid and complete, with high liver metabolism and subsequent excretion into urine or bile.

Prescribing

Topical NSAIDs

NSAIDs are ideally administered topically, rather than orally in the management of localized pain associated with OA, allowing pain relief, while minimizing systemic exposure and the associated toxicity, particularly with chronic use. The NSAIDs **diclofenac**, **ibuprofen**, **piroxicam**, **ketoprofen**, and **felbinac** are all available in topical formulations, e.g. gels, creams, and foams, all of which are licensed for use in OA. Clinically, there is little to choose between them, although the largest body of evidence exists for diclofenac and ibuprofen, which together with felbinac tend to be the more expensive options. All agents should be applied by gentle massage to the affected area.

Diclofenac is also available for topical administration via a spray device and gel patch; however, neither is licensed for use in OA nor recommended for use by the Scottish Medicines Consortium.

Oral NSAIDs

Where an oral NSAID is deemed necessary, **naproxen** or low-dose **ibuprofen** (less than 1200 mg/day) are the preferred choice, due to their decreased cardiovascular risk compared with **diclofenac** or high dose ibuprofen, although efficacy is likely to be inferior. In all instances, the lowest possible dose should be used for the shortest possible duration and a PPI should be co-prescribed to reduce the risk of GI ulceration.

Unwanted effects

Topical NSAIDs

Topical NSAIDs are well tolerated, although can cause local reactions, particularly when applied to inflamed or broken skin, or mucous membranes. Patients should therefore be advised to wash their hands after application, and avoid contact with broken skin or eyes.

Systemic effects are less likely than with oral therapy, although they should not be used in combination with oral NSAIDs and care should be taken when applying to large areas.

> **PRESCRIBING WARNING**
>
> **Systemic toxicity with topical NSAIDs**
>
> - Topical NSAIDs applied to large areas increase the risk of systemic toxicity; therefore, consideration should be given to alternatives in patients with multiple, large joints affected.
> - Patients prescribed oral NSAIDs should be advised to discontinue topical formulations.

Oral NSAIDs

Chronic use of oral NSAIDs is associated with a higher risk of toxicity; in particular, GI toxicity and increased cardiovascular risk (see 'Prescribing warning: cardiovascular safety of NSAIDs and COX-2 inhibitors'). **Diclofenac** is therefore best avoided in patients with ischaemic heart disease, peripheral artery disease, cerebrovascular disease, or congestive heart failure. Caution is also recommended in patients with pre-existing cardiovascular risk factors such as hypertension, hyperlipidaemia, diabetes, and smokers.

PRESCRIBING WARNING

Cardiovascular safety of NSAIDs and COX-2 inhibitors

- In June 2013 the MHRA and EMA issued statements on the use of diclofenac with regards to its cardiovascular risk.
- The statements acknowledged that, like COX-2 inhibitors, diclofenac is associated with a small increased risk in arterial thromboembolic events (stroke, MI).
- The risk is increased at high doses for extended periods.
- They advise that all NSAIDs and COX-2 inhibitors should be used at the lowest possible dose for the shortest possible duration.

The risk of GI toxicity can be in part overcome by co-prescribing with a proton pump inhibitor, as is recommended for all patients on chronic treatment. NSAIDs should be avoided in patients with a history of ulcers or severe gastritis.

NSAIDs are associated with an increased risk of renal toxicity, with the elderly and those with pre-existing renal impairment being at greatest risk. Patients on chronic treatment should have renal and hepatic function monitored, and treatment discontinued in severe impairment. Alternative analgesia should be considered in patients on low-dose **aspirin**.

COX 2 inhibitors

Cyclo-oxygenase-2 inhibitors are novel NSAIDs that can reduce prostaglandin production by selectively blocking cyclo-oxygenase 2, but not cyclo-oxygenase 1 activity. Examples include celecoxib, etoricoxib, rofecoxib, and valdecoxib

Mechanism of action

COX-2 inhibitors also act to inhibit prostaglandin synthesis, although unlike other NSAIDs, they are selective non-competitive inhibitors of the cyclo-oxygenase 2 enzyme. The COX-1 isoform of cyclo-oxygenase is mainly expressed ubiquitously and constitutively, having a role in the protection of GI mucosa. COX-2, on the other hand, is absent or has low expression in most tissues, but this is increased in response to inflammatory or tissue-injury signals. As a result, COX-2 inhibitors were developed to deliver anti-inflammatory/analgesic activity, without the

GI toxicity thought to be associated with COX-1 inhibition (see 'Unwanted effects').

Prescribing

There are currently only two COX-2 inhibitors on the market licensed for use in osteoarthritis, **celecoxib** and **etoricoxib**, following the voluntary withdrawal of **rofecoxib** and **valdecoxib** primarily due to concerns over increased cardiovascular risk. As this risk is considered to be a class effect, COX-2 inhibitors are generally reserved for patients at high risk of gastroduodenal ulceration and should only be continued after a trial period where a benefit has been demonstrated.

Unwanted effects

Although COX-2 inhibitors were originally developed to optimize anti-inflammatory effect while reducing the toxicity associated with NSAID therapy, it is now understood that the differences in roles of the various isoenzymes are not so easy to separate. In that respect, targeting of COX-2 does not produce the desired safety profile. In practice, the only clear advantage of the COX-2 inhibitors is the reduced risk of gastroduodenal ulceration; although this benefit is lost in any patients co-prescribed low dose **aspirin**. GI toxicity remains a common side effect to therapy and a proton pump inhibitor is still required. As a result, the side effect profile to COX-2 inhibitors is comparable with the non-selective NSAIDs, with the same warnings for cardiovascular and renal toxicity.

Furthermore, **celecoxib** is a sulfonamide, a class renowned for its hypersensitivity reactions, such as rash and blood dyscrasias; it should therefore be avoided in patients known to be hypersensitive to sulfonamides.

Drug interactions

As with oral NSAIDs, patients prescribed COX-2 inhibitors should have any topical NSAIDs discontinued and alternatives considered in patients requiring low dose **aspirin**.

Rubefacients

Capsaicin exhibits analgesic properties through its ability to desensitize nociceptive terminals. Examples: capsaicin

Mechanism of action

Capsaicin is the active ingredient of hot chilli peppers and can elicit burning pain through activation of a non-selective cation channel expressed on the endings of sensory nerves. This capsaicin receptor, or TRPV1, is a polymodal (sensitive to various types of stimuli) sensory transducer molecule in the pain pathway. It is predominantly expressed in dorsal root ganglia and peripheral sensory nerve endings. Although it can also be found in the CNS, this is to a much lesser extent. TRPV1 integrates different types of stimuli, including harmful heat, tissue acidosis, and chemical types, which are all identified to produce pain.

Although **capsaicin** can produce pain, it also has analgesic qualities, in particular in pain that is linked to diabetic neuropathy or arthritis. This apparent paradox is related to capsaicin's capacity to desensitize TRPV1 receptors and thus block nociceptive signals from capsaicin, as well as other stimuli.

Prescribing

Topical **capsaicin** is the only rubefacient advocated for use in OA, where it demonstrates modest efficacy. It is available for use in two different strengths, with the lower potency cream (0.025%) available for symptomatic relief of osteoarthritis, particularly where it affects the knees or hands. The cream should be rubbed in gently to the affected area until there is no remaining residue. It can be safely used as an add-on therapy to more conventional treatment and patients should be advised it may take up to 2 weeks to work.

Unwanted effects

Adverse effects to **capsaicin** tend to be localized, causing burning and irritation, particularly if used more frequently than four times a day or applied to broken skin. The burning sensation may be worse when used after a bath or shower. Patients should be advised to wash hands thoroughly after application (unless hand/fingers are being treated), and to avoid contact with the eyes and nose.

Tramadol

Tramadol is a centrally acting analgesic that is structurally related to codeine and morphine, consisting of two enantiomers that act via different mechanisms.

Mechanism of action

See Topic 8.3, 'Local anaesthetics'.

Prescribing

Tramadol may be considered as an alternative to opioid analgesics for pain relief in OA, preferred by some as the GI toxicity tends to be less pronounced. In OA, doses are administered orally, starting as always with a low dose to establish the lowest effective dose. For more information see Topic 8.3, 'Local anaesthetics'.

Opioids

Opioid receptors can be found throughout both the central and peripheral nervous system. Agonists for the μ-receptor subtype show the strongest analgesic activity, but also have the highest potential for abuse. Examples include codeine, dihydrocodeine, buprenorphine, morphine, and fentanyl.

Mechanism of action

For specific mechanism of action see Topic 8.3, 'Local anaesthetics'.

Prescribing

Codeine is the most commonly used opioid for pain management in OA, either alone or in combination with **paracetamol** (**co-codamol**), and is reserved for use as a second line of treatment due to its unfavourable toxicity profile. Less commonly, paracetamol is used in combination with a low dose of **dihydrocodeine** (**co-dydramol**). Stronger opioids such as **morphine** may, however, be necessary where pain is particularly severe such as those unsuitable for surgery or during a flare of symptoms. Doses should always be carefully titrated to achieve the minimum effective dose. Topical preparations, such as **buprenorphine** or **fentanyl** patches, may be useful in some patients with chronic pain to help reduce tablet burden.

Unwanted effects

With the exception of constipation and pruritus, the common side effects (drowsiness, nausea, and vomiting) to opioids tend to be transient and can be minimized by titrating doses to pain. Constipation is particularly problematic with chronic use, especially at high doses where prophylactic laxatives are recommended, ideally with a stimulant such as **senna** to antagonize the effects of opioids on GI transit time. For more information see Topic 8.2, 'Local anaesthetics'.

Corticosteroids (intra-articular)

The rapid onset of effect after intra-articular administration of corticosteroids suggests a direct anti-inflammatory action. Examples include hydrocortisone acetate, methylprednsiolone acetate, triamcinolone acetonide, and triamcinolone hexacetonide.

Mechanism of action

Glucocorticoids act directly on nuclear steroid receptors controlling gene transcription and thus the levels of specific proteins. This leads to changes in T and B cell functions, modifications of cytokines and enzyme levels, and inhibition of phospholipase A2, which results in decreased production of pro-inflammatory derivatives of arachidonic acid. Despite the theoretical basis, demonstration of in vivo anti-inflammatory action of intra-articular corticosteroids in osteoarthritis has proven difficult. Trials of intra-articular steroids, mostly in knee osteoarthritis, have continued to show positive effects, but this is of short duration and confounded by strong placebo effect.

Prescribing

Injections for intra-articular administration are formulated to prolong the time they remain within the joint, while minimizing systemic absorption. In the case of corticosteroids this is achieved through selection of poorly water soluble salts formulated into a suspension. Available preparations include **hydrocortisone acetate**, **triamcinolone acetonide/hexacetonide**, and **methylprednisolone acetate**; the latter also available in combination with **lidocaine** to reduce pain on administration. Doses vary according to the size of the affected joint.

There is limited evidence that suggests triamcinolone (in particular, the hexacetonide salt) is more effective than the other agents, which may in part be due to its longer duration of action (inversely proportional to water solubility), although it is considerably more expensive.

Unwanted effects

Intra-articular administration of corticosteroids can cause local reactions such as pain and irritation. More severe toxicity is associated with repeated use for extended periods where it can be associated with joint destruction, avascular necrosis, or joint infection. After treatment patients should be advised to rest and report any symptoms suggestive of septic arthritis such as local swelling, fever, and restricted joint movement.

The extent of systemic absorption following intra-articular administration of corticosteroids depends on the dose, drug, and duration of treatment. For more details on systemic toxicity see Topic 6.6, 'Inflammatory bowel disease'.

Interactions

Due to reduced systemic absorption, interactions with corticosteroids are less likely with intra-articular administration, unless high doses are used repeatedly.

Glucosamine

The rationale for the use of glucosamine is based on the supposed normalization of cartilage metabolism, which may favourably modify the natural progression of osteoarthritis.

Mechanism of action

Glucosamine sulphate is a naturally occurring amino monosaccharide, which is a component of the articular cartilage glycosaminoglycans. The role of glucosamine sulphate in osteoarthritis is largely based on in vitro studies and animal models, where it has been shown to normalize cartilage metabolism, rebuild experimentally damaged cartilage and show weak anti-inflammatory properties. Many of the studies conducted in humans are subject to controversy.

Prescribing

Many patients with OA are known to self-medicate with **glucosamine**, either on its own or in combination with **chondroitin**. It is classified as a nutritional supplement making it readily available and is advertised for use in OA, despite clinical trials remaining inconclusive regarding its overall benefit. Although not recommended for prescribing, any patients wishing to purchase their own should be advised to consider a 6-month trial period to ascertain if there is any clinical benefit. For most any reduction in pain is likely to be minimal.

Unwanted effects

Within the recommended dose, **glucosamine** is considered to be safe. Concerns that glucosamine may cause problems in diabetic patients, as glucosamine interferes with glucose metabolism and increases insulin resistance, remain theoretical.

Further reading

Goodwin JLR, Kraemer JJ, Bajwa ZH (2009) The use of opioids in the treatment of osteoarthritis: when, why and how? *Current Rheumatology Reports* 11(1), 5–14.

Hunter DJ (Ed.) (2009) Osteoarthritis. *Medical Clinics of North America* 93(1), 1–244.

Vincent TL, Troeberg L (2013) Pathogenesis of osteoarthritis. In: Oxford Textbook of Rheumatology (4 edn.), pp. 1163–96. Oxford: Oxford University Press.

Guidelines

EMA (2013) PRAC recommends the same cardiovascular precautions for diclofenac as for selective COX-2 inhibitors. http://www.ema.europa.eu/docs/en_GB/document_library/Press_release/2013/06/WC500144451.pdf [accessed 3 April 2019].

Hochberg MC, Altman RD, April AT, et al. (2012) American College of Rheumatology 2012 Recommendations for the use of nonpharmacologic and pharmacologic therapies in osteoarthritis of the hand, hip, and knee. *Arthritis Care Research* 64(4), 465–74.

McAlindon TE, Bannuru RR, Sullivan MC et al. (2014). OARSI guidelines for the non-surgical management of knee osteoarthritis. *Osteoarthritis Cartilage* 22, 363–388. https://www.oarsi.org/sites/default/files/docs/2014/non_surgical_treatment_of_knee_oa_march_2014.pdf [accessed 3 April 2019].

NICE CG177 (2014) Osteoarthritis: care and management in adults. https://www.nice.org.uk/Guidance/CG177 [accessed 3 April 2019].

Porcheret M, Healey E, Dziedzic K, et al. (2011) Osteoarthritis: a modern approach to diagnosis and management Arthritis Research UK; Practical advice for GPs on management of rheumatic disease Series 6, Hands on No 10 https://www.arthritisresearchuk.org/~/media/Files/Education/Hands-On/HO10-Autumn-2011-with-Exercise-sheet.ashx [accessed 5 April 2019].

MHRA Drug Safety Update (2013) Diclofenac: new contraindications and warnings after a *Europe-wide Review of Cardiovascular Safety* 6(11). http://www.mhra.gov.uk/Safetyinformation/DrugSafetyUpdate/CON286975 [accessed 3 April 2019].

The inflammatory arthropathies are a group of auto-immune conditions that include rheumatoid arthritis (RA), ankylosing spondylitis (AS), and psoriatic arthritis. Of these, RA is the most common, with a prevalence in adults of about 1%, affecting females three or four times more often than men. It typically affects the small joints of the hand and feet, with a peak onset of 25-50 years. AS is a chronic seronegative inflammatory arthropathy that tends to affect the lumbosacral region initially, before progressing to affect the whole spine. It is insidious in onset and usually presents before 30 years of age. The disease is three times more common in men, with higher rates in northern Europe, and a prevalence of 0.2%. Psoriatic arthritis is the least common inflammatory arthropathy; however, its precise prevalence is difficult to determine and varies considerably between countries (0.001–0.4%), in part due to the lack of universally accepted criteria. It typically affects synovial tissue, skin and enthuses, and is seronegative for rheumatoid factor. This chapter will focus on RA and AS.

Pathophysiology

Rheumatoid arthritis

RA is a common systemic autoimmune inflammatory disease that affects multiple synovial joints, and can lead to extra-articular and systemic inflammatory changes. The exact causes are unknown, but it is autoimmune in nature with a genetic component that is probably triggered by environmental factors. The HLA-DRB1 gene encodes the HLA class II histocompatibility antigen DRB1 beta chain protein. DRB1 encodes the most common beta subunit of HLA-DR, with several alleles of DRB1 being strongly associated with RA. The HLA DRB1 locus forms part of the binding groove of MHC Class II proteins present on antigen presenting and immune cells involved in the adaptive immune response (like in SLE; see Topic 7.4, 'Metabolic bone disease'). Environmental factors such as smoking, infection (e.g. Epstein–Barr virus or Rubella) or trauma may trigger the initial autoimmune reaction. Sex hormones may also be implicated, given the preponderance of RA in females.

The precise molecular and cellular mechanisms behind RA remain unclear, although it is believed that T helper cells drive the auto-immunity in RA. Specifically, Th-1 and, more recently, Th-17 cells, are believed to play a role in promoting release of interleukins, leading to a chronic inflammatory response and subsequent tissue damage. Th-17 have been shown to release IL-17, IL-21, and IL-22, through initial activation via the pro-inflammatory interleukin (IL-23). Both IL-17 and TNFα are highly expressed in the synovium and synovial fluid of RA patients. This increased presence of IL-17 leads to greater expression of receptor activator of nuclear factor kappa-B ligand (RANKL), which is present on the surface of osteoblasts and synoviocytes, thus activating osteoclast differentiation and causing bony destruction. This destruction typically occurs at or near the attachment of the joint capsule. The ongoing infiltration of inflammatory cells (macrophages, lymphocytes, and plasma cells), leads to a characteristic 'pannus' of inflammatory synovial tissue.

The presence of other mediator cells such as T cells, B cells, mast cells, and macrophages within the synovium, may also contribute towards autoimmunity through the secretion of pro-inflammatory cytokines, such as IL-1, IL-6, and TNFα. These cytokines can stimulate macrophages to secrete metalloproteinases (MMPs), which breakdown matrix proteins leading to cartilage destruction and further bony erosion. IL-6 may also be secreted by T-cells and stimulate osteoclast formation, or leave the joint space to initiate an acute phase reaction. Specific ligands targeted to modulate the action of TNFα, IL-1, and IL-6 have been shown to be efficacious in RA, and these are described below.

Humoral immunity through B cells can lead primarily to antibody formation, but also to cytokine release and modulation of T cells. In RA the crucial role of B-cells is in the production of autoantibodies to IgG molecules [rheumatoid factor (RF)] and to cyclic citrullinated proteins (i.e. anti-citrullinated protein antibodies (ACPAs). RF is present in approximately 75–80% of patients at some point in the course of their disease, although it is also present in other autoimmune conditions, such as SLE and primary Sjögren's syndrome. ACPAs have a higher specificity for RA and cyclic citrullinated peptides are used in the assay to detect these autoantibodies; RF measurements are still routinely carried out, as they provide a good marker for activity and prognosis. This link between ACPA and RA, has led to the theory that citrullinated proteins are likely implicated in the pathogenesis of RA through TNFα production. In brief, successful treatments for RA involve modulating pathways that interfere with immune signalling via IL-1, TNFα, IL-6, CD20, etc. In subtle, but significantly different forms of inflammatory arthritis there has also been success by intervening in IL-12/23 and IL-17 signalling.

Symptoms of RA are insidious and symmetrical in nature, characterized by warm painful joints that are particularly stiff in the mornings. As the local disease progresses there may be tendon rupture and increased joint deformity (e.g. in the hand, ulnar deviation, swan neck, Boutonnière's, and Z deformities). Progress may be primarily progressive or may follow a more relapsing-remitting pattern. The overall aim of treatment is to ameliorate disease activity; and hence, slow the structural destruction and improve a patient's quality of life. Thus, with the exception of localized mild disease where treatment with simple analgesics may suffice, patients are initiated early on immunomodulating disease-modifying anti-rheumatic drugs (DMARDs).

In the presence of extra-articular or systemic disease, more aggressive management therapies may be required to treat diseased arterial walls, granulomatous extravascular nodules and chronic inflammatory changes with the lung or pericardium. The arterial walls may show fibrous hyperplasia that can be seen as systemic vasculitis (e.g. Raynaud's, skin ulceration), and vessel obstruction can occur affecting coronary or pulmonary vessels, leading to serious treatment resistant complications such as rheumatoid interstitial lung disease.

Ankylosing spondylitis

AS is one of a number of conditions known collectively as the seronegative spondyloarthropathies, which are characteristically associated with HLA-B27 and involve, to varying degrees, the spine, e.g. juvenile enthesitis-related arthritis, psoriatic arthritis, reactive arthropathy, and enteropathic arthritis. AS affects men two to three times more commonly than women, typically presenting before the age of 30, although up to 20% of people affected will remain symptom free.

AS has a strong genetic component with 90% possessing the *HLA-B27* gene, although other genes have been associated, such as *HLA B60, HLA DR1, IL-1* gene cluster and *IL23R*. The prevalence of *HLA-B27* is significantly raised in AS, although the relevance of this to the pathogenesis of the disease remains unknown. It is significant, however, that *HLA-B27* encodes for an MHC class I protein and, hence, has a role in antigen presentation. A number of theories exist as to the pathophysiological mechanism, such as the presentation of a bacterial protein by B27 to CD8+ T cells. The *B27* gene is also associated with dysfunctional immune responses, so there may be decreased TNFα or IFNγ causing auto-inflammatory changes. The gene, *ERAP1*, also has a role in HLA-B27 antigen presentation and can lead to loss of TNF, IL-1, and IL-6 receptors. As with RA, more recently, the involvement of Th17 and the IL-17/ IL-23 pathway has been implicated in genetic studies.

Typical presentation of disease is inflammatory back pain of gradual onset that tends to improve with exercise rather than rest, together with other musculoskeletal manifestations, such as peripheral enthesis (inflammation at tendon or ligament insertions) in the heel and arthritis. Arthritis is typically asymmetrical and involves the lower extremities. Predictably, there is restricted lumbar spinal flexion/extension with progressive disease, reduced chest expansion, and around 50% of patients have a rising ESR and CRP; to date, serological markers like RF and ANA are unhelpful, but diagnosis can be confirmed by HLA-B27 testing. Around 30% of patients may have additional extra-articular manifestations such as uveitis, heart block from fibrosis of the conduction system, pulmonary fibrosis, and osteoporosis suggesting some pathophysiological parallels exists with RA.

For a full summary of the relevant pathways and drug targets, see Figure 7.4.

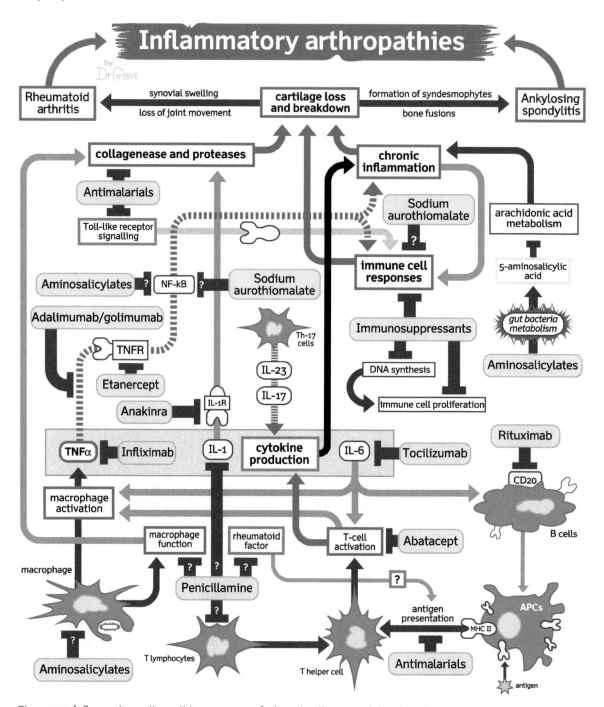

Figure 7.4 Inflammatory arthropathies: summary of relevant pathways and drug targets.

Management

Rheumatoid arthritis

Patients with rheumatoid arthritis are best managed by a specialist team within secondary care to ensure access to multi-disciplinary support, and appropriate initiation and management of complex treatment. Ideally, treatment should be initiated within 3 months of symptom onset; therefore, patients presenting beyond this time or those with disease that affect the small joints of the hands or feet, or multiple joints, should be referred urgently within 2 weeks. For initial management in primary care, corticosteroids are best avoided until a specialist assessment has been carried out, as they may interfere with diagnosis and subsequent treatment strategies. However, interim symptomatic treatment primarily with simple analgesia (**paracetamol** with or without **codeine**) may be started. Where these alone fail to manage symptoms, a NSAID (**ibuprofen** or **naproxen**) or COX-2 inhibitor may be started, in the absence of any contraindications (e.g. cardiovascular, GI, or renal). NSAIDs and COX-2 inhibitors should be prescribed with a proton pump inhibitor (PPI) and consideration given to minimizing use in high risk patients.

Initial investigations should include a clinical examination (pain scores, assessment of number of affected joints) and blood tests for rheumatoid factor, ESR, CRP, and anti-cyclic citrullinated peptide antibodies (ACPA), in order to confirm diagnosis and assess severity. Imaging should include X-rays of affected joints, including the hands and feet. Ultrasound scanning may be useful to detect sub-clinical synovitis. Disease Activity Scores DAS/DAS28 scores are calculated based on the number of affected joints, pain scores, and circulating inflammatory markers to assess level of disease activity (see Table 7.1). This is subsequently used to monitor and adjust treatment.

Table 7.1 Disease activity score (DAS28)

DAS28 (Disease activity score)	Activity
<2.6	Disease remission
2.6–3.2	Low activity
3.3–5.2	Moderate activity
>5.2	Severe activity

Reproduced from Prevoo ML, Van 't Hof MA, Kruper HH et al (1995) Modified disease activity scores that include twenty-eight joint counts. Development and validation in a prospective longitudinal study of patients with rheumatoid arthritis. *Arthritis Rheum*, 38 (1) 44-48. Copyright © 2005, John Wiley and Sons. https://doi.org/10.1002/art.1780380107

Active RA can have a significant impact on quality of life, due to pain, and its effect on physical activity, thus making everyday activities difficult and imposing social isolation. These issues should be addressed as part of treatment, by ensuring access to health professionals, including occupational therapists, physiotherapists, podiatrists, and specialist nurses to provide the necessary support. Regular exercise should be encouraged for general fitness, as well as improving joint flexibility and muscle strength to enable better function.

Current thinking in RA management is early initiation of DMARDs (see Table 7.2) preferably within 3 months of onset of symptoms, in order to prevent joint damage, and subsequent loss of function. At diagnosis, **methotrexate** is usually started, either alone or in combination with another DMARD, often alongside a short course of glucocorticoids to induce remission and NSAIDs to control flares. DMARD doses are generally escalated rapidly to achieve a clinical response and, once clinical remission is achieved, consideration given to dose reduction. With conventional DMARDs, once therapy has reached an optimal dose, addition of a further agent is more effective than switching between agents.

In the UK patients that fail to respond adequately to methotrexate and another DMARD, with a DAS28 score greater than 5.1, are eligible for treatment with a biologic agent (see Table 7.3). Biologics are initiated in addition to methotrexate, unless methotrexate is contraindicated or poorly tolerated, in which case some may be used as monotherapy (**adalimumab**, **etanercept**, **certolizumab pegol**, and **tocilizumab**). Choice is generally dictated by cost and patient preference, taking into consideration treatment schedules, and any contraindications. In all cases, it should be used for a period of 6 months to assess efficacy, and only continued where there is evidence of a moderate response, assessed using the European League Against Rheumatism (EULAR) criteria. Patients deemed unresponsive may be switched between agents, as combining two biologics is not currently recommended due to the high risk of toxicity.

In severe disease unresponsive to DMARDs, and at least one anti-TNFα, or in those where anti-TNFα treatment is unsuitable, **rituximab** may be considered. Although a further course should not be repeated before 6 months. In the UK, **anakinra** is currently reserved for use within the context of a clinical trial.

In some countries patients presenting with a high level of disease activity and poor prognostic factors (see Box 7.2), cytokine inhibitors may be initiated at first presentation. Globally, the introduction of biologics and the move to a more aggressive treatment strategy, has resulted in

Table 7.2 DMARDS used in RA

	Administration	Time to response	Notes
Methotrexate	Oral, IM, IV, SC Given weekly	6 weeks–3 months	Most widely used DMARD in RA
Sulfasalazine	Orally	> 3 months	Widely used in RA
Leflunomide	Orally	8–12 weeks	Often used second line, e.g. where response to methotrexate is inadequate
Hydroxychloroquine	Orally	6 weeks–6 months	Generally used in mild disease or as combination therapy
Sodium aurothiomalate	IM	Once cumulative dose >500 mg has been given	Discontinue of no response after 1000 mg cumulative dose, rarely used and largely discontinued
Penicillamine	Orally	3–6 months	Rarely used
Ciclosporin	Orally	3 months	Used less frequently in RA, usually second line
Azathioprine	Orally (IV rarely)	6 weeks–3 months	Used in the treatment of numerous inflammatory disorders, e.g. IBD, SLE
Cyclophosphamide	Orally, IV (in hospital)	6 weeks–3 months	Reserved for severe/refractory disease or in the presence of complications, e.g. vasculitis, scleroderma
Mycophenolate	Orally	6 weeks–3 months	Reserved for use in severe disease where other options have failed

Table 7.3 Biologics available for use in RA

Biologic	Target	Route of administration	Frequency of administration	Can be used as monotherapy
Adalimumab	Anti-TNFα	SC	Fortnightly	Y
Etanercept	Anti-TNFα	SC	Weekly/twice weekly	Y
Golimumab	Anti-TNFα	SC	Monthly	N
Infliximab	Anti-TNFα	IV infusion	8-weekly after loading	N
Certolizumab pegol	Anti-TNFα	SC	Fortnightly after loading	Y
Tocalizumab	Anti-IL-6	IV	Monthly	Y
Abatacept	Inhibits T-cell activation	SC	Weekly	N
Anakinra	Anti-IL-1	SC	Daily	N
Rituximab	Anti CD20	IV infusion	2 doses 2 weeks apart	N

Box 7.2 Poor prognostic risk factors

Presence of more than one of the following features

- Functional limitation (e.g. HAQ DI)
- Extra-articular disease (rheumatoid nodules, RA vasculitis, Felty's syndrome)
- Positive rheumatoid factor or anti-cyclic citrullinated peptide antibodies
- Bony erosions on radiograph

a decreasing need for joint replacement surgery, due to better joint preservation.

Glucocorticoids should ideally be limited to manage acute flares, for which they may be administered orally, IM, or by intra-articular injection depending on the size and number of joints affected. In progressive disease, however, once all other biological options have been exhausted, long-term use may become unavoidable. In these instances, patients should be made aware of the risks, and steps taken to minimize toxicity, such as prescribing bone protection and using the smallest effective dose.

Ankylosing spondylitis

As with RA, patients presenting with suspected AS will require referral to a rheumatologist. Treatment for symptom control with either an NSAID or COX-2 inhibitor maybe initiated in primary care, with the usual consideration given to cardiovascular, GI, and renal risk factors. Where NSAIDs are not deemed appropriate, alternative treatment with **paracetamol** plus or minus **codeine** maybe considered.

Diagnosis of AS is often delayed by 5–7 years due to its insidious onset. It commonly presents with chronic or recurrent lower back pain characterized by stiffness and fatigue, although in some instances, presence of extra-articular manifestations may lead to diagnosis, e.g. psoriasis, IBD, or anterior uveitis. Presence of the latter requires urgent referral to ophthalmology within 24 hours to prevent loss of sight. Diagnosis of AS can be confirmed by testing for inflammatory markers (CRP, ESR), although these may be not be raised, and FBC, in combination with X-rays of the sacroiliac joint. As it may take several years for changes to be seen on X-ray, an MRI may be useful following a normal X-ray, where there is a high index of suspicion, as this can pick up early changes to sacroiliac joints.

Regular exercise and patient education are essential in AS management in order to maintain function and minimize deformity. Exercises at home or in groups, aim to reduce stiffness, maintain range of movement and strengthen muscles, particularly around joints, and will include deep breathing exercises to maintain flexibility in the rib cage.

Patients who fail treatment with first-line anti-inflammatories should be referred to a rheumatologist for optimization of treatment. Unlike RA, there is little evidence to suggest a benefit with DMARDs, perhaps with the exception of **sulfasalazine** or possibly **methotrexate**. After failing two NSAIDs, patients are generally initiated on biologics. The anti-TNFs; **infliximab**, **etanercept**, **adalimumab**, **certolizumab pegol,** and **golimumab**, are recommended for use by NICE, as are newer anti-IL17 treatments such as **secukinumab**. Patients should be assessed after a period of 12–16 weeks to determine treatment response and those who fail treatment with one biologic or are intolerant, may be switched to a second agent. An adequate response is defined as a 50% reduction in Bath Ankylosing Spondylitis Disease Activity Index (BASDAI) score from pretreatment levels, or at least a 2-cm reduction in spinal pain visual analogue scale (VAS). Corticosteroids, although not recommended for systemic use, may on occasions be injected intra-articularly for sacroiliitis or enthesitis. If DMARDs are prescribed, this is usually in the context of peripheral arthritis. DMARDs are used only rarely in those with involvement limited to the axial spine.

Further pharmacological management may be required to address associated pathologies, i.e. to modify cardiovascular risk, or the use of bisphosphonates with calcium and vitamin D supplementation to reduce the risk of osteoporosis. Patients will also require immunization against pneumococcal and influenza infections.

Drug classes used in management

DMARDs: immunosuppressants

DMARDs, or Disease-Modifying Anti-Rheumatic Drugs, are a chemically heterogeneous group of drugs that have a slow onset of action and modulate distinct steps of the immune and inflammatory response. Examples: methotrexate, azathioprine, ciclosporin, cyclophosphamide, and leflunomide.

Mechanism of action

Methotrexate was originally developed as an anti-cancer drug, and only started to be used in immune-inflammatory diseases at a later stage, mainly in the field of rheumatology. Despite this commonality, the dose in oncology is several-fold higher than the one used in systemic immune-inflammatory rheumatological diseases. As a result, side effects are different, but rarely life-threatening when administered as long-term, low-dose therapy, as it is in the treatment of arthropathies. The anti-proliferative activity of methotrexate comes from its ability to inhibit folic acid reductase, which promotes the inhibition of DNA synthesis and cell division, although as with other DMARDs its precise mechanism in the management of RA is not completely understood. It is thought that methotrexate is brought into the cell and metabolized to polyglutamates (methotrexate-glu), which might be the true anti-inflammatory agent. It binds dihydrofolate reductase and has high affinity with enzymes that require folate co-factors, blocking tetrahydrofolate dependent steps in cell metabolism. In particular, they affect purine biosynthesis leading to adenosine over-production. Extracellular adenosine actions are mainly exerted via adenosine G protein A2a receptors, which augment intracellular cAMP and cause immunosuppression by inhibition of phagocytosis, and the secretion of TNF, IFNY, IL1, IL12, and others. In addition, it has been suggested that methotrexate can have an effect on decreasing proteinase production.

The soil fungi extract **ciclosporin** is a crucial drug in the prevention of rejection in organ transplant. A powerful immunosuppressant, it exerts inhibition of immunocompetent lymphocytes in the Go or G1 cell cycle phase, and inhibits production of lymphokine and interleukin release. It is also well established that ciclosporin can inhibit the phosphatase activity of calcineurin through formation of a complex with cyclophilin. In this way, it can regulate the nuclear translocation and subsequent activation of nuclear factor of activated T cells (NFAT) transcription factors, normally controlled by calcineurin. Ciclosporin can also block the activation of JNK and p38 signalling pathways that is triggered by antigen recognition, making it a specific inhibitor of T cell activation.

Azathioprine has systemic immunosuppressive actions and has been used in lupus erythematosus therapy. It is a purine analogue that is metabolized to 6-mercaptopurine and then enzymatically converted into 6-thiouric acid, 6 methyl-mercaptopurine and 6-thioguanine. Ultimately, it can become incorporated into replicating DNA and can also block the *de novo* pathway of purine synthesis. This latter action is thought to contribute to its relatively specificity to lymphocytes, due to their lack of salvage pathway.

Cyclophosphamide is an alkylating agent that can add alkyl groups to DNA bases disrupting its function and leading to cell death. It can decrease the immune system response to various conditions.

Leflunomide is rapidly absorbed and converted to teriflunomide, which acts as a selective inhibitor of the *de novo* pyrimidine synthesis. As a result, activated T cells that are dependent on this will be selectively more affected. Leflunomide appears to regulate autoimmune lymphocytes, interfering with cell cycle progression and preventing autoimmune lymphocytes expansion.

Prescribing

Aside from **methotrexate** the immunosuppressant DMARDs are generally reserved for use in patients failing treatment with alternative DMARDs due to their less favourable safety profile, and are used less frequently since the introduction of the biologics. Methotrexate is the DMARD of choice, due to its favourable efficacy/toxicity profile, being backed up with strong evidence, and well tolerated when adequately monitored.

In the treatment of inflammatory arthropathies, methotrexate can be administered orally, SC or IM on a weekly basis, with doses titrated to achieve an adequate clinical response. It is invariably prescribed concomitantly with **folic acid** (taken on a different day) to reduce toxicity.

PRESCRIBING WARNING

Errors with methotrexate frequency

● There have been a number of severe and even fatal outcomes where patients have been incorrectly prescribed or administered methotrexate on a daily basis.

● Prescribers should take care to ensure that methotrexate is prescribed on a weekly basis and the patients adequately counselled on this.

● Most centres advocate the use of 2.5 mg tablets only (not 10 mg) to prevent the risk of four times the overdose, when a switch has been made.

Where used, **azathioprine**, **leflunomide**, **ciclosporin**, and **cyclophosphamide** are administered orally OD, with doses titrated up for optimal response. Cyclophosphamide may also be administered IV to prevent organ damage, e.g. in the treatment of rheumatoid vasculitis.

Unwanted effects

In general, DMARD immunosuppressants often cause aphthous ulceration and minor bowel discomfort that is usually tolerated. Hypertension is also common with **leflunomide**, thus patients should have their blood pressure monitored while on treatment.

Beyond these common side effects, suppressive effects on bone marrow function, can lead to blood dyscrasias, a well-recognized phenomena with the immunosuppressants, with potentially life-threatening consequences. Patients on immunosuppressant treatment require a regular FBC and should be advised to report signs of haematological toxicity, such as unexplained bleeding, bruising, or sore throat. The risk of haematological toxicity with **azathioprine** may be more common in individuals deficient in TPMT, thus TPMT status is often checked prior to commencing azathioprine. Haematological toxicity necessitates immediate discontinuation of therapy, and in the case of **methotrexate**, rescue treatment with **folinic acid** may be required, while with leflunomide, a **colestyramine** wash-out may be requested. For leflunomide BP monitoring is required.

As immunosuppressants are hepatotoxic, it is also recommended that LFTs are monitored. The risk of toxicity is increased in elderly patients and in the presence of renal impairment or interacting drugs such as anti-folates (e.g. **trimethoprim**), other immunosuppressants or drugs that impair excretion such as penicillins). As possible teratogens, women of child-bearing potential should be advised of the risks and consideration given to using alternative agents where necessary. For more information see Topic 13.1, 'Haemato-oncology and malignancy'.

DMARDs: antimalarials

The antimalarial drug hydroxychloroquine is a lipophilic lysosomotropic amine also used as an anti-inflammatory drug in RA and lupus. For example, hydroxychloroquine.

Mechanism of action

The immunosuppressive properties of **hydroxychloroquine** appear to be related to its interference with antigen processing and presentation. This seems to relate to its ability to increase the pH of intracellular vacuoles in antigen presenting cells, leading to invariant chain dissociation from the major histocompatibility complex class II molecule and antigen binding inhibition. Failure to engage with antigen disrupts the signalling pathways that lead to T-cell activation. In addition, hydroxychloroquine has been found to inhibit Toll-like receptor signalling, preventing the activation of immune cell responses. It can also accumulate in white blood cells, inhibiting the

activity of collagenases and proteases involved in cartilage breakdown.

Prescribing

Hydroxychloroquine, although perhaps inferior in terms of efficacy compared with other DMARDs used in rheumatoid arthritis, has a favourable side effect profile, and thus may be considered in patients intolerant of other DMARDs. Doses are administered orally OD and may be escalated provided a maximum dose of 6.5 mg/kg/day is not exceeded, based on ideal body weight.

Unwanted effects

Hydroxychloroquine is generally well tolerated, although it can cause GI side effects, skin reactions (including pigmentary changes), hair bleaching and alopecia. Rarely, albeit more serious, alterations in pigmentation may occur in the eyes leading to visual field defects and retinopathy. Patients should have a baseline ophthalmology review, repeated at 12 months. The risk of haematological toxicity is low compared with other DMARDs. Anti-malarials are also associated with QT interval-prolongation, particularly when taken concurrently with other drugs known to have this effect, e.g. **halofantrine**, **amiodarone**, and **moxifloxacin**.

As antimalarials are largely metabolized in the liver they should be used cautiously in moderate/severe hepatic impairment. There is also an increased risk of haemolysis with G6PD deficiency, although this is not a contraindication to use.

Penicillamine

A heavy metal chelator, penicillamine is an α-amino acid metabolite of penicillin that has immunosuppressant properties.

Mechanism of action

Penicillamine can exist as two enantiomers, with D-penicillamine being the naturally occurring isomer and the only one used clinically. Once penicillamine is ingested, it transforms into disulfides (N- and S-methyl-D-penicillamine), which bind to albumin and are responsible for the slow elimination of the drug from plasma. In addition to being highly water soluble and degradation resistant, the molecular structure of penicillamine enables it to chelate metals such as copper and lead through stable complex formation by thiol group, allowing increased kidney excretion.

The immunosuppressive activity of penicillamine is due to a reduction in T-lymphocytes, inhibition of macrophage function, and a decreasing IL-1 and rheumatoid factor, but the mechanism of action is unknown. In addition, it also prevents collagen from cross-linking, by interfering with tropocollagen molecules. Unlike other cytotoxic immunosupressants, penicillamine can decrease IgM rheumatoid factor without a general effect on serum immunoglobulins.

Prescribing

Penicillamine is now rarely used in RA since the advent of newer, more effective agents. Response times to treatment can be slow (6–12 months) and the risk of side effects remains high, including haematological toxicity. Where used, doses are administered orally and titrated-up at monthly intervals to higher doses that are split over the day to improve tolerance.

Unwanted effects

Aside from GI side effects, **penicillamine** has the potential to cause severe haematological and renal (glomerulonephritis) toxicity. Elderly patents and those with pre-existing renal impairment are particularly susceptible, as are those on concomitant therapy with other immunosuppressive DMARDs, such as **hydroxychloroquine** or **gold**. While on treatment, regular monitoring should be carried out and patients advised to report signs of haematological toxicity (sore throat, fever, unexplained bleeding, or bruising). As with most drugs allergic reactions can occur, with the risk slightly increased in patients sensitive to penicillin or gold.

Aminosalicylates (sulfasalazine)

The anti-inflammatory drug sulfasalazine serves as a route to deliver sulfapyridine and 5-aminosalicylic acid (mesalazine) to the gut where inhibition of prostaglandin and leukotriene synthesis can occur during inflammation.

Mechanism of action

The exact mechanism of action of **sulfasalazine** and its metabolite sulfapyridine in RA is still unresolved, but the inhibition of folate-dependent enzymes, and the subsequent impairment of lymphocyte function could be

a factor. The induction of apoptosis in neutrophils and macrophages can have further contributory effects, while the ability to block TNFα mediated translocation of NF-κB is also a known property.

For more information see Topic 6.6, 'Inflammatory bowel disease'.

Prescribing

Sulfasalazine is one of the more widely used DMARDs, due to its good efficacy and reasonable tolerability, and is the only aminosalicylate licensed for this indication. Doses are administered orally, titrated at weekly intervals to achieve the desired clinical response. Only the enteric-coated tablets, designed to help reduce GI effects, are licensed for use in RA.

Unwanted effects

Side effects to **sulfasalazine** are relatively common and tend to occur within 3–6 months of starting treatment. Patients frequently complain of headaches and GI effects such as diarrhoea, pain, and nausea. Further side effects can be attributed to the sulfapyridine moiety, such as hypersensitivity reactions (including DRESS), fever, and rash. Haematological and hepatic toxicity is also widely reported with use and, for this reason, patients should have FBCs weekly for the first month and LFTs monitored while on treatment. For more details see sulfasalazine in Topic 6.6, 'Inflammatory bowel disease'.

Sodium aurothiomalate

The parenteral gold salts (aurothiomalate) have demonstrated broad immunosuppressant properties, but no central mechanism of action has been described yet.

Mechanism of action

In a similar way to other immunosuppressive agents, **gold** supresses NF-κB activity, producing a shift in the cytokine environment from pro- to anti-inflammatory. Although comparable with other DMARDs in terms of efficacy and inhibition of radiographic progression, toxicity related to skin, and mucosal irritation has been raised as an issue.

Prescribing

IM **gold** for the management of RA has been largely superseded by newer technologies, due to poor tolerability and high drop-out rates. Doses are administered weekly following an initial test dose. Onset of action is slow, such that the full benefit is unlikely to be seen until a cumulative dose of 300–500 mg (6–10 weeks) is reached. Treatment should be discontinued if no benefit is seen after 1 g. Once established on a maintenance dose the interval may be gradually increased to 4–6-weekly, which if tolerated, may be beneficial where compliance is an issue.

Unwanted effects

Anaphylactic reactions to **gold** are relatively common, often presenting within 10 minutes of administration and requiring immediate discontinuation of treatment. Other signs of toxicity include rash, pruritus, blood dyscrasias, albuminuria, or eosinophilia. Prior to starting treatment, any pre-existing conditions should be excluded, i.e. testing urine for albumin, checking skin for rashes and carrying out a FBC to identify blood dyscrasias. Monitoring should continue throughout treatment, as reactions such as blood dyscrasias are more likely to occur after 10–20 weeks. As with all immunosuppressive drugs, patients should be advised to report symptoms such as sore throat, fever, bruising, etc. The risk of toxicity is increased in renal or hepatic impairment, where **gold** is contraindicated. Concomitant therapy with ACE inhibitors can also increase the risk of toxicity.

Other, less common, but serious or even potentially life-threatening complications, include pulmonary fibrosis, peripheral neuropathy, and encephalopathy.

Anti-TNFα cytokine modulators

The finding that TNFα and other cytokines are upregulated in rheumatoid arthritis has prompted the development of various biological approaches to inhibit its inflammatory actions. Examples include adalimumab, etanercept, infliximab, certolizumab pegol, and golimumab.

Mechanism of action

Anti-TNFα agents are normally grouped within the so-called 'biological agents', due to their mode of manufacture. However, they possess different molecular mechanisms to disrupt inflammatory signals activated by TNFα-dependent signalling pathways.

The TNFα chimeric antibody, **infliximab** is made of human constant and murine variable regions. It has high affinity for the soluble and transmembrane forms of TNFα, preventing its binding with the receptor (see also Topic 6.6, 'Inflammatory bowel disease'). **Adalimumab** and **golimumab** are both human monoclonal antibodies against TNFα that also prevent the interaction with the receptor. **Certolizumab pegol** is a PEGylated Fab fragment that can bind to soluble and membrane-bound TNFα. It is also missing the Fc regions of a humanized TNFα monoclonal antibody.

Etanercept uses a different molecular approach to target the decrease of TNFα inflammatory actions. As a dimeric fusion protein composed by the ligand-binding domain of the TNF receptor and human IgG1, etanercept can bind two TNFα molecules and competes with the endogenous TNF receptor for binding with soluble TNFα.

Prescribing

The anti-TNFα agents are licensed for use in combination with **methotrexate** in the management of moderate to severe rheumatoid arthritis in patients failing therapy with combination DMARD therapy, although **adalimumab**, **certolizumab pegol**, and **etanercept** may be used as monotherapy, where methotrexate is not tolerated or contraindicated. The frequency of administration varies from twice-weekly with etanercept, to 8-weekly with **infliximab**, once patients are on a maintenance dose. Treatment is administered SC, except for infliximab, which is given by IV infusion, thereby requiring an outpatient hospital admission. Infliximab, adalimumab, and etanercept are the most widely used, although newer agents are being used with increasing frequency. In all cases, treatment should be reassessed after 6 months and discontinued where response is inadequate, i.e. a DAS28 decrease of less than 1.2 points.

Unwanted effects

As TNFα plays a key role in clearing infections, inhibition significantly increases the risk. In more severe cases, this may include sepsis, pneumonia, invasive fungal infections, and even tuberculosis. Consequently, any latent tuberculosis or pre-existing infections should be excluded prior to starting treatment, and at-risk patients closely monitored. Live vaccines should also be avoided while on treatment and for up to 5 months after.

TNFα also has anti-tumour effects so that the risk of developing a malignancy such as lymphoma, leukaemia, or melanoma, is potentially increased in patients receiving anti-TNFα treatment. Caution is recommended when prescribing for patients with a previous history of malignancy. Treatment is also predictably associated with haematological toxicity including blood dyscrasias, for which patients should be counselled on.

Hypersensitivity reactions are common with anti-TNFα therapy, administration of **infliximab** in particular is associated with acute infusion-related reactions that occur within 1–2 hours of infusion, usually related to the first or second dose. Patients complain of symptoms such as fever, chills, pruritus, chest pain, hypotension, and hypertension, which may be partially relieved by reducing the rate of the infusion and pretreating with antihistamines and **paracetamol**. Delayed reactions (after 3–12 days) occur less commonly, presenting as fever and muscle pain, and with the risk increased in those who have recently restarted treatment.

Neurological toxicity is a rare but serious adverse effect associated with treatment, either as exacerbation of pre-existing neurological pathologies, e.g. multiple sclerosis or precipitation of new demyelinating disease (e.g. Guillain–Barré syndrome).

Other non-specific side effects to anti-TNFα include GI toxicity, headaches, and dizziness.

Non-TNFα cytokine modulators

In addition to the direct block of TNF-α signalling, other non-TNF-α-mediated biological approaches have been developed to target inflammatory responses in rheumatoid arthritis. Examples include abatacept, rituximab, tocalizumab, and anakinra.

Mechanism of action

Rituximab is a chimeric human/murine monoclonal antibody against the CD20 antigen that is present on mature and pre-B cells. It can specifically deplete CD20+ B cells, which have numerous functions in the pathogenesis of the disease (such as antigen presentation and production of cytokines).

The pluripotent cytokine interleukin-6, activates T cells, B cells, macrophages, and osteoclasts, and is involved in the pathogenesis of RA. As a result, it has been a target for novel RA therapies. **Tocilizumab** is a humanized anti-interleukin-6 receptor monoclonal antibody that prevents binding of interleukin-6 and subsequent activation.

The recombinant fusion protein **abatacept** is made of the extracellular domain of human cytotoxic T-lymphocyte-associated antigen 4 (CTLA-4) and part of the Fc domain of human IgG1. It has high affinity for CD28 and thus interferes with T-cell activation by competing with CD80 and CD86.

Anakinra is a recombinant molecule that competitively binds to the interleukin-1 type receptor (IL-1R), blocking its biological activity. IL-1 is produced as a reaction to inflammatory stimuli and it has elevated levels in patients with RA, which can lead to cartilage degradation and bone resorption.

Prescribing

Like anti-TNFα agents, the non-TNF cytokine modulators are also used in combination with **methotrexate**. They are not, however, used in combination with each other. Each agent varies slightly in its route and frequency of administration, i.e. as an IV infusion or subcutaneously on a 2–4-weekly basis. **Anakinra** is infrequently used both in the UK (not recommended for use by NICE or SIGN, except within a clinical trial) and the USA, due to its high cost relative to its efficacy compared with other biologics.

Unwanted effects

Side effects to the non-TNF cytokine modulators are, on the whole, comparable with anti-TNFα agents, in particular the risk of causing infections, haematological, cardiovascular, and mild neurological toxicity, as well as hypersensitivity reactions. With **rituximab** it is recommended that patients are pretreated with **methylprednisolone** and an anti-histamine to reduce the risk of an infusion-related reaction. Response to live vaccines is likely to be impaired, although non-live vaccines may still be used. Treatment should be avoided in patients with an underlying severe infection, including tuberculosis. The risk of malignancy, although still a potential, appears to be less likely than it is with anti-TNF therapy.

The effects of combining two cytokine modulators remains largely unexplored and is not currently recommended due to the high potential for increased toxicity, particularly of severe side effects.

PRACTICAL PRESCRIBING

Monoclonal antibody resistance
Long-term use of monoclonal antibodies is associated with a reduction in efficacy due to an acquired resistance to therapy.

Further reading

Liu JT, Yeh HM, Liu SY, et al. (2014) Psoriatic arthritis: epidemiology, diagnosis and treatment. *World Journal of Orthopedics* 5(4), 537–43.

Maxwell LJ, Zochling J, Boonen A, et al. (2015) TNF-alpha inhibitors for ankylosing spondylitis (review), *Cochrane*

Database of Systematic Reviews 4, Art: CD005468. http://onlinelibrary.wiley.com/doi/10.1002/14651858.CD005468.pub2/epdf [accessed 3 April 2019].

McInnes IB, O'Dell JR (2010) State of the art: rheumatoid arthritis. *Annals of Rheumatic Diseases* 69(11), 1898–906.

Meier FMP, Hermann W, Muller-Ladner U (2013) Current immunotherapy in rheumatoid arthritis. *Immunotherapy* 5(9), 955–74.

Prevoo ML, Van 't Hof MA, Kruper HH, et al. (1995) Modified disease activity scores that include twenty-eight joint counts. Development and validation in a prospective longitudinal study of patients with rheumatoid arthritis. *Arthritis and Rheumatics* 38(1), 44–8.

Guidelines

Braun J, van den Berg R, Baraliakos X, et al. (2011) 2010 update of the ASAS/EULAR recommendations for the management of ankylosing spondylitis. *Annals of Rheumatic Diseases* 70, 896–904.

NICE CG79 (2015) Rheumatoid arthritis: The management of rheumatoid arthritis in adults. https://www.nice.org.uk/guidance/cg79 [accessed 3 April 2019].

NICE TA195 (2010) Adalimumab, etanercept, infliximab, rituximab and abatacept for the treatment of rheumatoid arthritis after the failure of a TNF inhibitor. https://www.nice.org.uk/guidance/TA195 [accessed 3 April 2019].

NICE TA375 (2016) Adalimumab, etanercept, infliximab, certolizumabpegil, golimumab, tocilizumab and abatacept for rheumatoid arthritis not previously treated with DMARDS or after conventional DMARDs only have failed. https://www.nice.org.uk/guidance/TA375 [accessed 3 April 2019].

NICE TA383 (2016) TNF-alpha inhibitors for ankylosing spondylitis and non-radiographic axial spondylitis. https://www.nice.org.uk/guidance/TA383 [accessed 3 April 2019].

SIGN 123 (2011) Management of early rheumatoid arthritis: a national clinical guideline. https://www.sign.ac.uk/assets/sign123.pdf [accessed 3 April 2019].

Singh JA, Furst DE, Bharat A et al. (2012) Update of the 2008 American College of Rheumatology Recommendations for the use of disease-modifying antirheumatic drugs and biologic agents in the treatment of rheumatoid arthritis. *Arthritis Care Research* 64(5), 625–39.

7.3 Gout and hyperuricaemia

Gout is the most common inflammatory arthritis in men, being three to four times more common than in women, although the difference declines with increasing age. It has a prevalence of approximately 2%. The condition involves deposition of monosodium urate monohydrate crystals in joints and soft tissues. It is often recurrent, associated with comorbidities (e.g. chronic kidney disease, hypertension) and chronically managed by reducing serum urate levels.

Pathophysiology

Hyperuricaemia is the key biochemical marker of gout. Rising serum urate levels, in the most part, are a result of failing renal excretion (i.e. due to renal failure and hypertension, which can further exacerbate renal function) and/or accumulation of purines, from nucleic acid biosynthesis breakdown or dietary purines directly. Urate is filtered at the glomerulus and reabsorbed by the proximal tubule, so that dysfunction of membrane urate transporters (e.g. SLC2A9, OAT) may account for reduced excretion. A diet high in purines such as red meat, seafood, and cheese that are not efficiently excreted, further contributes to urate accumulation. Once serum urate concentration reaches saturation point, crystal formation can occur in the synovium of joints.

Typically, acute attacks of gout result from a trigger such as trauma, alcohol, high purine intake, or dehydration. This attack often affects a lower limb joint, in particular the metatarsophalangeal of the great toe, and presents as erythema, tenderness, swelling, and reduced mobility. This acute inflammatory process is initiated through a number of processes including toll-like receptors activating complement, macrophages, and the release of IL-8 to cause neutrophil infiltration. As the neutrophils (and latterly monocytes) interact with the monosodium urate crystals, a number of pro-inflammatory events occur with the production of nitric oxide, eicosanoids, IL-1, IL-8, TNFα, and COX-2. The use of NSAIDs, which inhibit COX or selective COX-2 inhibitors (e.g. **etoricoxib**), reduce circulating prostaglandins to reduce the length and severity of an acute attack, although this should be offset by the increased cardiovascular risk associated with their use (see 'Prescribing warning: risk of cardiovascular toxicity with NSAIDS and COX2 inhibitors'). Likewise, **colchicine** may have anti-inflammatory effects acutely, by altering cellular cytoskeleton function and, hence, impairing neutrophil mobility and cell division required to mount an inflammatory response. Recently, the IL-1 inhibitor **canakinumab**, has been licensed for use in gout and has a role in resistant cases where other treatment options are contraindicated. A further member of the class **anakinra** is under investigation for use in gout. In most cases, acute attacks are self-limiting and usually resolve within 7–10 days.

Chronic hyperuricaemia and recurrent episodes of gout, can affect multiple joints and lead to the formation of tophi, which result in joint damage and morbidity. Gouty tophi are deposits of MSU crystals that form in joints, particularly in cooler regions (e.g. fingers, toes, and ears), and may lead to bony erosion or abnormal osteoclast/osteoblast function. Recurrent episodes are much more likely in those with comorbidities; recurrent gout should be a 'red-flag' for cardiovascular disease. The use of diuretics can also predispose to gout in those with heart failure. Current guidance recommends that, after a second attack within 12 months or if significant risk factors, long-term urate-lowering therapy, with a xanthine oxidase inhibitor (e.g. **allopurinol** or, second-line **febuxostat**) should be considered. Inhibitors help reduce serum urate levels by acting

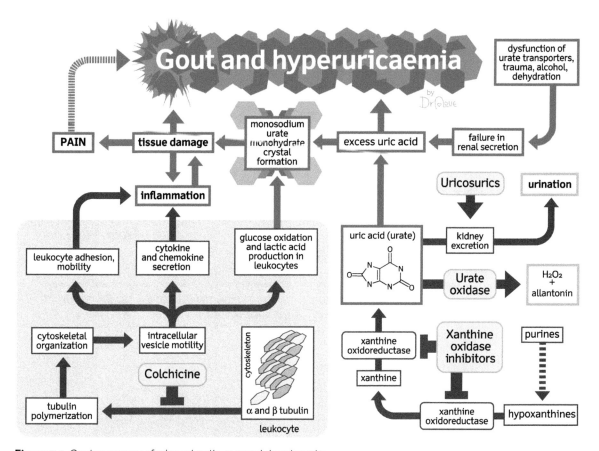

Figure 7.5 Gout: summary of relevant pathways and drug targets.

on the purine degradation pathway. Alternative urate lowering drugs include the urate oxidases (**rasburicase**, **pegloticase**) and uricosurics (e.g. **probenecid**).

For a full summary of the relevant pathways and drug targets, see Figure 7.5.

Management

A diagnosis of acute gout is based primarily on clinical history and examination, with identification of risk factors potentially helpful (see Box 7.3) in the presence of a hot, inflamed, and painful joint. Measurement of serum uric acid is not routinely recommended at diagnosis, as levels may be normal during an acute attack.

A differential diagnosis of septic arthritis should be considered, where patients will probably present as systemically unwell, as this requires urgent referral for treatment. The presence of tophi may aid diagnosis, but may not always be present as they can take 10 years to develop

Box 7.3 Risk factors for gout

- Excessive alcohol intake
- G6PD deficiency
- Obesity
- Renal impairment
- Diabetes mellitus
- Smoking
- Male sex
- Purine rich diet (red meat, seafood)
- Hyperlipidaemia
- Hypertension
- Hyperglycaemia
- Drugs that inhibit excretion, e.g. thiazides, ciclosporin, tacrolimus, low dose aspirin
- Drugs that promote production, e.g. cytotoxics

after the first acute attack. A definitive diagnosis of gout can only be made in the presence of urate crystals in the synovial fluid.

The aim of treatment is to resolve an acute attack and prevent recurrence by reducing serum urate levels, either by inhibiting production (e.g. xanthine oxidase inhibitors, urate oxidase), or promoting excretion (uricosurics; see Figure 7.6). Unless contraindicated, NSAIDS are the treatment of choice in the management of an acute attack (e.g. **naproxen**, **diclofenac**, and **indometacin**), and should be continued until 48 hours after the attack has resolved. In patients at high risk of GI toxicity, a proton pump inhibitor is frequently co-prescribed, and NSAIDs avoided in patients with high cardiovascular (see prescribing warning) or renal risk. In patients intolerant of, or unable to take NSAIDs, **colchicine** may be used, or failing that corticosteroids. Where only one or two joints are affected, intra-articular corticosteroids (with **triamcinolone acetonide** or **methylprednisolone acetate**) can be administered following initial joint aspiration; however,

where gout affects multiple joints, systemic corticosteroids are preferred (oral or IM). **Paracetamol** and **codeine** provide last-line options in patients where all other measures are unsuitable.

PRESCRIBING WARNING

Risk of cardiovascular toxicity with NSAIDs and COX 2 inhibitors.

- COX-2 inhibitors and NSAIDs are associated with an increased risk of a cardiovascular event such as an MI or stroke.

- The risk with NSAIDs is likely to be lower than with COX-2 inhibitors, with the exception of diclofenac and high dose ibuprofen.

- In all cases treatment with NSAIDs and COX-2 inhibitors should be used at the lowest possible dose for the shortest possible duration and a PPI co-prescribed in patients at risk of ulcers.

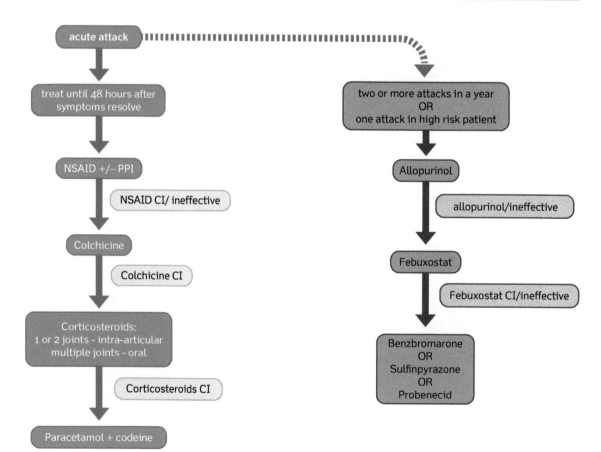

Figure 7.6 Management of gout.

In addition, all patients should be offered advice on life-style modifications by promoting healthy eating (low-fat dairy and vegetables), moderate alcohol consumption, and avoiding dehydration by drinking up to 2 L of water/day. Patients should be encouraged to consume a diet low in fat, protein, and purine rich food, e.g. avoid offal, sweetened drinks/juices, and limit red meat and shellfish.

Following a second acute attack within 12 months, the patient should be reviewed after a period of 4–6 weeks, at which point serum uric acid levels should be measured and consideration given to starting urate-lowering treatment, i.e. more than 2 attacks in a year or those at high risk of recurrence. Treatment with **allopurinol** should be started 1–2 weeks after swelling has subsided and doses titrated to achieve a serum uric acid level below 300 µmol/L. Concurrent treatment with NSAIDs for up to 6 weeks or colchicine for up to 6 months should be prescribed to prevent a recurrence. Where allopurinol is contraindicated or not tolerated, treatment with **febuxostat** may be considered. With either drug, treatment should be continued during an acute gout attack.

Other less commonly used drugs include **sulfinpyrazone**, **probenecid**, and **benzbromarone**; although the latter two have been largely discontinued worldwide and are only available through specialist importing companies. The urate oxidase **pegloticase** was launched for the treatment of severe tophaceous gout, possibly with joint erosion, where other treatment options have failed and is currently recommended for use by the American College of Rheumatology. This product was withdrawn from the UK.

Acute hyperuricaemia may also occur secondary to tumour lysis syndrome following initiation of chemotherapy in patients with a high tumour burden; usually associated with acute leukaemias or lymphomas. If left untreated, this can lead to acute renal failure, and therefore prophylaxis with **allopurinol** is routinely prescribed on initiation of some chemotherapy regimens where tumour lysis is likely to occur. In high-risk patients, e.g. those with a particularly high presenting white cell count, prophylaxis with the recombinant urate oxidase, **rasburicase** may be necessary.

Drug classes used in management

Colchicine

The tricyclic alkaloid colchicine has the ability to inhibit microtubule polymerization, producing a disruption in the cytoskeleton and altering the regulation of many cellular processes, including cell division, migration, and polarization.

Mechanism of action

Microtubules are long rigid polymers composed of α and β tubulin that extend through the cytoplasm and form the cytoskeleton. The binding of **colchicine** to one tubulin molecule prevents its incorporation into the polymer and microtubule elongation. Disruption of the cytoskeleton can inhibit many signalling pathways and cellular processes, such as intracellular vesicle motility, and the secretion of endogenous mediators like cytokines and chemokines. Colchicine affects leukocyte mobility, adhesion, and cytokine production, which is responsible for most of the anti-inflammatory effects. It can also inhibit urate crystal deposition, most likely via the inhibition of glucose oxidation and subsequent lactic acid production in leukocytes.

Effective at a dose of 0.015 mg/kg, colchicine is toxic in doses above 0.1 mg/kg and lethal in a dose of 0.8 mg/kg, which leaves a very narrow therapeutic window and provides a source of concern for prescribing practitioners.

Prescribing

The optimal dosing of **colchicine** in the acute management of gout is subject to some controversy. Although licensed at a dose of 1 mg stat followed by doses of 500 µg every 2–3 hours until pain relief (max 6 mg), there is increasing interest in the use of low dose regimens. Low dose regimens, e.g. 500 µg two to three times daily (600 µg in the USA), have the potential for providing the same relief with better tolerability, although the evidence for this is not robust. In all cases, treatment should be initiated ideally within 12–24 hours of an acute attack for optimal benefit

Low dose colchicine may be continued for the first 6 months of treatment with urate-lowering treatment as prophylaxis, although this is not without toxicity.

Unwanted effects

GI effects occur in nearly all patients receiving high dose regimens of **colchicine**, in particular severe diarrhoea and vomiting, invariably resulting in discontinuation of treatment. The risk of toxicity is significantly increased in renal impairment and elderly patients. Other common toxicities include rashes, abdominal pain, and renal and hepatic impairment. Rarely, treatment may be associated with blood dyscrasias, peripheral neuritis, alopecia, and myopathy.

Drug interactions

As a metabolite for the CYP3A4 enzyme and P-glycoprotein, and due to its narrow therapeutic index, **colchicine** should not be used in combination with potent inhibitors of these enzymes. This includes the CYP 3A4 inhibitors macrolides (**erythromycin**, **clarithromycin**), ARVs (**ritonavir**, **indinavir**, **atazanavir**), **simvastatin**, and azole antifungals (**itraconazole**); as well as the P-glycoprotein inhibitors; **ciclosporin, verapamil**, and **quinidine**. Ciclosporin also increases the renal toxicity of colchicine.

Xanthine oxidase inhibitors

Inhibitors of xanthine oxidase supress uric acid production, and have been the therapeutic cornerstone of gout and conditions associated with hyperuricemia for several decades. For example, allopurinol and febuxostat.

Mechanism of action

Xanthine oxidase and xanthine dehydrogenase are interconvertible forms of the same enzyme, xanthine oxidoreductase, which is widely distributed throughout various organs, including kidney, heart, lung, gut, liver, brain, and plasma. They take part in a variety of biochemical reactions such as the hydroxylation of aromatic heterocycles purines, pterins, and aldehydes, contributing to the detoxification or activation of endogenous compounds or xenobiotics. Among their primary role is the conversion of hypoxanthine to xanthine and xanthine to uric acid.

Allopurinol and its major active metabolite oxypurinol inhibit the activity of xanthine oxidase and supress uric acid production. In addition, it has been proposed that elevation of adenosine levels and activation of adenosine A1 receptors, could lead to antinociceptive effects.

Febuxostat has selective affinity for both the oxidized and reduced forms of xanthine oxidase. In contrast to allopurinol, further enzymes in purine and pyrimidine metabolic pathways are not inhibited by febuxostat, mainly because it lacks a purine-like backbone.

Prescribing

Allopurinol is widely used in gout due to its low cost and favourable tolerability. Treatment is reserved for use in patients who have experienced repeated attacks, or who have evidence of complications such as joint damage or tophi; and should not be initiated until the acute attack has resolved. Concurrent use of NSAIDs or **colchicine** is recommended for at least the first month of treatment.

Doses are started low and gradually titrated up every 2–3 weeks to a maintenance dose of 100–900 mg daily to achieve optimal serum urate levels, i.e. less than 300 µmol/L. Allopurinol is best taken with food to reduce the risk of GI toxicity; however, where patients remain intolerant, doses may be divided in the day.

The newer xanthine oxidase inhibitor **febuxostat** is more effective than allopurinol used at a fixed dose (i.e. not titrated to serum urate levels), but may not show benefit over allopurinol therapy that has been titrated to optimize efficacy. It is therefore reserved for second-line use in patients intolerant of allopurinol.

Unwanted effects

Xanthine oxidase inhibitors are generally well tolerated, causing few side effects of minor severity. Skin rashes tend to be the most common adverse effect and may occur at any time while on treatment. In more severe cases, this may include Stevens–Johnson syndrome or toxic epidermal necrolysis, requiring immediate discontinuation. Other non-specific toxicities include GI effects and headaches. Both **allopurinol** and **febuxostat** are cleared through renal and hepatic pathways; in particular, dose reductions are recommended in severe renal impairment where there is a risk of accumulation.

Febuxostat is cautioned in ischaemic heart disease and congestive heart failure following studies comparing it with allopurinol, which identified an increase in the rate of cardiovascular events.

Drug interactions

The enzyme urate oxidase is responsible for the activation (e.g. **theophylline**) and elimination of some drugs, (e.g. **mercaptopurine**) thus concomitant use of a xanthine oxidase inhibitor, may alter their efficacy.

Uricosurics

Uricosuric agents can increase the excretion of uric acid in the urine, producing a reduction in the concentration of plasma uric acid. For example, probenecid, sulfinpyrazone, and benzbromarone.

Mechanism of action

There are several drugs included in the uricosuric class, although these are not the only drugs capable of reducing blood uric acid. **Probenecid** is a well-established agent, which is thought to act in the kidney proximal tubes on an organic anion transporter, blocking urate absorption, and thus promoting uric acid excretion.

The drug **sulfinpyrazone** competitively inhibits the urate anion transporter 1 (hURAT1) and the human organic anion transporter 4 (hOAT4), decreasing the reabsorption of uric acid and facilitating excretion in the urine. Since it lacks analgesic and anti-inflammatory properties it is not used for the treatment of acute attacks.

Benzbromarone is a benzofuran derivative that reduces the proximal tubular reabsorption of uric acid. It also acts as a non-competitive inhibitor of xanthine oxidase, but shares no structural homology to **allopurinol** or hypoxanthine.

Prescribing

Despite their good efficacy and direct action in promoting urate excretion (the most common cause of hyperuricaemia), the uricosurics are infrequently used to prevent gout, due to their lack of extensive availability, poor tolerability, and relatively complex dosing regimens. They may, however, be of value in patients intolerant of **allopurinol** and **febuxostat**, or where xanthine oxidase inhibitors produce an inadequate response.

As with the xanthine oxidase inhibitors, doses are administered orally and titrated up to achieve the desired effect. Of the three, **benzbromarone** is possibly the most effective, although **probenecid** is more widely available as it is routinely used to optimize the efficacy of **cidofovir** by intentionally inhibiting its excretion.

Uricosurics must be taken with adequate fluid (2–3 L/day) to reduce the risk of uric acid renal calculi, and urinary alkalization should be considered. Treatment is unlikely to be effective in chronic renal failure.

Unwanted effects

The predominating risk associated with the uricosurics is the formation of uric acid renal calculi and the ability to induce renal impairment. Treatment should be avoided in patients with an underlying predisposition. GI side effects are relatively common with treatment and less frequently uricosurics can impair platelet function, thus increasing the risk of bleeding. Hypersensitivity reactions and rashes may also occur. Although these are unlikely to be of the same magnitude as those seen with **allopurinol**.

Urate oxidase

Urate oxidase, which is not present in humans, acts to oxidize soluble uric acid to oxidative intermediates, decreasing serum urate levels. For example, rasburicase and pegloticase.

Mechanism of action

The oxidative intermediates produced by the oxidation of uric acid by urate oxidase are slowly and non-enzymatically converted to allantoin, which is an inert and water soluble purine metabolite, with hydrogen peroxide produced as a by-product.

Rasburicase is a non-pegylated, recombinant, fungal urate oxidase enzyme that did not demonstrate sustainable tolerability in pilot studies. However, the pegylation of urate oxidases supresses immunogenicity and increases half-life. This led to the development of **pegloticase**, a recombinant porcine-like urate oxidase conjugated to polyethylene glycol, which has been introduced with better results for chronic gout in patients that are refractory to conventional therapy.

Prescribing

Although urate oxidases play little role in the management of gout, they are highly effective in managing severe hyperuricaemia. **Rasburicase** is reserved for use in preventing tumour lysis syndrome associated with chemotherapy in high-risk patients, where it is administered IV for the first 5–7 days of treatment. **Pegloticase**, although licensed in severe tophaceous gout is widely considered to be non-cost effective and not licensed for use in the UK.

> **PRACTICAL PRESCRIBING**
>
> **Blood sampling patients on rasburicase**
>
> When taking blood samples of patients on rasburicase for measuring serum urate, the tube must contain heparin and be pre-chilled to prevent further degradation ex vivo. Samples must remain chilled by immersing in an ice bath and be centrifuged at 4°C. Results should be analysed within 4 hours.

Unwanted effects

The urate oxidases should not be used in patients with G6PD deficiency, and those at high risk should be screened prior to starting treatment. As proteins, the risk of hypersensitivity reactions with **rasburicase** and **pegloticase** is relatively high, including anaphylaxis and fevers, particularly in patients with a history of atopic allergies. Less commonly, patients complain of GI toxicity.

Further reading

Choi HK, Mount DB, Reginato AM (2005) Pathogenesis of gout. *Annals of Internal Medicine* 143, 499–516.

Dalbeth N, Haskard DO (2005) Mechanisms of inflammation in gout. *Rheumatology (Oxford)* 44, 1090–6.

Smith HS, Bracken D, Smith J (2011) Gout: current insights and future perspectives. *Journal of Pain* 12(11), 1113–29.

Guidelines

Jordan KM, Cameron JS, Snaith M, et al. (2007) British society for rheumatology and British health professionals in rheumatology guideline for the management of gout. *Rheumatology* 46(8), 1372–4.

Khanna D, Fitzgerald JD, Khanna PP, et al. (2012) American College of Rheumatology Guidelines for Management of Gout. Part 1: systematic nonpharmacologic and pharmacologic therapeutic approaches to hyperuricemia. *Arthritis Care Research* 64(10), 1431–46.

Khanna D, Khanna PP, Fitzgerald JD et al. (2012) American College of Rheumatology Guidelines for Management of Gout. Part 2: therapy and anti-inflammatory prophylaxis of acute gouty arthritis. *Arthritis Care Research* 64(10), 1447–61.

NICE TA164 (2011) Febuxostat for the management of hyperuricaemia in people with gout. https://www.nice.org.uk/guidance/TA164 [accessed 4 April 2019].

NICE TA291 (2013) Pegloticase for treating severe debilitating chronic tophaceous gout. https://www.nice.org.uk/guidance/ta291 [accessed 4 April 2019].

7.4 Metabolic bone disease (Paget's, osteoporosis)

The most common disorders of the bones are osteoporosis and Paget's disease of bone. Osteoporosis (OP) describes a state in which the bone is prone to fracture. It occurs naturally in women after the menopause, with ~2 million affected in the UK, and is mainly due to a progressive reduction in bone mass, where bone resorption exceeds bone formation. In other situations, osteoporosis arises as a result of other causes, such as reduced sex hormone levels or long-term corticosteroid administration. Paget's disease of bone (PDB), first described in 1877, is a disease of bone turnover. Lytic loss of bone, followed by excessive formation results in bones that are highly vascular and mechanically weak (sclerotic). The disease affects men slightly more (3:2) and is most common in those over 40 years, affecting ~2% of adults over age 55. However, this varies with geographical location and with most patients being asymptomatic, often remains undiagnosed.

Pathophysiology

Osteoporosis

The physiology of bone production and maintenance means that a number of key cells are responsible for bone turnover and attainment of appropriate bone mass. Osteoclasts are responsible for the resorption of mineralized bone and perform this by attaching to bone matrix molecules with subsequent dissolution of bone-trapped minerals. On the other hand, osteoblasts aid in the formation and mineralization of bone matrix. These two key players are in dynamic equilibrium, under the influence of genetic and environmental factors in the process of healthy bone growth, repair, and adaptation to mechanical stresses through on-going bone remodelling. The sites of remodelling, 'bone multicellular units', are typically in equilibrium (i.e. formation = resorption) and as new bone matrix (osteoid) is laid down, it is subsequently mineralized. It takes months for osteoblasts to lay down new bone, as opposed to weeks for resorption by osteoclasts.

A final common mechanism in the resorption of bone involves the RANK/OPG (receptor activator of nuclear κ-B/osteoprotegerin) system. In this system, osteoblasts express RANK-ligand, which binds to RANK-receptor expressed on osteoclasts (precursor cells) and, hence, regulate cell survival and bone resorption. OPG is secreted by osteoblasts, binds to RANKL and prevents its interaction with RANK, stopping excessive bone resorption. The ratio of RANK/OPG can determine bone mineral density.

Peak bone mineral density (BMD) is generally attained by the age of 25 years and from the late 30s there is a natural gradual decline. A strong genetic component exists through genes (e.g. insulin-like growth factor, lipoprotein receptor-related protein 5 (LRP5), oestrogen receptor, parathyroid hormone) and sex hormones (e.g. oestrogen and testosterone) to establish and maintain BMD. Nutrition, through Ca^{2+} and vitamin D, and weight-bearing exercise in the young are also key to formation of a healthy BMD.

BMD decreases with age, particularly in females following menopause, at rates in the order of up to 1% per year. Loss in post-menopausal females occurs as a result of reduced circulating levels of oestrogen (see other risk factors Table 7.4) and despite being asymptomatic, bony changes can present solely with a low-impact traumatic fracture (typically femur). Up to 50% of post-menopausal women will experience a fracture. Lack of oestrogen means T-cells recruit osteoclasts (with IL-6 maintaining recruitment and IL-1 stimulating osteoclast production) so excessive bone resorption occurs with inadequate replacement. This mechanism is also in place, where drug-induced OP is seen with aromatase inhibitors (e.g. **exemestane**) or gonadotrophin-releasing hormone agonists used in hormone-sensitive cancers (e.g. breast). In many patients, poor dietary intake of Ca^{2+} through impaired GI uptake, or through vitamin D deficiency, can lead to secondary hyperparathyroidism (see Topic 4.4, 'Parathyroid disease'), where the PTH increases resorption of Ca^{2+} from bone, decreases renal loss, and up-regulates active vitamin D conversion (providing there is substrate precursor).

Bisphosphonates are the mainstay of treatment, causing either osteoclast apoptosis (e.g. **etidronate**), or modifying the mevalonate pathway and inhibiting osteoclast function and recruitment (e.g. **alendronic acid**, **risedronate**)—mechanism shown in 'Drug classes used in management, Bisphosphonates, Mechanism of action'. Co-prescribing these drugs with Ca^{2+} and vitamin D replacement is generally considered routine practice, although the evidence for this is somewhat controversial, as is the theory of increased cardiovascular risk with prolonged replacement. Historically, hormone replacement therapy was, as the pathophysiology would support, the preferred treatment—replacing the lost oestrogen so osteoclasts could function normally; however, since 2003 its use has greatly diminished due to increased risks of breast cancer, VTE, and stroke. It still has a role, however, in specific patient groups.

Paget's disease of bone (PDB)

Much like OP, PDB is a disease of bone remodelling. It is a localized disease characterized by osteoclast over-activity with subsequent compensatory osteoblast over-activity. The disease may affect a single bone or be multifocal (e.g. spine, pelvis, femur, skull), demonstrated as osteolytic lesions on plain radiographs. The increased osteoclast over-activity may result from viral (e.g. paramyoxviruses) or genetic triggers (e.g. gene TNFRSF11A on chromosome 18q21-22, which encodes RANK). These dysfunctional osteoclasts can produce osteotrophic factors, like IL-6, which maintain osteoclast recruitment, perpetuate bone resorption, and increase bone turnover, for which alkaline phosphastase is a marker. As a consequence of bone resorption there is up-regulation of osteoblasts, which over time, make new 'disorganized' woven bone that is sclerotic in appearance and weaker than normal.

Disorganized bone deposition is initially asymptomatic, but may latterly present with deep bone pain that is associated with other localized characteristics (i.e. with hip pain, there may be bowing of the femur, or with skull involvement there may be hearing loss, vertigo, or cranial nerve

signs). Treatment strategies involve the bisphosphonates and suppression of RANKL-induced bone resorption, with decreases in RANKL and increased osteoprotegerin production (see 'Pathophysiology, Osteoporosis').

For a full summary of the relevant pathways and drug targets, see Figure 7.7.

Management

Osteoporosis

Management strategies with osteoporosis have been developed to identify patients likely to have reduced bone mineral density, and therefore initiate treatment to reduce the risk of a fragility fracture. Initial investigations should include assessment of Ca^{2+} intake and vitamin D deficiency. Routine risk assessments should ideally be carried out in all women over 65 and men over 75 years of age, as well as those over 50 with risk factors (see Table 7.4).

Risk assessment for fragility fractures can be carried out using the tools, FRAX, or Fracture to determine the 10-year probability of a fracture; or by measurement of BMD using dual-energy X-ray absorptiometry (DXA). Professional body opinion differs in how the tools should be applied in clinical practice, with some opting to use FRAX to identify patients requiring prophylaxis and BMD in a select patient group (NOGG, NICE), while others use BMD in all at risk patients (NOF). FRAX can be carried out either with or without a BMD.

Preventative measures include advice on lifestyle modifications to reduce risk factors. Patients should be advised on smoking cessation, avoiding excessive alcohol, and undertaking regular weight-bearing exercise. In addition, intake of vitamin D should be optimized (800–1000 units/day) with supplementation, and Ca^{2+} through diet or supplementation (1–1.2 g/day), depending on status.

Pharmacological interventions should be initiated in patients considered to be at high risk of having a fragility fracture (based on FRAX score or BMD with a T-score less than –2.5SD). Primary treatment is with an oral bisphosphonates, usually **alendronic acid** first line, or **risedronate** in those intolerant. Oral bisphosphonates are favoured for their cost-effectiveness and have the added advantage of continuing benefit following cessation of treatment. In patients who are intolerant of oral bisphosphonates, alternatives include IV bisphosphonates (**zoledronic acid, ibandronic acid**), **raloxifene, teriparatide**, or **denosumab**; with choice in

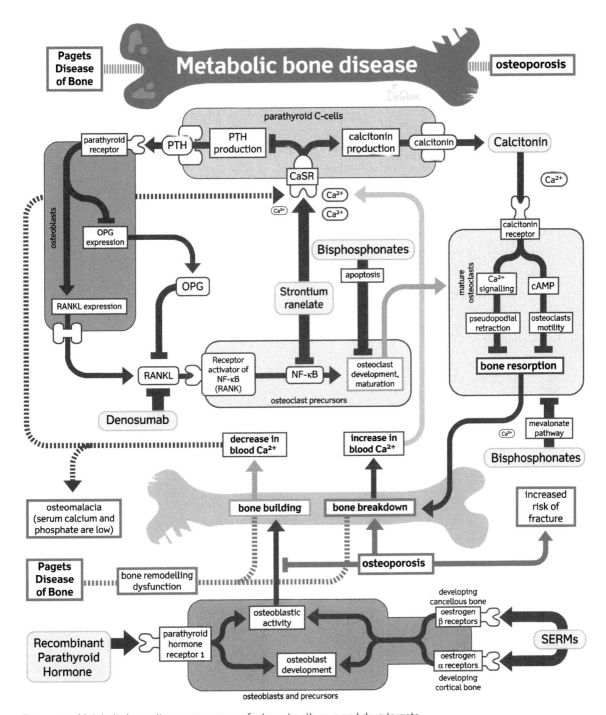

Figure 7.7 Metabolic bone disease: summary of relevant pathways and drug targets.

part determined by licensed indication (see Table 7.5). The use of **strontium** or **calcitonin** are no longer widely recommended in osteoporosis as the risk of cancer was felt to outweigh the benefits of treatment.

In all cases, treatment should be reviewed after a period of 3–5 years, depending on the drug used, and a repeat risk assessment carried out. In those at moderate risk, or with a T score greater than –2.5, a drug holiday

Table 7.4 Risk factors for osteoporosis

Risk factors for fragility fractures	Secondary causes of osteoporosis	Drugs can that affect BMD
Age	Diabetes mellitus	Proton pump inhibitors
Sex	Osteoarthritis	SSRIs
Previous fragility fracture	Rheumatoid arthritis	Anticonvulsants
History of falls	Untreated hypogonadism	Calcineurin inhibitors
Smoking	Prolonged immobility	GnRH antagonists and agonists
Excessive alcohol intake	Organ transplantation	Excessive levothyroxine
Current/frequent use of glucocorticoids	Liver disease	Thiazolidinediones
Family history of hip fracture	GI disease	Methotrexate
BMI <18.5 kg/m^2		Lithium
		Glucocorticoids
		Heparin

could be considered; while those at high risk or receiving denosumab should remain on treatment or switched to an alternative agent. That said repeat DXA scanning is not advocated routinely.

Paget's disease of the bone

As only about 5% of patients with Paget's disease present with symptoms, diagnosis is often made following an incidental finding on imaging, or a raised alkaline phosphatase (ALP), which is indicative of high bone turnover. In asymptomatic patients, treatment is unlikely to be warranted, and in those that are symptomatic with evidence of low disease activity according to imaging and ALP, symptomatic relief with simple analgesics may suffice.

Active treatment of Paget's is indicated in patients with severe bone pain and, in some instances, to prevent disease progression, e.g. hypercalcaemia and those at risk

Table 7.5 Licensed indications of bisphosphonates and other agents

	Post-menopausal women	Men	Corticosteroid-induced osteoporosis	Paget's disease
Alendronic acid	Y	Y (daily prep only)	Y (daily prep only)	N
Risedronate	Y	Y (weekly only)	Y (daily only in women)	Y
Zoledronic acid	Y (5 mg)	Y (5 mg)	Y (5 mg)	Y (5 mg)
Ibandronic acid	Y	N	N	N
Pamidronate	N	N	N	Y
Raloxifene	Y	N	N	N
Strontium	Y	Y	Y	N
Teriparatide	Y	Y	Y	N
Denosumab (Prolia®)	Y	Y (prostate cancer)	N	N
Calcitonin	N	N	N	Y

of spinal cord compression or bone deformity to the face. Treatment is with a bisphosphonate, which may also help prevent deafness associated with disease progression. As with osteoporosis, the use of **calcitonin** has largely been superseded, due to inferior efficacy relative to the bisphosphonates.

Of the bisphosphonates, **pamidronate**, **risedronate**, and **tiludronate** (no longer available in the UK), have shown equal efficacy in inhibiting bone turnover in Paget's; however, the effects of **zoledronic acid** are superior. While on treatment patients should be monitored clinically for bone pain and through measurements of serum alkaline phosphatase levels, to indicate extent of bone turnover and thus disease activity. Radiological imaging may be used to monitor for improvement in osteolytic lesions. Optimal treatment effect should be seen by 6 months, and in those failing to show an adequate response at this point, treatment may be repeated. Repeated courses may also be offered to those that relapse, as demonstrated by symptoms or biochemical evidence, although the risk of relapse with zoledronic acid IV is very low.

Drug classes used in management

Bisphosphonates

Analogues of naturally occurring compounds that contain a pyrophosphate, the stable bisphosphonates inhibit bone resorption after being taken up and adsorbed to mineral surfaces in bone. In this way, they can interfere with the action of osteoclasts. Examples include alendronic acid, ibandronic acid, pamidronate, risedronate, tiludronate, and zoledronic acid.

Mechanism of action

The non-hydrolysable P-C-P backbone structure and ability to chelate Ca^{2+} allows bisphosphonates to be rapidly targeted to bone mineral. This route puts them into close contact with osteoclasts, but prevents prolonged interaction with other cells. In the process of osteoclast-mediated bone resorption, the acidic pH causes the dissociation of bisphosphonates from the bone mineral surface. This is followed by intracellular uptake into osteoclasts as a complex with Ca^{2+}. Bisphosphonates affect the bone resorption mediated by osteoclasts in a variety of ways, including the perturbation of cellular metabolism and induction of apoptosis.

The simple bisphosphonates are several orders of magnitude less potent than those that contain a nitrogen moiety, i.e. **pamidronate**, **alendronic acid**, **ibandronic acid**, **risedronate**, and **zoledronic acid**. They can inhibit farnesyl pyrophosphate synthetase, an enzyme in the mevalonic acid pathway that produces cholesterol, as well as isoprenoid lipids synthesis.

Prescribing

There are a number of bisphosphonates on the market licensed for a range of indications. They are widely used in the prophylaxis and treatment of osteoporosis (including post-menopausal and glucocorticoid-induced), as well as Paget's disease of the bone, bone metastases, and hypercalcaemia of malignancy (see Table 7.6). Bisphosphonates are available for oral (see 'Practical prescribing: oral administration of bisphosphonates') and IV administration.

PRACTICAL PRESCRIBING

Oral administration of bisphosphonates

- Oral absorption of bisphosphonates is poor, although this may be improved by taking on an empty stomach.

- To improve absorption and reduce the risk of oesophagitis, doses should be swallowed whole before breakfast, with plenty of water on waking with the patient sat upright. Patients should remain sat upright for 30 minutes and avoid food and drink for this time.

- Patients with impaired/delayed swallowing, such as those with oesophageal abnormalities or strictures, should not receive oral treatment. Neither is treatment recommended in severe dementia, where the ability to comply with administration advice is likely to be impaired.

Unwanted effects

Adverse effects reported with bisphosphonate therapy varies with route of administration and relative potency. Orally administered bisphosphonates are associated with a high risk of GI toxicity and, in particular, oesophageal reactions, including oesophagitis (see 'Practical prescribing: oral administration of bisphosphonates'). Caution is also advised in patients with pre-existing GI disease, such as gastritis or peptic ulcer disease, which may be aggravated. Other common side effects include abdominal pain,

Table 7.6 Choice of bisphosphonates

Drug	Oral administration	IV administration	Comments
Alendronic acid	As a daily and weekly preparation	No	Drug of choice in the prevention and management of osteoporosis. License varies with preparation
Ibandronic acid	Taken once a month to prevent post-menopausal osteoporosis	Administered every 3 months to prevent post-menopausal osteoporosis	More commonly used in hypercalcaemia of malignancy and to prevent bone damage in metastatic breast cancer
Pamidronate	No	Administered weekly or every other week in Paget's to a dose of 210 mg per course	Once the favoured IV bisphosphonate, although largely replaced by zoledronate Also used widely in malignancy
Risedronate	Daily in osteoporosis and Paget's. May also be used weekly to prevent post-menopausal osteoporosis	No	Used second-line in osteoporosis in patients unable to tolerate alendronic acid. Oral bisphosphonate of choice in Paget's
Zoledronic acid	No	Given as a single IV dose in Paget's and annually in post-menopausal osteoporosis.	Accepted for use in patients with post-menopausal osteoporosis unable to take oral therapy by the Scottish Medicine Consortium in 2008

dyspepsia, and flu-like symptoms, the latter affecting up to 30% of patients on zoledronic acid and patients should be advised of the risk.

As bisphosphonates affect bone resorption, treatment can cause hypocalcaemia and hypophosphataemia. Any pre-existing hypocalcaemia should therefore be corrected prior to initiating therapy and patients at increased risk should be monitored while on treatment, e.g. those with hypoparathyroidism, vitamin D deficiency, or if taking corticosteroids.

Warnings have been issued about the risk of osteonecrosis of the jaw with bisphosphonate therapy. The risk is linked to potency and exposure, thus occurs more commonly with IV treatment; in particular, **zoledronic acid** administered at the higher doses used in malignancy, rather than osteoporosis or Paget's. Patients on regular IV treatment should be seen regularly by a dentist and good oral hygiene promoted to reduce the risk.

Prolonged bisphosphonate exposure also increases the risk of an atypical fracture, likely as a result of suppressed bone turnover and a subsequent alteration in bone matrix and mineral properties leading to the formation of 'brittle' bones. For this reason, it is recommended that bisphosphonate use is reviewed after 5 years and only continued where benefits outweigh the risks.

Bisphosphonates are renally cleared and as such should be avoided in severe renal failure. For some, dose adjustment may be necessary in moderate impairment. The risk of renal toxicity with treatment is again increased with use of the more potent bisphosphonates, e.g. zoledronic acid.

Calcitonin

Calcitonin is a 32-amino acid molecule produced by parafollicular cells of the thyroid gland and linked to mineral metabolism. It prevents bone removal by osteoclasts, while promoting bone formation by osteoblasts.

Mechanism of action

Calcitonin binds with high affinity to the calcitonin receptor, a seven-transmembrane domain G-protein coupled receptor that is mainly found in osteoclasts. This binding has two major effects: first, it inhibits osteoclast motility and induces a quiescent state via a cAMP-mediated mechanism; secondly, it triggers osteoclast pseudopodial retraction, which is mediated by intracellular Ca^{2+} signalling. These changes decrease the area of osteoclast contact with the bone surface. Receptor activation also leads to enhanced production of vitamin D-producing enzymes, which increases Ca^{2+} retention and bone density. In bone, calcitonin also reduces Ca²⁺ release into the plasma as a result of inhibition of bone resorption.

Ligand-induced internalization and inhibition of calcitonin receptor synthesis leads to desensitization of treated cells, a process commonly referred in the clinic as 'escape phenomenon'.

Prescribing

Following oral administration, **calcitonin** is rapidly inactivated, thus treatment is administered SC or IM, on a daily basis. Intranasal preparations, previously available on the market, were withdrawn by the MHRA in 2012 due to high carcinogenic risk. Although parenteral preparations remain available, calcitonin is no longer advocated for use in osteoporosis as the risks of treatment are felt to outweigh the benefits.

Unwanted effects

As **calcitonin** is a peptide, the risk of hypersensitivity reactions are relatively common, i.e. rashes, flushing, etc. Non-allergic local flushing may also occur. Other commonly reported side effects include GI effects (nausea, vomiting, diarrhoea), dizziness, headaches, and more disturbingly with prolonged use, malignancy.

Selective oestrogen receptor modulators

Unlike oestrogens, which are full agonists, selective oestrogen-receptor modulators (SORMs) are chemically diverse compounds that exert selective agonist or antagonist effects on different oestrogen target tissues. For example, raloxifene.

Mechanism of action

SORM/SERMs do not have the steroid structure of oestrogens, but their tertiary structure permits them to bind to the oestrogen receptor. Although some members have been known for decades, only recently has their tissue specificity been recognized. Their unique pharmacology can be understood by three mechanisms—differential tissue expression of oestrogen receptors, differential conformation of the receptor upon ligand binding and the differential expression of co-regulator proteins.

Both isoforms of oestrogen receptors are found in bone cells, with β subtype concentrations being higher in developing cancellous bone and α predominating in developing cortical bone. Oestrogen deficiency increases bone turnover, shifting the equilibrium in favour of bone resorption over bone formation, which leads to bone loss.

Raloxifene is a second generation SORM that has oestrogen *agonist* effects on bone and cholesterol metabolism, but acts as a receptor *antagonist* on oestrogen receptors on mammary gland and uterine tissue. Binding to the receptor results in the differential expression of multiple oestrogen-regulated genes, and the positive effects on bone mass is, in part, achieved through the modulation of transforming growth factor *TGF-β3* gene, which encodes a bone matrix protein with antiosteoclastic capabilities. Activation or repression of target genes is mediated through the AF-1 and AF-2 transactivation domains.

Prescribing

Raloxifene is the sole SORM licensed for use in the prevention and treatment of osteoporosis in post-menopausal women. Taken OD, it may be of value in those unable to take oral bisphosphonates; however, NICE only advocate its use in secondary prevention. Furthermore, evidence suggests there is only a benefit in reducing the risk of vertebral fractures, not non-vertebral fractures.

Unwanted effects

As an oestrogen receptor modulator, predictable side effects mirror those seen with oestrogen therapy. Of particular note is an increased risk of venous thromboembolism (VTE) and thus it is contraindicated in anyone with a current or recent history of VTE. A positive side effect of **raloxifene** treatment is its potentially protective effect against breast cancer, making it an attractive option in younger post-menopausal women; however, falling outside of the license, this benefit has not been quantified. Furthermore, it is associated with an increased risk of endometrial cancer. For more information see Topic 4.6, 'Female reproduction'.

Denosumab

The human monoclonal antibody denosumab is raised against the receptor activator of nuclear factor κB (NF-κB) ligand (RANKL), which reversibly inhibits osteoclast-mediated bone resorption.

Mechanism of action

The RANK receptor is a member of the TNF superfamily that has actions on bone turnover, but also affects the maturation and activation of the immune system. Receptor activation promotes a variety of downstream signalling pathways that stimulate osteoclast development (osteoclastogenesis). These intracellular pathways include NF-κB, protein kinase C, MAP-kinase, Src kinase, and phosphatidylinositol metabolism.

Denosumab acts by preventing the interaction of RANKL with its receptor RANK, which causes the inhibition of the formation, survival, and function of osteoclasts. This in turn causes a decrease in bone resorption and the growth of bone mass.

Prescribing

There are two licensed formulations of **denosumab**, of which only one (Prolia®) is indicated in the treatment and prevention of osteoporosis. Treatment is administered by SC injection every 6 months, in combination with oral calcium and vitamin D supplementation. Prior to administration, calcium status should be assessed and replaced as appropriate due to the risk of hypocalcaemia. Evidence for its use demonstrates benefit in reducing the risk of both vertebral and non-vertebral fractures.

Unwanted effects

The side effect profile to **denosumab** is similar to that seen with the bisphosphonates, although like IV bisphosphonates it is not associated with oesophagitis with it being administered SC. Of particular note is the risk of hypocalcaemia, hypophosphatemia, osteonecrosis of the jaw, and atypical fractures. Although the risk of these are rare, any underlying hypocalcaemia should be corrected prior to starting treatment and a dental examination considered in patients at high risk of dental disease. Other more common non-specific side effects include pain in extremities, constipation, sciatica, and infection (urinary and upper respiratory tract).

As denosumab is composed of peptides and amino acids, it is cleared as an immunoglobulin, by degradation. It therefore relies on neither hepatic metabolism nor renal clearance to be excreted, and can be used in both renal and hepatic impairment. Furthermore, drug interactions are unlikely.

Strontium ranelate

Strontium is a trace element that is chemically close to Ca^{2+} and can act on bone metabolism leading into positive effects on bone mass, quality, and resistance.

Mechanism of action

Early in vitro studies have shown that **strontium** can reduce osteoclast differentiation, activity, and bone resorption. Strontium ranelate reduces the bone adherence of osteoclasts by affecting the actin-containing sealing zone, and could decrease osteoclast differentiation by modulating NF-κB pathway. *In vitro*, strontium has also demonstrated the capacity to increase the replication of pre-osteoblastic cells and the activity of functional osteoblasts, which results in the augmented synthesis of bone matrix.

As a divalent cation that is structurally comparable to Ca^{2+}, strontium has actions on similar cellular signalling mechanisms. Thus, the involvement of the Ca^{2+}-sensing receptor (Car) in the strontium-induced effect has been advocated. Recent findings demonstrating that strontium activates AKT signalling via the CaSR, further support the notion that strontium might influence bone cells differentiation via this receptor. In addition, other signalling pathways that are relevant in bone cells are likely involved, such as Wnt, the RANKL-RANK, and FGF receptor signalling.

Prescribing

Strontium is packaged in sachets containing oral granules that are to be mixed with water and taken immediately OD. Oral bioavailability is poor and can be reduced further (by 60–70%) in the presence of food and milk; it is, therefore, best taken on an empty stomach between meals, usually at bedtime. Concurrent use of calcium and vitamin D is recommended in patients with poor dietary intake.

It is effective in reducing the incidence of both vertebral and non-vertebral fractures in men and post-menopausal women, although it is not licensed for use in the USA and use is generally limited by the high risk of toxicity.

Unwanted effects

Cautions and side effects

There are a number of significant toxicities reported with **strontium ranelate**, including increased risk of VTE and myocardial infarction. Treatment is therefore contraindicated in patients with a previous history of VTE and with a high cardiovascular risk. Severe life-threatening skin reactions are also associated with therapy including DRESS, Stevens–Johnson syndrome and toxic epidermal necrolysis, particularly in the first 6 weeks of treatment. Patients who develop a rash should be advised to seek advice urgently.

Other adverse effects include headaches and GI toxicity, which tend to be mild and transient, and alopecia, which usually reverses on drug withdrawal.

Excretion of strontium is by renal clearance; thus treatment is contraindicated in severe renal impairment, i.e. with a CrCl less than 30 mL/minute.

Drug interactions

Drug interactions with **strontium ranelate** can occur as a result of it forming a complex with other medication or food, thus impairing absorption. Drugs with the potential to form complexes with strontium include oral tetracyclines, quinolones, and aluminium- and magnesium-containing antacids. Interactions can be avoided by allowing an interval of at least 2 hours between drugs.

Recombinant parathyroid hormone

The biosynthetic human PTH 1-34 (teriparatide) was the first anabolic treatment used for diseases of the bone. It acts via the PTH-receptor-1 that is located in osteoblasts and renal tubular cells.

Mechanism of action

The molecular actions of **teriparatide** are via the membrane G-protein-dependent PTH receptor. Binding of the ligand activates adenylatecyclase and various phospholipases (A, C, and D) increasing the levels of cAMP and Ca^{2+} inside the cell.

Treatment with teriparatide augments the amount of osteoblasts and the formation of bone via activation of pre-existing osteoblasts, the differentiation of lining cells and a decrease in osteoblasts apoptosis. It can thus increase bone mass, structural integrity, bone strength, and diameter. The anabolic effects of teriparatide constitute a breakthrough in the treatment of bone disease and a change in several paradigms of bone physiology, which were mainly based on antiresorptive mechanisms.

Prescribing

Teriparatide is administered SC once a day for up to 24 months in the treatment of osteoporosis in men and post-menopausal women, including those with corticosteroid-induced disease. In the UK, it is reserved for use after the failure of other treatments, for instance in those unable to tolerate therapy due to GI toxicity, for the secondary prevention of osteoporosis. Treatment is effective in reducing the risk of vertebral and non-vertebral fractures with the exception of hip fractures. On cessation of treatment, bone loss can be rapid and, in the USA, follow-on treatment with an antiresorptive treatment is recommended.

Unwanted effects

The most widely reported adverse effects to **teriparatide** include headache, dizziness, pain in the injected limb, and nausea. Four to six hours following an injection, patients may experience transient effects such as an increase in serum Ca^{2+} (see 'Practical prescribing: transient hypercalcaemia following teriparatide therapy') and orthostatic hypotension. There is also a potential to exacerbate urolithiasis.

PRACTICAL PRESCRIBING

Transient hypercalcaemia following teriparatide therapy

- Administration of teriparatide can cause a transient increase in serum Ca^{2+}.
- Serum Ca^{2+} peaks 4–6 hours after dose and normalizes 16–24 hours later.
- Routine serum Ca^{2+} monitoring is not recommended.
- Where serum levels are required for other purposes, these should be taken at least 16 hours following the dose.

Unlike other drug therapies, teriparatide is contraindicated in metabolic bone disease (with the exception of primary or corticosteroid-induced osteoporosis), skeletal malignancies, or bone metastases. Any unexplained elevation in serum alkaline phosphatase should be investigated prior to initiation and treatment avoided in pre-existing hypercalcaemia.

Despite the lack of studies looking at the excretion and metabolism of teriparatide, it is thought to be eliminated through hepatic metabolism and renal clearance. Treatment is contraindicated in severe renal impairment, but no dose adjustment is required in hepatic impairment and there have been no reports of clinically significant drug interactions.

Further reading

De Paula FJA, Rosen CJ (2010) Back to the future: revisiting parathyroid hormone and calcitonin control of bone remodelling. *Hormone Metabolism Research* 42(5), 299–306.

Merlotti D, Gennari l, Martini G, et al. (2007) Comparison of different intravenous bisphosphonate regimens for Paget's disease of bone. *Journal of Bone and Mineral Research* 22(10), 1510–17.

Riggs Band Hartmann LC (2003) Selective oestrogen-receptor modulators—mechanism of action and application to clinical practice. *New England Journal of Medicine* 348(7), 618–29.

Rogers MJ, Crockett JC, Coxon FP, et al. (2011) Biochemical and molecular mechanisms of action of bisphosphonates. *Bone* 49(1), 34–41.

Saidak Z, Marie PJ (2012) Strontium signalling: molecular mechanisms and therapeutic implications in osteoporosis. *Pharmacological Therapy* 136(2), 216–26.

Selby PL (2006) Guidelines for the diagnosis and management of Paget's disease: a UK perspective. *Journal of Bone and Mineral Research*, 21(2), 92–3.

Selby PL, Davie MW, Ralston SH, Stone MD (2002) Guidelines on the Management of Paget's Disease of Bone. *Bone* 31 (3) 10–9.

Wada T, Nakashima T, Hiroshi N, et al. (2006) RANKL-RANK signalling in osteoclastogenesis and bone disease. *Trends in Molecular Medicine* 12(1), 17–25.

Guidelines

Cosman F, de Beur SJ, LeBoff MS (2014) Clinician's guide to prevention and treatment of osteoporosis. *Osteoporosis International* 25(10), 2359–81. https://www.nof.org/news/nofs-clinicians-guide-published-by-osteoporosis-international/ [accessed 9 April 2019].

National Osteoporosis Guidelines Group (NOGG) 2017: Clinical guideline for the prevention and treatment of osteoporosis. https://www.sheffield.ac.uk/NOGG/NOGG%20Guideline%202017.pdf [accessed 9 April 2019].

NICE CG146 (Aug 2012). Osteoporosis: assessing the risk of fragility fracture. https://www.nice.org.uk/guidance/cg146 [accessed 6 April 2019].

NICE TA160 (2011) Alendronate, etidronate, risedronate, raloxifene and strontium ranelate for the primary prevention of osteoporotic fragility fractures in postmenopausal women. https://www.nice.org.uk/guidance/ta161 [accessed 6 April 2019].

NICE TA161 (2011) Alendronate, etidronate, risedronate, raloxifene, strontium ranelate and teriparatide for the secondary prevention of osteoporotic fragility fractures in postmenopausal women. https://www.nice.org.uk/guidance/ta161 [accessed 6 April 2019].

NICE TA204 (2010) Denosumab for the prevention of osteoporotic fragility fractures in postmenopausal women. https://www.nice.org.uk/guidance/ta204 [accessed 6 April 2019].

Singer FR, Bone HG, Hosking DJ, et al. (2014) Paget's disease of bone: an endocrine society clinical practice guideline. *Journal of Clinical Endocrinology & Metabolism* 99(12), 4408–22. https://academic.oup.com/jcem/article/99/12/4408/2833929 [accessed 9 April 2019].

8.1 General anaesthetics and neuromuscular blockade

Anaesthesia is a state of reversible unconsciousness that comprises some or all of the 'triad of anaesthesia'—hypnosis, analgesia, and muscle relaxation. Safe and effective anaesthesia requires information of the drug's potency at effector sites and knowledge of administration concentrations, as well as an understanding of the degree of noxious stimulus and how a patient's physiology may modulate drug actions.

Historically, the first compounds used as anaesthetics were diethyl ether, nitrous oxide, and chloroform. Diethyl ether was demonstrated to the wider medical community in 1846 by William Morton in the removal of a jaw lump from Gilbert Abbot, and the introduction of chloroform followed within the year. It was noted by James Simpson, Professor of Obstetrics in Edinburgh in 1847, that chloroform was much more potent, but had a tendency to precipitate death in the anxious and could cause severe liver damage. This tendency demonstrates clearly that the depth of anaesthesia is critical. Too much circulating drug can lead to respiratory depression, cardiac arrhythmias, and death, while too little permits persistent consciousness, pain, and muscular spasm. This is of particular concern with regards to laryngospasm, which when combined with an unsecured airway can rapidly lead to hypoxia and death. Nowadays, death is incredibly rare, with signs of hypotension, tachy-, or bradycardia detected early and easily reversed by controlling drug dosage. The risk of drug-induced side effects when using anaesthetic drugs means that the depth of anaesthesia must be closely monitored. This is achieved subjectively with experience and training, in combination with objective clinical assessment, such as pulse, BP, and mean alveolar concentration. See Table 8.1 for ideal properties of anaesthetic agents.

There are many approaches to the application of general anaesthesia, and these depend on clinical situation, depth, and length of anaesthesia required, the type of surgical or interventional procedure to be undertaken and associated patient risk factors.

Stages of anaesthesia

The stages of anaesthesia (outlined in Table 8.2) was a concept introduced at a time when induction was routinely achieved through the use of inhalational anaesthetics. More recently the use of IV induction agents has meant that transition between these stages is smoother, resulting in a rapid induction with minimal excitation responses, compared with inhalation agents. Inhalation agents also carry the risk of airway irritation. Practically, however, inhalational agents are of great use when spontaneous ventilation can be maintained, such as in a partially obstructed airway, or when IV access is initially difficult to obtain (e.g. in a stressed child). Regardless of induction agent used, anaesthesia carries a risk of vomiting and aspiration. In light of this risk, patients are fasted for 6 hours prior to surgery, with clear fluids withheld from 2 hours pre-operatively. In addition to achieving hypnosis, further agents are required to achieve analgesia. Short-acting analgesics such as **fentanyl** and **remifentanil** may be given in combination with anti-emetic drugs including *ondansetron, to produce a comfortable peri- and post-operative experience.*

Table 8.1 Ideal properties of anaesthetic agents

Ideal properties of inhalational agent	Ideal properties of intravenous agent
Chemically stable	Simple preparation
Non-flammable	Compatible with other agents/fluids
Compatible with other agents/fluids	Painless on administration
Potent	High potency and efficacy
Non-irritant to airway	Predictable action within one arm:brain circulation time
Non-toxic	Analgesia
Analgesic	Non-cardiotoxic
Non-cardiotoxic	Depression of airway reflexes for intubation
Rapid and predictable offset of effect	Rapid and predictable offset of effect
Reversible	Rapid metabolism for minimal hangover

Additional drugs may also be required to achieve a neuromuscular blockade, facilitating tracheal intubation, and abdominal operations.

Routine induction of anaesthesia

Routine induction of anaesthesia is used in patients where there is little chance of aspiration, i.e. in elective surgery where patients have been appropriately fasted, and can involve the use of inhalational (e.g. **sevoflurane**) or IV induction agents (e.g. **propofol**). Typically, an induction agent like propofol can be used alone or in combination with a co-induction agent like **fentanyl** (an opiate; see Topic 8.3, 'Analgesia and pain management') or **midazolam** (a benzodiazepine; see Topic 10.1, 'Anxiety'). Co-induction agents may be used as an early premedication, so anxiety and recall is impaired, with the added benefit of smoother induction.

Rapid sequence induction

In emergency situations a technique known as rapid sequence induction (RSI) is the preferred approach, since it induces rapid unconsciousness and neuromuscular blockade, allowing swift control of the airway. As such, it can be used in those at risk of vomiting and aspiration. Anaesthesia is generally induced within 1 minute, using drug doses calculated by body weight, rather than titrated to effect as in controlled elective situations. Hypnosis is achieved by means of an IV induction agent, such as **propofol**, **thiopental**, or **ketamine**; of which propofol is most commonly used. At a dose of 1.5–2.5 mg/kg, it provides rapid onset of anaesthesia with recovery in 5–10 minutes. A downside of propofol is its capacity to induce vasodilation and decrease cardiac output, so it is prudent to have a vasopressor to hand, such as **metaraminol**. Etomidate was previously used in patients at risk of haemodynamic compromise, although its suppression of

Table 8.2 Stages of anaesthesia

Stages of anaesthesia	Definition
Stage 1	Also known as 'induction', is the period between the initial administration of the induction agents and loss of consciousness.
Stage 2	Also known as the 'excitement stage', is the period following loss of consciousness and marked by excited and delirious activity.
Stage 3	Or 'surgical anaesthesia'. During this stage, the skeletal muscles relax, vomiting stops, and respiratory depression occurs.
Stage 4	Also known as 'overdose'

Adapted from Guedel AE. *Inhalation Anaesthesia: a Fundamental Guide, Second Edition*, New York, 1951, Macmillan.

the steroid axis has resulted in its almost complete withdrawal from use.

Neuromuscular blockade

In a routine induction, where indicated, non-depolarizing neuromuscular blockers such as atracurium or rocuronium are used (bolus 0.5 mg/kg). As the patient is starved, manual ventilation can be performed, while the drug is taking effect prior to the insertion of a tracheal tube. In a rapid sequence induction, where the stomach may be full or there is a risk of reflux, faster-acting agents, such as suxamethonium or rocuronium (1.2 mg/kg) are required. In this case, thorough pre-oxygenation allows a period of apnoea prior to intubation, minimizing the risk of regurgitation. If intubation and ventilation cannot be achieved, the rapid offset of both induction agent and suxamethonium (approx 5 minutes) permits awakening of the patient before hypoxia ensues. If this occurs after administration of rocuronium, the specific reversal agent sugammadex must be given to produce the same effect (see Figure 8.1).

Use of general anaesthetics

Inhaled anaesthetics

Inhaled anaesthetics have almost no analgesic properties (except nitrous oxide), but are very effective at inducing unconsciousness and amnesia. The ability to achieve sufficient concentrations of inhaled drug to obtain anaesthesia is dependent on a number of factors, including the rate of absorption at lung alveoli, the rate at which the drug attains equilibrium in blood, the concentrations in blood and brain, and the delivery to the brain (i.e. cardiac output). For each inhaled drug these factors are influenced by their biophysical properties which define either relative solubility in blood/water (i.e. blood:gas partition coefficient) or lipid (i.e. oil:gas partition coefficient).

Blood:gas partition coefficient (water/blood solubility)

Potent **halothane** (which is no longer used) is relatively water soluble and as such may require delivery in high amounts to achieve high circulating concentrations. The high concentrations need to be administered in order to raise the partial pressure of the drug in plasma quickly, so that sufficient compound reaches the brain (and lipid

soluble regions) to cause anaesthesia. Agents with poor blood solubility will have a faster onset of action, for example **sevoflurane**, with its low blood:gas partition coefficient, rapidly achieves raised alveolar concentrations.

Oil:gas partition coefficient (lipid solubility)

Lipid solubility is related to drug potency. If a drug is more potent, then a lower concentration is required to achieve the desired clinical effect, thus the oil:gas ratio is high. On this basis, the low potency agent **nitrous oxide**, with its low oil:gas ratio of 1.4 (c.f. 224 for halothane), requires an incredibly high partial pressure of drug in the brain to achieve surgical anaesthesia. The difficulty here is that patients cannot be administered less than 21% oxygen, making it impossible to anaesthetize a patient solely with nitrous oxide. As a result, the most appropriate mixture of anaesthetic agents must be selected for any given case.

Second gas effect

Although **nitrous oxide** is in itself not potent, it has a low blood:gas partial coefficient. It is therefore rapidly absorbed from alveoli and is used for its 'second gas' effect to accelerate the rise in the alveolar concentrations of a second inhalational agent. Rapid absorption of nitrous oxide from the alveoli increases relative concentration of any inhalational agent also used, thus increasing the diffusion gradient for that agent and speeding up induction. During recovery, however, the rapid elimination of nitrous oxide from the alveoli can result in diffusional hypoxia, which can be overcome by the supplemental administration of oxygen.

Minimum alveolar concentration

Agent biophysical properties and patient physiology (e.g. comorbidities and drugs), dictate potency and as such inform the minimum alveolar concentration (MAC) of agent required to achieve anaesthesia. It is therefore inversely related to the oil:gas partition coefficient. 1 MAC is the concentration of vapour in the lungs that is needed to prevent a motor response in 50% of subjects in response to a standardized surgical stimulus; it is much like the EC_{50} of a drug (see Chapter 1, Principles of clinical pharmacology). MAC numbers assume no other sedative or analgesic drugs are circulating and it does not reflect an individual's changing physiology, as this will affect relative potency and, hence, MAC. MAC is decreased by benzodiazepines and opioids, hypotension, old age, metabolic acidosis, or pregnancy. Chronic alcoholics, infants, thyroid disease, and those with red hair have an increased MAC. Volatile anaesthetics produce dose-dependent relaxation of skeletal muscles and

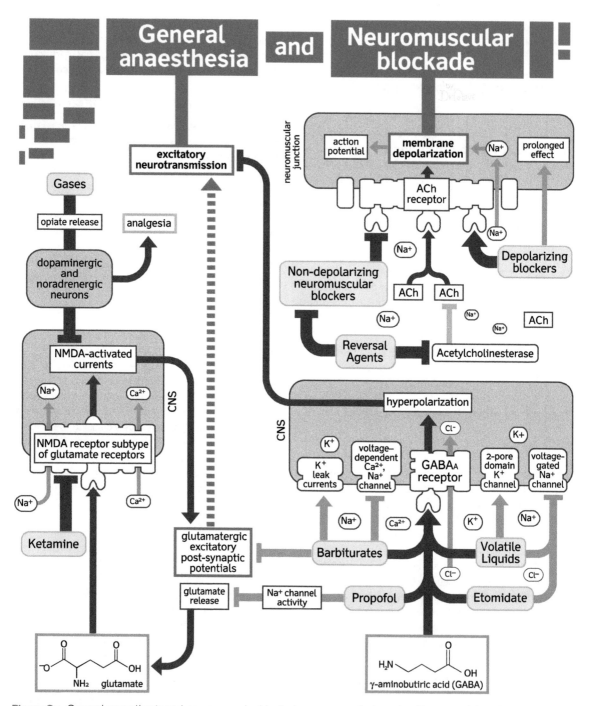

Figure 8.1 General anaesthesia and neuromuscular blockade: summary of relevant pathways and drug targets.

enhance ACh and non-depolarizing neuromuscular drugs (especially **desflurane**).

Intravenous anaesthetics: non-barbiturates

For most applications today, **propofol** is the IV anaesthetic drug of choice, used for both induction and maintenance by bolus or continuous infusion. It is highly lipid soluble and suitable for anything from light sedation through to full surgical anaesthesia, with the added advantage that is does not trigger malignant hyperthermia (see 'Depolarizing neuromuscular blockers, Malignant hyperthermia') and the incidence of nausea and vomiting is low. Its inhibitory effect on $GABA_A$, NMDA, ACh, and serotonin receptors induces hypnosis, as well as causing widespread vasodilation, cardiac output decline and respiratory depression. Dose ranges are well established for induction, maintenance, and sedation, with onset occurring within 90 seconds and offset after 5–8 minutes. The terminal half-life is around 10–12 hours, but the drug is rapidly redistributed so patients wake quickly. In the longer term, propofol is cleared from plasma by hepatic and extra-hepatic means. Like propofol, **etomidate** potentiates GABA activity and can be used in RSI, ECT, and cardioversion; it has no analgesic properties. Its side effect of adrenal suppression has dramatically reduced its popularity in the UK.

Ketamine is an alternative IV agent (as well as oral, rectal, intranasal, and IM), derived from phencyclidine, and hence, acts to antagonize NMDA receptors. This action causes dissociation of functional awareness within the brain's thalamus and cortex such that spontaneous respiration, swallow, cough, and reflexes are maintained when anaesthesia is induced; it has the added benefit in trauma patients that BP is maintained. Despite this, airway support may still be required and there is a risk of laryngospasm.

Intravenous anaesthetics: barbiturates

The barbiturates, like **thiopental** or **phenobarbital**, are rarely used since the introduction of **propofol**; however, they may be considered in patients requiring RSI or those with raised intracranial pressure. Drugs of this class are derived from barbituric acid; phenyl substitutions at the C5 position (i.e. **phenobarbital**) can confer anticonvulsant activities, while sulphur substitutions at C2 (i.e. thiopental) confers lipid solubility and added potency. Like some of the non-barbiturate drugs cited previously, sites

of action include enhanced GABA transmission, and inhibition of glutamate and ACh transmission, primarily within the reticular activating system; this junction within the brain stem can alter conscious level and induce hypnosis.

Use of neuromuscular blockers

As indicated previously, muscle relaxation is a key component to performing effective surgery and controlled anaesthesia; for this two classes of drug exist.

Depolarizing agents

The depolarizing agent **suxamethonium** is used in RSI and, when short duration or rapid onset muscle relaxation is required for short procedures (e.g. laryngoscopies, or in electroconvulsive therapy). It acts as an agonist at cholinergic receptors to cause muscle contraction by overwhelming endogenous ACh action, causing fasciculations, then a reversible but prolonged paralysis.

Non-depolarizing agents

The non-depolarizing blockers have a variable course of action and can be used to optimize intubation, ventilation, and surgical conditions and avoid the risk of fasciculations seen with **suxamethonium** contraction effects. These blockers competitively antagonize post-synaptic ACh receptors and halt neuromuscular transmission until the natural ligand ACh is replenished. Actions of non-depolarizing blockers may be short-acting (15–20 minutes), intermediate acting (20–50 minutes) or long-acting (>50 minutes).

Drugs used for anaesthesia

Detailed understanding of the mechanism of action of general anaesthetics remains incomplete. Once believed to be 'drugs without receptors', their low potency (micromolar to millimolar) impeded identification of their molecular targets for many years. Initially, attention focused on the hydrophobic nature of general anaesthetics and their apparent 'non-specific' effect on cellular membranes. More recent evidence established the enantiomeric selectivity exhibited by several anaesthetics and thus implicated specific binding sites on ion channels as the more likely mechanism for anaesthetic action (e.g. **isoflurane** and **propofol** at $GABA_A$ and/or GluR6 receptors).

Inhalational anaesthetics: nitrous oxide

The non-halogenated inhaled anaesthetics have little or no effect on the GABA$_A$ receptor subtypes tested so far, but depress excitatory glutamate-mediated synaptic transmission post-synaptically via blockade of NMDA glutamate receptors. For example, nitrous oxide.

Mechanism of action

The NMDA receptor subtype of glutamate receptors are ligand-gated channels permeable to Na$^+$ and Ca^{2+} that contribute to excitatory neurotransmission after glutamate release. They are known to have an important role in the CNS in learning, memory, and the sensitization of pain processing pathways. The relatively recent description of the ability of **nitrous oxide** to inhibit NMDA-activated currents has addressed some of its potential mechanism in anaesthesia.

Although the analgesic properties of nitrous oxide are attributed to the release of opioid peptide, the same underlying mechanism is thought to contribute to the anaesthetic mechanisms, at least partially, by interacting with dopaminergic and noradrenergic neurons. Studies have shown region-dependent effects of nitrous oxide on dopamine, and/or noradrenaline concentrations or turnover in the brain. Interestingly, opioid peptides have been shown to regulate catecholamine release in the CNS, providing a potential mechanism for the nitrous oxide effects on dopaminergic and noradrenergic pathways.

Prescribing

Nitrous oxide is the oldest of the anaesthetic agents still in use today, although its administration at high concentrations is limited by the necessity to co-administer oxygen in varying concentrations (50–66%). It possesses weak anaesthetic properties, but potent analgesic properties, and although insufficient to induce unconsciousness, it can be used for the purpose of conscious analgesia (**Entonox®**), e.g. during child birth or for minor painful procedures.

Nitrous oxide also acts to increase the speed of uptake at the alveolar blood interface. Consequently, when used as the carrier gas for the administration of anaesthetic gases, compared with oxygen alone, it increases the uptake into the blood across the alveolar wall concentration of anaesthetic gases, subsequently lowering the mean alveolar concentration and hastening onset of action.

Inhalational anaesthetics: volatile agents

Volatile ether anaesthetics (e.g. isoflurane, sevoflurane, desflurane, and enflurane) and some of the alkanes (e.g. halothane) act mainly by enhancing GABA$_A$ receptor function, increasing channel opening and leading to enhanced inhibition at both synaptic and extrasynaptic level. In addition, other ion channels are also targeted, including Na$^+$ and K$^+$ types.

Mechanism of action

Transient, inhibitory post-synaptic currents that are mediated by GABA$_A$ receptors generate fast synaptic inhibition. Volatile anaesthetics act to prolong these inhibitory post-synaptic potentials enhancing the net inhibitory effect. Facilitation at the inhibitory glycine receptor (also a Cl$^-$ permeable channel) also appears to contribute to the central mechanism of action of volatile anaesthetics.

In addition to GABA$_A$ receptors, volatile anaesthetics also affect the function of other ion channels. These include voltage-gated Na$^+$ channels, which are essential to axonal conduction, synaptic function, and overall neuronal excitability. Volatile anaesthetics also inhibit native Na$^+$ channels in dorsal root ganglia neurons and isolated nerve terminals at clinical concentrations.

The activation of K$^+$ channels has also been observed at clinical concentrations, so increased K$^+$ channel conductance occurs. This leads to hyperpolarization and reduced responsiveness to excitatory synaptic input.

Prescribing

The volatile agents are administered through a vaporizer where they are mixed with oxygen, with or without **nitrous oxide**. The agents may be used for induction (i.e. **sevoflurane**) and maintenance (i.e. **isoflurane** and **desflurane**) of anaesthesia, with doses titrated to achieve the desired response. Unlike nitrous, however, the volatile agents possess no analgesic properties.

Advantages and disadvantages of inhalational anaesthetics

Potency

Increasing halogenation (i.e. Cl- or Fl- groups) and molecular weight all affect potency; the oldest agent **halothane** is the most potent and volatile, but is no longer manufactured worldwide. Although it is not routine to perform inhalational inductions in anyone other than paediatric cases, **sevoflurane**, which is less potent, has a pleasant odour and is often used with **nitrous oxide** for efficient smooth induction and maintenance of anaesthesia. The potency of an inhaled anaesthetic is defined by its MAC (see 'Minimum alveolar concentration')

Significant adverse reaction

The volatile agents may trigger a rare life-threatening condition called malignant hyperthermia in patients with this autosomal dominant disorder (see 'Depolarizing neuromuscular blockers, Unwanted effects').

Cardiovascular effects

The inhaled anaesthetics tend to depress myocardial function and reduce peripheral resistance, leading to a decrease in BP. In some cases, however, compensatory sympathetic stimulation leads to tachycardia with sudden increases in inhaled concentration (see Table 8.3). **Isoflurane** or **desflurane** are associated with respiratory and airway problems much more than cardiac responses.

Respiratory effects

Inhaled anaesthetics affect both the airways and rate of ventilation. With the exception of **desflurane**, action on the airways causing bronchodilation, with **halothane** being the most potent. Desflurane, however, has been shown to cause either bronchoconstriction (particularly in smokers), or at least no bronchodilation. In terms of ventilation the volatile agents act to increase respiratory rate and decrease tidal volume, leading to a decrease in minute ventilation. Although **nitrous oxide** also increases respiratory rate when used alone, it causes a small decrease in tidal volume so that minute ventilation remains unchanged.

Cerebral effects

The inhalational anaesthetics act to increase cerebral blood flow, except for low doses of **sevoflurane,** which decreases blood flow. **Nitrous oxide** also increases cerebral blood flow, although these effects are lost in combination with another agent. As a class, the volatile agents induce EEG changes, which with **enflurane** can result in increased seizure activity, whereas **isoflurane** has anticonvulsant properties.

Haematological effects

Nitrous oxide interferes with the folate pathway by oxidizing the cobalt ion in vitamin B12, thus inhibiting methionine synthase, which normally acts to produce methionine and tetrahydrofolate. Prolonged exposure, particularly in patients with pre-existing B12 deficiency, can lead to megaloblastic anaemia and agranulocytosis, although with current usage strategies the risk is small. Volatile agents may also affect neutrophil or platelet function, but this is unlikely to be of clinical significance.

Hepatic effects

The inhalational agents act to reduce hepatic portal blood flow, although with the exception of **halothane**, there is a compensatory increase in hepatic arterial flow so as to maintain hepatic blood flow. Volatile agents can also give rise to a transient increase in hepatic enzymes, an effect not seen with **nitrous oxide**. Hepatitis and rises in transaminases are most likely with halothane, although in general effects tend to be mild and reversible, only rarely causing severe hepatitis.

Renal effects

The inhalational agents act to reduce renal blood flow, glomerular filtration rate, and urine production, but they are generally well tolerated clinically (Table 8.3).

Intravenous anaesthetics: barbiturates

Barbiturates suppress CNS activity by enhancing the function of $GABA_A$ receptors, decreasing excitatory amino acids and Na^+ channel responses, and interacting with membrane Ca^{2+} channels to decrease Ca^{2+} conductance. For example, thiopental.

Mechanism of action

Barbiturates are organized into four classes—long-, intermediate-, short-, and ultrashort-acting types. **Phenobarbital** is the prototype for long-acting barbiturates, with a peak plasma level at 6–18 hours and duration of action of about 24 hours. The intermediate- to short-acting barbiturates (**pentobarbital** and **secobarbital**), have higher lipid solubility that allows rapid crossing of the blood–brain barrier and sedation within 30 minutes. Peak plasma concentrations occurs 1–2 hours after ingestion. The ultrashort-acting barbiturates (**thiopental**) are so lipophilic that when administered IV they are absorbed by

Table 8.3 Summary of effects of inhalational anaesthetics

	Nitrous oxide	Isoflurane	Desflurane	Sevoflurane
MAC (%)				
In 100% O_2	104	1.15	5-10	1.7-2
With 70% NO	N/A	0.41	2.30	0.62
Onset of action	< 1 minute	7–10 minutes	2–4 minutes	<2 minutes
Cardiac effects				
Heart rate	↔	↑	↑	↑/↓
Cardiac output	↓	↓	↓	↓/↔
Peripheral resistance	↔	↓↓	↓↓	↓
Respiratory effects				
Airways	Dilation +	Dilation ++	Constriction	Dilation ++
Respiratory rate	↑	↑	↑	↑
Renal effects				
Renal blood flow	↓	↓	↓	↓
GFR	↓	↓	↓	↓
Urine production	↓	↓	↓	↓

Adapted from Moppett I (2012) Inhalational anaesthetics. *Anaesth Intens Care*, 13 (7) 348-353. Copyright © 2012 Elsevier Ltd. All rights reserved. https://doi.org/10.1016/j.mpaic.2012.04.003

the brain within one arm:brain circulation time. However, due to the rapid redistribution to other body tissues, primarily fat, they have relatively brief clinical effects.

The ionic mechanisms of barbiturate-induced depression of excitability include suppression of glutamatergic excitatory post-synaptic potentials, voltage-dependent Ca^{2+} and Na^+ currents, as well as activation of leak K^+ currents. Barbiturates enhance synaptic inhibition mediated by $GABA_A$ and enhance the duration of the channel opening, this leads to a greater degree of hyperpolarization and decreased neuronal excitability. In the absence of GABA, barbiturates can also activate $GABA_A$ receptors by direct agonism.

Barbiturates including thiopental are used for RSI and in patients with raised intracranial pressures; they may have neuroprotective effects by reducing cerebral metabolism.

Prescribing

Over the decades a number of barbiturates have been developed for the purpose of inducing anaesthesia, although only the ultrashort-acting agent **thiopental** remains widely used. Thiopental has a rapid onset of action, inducing anaesthesia within 30 seconds of injecting, although this may be increased in patients with poor cardiac

output. Like other barbiturates, it is a potent anaesthetic, but lacks analgesic properties.

The barbiturates are metabolized in the liver and can induce enzymes, most notably δ-aminolevulinic acid synthetase, which is involved in the porphyrin production. As such, porphyria is an absolute contraindication for barbiturates, as they may precipitate severe abdominal pain, nausea, vomiting, psychiatric disorders, and neurologic abnormalities.

Intravenous anaesthetics: non-barbiturates—propofol

The short-acting IV anaesthetic propofol is used for induction and maintenance of anaesthesia. Its mechanism of action involves a positive modulation of the $GABA_A$ receptor, with subsequent increase of inhibitory neuronal inputs.

Mechanism of action

Beyond the positive modulation of $GABA_A$ receptor function, it has been reported that at clinically relevant concentrations **propofol** inhibits glutamate release by targeting

Na⁺ channel blockade, or by activating GABA$_A$ receptors directly. It has also been suggested that propofol acts as a weak inhibitor of the NMDA receptor and can reduce Ca²⁺ influx through slow Ca²⁺ channels, while also modulating glycine and neuronal nicotinic acetylcholine receptors, with an EC$_{50}$ of approximately an order of magnitude higher than that of GABA$_A$ receptors.

Prescribing

Propofol is the most widely used intravenous anaesthetic agent for both induction and maintenance of anaesthesia. Being highly lipophilic it distributes rapidly into the CNS and acts within 20–40 seconds of administration. Propofol can induce involuntary movements during induction. Recovery is also rapid, so that propofol has less hangover effects compared with other anaesthetic agents.

Intravenous anaesthetics: non-barbiturates—ketamine

Ketamine is a versatile drug that can be used, in different doses, for analgesia, sedation, and induction of general anaesthesia. It is a phencyclidine derivative that acts by blocking the NMDA subtype of glutamate receptors, the main excitatory transmitter in the brain.

Mechanism of action

Ketamine produces a spectrum of anaesthetic action giving rise to a 'dissociative' anaesthesia. The effects have been described as comprising:

- Hypnosis, including psychotomimetic effects at low concentrations, followed by sedation and unconsciousness with higher doses.
- Intense analgesia.
- Increased sympathetic activity.
- Maintenance of airway tone and respiration.

Blockade of NMDA receptors and excitatory synaptic activity is the likely mechanism for the loss of responsiveness associated with clinical anaesthesia after ketamine.

At the molecular level, ketamine acts as an open channel blocker with a slow dissociation rate. Its mechanism of action is described through a phenomenon called 'trapping block' in which after glutamate has dissociated from its binding site, ketamine remains trapped in the now closed ion channel. This causes a prolonged tonic blockade that

disrupts physiological and pathological functions. In contrast, fast off-rate NMDA antagonists tend to have minimal sedative effects (e.g. **memantine**).

Unlike other induction agents/general anaesthetics ketamine does not interact with GABA$_A$ receptors, but in addition to NMDA receptor blockade, it is known to block other neuronal targets (e.g. HCN-1, nicotinic acetylcholine ion channels, voltage-operated Ca²⁺ channels). It has been shown to reduce cholinergic neuromodulation and increase the release of aminergic neuromodulators (dopamine and noradrenaline).

Ketamine has also been shown to have clinical effects in chronic pain and as an antidepressant, but these effects far outlast actual drug levels and are likely mediated by secondary changes in structural synaptic connectivity, induced by ketamine-evoked hyper-glutamatergic neurotransmission.

Prescribing

Ketamine has both anaesthetic and analgesic properties, which make its valuable in the emergency setting, but the emergence phenomena (psychosis on recovery) limit its value in elective cases. Dissociative anaesthesia increases the likelihood of psychiatric toxicity such as hallucinations, delirium, and psychosis on recovery. These effects may be aggravated when it is used in combination with opioids and may be partly managed by avoiding stimulus (verbal and tactile) during the recovery period. It has a relatively quick onset of action, inducing unconsciousness within 30–60 seconds of IV administration. The duration of action is dose related, with 2 mg/kg producing around 10–15 minutes of anaesthesia, although compared with other agents, effects are prolonged and recovery is slow.

Intravenous anaesthetics: non-barbiturates—etomidate

Etomidate is an imidazole derivative used as an ultrashort-acting non-barbiturate anaesthetic and hypnotic. It exerts a depressant effect on the CNS by targeting the GABA$_A$ receptor.

Mechanism of action

Extensive electrophysiological evidence has indicated that **etomidate** acts by enhancing the response of GABA$_A$ receptors to GABA, or by direct activation of these receptors. In addition, etomidate has an effect on voltage-gated Na⁺ channels, which are the main molecular basis of action potential firing in neurons. Inhibition of these channels can contribute to the presynaptic effects of general anaesthetics on nerve terminal excitability and neurotransmitter release. Etomidate was shown to reduce Na$^+$ channel conductance in a concentration-dependent manner by reducing current amplitude and enhancing inactivation.

Prescribing

Etomidate has a rapid onset of action, working within ~1–2 minutes, but due to extensive redistribution and rapid metabolism the effects wear off quickly, and thus lacks hangover effects. This made it useful for day case surgery, but it is rarely used now.

It should not be used for maintenance treatment as prolonged use suppresses adrenocortical function. Etomidate, like **propofol**, also induces involuntary movements, which can be reduced by pretreating with opioids or benzodiazepines.

Advantage and disadvantages of intravenous anaesthetics

Cardiovascular effects

The barbiturates have a depressive effect on myocardial contractility and induce peripheral vasodilation (Table 8.4). In healthy patients this is usually compensated for by a reflex tachycardia, although in patients with impaired cardiac function or hypovolaemia, it can result in profound hypotension. Similarly, **propofol** acts to reduce arterial BP, and although the effects are more profound, it can be in part overcome by reducing the rate of administration. **Etomidate** is less likely to cause hypotension compared with other IV anaesthetics. **Ketamine** has the opposite effect on cardiovascular function, increasing cardiac output and, therefore, arterial BP.

Respiratory effects

Thiopental reduces the sensitivity of the respiratory centre to carbon dioxide leading to respiratory depression, particularly when used in combination with opioids. Patients therefore will likely require assisted ventilation. Following administration with **propofol** respiratory rate decreases along with tidal volume; resulting in respiratory depression that is enhanced by opioid use. Respiratory depression tends to be less with **etomidate** compared with either propofol or thiopental, although apnoeas will occur after an induction dose and will require manual ventilation for a period followed by mechanical ventilation.

Apnoea is more common with propofol than thiopental. **Ketamine** is a profound bronchodilator, making it highly useful in asthma, although it may still cause apnoeas.

Cerebral effects

Thiopental, **propofol**, and **etomidate** act to reduce cerebral metabolic rate and blood flow, thereby reducing intracranial pressure. **Ketamine** has the opposite effect, causing an increase in intracranial pressure, also commonly causing hallucinations and vivid dreams. Thiopental is a potent anti-convulsant, as to a lesser extent is propofol. Etomidate can induce seizures albeit incredibly rarely.

Endocrine effects

Etomidate has a suppressive effect on cortisol production, especially when administered continuously. It should therefore not be used in maintenance anaesthesia where profound suppression can increase the risk of sepsis and therefore mortality.

Hepatic effects

Hepatic function is transiently impaired particularly with **propofol** as reduced cardiac output reduces hepatic perfusion. **Thiopental** induces hepatic enzymes so that clearance of other drugs may be accelerated and patients with severe hepatic dysfunction should receive thiopental more slowly. **Ketamine** is, in part, hepatically metabolized to inactive metabolites, so that effects are prolonged in hepatic impairment.

Renal effects

Thiopental and to a lesser degree **propofol** act to depress renal function. Effects tend to be mild and transient.

Other considerations

Propofol causes pain on induction and is contraindicated for continuous infusion in children. It can also dye urine green. **Thiopental** is dangerous if it extravasates or is injected intra-arterially, and is contraindicated in porphyric patients.

Drugs used for neuromuscular blockade

The nerve terminal in the neuromuscular junction is responsible for the synthesis, storage, mobilization,

Table 8.4 Summary of effects of intravenous anaesthetics

	Thiopental	Propofol	Ketamine	Etomidate
Cardiovascular effects				
Cardiac output	↓	↓	↑	↓
Peripheral resistance	↓	↓↓	↑	↓
BP	↓↓	↓↓↓	↑/↔	↓
Respiratory effects				
Respiratory rate	↓	↑	↔	↑
Tidal volume	↓	↓	↔	↓
Cerebral effects				
Blood flow	↓	↓	↑	↓
Metabolic rate	↓	↓	↑	↓
Intracranial pressure	↓	↓	↑	↓

release, and recycling of the neurotransmitter acetylcholine (ACh). Once an action potential arrives at the nerve terminal, ACh is released from the synaptic vesicles and crosses the junctional cleft to bind to post-junctional receptors. Binding of two molecules of ACh to the receptor causes it to open and Na^+ to flow down its concentration gradient, leading to a local depolarization of the muscle membrane.

Agents can modify neuromuscular transmission via different mechanisms:

- receptor occlusion, where a substance physically competes with ACh and blocks its binding to the receptor, thus preventing the channel from opening;
- closed channel block, in which a molecule physically obstructs the mouth of the channel and impedes the passage of cations;
- open channel block, where a positively charged molecule enters the channel once its opened, reducing current flow;
- presynaptic receptors, which can be targeted in order to modulate the release of ACh in the synaptic junction;
- membrane effectors, which can modify the integrity of the phospholipid cell membrane, thus influencing the function of the channel.

Although all of these are biologically important, only two mechanisms are exploited clinically to prevent the physiological action of ACh in the neuromuscular junction.

Depolarizing neuromuscular blockers

Depolarizing blockers occupy the ACh binding site and act as agonists that produce ACh nicotinic receptor activation and cell membrane depolarization. Unlike the effect of ACh, which is short, neuromuscular blocking agents have a more prolonged effect that leads to the receptor mechanism being rendered insensitive for a longer period of time. For example, suxamethonium.

Mechanism of action

Suxamethonium, the only depolarizing agent used clinically, is not hydrolysed by acetylcholinesterase and therefore has a longer duration of effect than ACh in the neuromuscular junction. The degradation of suxamethonium by butyrylcholinesterase is a much slower reaction than that observed by acetylcholinesterase for ACh. The prolonged activation of the receptor leads to sustained depolarization that does not allow the muscle cell to repolarize, inactivating the voltage-gated Na^+ channels in the muscle membrane adjacent to the motor end-plate and resulting in a temporary insulating zone of electrical inexcitability. Since Ca^{2+} is removed from the cytoplasm independent of repolarization, the muscle relaxes, and flaccidity, rather than tetany is observed.

Prescribing

Suxamethonium is the least potent, and therefore most rapidly acting of the neuromuscular blockers, producing a complete block within 1 minute of administration.

Recovery takes 5–10 minutes, although this is increased in patients who are malnourished, pregnant, or have an inherited abnormality of plasma cholinesterase (suxamethonium apnoea). Doses can be administered as an IV bolus or IM injection. Its rapid onset of action makes it a valuable option for RSI and emergency intubation.

Unwanted effects

Suxamethonium has numerous adverse effects, largely associated with its depolarizing actions. Stimulation of autonomic ACh receptors can cause arrhythmias, both tachycardic and bradycardic in nature. Effects are often dose-dependant and bradycardia more commonly associated with repeat doses. Prolonged muscle depolarization can also lead to hyperkalaemia (especially in renal failure and burns patients).

Malignant hyperthermia is a rare, but potentially fatal condition that can occur with trigger agents like suxamethonium or the volatile anaesthetics. It is an autosomal-dominant inherited condition with variable penetrance. Exposure to any trigger agent, alone or in combination, can provoke a reaction if the patient has the underlying condition. The mutation is in proteins responsible for managing intracellular Ca^{2+} levels; raised intracellular levels lead to muscle cell damage. It is characterized by tachycardia, a rising CO_2, muscle rigidity, tachypnoea, and a rapid rise in temperature (late sign). Treatment is with **dantrolene**.

Non-depolarizing blockers

The non-depolarizing neuromuscular blockers stop receptor activation by binding to the ACh site, acting as antagonists that prevent membrane depolarization. Examples include pancuronium, vecuronium, atracurium, cisatracurium, mivacurium, and rocuronium.

Mechanism of action

The non-depolarizing blockers bind in a reversible manner to the ACh binding sites on the α subunits of the ACh nicotinic receptor, preventing receptor activation. In the presence of non-depolarizing agents, a dynamic equilibrium exists that favours either the agonist or antagonist, depending on their relative concentrations. Thus, anticholinesterase agents that prolong the presence of ACh in the synaptic cleft can *usually* antagonize them.

Tubocurarine is an alkaloid extracted from the South American plant *Chondrodendron tomentosum* and was the first non-depolarizing blocker to enter clinical practice. It was the original drug against which all new agents were compared, although it is no longer available in the UK. Instead, agents in clinical use are all large, bulky molecules with one, two, or three positively charged nitrogen atoms. They are classified according to their duration of action, which is inversely related to their potency.

Long-acting agents

Pancuronium was the first steroid-based neuromuscular blocking agent used clinically. More potent than curare, but with less effect on the circulatory system and on histamine release. It has an onset time of about 3–4 minutes, with 50–60 minutes duration. Due to its extended duration of action it is associated with an increased risk of residual paralysis, compared with intermediate-acting agents.

Intermediate-acting agents

Atracurium, an ester with two positively charged nitrogen atoms and four asymmetric centres, has a total of 16 potential stereoisomers. Developed to exploit the Hoffman elimination reaction in its metabolism, the atracurium molecule spontaneously breaks down in a temperature and pH dependent process. Although it lacks cardiovascular effects, histamine release could be a problem when exceeding 0.5–0.6 mg/kg doses; it manifests as cutaneous reactions, but can lead to vasodilation, and hypotension/tachycardia or wheeze. **Cisatracurium** is a single isomer preparation of the main active ingredient in atracurium, which is almost three times more potent and with a slower onset. It has less effect on histamine release.

Vecuronium is a synthetic steroid almost devoid of cardiovascular side effects. It is metabolized by the hepatic route, and eliminated by the kidneys and in bile; accumulation has been reported with higher doses. **Rocuronium** is another steroid-based agent, with a short onset time by administering higher doses, making it a viable alternative to suxamethonium in experienced hands (see also 'Sugammadex'). It does not accumulate with repeated doses, and is again almost devoid of cardiovascular and histamine release effects.

Short-acting agents

Mivacurium belongs to the same **atracurium** family (benzylisoquinoliniums) and is the only non-depolarizing agent that can be metabolized by acetylcholinesterase in the plasma. Thus, reducing the activity of plasma cholinesterase can prolong its duration of action. Onset

Table 8.5 Summary of action of the non-depolarizing blockers

	Potency (ED$_{95}$)	Onset of action (minutes)	Duration of action (minutes) initial dose	maintenance dose	Histamine release
Atracurium	0.25	1.5	30–40	15–25	Yes
Cisatracurium	0.05	2	30–40	20	No
Mivacurium	0.08	2–2.5	15–30	15	Yes
Pancuronium	0.06	1.5-2.5	60–120	25–60	No
Rocuronium	0.4	1	30–40	15–20	No
Vecuronium	0.05	2-3	20–40	20–40	No

occurs in 3–5 minutes with a duration of 18–22 minutes. Recovery is very rapid and should not require reversal with anticholinesterase agents. Mivacurium metabolism is also prolonged with suxamethonium apnoea.

Prescribing

The neuromuscular blockers are used to relax skeletal muscle in various indications such as enabling intubation, during surgery, and also in the intensive care setting in the management of conditions such as respiratory distress or raised intracranial pressure. The choice of non-depolarizing neuromuscular blockers will vary according to the procedure to be carried out and selected, based on characteristics such as onset and duration of action, route of elimination, and side effects. The agents that act rapidly, for example, may be used in patients requiring urgent intubation, whereas those with a long duration of action used where extended neuromuscular blockade is required. Agents that induce histamine release are more likely to be problematic in patients with a cardiovascular history and brittle asthma.

Unwanted effects

Adverse effects vary between the non-depolarizing agents, based in part on their specificity for the nicotinic receptor and whether they act on muscarinic receptors. For example, the benzlisoquiniliniums (**atracurium**, **cisatracurium**, and **mivacurium**) are selective for the nicotinic-receptor, and therefore lack muscarinic or sympathetic activity; while the aminosteroids (**pancuronium** and **vecuronium**) act at nicotinic receptors in the pre-ganglionic neurons of parasympathetic pathways. The *reduction* in parasympathetic tone caused by pancuronium and at high doses, **rocuronium** leads to tachycardia and

hypertension, particularly in patients with pre-existing heart disease where dose reductions are advisable. **Suxamethonium** can also cause electrolyte disturbances, with the potential of aggravating cardiovascular toxicity. For this reason, any imbalances in fluids or electrolytes should be corrected prior to initiating treatment.

Drugs that are cleared via the kidney such as pancuronium, mivacurium, rocuronium, and vecuronium will require dose reductions in renal impairment. In severe impairment atracurium or cisatracurium may be preferred as their clearance is unaffected. Neuromuscular blockers should be used with considerable care in patients with pre-existing neuromuscular disorders, such as muscular dystrophy and myasthenia gravis, as effects may be significantly and unpredictably altered.

Reversal agents

Reversal agents are used for the restoration of normal neuromuscular function, an outcome that is achieved when the antagonist molecules leaves the neuromuscular junction. For example, **sugammadex** and anticholinesterases (**edrophonium**, **neostigmine**).

Mechanism of action

For some neuromuscular blocking agents, redistribution and/or slow elimination can be sufficient to reverse their actions, while for others, breakdown, either spontaneous (**atracurium**, **cisatracurium**) or by enzymatic processes (**suxamethonium**, **mivacurium**), can accelerate the process.

In the case of non-depolarizing agents, biasing the equilibrium within the neuromuscular junction towards

ACh can actively reverse their action. This is achieved by inhibiting acetylcholinesterase, reducing enzymatic breakdown of ACh, thereby increasing levels of neurotransmitter in the neuromuscular junction. Acetylcholinesterase is a large molecule with two active sites, the anionic, which binds the positively charged nitrogen in the ACh molecule, and the esteratic site, which binds the acetate component.

Edrophonium binds to the esteratic site in a competitive manner and is relatively short acting, thus suitable for reversing light to moderate block; it is almost never used in anaesthetics, but does have a role in myasthenia gravis. **Neostigmine** interacts with both the anionic and the esteratic site of the acetylcholinesterase molecule, inactivating the enzyme by carbamylation leading to a relatively slow enzyme reactivation process.

Recent research has identified a new family of reversal agents that can actively remove relaxant molecules by direct binding to them. In particular, the cyclodextrin **sugammadex** is the first selective relaxant binding agent that is used for the reversal of neuromuscular blockade by **rocuronium (or vecuronium)**. It has a lipophilic core and a hydrophilic periphery, and its encapsulation binding prevents rocuronium from interacting with the acetylcholine receptor. Since it can reverse neuromuscular blockade without inhibition of acetylcholinesterase it is devoid of autonomic instability and is very useful in failed intubation scenarios (with rocuronium or vecuronium).

Prescribing

The anticholinesterases, **neostigmine** and **edrophonium** have been used clinically to reverse the effects of non-depolarizing neuromuscular blocking agents, although the latter has now been largely discontinued. They are indicated where patients experience residual paralysis or when reversal is desired and are always administered with **atropine** or **glycopyrronium**, to overcome the effects of excess acetycholine action at muscarinic receptors (specifically, profound bradycardia). The reversal agents, however, are only effective if recovery is already established and when used too early can increase the risk of post-operative residual curarization (PORC). Furthermore, anticholinesterases actually prolong the effect of depolarizing NMBAs. Doses of anticholinesterase are administered by slow IV injection based on patient's weight and repeated where effects are inadequate.

Sugammadex can be used to reverse the effects of **rocuronium** and **vecuronium** most commonly in an emergency situation. Compared with anticholinesterases it produces a more rapid recovery and is better tolerated, lacking the muscarinic effects. Doses are again administered by IV injection based on patient weight and level of neuromuscular blockade to be reversed.

Unwanted effects

Unwanted effects to the anticholinesterase inhibitors are largely attributed to their muscarinic effects, i.e. nausea and vomiting, diarrhoea, bradycardia (followed by tachycardia and arrhythmias), sweating, urinary incontinence, hypersalivation, and QT interval prolongation. For this reason, they are always administered in combination with an anti-muscarinic agent (**glycopyrronium**) and should be avoided where such toxicity maybe problematic, e.g. urinary retention or intestinal obstruction. **Neostigmine** is renally cleared and dose reductions may be necessary in renal impairment.

In comparison, **sugammadex** is well tolerated, the incidence of side effects being rare, but occasionally causing hypersensitivity reactions, bradycardia, cardiac arrest, and possibly awareness during anaesthesia. As sugammadex acts by binding to **vecuronium** or **rocuronium**, drugs administered pre-operatively that cause displacement could result in a recurrence of neuromuscular blockade or delay in recovery, e.g. **toremifene** and **fusidic acid**.

Further reading

Bowman WC (2006) Neuromuscular block. *British Journal of Pharmacology* 147, S277–S286.

Claudius C, Garvey LH, Viby-Mogensen J (2009) The undesirable effects of neuromuscular blocking drugs. *Anaesthesia* 64 64(Sl Suppl. 1), 10–21.

Farooq K, Hunter JM (2011) Neuromuscular blocking agents and reversal agents. *Anaesthesia and Intensice Care* 12 (6), 267–70.

Greenberg SB, Vender J (2013) The use of neuromuscular blocking agents in the ICU: where are we now? *Critical Care Medicne* 41 (5), 1332–44.

Hemmings HC, Akabas MH, Goldstein PA, et al. (2005) Emerging molecular mechanisms of general anesthetic action. *Trends in Pharmacological Sciences* 26 (10), 503–10.

Kotani Y, Shimazawa M, Yoshimura S, et al. (2008) The experimental and clinical pharmacology of propofol, an anesthetic agent with neuroprotective properties. *Central Nervous System Neuroscience Therapy* 14 (2), 95–106.

Lambert DG (2014) Mechanisms of action of general anaesthetic drugs *Anaesth Intens Care* 15(7), 318–20.

Mashour GA, Forman SA, Campagna JA (2005) Mechanisms of general anesthesia: from molecules to mind. *Best Practice & Research in Clinical Anaesthesiology* 19 (3), 349–64.

Maze M, Fujinaga M (2001) Pharmacology of nitrous oxide. *Best Practice & Research in Clinical Anaesthesiology* 15 (3), 339–48.

Moppett I (2012) Inhalational anaesthetics. *Anaesth Intens Care* 13 (7) 348–53

Peck and Hill's Pharmacology for Anaesthesia and Intensive Care (2008) 3rd Edition. Cambridge.

Pollard B (2005) Neuromuscular blocking agents and reversal agents. *Anaesth Intens Care* 6 (6) 189–92.

Sleigh J, Harvey M, Voss L et al. (2014) Ketamine: More mechanisms of action than just NMDA blockade. *Trends Anaesthesia and Critical Care* 1–6.

Srivastava A, Hunter JM (2009) Reversal of neuromuscular block. *British Journal of Anaesthesia* 103 (1) 115–29.

Thomas G, Morgan M (2011) Monitoring neuromuscular blockade and depth of anaesthesia *Anaesth Intens Care* 12 (6) 271–4.

Guidelines

For general information see: The Association of Anaesthetists of Great Britain and Ireland www.aagbi.org [accessed 5 April 2019].

Robertson T (2011) Proposal for update of the anaesthesia and muscle relaxant sections of the WHO EML 18th Expert Committee on the Selection and Use of Essential Medicines. https://www.who.int/selection_medicines/committees/expert/18/applications/anaesthetic_proposal.pdf [accessed 5 April 2019]

8.2 Local anaesthetics

The main mechanism of action for local anaesthetics is the blockade of sodium (Na^+) channels (mainly voltage-gated), so that normal nerve depolarization and hence pain signal conduction, is reversibly blocked. **Cocaine**, isolated from coca leaves in 1860, was one of the first compounds considered for surgical local anaesthesia, as chewing of these leaves was known to numb the oropharynx. The uses of local anaesthetics are diverse and can be classified on the basis of site and technique of specific delivery, with certain specific compounds being beneficial due to their physiochemical and pharmacokinetic properties (e.g. hyperbaric **bupivacaine** used in spinal anaesthesia because of its predictable spread; see Figure 8.2).

Uses of local anaesthetics

The terminology of local anaesthetic usage can be unclear, but herein we discuss some of the important techniques and drugs that are used both locally (e.g. surface administration/application), regionally (e.g. peripheral nerve blocks), and centrally (e.g. epidural or spinal). Some texts categorize 'local' techniques as regional anaesthesia. The differing pharmacological properties of local anaesthetic drugs lend themselves to different administration techniques.

Local techniques

Topical/surface administration

Particular formulations of high dose drugs in a lipophilic medium, sucked as a lozenge, sprayed into mucous membranes or delivered by transdermal administration can be an extremely useful analgesic technique. Topical creams can contain **tetracaine** (e.g. Ametop), which blocks nociceptive transmission locally in a well-defined superficial region, hence its use in paediatrics and the needle-phobic prior to venepuncture. Equally, lidocaine sprayed onto mucous membranes can be used for airway procedures (e.g. to reduce the gag reflex in awake intubation). Local anaesthetic throat lozenges typically contain **benzocaine**, a weak and poorly absorbed ethyl ester that blocks surface pain transmission, thus making it useful in upper respiratory tract infections, in condoms to prevent premature ejaculation and in some ear drops (to reduce pain of otitis media). Local anaesthetic patches (e.g. 5% lidocaine) can also be useful in neuropathic pain and post-hepatic neuralgia where local skin application minimizes the amount of drug that enters the circulation.

Local field administration

This technique is probably the most common use of local anaesthetic drugs. Local injection of aqueous drug to skin, subdermis, around vessel nerves, and local structures can effectively reduce pain. At the superficial end, medium-acting drugs like **lidocaine** can be useful when a superficial laceration requires sutures in the emergency department. Equally, following more extensive surgery local anaesthetic administration to the wound closure will reduce postoperative pain and hasten patient mobility and discharge. During wound closure, deeper infiltration subfascially (e.g. in inguinal repair) will ensure a prolonged action post-operatively and generate better pain relief. Deeper localized injections may lead to field block per se and may isolate a specific area to pain transmission (e.g. for a single tooth extraction).

The local anaesthetic selected will depend on the required duration that sensation (and potentially motor) transmission is to remain suppressed (c.f. lidocaine versus **bupivacaine**) and whether or not an adjunct (e.g. **adrenaline**, Table 8.6) is required. Aspiration should be gently performed prior to injection of local anaesthetic, to avoid

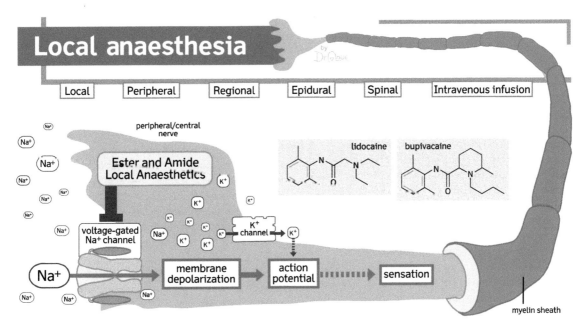

Figure 8.2 Local anaesthesia: summary of relevant pathways and drug targets.

Table 8.6 Commonly used local anaesthetic adjuncts.

Drug	Characteristics
Bicarbonate	Increases speed of onset by increasing pH of solution and therefore fraction of unionized LA, increasing transit across the nerve cell membrane. Add 1 mL 8.4% to every 10 mL lidocaine or 20 mL bupivacaine. Discard LA if precipitate forms
Adrenaline	Decreases vascular uptake through local vasoconstriction, thereby increasing duration of LA effect. Decreases peak plasma levels of lidocaine and mepivacaine. Little benefit if long-acting LAs used. Less effective in epidural than peripheral blocks. Do not exceed total dose of 200 µg in adult. Do not use for digital or penile blocks. Adding 1 mL of 1:10 000 solution (100 µg/mL) or 0.1 mL of 1:1000 solution (1 mg/mL) to 20 mL of LA produces a 1:200 000 dilution (5 µg/mL)
Clonidine	Acts on α_2 adrenergic receptors to prolong sensory and motor block and duration of postoperative analgesia. Effective in epidural, caudal, spinal, and peripheral nerve blocks. Use is limited by hypotension and sedation. Use 1–2 µg/mL
Ketamine	An NMDA receptor antagonist with weak LA properties. 0.5 mg/kg may extend and deepen caudal anaesthesia. S-ketamine has better side-effect profile
Opioids	Proven synergism with intrathecal and epidural LA. Beware delayed respiratory depression with intrathecal morphine in particular. All opioids have been used. Of doubtful benefit in peripheral blocks. Intra-articular morphine 2–5 mg in knee surgery is used in combination with LA by some surgeons. Evidence is weak for its efficacy
Glucose	Used to increase baricity of LA for intrathecal use. Hyperbaric bupivacaine contains 80 mg/mL dextrose, which allows more consistent spread of block and provides the opportunity to control spread by altering patient position. The increased baricity means it sinks, rather than rises in CSF, making it safer by preventing a high spinal block, and allowing manipulation by positioning the patient to direct the flow of anaesthetic

direct vascular injection with subsequent systemic side effects, particularly in the heart or brain.

Regional techniques

A number of benefits to regional administration exist, foremost of which is the ability to perform surgery in the absence of general anaesthesia and, hence, reduce complication rates in those at high risk (e.g. high BMI, cardiorespiratory disease). Regional anaesthesia reduces the need for airway interventions, improves analgesic control, reduces the body's surgery-induced stress responses, increases blood flow, and reduces the risk of thromboembolic events. However, some of these techniques are difficult to perform and may have higher failure rates leading to pain or nerve damage per se due to poor technique. They may also be painful when initially administered. Furthermore, blocks can lead to residual motor or sensory changes, which must be explained in the consenting process.

Peripheral nerve blockade

The principle of this technique is to produce a field of anaesthesia to a region distal to the nerve trunk that has

had its conduction blocked. One of the most common 'peripheral blocks' performed is to the femoral nerve. This block is particularly useful in total knee replacement and femoral shaft surgery for enhanced analgesia. As with many regional blocks the target nerve may be identified anatomically, with or without ultrasound, and/or by the use of a nerve stimulator. For example, the femoral nerve lies under the inguinal ligament about 1 cm lateral to the femoral artery and supplies the anterior muscles of the thigh. By means of a nerve stimulation device, the patella can be seen to contract and infusion of the local anaesthetic can remove this contraction effect, thus confirming femoral nerve blockade and analgesia. Depending on the type and location of block, a long- (e.g. **bupivacaine**) or medium-acting local anaesthetic (e.g. **lidocaine**) may be considered, with or without adjuncts to confer additional benefit (Table 8.6).

Central neural axis blockade

This includes the use of spinal anaesthesia techniques and epidural administration (Figure 8.3). Both of these techniques may be used alone or in conjunction with general anaesthesia, but their respective regions of drug site action are different; the epidural causes analgesia/

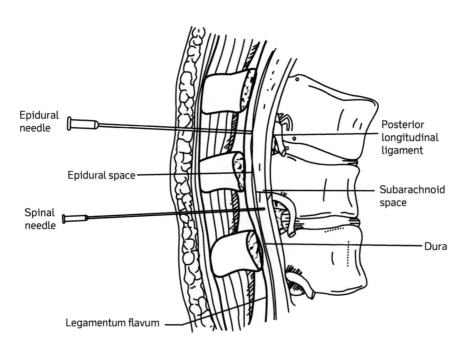

Figure 8.3 Subarachnoid and epidural spaces.

anaesthesia to nerve roots above and below the site of injection, while spinal injection within the subarachnoid space affects motor and sensory function below a spinal level (These are only performed below L2 due to the presence of nerve roots, i.e. cauda equina. Injection above L2 can cause damage to the solid spinal cord tissue present. A block, however, can be achieved up to T4 and higher for operations such as a caesarean section.)

Spinal anaesthesia

This is used most commonly for caesarean sections, inguinal hernia repairs, and perineal and lower limb surgery in those unsuitable for general anaesthesia. It involves injection of a 'heavy' local anaesthetic drug, which is administered to the subarachnoid space. The action of the drug is dependent on the baricity of the solution, posture of the patient, and the concentration of drug as it settles within the subarachnoid space. Thus, analgesia occurs bilaterally at a target spinal level, e.g. for C-section, a mid-thoracic block of T4–T6 would be desirable and achieved with 2–3.5 mL of hyperbaric **bupivacaine** with the patient supine. Continuous spinal anaesthesia is also possible where a catheter maintains drug delivery. Complications of high spinal anaesthesia drift can be serious and result in hypotension, bradycardia, and respiratory compromise.

Epidural anaesthesia

This may be used alone or in conjunction with general anaesthesia for procedure below the c-spine, and for post-operative and labour analgesia. Local anaesthetic, opioids, steroids, or combinations can be introduced to the epidural space by a catheter. The techniques can cause analgesia of sites above and below the site of injection, and thus produce segmental blockade depending on the volume and concentration of drug used. Generally, larger volumes of drug are used in epidural anaesthesia so the risks of systemic spread and drug complications exist, although this risk may be greater in spinal anaesthesia due to direct effects (e.g. hypotension, bradycardia). Furthermore, opioids around the epidural space may cause respiratory depression or puritis, but the highly synergistic effects reported with local anaesthetics combinations mean clinical use is routine and safe (Table 8.7). Differing degrees of sensory or motor analgesia may be attained with epidural anaesthesia.

Combined epidural and spinal anaesthesia can be used in labour to produce rapid effective analgesia with minimal motor blockade.

Intravenous regional anaesthesia

This techniques involves infusion of a local anaesthetic IV into an extremity that has been isolated by arterial and venous compression. Such techniques can be used in the forearm (Bier's Block), lower limb, and for sympathetic nerve blocks in chronic pain. The Biers block is most commonly used for the manipulation of minor fractures, and in forearm and hand surgery. It can only be used if the procedure is likely to last less than 30 minutes, and involves inflating a tourniquet cuff to twice the patients systolic BP and slowly injecting IV local anaesthetic (i.e. low dose **prilocaine** 0.5% or **lidocaine** 0.5%), so that motor and sensory blockade occurs within 5–10 minutes. The drug is thought to diffuse from the venous system to local nerve-ending blockade of neurotransmission. The obvious risk

Table 8.7 Epidural and local anaesthetics combinations

	Labour		Hip/knee surgery		Abdominal surgery	Thoracic surgery
Level of needle insertion	L3–L5		L3–L5		T8–T10	T5–T7
Height of block required	T8–T9	T10		T7	Relevant area	
Block type	Sensory		Motor, sensory		Sensory	Sensory
LA type concentration	Bupivacaine 0.1–0.25%	Bupivacaine 0.5%		Bupivacaine 0.25–0.5%	Bupivacaine 0.25–0.5%	
Opioid	Fentanyl		Diamorphine		Diamorphine	Diamorphine

with a Bier's block is that local anaesthetics may enter the systemic circulation and lead to cardiotoxicity. This is also why **bupivacaine**, **levobupivacaine**, and **ropivacaine** use should be avoided.

Drugs used for local anaesthesia

Ester and amide local anaesthetics

The block of Na^+ channels in nerve fibres by local anaesthetics renders them inactive, thus impeding depolarization currents and the propagation of action potentials. Examples include (esters) benzocaine, chloroprocaine, cocaine, procaine, tetracaine, and (amides) articaine, bupivacaine, levobupivacaine, lidocaine, prilocaine, and ropivacaine.

Mechanism of action

Local anaesthetics have a shared chemical structure that is made of a lipophilic aromatic ring, a link, and a hydrophilic amine group. Based on the structure of the link, they can be classified as:

- *amides* (-NH-CO-) such as **lidocaine**, **prilocaine**, **bupivacaine**, **ropivacaine**;
- *esters* (-O-CO-) e.g. **cocaine**, **procaine**, **chloroprocaine**, **tetracaine**, **benzocaine**.

Since they are weak bases, they are formulated as strong hydrochloride salts to make them soluble for injection.

It has been indicated that local anaesthetics can block Ca^{2+}, K^+, and G protein–regulated channels, but it is the blockade of Na^+ inward currents and subsequent inhibition of action potential propagation that is mainly responsible for their effects. The mechanism of action is dependent on the ionization state, predominantly delivered in the acidic form (pH 3–6), which dissociates in the relatively alkaline conditions of the perineural tissue (pH 7.4) to lipid-soluble free base. This allows these drugs to cross the cell membrane of the axon, where re-ionization occurs to the active moiety in the acidic axoplasm. In this way, they block the Na^+ channel from inside the cell *or* from the membrane lipid bilayer. When the channel is activated, ionized local anaesthetic can also gain access *via* the channel. Different types of nerve fibres demonstrate differential sensitivity to local anaesthetics, with motor fibres (e.g. type Aα) being least sensitive and type C (e.g. dorsal horn and post-ganglionic fibres) the most.

The potency and duration of action of local anaesthetic agents is linked to their lipid solubility, and the speed of onset of channel blockade is dependent on the concentration of local anaesthetic in the free base or non-ionized state (i.e. the dissociation constant (pKa) and the pH of the tissue). Alkaline conditions can accelerate the speed of onset, as the addition of bicarbonate makes the strong conjugate acidic ammonium ions dissociate and augments the concentration of the free base. In turn, intracellular diffusion of carbon dioxide makes the space inside the cell even more acidic, boosting re-ionization (a process called diffusion trapping). As such local anaesthetics are less effective when used in acidic tissues, e.g. inflamed and abscesses.

As weak bases, local anaesthetic agents become bound to $\alpha 1$-acid glycoproteins in the plasma. In turn, the site of metabolic degradation is determined by the type of drug linkage. Esters undergo fast ester hydrolysis by plasma pseudocholinesterases and thus have less potential for systemic toxicity, but an increased incidence of allergic reaction due to the formation of para-amino benzoic acid as a metabolite of hydrolysis.

Cocaine is a benzoic acid ester isolated from the leaves of *Erythroxylon coca* and employed for topical anaesthesia of the mucosa of the upper way due to its vasoconstrictor activity. It is the only local anaesthetic with vasoconstrictive properties, due to the blockade of noradrenaline re-uptake in the autonomic nervous system. **Procaine** is an ester with a slow onset and a short duration of action. In addition to its effects on Na^+ channels, it has also been shown to antagonize the function of NMDA receptors, as well as nicotinic acetylcholine receptors and the ionotropic serotonin receptor. **Cinchocaine** is an amide and one of the most potent and toxic of the long-acting local anaesthetics, thus nowadays its use is restricted largely to topical use for haemorrhoids.

Prescribing

The route of administration and clinical use of the various local anaesthetics is determined by their individual properties i.e. lipophilicity, duration of action, toxicity etc. (see Table 8.8). Due to their vasodilatory properties (with the exception of cocaine), they are sometimes administered in combination with adrenaline to produce a local vasoconstriction, to reduce blood flow and prolong anaesthetic effect.

Advantages and disadvantages

Toxicity to local anaesthetics is largely influenced by extent of systemic absorption. Topical administration of poorly absorbed anaesthetics such as **benzocaine** is

Table 8.8 Summary of properties and uses of local anaesthetics.

Local anaesthetic	Route of administration	Pharmacokinetics	Uses
Esters			
Benzocaine	Topical to mouth as gel, lozenge, or spray	Poor oral absorption	Sore throat
Cocaine	Topical (nasal spray)	Half-life prolonged by nasal spray, otherwise rapidly and extensively metabolized	Nasal spray for analgesia. Only legal route
Procaine		Medium onset and short duration of action	No longer used due to high risk of neurological toxicity
Tetracaine	Topical (spray, cream, eye drops)	Poor oral absorption with a slow onset and long duration of action	Primarily used as a topical anaesthetic applied to the oramucosa (spray), skin (cream) or eyes (drops)
Amides			
Articaine	Infiltration anaesthesia	Rapid onset and short duration of action	Dentistry in combination with adrenaline
Bupivacaine	Local infiltration, nerve block, epidural infusion and blockade	Slow onset and prolonged duration (3–9 hours) of action. Metabolized in the liver	Regional and local anaesthesia used alone or in combination with adrenaline and opioids (fentanyl)
Cinchocaine	Topical (cream)	Rapid onset and prolonged duration of action. Metabolized by esterases in plasma and liver	Haemorrhoids, either alone or in combination with a corticosteroid
Levobupivacaine	As for bupivacaine	As for bupivacaine	As for bupivacaine, but less cardiotoxic
Lidocaine	Topical (cream, sprays, gels, lozenges, patches), regional anaesthesia, nerve block, and local infiltration	Rapid onset and medium duration of action	Most widely used local anaesthetic for numerous indications including haemorrhoids, nerve pain (patch), dental pain, and regional and local anaesthesia. Used alone and in combination with other local anaesthetics or adrenaline. Lidocaine is also administered intravenously for the treatment of ventricular arrythmias
Mepivacaine	Infiltration anaesthesia and nerve block	Rapid onset and medium duration of action	Dentistry
Prilocaine	Topical (cream), local infiltration and nerve block	Medium onset and duration of action	Topical, regional, and local anaesthesia. Avoided in obstetrics due to risk of methaemoglobinaemias in infants
Ropivacaine	As for bupivacaine	Slow absorption and prolonged duration of action	As for bupivacaine with less cardiotoxicity and reduced potency

therefore generally well tolerated, although it may cause local irritation or hypersensitivity reactions. The risk of hypersensitivity reactions is higher with the ester-type anaesthetics than the amides.

Systemic toxicity most commonly affects well-perfused organs, thus increasing the risk of cardiac or neurological toxicity. The risk is greatest following inadvertent IV administration, delayed absorption from a depot, or when applied topically to broken or damaged skin. Topical agents should not therefore be applied to damaged/broken skin. The ester-type local anaesthetics are rapidly hydrolysed in the blood by cholinesterases thus have a short half-life, although the amides are metabolized in the liver so that the risk of toxicity is increased in hepatic impairment.

Cardiac toxicity

Local anaesthetics cause peripheral vasodilation and depress the cardiac action potential leading to hypotension, bradycardia, arrhythmias, and in severe cases, cardiac arrest. The risk of cardiac toxicity is high with **bupivacaine** due to its high lipid solubility and protein-binding capacity, which means it has a high affinity for binding to cardiac tissue. Despite this, bupivacaine is commonly used and well tolerated, but should be employed with caution IV in at-risk groups. The risk of cardiotoxicity is lower with **levobupivacaine** and **ropivacaine**, making them possible alternatives in high risk patients. Conversely, the use of adjunctive IV **adrenaline** in patients with cardiac disease is best avoided. As stated above, and unlike other agents, **cocaine** has a vasoconstrictive effect as it inhibits noradrenaline re-uptake.

Neurological toxicity

Neurological toxicity to local anaesthetics varies with serum levels, so that they produce a depressive effect at low levels and an excitatory effect at high levels. Depressive effects commonly present as a feeling of light-headedness, peri-oral tingling, and sedation, but in more severe cases can lead to loss of consciousness. Excitatory effects lead to agitation, restlessness, convulsions, and respiratory depression. The risk of neurological toxicity is especially great with **procaine**, thus its use has been largely superseded by other agents such as **lidocaine**. **Cocaine** can produce excitatory effects at lower doses and is not widely used.

Methaemoglobinaemia

High dose of some local anaesthetics (e.g. **prilocaine** and **benzocaine**) can induce methaemoglobinaemia, leading to shortness of breath and cyanosis. In more severe cases, patients can develop dysrhythmias and seizures, leading to coma and even death. Rapid identification and management with **methylthioninium chloride** is essential to reverse the effects of excessive methaemoglobin.

Overdose

At very high doses, local anaesthetics cause profound respiratory depression, which requires urgent treatment with assisted ventilation. **Naloxone** can also help reverse respiratory depression where concomitant opioids have been administered. In patients that present with seizures the treatment of choice is with **thiopental**, **propofol**, or a benzodiazepine such as **diazepam**. A bolus dose and infusion of **intralipid®** can also reverse both severe cardiovascular and neurological toxicity associated with local anaesthetic overdose. It is thought to work by binding to excessive circulating local anaesthetic due to their lipophilic nature, thereby reducing free-circulating levels.

PRESCRIBING WARNING

Local anaesthetics and adrenaline as adjunctive therapy

- Do not exceed body weight dose calculations for local anaesthetic administration:
  - Lidocaine (max without adrenaline 3 mg/kg, with adrenaline 7 mg/kg).
  - Bupivacaine (max 2 mg/kg).
  - Prilocaine (max 6 mg/kg).
- Adrenaline is used as an adjunct with a local anaesthetic for its vasoconstrictive effect this increases systemic absorption allowing for higher doses to be administered.
- Care should be taken to avoid IV administration and exceeding maximum doses.
- Co-administration of adrenaline should be avoided in cardiac disease due to the risk of hypertension or arrhythmias.

Further reading

Allman K, Wilson I (2015) *Oxford Handbook of Anaesthesia*, 4th edn. Oxford: Oxford University Press.

Beecroft C, Davies G (2013) Systemic toxic effects of local anaesthetics. *Anaesthesia and Intensive Care* 14(4), 146–8.

Columb MO, Hartley R (2014) Local anaesthetic agents. *Anaesthesia and Intensive Care* 15(2), 3–87.

Neal JM, Bernardscm, Hadzic A, et al. (2008). ASRA practice advisory on neurologic complications in regional anesthesia and pain medicine. *Regional Anesthesia and Pain Medicine* 33, 404–15.

Scholz A (2002) Mechanisms of (local) anaesthetics on voltage-gated sodium and other ion channels. *British Journal of Anaesthesia* 89, 52–61.

Scott NB. (2010) Wound infiltration for surgery [Review]. *Anaesthesia* 65(Suppl. 1), 67–75.

Sinatra RS, Froicu DB (2010) In: *Regional anesthesia complications in anesthesia emergencies* Ruskin K, Rosenbaum S (Eds). Oxford: Oxford University Press.

Spoors C, Kiff K (2010) *Training in Anaesthesia.* Oxford: Oxford University Press.

Subramaniam S, Tennant M (2005) A concise review of the basic biology and pharmacology of local analgesia. *Australian Dental Journal* 50(2), S23–30.

Guidelines

AAGBI Safety Guideline: The management of severe local anaesthetic toxicity (2010) http://www.aagbi.org/sites/default/files/la_toxicity_2010_0.pdf [accessed 5 April 2019].

8.3 Analgesia and pain management

Pain is an unpleasant sensory and emotional experience associated with actual or potential tissue damage, or described in terms of such damage. As such, it is a very personal event that may be subjective and based on an individual's perceptions. It is a complex phenomenon and not a linear, hard-wired, stimulation–response system, but influenced by central and peripheral neuroplasticity (e.g. phantom limb pain). It can, however, be broadly categorized under two main headings:

- Nociceptive pain: caused by trauma and injury.
- Neuropathic pain: caused by lesions or damage to the somatosensory system (i.e. nerves; e.g. diabetic neuropathy, disc prolapse).

The former is often a direct response to unpleasant stimuli and is commonly acute in onset (e.g. treading on a tack), but can be chronic, continuing for greater than 3 months (e.g. osteoarthritis). Nociceptive pain may be further subdivided according to the tissues that receives certain pain detecting fibres, and clues can be given to the origin of pain based on clinical history (e.g. in acute appendicitis).

Prescribers are more likely to be asked to treat pain than any other medical condition, with almost 21% of all people experiencing pain of some degree and 70% of them seeking medical advice and intervention. Within the community there is approximately 7% prevalence of neuropathic pain, which may be peripheral (e.g. trigeminal neuralgia, post-surgical pain or cancer-related pain) or central (e.g. stroke, MS) in origin. In general, pain is poorly managed, which can lead to long-term consequences on personal health and socioeconomic function, through decreased physical activity, insomnia, and depression.

Pathophysiology

Peripheral organs (e.g. bowel, skin) are innervated by *sensory nerve fibres*, which following noxious stimuli can send signals from the periphery to the brain. Mechanical, chemical, or thermal events increase action potential firing of these peripheral nerve fibres, projecting along ascending spinal cord tracts to thalamus and other brain regions. Two main classes of pain fibres exist peripherally and are termed the C-fibre, which is non-myelinated and slow conducting (0.5–2.0 m/s), and the Aδ-fibre, which is thin, myelinated and, hence, rapidly conducting (e.g. 3.0–30 m/s). During a stimulus, such as a burn, it is the Aδ-fibres that respond rapidly and are perceived as sharp localized pain, the C-fibres are also activated and generate the perception of a dull and more diffuse pain.

The cell bodies of these primary fibres, and those of visceral and muscle afferents, lie within the *dorsal root ganglia* where they connect to secondary afferents that can act as a 'gate'. The exact position of this synapse is variable, and stratified across the dorsal horn of the spinal cord, so that Aδ-fibres tend to synapse in the laminas I and V, while C-fibres synapse in I, II, and V; laminae I and V tend to be the main site of ascending pathways. Transmission within the dorsal horn involves numerous transmitters, which includes glutamate, substance P, and nitric oxide. Short interneurons that lie in lamina II and project to laminae I and V, constitute dense regions of opioid receptor expression. They are the source of modulation in ascending pathways, acting as an inhibitory gate up the spinothalamic tract. Other receptors are expressed in the region (i.e. 5-HT, adenosine, glycine, gamma-amino butyric acid (GABA), neurokinin-1, and α_2-adrenoreceptors), which may also modulate pain transmission.

Another important modulating influence in the 'gating' of pain transmission are the *descending pathways*. These project down from midbrain structures, peri-aqueductal grey, and nucleus raphe magnus, along the dorsolateral funiculus of the spinal cord, to form serotoninergic and noradrenergic synapses with the dorsal horn neurons, thus inhibiting pain pathways. These descending pathways are further sites of encephalin, serotonergic transmission, and expression of α_2-adrenoceptors; the latter may cause pain inhibition through sympathetic drive (i.e. the adrenaline of traumatic injury acting as an analgesic).

This arrangement of peripheral and spinal neurons, as well as being a feedback-gated system, is also significantly modulated by neuronal plasticity. One such phenomenon that modulates the pathway is *sensitization*, where a normally innocuous stimulus is interpreted as a heightened pain perception (i.e. allodynia). Within primary neurons, peripheral tissue damage or inflammation, and subsequent release of local mediators like substance P, ATP, bradykinin, and acidosis, can lower the thresholds of neuronal firing, thereby increasing the activity of *ascending pathways*. This enhanced ectopic firing is mediated through changes in Na^+ and Ca^{2+} flux, with the latter being targets for neuropathic agents like **gabapentin**. Enhanced firing from the primary neuron subsequently leads to increased release of glutamate and glycine, which may act on post-synaptic NMDA receptors of second order neurons. These ionotropic receptors are normally blocked by Mg^{2+}, but following augmented stimulation via other glutamate receptor channels, the subsequent intracellular depolarization leads to removal of the Mg^{2+} block. This, in turn, allows persistent and intense Ca^{2+} fluxes so that heightened ascending pain signalling occurs. This persistent abnormal stimulation leads to massive excitation, termed '*wind-up*' and is another mechanism involved in allodynia and the pathophysiology of neuropathic pain. Interestingly, potentiation of the post-synaptic pathway occurs with associated enhanced NO signalling and long-term changes in gene transcription, together with the reduction in the influence of inhibitory descending [e.g. serotonergic, noradrenergic (namely monoaminergic)] pathways. Much of the opioid action in pain relief is at primary presynaptic receptors, or at post-synaptic secondary receptors and is effective for simple pain. However, when a stimulus is strong, prolonged, or unusual and wind-up occurs, the effectiveness of opioids on the pathway are diminished, i.e. wind-up break through occurs.

Ascending pain pathways enter a complex pain matrix within the brain that is modulated by many other neural pathways, so that different levels of cognitive processing, mood and arousal states alter pain status, and make perception complex and diverse between individuals. However, key areas include the primary and secondary somatosensory cortex, prefrontal cortex, and thalamus.

Inflammatory mediators

To this end, there are multiple sites that may be targeted to modulate pain stimulus initiation, its transmission, and its subsequent central perception. At the local site of a stimulus (mechanical, thermal, or chemical), nociceptor stimulation is modulated by the presence of inflammatory mediators. Here, arachidonic acid (AA) up-regulates cyclo-oxygenase 2 (COX-2), an inducible form of the enzyme that converts AA to metabolites, including prostaglandin E2, prostaglandin G2, and prostaglandin H2. These prostaglandins lower the activation threshold of primary neurons, so inhibition of COX-2 with NSAIDs can reduce sensitization and inflammatory causes of pain. (Hence, the usefulness of NSAIDs, like **ibuprofen**, **diclofenac**, and **naproxen** in chronic inflammatory pain conditions.) Unfortunately, these non-specific NSAIDs also act at COX-1, which is a constitutive form that is located in many tissues (e.g. gastric mucosa) and cells (e.g. platelets), and can lead to a propensity of gastric ulcers and bleeding. There are specific COX-2 inhibitors (see 'NSAIDs/COX inhibitors'). The action of **paracetamol**, although poorly understood, appears to be upon the central and peripheral nervous system by inhibiting COX in a non-classical way (see 'Paracetamol'). Transmission of the pain stimulus to the spinal cord can also be modulated directly by introduction of local anaesthetics (see Topic 8.2, 'Local anaesthetics') so action potential propagation is reduced.

Therapeutic opioids

The therapeutic opioids are class agonists that act with differential activity at three transmembrane receptor subtypes—mu (μ), kappa (κ), and delta (δ). μ receptors are located in spinal and supraspinal regions (see 'Pathophysiology') and are responsible for analgesia, changes in respiratory rate and the feeling of euphoria. κ receptor types are also located spinally, and are responsible for analgesia and sedative effects, whereas δ receptor subtype acts to modulate the activity of μ receptors, potentiating spinal analgesia. All these receptor subtypes are G protein–linked and lead to a decrease in cAMP and K$^+$ fluxes, so that neurons are less likely to fire action potentials. Within the raphe magnus, μ receptor activation can also reduce GABA signalling onto descending serotonergic fibres (disinhibition) so augmentation of gating in the dorsal horn occurs and ascending pain signals are reduced. Further opioid receptors are centrally located (e.g. ε in the medulla, which modulate the descending pathways) and may be targets of opioid analgesia. The endogenous ligand, β-endorphin, is equipotent at all opioid receptor subtypes, but other opioid peptides show subtype preference (e.g. enkephlins for δ, dynorphins for κ). The exogenous opioid ligands also show receptor specificity and differential action. **Morphine** and **codeine**, for instance are full agonists acting primarily at μ, with weak activity at δ and κ. Interestingly, κ receptors can antagonize the action of μ-induced analgesia, so certain ligands (e.g. **buprenorphine**) with mixed agonist action at μ and antagonism at κ, potentially augment their own analgesic action. Other ligands, such as **tramadol** and **methadone**, have diverse action at both μ receptors, and also inhibit noradrenaline and serotonin uptake, thus are of benefit in some people insensitive to codeine.

Tolerance

This diversity of action of opiate drugs can be helpful, or troublesome when tolerance to certain ligands occurs and pain is poorly managed. *Tolerance* occurs when an increasing plasma concentration of drug is required for the same level of analgesic effect. It happens as a consequence of cellular adaptation, so that decreased levels of cAMP, from receptor activation, are overcome by gene up-regulation and increased synthesis of adenylate cyclase and G proteins. Some opiates show a great degree of 'cross-talk' so when tolerance to one drug occurs, the patient may be equally tolerant of another; so doses may need to be raised or an alternative opiate found.

A further site of action that can be modulated to produce analgesia is the monoaminergic descending inhibitory fibres, where tricyclic antidepressants, such as **amitriptyline**, and serotonin-noradrenaline reuptake inhibitors, such as **duloxetine**, can augment the gating process to reduce ascending pain signals; these are particularly useful in neuropathic and complex chronic pain where central effects can help by raising mood.

For a full summary of the relevant pathways and drug targets, see Figure 8.4.

Management

Acute pain

Acute pain management is most commonly indicated peri-operatively or following trauma, and when managed well can lead to reduced analgesic consumption, fewer side effects, and earlier discharge from hospital. More specifically, patients admitted for elective surgery (e.g. orthopaedic surgery) are increasingly being treated according to enhanced recovery pathways, with the aim of optimizing pain control, and thereby reducing the time to mobilization and discharge.

Prior to initiating analgesia, consideration should be given to the site and severity of pain, previous effective analgesia and any allergies or co-morbidities that the patient may have. Pain is best assessed using a pain scale, of which there are many. In most cases, a score of 0–10 is used, where 0 is defined as no pain and 10 the worst pain imaginable. A score of 7 or more is considered to be severe pain. The WHO analgesic ladder provides a useful starting point when initiating analgesia (see Figure 8.5). In all cases, pain relief should be administered orally, where possible, starting with the lowest effective dose and administered 'by the clock', to prevent breakthrough pain associated with on demand treatment.

Mild pain will usually respond to treatment with simple analgesia (**paracetamol** and NSAIDs) unless contraindicated, in which case a weak opioid may be necessary. In patients with moderate to severe pain, weak (e.g. **codeine**, **dihydrocodeine**) or strong opioids (e.g. **morphine**, **fentanyl**, **oxycodone**) should always be used in combination with simple analgesics in a multi-modal approach. In this way, pain control is optimized, while side effects are minimized. Where patients fail to respond to first-line options, adjuvant or targeted therapies, such as antidepressants, anti-epileptics, or local anaesthetics may be appropriate. While on analgesia, patients will require regular assessment of pain relief and side effects, so treatment may be optimized and side effects appropriately managed, e.g. dyspepsia, constipation, sickness, etc.

For acute severe pain in the prehospital and emergency department environment, **ketamine** is an option for analgesia-sedation (Topic 8.1, 'General anaesthesia'). It produces dissociative anaesthesia, and is characterized by a trance-like state and amnesia, making it particularly useful for short, but painful procedures (e.g. reduction of fractures/dislocations) especially with its relatively short half-life (~15 minutes). In specialist hands, low-dose ketamine is also an option for chronic pain management.

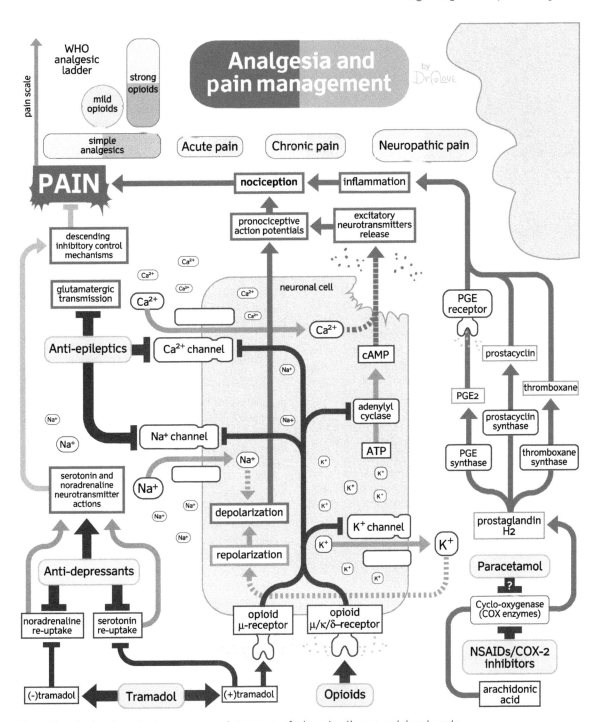

Figure 8.4 Analgesia and pain management: summary of relevant pathways and drug targets.

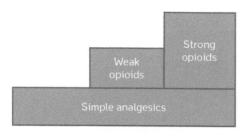

Figure 8.5 World Health Organization analgesic ladder.
Adapted from World Health Organization analgesic ladder.
© Copyright World Health Organization (WHO), 2016.

Chronic pain

Managing chronic pain is considerably more challenging than acute pain, due to its complex nature. As well as determining severity, type, and site of pain, assessments should consider the impact of chronic pain on emotional and physical function. Patients may benefit from psychological input, such as pain management programmes (including self-help) or tailored physical therapy. In all instances, therapy should be adapted to patient needs, ensuring that they are actively involved in any decisions made. There are numerous non-pharmacological interventions that can be of benefit and include *transcutaneous electrical nerve stimulation (TENS)*, implantable stimulators (e.g. peripheral nerve stimulators and spinal cord stimulators), and surgical neurolysis.

In terms of pharmacological management, the WHO analgesic ladder provides a useful starting point, despite the fact it was neither developed, nor adequately assessed for use in chronic pain. As with acute pain, doses should be started at the lowest effective dose and titrated up to response. Response to treatment in terms of efficacy and side effects can vary considerably between individuals, due either to the nature of the pain or genetic factors. For this reason, switching between drugs within a class (e.g. opioids) may be of benefit when the first fails to produce the desired response, with any ineffective treatment discontinued.

When prescribing analgesia for chronic pain management, consideration should also be given to toxicity associated with prolonged treatment. In particular, the risk of cardiovascular (myocardial infarction, stroke), GI (GI bleed, perforation), and renal toxicity is increased with chronic NSAID use. The risks of treatment should therefore be carefully weighed up against the benefits, and a PPI considered for gastro-protection. Chronic use of opioids for the purpose of pain relief is associated with an increase in the risk of addiction.

Neuropathic pain

Neuropathic pain can be an acute or, more commonly, a chronic phenomenon. As well as responding to more conventional therapy with opioids, a number of other drugs are advocated both within and outside of their license to manage neuropathic pain (i.e. antidepressants and anti-epileptics). Patients requiring pharmacological treatment should be offered **amitriptyline**, **duloxetine**, **gabapentin**, or **pregabalin** as first-line options, whereas **carbamazepine** may be useful for the management of trigeminal neuralgia. Drugs should be tried sequentially, titrated to optimal doses to establish the lowest effective dose and, where ineffective, a second agent introduced before the first drug is weaned and discontinued. In some instances, combination therapy may be necessary, although the evidence for this is somewhat lacking.

Complex regional pain syndrome

In complex regional pain syndrome (CRPS), patients suffer prolonged pain that is out of proportion to the initiating event and it is often reported as a burning, sharp, or 'electric shock'. It does not, however, relate to a specific dermatome or nerve distribution, is regional and associated with sensory, motor, autonomic, skin, and bone abnormalities. Its management is complex and involves both non-pharmacological and pharmacological methods. CRPS is normally managed by pain specialists and can include interventions such as physiotherapy and occupational therapy, with adjunct pharmacological interventions such as corticosteroids, bisphosphonates, tricyclic antidepressants, **gabapentin**, or other anticonvulsants, topical local anaesthetics or sympathetic nerve blocks.

Drug classes used in management

Paracetamol

Paracetamol, also known as acetaminophen, increases the pain threshold via indirect inhibition of cyclooxygenases, but has neither anti-inflammatory properties nor effect on platelet function.

Mechanism of action

Cyclo-oxygenase is the first enzyme involved in the conversion of arachidonic acid to prostaglandins, thromboxanes, and prostacyclin. Prostaglandins and PGE_2, in particular, are mediators of pain and inflammation. **Paracetamol** is an effective analgesic, but lacks anti-inflammatory actions, indicative of a restricted action in the central and peripheral nervous system. It has been suggested that, although paracetamol has no affinity for the active site of cyclo-oxygenase, it blocks activity by reducing the active oxidized form of cyclo-oxygenase to its inactive resting state. Inhibition would therefore be more effective under reducing conditions (low peroxide concentration). This might explain the selectivity of paracetamol for nerves, which actively reduce intracellular oxidation due to their high sensitivity to oxidants.

COX-3, a splice variant of COX-1, has been defined as a centrally located enzyme with a possible role in fever, and might be the molecular target for the mechanism of action of paracetamol. However, the clinical relevance of this is not yet clear.

Prescribing

Paracetamol can be administered orally, rectally, and more recently, IV. Oral paracetamol is widely available over the counter, sold in numerous formulations including tablets, capsules, caplets, soluble tablets, and liquid. Care should be taken to ensure patients do not exceed the maximum daily dose of 4 g/day by any route with consideration given to the possibility of self-medicating with paracetamol prior to seeking help. Where administered IV, a weight-based dose of 15 mg/kg/dose is recommended in patients under 50 kg.

Unwanted effects

Paracetamol is well tolerated within the maximum recommended dose of 4 g/day, with few reported side effects. It undergoes extensive hepatic metabolism with renal excretion and in overdose (greater than 15 g/day) causes significant and even fatal hepatic toxicity (see 'Prescribing warning: paracetamol overdose'). Despite this, it remains preferable to many analgesics for use in hepatic impairment, so long as the maximum dose is not exceeded.

PRESCRIBING WARNING

Paracetamol overdose

- Paracetamol accounts for the highest incidence of drug related overdoses, in part linked to ease of accessibility.
- Overdose is usually associated with an acute ingestion of excessive quantities, either intentionally or non-intentionally.
- Acetylcysteine can be administered up to 24 hours after ingestion, as three consecutive IV infusions in patients whose serum paracetamol levels exceed the recommended treatment line as advised by the MHRA.
- Increasingly chronic ingestion of paracetamol is being attributed to a higher risk of toxicity (e.g. cardiovascular, GI) than previously thought.

NSAIDs/COX 2 inhibitors

NSAIDs come from a wide range of chemical classes sharing anti-pyretic, anti-inflammatory, anti-uricaemic, and analgesic properties. This is attained via inhibition of COX-1 and COX-2. Examples include celecoxib, diclofenac, etodolac, etoricoxib, fenoprofen, flurbiprofen, ibuprofen, indometacin, ketoprofen, mefenamic acid, meloxicam, naproxen, piroxicam, and sulindac.

Mechanism of action

The blockade of prostaglandin production is intimately linked with the anti-nociceptive, anti-inflammatory, and anti-pyretic effects of NSAIDs. Inhibition of COX, however, can not only reduce inflammatory prostaglandin synthesis, but also decreases other eicosanoids with a protective physiological function, such as in platelets, the intestinal mucosa, and kidney; giving rise to a number of potentially severe adverse effects. Since the different types of NSAIDs have variable degrees of effects on each COX isoenzyme, they have diverse anti-inflammatory and adverse effects. Strategies to prevent these problems have included COX-inhibiting nitric oxide donors and compounds that can target COX-2 and thromboxane A2 receptors.

The adverse effects are mainly associated with the effects on constitutively expressed COX, and thus the

Table 8.9 Relative risks of major vascular events with coxibs and non-selective NSAIDs compared with placebo.

Regimen	Major vascular events (95% CI)	Major coronary events (95% CI)	Stroke (95% CI)	Hospitalization for heart failure (95% CI)
Coxibs	1.37 (1.14–1.66)	1.76 (1.31–2.37)	1.09 (0.78–1.52)	2.28 (1.62–3.20)
Naproxen	0.93 (0.69–1.27)	0.84 (0.52–1.35)	0.97 (0.59–1.60)	1.87 (1.10–3.16)
Diclofenac	1.41 (1.12–1.78)	1.70 (1.19–2.41)	1.18 (0.79–1.78)	1.85 (1.17–2.94)
Ibuprofen	1.44 (0.89–2.33)	2.22 (1.10–4.48)	0.97 (0.42–2.24)	2.49 (1.19–5.20)

Adapted from Michael Doherty et al. *Oxford Textbook of Osteoarthritis and Crystal Arthropathy, Third Edition*, Oxford, UK: Oxford University Press © 2016. Reproduced with permission of the Licensor through PLSclear.

incidence of renal impairment and gastric erosion is linked to inhibition of COX-1. The COX-2 specific antagonists (coxibs), however, have a relatively higher rate of cardiovascular complications that limits their clinical use, with only **celecoxib** and **etoricoxib** still available. The relative risks of major vascular events are outlined in Table 8.9.

Beyond the effects on COX inhibition, other biological targets have been suggested to contribute to the action of NSAIDs, such as the prostanoid DP_2-receptor, the multidrug-resistance protein MRP_4, which can transport prostaglandins, and peroxisome proliferator-activated receptors α and Y. More recently, evidence is also accumulating that NSAIDs include the endo-cannabinoid system in their analgesic actions, which might lead to the development of novel endocannabinoid-preferring COX inhibitors.

Prescribing

The efficacy of NSAIDs and other analgesics at different doses have been compared in work published by the Oxford Pain Group, in the Oxford League Table for analgesics in acute pain. Efficacy is based on the number of patients needed to treat (NNT) for one to achieve a 50% reduction in pain (see Table 8.10). NSAIDs compare favourably to other analgesics, although there are marked variations in the number of patients that were compared to derive an NNT value. Furthermore, the table does not take into consideration factors such as formulation or pain setting. Despite these limitations, the work does help to demonstrate the relative efficacy of NSAIDs for a given dose.

Unwanted effects

For more information see Topic 7.1, 'Osteoarthritis'.

Opioids

Opioids are the oldest and most potent drugs used for the treatment of severe pain. They act on opioid receptors, leading to the inhibition of sensory neuron excitability and pro-inflammatory neuropeptide release. Examples include weak (codeine, dihydrocodeine, meptazinol) and strong (alfentanil, buprenorphine diamorphine, fentanyl, methadone, morphine, oxycodone, pethidine, remifentanil, tapentadol).

Mechanism of action

Opioids act on heptahelical G protein–coupled receptors that are grouped in three different types—μ, δ, and κ. They are located and can be stimulated at all levels of the neural axis, including peripheral and central processes of primary sensory neurons (nociceptors), spinal cord (interneurons, projection neurons), brainstem, midbrain, and cortex. Opioid receptors couple to G proteins (Gi/Go), and promote the inhibition of adenylyl cyclase and/or opening of rectifying K^+ channels. This ultimately leads to decreased neuronal activity and the inhibition of action potential propagation in second order projection neurons. In addition, blockade of Ca^{2+} influx prevents the release of excitatory neurotransmitters that are pronociceptive. Opioids can also inhibit tetrodotoxin-resistant Na^+ channels, TRPV1 channels, and glutamate-evoked excitatory post-synaptic currents in the spinal cord.

Endogenous ligands are derived from the precursors of pro-opiomelanocortin, proenkephalin, and prodynorphin, which contain the 'opioid motif' at their amino terminals. Since they are susceptible to rapid enzymatic degradation once released, enkephalinase inhibitors have shown early promise as potent analgesic effectors in animal models and small human trials.

Table 8.10 Analgesics in acute pain

Analgesic	Dose	Number of patients in comparison	Percentage with at least 50% pain relief	NNT
Etoricoxib	180/240 mg	248	77	1.5 (1.3–1.7)
Etoricoxib	100/120 mg	500	70	1.6 (1.5–1.8)
Valdecoxib	40 mg	473	73	1.6 (1.4–1.8)
Ibuprofen	800 mg	76	100	1.6 (1.3–2.2)
Ketorolac	20 mg	69	57	1.8 (1.4–2.5)
Ketorolac (IM)	60 mg	116	56	1.8 (1.5–2.3)
Rofecoxib	50 mg	1900	63	1.9 (1.8–2.1)
Diclofenac	100 mg	411	67	1.9 (1.6–2.2)
Piroxicam	40 mg	30	80	1.9 (1.2–4.3)
Paracetamol/codeine	1000 mg/60 mg	197	57	2.1 (1.7–2.5)
Diclofenac	50 mg	738	63	2.3 (2.0–2.7)
Naproxen	440 mg	257	50	2.3 (2.0–2.9)
Ibuprofen	600 mg	203	79	2.4 (2.0–4.2)
Ibuprofen	400 mg	4703	56	2.4 (2.3–2.6)
Aspirin	1200 mg	279	61	2.4 (1.9–3.2)
Ketorolac	10 mg	790	50	2.6 (2.3–3.1)
Ibuprofen	200 mg	1414	45	2.7 (2.5–3.1)
Piroxicam	20 mg	280	63	2.7 (2.1–3.8)
Diclofenac	25 mg	204	54	2.8 (2.1–4.3)
Tramadol	150 mg	561	48	2.9 (2.4–3.6)
Morphine (IM)	10 mg	946	50	2.9 (2.6–3.6)
Paracetamol	500 mg	561	61	3.5 (2.2–13.3)
Paracetamol	1000 mg	2759	46	3.8 (3.4–4.4)
Codeine	60 mg	1305	15	16.7 (11–48)

The 2007 Oxford League table of Analgesic Efficacy. Copyright © 1994–2007 Bandolier.

The functional outcome of opioid receptor stimulation is the overall decreased transmission of nociceptive stimuli along the neural axis, and a profound reduction in the perception of pain. All opioid receptors mediate analgesia, but differ in their evoked side effects:

- μ-opioid receptors mediate respiratory depression, sedation, reward/euphoria, nausea, urinary retention, biliary spam, and constipation.

- κ-opioid receptors mediate dysphoric, aversive, sedative, and diuretic effects.

- δ-opioids mediate reward/euphoria, respiratory depression, and constipation.

Although immunosuppressive effects have been proposed, they have not been supported by clinical studies. The most widely available opioid drugs, **morphine**, **codeine**, **methadone**, **fentanyl**, and derivatives are agonists at μ-opioid receptors. Mixed agonists/antagonists, such as **buprenorphine** may act as agonists at low doses and as antagonists at higher doses. Novel ligands, which act exclusively in the periphery, are being developed using hydrophilic compounds with minimal ability to cross the blood–brain barrier (e.g. **loperamide**).

Prescribing

For the purpose of prescribing, opioids are broadly classed into weak (**codeine, dihydrocodeine, meptazinol**) and strong (**morphine, diamorphine, oxycodone, pethidine, fentanyl, buprenorphine, methadone**), with morphine being the most widely used. The strong agents that are pure opioid agonists lack the maximum doses seen with the weaker opioids, or those with mixed effects such as **tapentadol**.

Alfentanil, **remifentanil**, and **fentanyl** are most commonly used IV to optimize the effects of anaesthetics peri-operatively, although fentanyl patches in combination with sublingual tablets are useful in chronic pain with breakthrough symptoms.

In palliative care dose equivalents for opioids may need to be converted/calculated in order to optimize pain relief and route of administration, i.e. use of a syringe driver. For further information, see Table 8.11 and refer to NICE CG140.

> **PRESCRIBING WARNING**
>
> **Codeine metabolism**
> The ability to metabolize codeine to its active metabolite morphine, varies considerably between individuals so that:
> - Ultra-fast metabolizers are at increased risk of toxicity.
> - Slow metabolizers are less likely to respond.

Table 8.11 Opioids and route of administration.

Opioid	Route of administration	Pharmacokinetics	Uses
Alfentanil (predominantly μ receptors agonist)	IV	Rapid onset of action, faster than fentanyl. Hepatic metabolism and renal excretion	Peri-operative analgesia
Buprenorphine (partial μ agonist)	SL, TD, IM, IV	Onset of action varies with route of administration but generally slow. Undergoes extensive first pass metabolism hence SL administration	Acute and chronic pain. Treatment of addiction
Codeine	PO, IM	Weak analgesic, but metabolized to morphine, extent depending on status (see 'Prescribing warning: codeine metabolism')	Mild to moderate pain relief. Usually administered orally
Dihydrocodeine	PO, SC, IM	More potent analgesic than codeine, but metabolite less effective. More predictable activity	Mild to moderate pain relief. Usually administered orally
Diamorphine (predominantly μ, some κ agonist activity)	IV, SC, IM, IN, IT, Epid	Rapid onset of action, faster than morphine and more rapidly penetrates CNS. Half-life of 2–3 minutes (although has potent metabolites, including morphine). Metabolized in the liver and excreted via the kidneys	Favoured in syringe drivers for palliative care due to good solubility, allowing for high doses in small volumes

Table 8.11 Continued

Opioid	Route of administration	Pharmacokinetics	Uses
Fentanyl (predominantly μ, some κ and δ agonist activity)	TD, SL, IV	Rapid onset of action following IV administration, but rapidly metabolized, mainly in the liver, so plasma levels decrease rapidly	Peri-operative analgesia, also in chronic pain (patch) with acute (sublingual) use
Meptazinol (partial agonist on μ, lesser extent on κ and δ)	PO, IM, IV	Rapid onset of action following IV administration. Hepatic metabolism and renal clearance. Potency limited by partial agonist effects.	Moderate pain relief
Methadone (predominantly μ, some κ and δ)	PO, SC, IM	Slow onset of action and long half-life (12–18 hours), extended with regular dosing. Hepatic metabolism and renal clearance	Severe pain, cough in terminal disease and treatment of addiction
Morphine (predominantly μ, some κ agonist activity)	PO, SC, IM, IV, PR	Moderate onset of action following IV administration. Hepatic metabolism and clearance largely renal, but some (10%) in the bile	Acute and chronic pain, widely used
Oxycodone (μ, κ and δ agonist)	PO, SC, IV	Hepatic metabolism, excreted via the kidney and bile. Good oral bioavailability compared to morphine (80%)	Acute and chronic pain
Pethidine (predominantly μ agonist)	PO, SC, IM, IV	Short duration of action and associated with atropine-like effects. Accumulates in renal and hepatic impairment causing convulsions	Acute and chronic pain, administered by midwives in childbirth.
Remifentanil (μ agonist)	IV infusion	Onset of action comparable to alfentanil however rapidly metabolized in the blood to a weakly active metabolite so unlikely to accumulate in renal or hepatic impairment	Peri-operative analgesia
Tapentadol (μ agonist and inhibits noradrenaline reuptake)	PO	Rapid onset of action (20–40 minutes) following oral administration. Hepatic metabolism and renal excretion	Moderate to severe acute pain

Epid, epidurally; IM, intramuscular; IN, intranasal; IT, intrathecal; IV, intravenous; PO, oral; PR, rectal; SC, subcutaneous; SL, sublingual; TD transdermal.

Unwanted effects

On the whole, side effects to the different opioids are largely comparable, with slight variances based on their affinity for the different opioid receptor types, and the presence of other mechanisms of action. Other factors affecting tolerance include oral bioavailability, duration of action, route of administration and route of elimination, which can affect drug handling, and the risk of accumulation in renal or hepatic impairment. Orally administered drugs tend to be more likely to cause nausea and vomiting than those administered by other routes. Drugs with a prolonged duration of action tend to cause less sedative or euphoric effects associated with peak levels, e.g. **methadone**. For this reason, methadone is the drug of choice in the management of opioid withdrawal (see Topic 10.4, 'Drug abuse: addiction and dependency').

Gastrointestinal

GI side effects (nausea, vomiting, constipation, and dry mouth) are the most common side effects seen with opioid therapy, associated with action on μ and δ receptors, which leads to reduced GI motility. Although nausea and vomiting tend to subside with use, constipation will persist and requires proactive management, particularly with high or prolonged doses, ideally with a stimulant laxative. Post-operatively opioids are commonly prescribed with anti-emetics to reduce the risk of post-operative nausea and vomiting, probably aggravated where opioids are used peri-operatively.

Neurological

Neurological toxicity, such as drowsiness, confusion, and dizziness, also common with opioid therapy, tends to be dose related and become less pronounced with prolonged exposure. Less commonly, opioids can precipitate mood changes and hallucinations, linked to action on κ receptors.

Respiratory

Respiratory depression can be especially problematic with opioid use. Linked with μ receptor activity, opioids act to reduce respiratory rate and decrease sensitivity to increased CO_2 levels. This is more pronounced when used in combination with IV anaesthetic agents. Effects can occur at normal therapeutic doses and can be fatal in overdose. As such, caution/extreme caution must be used when dosing patients with respiratory failure, although this would not preclude their use in certain situations (e.g. rib fractures).

Histamine release

Some opioids, including **morphine**, stimulate the release of histamine leading to effects such as hypotension, bronchoconstriction, and itching. In patients for whom this is a problem, switching to an alternative agent that lack some of these effects [e.g. **fentanyl** (although can cause itching) or **pethidine**] should be considered.

Endocrine

Long-term use of opioids can depress pituitary function, by decreasing the secretion of gonadotrophin-releasing hormone from the hypothalamus. Clinically, this can impair fertility, libido, bone mineral density, and muscle mass.

Dependence/tolerance

Tolerance is outlined above, but with opioids there is also a risk of dependence after prolonged use, where patients experience withdrawal effects when treatment is discontinued

suddenly or a reversal agent used (**naloxone**). Signs of withdrawal include diarrhoea, tremor, agitation, weight loss, and personality changes. For this reason, opioids should be withdrawn gradually and doses carefully titrated to pain, to ensure that the lowest effective dose is used. If properly managed, addiction to opioids when used for analgesia is rare (see Topic 10.4, 'Drug abuse: addiction and dependency'), although it has been recognized in chronic pain and, for this reason, many recommend that opioids are not used in patients with non-malignant chronic pain.

Drug interactions

On the whole, drug interactions with opioids are the predictable increase in neurological toxicity, when used in combination with other drugs known to possess similar effects such as sedation, confusion, dizziness, etc. Other drug-specific interactions include the action of potent inhibitors of cytochrome P450 enzymes (e.g. **ritonavir** and **voriconazole**), which increase serum **alfentanil** levels. **Methadone** has been known to increase the risk of ventricular arrhythmias through QT interval-prolongation, particularly when used in combination with other drugs that can cause this effect.

Tramadol

Structurally related to codeine and morphine, tramadol is a centrally acting analgesic, consisting of two enantiomers that act via different mechanisms.

Mechanism of action

A 50:50 racemate of (+) and (−) enantiomers, (+) tramadol and its metabolite (+) O-desmethyl-tramadol are agonists of the μ opioid receptor. In addition (−) tramadol inhibits noradrenaline re-uptake, while (+) tramadol inhibits serotonin re-uptake. Despite the specificity for the μ subtype of opioid receptors, the affinity is several orders of magnitude less than that of **codeine** or **morphine**, which is probably not sufficient to explain the full extent of its analgesic properties. The ability to inhibit the neuronal re-uptake of noradrenaline and serotonin, monoamines involved in the anti-nociceptive effects of descending inhibitory pathways in the CNS, most likely contributes a significant proportion of the analgesic effects seen with treatment.

Prescribing

Tramadol can be administered orally or by injection (IM or IV) up to 4-hourly for the treatment of moderate to severe pain and provides a useful alternative where opioid-related side effects are problematic, e.g. constipation and respiratory depression. However, due to its mixed effects, unlike pure opioid agonists, doses are capped to a maximum of 600 mg/day. More recently, due to its potential for abuse, it has been reclassified as a schedule 3 controlled drug, thus subject to the prescription requirements in common with other strong opioids.

Unwanted effects

Tramadol is generally well-tolerated, although it commonly causes dizziness and headaches, and albeit reduced, still has the potential to cause opioid-like toxicities (constipation, drowsiness, confusion, tolerance, dependence, respiratory depression, etc.). Other undesirable effects are linked to its effects on noradrenaline and serotonin, includes mood changes and flushing. Tramadol should be avoided in patients with acute intoxication of alcohol or opioids, or those who have received an MAOI in the preceding 14 days due to the theoretical risk of severe neurological toxicity.

Rarely, tramadol can precipitate a seizure, especially in those with a history of fitting or taking concomitant drugs known to lower the seizure threshold, i.e. antidepressants or antipsychotics. Concurrent use in patients on drugs known to potentiate serotonin transmission (SSRIs, SNRIs) increases the risk of serotonin syndrome, presenting as spontaneous clonus, hypertonia, hyperreflexia, and raised temperature.

Drug interactions

Concomitant use of **tramadol** with other serotoninergic agents, has the potential to precipitate serotonin syndrome in combination with antidepressants, in particular MAOIs and other drugs that affect serotonin, e.g. **linezolid**. In combination with antidepressants, tramadol can also increase the risk of seizures.

Antidepressants

> In the control of pain and analgesia, antidepressants act by enhancing the descending inhibitory control mechanisms, through the increase in serotonin and noradrenaline neurotransmitter actions. For example, amitriptyline and duloxetine.

Mechanism of action

In neuropathic pain, tricyclic antidepressants (TCAs) show superior efficacy over the selective serotonin reuptake inhibitors, indicating that the noradrenergic component is a key factor in decreasing it. Despite the observed clinical

benefit, the processes by which these drugs act in the nociceptive system is still relatively unknown. Some of the mechanisms proposed, mainly from animal models, include inhibition of serotonin/noradrenaline uptake at spinal cord dorsal horn synapses, α-adrenergic blockade, anti-cholinergic and anti-histaminic effects, K^+, Ca^{2+} and Na^+ channel blockade, and NMDA receptor antagonism.

Noradrenaline can be released within supraspinal structures at the spinal level by descending noradrenergic pathways, and at the peripheral level in dorsal root ganglia, following neuropathy-induced noradrenergic sprouting of sympathetic nerve fibres. Local administration of β2-adrenoceptor antagonists suggest that the initial substrate for antidepressants anti-allodynic action might be localized at the spinal cord and/or dorsal root ganglia, rather than at the supraspinal level. Recent studies have indicated that antidepressants might, indeed, act on β2-adrenoceptors, inhibiting local TNFα production, and also reversing nerve injury-induced CREB and PLCY-1 phosphorylation.

Prescribing

There are two antidepressants recommended for use by NICE in the management of neuropathic pain. **Amitriptyline**, a dibenzocycloheptene-derivative TCA, is used off-license and prescribed at doses lower than that required for the treatment of depression. Doses are given at night, due to the associated sedative side effects and titrated up to a maximum daily dose of 75 mg; at this point, if there is no effect an alternative agent should be considered. The selective serotonin-noradrenaline reuptake inhibitor **duloxetine** is licensed for use in diabetic peripheral neuropathy, prescribed at doses equivalent to those used in depression or anxiety disorders. Patients should be started on the lower dose and increased as necessary. For both drugs treatment should be gradually weaned and discontinued if there is failure to respond after 8 weeks of therapy.

Unwanted effects

For further information see Topic 10.2, 'Depression'.

Anti-epileptics

> The mechanisms of analgesic action of anti-epileptic drugs are via Na^+ channel blockade (carbamazepine), Ca^{2+} channel blockade (pregabalin, gabapentin), suppression of glutamatergic transmission (gabapentin, pregabalin, carbamazepine), or a combination of these effects.

Mechanism of action

As stated above, the symptomatology of pain is associated with neuronal hyperexcitability within nociceptive pathways, which is expressed as a decrease in the threshold for nociceptive sensory stimulation. Anti-epileptic drugs normally reduce neuronal excitability via modulation of ligand-gated ($GABA_A$ and ionotropic glutamate receptors) and voltage-activated (Na^+ and Ca^{2+}) ion channel function, and can thus have marked analgesic actions.

Pregabalin and **gabapentin** share a novel and specific high-affinity binding site at α 2-δ proteins of voltage-gated Ca^{2+} channels, which are particularly localized at synapses in the superficial dorsal horn of the spinal cord. Their analgesic action is probably due to inhibition of excitatory neurotransmitter release.

Prescribing

Gabapentin and **pregabalin** are both advocated by NICE for the management of neuropathic pain. Gabapentin is licensed for use in diabetic peripheral neuropathy and post-herpetic neuralgia, whereas pregabalin has a more general license for use in peripheral and central neuropathic pain; despite this, gabapentin tends to be more widely used, based on experience and cost.

Both drugs are administered TDS, although gabapentin is increased from OD, to BD, to TDS over the first 3 days. Both drugs doses are titrated gradually to response, which takes longer with gabapentin due to its greater scope for dose escalation. As with the tricyclic antidepressants, treatment should be gradually withdrawn and discontinued where patients fail to respond, this time after 4 weeks of treatment. Gabapentin is increasingly being used as an adjunct in enhanced recovery protocols (e.g. for hip or knee replacements).

Carbamazepine is both recommended and licensed for pain relief associated with trigeminal neuralgia. Doses are again titrated to response, with total daily doses split and given BD to QDS to improve tolerance. Once pain relief is achieved doses may be gradually reduced to an effective maintenance dose.

Unwanted effects

Lower doses of **gabapentin** and **pregabalin** are recommended in renal impairment. For more information see Topic 9.2, 'Epilepsy'.

Further reading

Bandolier. The Oxford Pain Internet Site. http://www.bandolier.org.uk/booth/painpag/index.html [accessed 6 April 2019].

Bashir U, Colvin LA (2013) The place of pharmacological treatment in chronic pain. *Anaesthesia and Intensive Care Medicine* 14(12), 528–32.

Bohren Y, Tessier L-H, Megat S, et al. (2013) Antidepressants suppress neuropathic pain by a peripheral β2-adrenoceptor mediated anti-TNFα mechanism. *Neurobiological Diseases* 60, 39–50.

Cervero F, and Laird JM (2004) Understanding the signalling and transmission of visceral nociceptive events. *Journal of Neurobiology* 61, 45–54.

Davis MP (2011) Fentanyl for breakthrough pain: a systemic review *Expert Reviews of Neurotherapy* 11(8), 1197–216.

Fowler CJ (2012) NSAIDs: endocannabinoid stimulating anti-inflammatory drugs? *Trends in Pharmacological Sciences* 33(9), 468–73.

Hebbes C, Lambert D (2011) Non-opioid analgesics. *Anaesthesia and Intensive Care Medicine* 12(2), 69–72.

Kusuda R, Ravanelli MI, Cadetti F, et al. (2013) Long-term antidepressant treatment inhibits neurophatic pain-induced CREB and PLCY-1 phosphorylation in the mouse spinal cord dorsal horn. *Journal of Pain* 14(10), 1162–72.

Ong CKS, Lirk P, Tan CH, et al. (2007) An evidence-based update on nonsteroidal anti-inflammatory drugs. *Clinical Medicine and Research* 5(1), 19–34.

Paton F, Chambers D, Wilson P, et al. (2014) Effectiveness and implementation of enhanced recovery after surgery programmes: a rapid evidence synthesis. *British Medical Journal Open* 4(7), e005015.

Roberts E, Delgado Nunes V, Buckner S (2016) Paracetamol: not as safe as we thought? A systemic literature review of observational studies. *Annals of Rheumatic Diseases* 75, 552–9.

Stein C (2013) Opioids, sensory systems and chronic pain. *European Journal of Pharmacology* 716(1–3), 179–87.

Stein C, Lang LJ (2009) Peripheral mechanisms of opioid analgesia. *Current Opinions in Pharmacology* 9(1), 3–8.

Guidelines

American Society of Anesthesiologists Task Force (2012) Practice guidelines for acute pain management in the perioperative setting. *Anesthesiology* 116(2), 248–73.

Australian and New Zealand College of Anaesthetists (2013) Guidelines on acute pain management. Ancza guideline PS41. http://www.anzca.edu.au/resources/professional-documents/pdfs/ps41-2013-guidelines-on-acute-pain-management.pdf [accessed 6 April 2019].

NHMRC (2011) Emergency care acute pain management manual. file:///Users/lab/Downloads/cp135_emergency_acute_pain_management_manual.pdf [accessed 17 April 2019].

NICE (2019) Neuropathic pain overview. https://pathways.nice.org.uk/pathways/neuropathic-pain [accessed 6 April 2019].

NICE CG140 (2012) Palliative care for adults: strong opioids for pain relief. https://www.nice.org.uk/guidance/cg140 [accessed 6 April 2019].

NICE CG173 (2014) Neuropathic pain in adults: pharmacological management in non-specialist settings. https://www.nice.org.uk/guidance/cg173 [accessed 6 April 2019].

RCEM Guidance: Paracetamol overdose: new guidance on the use of intravenous acetylcysteine. (1986) https://www.rcem.ac.uk/RCEM/Quality-Policy/Clinical_Standards_Guidance/RCEM_Guidance.aspx?WebsiteKey=b3d6bb2a-abba-44ed-b758-467776a958cd&hkey=862bd964-0363-4f7f-bdab-89e4a68c9de4&RCEM_Guidance=6 [accessed 17 April 2019].

Royal College of Emergency Medicine (2013) MHRA Guidelines: paracetamol overdose.

Royal College of Physicians (2012) Complex regional pain syndrome guideline. https://www.rcplondon.ac.uk/guidelines-policy/pain-complex-regional-pain-syndrome [accessed 6 April 2019].

SIGN (2013) Management of chronic pain. SIGN 136. http://www.sign.ac.uk/pdf/SIGN136.pdf [accessed 6 April 2019].

Toxbase (2019) www.toxbase.org [accessed 17 April 2019].

9 Neurology

9.1 Cerebrovascular disease

Cerebrovascular disease encompasses all disorders that temporarily or permanently affect the way oxygen and glucose are delivered to the brain via cerebral blood vessels. *Stroke* is a sudden focal event that leads to neurological deficit, because of disturbed circulation. *Ischaemic strokes* account for around 80% of total numbers and are caused by inadequate blood flow secondary to occlusion by an atheroma, embolus, or less commonly, severe local vasospasm. The remaining 20% are *haemorrhagic strokes* that occur because of a bleed through ruptured vessels and may be defined by their location.

Historically, symptomatology in stroke exceeds 24 hours and where symptoms resolve before this, i.e. a transient vessel occlusion, is termed a *transient ischaemic attack* (TIA). More recently, however, a TIA has been defined by the American Heart Association and American Stroke Association (AHA/ASA) as a 'transient episode of neurologic dysfunction caused by focal brain, spinal cord or retinal ischaemia without acute infarction'. TIAs occur more commonly in men, increasing with age and affecting 35 per 100 000 people. It is also associated with an increased risk of stroke.

Stroke is a major health burden in the UK, with an annual incidence in excess of 150 000, accounting for approximately 40 000 deaths/year. Furthermore, there are approximately 1.2 million people in the UK living with the effects of a stroke. Modification of risk factors, rapid clinical diagnosis, and efficient early intervention is essential in reducing incidence and improving outcomes (see Figure 9.1).

Pathophysiology: ischaemic stroke

Ischaemic stroke, the most common form of cerebrovascular disease, results mainly from the enlargement or rupture of an atheromatous plaque, or from an embolus that travels from the systemic arterial system into the CNS vasculature. The subsequent reduction in oxygenated blood flow by 20–30% deprives brain tissues, normally completely dependent on aerobic metabolism, of glucose and oxygen.

At a cellular level the resultant anaerobic conditions trigger the ischaemic cascade, so that cells ultimately undergo apoptosis and die. Persistent ischaemia lasting more than 1 hour leads to local tissue necrosis, neuroinflammation, and oedema. Prior to cellular apoptosis, the normally maintained electrochemical gradient across the cell membrane is disrupted, such that intracellular Ca^{2+}, Na^+, and Cl^- levels rise uncontrollably, bringing with it an inflow of water causing neurons and glia to swell. In addition, the ischaemic cascade stimulates the release of excitatory neurotransmitters such as glutamate, which act on AMPA and NMDA receptors to further enhance intracellular Ca^{2+} levels. This process of excitotoxicity results in the formation of free radical species and up-regulation of cellular digestive enzymes (e.g. endonucleases and phospholipases), leading to irreversible cell membrane breakdown. Furthermore, the increase in glutamate concentrations can result in localized seizure activity in surviving proximal cells.

Given that different regions of the brain are supplied by different arterial territories (Figure 9.2), good knowledge of the vascular anatomy can identify which arterial branches are at the site of a lesion; these present clinically as stroke syndromes (see Table 9.1 for common presentations and the territories supplied). The common carotid and sites of bifurcation along its path are potential loci for atheroma formation in at risk patients (and present with a carotid bruits; a systolic sound over the carotid artery on auscultation). Emboli or occlusion occurring along the internal carotid artery will affect the brain, specifically the anterior circulation. Vertebrobasilar vessels supply the posterior circulation.

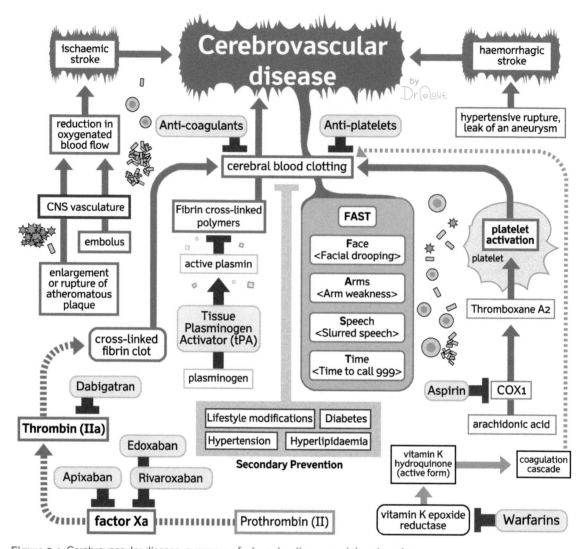

Figure 9.1 Cerebrovascular disease: summary of relevant pathways and drug targets.

Deficits caused by occlusive ischaemic stroke must be addressed rapidly with reperfusion interventions, either by IV thrombolytic therapy (e.g. t-PA, see 'Drug classes used in management, Tissue plasminogen activator: alteplase') or endovascular intervention, in order to limit diffuse tissue damage. Despite this, however, a stroke often results in significant morbidity and mortality, thus primary and secondary prevention strategies are fundamental in management.

Acute management

World-wide, advances in the acute management of cerebrovascular disease have focused on rapid diagnosis,

early introduction of thrombolysis and optimization of anti-platelet therapy, to improve treatment outcomes and minimize long-term sequelae (Figure 9.3). In the UK, national programmes (e.g. FAST see Table 9.2) have been used to promote early detection through education, to both the public and emergency services. Stroke is now widely accepted as a medical emergency and prioritized in the same way as MI, ensuring rapid access to appropriate care.

Validation tools, such as FAST, outside of hospital, and ROSIER, on presentation to the emergency department, are used to enable a rapid diagnosis and exclude differentials, such as hypoglycaemia, migraine, seizures, and trauma. Neurological symptoms that resolve within

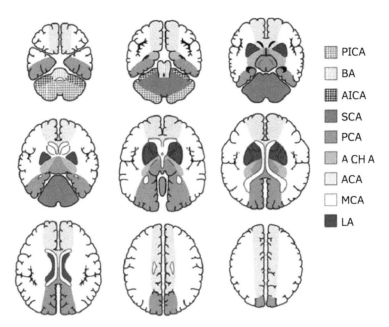

Figure 9.2 Territories of the main cerebral arteries supplying the supratentorial structures. PICA, posterior inferior cerebellar artery; BA, basilar artery; AICA, anterior inferior cerebellar artery; SCA, superior cerebellar artery; PCA, posterior cerebral artery; AChA, anterior choroidal artery; ACA, anterior cerebral artery; MCA middle cerebral artery; LA, lenticulostriate artery.

minutes/hours are suggestive of a TIA, although persisting symptoms should be considered a stroke and the patient admitted to specialist care within 4 hours. On admission, patients require a full examination, history, and routine tests (see Box 9.1). Brain imaging, by CT or MRI, should be performed as soon as possible (within half-an-hour of admission) to exclude haemorrhage and guide management. Once diagnosed, an ischaemic stroke requires urgent

Table 9.1 Common presentations of stroke and the territories supplied

Artery	Weakness	Sensory loss	Visual field deficit	Other
MCA	Contralateral face, arm more than leg	Contralateral face, arm more than leg	Contralateral hemifield	1. Impaired gaze in contralateral direction 2a. Dominant/left hemisphere MCA: aphasia, apraxia, 2b. Non-dominant/right hemisphere MCA: visuospatial impairment 3. Neglect (especially with non-dominant hemisphere MCA strokes)
ACA	Contralateral leg more than arm	Contralateral leg more than arm		Deficits of attention and/or motivation, urinary incontinence, mutism (abulia)
PCA			Contralateral hemifield	Dominant hemisphere PCA: alexia without agraphia, memory loss

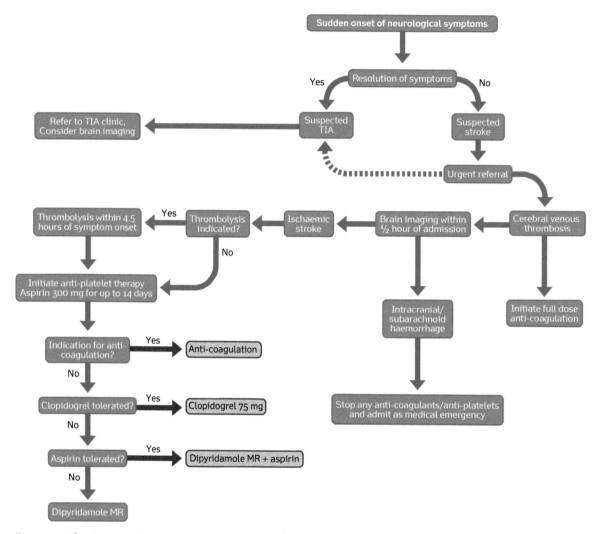

Figure 9.3 Cerebrovascular disease: management flow chart.

thrombolysis with **alteplase**, unless contraindicated. This should be administered as early as possible and at least within 4.5 hours of onset of stroke symptoms; administration beyond this time is unlikely to confer a benefit.

Table 9.2 FAST algorithm

Sign	Definition
Face	Facial drooping
Arms	Arm weakness
Speech	Slurred speech
Time	Time to call 999

In addition, endovascular thrombectomy is increasingly being carried out following thrombolysis, to remove the clot and re-establish cerebral blood flow. This can be done either under sedation or general anaesthesia using X-ray guidance, once the exact location of the occlusion has been identified by CT/MR angiography.

Antiplatelet treatment is routinely used for secondary prophylaxis, following a stroke or TIA, once an intracranial haemorrhage has been excluded. Treatment with high dose **aspirin** (300 mg) should be initiated as soon as possible, or 24 hours after thrombolysis, and continued for 2 weeks or until point of discharge, if this is sooner. In patients intolerant of aspirin, co-administration of a PPI may be considered, or the use

Box 9.1 Summary of work up in suspected stroke

History: onset of symptoms

- Co-morbidities (e.g. epilepsy, diabetes, alcohol/drug abuse, cardiac disease, TIA)
- Drug history

Examination: pulse, BP, temperature

- Oxygen saturation
- Signs of trauma
- Neurological exam
- Chest auscultation (e.g. arrhythmias, murmurs)

Blood tests: glucose

- Electrolytes
- Creatinine/urea
- LFTs
- Troponin
- APTT/prothrombin time/INR

Other tests: brain imaging (as soon as possible on presentation, CT preferred)

- ECG
- Pregnancy

of **clopidogrel** as an alternative. After 2 weeks of high-dose aspirin treatment, patients should be switched to clopidogrel for long-term management. Patients intolerant of clopidogrel may be treated with a combination of aspirin and **dipyridamole**, or dipyridamole monotherapy if intolerant of aspirin, too.

Atrial fibrillation is a major risk factor for stroke and these patients therefore require long-term anticoagulation. Patients already requiring anticoagulation will need to continue to receive an anticoagulant as maintenance therapy. In newly diagnosed AF, anticoagulant therapy should be started immediately following a TIA and about 2 weeks after an ischaemic stroke, depending on the risk of bleeding. Choice of anti-coagulant (**warfarin**, **apixaban**, **dabigatran**, **edoxaban**, or **rivaroxaban**) will depend on patient factors and local availability, and should be decided in conjunction with the patient. That said, many centres now favour the use of a NOAC as, unlike warfarin, there is no need for monitoring or dose adjusting. In patients diagnosed with a cerebral venous thrombosis, treatment dose anticoagulation should be initiated up front, with **LMWH** cover until oral anticoagulation is therapeutic.

Numerous drugs have been investigated for neuro-protection following a stroke, but to date, none have demonstrated a clear benefit, although withdrawal of a statin acutely following an ischaemic stroke may increase the risk of death. Primary management in acute stroke therefore remains close monitoring and optimization of interventions, as listed in Table 9.3.

Secondary prevention

Following an acute cerebrovascular event, the risk of a further episode is increased, particularly in the early days or weeks. Secondary prevention should be individualized to patients, so that modifiable risk factors are minimized using both pharmacological and non-pharmacological measures.

Lifestyle modifications

This includes smoking cessation, weight loss, exercise, dietary modifications (e.g. salt and fat restriction, increased fruit and vegetable consumption) and moderation of alcohol intake.

Hypertension

BP reduction in hypertensive patients should be initiated 24 hours post-stroke, using both pharmacological and non-pharmacological measures, as appropriate. No optimal BP has been identified specifically post-stroke, thus recommendations remain as they are for all hypertensive patients (see Topic 2.1, 'Hypertension').

Hyperlipidaemia

Statins are the only lipid-lowering drugs known to reduce cardiovascular risk and should be offered to all patients following a stroke or TIA, with cholesterol levels checked after 3 months to assess response. Doses should be adjusted to response and used in combination with dietary advice. In patients with a history of intracerebral haemorrhage, statins may increase the risk of a further haemorrhage, so should be used with caution.

Diabetes

Optimizing glycaemic control is likely to be beneficial in reducing the risk of recurrent stroke. Again, this can be achieved through dietary and pharmacological measures (hypoglycaemics, insulin), in line with standards for

Table 9.3 Supportive management post-stroke

Monitoring parameter	Intervention
Blood glucose	Aim for a concentration between 4 and 11 mmol/ L. In diabetic patients, this can be achieved through IV insulin and glucose infusions
Oxygen saturation	Oxygen is only recommended in hypoxic patients following a stroke to maintain saturations at 95% or higher
Blood pressure	Management of hypertension is only recommended in severe cases, in symptomatic patients, e.g. hypertensive encephalopathy or intracranial haemorrhage. Patients undergoing thrombolysis should have BP maintained below 185/100 mmHg to reduce the risk of intracranial haemorrhage
Temperature	In hyperthermic patients any underlying cause should be identified and treated. Antipyretics may be used to reduce temperature
Nutrition and hydration	Post-stroke patients should be assessed for dysphagia before commencing oral nutrition. In patients with dysphagia, a NG tube should be used to enable enteral feeding. In dehydrated patients isotonic IV solutions, such as NaCl 0.9% should be used for rehydration, as hypotonic solutions may exacerbate brain oedema

managing all diabetic mellitus patients (see Topic 4.5, 'Diabetes mellitus').

Pathophysiology: haemorrhagic stroke

Haemorrhagic stroke can occur because of a subarachnoid haemorrhage (SAH) or intracerebral haemorrhage (ICH; or intraparenchymal haemorrhage where rupture of intracerebral/brainstem arteries results in local parenchymal lesions). Collectively, they are less common than ischaemic stroke, present differently, and require very different management, thus emphasizing the need for a CT/MRI on presentation, to differentiate ischaemic from haemorrhagic causes.

After ischaemic stroke, ICH is the second most common cause of stroke and can occur secondary to hypertension, vascular malformations, tumours, bleeding disorders, and/ or drug therapy. Patients with ICH typically present with headaches, vomiting, and altered mental status, although can present much like an ischaemic stroke, with clinical signs determined by the size/location of the haemorrhage.

SAH typically occurs as a result of non-traumatic rupture of an aneurysm on the circle of Willis (Berry aneurysm) and accounts for about 5% of strokes. It is often reported as a sudden-onset agonizing 'thunderclap' headache, with declining mental state, neck stiffness, nausea, and seizures. Strong risk factors for SAH include hypertension, smoking and family history, although incidence

has also been linked to excessive alcohol consumption, oestrogen deficiency, and some drug therapies (e.g. anticoagulants). CT head is the first line investigation, which may demonstrate hyperdense areas in the basal cisterns, major fissures, and sulci. Should CT be unrevealing and/or medical attention sought after 24 hours, lumbar puncture may be required; this will demonstrate xanthochromia.

The effects of haemorrhagic stroke are multifocal, with rapid spread of blood into the cerebrospinal fluid (CSF) simultaneously, leading to raised intracranial pressure and a reduction in cerebral blood flow and neuronal ischemia, which in turn triggers the release of toxic excitatory amino acids (e.g. glutamate). Subsequently, this can lead to rebound systemic hypertension, vasospasm (secondary to products of cell lysis), hydrocephalus, and seizures. Pharmacological treatment strategies broadly aim to manage hypertension (anti-hypertensives) and control bleeding (peripheral vasodilators), as well as manage secondary effects such as vasospasm (antivasospastics) and seizures (anti-epileptics). Overzealous anti-hypertensive treatment, however, can be detrimental since it will reduce the already limited brain perfusion.

Management

Intracerebral haemorrhage

ICH is best managed in an ICU setting to ensure access to supportive management and intensive monitoring. For patients on oral anticoagulants, rapid reversal is recommended as appropriate for the anticoagulant, e.g. the use of vitamin K with **warfarin** (see Topic, 2.8, 'Venous thromboembolism'). Surgery may be indicated for the removal of haemorrhage, depending on the site and extent of bleed, in order to reduce the risk of hydrocephalus and subsequent neuronal damage. Raised blood pressure (>180 mmHg) should be managed with IV fluids and anti-hypertensive therapy (e.g. **labetalol**, **hydralazine**, **nicardipine**), with frequent monitoring to achieve an SBP of 140 mmHg. This has been shown to be safe and associated with better functional recovery. In addition, IV insulin therapy is used routinely to reduce the risk of increased mortality associated with high blood glucose, although hypoglycaemia can be similarly detrimental and should also be avoided, thus the need for frequent monitoring.

In a non-cerebellar bleed where the patient is decompensating and raised intracranial pressure is evident despite analgesia, tracheal intubation/ventilation, osmotic diuretic therapy with **mannitol** can be considered (see Topic 5.2, 'Acute kidney injury). In cerebral oedema, mannitol helps by causing water to be drawn out of cells to extracellular fluid into plasma; it therefore induces diuresis by elevating the osmotic pressure of glomerular filtrate so tubular reabsorption of water and solutes is reduced.

Antiepileptics are initiated IV in the case of a seizure, or where there is evidence of a change in mental status with associated EEG changes. They are not recommended for routine seizure prophylaxis following an ICH.

Long-term prevention of recurrence is through the management of identified risk factors, e.g. hypertension and excessive alcohol use. Where anticoagulant and antiplatelets need to be reinstated, this should not be done for at least 4 weeks following an ICH.

Subarachnoid haemorrhage

A subarachnoid haemorrhage is a medical emergency requiring rapid treatment to reduce the risk of rebleeding. This is primarily achieved through aneurysm obliteration, in combination with BP and haemodynamic control, using IV antihypertensives (e.g. **nicardipine**, **labetalol**, or **sodium nitroprusside**) and fluids to achieve an SBP < 160 mmHg. Excessive reduction, however, is associated with increased morbidity due to impaired cerebral perfusion. During surgery, blood glucose levels are closely monitored and managed with IV insulin/glucose, as hyperglycaemia during surgery is associated with poorer outcomes.

Following surgery, patients are at increased risk of infarction secondary to arterial vasospasm; IV **nimodipine**

and fluids to maintain normal circulating blood volume is therefore recommended in all patients following an SAH (secondary to an aneurysm), in order to optimize neurological outcomes. Additional treatment with anti-epileptics, used both as treatment and, in some cases, early on as prophylaxis, may also be beneficial.

Drug classes used in management

Tissue plasminogen activator: alteplase

> The tissue-type plasminogen activator (tPA) is a serine protease that cleaves plasminogen into active plasmin, which in turns digests fibrin in plasma and thus has a thrombolytic effect in the treatment of ischemic stroke. For example, alteplase

Mechanism of action

Thrombolysis is the dissolution of a thrombus (blood clot) by enzymatic breakdown. It is achieved by clearing the cross-linked fibrin and making the clot soluble, thus subjecting it to further enzymatic proteolysis. Endogenous tPA is widely expressed in the CNS and is involved in synaptic plasticity mechanisms. It facilitates Ca^{2+} influx following NMDA receptor activation, while other synaptic effects are achieved through plasmin, which converts precursor brain-derived neurotrophic factor (BDNF) into mature BDNF.

Crucially, beyond its clot dissolving properties, tPA can damage the basal lamina of the blood vessels, producing oedema, disruption of the blood–brain barrier or haemorrhage. **Alteplase** and plasmin can also affect non-fibrin molecular targets in the extracellular matrix of the brain, with damaging effects including interactions with NMDA receptors that could amplify toxic Ca^{2+} currents during ischaemic excitotoxicity.

Prescribing

Of the fibrinolytic drugs, only **alteplase** is licensed in acute ischaemic stroke; however, less than 5% of patients receive it due to the narrow therapeutic window (within 4.5 hours of stroke), limited access to expertise and facilities, and high risk of haemorrhagic complications. Treatment should be initiated as soon as possible under the supervision of a specialist, once intracranial haemorrhage has been excluded by brain scan. Use beyond 4.5 hours of onset of symptoms is not currently advocated.

Doses are administered based on patient's weight, with 10% administered as an IV injection and the remainder as an infusion over 90 minutes.

Unwanted effects

See Topic 2.5, 'Acute coronary syndrome'.

Antiplatelets

> Antiplatelet-aggregating therapy constitutes a valid therapeutic option in cerebrovascular disease, once the absence of intracranial haemorrhage has been confirmed. For example, aspirin, clopidogrel, and dipyridamole.

Mechanism of action

For further details on mechanisms of anti-platelet activity, see Topic 2.5, 'Acute coronary syndrome'.

Prescribing

Of the antiplatelets, **aspirin**, **clopidogrel**, and **dipyridamole** are used in stroke or TIA. High-dose aspirin is the recommended first line of treatment, started within 24 hours and continued for 2 weeks, before being switched to clopidogrel for long-term prophylaxis. In patients unable to swallow post-stroke, soluble aspirin can be administered down a nasogastric (NG) tube or failing that as a suppository for rectal administration.

The evidence for clopidogrel immediately post-stroke is limited, although it may be used in patients unable to tolerate aspirin. As it can take 2–3 days to achieve its full anti-platelet effect, a loading dose of 300 mg is recommended. Similarly, **dipyridamole** slow release is reserved for use in combination with aspirin in patients who have had a TIA, or as monotherapy in patients intolerant of aspirin.

The role of antiplatelets for primary prevention is less clear, although there is some rational for the use of **aspirin** in high-risk patients, i.e. those with a greater than 10% chance of having a cardiovascular event in the next 10 years. Use in low risk patients with or without diabetes, has not demonstrated a benefit with regards to stroke prevention.

> ### PRESCRIBING WARNING
>
> **Drug administration in patients with impaired swallow post-stroke**
>
> Following a stroke all patients will need their swallow reflex assessed prior to administering any drugs, foods, or drinks. Where swallow is impaired, a NG tube should be placed. Consideration should be given to drug administration via an NG tube. Where available, liquid or soluble formulations should be used via an NG tube.

Unwanted effects

See Topic 2.5, 'Acute coronary syndrome'.

Anticoagulants

> The immediate use of anticoagulants after stroke might reduce the infarcted cerebral tissue volume, thus lessening neurological deficit and disability, while the risk of thromboembolic stroke and DVT can also be diminished. However, augmented risk of intracranial haemorrhage needs to be considered before treatment. Examples include apixaban, dabigatran, edoxaban, and rivaroxaban.

Mechanism of action

For more details on mechanisms of anti-coagulant action, see Topic 2.8, 'Venous thromboembolism'.

Prescribing

Warfarin and the newer oral anti-coagulants—**apixaban**, **dabigatran**, **edoxaban,** and **rivaroxaban**, are recommended as treatment options for the secondary prevention of stroke in patients with atrial fibrillation. Choice of treatment depends on patient factors and local availability (see Topic 2.8, 'Venous thromboembolism').

Unwanted effects

See Topic 2.8, 'Venous thromboembolism'.

Further reading

Deb P, Sharma S, Hassan KH (2010) Pathophysiologic mechanisms of acute ischemic stroke: An overview with emphasis on therapeutic significance beyond thrombolysis. *Pathophysiology* 17(3), 197–218.

Guidelines

Connolly ES, Rabinstein AA, Carhuapoma JR, et al. (2012) Guideline for the management of aneurysmal subarachnoid haemorrhage: A guideline for healthcare professionals from the AHA/ASA. *Stroke* 43, 1711 37.

Hemphill JC, Greenberg SM, Anderson CS, et al. (2015) Guidelines for the management of spontaneous intracerebral haemorrhage: A guideline for healthcare professionals form the AHA/ASA. *Stroke* 46, 2032–60.

Kernan WN, Ovbiagele, Black HR, et al. (2014) Guidelines for the prevention of stroke in patients with stroke or transient ischemic attack: a guideline for healthcare professionals from the American Heart Association/American Stroke Association *Stroke* 45(7), 2160–236. http://stroke.ahajournals.org/content/early/2014/04/30/STR.0000000000000024.full.pdf+html [accessed 6 April 2019].

Meschia JF, Bushnell C, Boden-Albala B (2014) Guidelines for the primary prevention of stroke: a statement for healthcare professionals from the American Heart Association/American Stroke Association. *Stroke* 45, 3754–832. http://stroke.ahajournals.org/content/45/12/3754 [accessed 6 April 2019].

NICE CG68 (2008) Stroke and transient ischaemic attack in over 16s: diagnosis and initial management. https://www.nice.org.uk/guidance/cg68 [accessed 6 April 2019].

NICE CG162 (2013) Stroke in rehabilitation in adults. https://www.nice.org.uk/guidance/cg162 [accessed 6 April 2019].

NICE QS2 (2016) Stroke in adults (Updated Apr 2016). https://www.nice.org.uk/guidance/qs2 [accessed 6 April 2019].

NICE Stroke Pathway (2019) http://pathways.nice.org.uk/pathways/stroke [accessed 6 April 2019].

NICE TA249 (2012) Dabigatran etexilate for the prevention of stroke and systemic embolism in atrial fibrillation. https://www.nice.org.uk/guidance/ta249 [accessed 6 April 2019].

NICE TA264 (2012) Alteplase for treating acute ischaemic stroke https://www.nice.org.uk/guidance/ta264 [accessed 6 April 2019].

NICE TA275 (2012) Rivaroxaban for the prevention of stroke and systemic embolism in people with atrial fibrillation. https://www.nice.org.uk/guidance/ta256 [accessed 6 April 2019].

NICE TA275 (2013) Apixaban for preventing stroke and systemic embolism in people with nonvalvular atrial fibrillation. https://www.nice.org.uk/guidance/ta275 [accessed 6 April 2019].

NICE TA355 (2015) Edoxaban for preventing stroke and systemic embolism in people with non-valvular atrial fibrillation. https://www.nice.org.uk/guidance/ta355 [accessed 6 April 2019].

Powers WJ, Derdeyn CP, Biller J, et al. (2015) 2015 American Heart Association/American Stroke Association Focused update of the 2013 Guidelines for the early management of patients with acute ischemic stroke. *Stroke* 46, 3024–39. http://stroke.ahajournals.org/content/46/10/3020 [accessed 6 April 2019].

Royal College of Physicians (2012) National Clinical Guidelines for Stroke: prepared by the Intercollegiate Stroke Working Party, 4th edn. https://www.rcplondon.ac.uk/sites/default/files/national-clinical-guidelines-for-stroke-fourth-edition.pdf [accessed 6 April 2019].

9.2 Epilepsy (including status epilepticus)

Seizures are diagnosed on the basis of 'a transient occurrence of signs and/or symptoms due to abnormal excessive or synchronous neuronal activity in the brain' (Fisher et al. 2005). A diagnosis of epilepsy is made when two or more unprovoked episodes of neurological dysfunction (i.e. epileptic seizures) occur, at least 24 hours apart. A seizure results from synchronous bursts of neuronal activity, most frequently observed in the neocortex of the brain, but which can also arrive from subcortical structures. Abnormal firing can begin and remain localized within the brain, causing 'focal' seizures. Otherwise, synchronous firing may appear to arise in a manner that is immediately widespread throughout the brain, resulting in 'generalized' seizures, which include both absence seizures and tonic/clonic events. The pathophysiology of seizures is variable. Careful clinical history, examination, and in particular, witness descriptions (a collateral history) is vital in determining the semiology and ensuring the correct diagnosis. Establishing the seizure subtype helps to ensure that the most effective pharmacological agent is selected. The most recent International League Against Epilepsy (ILAE) classification (Fisher et al. 2017) recommends starting by discriminating between focal and generalized events, with a third 'unknown' group for patients in whom the distinction remains unclear.

This latest classification has replaced previous classifiers (dyscognitive, simple partial, complex partial, psychic, and secondarily generalized) and introduced more descriptive terminology for focal seizures. Subtypes include automatisms, autonomic, behaviour arrest, cognitive, emotional, hyperkinetic, sensory, and focal-to-bilateral tonic–clonic seizures. Atonic, clonic, epileptic spasms, myoclonic, and tonic seizures can be either focal or generalized. New generalized seizure types include absence with eyelid myoclonia, myoclonic absence, myoclonic–tonic–clonic, myoclonic–atonic, and epileptic spasms. It will take time for this new classification to be widely adopted. Arcane and poorly discriminating terms such as 'Grand mal' and 'Petit mal' are likely to persist in both medical and lay parlance, and so care will be required to avoid confusion.

Focal seizures may also spread to become generalized ('focal to bilateral tonic–clonic seizure', formerly termed 'secondary generalized'). Loss of or altered awareness may occur in focal cognitive or behavioural seizures (previously called 'complex partial' or 'focal dyscognitive' seizures) but, in general, loss of consciousness is the hallmark of a generalized event. Both antecedent/prodromal symptoms (aura) and post-ictal phenomena may give vital clues as to the diagnosis of epilepsy (especially with regard to excluding alternative diagnoses) and may also hint as to the likely focus. Historical details not apparently related to the event (and which the patient may not at all relate to it) can also be helpful. For example, a history of diurnal myoclonic jerks in a teenager who has had a generalized tonic–clonic seizure (GTC) support the possibility of juvenile myoclonic epilepsy, as does a history of childhood 'blank spells' (suggestive of previous absence seizures). Frequent 'déjà vu', complaints of poor memory and/or olfactory or gustatory aura may suggest temporal lobe epilepsy.

Epilepsy may be primary (genetic and/or resulting from congenitally abnormal anatomy) or secondary (acquired, e.g. traumatic brain injury, stroke, Alzheimer's disease; drugs or alcohol) in cause. In patients with primary epilepsy without structural lesions, the term idiopathic generalized epilepsy (IGE) is often used, and a genetic cause is probable in many such cases. In both primary and secondary epilepsy, seizures may be provoked by certain factors including fatigue, dehydration, metabolic disturbance, alcohol, or other drug use, and intercurrent illness or fever. Photosensitive epilepsy [seizures provoked by stroboscopic (flashing) lights] is both rare and suggestive of particular IGE subtypes. The prevalence of epilepsy approximates 5 per 1000 population with highest rates of new diagnosis in children and adults over 60 years (there is a 'bimodal' distribution of incidence). In older people, seizures are more likely to be secondary and attributable to the burden of cerebrovascular disease neurodegenerative disease, such as Alzheimer's disease (~30%), whereas primary epilepsies are the norm in younger patients. Except in young patients with very typical epilepsy syndromes, neuroimaging is required to exclude possible space-occupying lesions as the cause of seizures.

The majority of patients with epilepsy have a normal life expectancy, but seizures are associated with increased morbidity and mortality (e.g. due to drowning, injury, accidents) or sudden unexpected death in epilepsy (SUDEP). SUDEP is more common when seizures are poorly controlled (whether due to refractory epilepsy or poor medication adherence). The cause of death may include respiratory apnoea, airway obstruction, or heart dysrhythmia. Fortunately, SUDEP is rare with rates of 1:1000 in diagnosed epileptics. It is associated with generalized convulsions (*tonic–clonic* or '*grand mal*') seizures, and is more common in patients with childhood epilepsy.

Patients with epilepsy may require life-long treatment with anti-epileptic medication, therefore identifying the *correct drug* and *dose* to prevent seizures, while limiting side effects is critical to optimize quality of life.

Seizure types

Seizure types are divided (using either clinical semiology or electroencephalogram [EEG]) into focal onset, generalized or unknown onset sub-classes (see Table 9.4).

Focal seizures

Focal seizures originate from networks within one cerebral hemisphere and may be localized to a small brain volume or distributed more widely, giving rise to clinical events that depend on the site of onset and extent of spread (see Table 9.5 for examples). They are subdivided as to whether or not consciousness/awareness is maintained and then according to the semiology. Abnormal electrical activity may then spread to the contralateral hemisphere, leading to secondary generalized seizures.

Generalized seizures

Generalized seizures rapidly engage both hemispheres and are associated with a loss of consciousness without warning (neither aura nor focal motor prodrome). There are several types of generalized seizure of which tonic–clonic ('grand mal') is the most frequently described. Simultaneous loss of consciousness ensues with tonic flexion/extension, jaw clenching, and stiffening of the limbs followed by a convulsive episode with rhythmic limb and truncal jerking, laboured breathing, and sometimes, airway compromise. Autonomic features may also occur followed by a period of flaccidity. The patient then enters a post-ictal phase during which they may remain obtunded (confused) and/or demonstrate persistent focal deficits (e.g. Todd's paresis). Most episodes are self-limiting and initial interventions are conservative, ensuring airway patency and protecting the patient from physical injury. Prolonged seizure (> 300 seconds) requires urgent intervention—status epilepticus (> 30 min) is a medical emergency.

A pattern of clonic seizures alone may be seen in infants and the young, where clonic jerks are witnessed. Pure tonic seizures may be seen at all ages and present as neck and facial muscle spasms lasting 60 seconds, these are often associated with other seizure types. Absence seizures ('petit mal') are also generalized events. These are characterized by a sudden loss of awareness that typically lasts a few seconds, and may or may not be associated with a loss of muscle tone. They can occur frequently (up to hundreds/day), although they are not associated with easily identifiable post-ictal features.

Pathophysiology

The pathophysiology of epileptic seizures is complex and relates to cellular physiology (small cation fluxes), neurotransmitter systems (including GABA and glutamate), and neuro-anatomy. Treatment is partly guided by knowledge of the factors that may alter each of these at the genetic, molecular, neurotransmitter, and neuroanatomical level.

Anatomy

Within the cerebral cortex, there are *pyramidal cells*, which are excitatory and propagate action potentials through glutamate release (glutamatergic), and *interneurons*, of which most are inhibitory and where gamma-amino-butyric acid (GABA) is the main neurotransmitter (GABAergic).

Table 9.4 Classification of seizure types.

	Type	Subtype	Symptoms/signs
Generalized onset	Motor	Tonic–clonic	Abrupt loss of consciousness Muscular stiffening and/or limb shaking Urinary incontinence or tongue biting *may* occur
		Clonic	Clonic—repeated or rhythmic, jerking muscle movements
		Tonic	Tonic—stiffening of muscles. Often affect muscles in the back, arms, and legs
		Myoclonic, Myotonic–tonic–clonic, Myotonic–atonic	Sudden brief jerks or twitches of the arms and/or legs
		Atonic	Loss of muscle control-sudden collapse
		Epileptic spasms	
	Non-motor (absence)	Typical	Staring or subtle body movements (e.g. eye blinking or lip smacking). Clusters occur, brief loss of awareness
		Atypical	
		Myoclonic	
		Eyelid myoclonia	
Focal seizures—with or without impaired awareness			
	Motor onset	Automatisms	
		Atonic	
		Clonic	
		Epileptic spasms	
		Hyperkinetic	
		Myoclonic	
		Tonic	
	Non-motor onset	Autonomic	
		Behaviour arrest	
		Cognitive	
		Emotional	
		Sensory	
Unknown			

Adapted from Fisher, R. Operational classification of seizure types by the International League Against Epilepsy: Position Paper of the ILAE Commission for Classification and Terminology. Epilepsia, March 2017. Copyright © 2017, John Wiley and Sons. doi:10.1111/epi.13670.

Table 9.5 Characteristic features of focal seizures

Seizure focus	Characteristic features
Mesial temporal lobe	Aura, psychic phenomena (déjà vu), hallucinations (olfactory, gustatory), autonomic effects (flushing, tachycardia), vertigo, restlessness, agitation, aphasia, confusion, automatism (lip smacking, hand picking, shouting/grunting)
Lateral temporal lobe	Auditory auras, visual hallucinations, vertigo
Frontal lobe	Hyperkinetic bilateral motor movements (kicking, thrashing, clapping)
Motor strip	Contralateral tonic/clonic limb movements, Jacksonian march
Parietal lobe	Subjective sensory symptoms, e.g. pins and needles, numbness
Occipital lobe	Visual hallucinations/loss, flashing lights

Adapted with permission from Flemming, K., Jones, L. (Eds). Mayo Clinic Neurology Board Review: Clinical Neurology for Initial certification and MOC. New York, USA: Oxford University Press. © Copyright Mayo Foundation for Medical Education and Research. Reproduced with permission of the Licensor through PLSclear.

The cells of the cortex are organized in a layered structure and the two types of neurons are closely associated in space. Localized release of GABA from interneurons can therefore cause inhibition of other local projecting neurons such as those from the subcortical structures that project to the pyramidal cells, where the primary transmitter is glutamate.

The cortex is divided up into lobes: *frontal, temporal, parietal*, and *occipital*, each of which specializes in various cognitive tasks. Over-activity within a specific area may lead to distinctive symptoms and signs related to lobar functions; for example, a focal, localized, seizure within the visual cortex of the occipital region may generate a visual aura or hallucination. Conversely, more widespread neural dysfunction involving the motor cortex may be observed as a generalized, tonic–clonic seizure.

Physiology

Nerve cells typically have a resting membrane potential of −70 mV. The inside of the cell is electrically negative ('polarized') with respect to the outside. During neurotransmission, specific neurotransmitter-activated receptors open ion channels leading to an influx of Na^+ and Ca^{2+} ions, which are at high concentrations outside the cell. This leads to depolarization with subsequent generation of an 'action potential', further release of transmitter, and propagation of the neuronal signal. Following the positive deflection of the action potential, there is a period of hyperpolarization (Figure 9.4, ③) when the cell is unable to fire again: This is known as the 'refractory period' during which time the cell recovers its resting membrane potential by activation of outward K^+ currents and/or influx of Cl^- ions in order to regain an equilibrium state at -70 mV.

Alterations in the drivers of these currents may cause cells to be incompletely repolarized and therefore have a greater tendency to fire in response to a given stimulus. If Na^+ or Ca^{2+} channels have a tendency toward sustained or slow depolarization (i.e. paroxysmal depolarization shifts), there may be rapid bursts of action potentials that can spread locally, regionally, or to the whole brain. These may be captured on EEGs as interictal spikes.

One mechanism in epilepsy is described in *absence seizures*—voltage-dependent T-type Ca^{2+} channels mediate burst-firing of thalamocortical neuronal projections; seen as 3-second spike and wave patterns on EEG. **Ethosuximide**, an anti-epileptic drug, blocks these T-type Ca^{2+} channels fluxes. Conversely, other 'anti-epileptic' drugs, such as **carbamazepine** or **vigabatrin**, that increase GABA may actually *induce* absence seizures in these patients by increasing the pool of available T-type Ca^{2+} channels. This demonstrates the clinical importance of defining seizure subtype prior to selecting appropriate pharmacotherapy.

In *focal onset seizures*, failure of normal cell function may result from decreased GABAergic inhibition. Loss of inhibitory potentials, may be mediated by $GABA_A$ Cl^- channel dysfunction, or by indirect inhibition of presynaptic excitatory transmitter release through a $GABA_B$ mediated K^+ current.

Increased activation of excitatory cells also contributes to epileptiform activity. The N-methyl-D-asparate (NMDA) type glutamate-receptor, is a potential target for

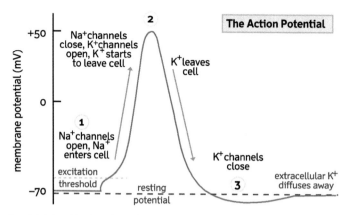

Figure 9.4 Neuronal ionic, which lead to depolarisation, release of neurotransmitter, and subsequent hyperpolarization when the cell can no longer be stimulated.

anti-epileptic therapies; it is permeable to Ca^{2+}, lies post-synaptically, and is prone to increasing responses to excitation over time ('potentiation'). Sustained activation of NMDA receptors is linked to excitotoxicity, cell death, and may be a hallmark of status epilepticus.

For a full summary of the relevant pathways and drug targets, see Figure 9.5.

Management

It is recommended that all cases of suspected epilepsy are referred to a specialist for confirmation of diagnosis and to ensure initiation of therapy that is appropriate to seizure type. Investigations on referral will include blood tests (glucose, electrolytes, etc.), an EEG and where necessary additional neuroimaging, either by CT or MRI, to identify any underlying structural abnormalities. Care should ideally be managed within a multidisciplinary team, with access to specialist nurses and other relevant support services.

Acute management/status epilepticus

Formally, status epilepticus has been defined as a seizure that lasts in excess of 30 minutes. However, as the majority of seizures are brief (lasting less than 5 minutes) and any prolonged seizures (lasting more than 5 minutes) are likely to continue, treatment protocols for managing status are based on seizures that last more than 5 minutes (Figure 9.6). This helps to ensure timely intervention and prevent any subsequent irreversible neuronal damage.

Primary management is to ensure the patient is safe by removing harmful objects and providing a cushioned surface. A prolonged or repeated (more than three in an hour) seizures will require urgent pharmacological management with a short-acting benzodiazepine. In the community this can be achieved with buccal **midazolam**, or rectal **diazepam**. For patients who have had a previous prolonged seizure, or who are known to have repeated seizures, this may be prescribed for administration by an appropriately trained family member or carer in the community. Patients who continue to fit beyond 5 minutes despite pharmacological intervention will require urgent transfer by ambulance to hospital.

Lorazepam or diazepam may be administered IV in first attempts to control status epilepticus. For continued seizures, a second dose may need to be administered, but repeated dosing risks causing respiratory depression. Where such measures fail to stop a seizure, second-line treatment options include IV treatment with **phenytoin, fosphenytoin, levetiracetam, phenobarbital**, or **valproic acid**, based on local management guidelines and availability. In refractory disease, treatment with anaesthetics agents (e.g. **propofol, midazolam**, or sodium **thiopental**) may be necessary. Once the seizure has finished patients should be placed in the recovery position and, where appropriate, transferred to secondary care, e.g. a first seizure.

Chronic management

The aim of pharmacological management in active epilepsy is to achieve a seizure-free state, while minimizing patient side effects, ideally with monotherapy. Treatment

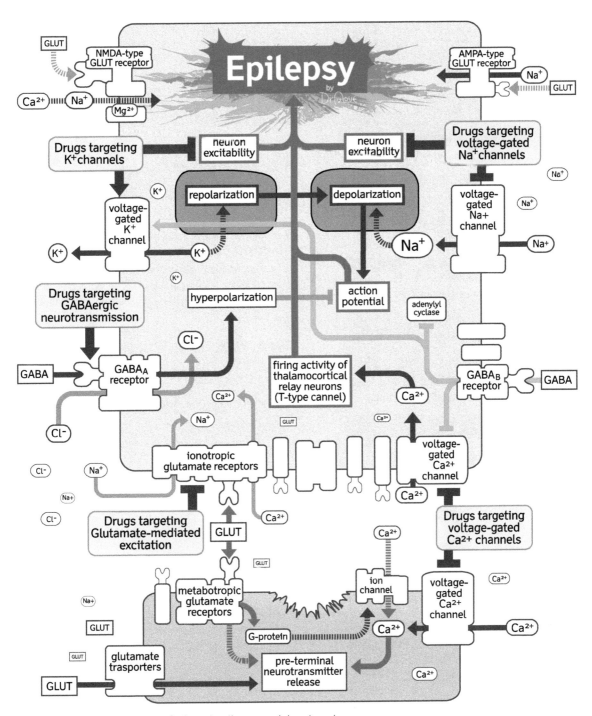

Figure 9.5 Epilepsy: summary of relevant pathways and drug targets.

is selected primarily according to seizure type, although it will also be influenced by age (child/adult/elderly) and any co-existing patient factors such as co-morbidities, drug intolerances/contraindications, interacting drugs,

and patient choice. Treatment should be initiated as soon as the diagnosis has been confirmed.

A large number of new AEDs have been introduced to the market, but comparative studies, such as the SANAD

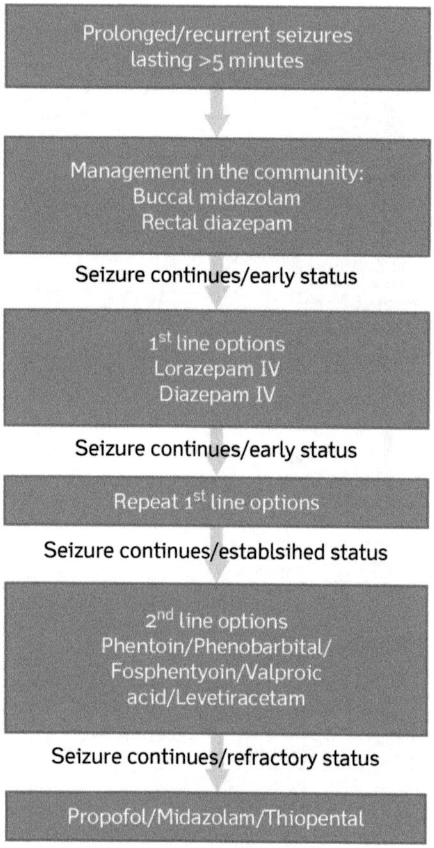

Figure 9.6 Management of status epilepticus.

Data from NICE CG137 Epilepsies: diagnosis and management (Updated April 2018) https://www.nice.org.uk/guidance/cg137 and Convulsive Status Epilepticus in Children and Adults, American Epilepsy Society Guideline (Feb 2016).

trial, suggest that the older agents, **sodium valproate** and **carbamazepine**, remain first-line options for generalized and focal seizures, respectively. **Lamotrigine**, however, may be used in place of carbamazepine for focal seizure, where it demonstrates both clinical and cost-effectiveness, and may have a more favourable side effect profile, particularly for women of child-bearing age and the elderly.

Patients are generally initiated on low doses of first-line drugs, which are then slowly titrated up to establish the minimum effective dose. Where treatment remains ineffective or is poorly tolerated, a second line drug may be introduced as an alternative or adjuvant therapy. The second-agent dose is again slowly titrated to effect before any previous therapy is discontinued. Although monotherapy is preferred, adjunctive therapy may be considered for patients failing on two consecutive drug treatments, but combined therapy is associated with greater toxicity and the risk of drug interactions.

Depending on seizure type, treatment will vary and should patients be experiencing multiple seizure types, certain therapies may even exacerbate seizures. Treatment options are (see NICE CG137, 2016):

Focal-onset seizures

- *First line*: carbamazepine or lamotrigine.
- *Second line*: levetiracetam, oxcarbazepine, or valproate.
- *Additional adjuncts*: clobazam, gabapentin, perampanel, retigabine, or topiramate.
- *If treatment failure with the above*: acetazolamide, eslicarbazepine acetate, lacosamide, phenobarbital, phenytoin, pregabalin, tiagabine, vigabatrin, or zonisamide.

Generalized seizures

Absence seizures

- *First line*: ethosuximide or valproate.
- *Second line*: lamotrigine.
- *If treatment failure with the above*: clobazam, clonazepam, levetiracetam, phenobarbital, topiramate, or zonisamide.
- *Drugs to avoid*: carbamazepine, eslicarbazepine acetate, gabapentin, oxcarbazepine, pregabalin, tiagabine, and vigabatrin.

Myoclonic seizures

- *First line*: valproate.
- *Second line*: levetiracetam or topiramate.
- *If treatment failure with the above*: clobazam, clonazepam, piracetam, or zonisamide.
- *Drugs to avoid*: carbamazepine, gabapentin, oxcarbazepine, phenytoin, pregabalin, tiagabine, and vigabatrin.

Tonic–clonic seizures

- *First line*: valproate.
- *Second line*: lamotrigine.

- *Third line*: carbamazepine or oxcarbazepine.
- *Additional adjuncts*: clobazam, levetiracetam, or topiramate.
- *If treatment failure with the above*: acetazolamide, clonazepam, phenobarbital, or phenytoin.
- *Drugs to avoid*: tiagabine and vigabatrin.

Tonic or atonic seizures

- *First line*: valproate.
- *Additional adjuncts*: lamotrigine.
- *Treatment failure with the above*: acetazolamide, clobazam, clonazepam, levetiracetam, phenobarbital, rufinamide, or topiramate.
- *Drugs to avoid*: carbamazepine, gabapentin, oxcarbazepine, pregabalin, tiagabine, and vigabatrin.

Drug classes used in management

Medications prescribed in the management of epilepsy aim to prevent abnormal paroxysmal neuronal discharge and there are three key anti-epileptic drugs (AED) mechanisms (Table 9.6; Rogowski and Loscher, 2004):

- Modulation of voltage gated cation channels (Na$^+$, K$^+$, and Ca^{2+}).
- Augmentation of inhibition (GABAergic transmission).
- Suppression of excitation (glutamatergic transmission).

Drugs targeting voltage-gated Na$^+$ channels

Several AEDs block voltage-gated Na$^+$ channels with different affinities for the channel's functional states or subtype selectivity. Therapeutic outcome depends upon fast channel inactivation and an increase in the number of channels in the inactivated state. Examples include carbamazepine, oxcarbazepine, eslicarbazepine, phenytoin, lamotrigine, lacosamide, and zonisamide.

Mechanism of action

The voltage-gated Na$^+$ channel is one of the principal regulators of the flow of cations across the cellular membrane. These channels are responsible for the up-stroke of the action potential (Figure 9.4). A multi-subunit structure forms the voltage-gated pore across the membrane, and this structure undergoes conformational modifications that regulate Na$^+$ conductance across the channel. An α-subunit, which forms the ion-conducting pore and provides voltage dependency, is associated with two auxiliary β subunits that modulate their expression and function.

Carbamazepine is widely prescribed in epilepsy with a half-life of 12–18 hours and is a Na$^+$ channel blocker, which reduces the rate of neuronal firing; it also has K$^+$ channel activator activity. Like most Na$^+$ blocking AEDs, **lamotrigine**, **felbamate**, **topiramate**, and **oxcarbazepine**, highest affinity of blockade occurs when the channel is in the inactivated state, causing frequency-dependent reduction in channel conductance. Lamotrigine also has both N- and P/Q-types CCB activity. **Lacosamide**, is a new AED used in focal seizures, with action modulating the Na$^+$-mediated slow-inactivation state.

Drugs targeting K$^+$ channels

The potentiation of voltage-sensitive K$^+$ channels, which are directly involved in neuron excitability, constitutes an important functional target for anti-epileptic drugs. For example, carbamazepine and retigabine.

Mechanism of action

At the neuronal level, K$^+$ channels are responsible for the repolarization of the plasma membrane after a Na$^+$-induced depolarization phase. Direct activation of voltage-dependent K$^+$ channels limits the firing of action potentials by hyperpolarizing the neuronal membrane. As such, activators of this channel have anticonvulsant effects in experimental seizure models, while blockers are able to induce seizures.

The clinical development of the first K$^+$ channel openers for epilepsy has been slow, despite the fact that the first preclinical assessments of compounds date from the 1980s. The demonstration of a K$^+$ channel modulatory link for **retigabine** (ezogabine) was later strengthened by findings demonstrating an interaction with KCNQ2–5 (Kv7.2–7.5) ion channels, which are important determinants of neuronal excitability.

Table 9.6 Overview of mechanisms of action of AEDs

Drug	Na$^+$ channel	Ca^{2+} channel	K$^+$ channel	GABA	Other
Carbamazepine	Stabilize inactive state	Antagonistic properties	Potential modulation	Potentiate GABA receptors	
Phenytoin	Stabilize inactive state				
Sodium valproate	Block			Inhibits GABA degradation, Increase GABA	
Eslicarbazepine	Block				
Phenobarbital		Block		Increase in GABA receptor function	
Gabapentin		Decrease trafficking/function		Increase GABA synthesis	NMDA binding
Lamotrigine	Bind to inactive state	Possible block			
Lacosamide	Increase slow inactivation				
Levetiracetam					Binding to synaptic SV2A, decrease release
Perampanel					Non-competitive antagonist AMPA receptors
Tiagabine				GABA re-uptake inhibitor	
Vigabatrin				Inhibits GABA degradation	
Zonisamide	Block	Decrease of T-type Ca^{2+} currents			
Rufinamide	Prolongs inactive state				
Retigabine			Positive modulator		
Ethosuximide		Block of T-type Ca^{2+} channels			
Felbamate				Positive modulator of GABA receptor	Blocker of NMDA receptors
Benzodiazepine				Potentiation of GABA receptor	
Pregabalin		Modulation of function			

Drugs targeting voltage-gated Ca²⁺ channels

Given their role in the regulation of the firing activity of thalamocortical neurons and pre-terminal neurotransmitter release, the blockade of voltage-gated Ca^{2+} channels constitutes an important functional target for the control of nervous system excitability. Examples include ethosuximide, sodium valproate, levetiracetam, lamotrigine, gabapentin, pregabalin, topiramate, phenytoin, and carbamazepine.

Mechanism of action

Sharing key structural similarities with the Na^+ channel counterparts, the ion conducting α-subunit of the Ca^{2+} channel also confers voltage dependency and associates with other subunits named β, γ, and δ, which can modulate gating. Depending on the membrane potential at which they are activated, voltage-sensitive Ca^{2+} channels can be classified into low or high threshold. Low voltage-activated channels of the T-type are predominantly expressed in thalamocortical relay neurons and contribute to bursting behaviour and abnormal oscillations during absence seizure activity. Therefore, they are important therapeutic targets for **ethosuximide** and **sodium valproate**, used in absence seizures. The high-voltage activated Ca^{2+} channels have been classified in further subgroups (L-, R-, P/Q-, and N-types). Several of these are located at presynaptic terminals where they can regulate neurotransmitter release. Their blockade might thus prevent excessive neurotransmission and provide a target for anti-epileptic therapy.

Drugs targeting GABAergic neurotransmission

As the most abundant and important inhibitory neurotransmitter, the modulation of GABA receptor function constitutes the oldest mechanism in the pharmacological treatment of epilepsy. In the pathological brain, variations in the expression and subunit composition of GABA receptors contribute to overall altered inhibition. Examples include carbamazepine, sodium valproate, gabapentin, phenobarbital, benzodiazepines, vigabatrin, tiagabine, felbamate, topiramate, and zonisamide.

Mechanism of action

The synaptic release of GABA in the brain leads to the activation of two subtypes of GABA receptors, identified by their structure, pharmacology, and function. The post-synaptic $GABA_A$ are pentameric ligand-gated ion channels that respond by increasing Cl^- conductance, resulting in neuronal hyperpolarization and reduced excitability. Importantly, disease-linked alterations in the Cl^- concentration gradients, possibly by changes in the expression of the K^+/Cl^- co-transporter, could switch the direction of Cl^- fluxes, resulting in depolarizing responses.

The pre- and post-synaptic $GABA_B$ receptors are metabotropic G protein–coupled receptors, their activation resulting in the inhibition of adenylyl cyclase, voltage-gated Ca^{2+} channels and activation of inwardly rectifying K^+ channels.

The GABAergic system is targeted by several AEDs, through increased GABA synthesis, release, receptor facilitation, and reduced inactivation. **Phenobarbital** potentiates GABA responses by binding to a specific site of the $GABA_A$ receptor complex and prolonging receptor opening times. The direct activation of $GABA_A$ at high phenobarbital concentrations explains the risk of overdose observed with barbiturates. **Benzodiazepines** bind to a specific site of the $GABA_A$ receptor, increasing binding affinity for the neurotransmitter and the probability of receptor opening. Since the effect is dependent on the binding of endogenous GABA pools, they do not share the barbiturates risk of fatal overdosing.

Vigabatrin is an irreversible inhibitor of GABA transaminase, which is responsible for the degradation of the neurotransmitter in pre-synaptic neurons and glia cells. Enzyme inhibition significantly increases GABA concentrations in the brain, potentiating tonic inhibition. **Tiagabine** has been designed as an inhibitor of neurotransmitter reuptake by the GABA transporter GAT-1, in both presynaptic neuron terminals and neighbouring glia. This only enhances the effect of endogenously released GABA, thus limiting the potential adverse effects. Sodium valproate and gabapentin (in addition to activities at Na^+ and Ca^{2+} channels) also influence GABA turnover by increasing neurotransmitter synthesis and/or release.

Drugs targeting glutamate-mediated excitation

Glutamate is the principal excitatory neurotransmitter in the mammalian brain and the inhibition of its neuronal release and blockade of its receptors constitute important therapeutic targets in epilepsy. Examples include felbamate, topiramate, phenobarbital, perampanel, and gabapentin.

Mechanism of action

The over-activation of glutamatergic neurotransmission, or the abnormal function of the glutamate receptors, has been observed in some models of experimental seizures and in epilepsy syndromes. Glutamate release at the synapse has pharmacological effects on various sub-types of glutamate receptors, classified into ionotropic (form an ion channel pore) and metabotropic (indirectly linked to ion channels through a system of secondary messengers) families. Several specific transporters, both at nerve terminals and surrounding glial cells, complete the removal of glutamate from the synapse.

The ionotropic glutamate receptors are ligand-gated ion channels permeable to Na^+ and depending on sub-type and subunit composition, Ca^{2+} ions. The α-amino-3-hydroxy-5-methyl-isoxazole-4-propionic acid (AMPA) and kainate subtypes are implicated in fast excitatory neurotransmission, while the NMDA, which requires initial depolarization to be activated, is recruited during periods of prolonged membrane depolarization. The metabotropic glutamate receptors are G protein–linked and they localize mostly at the presynaptic level, possible regulating neurotransmitter release.

So far, no specific antagonist for glutamate receptors has been developed for epilepsy, however, the blockade of ionotropic glutamate receptors is believed to contribute to the therapeutic activity of various anti-epileptic compounds with multiple molecular targets. **Felbamate** can inhibit NMDA receptors at therapeutic doses, while **topiramate's** complex pharmacology probably includes NMDA antagonistic activity. An interaction with AMPA has also been proposed for **phenobarbital**, although the functional implications have not been elucidated. More selective AMPA antagonists include **perampanel** and more are currently being developed.

Prescribing

There are a plethora of medications on the market to manage seizure control in epilepsy, used both within and outside of their product license (see Table 9.7). Selection of therapy should be evidence-based for the seizure type, but also take into consideration patient factors such as the presence of co-morbidities, previous therapy, concurrent drugs, likely compliance, etc. In all instances, doses are started at the lowest dose and gradually increased to achieve a seizure-free state. Where drugs have been escalated to the maximum tolerated dose and the patient continues to fit after the first drug, a second drug may be added in or used as an alternative.

Prescribers should be aware of any necessary dose modifications when drugs are used in combination, due to the high potential for interactions with AEDs and the need for prescribing by brand in some instances (see 'Prescribing warning: switching between brands').

PRESCRIBING WARNING

Switching between brands of AEDs

Due to the narrow therapeutic index of some AEDs, care should be taken when switching between brands. The MHRA has therefore divided AEDs into three classes to minimize risk of treatment failure:

- *Category 1*: maintain on specific brand, carbamazepine, phenobarbital, phenytoin, and primidone.
- *Category 2*: consider maintaining specific brand based on risk, clobazam, clonazepam, ezlicarbazepine, lamotrigine, perampanel, oxcarbazepine, sodium valproate, retigabine, rufinamide, topiramate, and zonisamide.
- *Category 3*: unnecessary to maintain on specific brand, ethosuximide, gabapentin, lacosamide, levetiracetam, pregabalin, tiagabine, and vigabatrin.

Unwanted effects

Side effects to anti-epileptic drugs (AEDs) are relatively common, in part due to their lack of specificity and narrow therapeutic index, but also due to their site of action. Many of the side effects can be predicted from the mechanism of action and are dose related, although idiosyncratic reactions, such as hypersensitivity reactions, are also common. Dose-related adverse effects could be partly managed through careful dose titration, or the use of slow release preparations to avoid large fluctuations in serum levels.

Central nervous system

In-line with their mechanism of action in supressing neuronal hyperexcitability, CNS toxicity (neurological, psychiatric, and altered seizure activity) is common with anti-epileptics. In particular, side effects such as drowsiness, somnolence, cognition, agitation, aggression, and psychosis are widely reported, especially with higher doses and when drugs are used in combination. The nature and extent of CNS toxicity varies between agents, for example, sedative effects are particularly pronounced with **phenobarbital** and **primidone**, whereas mood disturbances

Table 9.7 Summary of prescribing information and adverse reactions to AEDs

Drug	Dosing/ formulation	Licensed indication	Cautions and contraindications	Side effects	Interactions
Sodium valproate	Orally OD, BD: tablets, MR tablets and liquid IV BD, QDS	All forms of epilepsy as monotherapy or adjunctive therapy	*CIs*: severe hepatic dysfunction, porphyrias *Cautions*: withdraw gradually, monitor LFTs and FBC due to risk of severe toxicity Consider dose reduction in renal impairment Take care when switching between manufacturers	*CNS toxicity*: tremor, EPSEs, drowsiness, confusion, agitation *Haematological toxicity*: anaemia, thrombocytopenia *Hepatic toxicity*: deranged LFTs, severe liver damage etc. *Electrolyte disturbances*: e.g. hyponatramia, SIADH, oedema *Other*: nausea, vomiting, dysmenorrhea, rashes	Increased levels of lamotrigine, phenytoin, carbamazepine, phenobarbital, ethosuximide, rufinamide, anti-psychotics, anti-depressants, lithium, warfarin, benzodiazepines
Lamotrigine	Orally OD, BD: tablets, dispersible tablets	All forms of epilepsy as monotherapy or adjunctive therapy	*Cautions*: risk of severe skin reactions. Reduce dose in severe renal or hepatic impairment	*CNS toxicity*: headaches, dizziness, drowsiness, aggression and confusion. *Haematological toxicity*: rarely causes abnormalities *Other*: nausea, vomiting, rash, fatigue, diplopia, blurred vision	Reduces efficacy of OCs Levels reduced by rifampicin Levels increased by sodium valproate
Carbamazepine	Orally OD, BD: tablets, MR tablets, chewable tablets and liquid Rectally QDS: suppositories	All forms of epilepsy except absence and myoclonic. Monotherapy and adjunctive therapy	*CI*: AV block, bone marrow depression, hepatic porphyrias *Cautions*: monitor at baseline and during treatment: FBC (particularly platelets), LFTs. Risk of severe skin reaction increased in some ethnic groups. Use with caution in severe renal or hepatic impairment	*Haematological toxicity*: e.g. leucopenia, agranulocytosis, anaemia *Electrolyte disturbances*: e.g. hyponatramia, SIADH, oedema *CNS toxicity*: e.g. dizziness, confusion, drowsiness, headache *Other*: nausea, vomiting, deranged LFTs, skin reactions, diplopia, blurred vision	Reduces levels of ethosuximide, felbamate, lamotrigine, oxcarbazepine, sodium valproate, tiagabine, topiramate, zonisamide, levetiracetam, OCs, warfarin, apixaban, rivaroxaban, dihydropyridines, digoxin, simvastatin, atorvastatin, ciclosporin, tacrolimus, anti-psychotics, anti-depressants. Levels increased by erythromycin, clarithromycin, azoles, protease inhibitors

(continued)

Table 9.7 Continued

Drug	Dosing/formulation	Licensed indication	Cautions and contraindications	Side effects	Interactions
Ethosuximide	Orally BD: capsules, liquid	Absence seizures (including those with tonic clonic) and myoclonic seizures	Cautions in severe haptic and renal impairment May aggravate tonic clonic seizures	*Haematological toxicity:* uncommon but potentially severe/ fatal *Others:* diarrhoea, weight loss, rash, drowsiness, dizziness	Levels reduced by carbamazepine, phenytoin, phenobarbital, primidone. Levels increased by sodium valproate, felbamate, rufinamide
Eslicarbazepine	Orally OD: tablets	Refractory partial seizures +/– secondary generalization as adjunctive therapy	CIs 2nd or 3rd degree AV block *Cautions:* Reduce dose in moderate to severe renal impairment. Avoid in severe hepatic impairment	*CNS toxicity:* dizziness, drowsiness, headaches *Other:* nausea, vomiting, diarrhoea, rash, deranged LFTS	Weak inducer. Levels decreased by phenytoin and carbamazepine
Felbamate	Orally TDS, QDS: tablets	Partial seizures as monotherapy or adjunctive therapy Named patient basis only due to hepatic toxicity.		*CNS toxicity:* insomnia, headaches *Haematological:* Aplastic anaemia (30% fatal) *Hepatic toxicity:* risk of hepatic failure *Other:* nausea, vomiting, rash, weight loss	Increases levels of carbamazepine, phenytoin, sodium valproate, warfarin Reduces efficacy of OCs
Gabapentin	Orally TDS: capsules	Partial seizures +/– secondary generalization as monotherapy or adjunctive therapy	*Cautions:* may aggravate absence seizures, risk of DRESS. Reduce dose in renal impairment	*CNS toxicity:* altered mood/ thinking, emotional lability, hostility, fatigue *Haematological:* leucopenia *Other:* weight gain, hypertension, facial and peripheral oedema	Absorption decreased by Mg and Al containing antacids when given at the same time Increased risk of CNS depression
Lacosamide	Orally BD: tablets, liquid IV BD: intermittent infusion	Refractory partial seizures +/– secondary generalization as adjunctive therapy	CIs: 2nd or 3rd degree AV block *Cautions:* conduction problems or severe cardiac disease as can prolong PR interval Reduce dose in renal or hepatic impairment	*CNS toxicity:* dizziness, headache, confusion, insomnia, altered cognition *Cardiac toxicity:* AV block, bradycardia, AF *Other:* nausea, vomiting, constipation, rash, diplopia, blurred vision	Levels may be increased by azoles, macrolides and protease inhibitors. Levels reduced by phenytoin, carbamazepine and phenobarbital Increased risk of arrhythmias with drugs that cause PR prolongation

Levetiracetam	Orally BD: tablets, liquid IV BD: Intermittent infusion	Partial onset +/– secondary generalization as monotherapy and adjunctive therapy, Idiopathic generalized epilepsy, juvenile myoclonic epilepsy	*Cautions:* reduce dose in renal impairment	*CNS toxicity:* drowsiness, dizziness, headache, amnesia, emotional lability, agitation, aggression *Haematological toxicity:* thrombocytopenia, leucopenia, pancytopenia *Other:* nausea, vomiting, diarrhoea, diplopia, blurred vision, hepatitis	Unlikely
Oxcarbazepine	Orally BD: tablets, liquid	Partial seizures +/– secondary generalization as monotherapy and adjunctive therapy	*Cautions:* Risk of severe skin reaction increased in some ethnic groups, cardiac conduction disorders, monitor sodium in patients at risk of hyponatraemia, acute hepatic porphyria. Caution in severe hepatic impairment and reduce dose in severe renal impairment	*CNS toxicity:* drowsiness, dizziness, headache, confusion, apathy *Other:* nausea, vomiting, diarrhoea/ constipation, leucopenia	Weak inducer. Levels decreased by carbamazepine, phenytoin, and phenobarbital
Perampanel	Orally OD (at night): tablets	Refractory partial seizures +/– secondary generalization as adjunctive therapy	*Cautions:* risk of aggressive behaviour	*CNS toxicity:* drowsiness, dizziness, aggression, agitation *Other:* fatigue, nausea, diplopia, blurred vision, weight gain	Reduces efficacy of POP
Phenobarbital	Orally OD (at night): tablets, liquid IV: Slow injection	All forms of epilepsy except absence seizures Can be given IV in status epilepticus	*CIs:* acute intermittent porphyria, severe renal/ hepatic impairment, severe respiratory depression *Cautions:* use in the elderly. Narrow therapeutic index— may require therapeutic drug monitoring	*Haematological:* megaloblastic anaemia (folate deficiency), agranulocytosis, thrombocytopenia *CNS toxicity:* drowsiness, lethargy, paradoxical excitation/ hallucinations *Other:* rickets, osteomalacia, rash	See carbamazepine although effects slightly less pronounced

(continued)

Table 9.7 Continued

Drug	Dosing/formulation	Licensed indication	Cautions and contraindications	Side effects	Interactions
Phenytoin	Orally OD, BD: tablets, capsules, chewable tablets, liquid IV: slow injection, infusion	All forms of epilepsy, except absence seizures. Can be given IV for status epilepticus	*Cautions:* reduce dose in hepatic impairment, increased risk of severe skin reaction in some ethnic groups, avoid in acute porphyria, risk of osteomalacia—consider vitamin D/ calcium supplements in at risk patients Narrow therapeutic index—may require therapeutic drug monitoring especially with IV treatment	*CNS toxicity:* drowsiness, dizziness, headache *Haematological toxicity:* megaloblastic anaemia, leucopenia, thrombocytopenia, aplastic anaemia *Other:* hirsutism, coarsening of facial features, hepatic toxicity, nausea, vomiting, constipation	See carbamazepine, although effects slightly less pronounced
Pregabalin	Orally BD, TDS: capsules	Partial seizures +/- secondary generalization as adjunctive therapy	*Cautions:* severe heart failure, co-morbidities that predispose to encephalopathy	*CNS toxicity:* drowsiness, dizziness, irritability, amnesia *Other:* nausea, vomiting, dry mouth, constipation, weight gain, blurred vision, diplopia. Rarely QT interval prolongation and heart failure	Increased risk of CNS depression
Retigabine	Orally TDS: tablets	Refractory partial seizures +/- secondary generalization as adjunctive therapy	*Cautions:* patients at risk of or with known QT interval prolongation, risk of urinary retention, reduce dose in renal and hepatic impairment	*CNS toxicity:* drowsiness, dizziness, amnesia, psychosis, tremor, altered coordination *Other:* nausea, constipation, weight gain, dry mouth, blurred vision, diplopia	Unlikely
Rufinamide	Orally BD: tablets	Lennox–Gastaut seizures as adjunctive therapy	*Cautions:* high risk of severe hypersensitivity reaction on initiation, titrate carefully in mild to moderate haptic impairment, avoid in severe hepatic impairment	*CNS toxicity:* drowsiness, dizziness, headache, anxiety, altered coordination *Other:* nausea, vomiting, constipation, diarrhoea, weight loss, blurred vision, diplopia	Levels increased by sodium valproate. May reduce efficacy of OCs
Tiagabine	Orally OD,BD: tablets	Refractory partial seizures +/- secondary generalization as adjunctive therapy	*Cautions:* acute porphyria, reduce dose in hepatic impairment	*CNS toxicity:* drowsiness, tremor, impaired concentration, emotional lability, psychosis *Other:* diarrhoea, visual disturbances	Levels reduced by carbamazepine, phenytoin, phenobarbital, and primidone

Drug	Route/Form	Indication	Cautions/CIs	Toxicity	Interactions
Topiramate	Orally BD: tablets, capsules, sprinkle capsules	Generalized tonic clonic seizures and partial seizures +/- secondary generalization as monotherapy and adjunctive therapy	*Cautions*: Metabolic acidosis, nephrolithiasis (ensure adequate hydration). Reduce dose in renal and hepatic impairment	*CNS toxicity*: impaired attention and coordination, tremor, drowsiness, sleepiness, agitation *Musculoskeletal toxicity*: muscle pain/ weakness/ spasm *Other*: nausea, vomiting, diarrhoea, dry mouth, dry eyes, nephrolithiasis, rash	Levels reduced by carbamazepine, phenytoin, phenobarbital and primidone May reduce efficacy of OCs, particularly at higher doses
Vigabatrin	Orally OD, BD: tablets, sachets	Refractory partial seizures +/- secondary generalization as adjunctive therapy	*CIs*: visual field defects—test pre-treatment and then 6-monthly *Cautions*: elderly, history of mental health disorders Reduce dose in renal impairment	*CNS toxicity*: drowsiness, confusion, agitation, depression, aggression, increase in seizure frequency (rare) *Other*: nausea, oedema, visual field defects	Unlikely
Zonisamide	Orally BD: capsules	Refractory partial seizures +/- secondary generalization as adjunctive therapy.	*CIs*: hypersensitivity to sulphonamides *Cautions*: nephrolithiasis (ensure adequate hydration), metabolic acidosis, hyperthermia Reduce dose in renal and haptic impairment. Avoid in severe impairment	*CNS toxicity*: drowsiness, dizziness, confusion, agitation, amnesia, psychosis *Other*: nausea, diarrhoea, weight loss, nephrolithiasis, hypokalaemia, impaired sweating, hepatitis (rare)	Increased risk of toxicity with other carbonic anhydrase inhibitors, e.g. acetazolamide and topiramate (weak inhibitor)

and behavioural toxicity can be problematic with some of the newer drugs. Other psychiatric effects include an increased risk of suicidal ideation, which should be taken into consideration when prescribing in at risk patients.

Some anti-epileptics can actually exacerbate seizures e.g. **carbamazepine** in absence or myoclonic seizures, due to their effect in increasing GABA activity. It is therefore essential that patients are closely monitored and a choice made appropriate for seizure type. For all anti-epileptics, caution is essential when withdrawing therapy due to the risk of rebound seizures when medication is stopped suddenly.

Haematological

The incidence of haematological toxicity shows significant variation between AEDs, and unlike CNS toxicity, is unlikely to be dose related. Adverse effects include leucopenia, thrombocytopenia, agranulocytosis, pancytopenia, aplastic anaemia, and bone marrow depression, and is particularly pronounced with **carbamazepine**, **oxcarbazepine**, **ethosuximide,** and **sodium valproate**. As reactions are unpredictable, patients should be advised to report any symptoms suggestive of toxicity (e.g. unexplained bruising, bleeding, infection, etc.).

Endocrine

Hyponatraemia and oedema due to an increase in anti-diuretic hormone release from the pituitary, is widely reported with **oxcarbazepine,** and to a lesser extent with **carbamazepine** and **sodium valproate**. The effects are more pronounced in the elderly and in combination with other drugs known to cause SIADH.

Hypothyroidism can also occur secondary to AEDs, especially with **phenytoin**, but also **phenobarbital**, oxcarbazepine, carbamazepine, and sodium valproate. Weight gain is also problematic with both newer and older agents, in particular **gabapentin**, **pregabalin**, **topiramate**, and sodium valproate.

With continued use, AEDs are more likely to cause toxicity, such as osteomalacia and sexual dysfunction. Phenytoin is known to cause hirsutism and coarsening of facial features with long-term use and sodium valproate hair loss; these may be particularly problematic if prescribed for young women.

Hepatic

Nearly all of the AEDs are metabolized via the liver before being excreted by the kidney. As a result, dose modifications are often necessary in hepatic impairment and use contraindicated in severe impairment. Furthermore, the propensity for drug interactions is high, with many being both substrates for, and modulators of, cytochrome (CYP) P450 enzymes (see 'Drug interactions').

Hepatic toxicity tends to be idiosyncratic and of greatest concern with, although not unique to, **sodium valproate**, **phenytoin**, **phenobarbital**, and **carbamazepine**, where the risk of severe toxicity is increased. For this reason, baseline LFTs are recommended when initiating AED therapy and levels repeated intermittently while on therapy. More importantly, patients should be advised to report any symptoms suggestive of hepatic toxicity that might otherwise be missed with infrequent monitoring.

Gastrointestinal

Nausea, vomiting, and diarrhoea are widely reported side effects to nearly all AEDs, although, in general, these effects tend to be dose related and transient. Strategies such as the use of slow-release preparations or ingestion with food may help to alleviate some symptoms.

Cardiac toxicity

Although rare, cardiac toxicity in the form of altered conduction has been reported with AEDs. Caution is recommended with **retigabine**, which is known to cause QT interval prolongation and **lacosamide**, which is associated with PR prolongation. Other AEDs can rarely cause bradycardia or arrhythmias.

Hypersensitivity reactions

Skin reactions are the most common idiosyncratic reactions to AED therapy that typically present as reversible rashes, but in more severe cases, can progress to Stevens–Johnson syndrome or toxic epidermal necrolysis. The risk is greatest with **sodium valproate**, **carbamazepine**, **oxcarbazepine**, **phenytoin**, and **lamotrigine**, although can occur with all AEDs. More specifically, **gabapentin** has been associated with DRESS and **rufinamide** with a severe hypersensitivity syndrome.

Teratogenicity

Women planning to become pregnant should be counselled on the relative risks of AEDs and epilepsy in pregnancy, and reassured that 90% of pregnancies result in a good outcome. The risk of foetal malformations in women taking AEDs (4–6%) is twice that of those who do not. In particular, **sodium valproate** is associated with a significantly increased risk of neural tube defects, major malformations (cardiovascular, urogenital, etc.) and impaired cognitive development and it is therefore recommended to be avoided in pregnancy. The risk with sodium valproate is higher at doses in excess of 1100 mg/day.

Other high-risk anti-epileptics include **phenytoin**, **phenobarbital**, **carbamazepine**, and **topiramate**, although the safety of many other AEDs is not well established. **Lamotrigine** is associated with the lowest risk of foetal malformations, however this needs to be weighed up against the potential for inferior efficacy and the risk of uncontrolled seizures on the mother and foetus.

The risk of neural tube defects with the folate antagonists (carbamazepine, phenytoin, **primidone**, phenobarbital) or other anti-folates (sodium valproate) may, in part, be reduced with adequate supplementation (folic acid 5 mg/day) taken at least 1 month prior to conceiving and during the first trimester.

Drug interactions

Collectively, the AEDs have a high tendency for clinically significant drug interactions; the risk being greater with the older AEDs known to be potent enzyme inducers (**phenytoin**, **phenobarbital**, **carbamazepine**, **primidone**) or inhibitors (**sodium valproate**) of the CYP P450 enzymes. Contributing factors include a narrow therapeutic index, a high incidence of dose-related side effects and those that are modulators and/or substrates of the CYP P450 enzyme system. The risk of interactions varies between individuals, hence when co-prescribing AEDs with other therapy patients should be carefully monitored, particularly within 2–4 weeks of initiation or a dose change. There are a number of interactions to be aware of.

Interactions between AEDs

Carbamazepine, **phenytoin**, **phenobarbital**, and **primidone** can reduce plasma levels of other AEDs including **ethosuximide**, **felbamate**, **lamotrigine**, **oxcarbazepine**, **sodium valproate**, **tiagabine**, **topiramate**, **zonisamide**, and to a lesser extent **levetiracetam**. This is likely to be of greatest significance when treatment is being withdrawn or substituted, as clinically the addition of a second drug will in part compensate for the low serum levels. Other newer drugs with the potential to induce enzymes include felbamate, **eslicarbazepine**, oxcarbazepine, and topiramate, although probably of less clinical significance.

The enzyme inhibitors sodium valproate, felbamate, and **rufinamide** have the potential to increase serum levels of the older AEDs (phenytoin, carbamazepine, phenobarbital, sodium valproate, and ethosuximide), as well as some newer drugs including lamotrigine and rufinamide. Where a second interacting AED is added, patients should be closely monitored for the first 2–4 weeks for signs of toxicity.

Interactions with antimicrobials

The macrolides **erythromycin** and **clarithromycin** are potent enzyme inhibitors of CYP3A4, which can lead to raised and potentially toxic levels of **carbamazepine** and concurrent use should be avoided. Although also metabolized by the CYP isoenzyme the risk with **phenytoin**, **sodium valproate**, and **lacosamide** is likely to be of less significance, as these drugs are also metabolized by other pathways.

Other potent inhibitors of CYP3A4 that may increase carbamazepine levels include the azole anti-fungals (**fluconazole**, **ketoconazole** and to a lesser extent **voriconazole** and **itraconazole**) and the protease inhibitor, antivirals (e.g. **ritonavir**). Phenobarbital and phenytoin levels may again be altered by the same inhibitors.

Rifampicin, a potent enzyme inducer may reduce the serum levels and thus efficacy of carbamazepine, phenytoin, phenobarbital, and lamotrigine.

Interactions with oral contraceptives and in pregnancy

Women of child-bearing age should be carefully counselled on the risk of drug interactions between oral contraceptives and AEDs. Where possible, it is advisable to consider AEDs with a lower tendency for drug interactions, especially as many are known to be teratogenic. The enzyme-inducing AEDs can have significant effect on the efficacy of some oral contraceptives, rendering them ineffective, e.g. **carbamazepine**, **phenytoin**, **phenobarbital**, **oxcarbazepine**, **eslicarbazepine**, **topiramate** (at higher doses), and to a lesser degree **felbamate** and **lamotrigine**. **Perampanel** can reduce the efficacy of **progesterone-only pills**.

As AEDs can increase the risk of folate deficiency, pregnant women requiring treatment with the older AEDs are advised to supplement with higher doses of folic acid to prevent neural tube defects.

Interactions with oral anticoagulants

The oral anticoagulants **warfarin**, **apixaban** and **rivaroxaban** are all substrates for CYP_{450} and thus are likely to have altered efficacy in the presence of **carbamazepine**, **phenytoin**, and **phenobarbital**. **Dabigatran** and **edoxaban** are metabolized through alternative pathways so efficacy should be unaffected.

Other interactions

Other potential interactions to be aware of include the effects of the enzyme inducers on some cardiovascular drugs such as the (calcium channel blockers, statins, and digoxin), anti-psychotics, anti-depressants, anxiolytics, and immunosuppressants. Similarly, **sodium valproate** as an enzyme inhibitor can increase the effects of some antipsychotics and **antidepressants**.

Pharmacodynamic interactions with the AEDs are less well documented, although those agents that have the potential to cause PR (**lacosamide**) or QT prolongation (**retigabine**) should be used cautiously with other drugs that have the same risk.

Further reading

Ahmed R, Apen K, Endean C (2014) Epilepsy in pregnancy: a collaborative team effort of obstetricians, neurologists and primary care physicians for a successful outcome. *Neurology* 43(3), 112–16.

Johannessen SI, Johannessen, Landmark C (2010) Antiepileptic drug interactions—principles and clinical implications. *Current Neuorpharmacology* 8, 254–67.

Kennedy GM, Lhatoo SD (2008) CNS adverse events associated with antiepileptic drugs. *CNS Drugs* 22(9), 739–60.

Rogawski MA, Loscher W (2004) The neurobiology of antiepileptic drugs. *Nature Review Neurosciences* 5(7), 553–64.

Guidelines

Berg AT, Berkovic SF, Brodie MJ, et al. (2010) Revised terminology and concepts for organization of seizures and epilepsies: report of the ILAE commission on classification and terminology, 2005–2009. *Epilepsia* 51(4), 676–85.

Fisher RS, Cross JH, French JA, et al. (2017) Operational classification of seizure types by the International League Against Epilepsy: position paper of the ILAE Commission for Classification and Terminology. *Epilepsia*, 58(4), 522–30.

Fisher RS, van Emde Boas W, Blume W, et al. (2005) Epileptic seizures and epilepsy: definitions proposed by the International League Against Epilepsy (ILAE) and the International Bureau for Epilepsy (IBE). *Epilepsia* 46(4), 470–72.

Fisher RS, Acevedo C, Arzimanoglou A, et al. (2014) A practical clinical definition of epilepsy. *Epilepsia* 55(4), 475–82.

Glauser T, Ben-Menachem E, Bourgeois B, et al. (2013) Updated ILAE evidence review of antiepileptic drug efficacy and effectiveness as initial monotherapy for epileptic seizures and syndromes. *Epilepsia* 1–13.

Glauser T, Shinnar S, Gloss D, et al. (2016) Evidence-based guideline: treatment of convulsive status epilepticus in children and adults. Report of the guideline committee of the American Epilepsy Society. *Epilepsy Currents* 16(1), 48–61. http://www.epilepsycurrents.org/doi/full/10.5698/1535-7597-16.1.48 [accessed 7 April 2019].

Krumholz A, Wiebe S, Gronseth GS, et al. (2015) Evidence-based guideline: management of an unprovoked first seizure in adults. *Neurology* 84, 1705–13. https://www.ncbi.nlm.nih.gov/pubmed/25901057 [accessed 7 April 2019].

NICE CG137 (2016) Epilepsies diagnosis and management. https://www.nice.org.uk/guidance/cg137 [accessed 7 April 2019].

NICE Pathway epilepsy http://pathways.nice.org.uk/pathways/epilepsy [accessed 7 April 2019].

Trinka E, Cock H, Hesdorfer D, et al. (2015) A definition and classification of status epilepticus: report of the ILAE task force on classification of status epilepticus. *Epilepsia* 56(10), 1515–23. http://www.ncbi.nlm.nih.gov/books/NBK2513/ [accessed 7 April 2019].

9.3 Parkinsonism

Parkinsonism is a syndrome characterized by tremor, bradykinesia (slowness of movement), rigidity, and postural instability. Idiopathic (also known as primary) Parkinson's disease (PD) is the most common cause of Parkinsonism, but the syndrome also features with other neurological conditions. Although traditionally considered a motor disease, the non-motor symptoms predate the emergence of the motor phenomena, and cause greater impairment in quality of life throughout the disease progression.

PD is a neurodegenerative disease, with an insidious onset that peaks in 55–65-year-olds. It has an incidence of ~18 per 100 000, with men 1.5 times more likely to be affected. Genetic and environmental factors are important in the development of PD (Table 9.8), and although the majority of cases are sporadic, those with a first degree relative with PD are 2.5–3 times more likely to develop it.

Pathophysiology

The loss of the darkly pigmented neuromelanin neurons of the substantia nigra (SN) has long been associated with the symptoms of PD. In the 1950s, the understanding of the role of dopamine as a neurotransmitter gave further indications that the dopaminergic nigrostriatal pathway was involved in the disease pathophysiology.

The majority of PD cases are sporadic in nature and numerous studies have reported *environmental factors* that may contribute to this cohort, although no single causal factor has yet been identified. Metal ions (e.g. iron, manganese, and aluminium), organophosphates (present in some pesticides) or 1-methyl-4-phenyl-1,2,3,6-tetrahydropyridine (MPTP), may lead to oxidative stress mechanism through free radical formation. This, in turn, inhibits oxidative phosphorylation of NADH-dehydrogenase in mitochondria, resulting in reduced ATP and ultimately dopamine (DA) cell death.

The concept of a *genetic link* to PD is also clear, since the risk of being diagnosed with PD is 2.5–3 times greater in those with a first degree relative. To date, a number of genes have been identified, which fit an autosomal dominant or recessive pattern that may account for familial, juvenile, and also contribute to sporadic onset disease. SNCA on chromosome 4, is the first gene to be identified and encodes for the presynaptic neuronal protein α-synuclein, which is found within Lewy bodies. These major filamentous component may have an important role in the aetiology of PD (see 'Further reading'). Other genes that have been characterized include the autosomal recessive Parkin, which is associated with juvenile onset disease and acts via the ubiquitin pathway; and LRRK2, the leucine-rich repeat kinase that encodes for the protein dardarin and affects dendritic branching.

A pathological hallmark of PD is the presence of Lewy body inclusions within the cytoplasm, which is associated with the DA neuronal loss and can be found in the basal ganglia, brainstem, and cortex, depending on the stage of disease. The Braak hypothesis proposes that PD 'ascends' in six stages from the lower brainstem in the dorsal motor nucleus, to eventually reach the cerebral cortex, giving rise to Lewy pathology (see Table 9.9). This accounts for the progressive symptomatology, which starts initially as non-motor symptoms (e.g. olfactory loss, sleep disorders), with later development of motor symptoms (i.e. bradykinesia).

Parkinsonian symptoms only present when more than 50–80% of striatal DA terminals have been lost (Deumens et al., 2002). As a result, diagnosis of PD occurs relatively late in the pathophysiology of the disease, when DA neurons are lost within the basal ganglia. The neuronal pathways of the basal ganglia are highly complex, and influence both motor and non-motor functions. Two main pathways exist, one stimulatory (*direct*) and the other inhibitory (*indirect*), which have a net effect on the initiation of motor activity output from the cortex. As DA degeneration occurs, the nigrostriatal pathway influence is lost so

Table 9.8 Causes of Parkinsonism

	Examples
Neurodegenerative disorders	Parkinson's disease, Lewy body dementia, progressive supranuclear palsy, multisystem atrophy
Secondary Parkinsonism	Drug-induced: dopamine antagonists (e.g. metoclopramide, prochlorperazine), atypical anti-psychotics
	Toxins (e.g. carbon monoxide, cyanide)
	Metabolic disorders (e.g. Wilson's disease, hypoparathyroidism)
	Infection
	Head trauma (e.g. boxing)

that dynamic equilibrium shifts towards predomination of the *direct pathway*. This results in bradykinesia through over-excitation of the medial globus pallidus and subsequent enhancement of GABAergic thalamic inhibition (Figure 9.7), so that glutamatergic output to the cortex and spinal cord is decreased. The loss of DA neurons also results in over-excitation of the subthalamic nucleus and internal globus pallidus.

Pharmacological treatment of PD was largely ineffective until 1960, when therapy based on muscarinic receptors antagonism was introduced. Striatal neurons, which possess muscarinic receptors, receive inputs from striatal cholinergic interneurons and an inhibitory DA input originating in the substantia nigra pars compacta (SNc), which is lost in PD. Loss of this DA input disinhibits the cholinergic neurons, and therefore muscarinic antagonists reduce activity to normal levels.

As DA transmission is lost in PD, the use of the DA precursor dihydroxyphenylalanine (DOPA) was subsequently instigated (Cotzias et al., 1967). The L-isomer of DOPA was the first practical choice for pharmacological development of an oral agent, as it crosses the blood–brain barrier (before conversion to dopamine in the brain); DA itself does not. l-DOPA (**levodopa**) was initially hailed as a cure for PD, although numerous 'complications' of treatment, including motor fluctuations (such as 'on–off' phenomena, whereby response to medication can fluctuate at random intervals), writhing involuntary movements (dyskinesia), visual hallucinations, and confusion, were superimposed on the disease-related symptoms. In addition, side effects to levodopa were caused by the conversion of DA in the periphery, which led to the use of DOPA-decarboxylase inhibitors in conjunction with levodopa therapy. Inhibitors such as carbidopa and benserazide increase the amount of levodopa crossing the blood–brain barrier, while reducing peripheral side effects such as nausea and vomiting caused by actions at the chemoreceptor trigger zone (see Topic 6.1, 'Nausea and vomiting'). These combined therapies (e.g. levodopa/carbidopa) form the mainstay of treatment today (see 'Drug classes use in management, levodopa').

As the disease progresses, dopamine-modifying strategies may be less efficacious. In addition, 'swamping' the

Table 9.9 Summary of Braak staging

	Stage	Anatomy	Signs/symptoms
Pre-symptomatic	1	Dorsal motor nucleus (anterior olfactory nucleus)	Non-motor signs/autonomic dysfunction, e.g. bladder disorders, constipation
	2	Lower brainstem, i.e. locus ceruleus, intermediate reticular zone	Non-motor signs, e.g. insomnia, depression
Symptomatic	3	Midbrain structures, i.e. substantia nigra, amygdala, hippocampus	Motor signs, e.g. unilateral tremor, rigidity, akinesia
	4	Temporal mesocortex, thalamus	Motor signs, e.g. bilateral disease
	5	Neocortex high order association	Motor signs, e.g. poor balance, falls, emotional/cognitive decline
	6	Neocortex, primary, secondary	Dependency, dementia

Adapted from Braak, H. et al. Staging of brain pathology related to sporadice Parkinson's disease. *Neurobiol Aging* 24:2 197–211. Copyright © 1969, Elsevier. https://doi.org/10.1016/S0197-4580(02)00065-9

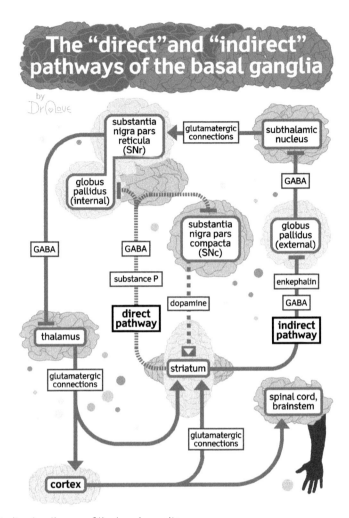

Figure 9.7 Direct and indirect pathways of the basal ganglia.

Data from *Trends in Neuroscience*, 13, 7, Garrett E, Alexander Michael D Crutcher, Functional architecture of basal ganglia circuits: neural substrates of parallel processing, pp. 266–71, 1990.

entire dopaminergic system means that diffuse central actions and side effects remain [e.g. dyskinetic involuntary movements, restlessness (akathisia)]. Where levels of precursor drug are insufficient, endogenous levels of DA can be increased through inhibition of the enzyme catechol-*O*-methyltransferase (COMT); responsible for the breakdown of DA, adrenaline, and noradrenaline. COMT inhibitors such as **entacapone** act to prolong synaptic levels of DA and enhance replacement efficacy in late stage disease.

A second generation and further development strategy of dopaminergic anti-Parkinson drugs has been based on direct DA receptor agonism. There are five DA receptor subtypes, with D_1 (excitatory) and D_2 (inhibitory) being most prominent in the striatum. Agonists such as

apomorphine or **bromocriptine** originally demonstrated inferior therapeutic potency to L-DOPA (Olanow et al., 1987). However, in individuals who respond well to trial agonist therapies, the long-term efficacy is good with a reduced risk of dyskinesia and 'off' side effects. As different DA agonists show differential activity at receptor subtypes, the choice of these can, with clinical awareness, be tailored to ameliorate certain symptom profiles (i.e. **pramipexole** with D3 agonism to ameliorate tremor and depression).

A further approach has involved the protection of neurons from the degenerative process. This strategy began with antioxidants and, in particular, MAO inhibitors. While somewhat controversial, MAO inhibitors (such as **deprenyl** and **selegiline**) are used frequently in early PD. Deprenyl, known to inhibit a dopamine-degrading enzyme, MAO, in the synaptic cleft, enhances the clinical effect of DA and patient quality of life by slowing dopamine's catabolism (Golbe et al., 1988). Other treatments that aim to have protective properties involve NMDA receptor antagonists, Ca^{2+} antagonists and iron-chelating agents, which can prevent excitotoxicity, iron-induced toxicity and MPTP-induced neurotoxicity (Kupsch et al., 1995). In addition to these potential treatments, neurotrophic factors such as brain-derived neurotrophic factor and nerve growth factor remain under investigation, although their therapeutic use is limited since direct infusion into the brain is required.

For a full summary of the relevant pathways and drug targets, see Figure 9.8.

Management

A diagnosis of Parkinsonism is made in the presence of typical signs and symptoms (rigidity, tremor, and bradykinesia), with or without non-motor features (sleep disturbance, constipation, impaired olfaction, cognition, and depression). Postural instability is a cardinal feature that tends to occur as the disease progresses and early emergence of this feature should prompt consideration of alternative diagnosis such as progressive supranuclear palsy. Primary investigations aim to identify any underlying causes such as drug- or toxin-induced, and vascular Parkinsonism. As there is no specific test available for idiopathic PD the diagnosis is made clinically. Features that suggest a potential alternative diagnosis include symmetry of motor signs, lack of response to levodopa, early emergence of postural instability and falls, and early dysautonomia (postural hypotension, erectile dysfunction, and impaired sweating).

Treatment is frequently initiated at diagnosis. Whereas historically treatment was often deferred until quality of life was significantly impacted (in an effort to avoid the emergence of, e.g. dyskinesia), more recent evidence supports initiating treatment early to improve and maintain quality of life.

Management of motor features

Choice of treatment at presentation will depend on the nature and severity of symptoms, patient needs and the age of onset (Table 9.10). Treatment should be optimized to provide symptomatic relief and improve quality of life, whilst minimizing side effects. Three main classes of drug

exist, in order of efficacy—**levodopa**, dopamine agonists, and MAOB. As the disease progresses these drugs are frequently used in combination. COMT inhibitors are added when patients are taking levodopa to extend the duration of action and can be administered with each dose (**entacapone**) or once a day (**opicapone**). **Amandatine** is often trialled for dyskinesia. Lastly, anticholinergic drugs (e.g. **trihexyphenidyl**) can be used for tremor, but increasing recognition of the cognitive vulnerability of patients with PD is such that it is rarely used in older people or in those with evident cognitive dysfunction.

MAOB inhibitors possess only modest anti-PD effect, but they are beneficial in helping to delay the need for **levodopa**, and when used in combination they can reduce the incidence of motor fluctuations. As monotherapy they are therefore beneficial for early treatment of mild symptoms, particularly in younger patients (less than 70). **Rasagiline** is approved for monotherapy or use in combination with other agents, while **selegiline** is only approved for adjunctive use. Studies looking at whether they have additional neuroprotective effects have to date been inconclusive.

Levodopa provides the most effective relief against dopaminergic-related symptoms, i.e. bradykinesia, rigidity, and tremor, thus improving quality of life. It is, however, unlikely to be of benefit against non-dopaminergic symptoms, such as speech disturbance or postural instability. Although very effective in early disease, long-term effects tend to 'wear off', so that doses are required more frequently and patients develop motor complications such as dyskinesias. The use of a modified release preparation has not been shown to ameliorate this effect, so dose levels may need to be reduced or addition of amantadine can be considered. Administered on its own, **levodopa** is rapidly metabolized peripherally by dopa decarboxylase; therefore, it is always administered with a dopa decarboxylase inhibitor (**carbidopa** or **benserazide**) to promote uptake across the blood–brain barrier.

COMT inhibitors may be used as adjuvant therapy to manage motor complications associated with **levodopa**, particularly where the effects of levodopa 'wear off' prematurely between doses. They will, however, increase the risk of dopaminergic side effects (nausea, vomiting, and dyskinesia), and particular care should be taken with **tolcapone** due to associated liver toxicity.

Dopamine agonists may be used as either monotherapy or adjunctive therapy in PD. They can be subdivided into two groups—ergot and non-ergot alkaloids—with the former now very rarely used due to the risk of infrequent, but serious serosal reactions associated with ergot alkaloids (pleural, pericardial, or peritoneal effusions or fibrosis). Collectively, they tend to be less effective than **levodopa**, but still beneficial in improving symptoms and

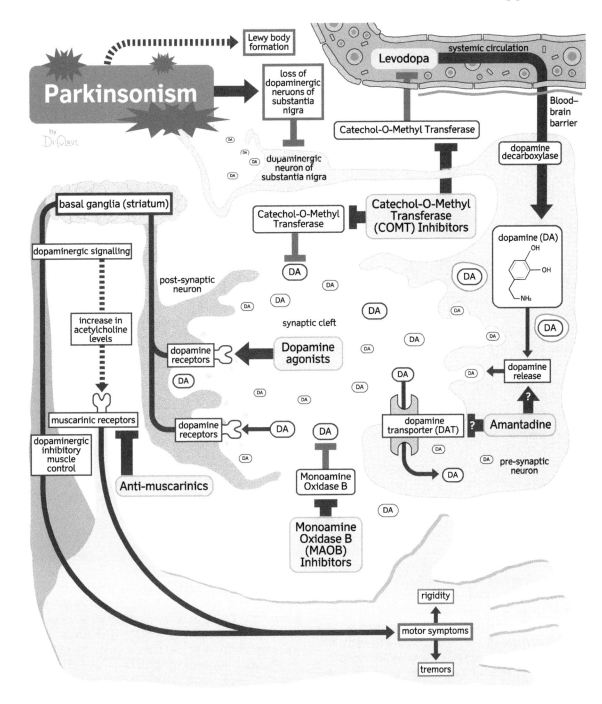

Figure 9.8 Parkinsonism: summary of relevant pathways and drug targets.

quality of life. Dopamine agonists are less likely to cause motor complications with long-term use, so may be used in combination with levodopa to help manage this. As disease progresses, those initially treated with monotherapy will require supplementary levodopa. When considering treatment it is important to counsel patients about the potential occurrence of impulse control disorders (ICD's). These are most commonly encountered with agonist use and comprise addictive behaviours manifesting as, e.g. troublesome gambling, hypersexuality, or binge eating.

Table 9.10 Summary of anti-PD treatment and their place in therapy

Drug	Initial therapy option	Adjuvant therapy with levodopa	Advanced PD
MAOB inhibitors	Y	Y (1st line)	Y
Levodopa	Y	N/A	Y
Dopamine agonists	Y (non-ergot 1st line)	Y (non-ergot 1st line)	Y
Anti-muscarinics	Y (not 1st line)	N	N
Amantadine	Y (not 1st line)	Y	Y
COMT inhibitors	N	Y (1st line)	Y
Apomorphine	N	N	Y

PRESCRIBING WARNING

Impulsive control disorder with dopamine agonists

- Dopamine agonists and less commonly levodopa are associated with impulse control disorders.
- The disorder is characterized by impulsive behaviour such as gambling, hypersexuality and binge eating.
- Patients and carers should be advised of the risks.
- Switching between agents in the class is unlikely to reverse the effects.
- Where it occurs treatment should be gradually withdrawn and stopped.

Anti-muscarinics have been used historically to reduce symptoms of PD, although their use is largely outdated due to their adverse effects, particularly on cognitive function in older patients that comprise the majority of people with PD. Their role is largely limited to use in young patients with severe tremor and in the absence of cognitive impairment.

Amantadine was originally developed as an anti-viral, and found by chance to be effective in PD, although with inferior efficacy compared with other treatment options. Clinically, it may be offered second line as an option in mild, early disease, or as adjuvant therapy in advanced disease to reduce dyskinesias associated with **levodopa**.

As the disease advances patients are often taking (or have trialled) levodopa, MAOB as well as agonists. At this juncture, three further treatments are often considered. *Apomorphine* is a dopamine agonist given SC. It can be used for sudden motor 'offs' as a self-administered injection or as a continuous infusion in an effort to reduce motor fluctuations. Being profoundly emetogenic, patients using **apomorphine** should be initiated on **domperidone**

first as prophylaxis, with ongoing consideration and monitoring of the QTc interval.

Once stabilized on PD treatment, therapy should not be interrupted or suddenly withdrawn due to the risk of developing acute akinesia or neuroleptic malignant syndrome. This should be taken into consideration when patients are hospitalized, ensuring timely access to medication and that administration is not disrupted due to malabsorption or fasting states.

Management of non-motor features

Non-motor symptoms of PD tend to occur throughout the disease, often pre-dating motor features and can have a major impact on quality of life.

Cognitive changes

Depression in PD is common and can co-exist with significant anxiety. Where anti-depressants are used, choice is determined by patient factors including drug interactions (particularly with the MAOIs), and doses carefully titrated. Cognitive behavioural therapy may also be useful. Patients presenting with psychosis should have any underlying causes excluded, such as dementia or drug-induced (e.g. by anti-PD therapy), and where necessary managed with atypical anti-psychotics, clozapine being most effective. There is high prevalence of cognitive impairment, with 80% of patients developing dementia. In early stage disease mild cognitive impairment tends to cause dysexecutive syndrome, whereby patients will have problems organizing complex goal related behaviour.

Sleep disturbances

In PD, these are largely managed conservatively, with patients offered advice on good sleep hygiene (avoiding stimulants, regular sleep patterns, exercise, etc.). Those affected by sudden sleep onset or excessive daytime somnolence should be advised not to drive or operate heavy machinery, and in some extreme cases offered treatment with **modafinil**. Modified-release **levodopa** may be helpful with nocturnal akinesia. **Selegiline** can be useful in younger patients as it is metabolized to amphetamine like substances, which can help with wakefulness, but conversely can worsen confusion in older people.

Falls

These are very common in moderate to later stage disease, particularly in advanced disease or in patients taking sedative drugs. All patients should be asked about falls and near falls to identify common risk factors such as freezing of gait, cognitive impairment, dyskinesia, postural hypotension, anticholinergic medication and environmental factors. (See Topic 1.1, 'Principles of clinical pharmacology, Part 3: evidence-based prescribing, Prescribing in patient groups, Elderly').

Autonomic disturbance

These results in numerous complications including constipation, dysphagia, urinary dysfunction, sexual dysfunction, orthostatic hypotension, sialhorrea, and excessive sweating. Special consideration should be given to patients with dysphagia prior to administering oral drug therapy (see 'Prescribing warning: drug administration in patients with dysphagia').

PRESCRIBING WARNING

Drug administration in patients with dysphagia

- Patients with dysphagia should be referred to speech and language therapy for assessment.

- In those where oral administration is deemed unsafe, drugs may be applied as a patch or by injection, or an NG tube placed.

- Ideally, only liquids or soluble tablets should be administered via a NG tube.

- Where these do not exist, tablets should only be crushed and capsules opened once it has been established this will neither affect bioavailability (e.g. MR preparations) nor cause harm to the patient (e.g. bisphosphonates).

- Tablets or capsules that have been manipulated are no longer within their product license and use is 'off-label'.

Pain

In PD, pain is often associated with rigidity and thus best managed by optimizing treatment of motor effects, as previously discussed.

Drug classes used in management

The main pharmacological treatments available either boost the levels of DA in the brain or mimic the effects of DA. To date, therapies can neither significantly arrest nor reverse the progression of the disease.

Monoamine oxidase B inhibitors

Inhibition of MAOB prevents the breakdown of dopamine in the brain, increasing the levels of available dopamine and prolonging its synaptic effects. It can be used in combination with levodopa, to enhance its anti-Parkinsonian effects and allowing a reduction in levodopa dose. For example, rasagiline and selegiline

Mechanism of action

MAOB localizes in mitochondrial membranes throughout the body; in nerve terminals, brain, liver, and intestinal mucosa. It catalyses the oxidative deamination of biogenic and xenobiotic amines, and has an important role in the metabolism of neuroactive amines in the CNS and peripheral tissues. Inhibition of MAOB therefore increases DA availability with a subsequent increase in dopaminergic neurotransmission. Since the normal enzymatic activity of MAOB creates reactive oxygen species that can lead to neuronal damage, MAOB inhibitors were originally indicated as 'neuroprotective' agents in the treatment of PD. Although much debated, this latter property has not been convincingly demonstrated in human patients.

Rasagiline is a propargylamine and a potent, selective, and irreversible inhibitor of MAOB. **Selegiline** is a selective and irreversible inhibitor of MAOB, which has been shown to have only a mild therapeutic effect on the management of PD when used alone. It can also inhibit monoamine oxidase A (MAOA) at higher doses, which allows for its use in the treatment of depression.

Prescribing

Selegiline and **rasagiline** are administered orally either as monotherapy up-front in patients with mild symptoms of

PD, or as adjunctive therapy to help reduce the fluctuations seen with continued levodopa therapy. They are effective at doses sufficiently low so as not to cause the 'cheese reaction' seen with the non-selective MAOIs. Both drugs are administered OD, with selegiline best taken in the morning as it is metabolized to L-amphetamine and thus likely to cause insomnia. If poorly tolerated, the dose of selegiline may be split, with the second dose given at lunchtime.

Unwanted effects

Compared with the non-selective MAOIs, the MAOB inhibitors tend to be better tolerated, particularly as they are less likely to cause hypertension when taken in combination with tyramine rich food. **Selegiline** is the least well tolerated of the two as it is metabolized to L-amphetamine and can thus induce sympathomimetic side effects, including insomnia, hypertension, tachycardia, sweating, etc. Caution is therefore recommended in patients with underlying cardiovascular disease.

Selegiline and **rasagiline** should be used with caution in severe renal impairment, whereas in severe hepatic impairment selegiline may be used with care, but rasagiline avoided.

Drug interactions

As MAOB inhibitors augment the effects of **levodopa**, the risk of side effects is increased when used in combination, in particular dyskinesias and hypotension. Other interactions of note are those with anti-depressants (see Topic 10.2, 'Depression'). For example, MAOB inhibitors should not be used in combination with a second MAOI, including **linezolid**, or some antidepressants (SSRIs, SNRIs), while with other antidepressants, care should be taken as the risk of an interaction is still high. Concurrent use of **pethidine** and MAOB inhibitors is also contraindicated due to the risk of hyperpyrexia.

Rasagiline is a substrate on CYP 1A2 and may show increased toxicity in combination with inhibitors of this enzyme such as **ciprofloxacin**.

Neither drug should be taken concurrently with sympathomimetics, although the risk is greater with **selegiline**.

Levodopa

Levodopa non-specifically increases the concentration of dopamine in the brain and relieves one of the key neurotransmitter imbalances observed in PD. For example, levodopa plus benserazide and levodopa plus carbidopa.

Mechanism of action

Levodopa acts as a dopamine precursor that is able to cross the blood–brain barrier. It is subsequently converted to dopamine by the enzyme dopamine decarboxylase, increasing the neuron capacity for dopamine release and subsequent stimulation of dopamine receptors. Since oral administration leads to rapid peripheral decarboxylation, levodopa is administered as a pro-drug with a peripheral dopamine decarboxylase inhibitor, thus avoiding conversion in the stomach and the periphery.

It is now recognized that the significant benefits are limited to an average of approximately 10 years. This is due to the progressive degeneration of dopaminergic neurons, with subsequent decrease in the ability to regulate the release of levodopa-derived dopamine in the striatum. Importantly, the concentration of levodopa in the brain is dependent on plasma levels, which can fluctuate markedly following long-term treatment. Although the *in vitro* autoxidation of levodopa can lead to the generation of oxidative stress and necrotic neuronal death, *in vivo* studies have thus far not shown sufficient evidence to indicate that levodopa can accelerate neuronal degeneration.

Prescribing

There are two **levodopa** preparations widely available for use in the management of PD—**co-beneldopa** (levodopa plus benserazide) and **co-careldopa** (levodopa plus carbidopa). More recently, co-careldopa has been formulated in combination with **entacapone** to aid compliance.

The timing of **levodopa** doses is essential in optimizing symptom control, so that doses should be spaced out equally through the day.

Unwanted effects

As dopamine receptors exist throughout the body, **levodopa** can induce a broad spectrum of unwanted effects. Particular care is recommended in patients with underlying cardiovascular disease (due to the risk of hypotension, or more rarely arrhythmias), pulmonary disease, convulsions, endocrine disorders, peptic ulcer disease, or psychiatric illness. Treatment is contraindicated in severe psychosis and in narrow-angle glaucoma.

The most common side effects to treatment are nausea and vomiting. Although usually self-limiting, this may be overcome by the use of **domperidone** (caution QTc) to antagonize peripheral effects. Other side effects tend to be neurological (dizziness, depression, drowsiness, and sudden onset of sleep), cardiovascular (hypotension, arrhythmias) or anti-muscarinic (constipation, dry eyes, blurred vision). Behavioural conditions, such as impulse control disorders, have also been reported to therapy.

In general, long-term effects of **levodopa** tend to be the most problematic for patients, as continued use leads to a wearing off effect and dyskinesias. This may be delayed by starting treatment at low doses and titrating up slowly, or with the addition of other PD treatment options to minimize the effects.

PRESCRIBING WARNING

Sudden onset of sleep

- Levodopa and dopamine agonists are both known to cause sudden sleep onset and excessive daytime sleepiness.
- Patients should be counselled on the risks and where affected advised not to drive or operate heavy machinery.

Drug interactions

Care should be taken when prescribing **levodopa** with other drugs that have a similar side effect profile, such as anti-hypertensives, anti-muscarinics, and anti-depressants. Although widely prescribed with selective MAOB inhibitors, levodopa should not be used in combination with non-selective MAOI anti-depressants. Predictably, concurrent use with centrally acting dopamine antagonists has the potential to reduce the efficacy of levodopa and is best avoided.

Dopamine agonists

The members of this drug class mimic the natural action of dopamine in the brain by stimulating dopamine receptors directly. Examples include apomorphine, bromocriptine, cabergoline, pergolide, pramipexole, ropinirole, and rotigotine.

Mechanism of action

Initially utilized as adjunctive therapy with **levodopa**, dopamine receptor agonists have now been shown to be effective in early and moderate disease, allowing for an important delay in the start of levodopa therapy.

There are five different types of dopamine receptors identified in the brain, with D_1 and D_2 present in the basal ganglia, and D_3, D_4, and D_5 also found in other areas of the brain, like the limbic system. Stimulation of dopamine receptors in the dorsal striatum, such as D_2 receptors, is the primary mechanism by which these drugs ameliorate the motor symptoms associated with PD. The D_3 receptor appears to be a likely target for the treatment of non-motor features associated with PD.

The dopamine agonists can be divided into the ergot alkaloids (**bromocriptine**, **cabergoline**, and **pergolide**) and the non-ergot alkaloids (**pramipexole**, **ropinirole**, **rotigotine**, and **apomorphine**).

Cabergoline and bromocriptine exhibit potent agonist activity on D_2 receptors, with some affinity for 5-HT and D_3 receptors. Pergolide acts as an agonist at D_2 and D_1 receptors, D_3, and some of the 5-HT receptors. Ropinirole binds to D_3 and D_2 receptors. Pramipexole has higher affinity for D_3 than for D_2 receptors, and in addition to improving motor symptoms via D_2, can alleviate PD-related depression, probably through activation of D_3 receptors in the nucleus accumbens. Rotigotine can act as an agonist on all dopamine receptors, but has the highest affinity for the D_3 receptor subtype. Apomorphine is a non-selective DA receptor agonist, with highest affinity for D_1 receptors.

Prescribing

The ergot alkaloids are largely avoided due to the risk of severe fibrotic reactions (see 'Prescribing warning: conversion to rotigotine patches'). Apart from **rotigotine** and **apomorphine**, the dopamine agonists are administered orally, with doses started low and gradually titrated up to effect. **Pramipexole** and **ropinirole** are also available in slow-release preparations to enable OD dosing.

Rotigotine is administered as a transdermal patch every 24 hours, which may be of particular benefit in patients where compliance is an issue or the oral route is unavailable (see 'Practical prescribing: conversion to rotigotine patches').

PRACTICAL PRESCRIBING

Conversion to rotigotine patches

Patients with acute difficulties in swallowing, e.g. following a stroke or peri-operatively, may be switched from their usual regime to a rotigotine patch, up to a maximum dose of 16 mg in 24 hours. Conversion should take into consideration all relevant anti-PD medication. Patches come in a number of strengths, but cannot be cut. Approximately 10 mg per 24 hours of rotigotine is equivalent to:

- Co-careldopa/co-beneldopa 125 mg QDS.
- Co-careldopa + entacapone 100/25/200 mg TDS.
- Pramipexole 1 mg TDS.
- Ropinirole 4 mg TDS/12 mg MR OD.

Apomorphine is generally reserved for severe advanced PD, where other measures have failed to control symptoms. As it undergoes extensive first-pass metabolism, it has poor oral bioavailability and is, therefore, administered SC as intermittent bolus doses or as a continuous infusion if patients experience frequent 'off' periods. Patients should be trained to use the prefilled pens that are easier to use in an 'off' period. Apomorphine is no longer advocated for use as a challenge test in the diagnosis of PD.

Unwanted effects

Side effects and cautions to the dopamine agonists are much the same as those to **levodopa**, although the risk and severity of side effects tends to be greater. Side effects such as nausea, dizziness, and drowsiness (including sudden onset of sleep) tend to be self-limiting and thus managed by slow dose titrations to achieve the desired effect. The emetic effects of **apomorphine** are so severe that all patients should be initiated on **domperidone** first TDS. Motor complications such as wearing-off effects and dyskinesias are less problematic with the dopamine agonists, although the risk of psychiatric disorders such as impulsive control disorders is greater for both the ergot and non-ergot derivatives.

Of greatest concern with the ergot alkaloids is their ability to cause fibrotic reactions (see 'Prescribing warning: fibrotic reactions with ergot alkaloids') and therefore they are contraindicated in all patients with a history of fibrosis (pulmonary, pericardial, or peritoneal) or valvulopathy.

PRESCRIBING WARNING

Fibrotic reactions with ergot alkaloids

- The ergot alkaloids have been known to cause severe fibrotic reactions affecting primarily serous membranes, i.e. pleura, pericardium, and peritoneum.
- Prior to initiation an ECG should be carried out to exclude any cardiac valvulopathy.
- While undergoing treatment, patients should be monitored for dyspnoea, persistent cough, chest pain, heart failure, and abdominal pain or tenderness.
- ECG should be repeated every 6–12 months and lung function tests carried out.

Drug interactions

As with levodopa the therapeutic effects of dopamine agonists are likely to be reversed in the presence of a centrally acting dopamine antagonist, thus concomitant use should be avoided. In addition, **erythromycin** can increase levels of ergot alkaloids increasing the risk of toxicity.

Catechol-O-methyl transferase inhibitors

Since the presence of a decarboxylase inhibitor leads to a significant quantity of orally administered levodopa being metabolized by COMT in the GI tract, COMT inhibitors are used to increase the proportion of each levodopa dose that can enter the brain. For example, entacapone and tolcapone.

Mechanism of action

COMT is one of several enzymes involved in the inactivation of catecholamines, such as dopamine, and noradrenaline, and some other hydroxylated metabolites. It is distributed throughout various organs, including liver, kidney, heart, lung muscle, neuronal tissues, and intestinal tract. COMT inhibitors maintain improved stable blood levels of levodopa with less pulsatile dosing, which results in more constant dopaminergic stimulation in the brain. Both **tolcapone** and **entacapone** are selective and reversible COMT inhibitors used as an adjunct to levodopa therapy.

Opicapone is a novel, long-acting, and potent third-generation COMT inhibitor, which has been recently approved as adjunctive treatment to levodopa. It has shown a significant improvement in off-time in fluctuating PD patients, and offers the possibility of convenient OD dosing.

Prescribing

Entacapone and **tolcapone** are both administered orally and licensed for use in combination with **levodopa**, with entacapone now formulated in combination with **co-careldopa** to help aid with compliance. Entacapone is taken at the same time as each levodopa dose and tolcapone taken with the first levodopa dose, then 6 and 12 hours later. **Opicapone** is taken OD. As the COMT inhibitors optimize the effects of levodopa, it may be necessary to adjust levodopa doses on initiation or cessation according to response. At the time a COMT inhibitor is added, however, higher levels of levodopa are often welcomed. With tolcapone the dose may be doubled if ineffective, although this is at the increased risk of hepatotoxicity and should be done with care in the absence of any underlying hepatic disease. Tolcapone tablets are bitter tasting and it is recommended that they are swallowed whole. Entacapone is used in preference to tolcapone as the risk of hepatic and cardiac toxicity with tolcapone warrants monitoring of liver function and cardiac function with echocardiograms.

Unwanted effects

As COMT inhibitors augment the effects of **levodopa**, levodopa-related toxicity is also increased, including nausea, dyskinesias, dystonia, sudden onset sleep disorders, and less commonly, impulse control disorders. Patients should be made aware of this risk prior to starting treatment. As with other anti-PD therapy, sudden cessation can cause malignant neuroleptic syndrome. The main risks are of diarrhoea and discolouration (orange tinge) of body secretions (tears, urine).

Although rare, **tolcapone** is known to cause severe and potentially fatal hepatic injury. The risk is greatest in the first 1–6 months and more commonly affects females. LFTs should be monitored at initiation and repeated every 2 weeks for the first year, then 4-weekly for 6 months, and thereafter 8-weekly. Both drugs are contraindicated in hepatic impairment.

Drug interactions

Drug interactions with COMT inhibitors are uncommon. They may be taken in combination with MAOB inhibitors, although this is likely to increase toxicity as it does with other anti-PD therapy. **Entacapone** can bind to iron in the GI tract, thereby reducing absorption, which can be avoided by spacing the two by 2–3 hours.

Anti-muscarinics

> These drugs act by blocking centrally active muscarinic receptors, and although they were the first accepted treatment for PD, their current role is largely limited to patients with tremor that are resistant to dopaminergic agents. For example, orphenadrine, procyclidine, and trihexyphenidyl.

Mechanism of action

The rationale for the use of anti-muscarinic drugs in PD is that the progressive loss of dopaminergic innervation to the striatum correlates with an increase in acetylcholine levels, which contributes to the development of motor symptoms.

Muscarinic receptor antagonists are normally associated with neuropsychiatric and cognitive disturbances,

probably due to their non-specificity for a muscarinic subtype or brain region. Since experimental data suggests that M_4 autoreceptors in cholinergic striatal interneurons are responsible for the elevated acetylcholine release in the striatum, they could potentially offer a more specific therapeutic approach.

Procyclidine and **orphenadrine** are non-selective muscarinic receptor antagonists with predominantly central effects, the latter also having mild anti-histaminic and local anaesthetic properties. **Trihexyphenidyl** is a selective M_1 muscarinic receptor antagonist.

The cholinergic system in the striatum has also been considered as a therapeutic target through the development of specific nicotinic receptor agonists selective for $α6β2$ and $α4β2$ nAChR subtypes, which play a key role in the release of dopamine from dopaminergic terminals. The targeting of nicotinic Ach receptors might also offer improvements in memory and emotional disturbances, sleep perturbations, and other features of PD.

Prescribing

There are three anti-muscarinic agents that are indicated for the treatment of PD; **orphenadrine**, **procyclidine**, and **trihexyphenidyl**. Doses are administered orally BD–QDS, depending on the drug used, starting at the lowest dose and gradually increasing to achieve an optimal response. All three agents may also be used to reverse extrapyramidal side effects induced by other drugs such as **metoclopramide** or **phenothiazines**.

Unwanted effects

The role of anti-muscarinics in the treatment of PD has largely been replaced by newer agents, primarily due to their poor tolerability. Anti-muscarinic drugs induce side effects in 30–50% of patients, most commonly causing constipation, dry mouth, blurred vision, confusion, and cognitive impairment; the latter most pronounced in elderly patients, in whom they are best avoided. They should be used with caution in glaucoma, prostatic hyperplasia and intestinal obstruction, as they can aggravate symptoms. Particular care is required when using in combination with other anti-muscarinics or drugs with anti-muscarinic activity, where side effects are more pronounced.

Amantadine

> Originally used as an antiviral agent in the treatment of influenza A, amantadine appears to exert an enhancing effect on dopamine release from presynaptic terminals.

Mechanism of action

The mechanisms for the therapeutic effects of **amantadine** in PD have not been fully elucidated, but seem to involve an increase in dopamine release and block of dopamine re-uptake, which leads to an overall augmentation of dopaminergic neurotransmission. Evidence has also been presented supporting a role for amantadine as an NMDA-glutamate receptor antagonist, which could have a potential neuroprotective effect through the decrease of NMDA-mediated excitotoxicity. The antiviral mechanism appears to be unrelated to its role in PD.

Prescribing

As **amantadine** was originally developed as an antiviral, not all brands are licensed for PD. Although it may be used up front in PD, its efficacy is limited and tends to wear off over time; it is therefore more commonly prescribed in combination with levodopa to minimize fluctuations and reduce dyskinesias. In all instances, doses are started low and increased weekly according to signs and symptoms. As with other anti-PD drugs, amantadine should not be stopped abruptly due to the risk of neuroleptic malignant syndrome.

Unwanted effects

Amantadine is generally well tolerated as side effects tend to be mild and transient. More common reactions include neurological toxicity such as headaches, anxiety, mood disturbances, insomnia, and confusion; as well as ankle oedema and GI effects (nausea, vomiting, and constipation). Doses should be reduced in mild to moderate renal impairment and treatment avoided in severe impairment. Caution is also recommended in hepatic impairment.

Interactions with amantadine are infrequent, although some diuretics may impair clearance leading to increased toxicity.

Further reading

Braak H, Del Tredici K, Rub U, et al. (2003) Staging of brain pathology related to sporadice Parkinson's disease. *Neurobiological Aging* 24, 197–211.

Brichta L, Greengard P, Flajolet M (2013) Advances in the pharmacological treatment of Parkinson's disease: targeting neurotransmitter systems. *Trends in Neurosciences* 36(9), 543–54.

Cotzias GC, Van Woert MH, Schiffer LM, et al. (1967) Aromatic amino acids and modification of parkinsonism. *New England Journal of Medicine* 276, 374–9.

Devos D, Defebvre L, Bordet R. (2010) Dopaminergic and non-dopaminergic pharmacological hypotheses for gait disorders in Parkinson's disease. *Fundamental Clinical Pharmacology* 24, 407–21.

Deumens R, Blokland A, Prickaerts J. (2002) Modeling Parkinson's disease in rats: an evaluation of 6-OHDA lesions of the nigrostriatal pathway. *Experimental Neurology* 175(2), 303–17.

Edwards M, Quinn N, Bhatia K (2008) *OSH Parkinson's Disease and Other Movement Disorders*. Oxford: Oxford University Press.

Golbe LI, Farrell TM, Davis PH. (1988) Case-control study of early life dietary factors in Parkinson's disease. *Archives of Neurology* 45(12), 1350–3.

Kupsch A, Gerlach M, Pupeter SC, et al. (1995) Pretreatment with nimodipine prevents MPTP-induced neurotoxicity at the nigral, but not at the striatal level in mice. *Neuroreport* 6(4), 621–5.

Olanow CW, Alberts MJ (1987) Double-blind controlled study of pergolide mesylate as an adjunct to Sinemet in the treatment of Parkinson's disease. *Advances in Neurology* 45, 555–60.

Olanow C, Brundin P (2013) Parkinson's disease and alpha synuclein: is Parkinson's disease a prion-like disorder? *Movement Disorders* 28(1), 31–40.

Seppi K, Weintraub D, Coelho M (2011) The Movement Disorder Society Evidence-Based Medicine Review Update: treatments for the non-motor symptoms of Parkinson's disease. *Movement Disorders* 26(Suppl. 3), S42–80.

Guidelines

AAN (2006a) Practice parameter: neuroprotective strategies and alternative therapies for Parkinson disease (an evidence-based review) *Neurology* 66 (7), 976–82.

AAN (2006b) Practice parameter: treatment of Parkinson disease with motor fluctuations and dyskinesia (an evidence-based review). *Neurology* 66 (7), 983–95.

AAN (2010) Treatment of nonmotor symptoms of Parkinson's disease *Neurology* 74, 924–31

NICE CG35 (June 2006) Parkinson's disease in over 20's: diagnosis and management. https://www.nice.org.uk/guidance/cg35 [accessed 7 April 2019].

NICE Pathway (2019) Parkinson's disease https://pathways.nice.org.uk/pathways/parkinsons-disease [accessed 7 April 2019].

Parkinson Society Canada (2012): Canadian Guidelines on Parkinson's disease. *Canadian Journal of Neurological Sciences* 39 (4), Suppl. 4. http://www.parkinsonclinicalguidelines.ca/sites/default/files/PD_Guidelines_2012.pdf [accessed 7 April 2019].

SIGN 113 (2010) Diagnosis and pharmacological management of Parkinson's disease: A national clinical guideline. https://www.sign.ac.uk/sign-113-diagnosis-and-pharmacological-management-of-parkinson-s-disease.html [accessed 24 April 2019].

9.4 Dementia and Alzheimer's disease

Dementia is a process of altered mental state, which is insidious in onset and chronic in nature. It typically comprises cognitive impairment (e.g. affecting short-term memory, language, attention, problem-solving), with personality and behavioural changes that lead to difficulties in performing daily living activities. Strictly speaking, dementia is a syndrome and is classified into several diseases of different aetiology and dominant pathology/pathophysiology. The most common dementia is Alzheimer's disease (AD), which accounts for 50% of dementias, and results from degeneration of the cerebral cortex with deposition of amyloid and neurofibrillary tangles (proteins; see 'Pathophysiology, Alzheimer's disease'). *Vascular dementia* accounts for a quarter of dementias, and occurs as a result of brain damage secondary to microscopic bleeds or clots e.g. in cerebrovascular disease. A third type of dementia is *dementia with Lewy bodies* (DLB) (~15%), where protein is deposited in the brainstem and neocortex, and is associated with Parkinsonism (in effect, a spectrum of disease and pathology exists from Lewy Body to Parkinson's disease).

The prevalence of dementia doubles every 5 years beyond 60 years old, starting at levels of 1.5%, rising to 13% amongst 80-year-olds and to >25% in those over 90. Alzheimer's disease is more common in females, with global variations, suggesting some genetic or environmental risk factors.

Pathophysiology

Alzheimer's disease

Alzheimer's disease is the most common form of dementia seen in those over 65 years old, and has genetic- and sex-linked risk factors. The slightly increased risk of developing AD in females may be due to the loss of circulating oestrogen levels in the post-menopause period, as this hormone possesses antioxidant activity and shows neuroprotective properties. Age is still the most important risk factor, with family history also being significant, albeit only predicting a small increase in risk (3.5-fold from a first-degree relative).

Despite this small autosomal dominant carry-through, three causative genes have been identified in the pathophysiology: presenilin I and II, and amyloid precursor protein (APP). Mutations in these genes modify the way in which the APP is processed, although collectively these account for only about 1% of AD. In sporadic disease, there appears to be a substantial genetic effect, probably mediated through the presence or absence of APoE4 alleles, plus other factors not yet fully characterized.

The principal mechanistic hypothesis underlying AD is centred on the pathological presence of amyloid plaques within the brain. These plaques are composed of numerous proteins, with one of the dominant components being amyloid β protein (Aβ), a cleavage product from APP. APP is an integral membrane bound protein, whose function is thought to involve synapse formation, neuroplasticity, and iron export. Enzymes, called secretases (α, β and γ), cleave APP leading to the formation of Aβ. The γ-secretase, a transmembrane protein, is composed of 4 protein subunits including presenilin I and II, which act as proteases. Mutations in the presenilin gene therefore affects proteolytic activity, leading to altered ratios of Aβ42 and Aβ40 subunits. Interestingly, there is growing evidence for the role of cholesterol and lipid raft maintenance by APP in AD, and the presence of certain lipoproteins [via apolipoprotein E (ApoE) genes] in serum and CSF, constitute an increased risk factor. The formation of Aβ42 in particular is highly amyloidogenic, and leads to plaque formation and accumulation within the hippocampus and cerebral cortex. Certain genotypes of ApoE may increase Aβ production and failure of its clearance greatly enhances the risk of AD.

Aβ itself can affect neuron functioning, leading to changes in apoptosis, plasma membrane, and DNA stability; and when formed into fibrils (accumulating Aβ), can also alter the status of another key structural protein (Tau). Tau is found in neurofibrillary tangles, another characteristic pathological observation, where hyperphosphorylated Tau protein aggregates within neurons throughout the brain. Levels of these deposits tend to closely correlate with clinical symptoms and signs and are also present in other forms of dementia (e.g. frontotemporal dementia). The correlation between Aβ accumulation and symptoms is less evident.

As AD progresses, there is failure and loss of cholinergic innervation (e.g. from nucleus basalis of Meynert) to the hippocampus, amygdala, and neocortex, with concomitant decline in enzymes responsible for the manufacture of ACh (choline acetyltransferase; ChAT) and its breakdown enzyme (acetylcholinesterase; AChE).

Aβ itself can also modify the functioning of NMDA receptors and affect the passage of Ca^{2+} through this channel. Moreover, NMDA receptor activity can influence the hyperphosphorylation of Tau, so that enhanced function can increase deposition of neurofibrillary tangles. The NMDA receptor is important for learning and memory, and its over-stimulation, with associated Ca^{2+} influxes, may cause oxidative stress, which contributes to disease progression, and the decline in hippocampal and cortical functioning. The use of **memantine**, an NMDA open-channel receptor blocker in AD, reduces the Ca^{2+} fluxes in over-stimulation, while enabling these receptors to continue to function in a normal physiological pattern (see 'Drug classes used in management, NMDA receptor antagonists').

One of the early symptoms in AD is the loss of new day-to-day memories (episodic memory), a consequence of medial temporal lobe dysfunction. Where symptoms are mild and do not disrupt normal daily function, this is described as mild cognitive impairment. However, as the pathological changes progress to encompass the hippocampus and cortex, severe short-term memory loss occurs accompanied by impairment in other cognitive domains, which can lead to difficulties in word finding, loss of spatial awareness, attention deficit and social functioning. The fibrillogenic loss of cholinergic innervation to the hippocampus and cortex is thought to be responsible for many of these symptoms and the associated decline in ChAT

and AChE; thus, one way to stabilize cholinergic transmission is to generate a net increase in synaptic levels of ACh through inhibition of AChE (see 'Drug classes used in management, NMDA receptor antagonists'). This can help in the short term to stabilize some CNS function but ultimately disease progression cannot be reversed. Oestrogen, other antioxidants, antibodies against Aβ, and fibril-destructing compounds, have all been investigated unsuccessfully as means to stabilize/prevent the neural loss. Failure to demonstrate an effect may, in part, be due to poor early, reliable, diagnostic tests, so that the disease may have progressed beyond an efficacious treatment window.

Dementia with Lewy bodies

Dementia with Lewy bodies (DLB) is distinct from AD in both presentation and pathophysiology, but it is often mistaken for the latter. DLB occurs as a result of neurodegeneration, with progressive loss of neurons and the neurotransmitters produced, i.e. ACh, dopamine, and glutamate. Degeneration of the substantia nigra leads to a decrease in dopamine production, accounting for its historical overlap with Parkinson's disease and the presence of Parkinson symptoms in most patients. Neurodegeneration is believed to occur as a consequence of α-synuclein aggregation. Lewy bodies are spherical neuronal inclusions made up of abnormal neurofilament proteins that are present in the cerebral cortex, and are believed to be formed as a cytoprotective response to α-synuclein aggregation. Diagnosis of DLB is based on clinical criteria, i.e. fluctuating attention, visual hallucinations, and spontaneous Parkinsonian motor signs. DLB is also diagnosed when dementia emerges within a year of onset of Parkinson's disease. As with AD, acetylcholinesterase inhibitors have a role to play in DLB by ameliorating the impaired cholinergic activity. Similarly, NMDA inhibitors have been shown to be effective in some patients in managing symptoms. Levodopa therapy may also be effective in managing associated parkinsonian symptoms.

For a full summary of the relevant pathways and drug targets, see Figure 9.9.

Management

A diagnosis of dementia is primarily made from a thorough clinical history taken from both the patient and, ideally, from someone who knows them well, followed by a mental

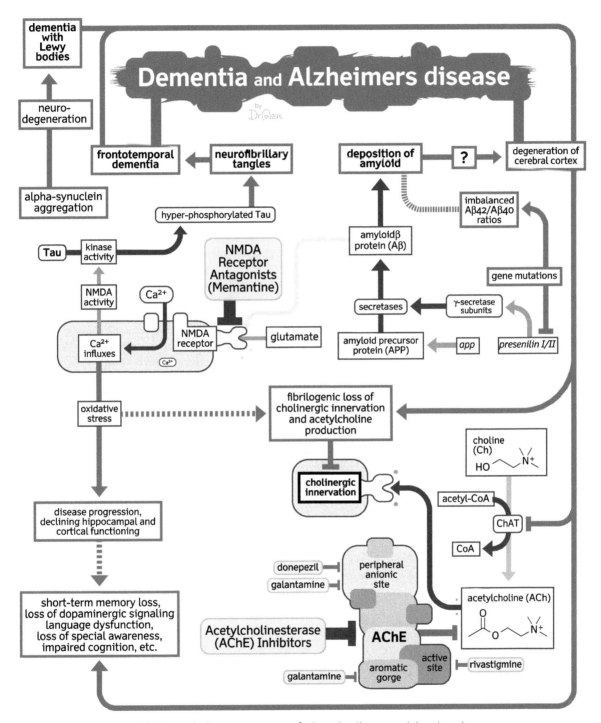

Figure 9.9 Dementia and Alzheimer's disease: summary of relevant pathways and drug targets.

test to assess cognitive function. The Montreal Cognitive Assessment (MoCA) or Mini Mental State Examination (MMSE) are widely used for this, although other tests such as the six-item cognitive impairment test (6-CIT) and the General Practitioner Assessment of Cognition (GPCOG) may also be used.

Investigations (see Table 9.11) and a comprehensive drug history (including self-medicated or illicit drug use), are undertaken to exclude differential diagnoses or identify the rare, but treatable causes of dementia. Drugs such as those with antimuscarinic properties are widely known to impair cognition and should be pro-actively stopped and/or avoided in anyone with dementia or at risk, i.e. particularly older people. Testing for HIV or syphilis is not routinely recommended, but may be considered in 'at-risk' patients.

Imaging techniques such as MRI, CT, amyloid positron emission tomography (PET), and single-photon emission computed tomography (SPECT) can help in the diagnosis of dementia by excluding other pathologies or identifying changes consistent with some dementia subtypes. Differentiation between the types of dementia is based on standardized criteria, i.e. Alzheimer's, Lewy bodies, vascular, and frontotemporal dementia, and is best undertaken by a specialist in the field. Increasingly, biomarkers such as amyloid levels have been developed to aid with differentiation.

As there is no cure for the neurodegenerative diseases that cause dementia; much of the care focuses on recognizing patient needs so that they are provided with the necessary support. Pharmacological management may be offered to slow the progression of cognitive impairment, and behavioural and functional symptoms, although with limited success. As drug treatment carries its own risks, the decision to treat should be based on individual factors and should be made in collaboration with the patient and/or carer(s). Furthermore, response to treatment varies markedly between patients, so it is recommended that treatment is reviewed every 6 months.

The AChE inhibitors (**donepezil**, **galantamine**, and **rivastigmine**) are recommended for first-line use in mild to moderate Alzheimer's disease and should be considered in DLB, particularly in patients with distressing behavioural changes. For patients with AD who are intolerant or in more severe disease, **memantine** may be considered. Due to the underlying pathology in vascular dementia the AChE inhibitors are unlikely to be of benefit and thus not recommended for use.

Some patients may require additional drug treatment to manage associated behavioural disturbances such as aggression, agitation, or depression. Antipsychotics may be considered, although due to their anticholinergic effects, they should be avoided unless initiated by a specialist in DLB, as they are likely to further impair cognition, can induce orthostatic hypotension, increase the risk of stroke, and lead to severe extrapyramidal side effects. Similarly, other anticholinergic medication should be withheld in this patient group.

Treatment with **levodopa** in DLB may be of benefit in the presence of Parkinsonism, although response rates tends to be lower than in patients with PD alone (30–50%). Where used doses should be started low and gradually titrated to effect.

Drug classes used in management

Acetylcholinesterase inhibitors

Inhibition of AChE, the enzyme that hydrolyses the neurotransmitter acetylcholine aims to increase impaired cholinergic neurotransmission and prevent some of the non-catalytic cytotoxic actions of AChE. For example, donepezil, galantamine, and rivastigmine.

Mechanism of action

Acetylcholinesterase is responsible for the termination of the cholinergic nerve transmission after acetylcholine release into the synapse. AChE's structure is that of a narrow gorge that has two separate sites—the catalytic and the peripheral anionic site. Located at the bottom

Table 9.11 Investigations in suspected dementia

Investigation	Differential
Full blood count	Anaemia, infection
ESR/CRP	Infection
TFTs	Hyper/hypothyroidism
Serum biochemistry (electrolytes, calcium, phosphate, creatinine, glucose)	Electrolyte imbalance, dehydration, parathyroid disorders, renal impairment, hypoglycaemia
LFTs	Hepatic impairment
Serum B12/folate	B12/folate deficiency

of the cavity, the catalytic site is mainly responsible for the interaction with the substrate. The peripheral anionic site is found at the entrance of the catalytic gorge, and its interaction with ligands can change the conformation of the active centre. This site binds to the substrate transiently, as a first stage of the catalytic pathway that enhances the efficiency of the reaction.

Studies have indicated that the activity of AChE is increased in AD patients, augmenting ACh hydrolysis, as well as enhancing various non-catalytic actions, such as the pro-aggregating activity of Aβ to form a complex with the growing fibrils that has higher cytotoxicity than the β-amyloid fibrils alone. The peripheral anionic site has been identified as the structural domain that promotes β-amyloid peptide aggregation. The AChE inhibitors therefore not only promote cholinergic transmission through the increase of available ACh, but can also affect the synthesis, deposition, and aggregation of toxic Aβ–peptide. In effect, the design of dual binding site inhibitors of the AChE constitutes the main goal in the development of novel agents with extended pharmacological profile.

Donepezil is a centrally active, potent, specific, non-competitive, and reversible cholinesterase inhibitor that can bind to the peripheral anionic site. **Rivastigmine** is a carbamate derivative that is structurally associated to **physostigmine**, but not to donepezil or **tacrine** (withdrawn from the market). It is a powerful, slow-reversible inhibitor that binds at the active site. Unlike donepezil, which can selectively inhibit AChE, rivastigmine inhibits both AChE and butyrylcholinesterase. The alkaloid **galantamine** interacts with the anionic site and the aromatic gorge, and is recognized as a selective, competitive, and rapidly reversible AChE inhibitor. Moreover, galantamine acts as an allosteric ligand when binding to nicotinic cholinergic receptors, inducing their positive modulation and enhancing their function in the presence of ACh. Since the cognitive impairment seen in AD has been correlated with a decrease in nicotinic receptors, their allosteric modulation by galantamine may be beneficial for treatment.

Prescribing

Donepezil and **galantamine** are only licensed for use in Alzheimer's disease, whereas some formulations of **rivastigmine** are also licensed for use in Parkinson's disease dementia (PDD). All drugs are administered orally, with rivastigmine also available as a patch to aid the pharmacokinetic profile. Alternatively, in patients unable to manage tablets or capsules, soluble tablets (donepezil) or solutions (rivastigmine, galantamine) may be used. To promote compliance, donepezil (due to its long half-life) and galantamine *slow release,* may be administered OD.

Unwanted effects

Side effects most widely reported with AChE inhibitors tend to be GI, including nausea, vomiting, dyspepsia, and diarrhoea.

Non-specific inhibition of AChE can impact on multiple systems, inducing effects such as bradycardia and respiratory depression. Particular care is therefore necessary when prescribing in patients with underlying cardiovascular disease or respiratory compromise. Treatment is also associated with neurological toxicity, such as dizziness, tremor, headache and sleep disturbances, which can limit its use in practice.

Although predictably AChE inhibitors antagonize the effects of anticholinergics, drug interactions of clinical significance are unlikely.

NMDA receptor antagonists (memantine)

The non-competitive and voltage-dependent NMDA receptor antagonist memantine can prevent the effects of tonic and pathologically high concentrations of the neurotransmitter glutamate, which could promote neuronal dysfunction.

Mechanism of action

The binding sites of **memantine** are located within the ion channel of the NMDA subtype of glutamate receptors, overlapping with the binding sites of the endogenous NMDA antagonist Mg^{2+}. This antagonism is voltage dependent as memantine channel block can be removed by sustained membrane depolarization.

Memantine acts to reduce the raised levels of potentially abnormal Ca^{2+} influx observed in the presence of slightly augmented glutamate levels, without affecting transient physiological activation by the much higher concentrations of glutamate released in the synapse, essential for learning and memory processes. Thus, memantine mainly reduces the background 'noise' of Ca^{2+} influx through NMDA receptors under pathological conditions. In addition, the potentially neuroprotective role of memantine is derived from its ability to block glutamate-induced excitotoxicity that occurs in many neurodegenerative diseases, and is mainly mediated by an increase in NMDA-dependent Ca^{2+} influx.

Prescribing

Memantine is the only NMDA receptor antagonist licensed for use in AD, but only in moderate to severe disease, as evidence of a benefit in terms of cost-effectiveness over the AChE inhibitors in mild to moderate disease, has not been established. Doses are administered orally OD as either a tablet or a liquid, increased every 7 days to achieve a maintenance dose.

Unwanted effects

Compared with the AChE inhibitors, **memantine** is more likely to cause CNS, rather than GI toxicity, in particular, dizziness, headache, and drowsiness, although incidence is reported to be little more common than placebo. Rarely, memantine has been known to induce seizures and, as such, should be used cautiously in patients with a history of epilepsy. Other side effects include constipation, hypertension, and dyspnoea.

Drug interactions

Interactions with **memantine** tend to be pharmacodynamic in nature. In particular, its effects are augmented in combination with other NMDA antagonists (e.g. **ketamine**, **amantadine**, and **dextromethorphan**) and to a lesser extent with anticholinergics and dopaminergics. Conversely, the effects of barbiturates and neuroleptics may be reduced.

Further reading

Ballard C, Gauthier S, Corbett A, et al. (2011) Alzheimer's disease. *Lancet* 377, 1019–31.

Burns A, Iliffe S (2009) Alzheimer's disease. *British Medical Journal* 5, 338.

Colovic M, Krstic DZ, Lazarevic-Pasti TD, et al. (2013) Acetylcholinesterase inhibitors: pharmacology and toxicology. *Current Neuropharmacology* 11(3), 315–35.

Hasselmo ME. (2006) The role of acetylcholine in learning and memory. *Current Opinions in Neurobiology* 16, 710–15.

Peng D, Yuan X, Zhu R (2013) Memantine hydrochloride in the treatment of dementia subtypes. *Journal of Clinical Neurosciences* 20(11), 1482–85.

Singh M, Kaur M, Kukreja H, et al. (2013) Acetylcholinesterase inhibitors as Alzheimer therapy: from nerve toxins to neuroprotection. *European Journal of Medical Chemistry* 70, 165–88.

Guidelines

American College of Physicians (2008) Current pharmacologic treatment of dementia: a clinical practice guideline from the American College of Physicians and the American Academy of Family Physicians *Annals of Internal Medicine* 148, 370–8.

Birks J (2006) Cholinesterase inhibitors for Alzheimer's disease *Cochrane Database of Systematic Reviews* (1), CD005593. https://www.cochranelibrary.com/cdsr/doi/10.1002/14651858.CD005593/abstract [accessed 9 April 2019].

NICE CG42 (2014) Dementia: supporting people with dementia and their carers in health and social care. https://www.nice.org.uk/guidance/cg42 [accessed 9 April 2019].

NICE Pathway (2019) Dementia http://pathways.nice.org.uk/pathways/dementia [accessed 9 April 2019].

NICE TA217 (2011) Donepezil, galantamine, rivastigmine and memantine for the treatment of Alzheimer's disease. https://www.nice.org.uk/guidance/TA217 [accessed 9 April 2019].

SIGN 86 (2006) Management of patients with dementia: A national clinical guideline. http://umh1946.edu.umh.es/wp-content/uploads/sites/172/2015/04/Management-of-patients-with-dementia-NHS.pdf [accessed 9 April 2019].

9.5 Multiple sclerosis

Multiple sclerosis (MS) is an inflammatory demyelinating disease of the CNS (brain and spinal cord), which despite lacking a clear known cause has much evidence suggesting it is predominantly a cell-mediated autoimmune condition. Repeated episodes of inflammation lead to focal plaques of demyelination in the white matter, blocking conduction and impairing action potential propagation. MS is believed to be multifactorial in origin, made up of genetic predisposition and environmental factors such as infection, chemical exposures, and/ or reduced vitamin D levels. Risk is also influenced by place of birth and residence, although those that migrate before the age of 15 will have a risk more in line with that of their adopted country. Incidence and prevalence rates are typically higher away from the equator and highest in northern countries. In the UK, prevalence is approximately 120/100 000. There is a female predominance (3:1), with Caucasians being most at risk, and diagnosis typically made in young adulthood. Clinically, there are three *main* phenotypes of MS—relapsing and remitting, benign relapsing-remitting, and primary progression (see 'Clinical presentation and management'); however, rarely patients may experience a single focal event, termed clinically isolated syndrome (CIS).

Pathophysiology

Genetic susceptibility and environmental exposure appear to be the strongest risk factors that lead to MS and influence its course.

Genetic factors

To date, the strongest genetic evidence is linked with the *DRB1* allele of the *HLA* genes (part of the MHC), which are responsible for presentation of antigens to immune cells (i.e. the differential between self and non-self); however, 45% of those with MS do not possess this allele.

Environmental factors

Two mainstream environmental factors have evidence in the aetiology of MS also:

- *Vitamin D*: low levels of vitamin D have been found in patients with relapsing-remitting MS, while high levels of 25-hydroxyvitamin D can be protective. This finding is consistent with the geographical distributions of MS patients, whose UV(B) exposure levels may be less than those closer to the equator. Vitamin D levels can affect immune responses and decrease inflammatory cytokine levels, an action that is of benefit in neuro-inflammation. Interestingly, vitamin D can affect the regulation of HLA-DRB1 and may provide a link between the environment and the genetic contribution to MS.

- *Epstein–Barr virus (EBV)*: this DNA virus causes infectious mononucleosis and has been linked to numerous autoimmune diseases (e.g. SLE, Sjorgens syndrome, and RA) and cancers (e.g. Hodgkin's lymphoma, nasopharyngeal carcinoma) and may have a role in MS. More than 99% of patients with MS have previously been infected with EBV and the risk of developing MS is increased in those with a higher-titre of anti-EBV antibodies. It has been suggested that EBV infection of B-lymphocytes converts them to long-lived memory B-cells. Subsequently, dysregulation of cytotoxic T-cells against these B-cells may cause autoimmune dysfunction.

Immunology

MS pathology is likely autoimmune in origin although the exact auto-antigen or foreign antigen responsible remains elusive. Very early in the disease process, breakdown of the blood–brain barrier occurs and immune cellular infiltration ensues. This is mediated by naïve T cells, which differentiate into Th1 cells (CD4+) as part of cell-mediated immunity, so that γ-interferon, TNFα, and IL-2 are key cytokines and macrophage infiltration occurs. The macrophages may then attack myelin antigens, leading to the breakdown of the sheath and latterly disturb axonal function. These antigens and IL-17 producing cells such as CD4+ and CD8+ T-cells, are found within active MS lesions in the CNS and the CD8+ T-cells (cytotoxic T-cells) may be responsible for direct acute axonal damage. Much like Y-interferon, IL-17 is associated with delayed-type reactions and can recruit neutrophils and monocytes to inflammatory sites. The exact role of B-cells in MS remains unclear, but it is apparent they are not extensive in acute early inflammation, although latterly clonal proliferation occurs (especially in the intrathecal space) with associated oligoclonal IgG production; a key diagnostic marker in MS. It is unclear whether the B cells themselves act in an antigen-presenting role or maintain the myelin injury process. Either way, in the acute inflammatory milieu microglia are recruited and release oxygen reactive species that are additionally cytotoxic to the oligodentrocytes.

Clinical presentation and management

There are three main phenotypes of disease in MS, the most common being relapsing-remitting (RRMS) (~70%), characterized by periods of demyelination separated by periods of complete or partial remission. Over time, remission becomes incomplete, until ultimately the patient enters a secondary progressive phase where symptoms are continuous and increasingly severe. Less commonly (~20%), patients present with a primary progressive phenotype, where symptoms are continuous and of increasing severity from first onset. Latterly relapses may occur infrequently. 10% of patients are affected by benign relapsing-remitting where relapses are interspersed with periods of complete remission without progressive disease.

Initial symptom presentation (Table 9.12) will depend on the site of inflammation within the CNS. Around 20% of patients initially present with an optic neuritis due to demyelination of the optic nerve, characterized by progressive unilateral vision reduction and eye pain. Another common presentation is acute transverse myelitis where partial motor, sensory, autonomic, or reflex function is denuded below the spinal level of the lesion. Characteristic symptoms include Lhermitte's symptom (electric shock/tingle down back/legs when head is bent forward).

A diagnosis of MS is made using MacDonald criteria, i.e. at least two separate episodes of neurological symptoms that can be attributed to demyelination, in conjunction with an MRI; 30 days apart and different CNS sites.

The diverse clinical presentations can be managed with systematic pharmacological approaches to improve symptoms Figure 9.10 and (Table 9.13). Given the pathophysiology in acute presentations or relapses, corticosteroids are particularly useful, as they can be both immunosuppressive and anti-inflammatory, reducing cytokine levels, lymphocyte up-regulation, T-cell function, and macrophage activation. Steroids, however, have no long-term effect on the disease so other therapies that intervene in the autoimmune inflammatory pathways are used to reduce relapses and lesions; the so-called disease-modifying therapies (DMT). The first of these treatments available for use in MS were **interferon beta** and **glatiramer acetate**, which despite showing a modest benefit, are being largely replaced with alternative agents due to their unacceptable toxicity and high-cost per quality-adjusted life-year (QALY). Increasingly, the DMT **dimethyl fumarate** is being used first line or alternatively **teriflunomide** and **fingolimod**. In highly active disease, **alemtuzumab** and **natalizumab** are treatment options. Clinical trials continue with other immunotherapies, e.g. **daclizumab** and **ocrelizumab**.

Acute management

Acute episodes are managed with corticosteroids reducing time to remission. **Methylprednisolone** orally, or if necessary, IV for 3–5 days. Dose tapering is not considered necessary. Although other drugs have been investigated in acute attacks, including immunoglobulin, the only other treatment modality shown to have any effect is plasma exchange in those that fail to respond to methylprednisolone.

Disease-modifying therapy

Current recommendations are to initiate DMT as early as possible in eligible patients, although evidence of effectiveness is limited and decisions should be made between patient, neurologist considering disease activity and treatment risks. There are currently seven licensed DMT options in MS of which **interferon beta**, **glatiramer acetate**, **dimethyl fumarate**, **fingolimod**, and **teriflunomide** are considered to be of moderate efficacy (category 1) in reducing relapse rate and number of lesions, and **natalizumab** and **alemtuzumab** of high efficacy (category 2).

Table 9.12 Symptoms of MS and their cause

	Symptom	Causes
Motor dysfunction	Gait	Secondary causes, e.g. ataxia, weakness, spasticity
	Tremor	Primary lesions/inflammation (brainstem)
	Weakness	Primary lesions/inflammation
	Spasticity	Secondary to paraplegia
Autonomic dysregulation	Neurogenic bladder (overactive/retention)	Primary lesions/inflammation
	Bowel dysfunction (constipation/incontinence)	Primary lesions/inflammation Secondary causes, e.g. decreased mobility
	Temperature dysregulation	Primary lesions/inflammation
	Sexual dysfunction	Primary lesions/inflammation Secondary causes, e.g. fatigue, medication, depression
Cognitive/behavioural dysfunction	Attention deficit Long-term memory impairment Delayed information processing	Significant lesions and atrophy Secondary causes, e.g. sleep disturbance, fatigue
General	Fatigue	Primary lesions/inflammation Secondary causes, e.g. sleep disturbances, interferon beta, or glatiramer acetate
	Sleep disturbances	Primary lesions/inflammation Secondary causes, e.g. restless leg syndrome
	Pain	Primary lesions/inflammation (e.g. optic neuritis) Secondary causes, e.g. immobility, spasticity
	Depression	Primary lesions/inflammation (in frontal lobe) Secondary causes, e.g. fatigue, cognitive impairment, medication, psychosocial

Active relapsing-remitting multiple sclerosis

Patients with active relapsing-remitting multiple sclerosis (RMMS) should be offered a category 1 DMT (e.g. **dimethyl fumarate**) or in more active disease **fingolimod**. **Teriflunomide** is an option in needle phobic patients, although its efficacy is more comparable with **interferon beta** and **glatiramer acetate**, i.e. likely to be of inferior efficacy to fingolimod and dimethyl fumarate. Furthermore, unlike other licensed treatments, interferon beta and glatiramer acetate are not advocated for use by NICE.

Highly active RRMS

In RRMS, **natalizumab** or **alemtuzumab** (category 2) are preferred agents. **Mitoxantrone** is not licensed in the UK and, although used off-label, this should be reserved for second-line due to high toxicity and no clear evidence of superior efficacy compared with the newer licensed drugs. There are currently no treatment options available for use in progressive MS.

For a full summary of the relevant pathways and drug targets, see Figure 9.11.

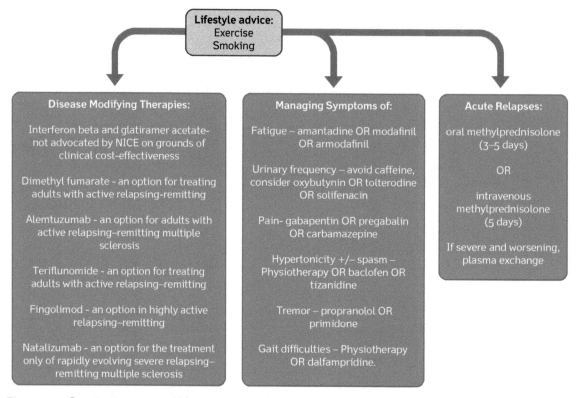

Figure 9.10 Overview management of multiple sclerosis.

Drug classes used in management

Interferon beta

Interferon beta was the first available treatment for relapsing remitting multiple sclerosis, although the mechanism of action is still poorly understood due to the complex biological response to interferon injections. For example, interferon beta 1a and 1b.

Mechanism of action

Interferons belong to the large class of glycoproteins known as cytokines and are key components of the innate immune system. Ten distinct interferons have been identified and they are classified according to the type of receptor through which they signal. Interferon beta belongs to the interferon type I group, based on its ability to bind to the interferon-α receptor on the cell surface. Type I interferons are single-chain polypeptides with compact, ordered structures with α helices and β pleated sheets.

The interferon-β receptor is composed of a signalling (IFNAR1) and a binding (IFNAR2) chain, both necessary for interferon beta cellular effects and constitutively expressed on the surface of virtually all cells. In the sequence of events leading to its biological activity, interferons bind to the binding chain of the receptor and engage with the signalling chain to form a high-affinity receptor-ligand complex, this allows the intracellular domains of the two receptor chains and associated proteins to interact. This association includes the JAK1/STAT signalling pathway, where activated STATS form a complex with other cytoplasmic proteins and translocate to the nucleus to bind to interferon sensitive responsive elements and regulate the expression of many genes.

The specific transcripts mediating the therapeutic benefit of interferon beta in multiple sclerosis are unknown, but involve the alteration of populations or functions of cells involved in the immune response, such as Type 2 dendritic cells, monocytes, regulatory T-cells, and CD56 bright NK cells.

Table 9.13 Symptom control in MS

Symptom	Non-pharmacological options	Pharmacological options
Spasticity	Physiotherapy, splints with severe contractures	*1st line*: baclofen, gabapentin (individually or in combination if needed) *2nd line*: tizanidine or dantrolene
Oscillopsia		*1st line*: gabapentin *2nd line*: memantine
Bladder dysfunction	Catheterization	Anti-muscarinics (see disorders of micturition)
Bowel dysfunction	Fluid intake, dietary advice	Laxatives
Sexual dysfunction	Identify and manage any underlying factors, e.g. depression	Sildenafil
Fatigue	Encourage good sleep hygiene, exercise, avoid drugs that may exaggerate fatigue	Amantadine
Tremor	Physiotherapy, surgery	β-blockers (propranolol), benzodiazepines
Depression/ mood	Psychotherapy	Anti-depressants Amitriptyline for emotional lability
Swallowing difficulties	Speech and language therapist assessment, gastrostomy	
Neuropathic pain		Anti-depressants (amitriptyline), anti-convulsants (gabapentin, pregabalin, carbamazepine)
Musculoskeletal pain	Physiotherapy	Analgesics, anti-depressants, anti-convulsants

Prescribing

Interferon beta is licensed as a DMT in relapsing/remitting and secondary progressive MS with evidence of relapse. Its use, however, is increasingly being superseded by newer, more effective agents and it is not recommended for use by NICE.

Unwanted effects

The most commonly reported side effects to treatment include flu-like symptoms (headache, fever, arthralgia, nausea, etc.) and injection site reactions (redness, swelling, pain, hypersensitivity, etc.). Tolerance can be improved by gradual dose titration and the use of pre-treatment with NSAIDs to reduce flu-like symptoms. The **interferon betas** are formulated in devices designed to reduce the risk of injection site reactions and the site of injection should be rotated.

Other effects include predictably hypersensitivity reactions and blood disorders, although it is also known to affect mood and personality, as well as cause fatigue. Use is therefore not recommended in those with severe depression or suicidal ideation. Caution is also recommended in cardiac disorders and hepatic impairment, which may be aggravated with interferon beta.

Glatiramer acetate

Glatiramer acetate is a copolymer made of the acetate salts of synthetic polypeptides and contains four naturally occurring amino acids: L-glutamic acid, L-alanine, L-tyrosine, and L-lysine. It acts as an immunomodulator by binding to major histocompatibility complex (MHC) molecules, competing with various myelin antigens for T-cell presentation.

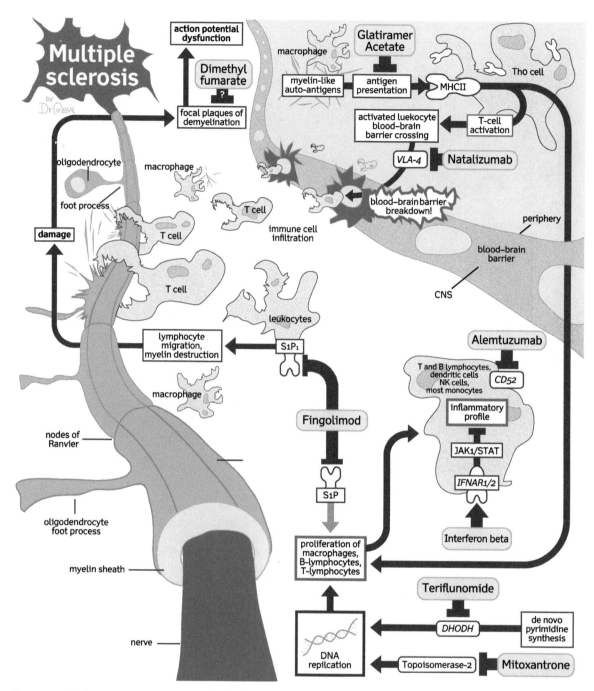

Figure 9.11 Multiple sclerosis: summary of relevant pathways and drug targets.

Mechanism of action

Initially developed to mimic a major component of the myelin sheath [myelin basic protein (MBP)] in order to induce the experimental animal model of MS [autoimmune encephalomyelitis (EAE)], **glatiramer acetate** (GA) unexpectedly protected against EAE. Moreover, in patients with relapsing-remitting MS, GA-reduced relapse rate, and delayed progression of disability. GA is the first therapeutic agent ever to have a copolymer as its active ingredient.

Due to the complexity and variability of its polypeptide mixture, it has been suggested that the total 'pool' of various amino acid sequences creates a multiple way of action required for therapeutic activity.

GA's initial step is to bind to MHC class II molecules, thus hindering T-cell presentation and inducing a shift to an anti-inflammatory Th2 type of T cell response. It has been also shown that GA induces alterations in various antigen-presenting cells, so that they skew responses from the pro-inflammatory to the protective anti-inflammatory pathway.

The initial immunological activity of GA appears to occur in the periphery and since GA is rapidly degraded, it is unlikely that sufficient amounts can reach the CNS to compete with myelin agents or modulate the immune response. It is thus accepted that the GA-induced immune cells that penetrate the CNS achieve the therapeutic effect.

Prescribing

Glatiramer acetate, like **interferon beta**, is licensed for use in relapsing/remitting MS, as well as in those at high risk of developing it in order to delay onset of clinically definite MS (CDMS), although again lacks NICE endorsement. It is administered OD by SC injection. Unlike some interferon beta formulations, however, it is not licensed for use in secondary progressive MS with active relapses.

Unwanted effects

Injection site reactions are the most widely reported adverse effects to **glatiramer acetate**, i.e. redness, pain, swelling, inflammation, and hypersensitivity reactions. Patients should be advised to rotate the site of injection to help minimize these effects, and following the first injection, be observed for a period of 30 minutes to detect any adverse reaction. Hypersensitivity reactions following administration are relatively common.

As with interferon beta treatment, it can aggravate depression and cardiac disorders, thus caution is recommended.

Dimethyl fumarate

Dimethyl fumarate is a simple molecule derived from fumaric acid that activates the nuclear factor (erythroid-derived 2)-like (Nrf2) pathway involved in cellular response to oxidative stress, causing immunomodulatory and neuroprotective effects. For example, dimethyl fumarate.

Mechanism of action

Initially developed for the treatment of psoriasis, it quickly became clear **dimethyl fumarate** had broad immunomodulatory actions. These properties are achieved through the ability to divert cytokine production toward a Th2 profile, both on lymphocytes and microglial cells. More, importantly, **dimethyl fumarate** can have an impact on the anti-oxidative stress cell machinery, promoting the transcription of genes that are downstream of the Nrf2 pathway, which besides immunomodulatory actions has the capacity for cytoprotection on glial cells, oligodendrocytes, and neurons.

Prescribing

In the absence of robust comparative data, extrapolation infers that **dimethyl fumarate** is more effective than **interferon beta** and **glatiramer acetate** in reducing relapses and lesion formation. Increasingly, it is being used first-line in RRMS, with NICE advocating its use.

Dimethyl fumarate has the added advantage of being taken orally. Doses are taken BD with food to improve tolerance. It is also formulated in capsules containing microtablets that are coated to help reduce gastric irritation and, therefore the capsule should be swallowed whole and the contents not manipulated in any way that may damage the coating. Doses are started low and doubled after 7 days.

Unwanted effects

Side effects to **dimethyl fumarate** are relatively common and potentially severe. Treatment is associated with hepatic and renal toxicity, as well as a risk of lymphopaenia. Patients will require baseline bloods (FBC, U&Es, and LFTs), repeated every 3–6 months.

Flushing and GI toxicity (diarrhoea, nausea, and abdominal pain) occur very commonly with treatment and may be managed through dose reductions and by ensuring doses are taken with food. Other relatively common side effects include skin rashes and hypersensitivity reactions.

Drug interactions with dimethyl fumarate are unlikely to be of clinical significance, although concurrent use with other nephrotoxic drugs may increase the risk of renal toxicity.

Monoclonal antibodies

The use of monoclonal antibodies as therapeutic agents allows the precise targeting of molecules involved in the pathology of multiple sclerosis. Although they can be grouped as a class, their mechanism of action is dependent on the specific target. For example, alemtuzumab and natalizumab.

Mechanism of action

The new-generation therapeutic monoclonal antibodies consist of chimeric proteins, in which only the antigen-specific highly variable part is mouse-derived, but all other regions are of human origin. This minimizes adverse immune reactions from foreign protein antigens. Monoclonal antibodies have distinct modes of action, involving different functional approaches towards the mechanisms of pathological cellular processes.

The monoclonal antibody **alemtuzumab** is a humanized IgG1k and a common example of a cell-depleting antibody. It targets human CD52, a 12-amino acid glycosylated glycosylphosphatidylinositol-linked surface protein, which is expressed on T and B lymphocytes, natural killer cells, dendritic cells, and most monocytes, but not on haematopoietic precursors. Treatment with alemtuzumab produces a rapid and almost complete depletion of CD52-bearing cells in the circulation, in a process mediated by antibody-dependent cellular cytotoxicity.

Natalizumab is a monoclonal antibody against the α4 subunit of the very late antigen (VLA-4 a dimer of the integrins α4 and β1). VLA-4 is expressed on virtually all activated leukocytes, enabling them to cross the blood–brain barrier, a process that is blocked by natalizumab.

Prescribing

Natalizumab is recommended for use in patients with highly active RRMS, despite treatment with first-line disease-modifying therapy, or in patients who present with rapidly evolving, severe relapsing/remitting MS. It is administered as an IV infusion over an hour every 4 weeks and should only be continued beyond 6 months where a benefit has been shown.

There is a risk of toxicity (Grave's disease, opportunistic infections, and potentially fatal thrombocytopenia). As with natalizumab it is reserved for use second-line, being more potent than the other DMTs, but significantly more toxic.

Alemtuzumab is administered as an IV infusion over 4 hours daily for 5 days, repeated 12 months later for 3 consecutive days. Patients should receive pretreatment with corticosteroids ± antihistamines and antipyretics to reduce the risk of adverse reactions. Patients also require prophylactic treatment with **aciclovir**.

Unwanted effects

As monoclonal antibodies, the adverse effects of greatest concern are immunological in nature, including hypersensitivity reactions, autoimmune-mediated reactions, malignancy, and infections, including opportunistic infections. Most common reactions are rash, headaches, pyrexia, and respiratory tract infections, affecting more than 20% of patients on treatment.

Due to the potential for severe toxicity, monitoring is an essential part of treatment with monoclonal antibodies; FBCs, U&Es (including creatinine), TFTs, and urinalysis.

Progressive multifocal leukoencephalopathy (PML) is a potentially fatal opportunistic infection caused by the JC virus that has been associated with **natalizumab** therapy (see 'Prescribing warning: PML and IRIS with natalizumab').

PRESCRIBING WARNING

PML and IRIS with natalizumab

- Natalizumab is associated with an increased risk of progressive multifocal leukoencephalopathy (PML).
- PML is a potentially life-threatening opportunistic infection caused by the JC virus
- Risk is increased in:
  - The presence of anti-JCV antibodies.
  - Patients who have received natalizumab for more than 2 years.
  - Patients who have received previous immunosuppressant therapy.
- Patients and carers should be made aware of the risks and advised on symptoms.
- Prior to treatment an MRI should performed; baseline and repeated annually.
- Where PML is suspected, treatment should be discontinued immediately.
- Nearly all patients with PML go on to develop immune reconstitution inflammatory syndrome (IRIS) on discontinuation of natalizumab.
- This again can lead to serious and even fatal neurological complications.
- Patients should therefore be closely monitored following withdrawal of natalizumab and any inflammation managed accordingly.

Alemtuzumab therapy is particularly associated with auto-antibody formation and a high risk of autoimmune diseases. Typical autoimmune conditions seen with treatment include thyroid dysfunction and idiopathic thrombocytopenic purpura (ITP), affecting approximately 36% and 1% of patients, respectively. Less commonly, treatment has been known to induce autoimmune nephropathies. Patients on treatment will require baseline measurements and frequent monitoring of thyroid function tests, U&Es, and FBC, while on treatment.

Further reading

Ascherio A, Munger KL, Simon KC (2010) Vitamin D and multiple sclerosis. *Lancet: Neurology* 9(6), 599–612.

Bomprezzi R (2015) Dimethyl fumarate in the treatment of relapsing-remitting multiple sclerosis: an overview. *Therapy in Advanced Neurology Disorders* 8(1), 20–30.

Coles A (2009) Multiple sclerosis: the bare essentials. *Practical Neurology* 9, 118–26.

Haghikia A, Hohlfeld R, Gold R, et al. (2013) Therapies for multiple sclerosis: translational achievements and outstanding needs. *Trends in Molecular Medicine* 19(5), 309–19.

Ingwersen J, Aktas O, Kuery P, et al. (2012) Fingolimod in multiple sclerosis: mechanism of action and clinical efficacy. *Clinical Immunology* 142, 15–24.

Klotz L, Meuth S, Wiendl H (2012) Immune mechanisms of new therapeutic strategies in multiple sclerosis: a focus on alemtuzumab. *Clinical Immunology* 142(1), 25–30.

Martinelli Boneschi F, Vacchi L, Rovaris M, et al. (2013) Mitoxantrone for multiple sclerosis. *Cochrane Database of Systematic Reviews* 31(5), CD002127.

Munger KL, Levin LI, Hollis BW, et al. (2006) Serum 25-hydroxyvitamin D levels and risk of multiple sclerosis. *Journal of the American Medical Association* 296(23), 2832–8.

Oksenberg JR, Baranzini SE, Sawcer S, et al. (2008) The genetics of multiple sclerosis: SNPs to pathways to pathogenesis. *Nature Review: Genetics* 9(7), 516–26.

Rudick R, Goetz S (2011) Beta-interferon for multiple sclerosis. *Experimental Cell Research* 317(9), 1301–11.

Warnke C, Stuve O, Kieseier B (2013) Teriflunomide for the treatment of multiple sclerosis. *Clinical Neurology and Neurosurgery* 115, S90–4.

Guidelines

Goodin E, Frohman M, Garmany GP, et al (2002) Disease modifying therapies in multiple sclerosis: Subcommittee of the American Academy of Neurology. *Neurology* 58, 169–78. http://www.neurology.org/content/58/2/169.full [accessed 9 April 2019].

NICE Pathways: Multiple sclerosis http://pathways.nice.org.uk/pathways/multiple-sclerosis [accessed 9 April 2019].

NICE QS108 (2016) Multiple sclerosis. https://www.nice.org.uk/guidance/qs108 [accessed 9 April 2019].

NICE TA32 (2002) Beta interferon and glatiramer acetate for the treatment of multiple sclerosis. https://www.nice.org.uk/Guidance/TA32 [accessed 9 April 2019].

NICE TA127 (2007) Natalizumab for the treatment of adults with highly active relapsing-remitting multiple sclerosis. https://www.nice.org.uk/guidance/ta127 [accessed 9 April 2019].

NICE CG186 (2014) Multiple Sclerosis in adults: management. https://www.nice.org.uk/guidance/cg186 [accessed 9 April 2019].

NICE TA254 (2012) Fingolimod for the treatment of highly active relapsing-remitting multiple sclerosis. https://www.nice.org.uk/guidance/ta254 [accessed 9 April 2019].

NICE TA303 (2014) Teriflunomide for treating relapsing-remitting multiple sclerosis. https://www.nice.org.uk/guidance/ta303 [accessed 9 April 2019].

NICE TA312 (2014) Alemtuzumab for treating relapsing-remitting multiple sclerosis. https://www.nice.org.uk/guidance/ta312 [accessed 9 April 2019].

NICE TA320 (2014) Dimethyl fumarate for treating relapsing-remitting multiple sclerosis. https://www.nice.org.uk/guidance/ta320 [accessed 9 April 2019].

Scolding N, Barnes D, Cader S, et al (2015) Association of British Neurologists: revised (2015) guidelines for prescribing disease-modifying treatments in multiple sclerosis *Practical Neurology* 15, 273–9.

9.6 Myasthenia gravis

Myasthenia gravis (MG) is an autoimmune disease in which autoantibodies target post-synaptic nicotinic receptors within the neuromuscular junction. It was first described in 1672 by Thomas Willis, who reported a condition where patients showed increased muscle fatigability during the day. Symptoms occur as a result of failing cholinergic neurotransmission within muscles, secondary to a reduction in the pool of nicotinic receptors available to respond to acetylcholine.

There are two predominant presenting patterns of symptoms: ocular (15%) and generalized (85%), the latter appearing as a more progressive and generalized weakness and fatigability. Most cases of ocular MG, however, will convert to generalized MG within 13 months of presentation. Collectively, prevalence is in the order of 15 per 100,000 and is bimodal, with a peak prevalence at 40 years of age in females, and 70 years of age in males. The incidence of late onset MG is increasing, although the reasons for this are poorly understood. While the exact aetiology is unknown, 10% of MG patients (mainly early onset) have an associated thymoma. Genome-wide scanning has shown a weak genetic link (35% concordance in monozygotic twins) and an association with the HLA-DR1 haplotype.

Pathophysiology

At the neuromuscular junction (NMJ), a neuron activates a muscle, causing it to contract. Activation involves an electrical impulse that travels down the presynaptic nerve and generates a change in the ionic gradient at the motor neuron terminal. This leads to the depolarization and entry of Ca^{2+} via the opening of presynaptic voltage-gated channels. The rise in presynaptic Ca^{2+} concentration triggers SNARE proteins (e.g. syntaxin 1), so that neurotransmitter vesicles fuse with the presynaptic membrane and release ACh into the neuromuscular cleft. This all-or-nothing response is what dictates transmission from electrical, to chemical, to muscular contraction, and ultimately depends on the presence of sufficient post-synaptic nicotinic receptors. These ligand-gated channels are ionophores that open after the binding of two ACh molecules. This binding triggers Na^+ entry and muscle depolarization, with Ca^{2+} influx activating Ca^{2+} release from the sarcoplasmic reticulum, so that actin and myosin muscle contraction ensues. For effective muscle contraction nicotinic acetylcholine receptors (nAChRs) must be 'clustered' together, a process that can be impaired by dysfunction in muscle-specific kinase (MuSK), rapsyn, and DOK7 proteins. Importantly, MuSK is also implicated in MG.

A number of enzymes and receptors at the pre- and post-synaptic sites can modify the levels of ACh within the cleft, and hence alter the post-synaptic effect. In the case of released ACh, the excess that persists in the cleft is rapidly broken down by the serine protease, acetylcholinesterase (AChE). Reversible AChE inhibitors transiently augment synaptic levels of ACh within physiological concentrations, and therefore have a role in the management of MG. **Pyridostigmine**, in particular is a reversible inhibitor of AChE that acts to overcome the functional consequences of failing nAChR, by transiently raising synaptic ACh levels in MG.

In MG, autoantibodies against nAChR themselves and/or MuSK are pathognomonic hallmarks of the disease, responsible for failing neuromuscular transmission. The targeting of nAChR by the immune system reduces the functional effectiveness of receptors by directly inhibiting their ion channel function, inducing complement-mediated dysfunction of the post-synaptic architecture and altering the rates of nAChR internalization and turnover. The auto-antibodies found in MG are predominantly complement-fixing types (e.g. IgG 1, 3, and 4 types), which means that the antigen-antibody complex is destroyed via the complement pathway, in a process that is poorly understood. Rising auto-antibody titres against both nAChR and/or MuSK, result in failing post-synaptic function and, in the case of MuSK, may lead to pre- and post-synaptic NMJ architectural disassembly and failed nAChR clustering. AChR clustering of receptors is a sign of post-synaptic specialization in the NMJ and is induced by agrin; MuSK is a receptor tyrosine kinase and component of the agrin receptor, and rapsyn, an AChR-associated anchoring protein.

The role of the thymus in MG has been the focus of much research, as most patients with AChR positive MG have an underlying thymus abnormality, either hyperplasia (60–70%) or a thymoma (10–15%), although patients with MuSK positive MG show no histological thymic changes.

In early-onset MG, the thymus is typically hyperplastic and possesses all the components necessary to initiate immune sensitization to nAChR (e.g. nAChR expressing myoid cells that 'would' become striated muscle cells, antigen presenting dendritic cells, and T cells). Auto-immunized T cells target AChR, giving rise to germinal centres in which B cells produce AChR antibodies.

In late-onset MG, the thymus is typically atrophic, lacking the germinal centres. Patients are more likely to have a thymoma, a capsulated epithelial tumour that possesses autoreactive T cells, which enter the peripheral circulation and lead to a self-perpetuating auto-immune response.

As the auto-antibodies in MG are heterogeneous in nature, they are thought to occur as a result of polyclonal B-cell activation; therefore, a non-specific immunosuppression treatment strategy using various agents that target different immune cells is of value, e.g. corticosteroids, **azathioprine**, **ciclosporin**, and **mycophenolate**. More recently, targeted therapy against B cells such as **rituximab** have also demonstrated a benefit in refractory MG, although these effects appear to be greater in MuSK-positive MG. In the short-term, IV **immunoglobulin** (IVIg) or plasmaphoresis can show marked clinical improvement in those with nAChR/MuSK positive markers (see 'Management') by decreasing circulating autoantibody levels (see 'Immunosuppressants, IV immunoglobulin').

The interventions outlined here must be considered in the context of comorbid disease and other medications. Furthermore, some drugs can exacerbate or even induce symptoms and should be avoided in MG if possible (see Table 9.14); for example, it has been reported that statins may prompt or unmask MG through an unknown mechanism, and that stopping the offending drug restores pre-morbid function. It is also noteworthy that MG patients are prone to respiratory tract infection due to their low tidal volume, prescribers should therefore be aware of

Table 9.14 Drug that can exacerbate MG symptoms/signs

Drug group	Examples
Neuromuscular blocking agents	Atracurium
	Vecuronium
Antibiotics	Aminoglycosides like gentamicin
	Macrolides like erythromycin
	Ciprofloxacin
	Clindamycin
Beta-blockers	Propranolol
	Atenolol
	Timolol eyedrops
Anti-arrhythmic drugs	Verapamil
	Quinidine and procainamide (both withdrawn)
Other drugs	Lithium
	Penicillamine
	Opiates, e.g. pethidine
	Phenytoin
	Statins
	Prednisolone

Data from Pascuzzi RM (2007) Medications and Myasthenia Gravis (A reference for health care professionals). Myasthenia Gravis Foundation of America.

antibiotics that can affect neuromuscular function (see Table 9.14).

For a full summary of the relevant pathways and drug targets, see Figure 9.12.

Management

Patients with myasthenia gravis typically present with muscle weakness and fatigue that worsens with sustained or repeated use, and improves with rest. Weakness tends to be more pronounced towards the end of the day and can be exacerbated by factors such as heat, exercise, emotional stress, pregnancy, and infections. In some instances, however, the disease is first revealed following exposure to drugs that exacerbate symptoms (see Table 9.14), such as general anaesthesia, antimalarials or β-blockers. Patients receiving **penicillamine** can also develop a penicillamine-induced autoimmune disease that usually resolves within weeks of stopping the drug.

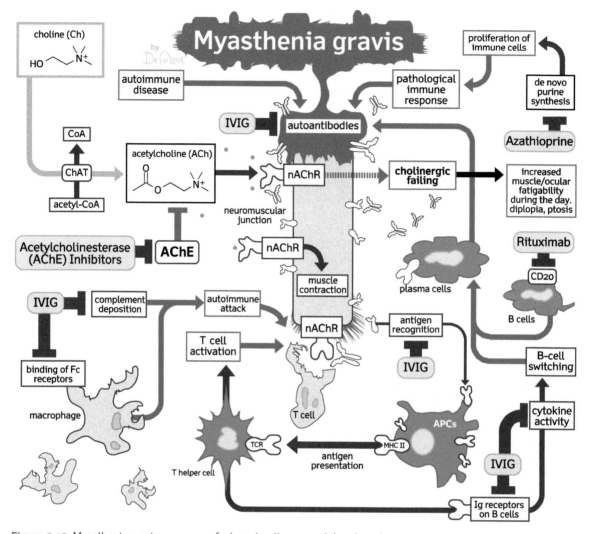

Figure 9.12 Myasthenia gravis: summary of relevant pathways and drug targets.

Diagnostic tests primarily include serum antibody testing, first for AChR antibodies, or in those that test negative, MuSK antibodies. In the absence of serum antibodies, neurophysiology, especially the single fibre electromyography (EMG) carried out by a specialist, can help with diagnosis if MG is still suspected. Diagnostic imaging of the thymus can determine any thymic involvement, and a brain MR scan can detect the presence of any alternative structural brain disease. In the case of diagnostic uncertainty the 'Tensilon'® or **edrophonium** test (see below) may be carried out by an MG specialist (see 'Practical prescribing: the "Tensilon"® or edrophonium test'), due to the risk of cardiovascular collapse. The test should not, however, be used in isolation, due to the risk of false positives/negatives.

> **PRACTICAL PRESCRIBING**
>
> **The 'Tensilon'® or edrophonium test**
>
> - Draw the contents of an ampoule (10 mg) into a syringe.
> - Administer a dose of 2 mg IV.
> - If patients fails to show an improvement in muscle tone within 30 seconds, repeat the dose.
> - The dose is repeated until patient responds, up to a maximum total dose of 10 mg.

In patients with ptosis where the Tensilon® test is unsuitable, the ice pack test may be a viable alternative, although only 80% effective and still susceptible to false positive and negative results. It works through application of an ice pack directly to the closed eyelid, as lowering muscle temperature helps improve neuromuscular transmission. After 2 minutes the ice pack is removed and the eyelid immediately assessed for improvement in muscle tone.

Work-up includes assessments of affected muscles for the purpose of disease classification, determined by severity, extent, age of onset, and presence of antibody type (see Table 9.15). In patients with signs of respiratory involvement (dyspnoea initially on exertion, but in severe disease at rest), FVC is a more reliable measure than peak flow and is used in conjunction with arterial blood gases.

Thyroid function tests are recommended in all patients, due to the increased risk of thyroid dysfunction. In patients with a thymoma, a thymectomy may be offered. The evidence for benefit in non-thymomatous myasthenia gravis however, is lacking and its role is therefore controversial.

Once diagnosed, patients should be made aware of factors that may precipitate a crisis, such as infections, surgery, pregnancy, childbirth, and certain drugs (see Table 9.14). It is essential that patients are empowered to advise anyone prescribing for them that they have MG, so as to avoid exposure to drugs that may precipitate a crisis. MG is a rare, complex disease, and a suitably experienced neurologist should lead on treatment where available.

Primary treatment of myasthenia gravis requires therapy to manage symptoms (AChE inhibitors), usually in combination with immunosuppressive therapy (corticosteroids and immunosuppressants) to induce and maintain a remission. Treatment strategy will depend on whether the patient presents with ocular or generalized disease, and severity of symptoms dictating whether or not they can be managed in an outpatient or inpatient setting

Outpatient management of myasthenia gravis

Primary treatment of myasthenia gravis is with the acetylcholinesterase inhibitor, **pyridostigmine**, with doses titrated up to establish the lowest effective dose. With dose escalation, the risk of muscarinic side effects is increased, excessive doses leading potentially to a cholinergic crisis and a paradoxical worsening of muscle weakness. Milder side effects, especially diarrhoea, can be managed with the anticholinergic, **propantheline**, without adversely affecting activity at the nicotinic

Table 9.15 Myasthenia Gravis Foundation of America Clinical Classification

Class	Muscle affected
I	Any eye muscle weakness (ptosis), all other muscles unaffected
II	Mild weakness of non-ocular muscles +/– ocular muscle weakness of any severity IIa Predominantly limb and/or axial muscles IIb Predominantly oropharyngeal and/or respiratory muscles
III	Moderate weakness of non-ocular muscles +/– ocular muscle weakness of any severity IIa Predominantly limb and/or axial muscles IIb Predominantly oropharyngeal and/or respiratory muscles
IV	Severe weakness of non-ocular muscles +/– ocular muscle weakness of any severity IIa Predominantly limb and/or axial muscles IIb Predominantly oropharyngeal and/or respiratory muscles. Feeding tube required, but not intubation
V	Intubation required to maintain airway
MuSK	MuSK antibodies present
Non-MuSK	MuSK antibodies not present

Adapted from *The Annals of Thoracic Surgery*, 70, 1, Alfred Jaretzki III, Richard J. Barohn, Raina M. Ernstoff, Task Force of the Medical Scientific Advisory Board of the Myasthenia Gravis Foundation of America, et al., Myasthenia gravis: recommendations for clinical research standards, pp. 327–334. Copyright © 2000 The Society of Thoracic Surgeons/Elsevier. Published by Elsevier Inc. All rights reserved. https://doi.org/10.1016/S0003-4975(00)01595-2

receptors. **Mebeverine** can also be used to manage adverse effects. Patients under the age of 45 years with generalized MG who test positive for AChR, may be offered a thymectomy.

Patients who fail to respond adequately to pyridostigmine after a few weeks at the maximum tolerated dose should be started on **prednisolone**, and pyridostigmine withdrawn gradually. Prednisolone doses are started low to prevent an initial worsening of symptoms, and gradually increased to a maximum dose of 50 mg alternate days in ocular MG, and 100 mg alternate days in generalized MG, until symptoms improve. Response time tends to be slow particularly in the case of generalized MG, where it may take months to achieve a remission, defined as the resolution of symptoms following withdrawal of pyridostigmine. Patients that remain symptomatic after 3 months, are intolerant of corticosteroids or require doses of 15–20 mg prednisolone on alternate days to maintain remission, should be referred for immunosuppression therapy.

Azathioprine is the immunosuppressant of choice in MG, although as with corticosteroids, response times tend to be slow. Treatment should be initiated once TMPT status has been assessed, as patients with very low activity are at high risk of toxicity and treatment should therefore be avoided. Azathioprine is escalated gradually over a period of 1 month to a maintenance dose, with the aim of reducing corticosteroid doses to less than 20 mg alternate days. Patients on treatment will require weekly blood tests (FBC, LFTs, and U&Es) to monitor for toxicity. Alternative immunosuppressants, such as **ciclosporin**, **mycophenolate mofetil**, and **methotrexate** may be considered in non-responders or as an alternative where azathioprine treatment is unsuitable.

Rituximab and **etanercept** are newer therapeutic options reserved for refractory disease, particularly as the value of **etanercept** in MG lacks any robust data. Other options in refractory disease include the use of **cyclophosphamide** with bone marrow transplant or with monoclonal Ab against the B cell surface marker CD20.

Inpatient management of myasthenia gravis—'myasthenic crisis'

Patients with severe symptoms (significant bulbar symptoms, low vital capacity, and respiratory symptoms) or progressive deterioration will need to be admitted for urgent escalation of therapy. **Immunoglobulins** in combination with corticosteroids are the main stay of treatment for severe bulbar and respiratory symptoms, the former given according to local treatment guidelines. Plasma exchange, however, may be considered if immunoglobulin therapy is deemed unsuitable. Patients with compromised respiratory function or difficulty swallowing, may require intubation or mechanical ventilation delivered within an intensive care setting. Ventilated patients should have any anticholinesterase inhibitors held as this can increase secretions.

Drug used in management

Acetylcholinesterase inhibitors

Treatment with AChE inhibitors is based on the attempt to partially restore the cholinergic neuromuscular transmission through the prolongation of post-synaptic receptor stimulation. Although they fully relieve symptoms in only a small proportion of patients, they still help improve myasthenic symptoms in almost all patients. For example, pyridostigmine, neostigmine, and edrophonium

Mechanism of action

The inhibition of acetylcholine esterase, the enzyme that normally degrades ACh in the neuromuscular synapse, has a symptomatic effect in MG, especially AChR positive MG. Both the therapeutic and toxic actions of acetylcholinesterase inhibitors occur secondary to accumulation of synaptic ACh levels and enhanced stimulation of cholinergic receptors in the central and/or peripheral nervous system. In MG treatment, side effects arise from raised ACh levels in the non-neuromuscular cholinergic synapses of the autonomic system, which also have exacerbated stimulation. Although alternative ways to increase acetylcholine neurotransmission in the neuromuscular synapse have been tried, all have shown inferior efficacy to the cholinesterase inhibitors.

Prescribing

Pyridostigmine is the acetylcholinesterase inhibitor of choice in the management of myasthenia gravis. In mild disease doses are started low (30 mg TDS) and gradually titrated to a maximum dose of 90 mg five times a day to achieve optimal symptom control. In some countries (not the UK), it is also available as a slow-release preparation that may be useful for night time administration in patients with mild weakness on wakening. For most patients, however, symptoms improve after a night's sleep and thus its value is limited. Furthermore, daytime use of slow-release preparations is not recommended due to the unpredictable release profile, leading to suboptimal symptom control. **Neostigmine** is a licensed alternative, but with its shorter half-life (50–90 minutes versus 3–4 hours for **pyridostigmine**), it requires more frequent administration, making it less favourable. It is however available in an IV formulation that may have a role short term in patients unable to take medication orally.

Edrophonium is a very short-acting acetylcholinesterase inhibitor used in the 'Tensilon'® test (see 'Practical prescribing: the "Tensilon"® or edrophonium test') for the purpose of diagnosis, due to its rapid onset of action, which enables an effect to be seen within 30–60 seconds of administration, persisting for 5–10 minutes. The rapid onset of action also increases the risk of cardiovascular collapse and so patients will need careful monitoring, and access to appropriate facilities and expertise.

Unwanted effects

Unwanted effects of AChE inhibitors occur as a result of cholinergic overactivity, typically causing diarrhoea, nausea, vomiting, stomach cramps, hypersalivation, increased lacrimation and bronchial secretions, bradycardia, and AV block. GI symptoms and excessive secretions can be controlled with anticholinergic therapy (e.g. **propantheline**, **glycopyrronium bromide**), and diarrhoea also managed with **loperamide**. **Mebeverine** may also be of value in managing gastrointestinal symptoms. Caution is recommended in patients with preexisting cardiac (e.g. AV block, arrhythmias) or respiratory (e.g. COPD, asthma) conditions, with elderly patients being more susceptible to toxicity.

In the case of a cholinergic crisis, treatment should be discontinued and patients managed urgently with rapid-onset anticholinergic drugs (e.g. **atropine**) and, where necessary, respiratory support.

PRESCRIBING WARNING

Cholinergic crisis versus myasthenic crisis

Prescribers should be aware that excessive doses of acetylcholinesterase inhibitors can induce a cholinergic crisis that leads to a paradoxical worsening of muscle strength, making it difficult to distinguish from a deterioration of disease.

Immunosuppressants

For information on the mechanism of action and prescribing of immunosuppressants see Topic 6.6, 'Inflammatory bowel disease', and Topic 7.2, 'Inflammatory arthropathies'.

IV immunoglobulin

IV immunoglobulin (IVIG) preparations are made of the pooled fraction of serum IgG from ~3000–60 000 blood donors and, although it is predominantly employed as a replacement therapy in immunodeficient individuals, it is also used to supress the pathological immune response in patients with autoimmune disease.

Mechanism of action

As a pooled source of IgG, the role of IVIG in MG is somewhat counter-intuitive, seeing that IgG (auto-antibodies) are responsible for the loss of nicotinic receptors. As MG is a T cell-dependent, antibody-mediated autoimmune disease, however, IVIG has been used in treatment and demonstrated efficacy on a long-term basis, with minor side effects. Despite the wide-ranging efficacy of IVIG treatment, the specific mechanism(s) of action have not been elucidated, but are likely to include cytokine inhibition, auto-antibody competition and the inhibition of complement deposition. Studies suggest it may also lead to interference with binding of Fc receptors on macrophages and Ig receptors on B cells, together with the obstruction of antigen recognition by sensitized T cells.

The IgG constant fragment (Fc) that links the adaptive and innate immune systems is key in the pro-inflammatory IgG activity. The threshold at which activation occurs is determined by the co-expression of activating and inhibitory Fc receptors that are expressed by the majority of cells of the innate immune response, e.g. macrophages, mast cells, basophils eosinophils, etc. This, in turn, determines the effector response strength that happens in cells after binding of IgG molecules. In this way, altering this balance can either augment or ameliorate the IgG binding immunomodulatory effects. The most convincing evidence to support the role of the Fc fragment of IgG in the immunomodulatory effects of IVIG, comes from studies that show how isolated IVIG Fc fragments can ameliorate autoimmune disease (e.g. ITP) in humans.

Prescribing

The use of IVIG can be beneficial to those patients with an acute period of myasthenic weakness, often called a 'myasthenic crisis' and can produce rapid and profound clinical benefit in those who are clinically stable. It is administered as an IV infusion, started at a slow rate that is increased incrementally every 30 minutes so long as it is tolerated. Doses are calculated according to body weight and often administered over 5 days. Where tolerated it can improve strength within several days. Its use is specialist and high cost.

Unwanted effects

Side effects to IVIG are generally infusion-related, hence the requirement to start the rate slowly and only increment if tolerated. Patients should be monitored for signs of a hypersensitivity reaction and falls in BP. Common side effects include headache, dizziness, nausea, tachycardia, and hypotension, which may be minimized by slowing down the rate of infusion.

Less commonly, IVIG therapy can, given the high molecular weights of molecules, lead to fluid overload and acute renal failure, as well as increase the risk of a thromboembolism, probably due to raised blood viscosity following infusion. High risk patients (e.g. obesity, hypertension, diabetes, previous VTE, thrombophilia) should receive treatment at the minimum infusion rate to reduce the risk of a thromboembolic event and renal complications.

As IVIG can impair the efficacy of live vaccines for up to 3 months (1 year with measles) following administration, live vaccines should be avoided in this time, e.g. measles, mumps, rubella vaccine (MMR).

Further reading

Berrih-Aknin S, Rgaheb S, Le Panse R, et al. (2013) Ectopic germinal centers, BAFF and anti B-cell therapy in myasthenia gravis. *Autoimmunitiy Reviews* 12, 885–93.
Carr AS, Cardwell CR, McCarron PO, McConville J et al. (2010) A systematic review of population based epidemiological studies in myasthenia gravis. *BMC Neurology* 10, 46.

Cea G, Benatar M, Verdugo RJ, Salinas RA et al. (2013) Thymectomy for non-thymomatous myasthenia gravis (Review). *The Cochrane Collaboration*, Issue (10).
Dalakas MC. (2004) The use of intravenous immunoglobulin in the treatment of autoimmune neuromuscular diseases: evidence-based indications and safety profile. *Pharmacological Therapy* 102(3), 177–193, 2004.)
Gajdos P, Chevret S, Toyka KV (2012) Intravenous immunoglobulin for myasthenia gravis (Review). *The Cochrane Collaboration*, Issue (12).
Gilhus NE, Owe JF, Midelfart Hoff J, et al. (2011) Myasthenia gravis: A review of available treatment choices. *Autoimmune disease* Article ID 847393.
Hilton-Jones D, Turner MR (Eds) (2014) *Oxford Textbook of Neuromuscular Disorders (Ed David Hilton-Jones and Martin R. Turner)*. Oxford: Oxford University Press. May 2014
Maddison P, McConville J, Farrugia ME, et al. (2011) The use of rituximab in myasthenia gravis and Lambert–Eaton myasthenic syndrome. *Journal of Neurology, Neurosurgery and Psychiatry* 2011; 82, 671–3.
Mehndiratta MM, Pandey S, Kuntzer T (2014) Acetylcholinesterase inhibitor treatment for myasthenia gravis (Review). *The Cochrane Collaboration* (10).
Schwab I, and Nimmerjahn F (2013) Intravenous immunoglobulin therapy: how does IgG modulate the immune system? *Nature Reviews Immunology* (13), 176–89.
Turner C (2007) A review of myasthenia gravis: pathogenesis, clinical features and treatment. *Current Anaesthesia and Critical Care* 18, 15–23.
Vincent A, Palace J, Hilton-Jones D (2001), Myasthenia gravis. *Lancet* 357, 22112121–128.

Guidelines

Pascuzzi RM (2007) *Medications and Myasthenia Gravis (A reference for health care professionals)*. New York, NY: Myasthenia Gravis Foundation of America.
Sussman J, Farrugia ME, Maddison P, et al. (2015) Myasthenia gravis: Association of British Neurologists' management guidelines. *Practical Neurology* 15, 199–206.

10 Psychiatry

10.1 Anxiety

Anxiety disorders

Anxiety disorders fall mainly into the category of neurotic, stress, or somatoform disorders, as defined by the international classification of disease system (ICD-11, WHO, 2018). They refer to several disorders that include generalized anxiety disorder (GAD), phobic anxiety disorders, panic disorder (± agoraphobia), obsessive compulsive disorder (OCD) and post-traumatic stress disorder (PTSD). Collectively, anxiety disorders affect almost 30% of people in the western world during their lifetime, with PTSD and GAD amongst the most prevalent. In general, anxiety disorders are associated with neurotransmitter dysregulation and amygdala hyperactivity.

Insomnia

Insomnia is the unsatisfactory quantity and/or quality of sleep, which persists for sufficient time to affect quality of life. It is often associated with other mental health (e.g. depression, anxiety, alcohol dependence) and physical (e.g. pain, neoplasms) pathologies, or iatrogenic effects (e.g. diuretic, β-blockers, statins, levodopa). It may require treatment if symptoms are troublesome. Chronic insomnia can last for years, and affects almost 10% of the population. Around 30% have symptoms that are occasionally worse, with higher prevalence in older age.

Pathophysiology of anxiety disorders

Many factors interplay to generate a state of anxiety, but from a biological perspective one of the key central brain pathways involved in this process is the limbic system, which regulates an array of functions, including emotion, fear, behaviour, and memory. One vital brain area that processes fear reactions from the thalamus and cortex is the amygdala, with connections to the hypothalamus, which can activate sympathetic reactions and the hypothalamic–pituitary axis (HPA). Activation/inhibition within this pathway leads to altered neurotransmitter activity.

Corticotrophin-releasing factor (CRF) is known to be released from the hypothalamus in response to stress, under the regulation of the amygdala. CRF acts to drive the HPA, promoting the release of ACTH from the pituitary and then cortisol from the adrenal gland. In effect, sustained CRF exposure may lead to limbic system up-regulation and the heightening of anxiety states. Moreover, dysregulation in this system and changes in central cortisol sensing systems (e.g. decreased receptor expression) may cause chronic anxiety.

The locus coeruleus (LC), is another brain region partly responsible for regulating the sympathetic effects of stress, again under the control of CRF. Here, CRF neurons activate the release of noradrenaline, accounting for the noradrenergic stress response.

GABA, The central neurons within the amygdala, nucleus stria terminalis, and hypothalamus are mostly GABAergic. Underactivity within this pathway can lead to modulation of the HPA-axis, cortisol levels, and hence anxiety. The role of GABA in anxiety is supported by the fact that agents that antagonize $GABA_A$ receptor function can induce symptoms of anxiety, as well as produce flashbacks of traumatic memories, while positive allosteric modulators of the $GABA_A$ receptors provide effective treatment in anxiety disorders.

The $GABA_A$ receptors are pentameric transmembrane complexes composed of different subunits (mainly α, β, and γ subtypes), which form a Cl⁻ permeable channel. It is thought that most GABA$_A$ receptors harbour a single type of α- and β -subunit variant, with the site for the natural ligand in GABA$_A$ receptors located at the interface between the α and β subunits. A separate site exists for allosteric ligands such as the benzodiazepines, which can enhance the Cl$^-$ flux in the presence of the agonist (positive allosteric modulation).

GABA$_A$ receptors may also be found peripherally on lymphocytes that are found to be abnormally low in those with GAD, with corresponding low mRNA levels. It is believed that in acute stress, the high levels of cortisol that are attained can, with time, chronically down-regulate the peripheral receptors. The central action of GABA$_A$ allosteric modulators can therefore decrease circulating cortisol, re-establishing peripheral receptors to normal levels.

Serotonin (5-HT) transmission is also known to play a key role in the pathogenesis of anxiety, although the exact mechanism is poorly understood. Contrary to noradrenaline, it is believed to increase 'resilience' in a traumatic/aversive experience through regulation of the limbic system. It is released from the raphe nuclei (RN), where predominant serotonergic afferents lie, usually in response to 'rhythmic' behaviour that often involves the head or neck (e.g. chewing/licking/grooming) or the trunk (e.g. running). Drugs that promote serotonin levels, such as the selective serotonin re-uptake inhibitors, have good efficacy in the treatment of GAD.

Melatonin is a hormone released in a circadian rhythm by the pineal gland to promote and maintain sleep, by evoking changes in neuronal firing rates in the suprachiasmatic nucleus (SCN). It acts through melatonin receptors in the pituitary and hypothalamus, modulating body temperature, metabolism, and alertness. Structurally similar to serotonin, with both derived from tryptophan.

Generalized anxiety disorder

GAD is a chronic and excessive worrying that is multifactorial in origin, and results from genetic, biological, psychological, and environmental factors. To date, although very few genetic studies have been performed, a mutation of the gene encoding glutamic acid decarboxylase (GAD1), which normally converts GABA to glutamate, has been implicated in disease pathology. In this condition, activation of central GABA$_A$ receptors can modulate the hypothalamic–pituitary axis to elevate the levels of the stress hormone cortisol. Elevated levels of cortisol are believed to act to reduce the number of peripheral GABA receptors, therefore, reducing the inhibitory effects of GABA in patients with GAD.

Chronic stimulation of the HPA axis in GAD is thought to lead to a reduction in corticosteroid receptors in the hippocampus, normally responsible for suppressing cortisol release, thus cortisol suppression may be reduced. Furthermore, some patients with GAD have been shown to have increased amygdala volume and demonstrated hyperactivity, again modulating the HPA axis and producing a heightened 'stress' response. Conversely, serotonin levels in patients with GAD tend to be low, and are again implicated as a contributory factor in GAD. Although levels of circulating NA remain normal in patients with GAD, α$_2$ adrenoceptors may have a dysfunctional response to fluctuating levels and thus produce diminished autonomic responses.

Post-traumatic stress disorder

PTSD is an anxiety disorder triggered by a traumatic event, and aside from severe anxiety, is associated with flashbacks and nightmares where the person relives the event. Typically, patients will have increased levels of adrenaline/noradrenaline with subsequent elevated BP and heart rate. Conversely, serotonin levels and sensitivity is likely reduced. HPA response also appears to be elevated in PTSD leading to excessive levels of CRF.

Obsessive compulsive disorder

OCD is characterized by repetitive urges/compulsions, associated with anxiety, and influenced by environmental and genetic factors. Its aetiology has long been attributed to serotonin, largely due to its response to SSRIs, as well as the association of serotonin with repetitive behaviour. However, preclinical, neuroimaging, and neurochemical studies have also demonstrated that the dopaminergic system is involved in inducing or aggravating symptoms, although the precise mechanism remains unknown. The involvement of dopamine transmission may indicate why up to 50% of patients fail to respond to SSRI monotherapy or the TCA, **clomipramine**, and why higher doses may be required than in depression; to reveal dopaminergic modulatory effects. Antipsychotics, such as **aripiprazole** and **risperidone** at low doses, (see Topic 10.3 'Schizophrenia and psychoses') have been used with some success in augmenting SSRIs in patients with OCD, particularly in patients with comorbid Tourette disorder or other tic disorders. Glutamate also has a potential role to play.

Phobias

Phobias are defined as exaggerated fear responses and avoidance that interferes with normal daily living. Little is known or understood about the underlying pathophysiology and pharmacotherapy is of limited value.

Pathophysiology of insomnia

Sleep architecture is composed of non-rapid eye movement (N-REM) and REM, and involves different complex neurochemical systems that can control the level of wakefulness. The timing and regulation of sleep, involves a brain region called the SCN, which feeds into the hypothalamus, and contributes to cortisol production and temperature regulation. The SCN receives innervation from the optic tract, and it can sense, together with the pineal gland, light–dark cycles that regulate levels of melatonin.

The development of insomnia is multifactorial, and most likely to be troublesome in those who are predisposed and/or undergo stress of some sort. Patients who suffer with insomnia tend to have previously been light sleepers who have undergone a trigger generating chronic hyperarousal. There is some evidence that in these groups high cortisol levels may be found to act through the HPA axis, leading to an ongoing sleep-related worry, with the limbic system intimately involved. As outlined above, the LC (NA) and raphe (5-HT) can modulate arousal states, via neurons that can be inhibited by GABAergic transmission. Allosteric modulation of the GABA$_A$ receptors with non-benzodiazepine ligands, like **zopiclone**, may be particularly useful in insomnia.

For a full summary of the relevant pathways and drug targets, see Figure 10.1.

Management

Anxiety disorders

In general, anxiety disorders are primarily managed non-pharmacologically through education, help-groups, and individualized psychological intervention such as cognitive behavioural therapy (CBT). The role of drug treatment is limited to those whose symptoms have not responded to non-pharmacological interventions, or for acute crisis management.

Benzodiazepines are the most widely used anxiolytics and although useful in an acute crisis, are not recommended in patients suffering from panic attacks or for chronic anxiety management. Long-term use is associated with dependence and tolerance (leading to problems on withdrawal), as well as increased anxiety, cognitive impairment, emotional blunting, falls, disinhibition, and paradoxical stimulation.

SSRIs, SNRIs, and **pregabalin** are recommended first-line in patients requiring pharmacological management for GAD, with treatment continued for a period of 6–24 months to prevent a relapse of symptoms. SSRIs are also the preferred drugs in managing panic disorders, although **venlafaxine** (unlicensed use) or a tricyclic anti-depressant may also be used. When prescribing, consideration should be given to licensed indications as these vary considerably between agents, although NICE advocates **sertraline** off-label for use first-line in GAD.

Prior to starting treatment, patients should be advised that it can take 2–4 weeks to see any benefit, and that there is likely to be a transient increase in anxiety following initiation. Doses are started low and only increased where patients fail to respond, at an interval of 4–6 weeks. Most patients will require low doses, but higher doses may be necessary for some, particularly those with obsessive compulsive, or post-traumatic stress disorder.

In patients with more complex disease, such as those at high risk of self-harming or with marked functional impairment, referral to secondary care for further intervention is essential. Management is likely to require a combination of intensive psychological intervention and drug therapy, which may include anti-psychotics.

Insomnia

Diagnosis of insomnia should include the identification of any underlying cause such as anxiety, depression, sleep apnoeas, alcohol consumption, and poor sleep hygiene. In the absence of an underlying cause about 30% of patients will respond to improvements in sleep hygiene, such as limiting caffeine intake, avoiding daytime naps, regular exercise, and appropriate sleep environment. Other interventions include behavioural and pharmacological measures, such as restricting the time spent in bed, relaxation, or the use of CBT. Although pharmacological management of insomnia is effective in inducing sleep, it is unlikely to confer

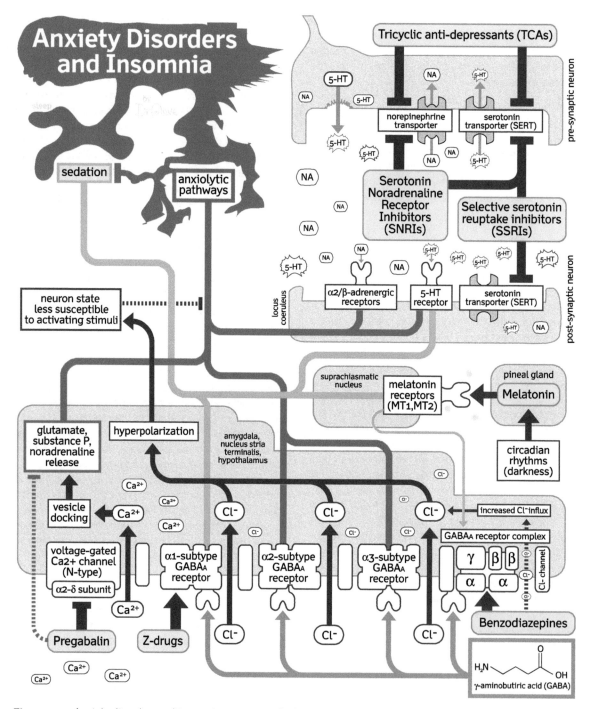

Figure 10.1 Anxiety disorders and insomnia: summary of relevant pathways and drug targets.

a benefit once treatment is stopped, unlike psychological intervention. Furthermore, hypnotics are associated with dependence, tolerance, and side effects that can impair function.

Treatment with hypnotics should be reserved for patients with infrequent or acute symptoms. When selecting between the benzodiazepines and 'z-drugs', consideration should be given to duration of action, with short-acting agents preferred in patients having trouble getting off to sleep, while intermediate-acting agents are preferred in those waking at night. **Melatonin** may be a useful option in patients where insomnia is caused by disturbances in circadian rhythm, such as shift workers or jet lag.

Drug classes used in management

Benzodiazepines

Benzodiazepines are a group of psycho-active drugs that act as allosteric modulators of the inhibitory GABA receptors in the CNS. Introduced in the 1960s, they still are the most widely used group of drugs for the treatment of anxiety. Examples include alprazolam, chlordiazepoxide, clonazepam, diazepam, flurazepam, loprazolam, lorazepam, lormetazepam, nitrazepam, oxazepam, and temazepam.

Mechanism of action

GABA is the main inhibitory neurotransmitter in the CNS and acts on two types of receptors—a metabotropic G protein–coupled receptor with pre- and post-synaptic functions, and a post-synaptic ionotropic receptor, which is selectively permeable to the negatively charged Cl^-. The latter is the most abundant in the CNS, and is allosterically modulated by different drugs such as benzodiazepines, barbiturates, and ethanol. As previously stated, this receptor is a heteropentameric ion channel, with a most frequent stoichiometry formed by two α subunits, two β and one Y. The $GABA_A$ receptors can mediate various physiological effects, such as sedation, amnesia, and other cognitive functions, anxiolysis, and muscle relaxation. Transgenic genetic studies with mice have indicated that the α1 subtype of $GABA_A$ receptors selectively mediates sedation and amnesic effects, while receptors that contain α2 and α3 subunits can influence anxiolytic processes.

Benzodiazepines bind to the $GABA_A$ receptor at a specific binding site ('benzodiazepines binding site'), where it generates an increment in the opening frequency of the ionic channel following activation by the endogenous GABA ligand. Classic benzodiazepines demonstrate equivalent binding affinity for all the GABA receptors subtypes that contain the Y2 subunit. The potentiation of the effect of endogenous GABA increases the flow of negatively charged Cl^-. This favours hyperpolarization of the membrane potential and a neuron state less susceptible to activating stimuli.

Prescribing

There are multiple benzodiazepines available worldwide for use in insomnia, anxiety, alcohol withdrawal, status epilepticus, or as a premedication prior to induction of anaesthesia. Choice will depend on licensed indication and duration of action relative to individual's requirements (see Table 10.1).

Unwanted effects

Prolonged use of benzodiazepine therapy leads to altered receptor function, so that the effects of agonists are reduced and antagonists enhanced. Consequently, chronic use, particularly at high doses, leads to tolerance and dependence, which can develop after as little as 2 weeks of treatment. Decreases in prescriptions for benzodiazepines suggests that avoiding long-term use is now widely accepted. In patients who have received extended courses, abrupt withdrawal commonly induces a rebound of symptoms that may be worse than the original insomnia, and is often associated with mood changes and agitation.

In some patients benzodiazepines exert paradoxical excitatory effects, particularly in the elderly, causing irritability, hallucinations, delusion, aggression, and nightmares. Others using benzodiazepines for insomnia report sleep-walking and carrying out activities, such as preparing food or driving in a semi-conscious state that they cannot later recall. In both instances, discontinuation is advised.

'Hangover' effects to benzodiazepines are more likely to occur with intermediate or long-acting agents, where the effects last into the next morning, and patients should be made aware of the risk.

Muscle weakness has been reported with benzodiazepine treatment, so use is cautioned in patients with pre-existing weakness or myasthenia gravis, although the risk of harm is rare.

At higher doses, such as IV doses or in overdose, the effects of benzodiazepines can be sufficient to cause respiratory and CNS depression. Although the incidence of fatalities is rare, the use of higher doses should be restricted to those with sufficient expertise and access to appropriate monitoring facilities and the reversal agent **flumazenil**.

Most benzodiazepines are hepatically metabolized via various pathways to a combination of active and inactive metabolites, before being renally cleared. Consequently,

Table 10.1 Summary of commonly used benzodiazepines and their uses

Benzodiazepine	Administration	Duration of action	Indication
Alprazolam	Orally TDS	Short-acting, peaks in 1–2 hours, half-life of 11–15 hours	Anxiety
Chlordiazepoxide	Orally TDS–QDS	Long-acting, peaks in 1–2 hours, half-life of active metabolite 201503 days	Anxiety, alcohol withdrawal
Clonazepam	Orally, IM	Long-acting, peaks in 3 hours, half-life 20–60 hours	Acute behavioural disturbance/agitation (IM)
Diazepam	Rectal, IV, oral	Long-acting, peaks in 30–60 minutes, prolonged half-life of 2–5 days	Anxiety, insomnia, muscle spasm, status epilepticus
Flurazepam	Orally at bedtime	Long-acting, acts in 30–60 minutes, half-life of active metabolite up to 100 hours	Insomnia
Loprazolam	Orally at bedtime	Intermediate-acting, peaks in 4 hours, half-life of about 12 hours	Insomnia
Lorazepam	Orally, IV, IM	Short-acting, acts in 2 hours, half-life of 10–20 hours	Anxiety, insomnia, pre-med, status epilepticus, acute mania, rapid tranquilization
Lormetazepam	Orally at bedtime	Short-acting, acts in 1.5 hours, half-life of 11 hours	Insomnia
Midazolam	IV and buccal. Unlicensed preparations for oral and intranasal use	Short-acting, peaks in 20–60 minutes, half-life of 1.5–2.5 hours (depending on route of administration)	Pre-med, conscious sedation, status epilepticus
Nitrazepam	Oral	Intermediate-acting, peaks in 2–3 hours, half-life of 30 hours	Insomnia
Oxazepam	Orally TDS–QDS	Short-acting, peaks in 2–3 hours, half-life of 6–20 hours	Anxiety
Temazepam	Orally at bedtime	Short-acting, peaks in 1 hour, half-life of 8–15 hours or more	Insomnia

effects are increased in impaired hepatic and renal function, as well as in the elderly. Consideration should be given to their use in alcohol withdrawal where patients often have liver damage.

Interactions

Drug interactions with benzodiazepines often occur because of enhanced effects in combination with other sedative drugs, or where metabolism is altered. Increased sedative effects and risk of respiratory depression is common with antihistamines, antidepressants, antipsychotics, opioids, and anaesthetics. Concomitant use with alcohol can also increase the risk of sedation and impair ability to drive.

Many of the benzodiazepines are metabolized in the liver via the cytochrome P450 enzyme system and thus have the potential for drug interactions; in particular, **midazolam**, **diazepam**, and **alprazolam**, and to a lesser extent **lorazepam**, **oxazepam**, and **temazepam**. Interactions of possible clinical significance with these include increased levels when taken with some antiretro-virals (avoid use with **ritonavir**, **indinavir**, **nelfinavir**, **saquinavir**, **delaviridine**, and **efavirenz**), macrolides, **sodium valproate**, **cimetidine**, **omeprazole**, and azole antifungals. Conversely, the inducers **rifampicin** and the xanthines are likely to reduce effects.

Z-drugs

Non-benzodiazepine hypnotics also increase the inhibitory Cl^- currents through the $GABA_A$ receptor via an allosteric mechanism. They are largely preferred over classical benzodiazepines due to better binding selectivity and pharmacokinetic profile. For example, zaleplon, zolpidem, and zopiclone.

Mechanism of action

Since GABA is the main inhibitory neurotransmitter in the human CNS, it is not surprising that the treatment of insomnia has been dictated by the use of drugs that augment the capacity of the $GABA_A$ receptor to decrease neuronal activity. Z-drugs have different pharmacological profiles to the benzodiazepines and, although they can still bind to the site for the benzodiazepine, have some se-lectivity for the α1 receptor subtype.

The short-acting and α1 selective imidazopyradine, **zolpidem**, has intermediate potency at α2 and α3 recep-tors, and minor activity at α5 receptors. It reduces sleep latency and night-time awakenings, improving total sleep duration. The pyrazolopyrimidine, **zaleplon**, has superior potency at the α1β2γ2 receptor subtype than the α2- and α3-containing subunits. Like **zolpidem**, it significantly de-creases latency to sleep onset, but is less consistent with sleep maintenance. However, it seems to have improved psychomotor profile with less cognitive effects.

Zopiclone is part of the cyclopyrrolone family with a binding spectrum similar to classic benzodiazepines. It can effectively decrease the latency to sleep and the quan-tity of night-time awakenings.

Prescribing

The z-drugs are licensed solely for use in the short-term management of insomnia that is sufficiently severe. In terms of clinical efficacy, there is little to distinguish be-tween them and the short-acting benzodiazepines.

All three drugs are available in two strengths, the lower of which is recommended for use in elderly patients or those with hepatic impairment. A lower dose of **zopiclone**

is also recommended in renal impairment. Doses are ad-ministered at night.

Unwanted effects

As the z-drugs act on the $GABA_A$ receptor in a similar way to benzodiazepines, they exhibit a comparable toxicity pro-file, including their propensity for inducing dependence, tolerance, and withdrawal symptoms, particularly with prolonged use and high doses (see 'Benzodiazepines'). **Zopiclone** is also commonly reported to cause a bitter or metallic taste.

Similarly, z-drugs have the same tendency for inter-actions both in terms of enhanced adverse effects when taken with drugs known to cause sedation and respiratory depression, etc., and by being metabolized by the cyto-chrome P450 enzyme system. The effects on the z-drugs, however, are less widely reported and likely to be of lesser clinical significance.

Melatonin

A lipophilic hormone that mainly originates from the pineal gland, melatonin is released into the blood and helps in the regulation of sleep–wake cycles. Its production is stimulated by darkness and high levels can induce sleep.

Mechanism of action

Beyond its role in circadian rhythm control, **melatonin** is involved in the regulation of many physiological pro-cesses, such as BP, ovarian and retinal physiology, oncogenesis, and osteoblast differentiation. The highly expressed melatonin receptors in the SCN of the hypo-thalamus are the main mediators of the role of melatonin in the sleep-wakefulness cycle.

There are two main types of melatonin receptors MT_1 and MT_2, both of which are G protein–coupled and pre-sent in a variety of tissues. MT_1 is expressed in the SCN of the hypothalamus and cardiac vessels, plus other brain areas and peripheral tissues, and is involved in circa-dian rhythm regulation and vessel constriction. MT_1 re-ceptors can link to an extensive diversity of G proteins and trigger numerous intracellular signalling processes, including inhibitory effects on cAMP cascade, a decrease in PKA activity and CREB phosphorylation, activation of PKC, K^+ channels, and stimulation of PLC-dependent signalling. The MT_2 receptors are known to be involved in retinal physiology, circadian rhythm, and dilation of cardiac vessels. They have a more restricted localization, including the cerebellum, SCN, retina, kidney, and cardiac cells. They also couple to the inhibition of cAMP formation and stimulation of protease inhibitor hydrolysis.

The suppression of neuronal activity by melatonin, possibly by changing GABA receptor complex functions, is one of the probable mechanism by which this hormone can help in the control of sleep. Because it is a natural hypnotic, with low toxicity and limited side effects, it has been used long term; this is, however, controversial.

Agomelatine is closely related to melatonin, and acts as a potent agonist at melatonin receptors (MT_1 and MT_2) and antagonist at $5\text{-}HT_{2C}$ receptors. It resynchronizes circadian rhythms and is mainly indicated for the treatment of major depressive episodes.

Prescribing

Melatonin is widely available world-wide as a 'food' supplement, although in the UK there is a single formulation licensed for sleep disturbances in people over 55 (Circadian®) and it is also manufactured in different formulations by various 'specials' manufacturers. As a food supplement or unlicensed special, these products may demonstrate marked variation in content and quality.

Unwanted effects

Melatonin is generally well tolerated with the most commonly reported side effects including headaches, nasopharyngitis, back pain, and arthralgia. Manufacturers of Circadin® recommend caution in patients with auto-immune disease. Metabolism is via the cytochrome P450 enzyme system and therefore, in principle, may be affected by inducers or inhibitors of the same enzymes.

Selective serotonin re-uptake inhibitors

> SSRIs act by selectively blocking the re-uptake of serotonin after its neuronal release, thus prolonging its effect on serotoninergic receptors. Examples include citalopram, escitalopram, fluoxetine, fluvoxamine, paroxetine, and sertraline

Mechanism of action

Serotoninergic neurotransmission has a key functional part in various physiological processes and pathological conditions, including the regulation of mood, control of impulses, sleep, libido, vigilance, and cognitive functions.

In addition, anxiety and fear can also be modulated by serotonin transmission.

SSRIs are the first-line treatment in anxiety disorders, mainly through enhancing serotoninergic neurotransmission and subsequent activation of the $5\text{-}HT_{1A}$ subtype of serotonin receptor. This is a G protein–coupled receptor that mediates inhibitory neurotransmission, and is expressed at high levels in limbic, temporal and prefrontal cortices. For more details see Topic 10.2, 'Depression').

Prescribing

Although all SSRIs are licensed for use in depression, they vary considerably in their secondary licensed indications (see Table 10.2). All agents have evidence to support their use in the management of panic disorders, whereas for GAD only **escitalopram**, **paroxetine**, and **sertraline** are indicated. In all cases, doses are started low and gradually increased to achieve a response to reduce the risk of unwanted effects, such as an initial increase in anxiety symptoms, insomnia and headaches. Patients are unlikely to see a benefit for at least 2–4 weeks and should continue for at least 12 weeks at the maximum-tolerated dose to determine efficacy.

Unwanted effects

See Topic 10.2, 'Depression'.

Serotonin-noradrenaline re-uptake inhibitors

> Serotonin-noradrenaline re-uptake inhibitors (SNRIs) act by blocking the re-uptake of serotonin and noradrenaline after its neuronal release, thus extending serotoninergic and noradrenergic effects on their receptors. For example, duloxetine and venlafaxine.

Mechanism of action

The use of antidepressants such as SSRIs and SNRIs in the treatment of anxiety are now established as effective alternatives to benzodiazepines. Like serotonin, noradrenaline neurotransmission is also involved in anxiety and depressive disorders, mainly via the α2-adrenergic receptors.

Duloxetine is a potent and selective SNRI, with much less activity at dopamine re-uptake. It is used in the treatment of major depressive disorder, as well as the acute management of GAD. Duloxetine has no significant affinity

Table 10.2 Licensed indications of SSRIs

SSRI	Generalized anxiety disorder	Panic disorder	Obsessive compulsive disorder
Citalopram	No	Yes	No
Escitalopram	Yes	No	Yes
Fluoxetine	No	No	Yes
Fluvoxamine	No	No	Yes
Paroxetine	Yes	Yes	Yes
Sertraline	No (social anxiety)	Yes	Yes

for dopaminergic, adrenergic, cholinergic, histaminergic, opioid, glutamate, and GABA receptors.

Venlafaxine and its metabolite O-desmethylvenlafaxine (ODV) potently inhibit the re-uptake of noradrenaline and serotonin, with only a weak inhibition of dopamine re-uptake. They are not active at histaminergic, muscarinic, or α1-adrenergic receptors.

See Topic 10.2, 'Depression' for details.

Prescribing

Both **venlafaxine** and **duloxetine** are available for use in GAD and, although unlicensed, venlafaxine has been shown to be effective in panic disorders. As with SSRIs, treatment can cause restlessness, headaches and agitation on initiation, and can take 2–4 weeks to be effective.

Unwanted effects

See Topic 10.2, 'Depression'.

Tricyclic anti-depressants

Tricyclic antidepressants (TCAs) are a heterogeneous group of drugs with anxiolytic activity mainly mediated by the inhibition of serotonin and noradrenaline re-uptake. For example, clomipramine and imipramine.

Mechanism of action

TCAs also have analgesic properties for neuropathic and neuralgic pain which might contribute to their therapeutic role in anxiety disorders. Although a mechanism for the analgesic action is not known, it might be due to an indirect action on opioid receptors via the serotoninergic route. TCAs side effects are mainly mediated by their antagonistic actions at other receptors, such as H_1-histamine, α_1-adrenoceptors, and cholinergic receptors.

The prototypical tricyclic antidepressant **imipramine**, acts by increasing the concentration of noradrenaline and serotonin in the synaptic cleft. With chronic use, imipramine can also down-regulate β-adrenergic receptors in the cerebral cortex and sensitize post-synaptic serotonergic receptors, which also contributes to increased serotonergic transmission.

Clomipramine is the 3-chloro-derivative of imipramine and a tricyclic antidepressant. It is a strong, but not entirely selective serotonin re-uptake inhibitor (SRI), with the main metabolite desmethyclomipramine being active as an inhibitor of noradrenaline reuptake.

For details see Topic 10.2, 'Depression'.

Prescribing

Although off-label, the TCAs **clomipramine** and **imipramine** have been shown to be effective in the management of panic disorders. Furthermore, the SRI properties of clomipramine, means that unlike other TCAs, it is effective in the management of OCD. As they have a less favourable side effect profile to the SSRIs or SNRIs, particularly in terms of cardiovascular toxicity in overdose, they are generally reserved for use second-line. They are also more likely to cause sedation, which may be beneficial in some patients. Intolerance may, in part, be overcome by starting with low doses and gradually increasing every 3–5 days to a therapeutic dose.

Unwanted effects

See Topic 10.2, 'Depression'.

Pregabalin

The GABA neurotransmitter structural derivative pregabalin binds to the α2-δ subunit and inhibits of the voltage-gated Ca^{2+} channel (N-type) in the CNS, which might explain its role as antinociceptive and antiseizure drug.

Mechanism of action

Despite the similarities with the GABA neurotransmitter, **pregabalin** does not bind directly to GABA receptors and does not augment GABA responses in cultured neurons.

However, prolonged stimulation leads to an increase in GABA receptor density in *in vitro* experimental models.

Instead, through high-affinity binding to voltage-gated Ca^{2+} channels, pregabalin decreases presynaptic vesicle docking and thus reduces the release of various neurotransmitters that have been implicated in anxiety disorders, such as glutamate, substance P, and noradrenaline.

Treatment with pregabalin is also associated with a positive effect in all forms of insomnia, which is relevant to its effectiveness given the fact that sleep disturbances are a common component of the clinical presentation of GAD.

Prescribing

Pregabalin has been shown to be effective in the management of GAD, with the added advantage of being effective within a couple of days of starting therapy. NICE advocate its use as a second-line in patients intolerant of an SSRI or SNRI, although other groups recommend it as first-line treatment. There is also emerging evidence of its role in OCD.

Unwanted effects

See Topic 9.2, 'Epilepsy (including status epilepticus)'.

Further reading

Aubry JM (2013) CRF system and mood disorders. *Journal of Chemical Neuroanatomy* 54, 20–4.

Buoli M, Caldiroli A, Caletti E, et al. (2013) New approaches to the pharmacological management of generalized anxiety disorder. *Expert Opinions in Pharmacotherapy* 14 (2), 175–84.

Falloon K, Arroll B, Raina Elley C, et al. (2011) The assessment and management of insomnia in primary care. *British Medical Journal* 342, d2899.

Herman JP, Ostrander MM, Mueller NK, et al. (2005) Limbic system mechanisms of stress regulation: hypothalamo-pituitary-adrenocortical axis. *Progress in Neuropsychopharmacology and Biological Psychiatry* 29(8), 1201–13.

Jetty PV, Charnet DS, Goddard AW (2001) Neurobiology of generalized anxiety disorder. *Psychological Clinics of North America* 24, 71–97.

Olivier JD, Vinkers CH, Olivier B (2013) The role of the serotonergic and GABA system in translational approaches in drug discovery for anxiety disorders. *Frontiers in Pharmacology* 11, 4–74.

Sateia MJ, Nowell PD (2004) Insomnia. *Lancet* 364, 1959–73.

Thoeringer CK, Ripke S, Unschuld PG, et al. (2009) The GABA transporter 1 (SLC6A1): a novel candidate gene for anxiety disorders. *Journal of Neural Transmission* 116, 649–57.

WHO (2018) International Classification of Disease, 11th revision. https://icd.who.int/en/ [accessed 23 April 2019].

Guidelines

Bandelow B, Sher L, Bunevicus R, et al. (2012) Guidelines for the pharmacological treatment of anxiety disorders, obsessive–compulsive disorder and posttraumatic stress disorder in primary care; WFSBP task force on mental disorders in primary care and WFSBP task force on anxiety disorders, OCD and PTSD. *International Journal of Psychiatry in Clinical Practice* 16, 77–84.

Baldwin DS, Anderson IM, Nutt DJ, et al. (2014) Evidence-based pharmacological treatment of anxiety disorders, post-traumatic stress disorder and obsessive-compulsive disorder: a revision of the 2005 guidelines from the British Association for Psychopharmacology. *Journal of Psychopharmacology* 28(5), 403–39. doi: 10.1177/0269881114525674.

NICE CG113 (2011) Generalised anxiety disorder and panic disorder in adults: management. https://www.nice.org.uk/guidance/cg113 [accessed 10 April 2019].

NICE TA77 (2004) Guidance on the use of zaleplon, zolpidem and zopiclone for the short-term management of insomnia. https://www.nice.org.uk/guidance/ta77 [accessed 10 April 2019].

Taylor D, Paton C, Kapur S (2015) *The Maudsley Prescribing Guidelines in Psychiatry*. Oxford: Wiley-Blackwell.

10.2 Depression

Depression is one of the most common disorders affecting mental health and has a significant impact on patients' physical, emotional, cognitive, and environmental function, and in some extreme cases can result in self-harm and suicide. Depression can be part of other psychiatric illnesses (e.g. other mood disorders, such as bipolar disorder) or co-exist with other conditions, such as anxiety disorders or schizophrenia. Under the ICD-10 classification, depressive episodes are considered as either single or recurrent events of varying severity (mild, moderate, severe), characterized by a depressed mood, loss of interest and enjoyment, and reduction in energy/activity. Rarely, in severe cases, patients may need to be placed under section of the Mental Health Act to protect them from causing harm to themselves or others. Over 90% of cases are managed in primary care with a combination of psychological therapies and/or pharmacological intervention.

Rates of major depressive disorder (MDD) are higher in those aged 25–44 years and amongst females (14%), with an overall prevalence in the order of 13% and a typical incidence of 15.5/1000. In particular, the rate of suicide is highest in men aged 40–50. Most presentations are episodic in nature and the risk of recurrence is greater where prognostic factors (e.g. psychosocial factors in childhood, social isolation) are poor. Patients with long-term conditions such as diabetes (19%) or Parkinson's disease (19%) are at higher risk.

Pathophysiology

The pathophysiology of MDD is a complex interplay of biological, psychological, and social factors that influence neurochemical change and neuroplasticity, but it is not yet entirely clear how neurochemical changes lead to symptomatology.

Genetics

MDD is heterogeneous in nature, with familial studies demonstrating moderate genetic influence. Candidate genes include a serotonin transporter gene, polymorphism in tryptophan hydroxylase-2 (the enzyme that is a rate-limiting step in the production of serotonin), cAMP response element-binding protein (CREB) and brain-derived neurotrophic factor (BDNF).

Neurochemical basis of depression

Much of the understanding of the neurochemical basis and brain pathways involved in MDD stem from historical observations, showing the beneficial effects of monoamine oxidase inhibitors (e.g. **isoniazid**) and tricyclic antidepressants (e.g. **imipramine**). This monoamine model proposes that there are deficiencies of serotonin (5-HT) and noradrenaline (NA); however, true depletion has been difficult to prove clinically, and as the benefit of these treatments is delayed, efficacy is not just a case of increasing 'synaptic levels' of neurotransmitters. The slow response to treatments may be explained through delayed desensitization of presynaptic 5-HT_{1A} autoreceptors and the subsequent post-synaptic down-regulation of receptors (i.e. 5-HT_2 and/or α_2 adrenoceptors). In MDD, it is likely that decreased 5-HT signalling leads to up-regulation of both pre- and post-synaptic receptors.

Serotonin is released from terminals to act at receptors (pre- or post-), or is taken back up into the cell via 5-HT uptake transporter (SERT). Acting at presynaptic receptors 5-HT can control its own release to modify synaptic levels and hence neurotransmission. Synaptic 5-HT can be metabolized by monoamine oxidase A (MAO A), which can indirectly affect re-uptake of neurotransmitter for subsequent release. *Serotonergic neurons* predominantly lie within the raphe nucleus and project to the hippocampus, thalamus, basal ganglia, and cortex, where they can affect emotional processing or memories.

Noradrenergic neurons project from the locus coeruleus and, when released, NA acts both pre- and post-synaptically to modulate mood and emotion. Presynaptic α2-adrenoceptors are inhibitory and reduce the release of NA from terminals, thus acting as a local feedback loop. In MDD, the reduction of NA concentrations at the synapse and CSF level, leads to an up-regulation of post-synaptic receptors in the cortex. The levels of synaptic neurotransmitter are also influenced by the NA re-uptake transporter (NRI) and its metabolising enzyme MAO (A and B), the latter with increased activity in MDD. Post-synaptic second messenger pathways, through cAMP and PKA, can also affect CREB and subsequent BDNF expression, with consequences in neuronal connectivity in projection regions like the hypothalamus and hippocampus.

Regulation of neurotransmitter levels

There are numerous targets that can modulate synaptic levels of transmitters, and their discovery has not only enabled improvements in symptomatology, but also contributed to pathophysiological understanding.

Elevating monoamine levels by inhibiting the breakdown enzyme MAO has been shown to improve symptoms in MDD. There are two types of MAO—MAO-A, which deaminates 5-HT and NA, and MAO-B, which deaminates dopamine, tyramine, and inhibitors of these. The use of MAOIs, however, is limited by their significant and serious side effects (see 'Monoamine oxidase inhibitors, Unwanted effects'). Another mechanism to elevate monoamine levels is with neurotransmitter re-uptake inhibitors such as tricyclic anti-depressants (TCAs) or SSRIs.

Although restoring monoaminergic transmission is the key step for therapeutic treatment, other more complex neuroplastic events are involved, including changes in receptor density and intracellular signalling, modulation of synaptic transmission, alteration of neuronal networks, and neurogenesis. A recent model based on an alternative 'cognitive' approach has been proposed to explain the delayed effect of antidepressant therapy. In this model, antidepressants produce fast changes in emotional-processing, although improvements in mood are slow because emotional associations must be re-learnt. Single

administrations of SSRI or SNRIs can increase the processing of positive information, so backing this hypothesis (see review by Willner et al., 2013).

In clinical practice, most antidepressants have *delayed onset* of effectiveness, a phenomenon that in neurochemical terms is mainly ascribed to the somatodendritic actions of 5-HT, leading to down-regulation of the 5-HT$_{1A}$ autoreceptors over weeks. The lower expression of these autoreceptors disinhibits the neuron once again, so that it can release more 5-HT into the cleft. Such slow protein expression changes may also account for the observation of increased suicide and self-harm risk when starting and stopping some antidepressants.

Stress and depression

The hypothalamic pituitary axis also has a strong influence over the risk of developing MDD. Chronic stress leads to sustained release of CRF from the hypothalamus, which in turn elevates levels of ACTH from the anterior pituitary gland (see Topic 4.1, 'The pituitary gland') and cortisol from the adrenal glands. In MDD, but also in other severe and enduring mental health conditions, it is believed that the stress-induced sustained release of CRF leads to dysregulation in the normal negative feedback pathways. This, in turn, provokes the decreased expression of CRF-1 receptors and glucocorticoid receptors in the hypothalamus and cortex. In suicide cases, subnormal CRF-1 expression levels have been noted. It is thought that around 50% of depression cases show high or dysfunctional rhythmicity of cortisol and, as such, dexamethasone-mediated negative feedback resistance can be demonstrated by a suppression test (see Topic 4.2, 'The adrenal gland'). Circulating cortisol will act at glucocorticoid receptors (as does dexamethasone) within the hippocampus, hypothalamus, and cortex, where it has been shown to cause neuronal atrophy in animal models. This atrophy is consistent with clinical MRI studies that demonstrate smaller hippocampal volume in MDD. As outlined previously, this chronic stress can ultimately deplete levels of BDNF and, hence, negatively impact on synapse formation and neuroplasticity. It is important to mention, however, that the dexamethasone suppression test is *not* a reliable marker for identifying depression.

For a full summary of the relevant pathways and drug targets, see Figure 10.2.

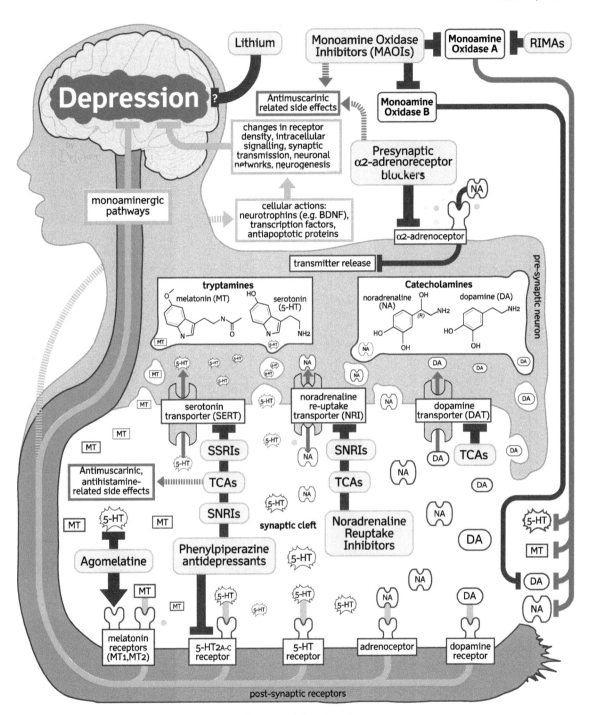

Figure 10.2 Depression: summary of relevant pathways and drug targets.

Table 10.3 Symptoms of depression

Typical symptoms	Common symptoms	Atypical symptoms
Low mood	Reduced concentration/attention	Weight gain
Anhedonia (loss of interest/pleasure)	Insomnia/hypersomnia	Increased appetite
Fatigue/low energy	Reduced self-esteem/self-confidence	Excessive sleepiness
	Excessive guilt/unworthiness	
	Loss of appetite/weight	
	Bleak pessimistic view of the future	
	Suicidal ideation	

Management

A diagnosis of depression is made based on the ICD-10 criteria for mild, moderate, or severe depression, either as a single or recurrent episode. Patients will usually present with two typical symptoms plus additional symptoms depending on severity (see Table 10.3)

Routine serum biochemistry, including TFTs and LFTs, as well as FBC, may be required to exclude any suspected differential diagnoses, such as hypothyroidism or anaemia.

The choice of intervention is guided by NICE Clinical Guidelines 90 and 91 (presence of chronic physical health problems) and follows a step-wise process, with most patients successfully managed in primary care (Figure 10.3). Severe cases, however, e.g. presence of severe self-neglect, self-harm, suicidal ideation, or psychotic episodes, will require specialist mental health services.

For the emergency situation in the high acuity, non-pregnant, psychotic, suicidal individual, hospitalization with psychiatric referral ± electroconvulsive therapy (ECT) may be required with initiation of

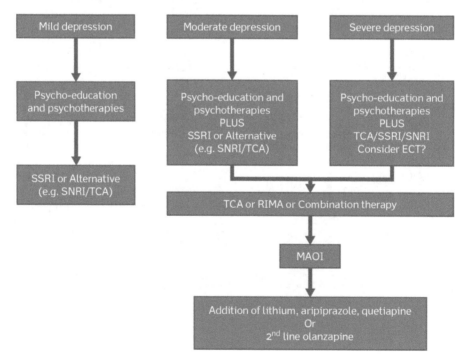

Figure 10.3 Management of depression.

Data from NICE CG90 Depression in adults: recognition and management (Updated April 2018) https://www.nice.org.uk/guidance/cg90

an SSRI. Other therapeutic options include the use of lorazepam for immediate emergency symptom management in a catatonic patient, with additional use of antipsychotics.

In the case of mild depression, pharmacological treatment is generally avoided up-front due to the relative risk–benefit and so active monitoring is recommended, with follow-up made after a period of 2 weeks. In mild–moderate severity, low intensity psychological intervention is preferred, delivered individually, or through support groups, or self-help programmes. Drug therapy may, however, be necessary, especially in those with a history of moderate to severe depression, or where symptoms have persisted for several years. Drug therapy, in combination with high-intensity psychological intervention (e.g. individual or group CBT), should be offered in severe depression.

Choice of drug therapy is influenced by patient factors, such as the presence of co-morbidities, patient preferences (influenced by side effect profile) or previous effective anti-depressant use; however, SSRIs are normally preferred due to their favourable side effects. Doses should be started at the lowest therapeutic dose and reviewed after 4 weeks to assess response. On initiation patients should be advised that, although they should see some benefit in the first 1 or 2 weeks, it will take longer (4–6 weeks) for them to realize the full benefit. Initially, they may experience a worsening of some symptoms, such as increased anxiety with SSRIs for around 1 or 2 weeks. Treatment should be continued for at least 6 months in a first episode of depression after resolution of symptoms, to minimize relapse. Care should be taken in patients considered to be at risk of overdose, e.g. by prescribing small quantities and avoiding antidepressants that are toxic in overdose, i.e. TCAs or **venlafaxine**.

In patients failing to respond within 3–4 weeks, consideration should be given to increasing the dose or switching to an alternative agent, considering drug half-life and the risk associated with using two agents concomitantly (see 'Prescribing warning: switching between antidepressants'). In general, the older drugs such as TCAs or MAOIs have been largely superseded by newer drugs such as venlafaxine or **mirtazapine**. In some instances, combination therapy may be deemed appropriate, such as in patients who demonstrate a small, but inadequate response to monotherapy, for whom **lithium** augmentation is not an option. NICE do not advocate the use of **dosulepin** in the management of depression due to the unacceptably high cardiac risk.

> ## PRESCRIBING WARNING
>
> ### Switching between antidepressants
>
> - There is limited evidence of the benefit of switching within or between classes
> - Switching between antidepressants can increase the risk of toxicity, particularly if:
>   - the original drug has a long half-life (e.g. fluoxetine);
>   - the original drug is known to inhibit metabolism of the new agent, e.g. fluoxetine/paroxetine can inhibit clearance pf TCAs;
>   - both agents have serotonergic activity—this will increase the risk of serotonin syndrome;
>   - switching from a non-reversible MAOI, here a 2-week washout period is required before starting a new antidepressant.
> - In all cases caution is required when switching between agents and manufacturers advice should be adhered to.

In complex depression, other treatment options include antipsychotic therapy (e.g. **olanzapine**, **risperidone**, **quetiapine**, **aripiprazole**). In severe depression ECT may be used and can be highly effective pending antidepressant medication delivering its benefit.

Antidepressants do not meet the criteria for being addictive, as there is no need to increase dose to maintain benefit and no primacy of drug-taking over other activities. However, it is recognized that discontinuation reactions may occur if a course of treatment (i.e. continuous taking beyond 8 weeks) is stopped abruptly. Step down the dose over a 4-week period to minimize any discontinuation events.

Drug classes used in management

Almost all currently available treatments for depression aim to restore the compromised neurotransmitter activity of monoaminergic cortico-limbic pathways.

Selective serotonin reuptake inhibitors

> SSRIs selectively inhibit the neuronal transporter for serotonin thus increasing the concentration of the neurotransmitter at the synapse and promoting receptor activation. This starts a cellular and molecular signalling cascade that results in adaptive responses leading to antidepressant action. Examples include citalopram, escitalopram, fluoxetine, fluvoxamine, paroxetine, and sertraline.

Mechanism of action

The acute short-term action of SSRIs is to produce the negative allosteric modulation of the pre-synaptic serotonin transporter, a molecular complex that includes an enzymatic component (energy producing Na^+/K^+ ATP), and separate binding sites for serotonin and SSRIs. Binding of SSRIs to the complex decreases the affinity of the transporter for binding serotonin (negative allosteric modulation), thereby reducing the rate of uptake. As a result, when SSRIs bind to the transporter there is an immediate accumulation of serotonin in the synapse and a subsequent increase in the activation of pre- and post-synaptic serotonin receptors. The presynaptic receptor activation results in inhibition of neuronal firing rates and a subsequent decrease in serotonin release. Thus, during SSRI treatment, there is an initial decrease in serotoninergic neuron firing, which gradually increases in subsequent weeks until it reaches therapeutic levels. This is likely a result of the desensitization of the presynaptic inhibitory receptors, and is one of the molecular explanations for the *delay* in beneficial effects observed in the clinic. However, a role for synaptic remodelling, together with changes in gene expression and neurogenesis has also been postulated.

Citalopram has the highest selectivity for serotonin inhibition over noradrenaline uptake. It also has some affinity for α-adrenoceptors and a small potency at blocking H_1-histamine-receptors. **Paroxetine** is the most potent blocker of serotonin re-uptake, but has a relatively low selectivity as it blocks muscarinic acetylcholine receptors almost as much as the tricyclic antidepressants imipramine and doxepin. Furthermore, is has a very short half-life, which can be problematic on withdrawal. **Sertraline** is the second most potent inhibitor of serotonin re-uptake and the second most selective over noradrenaline. It is the solitary SSRI that can bind to dopamine transporters, but its affinity for the neurotransmitter receptors is low and of no clinical significance. **Fluoxetine** was the first SSRI to become clinically available, and has, through its primary active metabolite **norfluoxetine**, a very long half-life (~7 days).

Prescribing

Of all the antidepressants, SSRIs are the most widely prescribed, with the advantage of being taken OD (except **fluvoxamine**). Doses are started at a therapeutic antidepressant dose and may subsequently be increased after an interval of 2–4 weeks if patients fail to show an adequate response. However, consideration should be given to the flat dose–response curve that SSRIs show in depression (higher doses of SSRIs are indicated in anxiety-related disorders), the potential for drug interactions and the presence of comorbidities.

Where treatment is to be stopped, higher doses require gradual withdrawal; particularly with shorter-acting agents such as **paroxetine**. Conversely, SSRIs with a longer half-life, e.g. **fluoxetine**, are more likely to be problematic with regards to drug interactions when switching between antidepressants.

Unwanted effects

Although generally better tolerated than TCAs, SSRIs still require caution in some patient groups, notably those at risk of seizures or co-existing cardiovascular morbidities. Following initiation, there is often an initial worsening of symptoms, resulting from neurological side effects, i.e. headache, nervousness, agitation, anxiety, insomnia, and fatigue. The risk of suicide and self-harm is increased during this period, when alerting effects can kindle sufficient energy to act on these impulses, necessitating close monitoring. Patients should be advised to seek immediate help if they are experiencing suicidal thoughts. Unlike some antidepressants, however, SSRIs are unlikely to be lethal in overdose.

The risk of seizures is potentially increased with SSRIs, and although this risk is small, treatment should be discontinued if patients demonstrate an increase in seizure frequency. Patients on SSRIs receiving ECT may also experience prolonged seizures.

Cardiovascular toxicity with SSRIs is considerably less than with TCAs and with lower severity, although they may still cause palpitations, flushing, and orthostatic hypotension. **Citalopram** and **escitalopram**, have been associated with prolongation of QT interval and *torsades de pointes*, and are contraindicated in at risk patients. Doses should be reduced in patients over 65 years and those with hepatic dysfunction. Metabolic effects of SSRIs include hyponatraemia and altered glycaemic control. Diabetic patients may require additional monitoring.

GI toxicity with SSRIs is relatively common, e.g. nausea, diarrhoea (particularly **sertraline**), dyspepsia, and GI bleeding, although these effects are likely to reduce with continued treatment. Sexual dysfunction is also widely reported, particularly with **paroxetine**.

Drug interactions

Of the interactions reported with SSRI treatment, the interaction with MAOIs is the most widely documented. Concurrent use of an SSRI with an MAOI significantly increases the risk of serotonin syndrome, which presents as palpitations, hypertension, hypothermia, rigidity, myoclonus, confusion, irritability, and delirium. The onset of symptoms can be rapid and in extreme cases, result in death. Concurrent use of an SSRI with another serotonergic drug including the triptans and **St John's Wort**, also increases the risk of serotonin syndrome. SSRIs may increase the risk of bleeding with anti-platelet (**aspirin**, other NSAIDs) or anti-coagulants (**warfarin**, NOACs).

SSRIs are largely metabolized via the cytochrome P450 enzyme. **Sertraline,** for example, is a mild-moderate inhibitor of CYP 2D6 and a substrate for CYP 3A4; clinically, however, this is only likely to affect **sertraline** levels in the presence of a potent enzyme inhibitor, such as **grapefruit juice**. **Fluoxetine** is a substrate for, and a potent inhibitor of, CYP 2D6; thus there is an increased potential for clinically relevant interactions, particularly on initiation or discontinuation of therapy, e.g. **warfarin** (increased risk of bleeding), **tamoxifen** (reduced activation). **Citalopram** is metabolized by multiple CYP isoenzymes thus minimizing the potential for a clinically significant interaction.

Serotonin noradrenaline reuptake inhibitors

SNRIs can block the uptake of both serotonin and noradrenaline transporters, increasing the availability of these neurotransmitters at the synapse. For example, duloxetine and venlafaxine.

Mechanism of action

In parallel with the serotoninergic system, hypofunction of the noradrenergic neuronal pathways, and of the α_2-adrenergic and β-adrenergic receptors in the frontal and prefrontal cortex, has been closely associated with depression.

Although all SNRIs inhibit serotonin and noradrenaline transporters, they do so with considerable variations in terms of affinity and selectivity. **Venlafaxine** has high affinity for the serotonin transporter, but not the noradrenaline one, and at low concentrations can act as an SSRI. As doses are increased, venlafaxine adopts a true SNRI profile and at maximum BNF dose it additionally adopts some dopamine re-uptake inhibitory properties. **Duloxetine** has a more balanced affinity, with slightly more selectivity for the serotonin transporter. **Milnacipran**, a third agent not licensed in the UK, is the most balanced of the three, and might be marginally more selective for the noradrenaline transporter.

In contrast to most SSRIs, all SNRIs are beneficial in relieving chronic pain associated with and independent of depressive states of mood. This is a significant clinical advantage, considering that pain is increasingly perceived as an integral part of depression. In common with SSRIs, SNRIs are also efficacious in several anxiety disorders.

Prescribing

Venlafaxine is increasingly gaining popularity in more severe disease, resistant to SSRI therapy, where it is likely to be more effective than SSRIs or **duloxetine**. As with SSRIs, doses are started low and may be administered OD if a modified-release preparation is used. Where necessary, doses may be escalated at 2-weekly intervals to optimize response. Dose adjustments are recommended in hepatic and severe renal impairment.

Unwanted effects

The side effect profile and cautions of SNRIs are predictably similar to that of SSRIs, although they tend to occur more frequently with SNRIs and are more likely to lead to discontinuation of therapy. In common with SSRIs, SNRIs are most likely to induce gastrointestinal and neurological side effects; increasing the risk of serotonin syndrome and suicidal ideation on initiation (more pronounced in patients under the age of 25 years).

Cardiovascular toxicity (e.g. arrhythmias), although uncommon, occurs more frequently with SNRIs compared with SSRIs, with risk increased in patients with pre-existing risk factors or in overdose. Hypertension occurs relatively often with treatment and can be so significant as to require treatment cessation. Hyponatraemia is also more common with SNRI therapy, secondary to syndrome of inappropriate anti-diuretic hormone (SIADH), and most likely to affect elderly patients or those who are dehydrated/volume-depleted, e.g. with diuretic use.

Drug interactions

Concomitant use of an SNRIs with a second serotonergic agent increases the risk of serotonin syndrome, e.g. MAOIs/reversible inhibitors of monoamine oxidase A (RIMAs), **lithium**, SSRIs, triptans, and **St John's Wort**. Neurological toxicity is also increased in the presence of alcohol. Other relevant pharmacodynamics interactions include increased risk of bleeding with antiplatelets and anticoagulants.

Metabolism of **venlafaxine** is mediated through the cytochrome P450 enzymes 2D6 and 3A4, to produce active and inactive metabolites, respectively. Drugs known to be potent inhibitors increase levels and the risk of toxicity, e.g. **ketoconazole**, **itraconazole**, **indinavir**, **ritonavir**, **clarithromycin**, and **telithromycin**. In contrast, **duloxetine** metabolized via 1A2 and a moderate inhibitor of 2D6, is less likely to cause clinically significant pharmacokinetic interactions.

Tricyclic anti-depressants

Tricyclic anti-depressants (TCAs) act by inhibiting the re-uptake of serotonin and noradrenaline with varying selectivity, together with dopamine to a lesser degree. Although their efficacy is indisputable, their large list of additional targets can lead to serious secondary effects. Examples include amitriptyline, clomipramine, dosulepin, doxepin, imipramine, lofepramine, and nortriptyline.

Mechanism of action

Despite their useful antidepressant action, due to their monoaminergic effect, which is similar to SNRIs, the ability of TCAs to also block the muscarinic-acetylcholine, α_1-adrenergic, and H_1-histamine receptors, is responsible for the long list of secondary effects (see 'Unwanted efforts') that has reduced their current use. The list of secondary targets also includes Ca^{2+}-activated and voltage-gated K^+ channels, L-type Ca^{2+} channels, and the cardiac and neuronal Na^+ channels.

In addition to their early use as first-line antidepressants, their capacity to regulate the descending serotoninergic and noradrenergic inhibitory pathways originating from the brainstem to the spinal cord, has prompted their use in the treatment of neuropathic pain. Importantly, their anti-neuralgic action is independent of their antidepressant effect and achieved at much lower doses.

In terms of selectivity, **desipramine** is one of the most potent at blocking noradrenaline re-uptake, but is far less potent as a serotonin re-uptake inhibitor. **Amitriptyline**, although a less potent inhibitor of noradrenaline re-uptake than desipramine, acts on both systems with similar efficacy. **Clomipramine** is a potent and fairly selective inhibitor of serotonin re-uptake.

Prescribing

The use of TCAs in the management of depression is largely limited to complex depression, when the newer generation of antidepressants have failed to improve symptoms. Similar efficacies means that choice is largely driven by side effect profile, as some agents are more sedating (**amitriptyline, clomipramine, dosulepin, doxepin**), while others have more profound antimuscarinic effects (**imipramine**). They also vary in their tendency to cause toxicity in overdose. Dosulepin should no longer be initiated in any new patients.

Treatment with TCAs is often initiated at doses lower than that required to achieve a clinical effect and slowly titrated up to an effective dose, to reduce the incidence of adverse effects. Doses can be administered OD and are generally best taken at night due to their sedative effects.

Unwanted effects

The additional inhibitory effects of tricyclic antidepressants on muscarinic and histamine receptors, accounts for their numerous adverse effects. Antimuscarinic (constipation, blurred vision, urinary retention, dry mouth, etc.) and antihistamine (sedation, weight gain) are the most common side effects. These effects tend to subside with time and can be minimized by starting with low doses, although the drop-out rate remains high, with few patients able to achieve therapeutic doses due to toxicity. Compared with other antidepressants, TCAs are associated with the greatest risk in overdose, except for **lofepramine**, further limiting their use.

TCAs should be used cautiously in patients with pathologies that may be aggravated by antimuscarinic activity, such as narrow angle glaucoma, urinary retention or benign prostatic hypertrophy. Effects tend to be more pronounced in the elderly.

Like with SSRIs, the risk of suicide is increased on initiation of treatment, particularly in those with a history of suicidal ideation. This is more pertinent with TCAs, due to their greater potential for severe and even fatal cardiovascular toxicity in overdose, e.g. hypotension, arrhythmias, MI, or heart block; they should therefore not be initiated in patients at high risk of cardiac arrhythmias or post-MI (except **lofepramine**). Again, like other antidepressants, treatment is associated with discontinuation effects following abrupt cessation of treatment, such as irritability and sleep disturbances.

Neurological toxicity, aside from sedation, is common with TCAs, and may include confusion, headache, and less commonly seizures and extrapyramidal side effects. Symptoms may be indicative of hyponatraemia, which is infrequently associated with therapy due to inappropriate secretion of antidiuretic hormone.

Drug interactions

Aside from the potential to interact with other antidepressants (see 'Prescribing warning: switching between antidepressants'), side effects of TCAs are more pronounced in combination with other agents that possess antimuscarinic or antihistamine properties. The risk of cardiovascular toxicity (arrhythmias, hypotension) may be potentiated in combination with antipsychotics, anaesthetics, or anti-arrhythmics.

Clomipramine as a substrate for the cytochrome P450 enzyme system (3A4 and 2C19), has a greater potential to interact with inducers or inhibitors of these enzymes, including **St John's Wort** (a potent enzyme inducer).

Monoamine oxidase inhibitors (MAOIs)

Inhibition of monoamine oxidase, an enzyme that is responsible for the oxidative deamination of endogenous and xenobiotic amines including serotonin, noradrenaline, and adrenaline, allows the accumulation of these neurotransmitters at the nerve terminal. For example, phenelzine, tranylcypromine, and isocarboxazid.

Mechanism of action

There are two isoforms of MAO enzymes, MAO-A, and MAO-B, which vary in terms of substrate preference, inhibitor specificity, and tissue localization. MAO-B preferentially deaminates phenylethylamine and trace amines, while MAO-A mainly affects those monoamines considered important in depression—serotonin and noradrenaline. Adrenaline and dopamine are deaminated by both MAO isoforms.

MAO enzyme inhibition increases the availability of monoamine neurotransmitters at the nerve terminal and thus positively affects the monaminergic axis relevant for the regulation of mood disorders. MAOIs are subdivided between non-selective inhibitors of both MAO isoforms (**phenelzine**,

tranylcypromine), and those selective for either MAO-A (**moclobemide**) or MAO-B (**selegiline**). The MAOIs initially developed for therapy could irreversibly interact with the enzyme, permanently deactivating it; therefore, synthesis of new enzyme is required to restore MAO function. More recently, a new generation of inhibitors were developed with the capacity to detach from the enzyme, allowing normal catabolism to resume (reversible MAOIs).

Through the inhibition of both MAO-A and MAO-B, the classical, non-selective, and irreversible MAOIs inhibit the first-pass metabolism of ingested tyramine, leading to its accumulation and the potential to develop severe hypertension.

Prescribing

Due to their effect on the inhibition of tyramine metabolism, the traditional MAOIs have a high potential for food and drug interactions. They are generally reserved for use when other options have failed. Particular care is required when switching from, or to another anti-depressant (see switching between antidepressants).

All are administered orally and require at least BD dosing due to their short half-life; best taken no later than 16.00 hours (see 'Drug and food interactions').

Unwanted effects

Insomnia is the most widely reported side effect to the MAOIs, followed by movement disorders, such as twitching or myoclonic movements. Besides these, adverse effects are generally comparable with those seen with other antidepressants. Neurological toxicity, such as agitation, can be more pronounced with the MAOIs and they should be avoided in patients with mania or acute confusion, where they can aggravate symptoms.

Drug and food interactions

Of greatest concern with the irreversible non-selective MAOIs, is their inhibitory effect on tyramine metabolism, leading to potentially harmful interactions with some foods (see 'Prescribing warning: food to avoid while on MAOIs') and drugs containing amines that are normally metabolized by the monoamine oxidase enzymes. Raised amine levels can induce a hypertensive crisis that, in severe cases, may be fatal. Due to the risk of profound hypertension, MAOIs are contraindicated in patients with heart failure, cerebrovascular disease, thyrotoxicosis, or phaeochromocytoma.

In terms of drug interactions, MAOIs should not be used in combination with or within 14 days of a second MAOI, TCA, SSRI, or SNRI. Caution is also recommended with other drugs that have selective or weak MAOI activity, e.g. the anti-Parkinson drug **selegiline** (MAOB inhibitor) and **linezolid** an antibiotic with weak MAOI activity.

Similarly, the use of CNS depressants, alcohol, or narcotics is best avoided. Other drugs that may potentiate the effects of MAOIs include antihypertensives, hypoglycaemics, anti-Parkinson drugs, or antimuscarinics. Patients on MAOIs should be advised to inform anyone prescribing for them, that they are on an MAOI with similar caution applied to the use of over the counter or herbal remedies, including **St John's Wort**.

PRESCRIBING WARNING

Foods to avoid while on MAOIs

Patients receiving MAOIs should be advised to consume a diet low in tyramine due to the risk of potentially severe hypertension. Foods that tend to be rich in tyramine are be those that have undergone breakdown by fermentation, smoking, curing, ageing, etc., and include:

- Mature cheeses e.g. blue cheeses, mature cheddar, unpasteurized cheeses, camembert
- Smoked/ cured meats and fish e.g. salami, pepperoni, pickled herring, shrimp paste
- Hung game
- Soy/ fish sauce
- Yeast extract e.g. marmite
- Yoghurt.
- Alcohol, e.g. wines and beers.
- Excessive tea/coffee/chocolate.
- Bean curd/soya bean paste or fermented.
- Sauerkraut.
- Broad (fava) beans (due to dopamine content).
- Protein supplements (check tyramine content).
- Ginseng may increase anxiety and insomnia.

Reversible inhibitors of monoamine oxidase A

The ability of RIMAs to selectively and reversible inhibit MAO-A has significantly improved their safety profile, while still increasing the monoaminergic transmission that is relevant for the amelioration of mood disorders. For example, moclobemide.

Mechanism of action

The selective inhibition of MAO-A by RIMAs leads to the more specific accumulation of those monoamines relevant for the neuronal regulation of mood disorders. The most common, **moclobemide** is a benzamide derivative that does not interact with neurotransmitter receptors, and has no effect on the synthesis, re-uptake, or release of neurotransmitters.

Prescribing

Due to its limited efficacy compared with other antidepressant drugs, **moclobemide** is ideally reserved for use when other options have failed. Doses are administered in divided doses and titrated up to achieve the desired response.

Unwanted effects

The adverse effects seen with the RIMAs are comparable with those seen with MAOIs, albeit to a lesser extent. Neurological toxicity tends to be the most common adverse effect, causing agitation, sleep disturbances, confusion, and headaches, although sedation is unlikely to be a problem with **moclobemide**. Like the MAOIs, moclobemide should not be used in mania or acute confusion, or in those at risk of a hypertensive crisis. RIMAs carry the same medicine management issues around discontinuation and suicidal ideation as other antidepressants, but they are unlikely to cause significant toxicity in overdose. Since RIMAs are displaced from MAO-A in the presence of tyramine, and MAO-B is not inhibited, the risk of developing tyramine-mediated hypertensive crisis is rare, although patients should still avoid consuming excessive amounts of tyramine.

Drug interactions

Interactions with RIMAs tend to be pharmacodynamic in nature, potentiating toxicity when prescribed with drugs, such as other MAOIs and sympathomimetics, or those that increase the risk of serotonin syndrome. **Moclobemide** should therefore not be used in combination with **dextromethorphan**, other MAOIs (including **selegiline**), SSRIs, SNRIs, or **pethidine**. Caution is also recommended in combination with **linezolid** due to its weak MAOI properties.

Noradrenaline specific serotonin agonists

> Noradrenaline specific serotonin agonists (NaSSA) can increase the neurotransmitter release of noradrenaline and serotonin, and thus contribute to the monoaminergic control of depressive states. For example, mirtazapine.

Mechanism of action

The NaSSA **mirtazapine** is a selective antagonist of the α2-adrenergic presynaptic receptors that are involved in the regulation of noradrenaline and serotonin neurotransmitters release. Blockade of α2-adrenoceptors on noradrenergic neurons, prevents the negative effect they have on presynaptic terminal release and causes an increase in noradrenaline release. Moreover, the blockade of α2-adrenoceptors on serotoninergic neurons, also promotes the release of serotonin and subsequent activation of post-synaptic 5-HT$_1$ receptors that are known for their role in the regulation of mood disorders. Because mirtazapine can also potently block 5-HT$_2$ and 5-HT$_3$ receptors, serotoninergic-mediated activation of 5-HT$_1$ receptors is enhanced. Blockade of 5-HT$_2$ receptors might also explain the lower incidence of adverse effects observed with mirtazapine, while antagonism of H$_1$-histamine receptors can contribute to its sedative effects.

Prescribing

After **citalopram** and **venlafaxine**, **mirtazapine** is fast becoming a widely-prescribed antidepressant. Doses are titrated up to an effective dose that is administered OD, ideally at night.

Unwanted effects

Common side effects to **mirtazapine** include increased appetite, weight gain, and sedation, making it a useful option in patients suffering from sleep disturbances and loss of appetite. Sedative effects tend to be transient, resolving after the first few weeks of treatment and are most pronounced with the 30-mg dose. At higher doses (45 mg) the antihistamine effects are counteracted, thus sedation can be less of a problem. It is less suitable in overweight or obese patients, or in those required to drive or operate heavy machinery as part of their work.

In common with many other antidepressants, mirtazapine may expose the risk of suicidal ideation on initiation and carry a risk of serotonin syndrome, hyponatraemia, seizures, and cardiovascular toxicity. It also has the potential to cause a rebound of symptoms if stopped suddenly and is associated with antimuscarinic effects, to which the elderly are particularly susceptible. Specific to mirtazapine is a small risk of bone marrow depression, thus patients are advised to report symptoms such as a sore throat or unexplained bruising or bleeding. Caution is recommended in severe renal or hepatic impairment, where clearance is likely to be impaired.

Drug interactions

Mirtazapine has the potential to induce both pharmacodynamic and pharmacokinetic drug interactions, the latter due to its clearance via the cytochrome P450 enzyme pathway. Mirtazapine should not be used with MAOIs and the risk of serotonin syndrome is increased in combination with other serotoninergics, e.g. SSRIs; that said, mirtazapine is often used in combination therapy.

Although co-administration of mirtazapine with potent enzyme inducers or inhibitors may alter serum levels, this is unlikely to be of clinical significance, in part since mirtazapine is metabolized by multiple isoenzymes.

Phenylpiperazine anti-depressants

> Phenylpiperazine drugs belong to the class of antidepressants that act as serotonin 5-HT$_{2A-C}$ receptor antagonists and serotonin re-uptake inhibitors (SARIs). This dual action may overcome some of the tolerability issues associated with second-generation antidepressants. For example, trazadone and nefazodone.

Mechanism of action

This is the first class of antidepressants capable of serotonin transporter inhibition, combined with antagonism at the 5-HT$_2$ subtype of serotonin receptors. Since the 5-HT$_{2A-C}$ receptors are thought to be responsible for the adverse effects linked to SSRIs and SNRIs therapy, 5-HT$_{2A-C}$ receptor antagonism can improve drug tolerability, while the increased serotonin levels observed after serotonin uptake blockade can still activate 5-HT$_{1A}$-mediated serotoninergic transmission.

Trazadone also exerts antagonistic properties on α1 and α2-adrenoceptors and H$_1$- histamine receptors, while possessing minimal anti-cholinergic actions. **Nefazodone** antagonizes α1-adrenergic receptors, while its affinity for α2-adrenergic, histaminic, benzodiazepine, dopaminergic, and cholinergic receptors is not significant.

Prescribing

Of the phenylpiperazine antidepressants, only **trazodone** is widely available, **nefazodone** being largely discontinued due to the risk of hepatic toxicity. Despite showing a favourable side effect profile compared with TCAs, toxicity is likely to be greater than with SSRIs; thus **trazodone** is infrequently used. Doses are started low and titrated up, divided into multiple daily dosing with the larger dose given at bedtime. Trazodone is sometimes used in lower doses for its anxiolytic properties, particularly in older adults. Priapism is occasionally problematic due to its alpha-blocking properties.

Unwanted effects

Trazodone demonstrates a side effect profile comparable with other antidepressants. As a second-generation antidepressant, it is thought to be less toxic than TCAs, particularly in terms of cardiac toxicity, toxicity in overdose, and antimuscarinic effects. However, it still is known to cause arrhythmias and heart block, and thus should be used cautiously in patients with a cardiac history and avoided following an MI.

Like **nefazodone**, trazodone is associated, albeit rarely, with severe hepatic toxicity. It is therefore advisable to monitor liver function and avoid in severe hepatic impairment. Other more common effects tend to be GI or neurological.

Drug interactions

Trazodone is part metabolized via CYP3A4 and, as such, has the potential to be affected by potent inducers (e.g. **carbamazepine**) and inhibitors of this enzyme (e.g. **ritonavir**, **saquinavir**, **erythromycin**, and **clarithromycin**).

In terms of pharmacodynamics interactions, the risk of serotonin syndrome is increased in combination with TCAs, MAOIs, SSRIs, and SNRIs. Care is recommended when co-prescribing with other drugs known to cause QT prolongation or sedation (including alcohol).

Noradrenaline re-uptake inhibitors

This drug class can increase extracellular levels of noradrenaline by selectively blocking its re-uptake, without affecting the serotoninergic system. For example, reboxetine.

Mechanism of action

The role of noradrenaline in the regulation of mood disorders is less prominent than that of serotonin. However, a defective regulation of noradrenergic neurons has been found in various areas of the brain linked with depression (cortex, thalamic-hypothalamic areas, and limbic system). **Reboxetine**, the main selective noradrenaline reuptake inhibitor used in the clinic, does not inhibit serotonin or dopamine re-uptake, and has only weak affinity for α-adrenergic, histamine H_1, and muscarinic-cholinergic receptors.

Prescribing

The efficacy of **reboxetine** as an antidepressant is considered inferior to other options, with some studies showing it to be little better than placebo. Oral doses are started small and titrated up to achieve a response.

Unwanted effects

Reboxetine is better tolerated than TCAs, showing a side effect profile more comparable with SSRIs. It is therefore less likely to be toxic in overdose or cause sexual dysfunction. Despite this, it is commonly associated with insomnia, agitation, tachycardia, postural hypotension, dizziness, and headaches. Reboxetine has antimuscarinic properties, thus causing dry mouth, blurred vision, constipation, and urinary retention, and should be used cautiously in at-risk patients, e.g. those with narrow angle glaucoma, benign prostatic hypertrophy, or the elderly, where dose reductions are recommended.

Like **trazodone**, **reboxetine** is a substrate of CYP3A4 and, therefore, prone to the effects of potent inducers or inhibitors of this enzyme (see 'Phenylpiperazine anti-depressants, Trazodone, Drug interactions'). Interactions of clinical significance with **reboxetine** are, however, rare.

Lithium

The alkali metal lithium is prescribed as lithium 'salts' and has a long history in the management of bipolar disorder, where it acts as a mood stabilizer, and in complex depression, where it can augment existing antidepressant medications.

Mechanism of action

Despite its long clinical history, the precise mechanisms by which it exerts its effects are not entirely known. It has been reported that chronic lithium use can enhance electro-physiological and behavioural responses mediated by $5-HT_{1A}$ receptors, most likely through an increase in serotonin release. This effect is postulated to occur at various levels, including serotonin synthesis and turnover, but also through the regulation of second messenger systems, neurotrophic signalling and gene expression.

Prescribing

Lithium is a drug with a narrow therapeutic index that requires careful monitoring to ensure levels are kept within the therapeutic range. Levels outside of this range are associated with inefficacy or toxicity. It is generally used in the management of treatment-resistant depression combined with a first-line antidepressant, or in bipolar disorder to help stabilize mood swings, with doses titrated to achieve a plasma level between 0.4 and 1 mmol/L. However, this can lead to marked differences in doses between patients. As bioavailability varies between products, lithium should be prescribed by brand name, and care taken if switching from lithium carbonate tablets to liquid formulations. Due to the poor water solubility of lithium carbonate, lithium citrate is used in liquid preparations. For clinical purposes, 520 mg lithium citrate can be considered equivalent to 200 mg lithium carbonate.

Unwanted effects

At therapeutic doses, side effects to **lithium** are generally mild and self-limiting, i.e. nausea, vertigo, thirst, polyuria, and fine tremors. Side effects to lithium become more pronounced with high plasma levels, so that levels over 1.5 mmol/L are considered toxic and above 3.0 mmol/L probably require dialysis treatments. Intermediate toxic levels may be managed by flushing lithium from the body using **mannitol** and ensuring the patient is well hydrated. Patients should be advised to report any symptoms of overdose (see prescribing warning).

As lithium can substitute for sodium or potassium at a cellular level, it can be transported intracellularly, leading to accumulation and significant toxicity, particularly in overdose. Toxicity predominantly affects the heart, muscles, thyroid, nervous system, and kidneys. The risk of toxicity is increased in the elderly, and in patients with fluid or electrolyte, e.g. secondary to prolonged vomiting or diarrhoea.

Treatment is contraindicated in the presence of pre-existing co-morbidities that may be potentiated by toxicity, i.e. cardiac disease, hypothyroidism, renal impairment, Addison's disease, or hyponatraemia. Prior to starting therapy, patients require baseline assessment of renal, cardiac, and thyroid function, and these repeated initially 3-monthly then 6–12-monthly during treatment. In addition, lithium levels should be checked 5 days after a dose change, once steady state has been reached. Lithium can reduce the output of thyroid hormone so that some patients present with a goitre that can be easily corrected with levothyroxine. Often any reduction in thyroid activity, however, should be picked up by blood tests before the patient notices any discomfort. The NPSA lithium resource pack should be made available to all patients prescribed lithium. Weight gain is a significant side effect of lithium therapy.

PRESCRIBING WARNING

Symptoms of lithium levels being too high

- *Mild*: nausea, diarrhoea, muscle weakness, fine resting tremor, polyuria, drowsiness.
- *Moderate*: myoclonic twitches/jerks, increased deep tendon reflexes, increased confusion/restlessness, slurred speech, urinary/faecal incontinence, hypernatraemia (related to drug-induced diabetes insipidus).
- *Severe*: coma, convulsions, arrhythmias, heart block, renal failure.

PRESCRIBING WARNING

Avoiding lithium toxicity in clinical practice— the 3 Ds of lithium toxicity

- Lithium levels may become unintentionally high for one of three reasons:
  - *Dehydration*: extreme fluid loss (e.g. vomiting, fever, diarrhoea) should prompt stopping lithium until patient is clinically better.
  - *Diet*: extreme changes to salt intake, particularly the exclusion of salt from the diet can promote lithium retention to compensate for salt loss.
  - *Drugs*: some medications, both prescribed, e.g. bendroflumethiazide, or available over the counter, e.g. ibuprofen, should be avoided as they can inhibit lithium clearance. Patients should be advised to consult the pharmacist before purchasing any over the counter medication.
- To reduce the risk:
  - Patients should be counselled on the above risks.
  - Monitoring is recommended initially every 3 months and then 6-monthly after a year if levels are stable and there are no confounding co-morbidities.

Drug interactions

Lithium is renally excreted in much the same way as sodium. Therefore, factors that affect sodium excretion or re-uptake, will impact similarly on lithium, affecting serum levels. Small alterations in clearance can result in changes in serum levels that causes therapeutic failure or toxicity. Drugs known to inhibit lithium excretion include NSAIDs, thiazide diuretics, ACE inhibitors, ARBs, **metronidazole**, and drugs that affect electrolyte balance, such as corticosteroids. Other drugs can enhance excretion, such as xanthines, some diuretics and sodium bicarbonate.

Pharmacodynamic interactions can also occur with lithium, in particular, more pronounced neurotoxicity in combination with antipsychotics and other serotonergic agents. As lithium has the potential to lower the seizure threshold, concomitant use with other drugs, such as other antidepressants or antipsychotics with the same potential should be done with caution.

Agomelatine

> Structurally related to melatonin, agomelatine is a melatonergic agonist with significant affinity to MT_1 and MT_2 receptors and which also antagonizes $5\text{-}HT_{2C}$ and $5\text{-}HT_{2B}$ receptors.

Mechanism of action

At least in part, the desynchronization of various bodily rhythms has been suggested to contribute to depression. The pineal gland hormone melatonin has been shown to regulate the sleep–wake cycle and this has promoted the development of therapeutic agents capable of stimulating the melatonergic receptors in the suprachiasmatic nucleus of the anterior hypothalamus.

Agomelatine is one such agent, which acts as an agonist on MT_1 and MT_2 receptors, as well as antagonizing $5\text{-}HT_{2C}$ and $5\text{-}HT_{2B}$ receptors. The specific role of MT_1 and MT_2 melatonergic receptors in the antidepressant actions of agomelatine was tested in experimental models of depression, where concomitant administration of a MT_1 and MT_2 receptor antagonist inhibited the antidepressant effect of both melatonin and agomelatine.

Prescribing

Agomelatine is indicated for use in severe depression where it has shown good efficacy and is usually well tolerated. Doses are generally started low and doubled after two weeks where response is insufficient.

Unwanted effects

Overall, side effects to **agomelatine** occur little more frequently than with placebo, the most commonly reported being nausea and dizziness, which tend to be transient.

Agomelatine does however have the potential to cause hepatic toxicity, most commonly causing deranged LFTs and, more rarely, hepatitis or hepatic failure. It is therefore recommended that LFTs are carried out prior to initiation, and rechecked at 3, 6, 12, and 24 weeks, to coincide with the period of greatest risk. Patients with pre-existing hepatic impairment or raised transaminases more than three times the upper limit of normal, should not receive agomelatine and, in those at risk of developing liver disease, caution is advised. Once metabolized in the liver, the metabolites of agomelatine are primarily renally excreted and can therefore accumulate in renal impairment.

Drug interactions

Agomelatine is a substrate primarily for CYP1A2, and to a lesser extent CYP2C19 and CYP2C9. Potent inhibitors of CYP1A2 such a **fluvoxamine** and **ciprofloxacin** should not be used in combination with agomelatine. Smoking and **rifampicin** will decrease agomelatine levels, and might reduce efficacy. As the risk of interactions with other antidepressants is negligible, treatment can be overlapped, making switching to/from agomelatine easier.

Vortioxetine

> The mechanism of action of vortioxetine is thought to be related to its direct modulation of serotonergic receptor activity and inhibition of the serotonin (5-HT) transporter

Mechanism of action

Non-clinical data indicate that vortioxetine is a $5\text{-}HT_3$, $5\text{-}HT_7$, and $5\text{-}HT_{1D}$ receptor antagonist, $5\text{-}HT_{1B}$ receptor partial agonist, $5\text{-}HT_{1A}$ receptor agonist, and inhibitor of the 5-HT transporter. This leads to modulation of neurotransmission in several systems, including predominantly serotonin, but probably also noradrenaline, dopamine, histamine, acetylcholine, GABA, and glutamate systems.

Prescribing

Vortioxetine is indicated for the treatment of major depressive episodes in adults. The more complex serotonergic pharmacology is thought to provide vortioxetine with improved cognitive outcomes following remission of the depression. NICE has approved this antidepressant as a third-line treatment option.

While lithium may be added to augment effect, vortioxetine should not be used alongside any MAOIs, including MAO-A inhibitor **moclobemide**. Vortioxetine can be stopped abruptly without the need for a gradual reduction in dose.

Unwanted effects

Common side effects include nausea, GI upset, and dizziness. There is little direct effect on reaction time and only at higher doses is sexual dysfunction identified.

Drug interactions

Vortioxetine is extensively metabolized in the liver, primarily through oxidation catalysed by CYP2D6 and, to a minor extent, CYP3A4/5 and CYP2C9, and subsequent glucuronic acid conjugation. Depending on the individual patient's response, a lower dose of vortioxetine may be considered if a strong CYP2D6 inhibitor (e.g. **bupropion**, **quinidine**, **fluoxetine**, **paroxetine**) is added to treatment. A dose increase of vortioxetine may be considered if a broad cytochrome P450 inducer (e.g. **rifampicin**, **carbamazepine**, **phenytoin**) is introduced.

Further reading

Duman RS (2014) Pathophysiology of depression and innovative treatments: remodeling glutamatergic synaptic connections. *Dialogues in Clinical Neurosciences* 16(1), 11–27.

Goldberg D (2006) The aetiology of depression. *Psychological Medicine* 36, 1341–7.

Jacobsen, J, Medvedev, IO, Caron MG (2012). The 5-HT deficiency theory of depression: perspectives from a naturalistic 5-HT deficiency model, the tryptophan hydroxylase 2Arg439His knockin mouse. *Philosophical Transactions of the Royal Society London B Biological Sciences* 367(1601), 2444–59.

Lorenzetti V, Allen NB, Fornito A, et al. (2009) Structural brain abnormalities in major depressive disorder: a selective review of recent MRI studies. *Journal of Affective Disorders* 117(1–2), 1–17.

Manji HK, Quiroz JA, Sporn J, et al. (2003) Enhancing neuronal plasticity and cellular resilience to develop novel, improved therapeutics for difficult-to-treat depression. *Biological Psychiatry* 53(8), 707–42.

McPherson S, Armstrong D (2012) General practitioner management of depression: (2012) Aa systematic review. *Qualitative Health Research* 22(8), 1150–1159.

Srinivasan V, Zakaria R, Othman Z, et al. (2012) Agomelatine in Depressive disorders: its novel mechanisms of action. *Journal of Neuropsychiatry and Clinical Neurosciences* 24(3), 290–308.

Taylor C, Fricker AD, Devi LA, et al. (2005) Mechanisms of action of antidepressants: from neurotransmitter systems to signaling pathways. *Cellular Signalling*, 17(5), 549–57.

Taylor D, Paton C, Kapur S (2015) *The Maudsley Prescribing Guidelines in Psychiatry*, 12th edn. Hoboken, NJ: Wiley.

Willner P, Scheel-Kruger J, Belzung C (2013) Neurobiology of depression and antidepressant action. *Neuroscience and Biobehavioral Reviews* 37, 2331–71.

Guidelines

Anderson IM, Ferrier IN, Baldwin RC, et al. (2008) Evidence-based guidelines for treating depressive disorders with antidepressants: a revision of the 2000 British Association for Psychopharmacology guidelines. *Journal of Psychopharmacology* 22(4), 343–96.

Bauer M, Penning A, Severus E, et al. (2013) World federation of societies of biological psychiatry (WFSBP). Guidelines for biological treatment of unipolar depressive disorders, Part 1: update 2013 on the acute and continuation of unipolar depressive disorders. *World Journal of Biological Psychiatry* (14), 334–85.

Cleare A, Pariante CM, Young A (2015) Evidence-based guidelines for treating depressive disorders with antidepressants: a revision of the 2008 British Association for Psychopharmacology guidelines *Journal of Psychopharmacology* 29(5), 459–525.

Gelenberg AJ, Freeman MP, Markowitz JC, et al. (2010) American Psychiatric Association: *Practice Guideline for the Treatment of Patients With Major Depressive Disorder*, 3rd edn.American Psychiatric Association. https://psychiatryonline.org/pb/assets/raw/sitewide/practice_guidelines/guidelines/mdd.pdf [accessed 23 April 2019].

NICE CG90 (2016) Depression in adults: the treatment and management of depression in adults. https://www.nice.org.uk/guidance/cg90 [accessed 11 April 2019].

NICE CG91 (2009) Depression in adults with a chronic physical health problem. https://www.nice.org.uk/guidance/CG91 [accessed 11 April 2019].

NICE TA367 (2015) Vorioxetine for treating major depressive episodes https://www.nice.org.uk/guidance/ta367 [accessed 11 April 2019].

SIGN 114 (2010) Non-pharmaceutical management of depression in adults. https://www.sign.ac.uk/sign-114-non-pharmaceutical-management-of-depression.html [accessed 11 April 2019].

10.3 Schizophrenia and psychosis

Schizophrenia is a disorder of the mind that affects the way someone thinks, feels, and behaves. It is described as a psychotic illness, and is the most common and disabling form of psychoses. The exact incidence of true psychosis is difficult to estimate, but is believed to be in the order of 50 per 100 000, with prevalence higher in some communities, e.g. Afro-Caribbeans and urban dwellers. Schizophrenia has a median incidence of 15 per 100 000 with most patients presenting between the ages of 16–30. However, late onset variant can occur after 40 years and very late onset schizophrenia-like psychosis after 60 years, albeit with slightly different symptoms and a higher incidence in women.

A psychotic episode typically involves hallucinations, delusions, and disruptions in thought, and may be associated with a variety of disorders including schizophrenia, depression, bipolar disorder, puerperal psychosis, schizo-affective disorders, and alcohol withdrawal. A *delusion* is a fixed unshakable belief that is maintained despite being contradicted by reality or rational argument amongst peers of the same community, whereas a *hallucination* is a sensory perception when the usual stimulus is absent (e.g. hearing a voice when nobody is present). Although visual hallucinations are common, hallucinations can involve any of the senses, and can be intrusive and instructive.

A diagnosis of schizophrenia is made in the presence of persisting symptoms as defined for example by ICD-11 (WHO, 2018) in most European countries, or DSM5 in the USA. Symptoms are classified into *positive* or *negative* (see Table 10.4), although a more current approach of describing schizophrenia has started to define five dimensions of symptoms, including the previously described *positive* and *negative*, but also *cognitive, aggressive*, and *affective* symptoms. In most patients, it is a lifelong condition with a higher incidence in men that accounts for almost a quarter of mental health admissions of younger patients.

Pathophysiology

The risk factors for developing schizophrenia stem from a complex interplay of genetic and environmental influences. One of the strongest risk factors is having one (10% chance) or two (50% chance) first-degree relatives with the condition. Furthermore, twin studies show that concordance rates are higher in monozygotic (40–50%) relative to dizygotic (10%) twins. Although there is a strong genetic influence, it is not truly Mendelian in its inheritance, with a number of gene-linkage studies identifying particular genes that can have an influencing role, including neuregulin, dysbindin, and a *COMT* mis-sense mutation. The latter *COMT* gene mutation leads to synthesis of an unstable enzyme that has reduced ability to breakdown the neurotransmitter dopamine (excessive levels of which are associated with acute psychosis), and in the presence of the right environmental triggers, can significantly increase the risk of schizophrenia.

Maternal obstetric complications are thought to influence the risk of developing schizophrenia, such as foetal or perinatal hypoxia, maternal disengagement with the pregnancy (e.g. continuing to smoke or failing to attend appointments due to their own mental state difficulties), or poor socioeconomic status. In childhood, developmental difficulties and delay, along with immigration status and geographic location are considered potential risk factors. Patients with a predisposition to schizophrenia and background-negative symptom patterns (see Table 10.5), are also at higher risk of developing or relapsing to a

Table 10.4 Classification of positive and negative symptoms associated with schizophrenia

	Definition	Response to treatment	Examples
Positive	Unusual behaviours or thoughts that can be an excess of normal function, are normally dramatic and often emphasized. They are typically the reason for bringing a patient to the attention of medical professionals	Major targets of antipsychotic drug treatments	Hallucinations, delusions, disorganization
Negative	Withdrawal or lack of function normally associated with a healthy individual. Symptoms are associated with extended periods of hospitalization and normally determine the degree of social capacity to function and overall prognosis	Available drug treatments have limited capacity to treat	Emotional withdrawal, poor rapport, passivity, apathetic social behaviour, difficulty with abstraction and lack of spontaneity

psychotic period when exposed to significant life events, high emotion, or substance misuse (e.g. cannabis).

Neurotransmitter dysregulation

The different symptoms that have been described for schizophrenia have been linked to dysregulation of neurotransmitters in relatively specific brain areas. Positive symptoms have been associated with malfunctioning mesolimbic circuits, including the nucleus accumbens, which is part of the reward circuits, and whose disruption might explain problems with reward and motivation.

Table 10.5 Symptoms of schizophrenia

Positive symptoms: change in behaviour or thought	Negative symptoms: withdrawal or loss of function
Hallucinations (usually auditory)	Memory loss
Agitation	Loss of concentration
Delusions	Apathy
Confused thoughts	Social withdrawal
Behavioural disturbances	Flat affect/paucity of speech
Catatonia	Blunted emotional response

Each of the remaining symptoms is dependent on the malfunctioning of the prefrontal cortex. Affective and negative symptoms are linked with mesocortical and ventromedial prefrontal cortex, while cognitive symptoms are associated with dorsolateral prefrontal cortex. Aggressive and impulsive conducts are thought to be linked with malfunctioning orbitofrontal cortex and its connections to the amygdala.

Dopamine

Genetic and epidemiological studies over the last 60 years have firmly established the role of the dopaminergic system in schizophrenia. In the early 1970s, several discoveries on the effects of antipsychotic drugs and the observation that amphetamine intake could produce schizophrenia-like symptoms in human volunteers, indicated that the underlying abnormality in the schizophrenic brain was an over-activity of dopaminergic mechanisms. More recent observations have confirmed that at least the more positive symptoms of schizophrenia can be linked with an increase in dopamine's synaptic release, in conjunction with a possible sensitization to the actions of dopamine at D_2 receptors.

Despite this recognition of the role of anti-D_2 mechanism as an antipsychotic target, the link with the phenomenological nature of psychosis has not been fully established. There is, however, a general agreement that dopamine plays a central role in 'reward' and 'reinforcement'. This involves increased dopaminergic firing in limbic regions, which is linked to 'reward prediction' after encountering novel stimuli. Increases in dopamine have also been related to rewarding mechanisms with longer timescales, which mediate the motivational salience of stimuli and their associations. In particular, this refers to how stimuli become attention grabbing and the focus of goal-directed behaviour, leading to reward-learning, which shapes future behaviour.

Serotonin

Changes in serotonin receptor (i.e. reduced $5-HT_{2A}$) expression within the frontal cortex are also seen in schizophrenia and offer an insight as to why some individuals fail to respond to first generation (typical) antipsychotics, whose action primarily targets dopamine blockade. $5-HT_{2A}$ regulates dopamine release in the striatal areas and affects voluntary motor control. In addition to acting as dopaminergic antagonists, second generation (atypical) antipsychotics act as partial agonists on serotonin receptors.

Glutamate/GABA

The role of glutamatergic signalling cannot be ignored in the pathophysiology of schizophrenia when drugs such as **ketamine** or **phencyclidine** (NMDA receptor antagonists) lead to psychotic and schizophreniform symptoms. Furthermore, unlike with other neurotransmitters, inhibition of glutamate also induces negative and cognitive symptoms in addition to psychotic effects. Modulation/dysfunction of NMDA receptors is therefore believed to play a role in schizophrenia and related disorders. In particular, an under-firing of NMDA receptors on inhibitory GABAergic interneurons, results in a paradoxical increase in secondary glutamatergic activity and subsequent increase in dopamine release. Furthermore, glutamate-mediated excitotoxicity may explain the structural neuroanatomical changes seen in schizophrenia.

Negative symptoms may result from subsets of this pathway, that contain further GABAergic interneurons, affecting ventral tegmental area (VTA) ascending pathways, so glutamate neuron over activation leads to greater firing of the second GABA neuron which supresses the final mesolimbic DA output. Certain genes (e.g. *GRIN1*) can contribute to NMDA receptor dysfunction so hyposensitivity of the receptor results, and depending on where in the neural circuit these lie, can lead to predomination of positive or negative symptom profiles. To this end, D-serine, glycine, and sarcosine, which modulate NMDA receptors, have been shown to confer therapeutic benefit, especially with respect to negative symptoms.

For a full summary of the relevant pathways and drug targets, see Figure 10.4.

Management

Although schizophrenia may be first suspected in primary care, a formal diagnosis requires specialist referral. Symptoms (Table 10.5), and the pattern in which they present, can vary markedly between individuals, although there is typically an initial prodromal phase characterized by mild psychotic-like symptoms, associated with symptoms of anxiety/altered mood and a gradual deterioration in social functioning. This prodromal period tends to develop insidiously over a period of days to years, interspersed with transient periods of psychotic symptoms that often resolve spontaneously.

A clinical history should identify symptoms (positive and negative) and any possible precipitating/risk factors, such as substance misuse and current medication. Any pre-existing medical conditions, e.g. epilepsy, stroke, and family history, should also be identified to exclude differential diagnoses and establish the presence of any contraindications to pharmacological therapy. Diagnosis in most European countries is based on the International Classification of Diseases-10 (ICD-10) criteria (see Box 10.1).

Antipsychotics (previously described as 'major tranquillizers' or 'neuroleptics') form the mainstay of pharmacological treatment in schizophrenia, and are selected according to patient choice and suitability. Doses are titrated up every 2 weeks within BNF limits to an effective, tolerated level. In patients that fail to respond after 4–6 weeks at optimum dose, a switch to an alternative agent from a different class may be necessary. Physical health care monitoring is also important in the management of the patient, both prior to starting and while on treatment, with routine testing essential (see Table 10.6). These may be carried out in primary care.

In some emergency situations, where patients present a risk to themselves or others due to overwhelming symptoms, they may require 'rapid tranquilization' with a benzodiazepine, such as **lorazepam**, an antipsychotic, or a combination of the two, ideally administered orally. Most hospital trusts have their own rapid tranquillization policy or protocol.

Patients with treatment refractory disease (failure of two different antipsychotics from two different classes, of which one should be a second generation antipsychotic), should be offered treatment with **clozapine**. Some patients may not want to take this agent due to the high burden of side effects, or the need for regular blood testing that is mandatory with this agent, due to the high risk of agranulocytosis (see 'Antipsychotics, Prescribing').

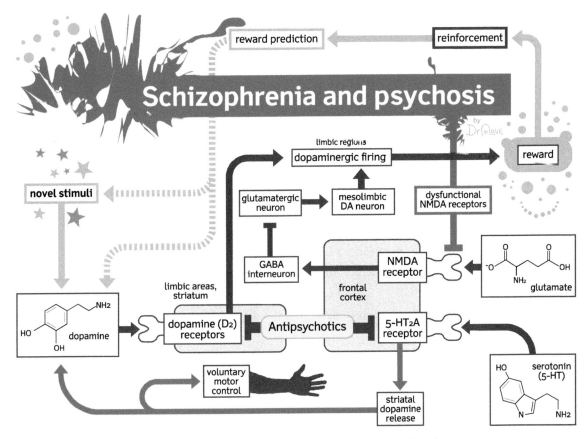

Figure 10.4 Schizophrenia and psychosis: summary of relevant pathways and drug targets.

Box 10.1 ICD-10 criteria for schizophrenia diagnosis

ICD-10: a diagnosis of schizophrenia is made where the following symptoms are present for the majority of time over at least a 1-month period, i.e.

- *One or more of*:
  - hallucinatory voices;
  - thought echo/insertion/broadcasting;
  - delusions of thought/actions/sensations or persistent delusions that are entirely impossible (e.g. adopting religious/political/superhuman identity).
- *Or any two of*:
  - persistent hallucinations of any form with associated delusions;
  - interrupted train of thought;
  - catatonia;
  - negative symptoms;
  - significant change in personal behaviour, e.g. self-care.

The evidence for combination therapy with two or more antipsychotics, however, is limited, and NICE only advocate it being done for an acute period, for example, when switching between agents. Some patients may require additional treatment with an antidepressant or sedative, depending on symptoms. Where adherence is an issue, depot injections provide a useful option.

Pharmacological therapy is used in combination with psychological (e.g. cognitive behavioural therapy) and psychosocial interventions, adjusted to patient's symptoms, ideally involving family members to optimize support and help prevent harm. Once the patient is in remission, consideration may be given to withdrawing antipsychotics gradually, although the risk of relapse within 2 years of a first episode is high and a second episode is likely to be more damaging and take longer to recover from. Close attention should therefore be paid to prognostic indicators and treatment only withdrawn under specialist advice. Only around 10–20% patients who recover after a first episode are able to successfully come off

Table 10.6 Recommended monitoring with antipsychotics

Test	Frequency
Weight	Baseline, frequently for 3 months then 12-monthly unless rapid weight gain
Blood glucose	Baseline, at 4–6 months then every 12 months (every 4–6 months with clozapine and olanzapine)
Serum prolactin	Baseline at 6 months then every 12 months
Serum lipids	3 months after starting treatment then every 12 months
BP	Baseline and frequently with dose changes
ECG	Baseline, after dose changes then every 12 months for high risk drugs, i.e. haloperidol, pimozide, and sertindole or in high risk patients
U&Es	Baseline then every 12 months
LFTs	Baseline then every 12 months
FBC	Baseline then every 12 months, except clozapine which is done weekly for first 18 weeks, 2-weekly for next 18 weeks then 4-weekly (secondary care only)
CRP	Baseline then only if malignant neuroleptic syndrome considered

medication. In relapse, choice of antipsychotics will be influenced by previous effective therapy and patient choice.

Drug classes used in management

Since the introduction of **chlorpromazine** in the 1950s, many other antipsychotic drugs have been developed and brought to the market. The blockade of dopaminergic transmission achieved with antipsychotics suppresses much of the positive symptomology that the patient experiences. This property does not automatically erase the specific mechanistic background of a delusional content, but may allow the patient with support of psychological interventions to revisit some of their beliefs and experiences. D_2 transmission blockade, however, can also diminish motivation and drive, which can explain the description by many patients of antipsychotics as 'dysphorics', and contribute to poor adherence.

Although the block of dopamine neurotransmission happens within hours of starting treatment, it has long been claimed that antipsychotic response can be delayed by 2–3 weeks, also known as the 'paradox of delayed onset'. More recent observations, however, seem to reject this theory, indicating that antipsychotic effects are evident within the first 24 hours to 1 week of treatment. It should

also be noted that many antipsychotics require titration to an effective dose, which at the outset is uncertain and can take time. There are no robust target therapeutic levels in place for antipsychotics, although **clozapine** has some markers for optimum outcomes.

Antipsychotics

The common characteristic of all antipsychotics is the blockade of dopamine D2 receptors, albeit most drugs have different binding affinity and dissociation constants. These properties, together with potential differences in the interaction with other receptor systems are behind most of the distinctions observed in antipsychotic therapy.

Mechanism of action

The antipsychotic effects for most drugs can be correlated with dopamine receptor occupancy, which can also predict the appearance of extrapyramidal side effects. As shown by PET and SPECT, conventional antipsychotics require a striatal D_2 receptor occupancy of 65–70% for antipsychotic efficacy, while surpassing 80% levels increases the risk of extrapyramidal symptoms. Therapeutic doses of antipsychotics seem to produce equally high levels of D_2 blockade in limbic areas and the striatum. While the effect in limbic areas is associated with the antipsychotic properties, blockade of dopamine receptors in the nigrostriatal pathways, which controls motor function, is responsible for developing extrapyramidal side effects (EPS).

The term first- and second-generation antipsychotics was used in the last decades to classify the drug classes used in the treatment of psychosis. However, more recent findings have established that, although antipsychotic drugs differ in their antagonist potency and adverse effect profiles, there is no defined atypical characteristic that separates first- from second-generation drugs. For this reason, we are not separating the mechanistic analysis of drug actions on those parameters, but providing a more general view of the receptor interactions that are relevant for antipsychotic treatment and reduced extrapyramidal symptoms.

The separation of dosage between antipsychotic effects and the ability to induce EPS has been a driver behind the development of novel antipsychotic drugs. As such, although high receptor occupancy is normally required for antipsychotic effects, some drugs (such as **clozapine** and **quetiapine**) manage to have therapeutic benefits at far lower levels of receptor occupancy. This may be the result of a stronger affinity for other dopaminergic subtypes (e.g. D_3) present in brain limbic and cortical regions linked with schizophrenia. Also, a relative low affinity for D_2 receptors and faster dissociation rates can be correlated with therapeutic efficacy.

In addition to the binding properties on dopaminergic receptors, antipsychotic drugs can also have varied effects on other neurotransmitter systems (Table 10.7). As such, antagonism of muscarinic receptors can be linked to the amelioration of EPS, although the often non-selective muscarinic receptor antagonism can also lead to cognitive side effects. Partial agonistic activity at 5-HT_{1A} serotoninergic receptors (e.g. clozapine) can offset cognitive and negative symptoms, while also potentiating the antipsychotic activity and counteracting the development of EPS. The blockade of 5-HT_{2A} has also been proposed to contribute towards the amelioration of the negative symptoms of schizophrenia, and upregulation of nigrostriatal dopamine function might decrease the liability of EPS. Some studies have proposed the concept of $D_2/5\text{-HT}_2$ receptor antagonism as an essential pharmacological effect underlying atypicality in antipsychotic action.

The development of schizophrenia-like symptoms after administration of non-competitive antagonists of the NMDA subtype of glutamate receptors, led to the hypothesis that hypofunction of this glutamatergic subtype can contribute to the pathophysiology of the disease. Some anti-psychotic drugs (clozapine, **olanzapine**), but not others (**haloperidol**), can attenuate NMDA antagonist-induced deficits in preclinical paradigms, raising the possibility that therapeutic efficacy might be, at least in part, associated with counteracting NMDA receptor hypofunction.

Prescribing

Although second-generation antipsychotics (SGAs) were previously recommended for use in preference to first-generation antipsychotics (FGAs), it is now widely accepted that as a whole they show comparable efficacy and tolerability, so are considered as a single heterogeneous group. Selection is therefore based on individual drug properties (see Table 10.8). Choice is directed by patient factors and ideally agreed in a shared decision model with the patient. Consideration should be given to side effect profiles, pre-existing co-morbidities, and adherence. Long-acting injections (depots), form part of the choice agenda and should not be seen as the formulation that represents a circumstance of legally imposed medication in a patient who would not otherwise agree to treatment.

Some of the FGAs are also used for other indications, such as anti-emetics, analgesics (neuropathic pain), and anxiolytics. In these circumstances, doses tend to be lower than those used to treat psychotic disorders.

Unwanted effects

The risk of toxicity with antipsychotics is high and requires consideration when prescribing for an individual. In comatose patients, and in those with CNS depression or phaeochromocytoma, antipsychotic use is contraindicated. Particular care is necessary in older patients who are more susceptible to adverse effects and is therefore reserved for use in severe disease at reduced doses. Side effects are wide-ranging and summarized in Table 10.9.

Extrapyramidal side effects

EPS occur as a result of dopamine blockade, and thus are more commonly observed with the higher potency FGAs (e.g. **haloperidol**, **pimozide**, **flupentixol**, **zuclopenthixol**, and the piperazine phenothiazines) and infrequently with SGAs or low-potency FGAs (e.g. aliphatic phenothiazines). Types of reactions can be divided into four sub-groups:

- *Parkinsonian-like*: symptoms such as tremor, rigidity, monotone voice, reduced facial expression, and hypersalivation, as seen in Parkinson's disease. These may be managed by reducing the dose, switching therapy, or using an antimuscarinic, e.g. **procyclidine**.

Table 10.7 Summary of receptor interactions of anti-psychotics relevant for therapeutic action

Antipsychotic	Receptor interaction
Amisulpride	Selective D_2-like antagonism
Aripiprazole	D_2 partial agonism; $5\text{-}HT_{1A}$ partial agonism; $5\text{-}HT_2$ antagonism
Clozapine	Low D_2 antagonism; $5\text{-}HT_2$, muscarinic and α_2 antagonism; $5\text{-}HT_{1A}$ partial agonism
Lurasidone	D_2 partial agonism; $5\text{-}HT_{1A}$ partial agonism; antagonism of $5\text{-}HT_{2A}$, $5\text{-}HT_7$ and α_2; no muscarinic effects
Olanzapine	D_2, $5\text{-}HT_2$, selective muscarinic antagonism
Quetiapine	Low D_2 antagonism; $5\text{-}HT_{2A}$ and α_2 antagonism, weak $5\text{-}HT_{1A}$ partial agonism
Risperidone	D_2, $5\text{-}HT_{2A}$, α_2 and α_1 antagonism (minimal M1 activity)
Ziprasidone	D_2, $5\text{-}HT_2$ antagonism, $5\text{-}HT_{1A}$ partial agonism, weak $5\text{-}HT$, NA uptake inhibition
Haloperidol	High D2 antagonism; 5-HT1A agonism, low affinity for histamine and muscarinic receptors

Adapted from Reynolds G.P. (2004) Receptor mechanisms in the treatment of schizophrenia. *Journal of Psychopharmacology*, 18:3 340-345. Copyright © 2004, © SAGE Publications. https://doi.org/10.1177/026988110401800303.

Table 10.8 Summary of anti-psychotics in clinical use

Pharmacological class	Examples	Route of administration	Comments
Phenothiazines Grp 1 (aliphatic)	Chlorpromazine Levomepromazine Promazine	PO, IM, PR PO, SC PO	Of these, only chlorpromazine tends to be used for psychosis and even this infrequently except in developing countries due to high risk of side effects. Chlorpromazine also used for intractable hiccups. Levomepromazine more commonly used as anti-emetic or in palliation for agitation and sickness. Evidence for efficacy of promazine is lacking
Phenothiazines Grp 2 (piperidine)	Pericyazine Pipotiazine	PO IM depot	Thioridazine has been largely withdrawn world-wide due to cardiovascular toxicity. Pipotiazine recently discontinued
Phenothiazines Grp 3 (piperazine)	Fluphenazine Perphenazine Prochlorperazine Trifluoperazine	IM depot PO PO, IM PO	Although marginally less sedating than other phenothiazines, still infrequently used. Prochlorperazine more commonly used at low doses as an anti-emetic
Thioxanthenes	Flupentixol Zuclopenthixol acetate Zuclopenthixol deconate	PO, IM depot IM IM depot	Largely used in their depot formulations

Table 10.8 Continued

Pharmacological class	Examples	Route of administration	Comments
Butyrophenones	Benperidol Haloperidol	PO PO, IM, IM depot	Haloperidol is still widely prescribed, including short-term use in delirium. Droperidol returned to the market for anti-emetic use only. Concerns over QT prolongation led to its original removal from the market where it was used in rapid tranquillization. ECG should be carried out on initiation and monitored while on long-term haloperidol. Benperidol historically used to suppress sexual deviancy
Diphenylbutylpipiridines	Pimozide	PO	Rarely used, relatively high risk of sudden death associated with QT interval prolongation thus routine ECG monitoring essential
Substituted benzamides	Sulpiride	PO	Most 'atypical' of the 'typicals'. Renally excreted, consider dose adjusting in renal impairment
Second generation anti-psychotics	Amisulpride Aripiprazole Asenapine Clozapine Lurasidone Olanzapine Paliperidone Quetiapine Risperidone Sertindole Ziprasidone	PO PO SL PO PO PO, IM depot PO, IM depot PO PO, IM depot PO PO	Chemically related to sulpiride, but more lipid soluble. Low metabolic burden. Partial agonist at D_2 receptors. Licensed only in management of mania. Note sub-lingual route. Treatment refractory use only. Has anti-violence and anti-suicide effects. Akathisia and somnolence are most common side effects. Of the remaining atypicals, risperidone, olanzapine, and quetiapine are the most widely prescribed first line in the treatment of schizophrenia. Conversely, clozapine is not licensed for first-line use, but widely acknowledged as the most effective agent in treatment refractory schizophrenia. The use of sertindole and ziprasidone are reserved for second-line use due to the greater risk of cardiac toxicity and sudden death. Neither are UK licensed

- *Dystonia*: abnormal movement due to uncontrolled muscle spasm, including oculogyric crisis. In acute/severe cases, patients will require treatment with parenteral antimuscarinic and subsequently switch to an agent less likely to induce EPS.
- *Akathisia*: intense restlessness that may be confused with agitation. Patients can be managed with dose reductions or changes in therapy. For some patients, the addition of a low-dose β-blocker, e.g. **propranolol**, may be of benefit.
- *Tardive dyskinesia*: develops in the longer term, and manifests as involuntary and repetitive movements, usually of the tongue or lips, but may also affect other parts of the body. In about half of cases it is irreversible, even

Table 10.9 Summary of unwanted effects and relevant SPCs

	Sedation	Hypotension	Anti-cholinergic effects	EPS	Raised prolactin	Weight gain	QT interval prolongation
First generation antipsychotics (FGAs)							
Phenothiazines							
Group 1 aliphatic	+++	+++	++	++	++	++	++
Group 2 piperidines	++	++	++	++	++	++	++
Group 3 phenothiazines	++	++	++	+++	++	++/+	++
Thioxanthines	+	+	+	+++	+++	+	+
Butyrophenones	+	+	+	+++	+++	+	+
Diphenylbutylpipiridines	+	+	+	+++	+++	+	+
Substituted benzamides	+	+	+	+	+++	+	+
Second generation antipsychotics (SGAs)							
Amisulpride	+	0	0	+	+++	+	+
Aripiprazole	0	+	0	+	0	+	0
Asenapine	+	0/+	0/+	0/+	+	+	0/+
Clozapine	+++	++	++	0	0	+++	+
Lurasidone	+	0/+	0/+	0/+	+	0/+	+
Olanzapine	++	+	0/+	+	+	+++	+
Paliperidone	+	++	+	+	++	++	+
Quetiapine	++	++	0	+	+	++	+
Risperidone	+	++	+	+	++	++	+
Sertindole	+	+	0	+	+	++	+++
Ziprasidone	+	0	0/+	+	0	+	++

Data from: Hasan A, Falkai P, Wobrock T et al (2012) World Federation of Societies of Biological Psychiatry (WFSBP) Guidelines for Biological Treatment of Schizophrenia, Part 1: Update 2012 on the acute treatment of schizophrenia and the management of treatment resistance, The World Journal of Biological Psychiatry, 13 318–378; Taylor D, Paton C, Kapur S (2015) *The Maudsley Prescribing Guidelines in Psychiatry 12th Edition*

when therapy is discontinued. Anticholinergics should not be administered, as these will make the situation worse. **Tetrabenazine** may be helpful in some patients.

The risk of side effects is largely dose related, and aside from tardive dyskinesia, tend to occur within the first few weeks of initiation or dose change.

Neuroleptic malignant syndrome

This is a rare, but potentially fatal consequence of antipsychotic agents, associated with D_2 receptor blockade. It is estimated to affect between 0.02 and 0.2% of patients treated with antipsychotics, although the mortality rate in untreated patients can be as high as 20%. Onset may be acute or insidious, and the course fluctuating. It is predominately associated with the older, typical agents, but has also been reported with some of the newer antipsychotics. High dose, combination therapy, co-morbidities (see Box 10.2), and the use of depot formulations are believed to increase the risk of NMS developing. NMS is essentially a diagnosis of exclusion, although five classic domains of symptoms suggestive of NMS include:

Box 10.2 Risk factors of developing neuroleptic malignant syndrome

- Organic brain disease
- Dementia
- Parkinson's disease
- Hyperthyroidism
- Alcoholism
- Agitation
- Recent exercise
- Dehydration
- A history of catatonia

- Altered mental state including confusion.
- Autonomic dysfunction with fluctuating BP and tachycardia; excessive sweating, incontinence.
- Muscle rigidity and/or tremor.
- Pyrexia with temperatures as high as 41°C.
- Biochemical markers of raised creatinine phosphokinase (CPK) and white cells.

Treatment
Treatment includes withdrawing the antipsychotic immediately and applying general supportive measures in a medical ward environment. Patients will probably require rehydration and short-acting benzodiazepines may be administered to manage agitation. **Dantrolene** is an effective agent for reducing high body temperature, while dopamine agonists such as **bromocriptine**, **levodopa**, or **apomorphine** can help manage some of the other syndromal effects. **Propranolol** may be helpful in managing tachycardia unless otherwise contraindicated.

The *reintroduction of antipsychotic therapy* following NMS is considered to be an acceptable risk for most patients. A period of 5–14 days should elapse between recovery from NMS and any re-introduction—the success of which is unlikely to be compromised by age or gender. Most patients are unlikely to want the original antipsychotic restarted (although challenge has been shown to be without incident) and many practitioners prefer structurally dissimilar agents at low dose. Depot preparations should be avoided and agents with less potent D_2 receptor blockade at therapeutic doses are recommended.

Metabolic/weight gain

The risk of weight gain and metabolic side effects, such as hyperlipidaemia and DM, is increased both by schizophrenia and the antipsychotics used to treat it. Although all antipsychotics have the potential to cause these effects, the risk is most pronounced with **olanzapine** and **clozapine,** and is possibly linked to inhibition of 5-HT_{2A} and 5-HT_{2C}.

Glucose intolerance can vary in severity from a mild intolerance to diabetic ketoacidosis. In patients with pre-existing diabetes, glucose intolerance is likely to be increased, so consideration should be given to using lower risk drugs, e.g. non-phenothiazine FGAs, **risperidone**, **aripiprazole**, or **amisulpride**. However, effective diabetes management can only be achieved when mental state is at its best. Patients should be advised to report symptoms of hyperglycaemia, such as excessive thirst or polyuria for appropriate follow-up. During treatment patients should have blood glucose and lipids monitored, as well as their weight. Optimizing control is paramount, as weight gain, hyperlipidaemia, diabetes, and schizophrenia are all independent risk factors for increased cardiovascular mortality.

Cardiovascular/hypotension

All antipsychotics have the potential to cause QT prolongation, leading to ventricular arrhythmias and potentially causing sudden death. The risk is increased with higher doses, pre-existing cardiac disease, deranged electrolytes, and for certain antipsychotics (e.g. phenothiazines, **sertindole**, and **ziprasidone**). In all cases, co-prescribing alongside other drugs known to cause QT prolongation is best avoided.

Orthostatic hypotension, secondary to α-blockade is mainly linked to the use of the low potency FGAs (e.g. phenothiazines) and **clozapine**. The risk of orthostatic hypotension is increased in the elderly, which may be managed by dividing doses and applying a more careful dose titration.

Clozapine is also associated with an increased risk of myocarditis, which in some cases can be fatal. The risk is greatest in the first 2 months of treatment, but can occur at any time. Patients should be advised to seek help in the event of persistent tachycardia, palpitations, or chest pain.

Antimuscarinic effects/sedation

Antimuscarinic effects to antipsychotics occur more commonly, but not exclusively, with the phenothiazines and **clozapine**. Effects include urinary retention, constipation, blurred vision, dry mouth, and impaired cognition. Similarly, these drugs are more likely to cause sedation, in part due to their additional antihistamine properties. Sedative effects tend to reduce over time and may be managed by promoting night-time administration, dividing or reducing doses, or failing that switching to a less sedating antipsychotic.

Sexual dysfunction/hyperprolactinaemia

In the tubero infundibular pathway, dopamine antagonism can lead to enhanced secretion of prolactin, which occurs most commonly with antipsychotics that have a higher affinity for D_2 receptors, i.e. all FGAs (particularly high potency), **risperidone** and **paliperidone**. In some cases, this may lead to galactorrhoea and sexual dysfunction in men and women alike. Effects are dose-related and, over time, prolonged exposure has the potential to increase the risk of reduced bone mineral density and possibly even increase the risk of breast cancer. As well as physically affecting sexual function, antipsychotic therapy can impair both libido and arousal.

Haematological

Although all antipsychotics may carry some haematological toxicity, the risk is considerably higher with **clozapine**, which is associated with neutropaenia and agranulocytosis. Consequently, clozapine is always initiated under specialist supervision and a FBC carried out weekly for the first 18 weeks of treatment, reducing to fortnightly for the rest of the first year on treatment. Thereafter 4-weekly blood testing remains in place during ongoing treatment and weekly testing resumed for a period of 6 weeks should a dose be missed for more than 48 hours. Furthermore, after 48 hours of missed doses, treatment will need to be retitrated. All patients on antipsychotics should be advised to report any symptoms suggestive of haematological toxicity, such as unexplained bruising or bleeding, or a sore throat.

Drug interactions

Antipsychotics have a high potential for drug interactions, as a result of both pharmacodynamic and pharmacokinetic interactions. Those of greatest significance include:

Increased risk of ventricular arrhythmias/QT prolongation The risk of QT prolongation may be enhanced in combination with other drugs that prolong QT interval (e.g. anti-arrhythmics, **atomoxetine**, antidepressants) or cause hypokalaemia (e.g. diuretics). The risk is also increased for antipsychotics that are metabolized via the cytochrome P450 enzyme system (e.g. **aripiprazole**, **quetiapine**) when used in combination with enzyme inhibitors such as azole antifungals, macrolides, and antiretrovirals.

Increased risk of CNS toxicity EPS is likely to be enhanced in combination with other drugs known to inhibit dopamine, such as **metoclopramide**, and will be more pronounced with the high potency agents. Caution is recommended when using antipsychotics in combination with drugs that cause sedation or seizures as antipsychotics act to lower the seizure threshold. In patients already on anti-epileptics, their efficacy may be impaired; furthermore, many anti-epileptics are known to impact on cytochrome P450 activity, thus affecting serum levels of antipsychotics metabolized by this pathway.

Hypotension The antihypertensive effects of α-blockers will likely be increased by antipsychotics, in particular the phenothiazines, **clozapine**, **risperidone**, and **quetiapine**.

Dopamine agonists As dopamine antagonists, antipsychotics can reverse the effects of **levodopa** and other drugs used in the treatment of Parkinson's. Managing psychotic symptoms in patients with Parkinson's is best undertaken with quetiapine as it least compromises the treatment goal of increasing dopamine activity in the nigrostriatal tract.

Antimuscarinic effects Antipsychotics with significant antimuscarinic effects (e.g. aliphatic phenothiazines and **olanzapine**) should be used cautiously alongside other drugs that possess antimuscarinic properties, particularly in older patients who are more susceptible to enhanced effects of dry mouth, blurred vision, constipation, and confusion.

Agranulocytosis **Clozapine** should not be routinely used in combination with drugs that cause bone marrow suppression due to the increased risk of agranulocytosis, e.g. cytotoxics, immunosuppressants. This includes avoiding concurrent administration of carbamazepine and phenothiazines. Antipsychotic combinations with clozapine including depot injections are sometimes employed, but this should be carried out under specialist supervision.

Further reading

Caspi A, Moffitt T E, Cannon M, et al. (2005). Moderation of the effect of adolescent-onset cannabis use on adult psychosis by a functional polymorphism in the catechol-O-methyltransferase gene: longitudinal evidence of a gene X environment interaction. *Biological Psychiatry* 57, 1117–27.

Emsley R., Bonginkosi C., Asmal L., et al. (2013) The nature of relapse in schizophrenia. *BMC Psychiatry* 13, 50.

Kapur S., Mizrahi R., Li M (2005) From dopamine to salience to psychosis: linking biology, pharmacology and phenomenology of psychosis. *Schizophrenia Research* 79(1), 59–68.

McDonald C, Bullmore ET. Sham PC, et al. (2004). Association of genetic risks for schizophrenia and bipolar disorder with specific and generic brain structural endophenotypes. *Archives of General Psychiatry*, 61, 974–84.

McGuire P, Jones P, Harvey I, et al. (1994). Cannabis and acute psychosis. *Schizophrenia Research*, 24, 995–1011.

Miyamoto S, Duncan GE, Marx CE, et al. (2005) Treatments for schizophrenia: a critical review of pharmacology and mechanisms of action of antipsychotic drugs. *Molecular Psychiatry*, 10, 79–104.

Muench J, Hamer AM. Adverse effects of antipsychotic medications March 1, 2010 *American Family Physician* 81(5), 617–22.

Pitman E, Nkajuma S, de la Fuente-Sandoval C, et al. (2014) Glutamate-mediated excitotoxicity in schizophrenia: a review. *European Neuropsychopharmacology* 24, 1951–605.

Reynolds GP (2004) Receptor mechanisms in the treatment of schizophrenia. *Journal of Psychopharmacology*, 18, 340–5.

Ross CA, Margolis RL, Reading SA, et al. (2006) Neurobiology of schizophrenia. *Neuron* 52(1), 139–53.

Schwartz TL, Sachdeva S, Stahl SM (2012) Glutamate neurocircuitry: theoretical underpinnings in schizophrenia. *Frontiers in Pharmacology* 3, 195.

WHO (2018) International Classification of Disease, 11th revision. https://icd.who.int/en/ [accessed 23 April 2019].

Guidelines

Hasan A, Falkai P, Wobrock T, et al. (2012) World Federation of Societies of Biological Psychiatry (WFSBP) Guidelines for Biological Treatment of Schizophrenia, Part 1: Update 2012 on the acute treatment of schizophrenia and the management of treatment resistance. *World Journal of Biological Psychiatry* 13, 318–78.

Hasan A, Falkai P, Wobrock T, et al. (2013) World Federation of Societies of Biological Psychiatry (WFSBP) Guidelines for Biological Treatment of Schizophrenia, Part 2: Update 2012 on the long-term treatment of schizophrenia and the management of antipsychotic-induced side effects. *World Journal of Biological Psychiatry* 14, 318–78.

NICE CG178 (2014) Psychosis and schizophrenia in adults: prevention and management. https://www.nice.org.uk/Guidance/CG178 [accessed 11 April 2019].

NICE NG10 (2015) Violence and aggression: short term management in mental health, health and community settings. https://www.nice.org.uk/guidance/ng10 [accessed 11 April 2019].

NICE Pathway (2019) Psychosis and schizophrenia. https://pathways.nice.org.uk/pathways/psychosis-and-schizophrenia [accessed 11 April 2019].

Taylor D, Paton C, Kapur S (2015) *The Maudsley Prescribing Guidelines in Psychiatry*, 12th edn. Oxford: Wiley Blackwell.

10.4 Drug abuse, addiction, and dependence (alcohol, nicotine, opioids)

Addictive disorders, drug dependence, and substance abuse have a major impact on health, society, families, and the economy. *Drug abuse* refers to intentional misuse or over-use of drugs, while being able to maintain behavioural control. The latter, *drug dependency,* implies 'impaired control' in drug use.

Pathophysiology

Drugs of addiction motivate individuals via reward pathways in the CNS (dopaminergic, GABAergic, and glutamatergic). Changes in the dopaminergic system can explain some social aspects of addiction and it is critical in compulsive drug use, as treatment-resistant addicts tend to have lower dopamine function. Early changes in addiction are mediated through dopamine neurotransmission, while long-term repeat exposures and withdrawal are mediated via glutamatergic signalling.

The key pathways involved in reward and addiction are located within the medial forebrain bundle, and include the nucleus accumbens (NAc) and ventral tegmental area (VTA); with ascending dopaminergic projections to the limbic system (amygdala, hippocampus) and prefrontal cortex (PFC).

Cocaine and amphetamines, through actions at the dopamine uptake transporter, reduce removal of DA from the synapse, so reward pathways are stimulated. Likewise, opiates acting through μ, κ, and δ receptors will reduce the tonic inhibition of dopaminergic neurons, so DA levels rise. Repeated stimulation of this pathway can lead to reward reinforcement and upregulation of pathways through synaptic plasticity.

In the case of alcohol, ethanol effects on the CNS are depressive, primarily through enhanced effects of GABA, although wide ranging acute and chronic effects may be seen.

For a full summary of the relevant pathways and drug targets, see Figure 10.5.

Management

Alcohol

Initial assessment can be carried out using the Alcohol Use Disorders Identification Test (AUDIT), for identifying and classifying excessive drinking. Alcohol consumption is classified into hazardous (risk of harmful consequences), harmful (causing harm to physical or mental health), or dependence (consumption associated with a strong desire and loss of control). Patients scoring more than 15 are deemed to have harmful drinking, while a score of 20 or more is indicative of dependence.

Primary management of harmful or hazardous drinking is through advice and goal-setting, with some patients requiring referral to a specialist. Drug therapy for hazardous or harmful drinking is limited to the possible need for

Drug abuse, addiction and dependence

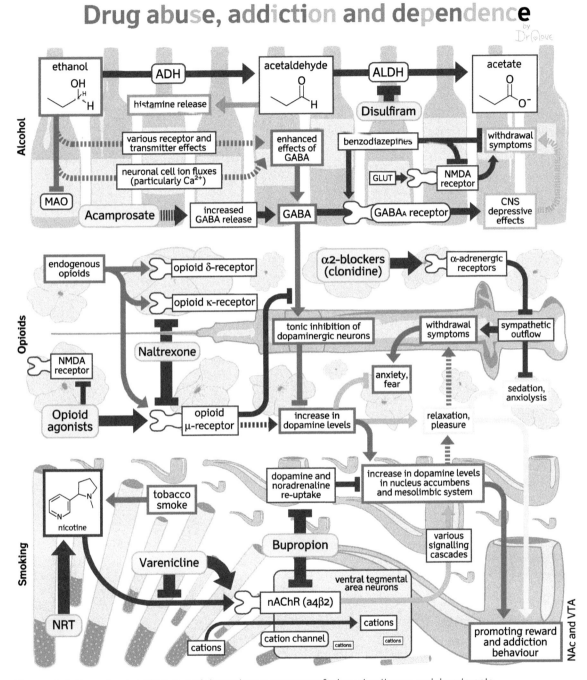

Figure 10.5 Drug abuse, addiction, and dependence: summary of relevant pathways and drug targets.

thiamine and **vitamin B Co Strong** in malnourished patients or those on antidepressant therapy.

In alcohol dependence, specialist intervention is essential to provide support with withdrawal, due to the risk of severe morbidity such as seizures, delirium tremens, and autonomic over-activity. Therapy may also be necessary to treat suspected Wernicke's encephalopathy or other complications of excessive use such as pancreatitis.

Interventions such as **acamprosate**, oral **naltrexone**, **disulfiram**, and, more recently, **nalmefene** may be considered to aid with abstinence.

Assisted withdrawal is usually carried out with a long-acting benzodiazepine; commonly, **chlordiazepoxide** or **diazepam** (for mechanism see Topic 10.1, 'Anxiety'). Those at risk of Wernicke's encephalopathy will also require supplementation of vitamin B, usually as oral **thiamine** plus **vitamin B Co Strong** or, acutely as parenteral vitamin B therapy.

Opioids

Opioid dependence is managed initially in much the same way as alcohol dependence. Pharmacological management should only be carried out under specialist supervision, with an opioid agonist given as maintenance treatment, invariably **methadone**, although **buprenorphine** (or Suboxone®—buprenorphine plus **naloxone**) may also be used. Monitoring should include blood/urine tests to identify continued substance misuse. Reduction should be gradual to reduce the risk of relapse. **Naltrexone** may be useful to prevent relapse.

Smoking

Smoking cessation is predominantly managed in primary care. Those smoking more than 20 a day, or needing a cigarette within 30 minutes of waking, are considered to be heavily dependent smokers and will likely require more intensive intervention. The preferred method of intervention is with referral to a support service.

There are three main pharmacological options for smoking cessation; **nicotine replacement therapy**, **bupropion**, and **varenicline**. In terms of efficacy, there is little to choose between them and patients should be allowed to select their preferred option.

Drug classes used in management

Acamprosate

Acamprosate is a synthetic compound with a chemical structure similar to the neurotransmitter GABA and the neuromodulator taurine, and is thought to stabilize the neurochemical balance that is disrupted during alcohol withdrawal.

Mechanism of action

One of the mechanism of action of **acamprosate** appears to be the capacity to act as a 'partial co-agonist' at the glutamate NMDA receptor. This could modulate the neurochemical effects of a surge in the release of excitatory neurotransmitter like glutamate, which is observed during alcohol withdrawal. Based on the similarities in structure to GABA, acamprosate has been also shown to interact with presynaptic GABA$_B$ receptors, increasing the release of GABA from presynaptic terminals.

Prescribing

Acamprosate can be prescribed to aid with abstinence, as part of a programme involving psychological support. Treatment is administered orally usually for up to 6 months.

Unwanted effects

The most common side effects to treatment with **acamprosate** are GI. Treatment is also thought to have an adverse effect on libido and can cause rashes.

Disulfiram

The anti-alcoholism drug disulfiram is an inhibitor of aldehyde dehydrogenase that is capable of inducing an aversive reaction to the consumption of alcohol. In this way, it can help patients reduce alcohol intake.

Mechanism of action

The high levels of acetaldehyde that accumulate after alcohol ingestion in those patients that have taken disulfiram cause mild/moderate symptoms [flushing of the face, nausea, vertigo, headache, and hypotension (now known as 'disulfiram-ethanol reaction')]. The direct association of these aversive reaction with the consumption of alcohol leads to a psychological deterrent.

Prescribing

Disulfiram is administered orally OD, initiated at least 24 hours after the last alcoholic drink. Doses are typically started high and reduced daily over 4–5 days to a maintenance dose. While on treatment, patients will require adequate monitoring/supervision to ensure efficacy.

Unwanted effects

Common side effects to **disulfiram** tend to be GI or neurological. Psychiatric reactions may also occur with treatment and it is therefore contraindicated in patients with suicidal ideation or at risk of psychosis. In overdose, patients can experience significant cardiovascular effects such as tachycardia and hypotension, which in severe cases can lead to cardiovascular collapse. Higher doses are also associated with hyperglycaemia and hepatic toxicity, thus caution is advised in diabetic patients, or those with hepatic or renal impairment.

Opioid agonists

Methadone and buprenorphine are synthetic opioids that act on the μ-opioid receptor expressed in all brain circuits of addiction, including the mesolimbic dopaminergic neurons projecting to the nucleus accumbens, and is essential for all activities elicited by opioids intake. For example, buprenorphine and methadone.

Mechanism of action

Three types of G protein–coupled receptors (μ, δ, and κ) are activated by endogenous opioid peptides. However, the discovery that the analgesic and addictive properties of **morphine** can be eliminated in mice missing the μ-opioid receptor, showed that this receptor mediates both the therapeutic and adverse activities of opioid compounds. Activation of μ-receptors inhibits GABA-mediated tonic inhibition of dopaminergic neurons in the ventral tegmental area.

The persistent alteration of dopaminergic, opioidergic, and stress responsive pathways observed in opiate addiction, motivates the need for long-term pharmacological treatment approaches through partial activation of μ-receptors (**methadone, buprenorphine**) or blockade (**naloxone, naltrexone**).

Methadone is commonly used as a racemic mixture (levo and dextromethadone), with levomethadone binding to the μ-opioid receptor as a full μ-opioid agonist. Dextromethadone, however, is inactive or weak as an opioid and has antagonist activity at the NMDA subtype of glutamate receptor. Administration of d-methadone has been shown to prevent systemically induced morphine tolerance in mice models and blocks NMDA-induced hyperalgesia. The NMDA blocking activity might be one of the contributing mechanisms by which methadone treatment can decrease opioids cravings and dependency. Although still addictive, the methadone abstinence has less severe symptoms compared with that of **morphine**.

Buprenorphine is a partial agonist on μ-receptors, combining agonistic and antagonistic properties so that the maximal response is below the maximum possible for the system. Buprenorphine is also an antagonist on κ- and δ-opioid receptors, but this is too weak to contribute to treatment effectiveness.

Prescribing

Opioids used for the management of opioid dependency either for withdrawal or maintenance therapy, have a long half-life in order to minimize withdrawal symptoms, without providing the 'high' associated with a rapid onset of action.

Methadone is available in liquid formulations, and it is given on a OD basis. Doses are initiated low (10–30 mg) and gradually increased to a dose at which patients no longer exhibit signs of withdrawal. Patients are then either maintained at this dose (maintenance treatment) or reduced (withdrawal treatment), based on patient and clinician preference.

Buprenorphine is available as sublingual tablets, administered OD. As the receptor affinity properties of buprenorphine might displace high efficacy opiate ligands and induce withdrawal symptoms, the first dose should be given no sooner than 12–24 hours of other agonists. As with methadone, initial doses are gradually increased to the point at which the patient no longer experiences withdrawal effects.

Unwanted effects

As both drugs undergo hepatic metabolism, the effects may be prolonged in hepatic impairment and use should be avoided in severe hepatic impairment. For further information, see Topic 8.3, 'Analgesia and pain management'.

α₂-blockers

The α-adrenergic specific agonists act on the CNS and can decrease sympathetic outflow, promoting sedation and anxiolysis. The systemic effects also include bradycardia and decreased sweating. For example, clonidine and lofexidine.

Mechanism of action

The stimulation of α-adrenoceptors can produce numerous cellular effects mediated by activation of multiple Gi proteins. These include inhibition of adenylyl cyclase, stimulation of phospholipase D and K^+ currents, and inhibition of Ca^{2+} currents. **Clonidine** stimulates all three of the α-adrenergic receptors subtypes with similar potency, and its efficacy is associated with its capacity to counteract the CNS properties of drug withdrawal.

Lofexidine is another $α_2$-adrenoceptor agonist that is believed to have higher affinity for the 2A receptor, resulting in less antihypertensive activity than clonidine, a non-selective $α_2$ agonist.

Prescribing

Clonidine is more commonly used in patients with high opioid requirements, e.g. following an admission to intensive care or in neonatal abstinence; however, it can be used in patients with drug addiction, although **lofexidine** tends to be preferred for this indication. Lofexidine is administered orally in divided doses to a maximum of 0.8 mg TDS, adjusted to mask withdrawal, without inducing excessive toxicity.

Unwanted effects

As an $α_2$-adrenergic agonist, side effects to **clonidine** and **lofexidine** predictably include hypotension, bradycardia, dry mouth, and sedation. For more details, see Topic 2.1, 'Hypertension'.

Naltrexone

Naltrexone is a semi-synthetic competitive μ and κ-opioid receptor antagonist that can prevent the effect of superimposed opiates for approximately 24–48 hours and achieves approximately 95% μ-receptor occupancy after steady-state oral administration.

Mechanism of action

The theoretical basis for the use of a μ-receptor antagonist in the treatment of addiction is the elimination of a response to the use of opiates. In this paradigm, if an antagonist prevents the relief of negative reinforcement following detoxification, then the addictive behaviour of turning to opiates would eventually cease. The lack of intrinsic opiate activity implies that naltrexone poses minimal risk of abuse, thus extended release delivery regimens might be used to improve treatment outcome.

Nalmefene is an antagonist of μ- and δ-opioid receptors, and a partial agonist of the κ-receptor subtype. It has a chemical structure comparable to naltrexone, but has been described to have a number of potential advantages, including more effective binding to central opioid receptors, higher bioavailability, and the absence of a dose-dependent association with liver toxicity.

Prescribing

Naltrexone can be used in opioid- or-alcohol dependent patients following withdrawal, to help maintain abstinence. Treatment should only be initiated once abstinence has been confirmed.

Doses can be administered orally OD (as a single tablet, 50 mg), but may be given as infrequently as three times a week. Treatment should be discontinued where there is evidence of continued substance misuse (see warnings in 'Unwanted effects'). Patients using naltrexone for alcohol dependence should discontinue treatment if drinking continues for 4–6 weeks after treatment has started.

Unwanted effects

As **naltrexone** is extensively metabolized in the liver before being predominantly renally excreted, it is contraindicated in severe renal and hepatic impairment, with care recommended in less severe impairment. LFTs and serum biochemistry should be routinely carried out at baseline.

On initiation, there is a risk of acute withdrawal symptoms, particularly if the patient has not been adequately detoxified; hence, the recommendation to carry out a dose/drug testing before starting treatment. Patients should be warned of the risk of withdrawal symptoms and, where necessary, treatment offered. They should also be warned of the risks in taking high doses of opioids to overcome the 'blockade' effects of naltrexone, as when the effects of naltrexone wear off, these can be fatal. In patients who relapse following naltrexone treatment, sensitivity to opioids may be increased, thus again increasing the risk of overdose.

Common side effects to naltrexone are neurological or GI in nature. Other effects include tachycardia and chest pain.

Nicotine replacement therapy (NRT)

Nicotine replacement therapy (NRT) acts by partially replacing the nicotine that was formally administered through smoking, thus decreasing the severity of withdrawal symptoms and cravings. It also decreases the reinforcing actions of tobacco's nicotine, offering an alternative for the reinforcing and cognitive actions.

Mechanism of action

The main problem with NRT is the inability to replicate the efficient nicotine delivery system provided by cigarette inhalation, thus failing to eliminate all withdrawal symptoms. Despite the drawbacks, all types of NRT can nearly double the chances of long-term abstinence.

E-cigarettes are designed for users to inhale nicotine in the absence of most of the harmful effects of smoking. The delivery of nicotine is achieved by heating and vaporizing a solution that contains nicotine, propylene glycol, and/or glycerine, plus added flavourings. E-cigarettes do not produce tar and carbon monoxide, although some low levels of toxicants have been found in the vapour. Recent reports have indicated that e-cigarette users are more likely to report abstinence than either those who used NRT bought over the counter or no aid.

Prescribing

The numerous available formulations of NRT allows for treatment to be tailored to individual needs, thus improving patient acceptability and adherence.

Unwanted effects

Cautions and side effects to NRT generally mimic those associated with the effects of nicotine obtained through smoking/chewing tobacco, although the overall risks with NRT are less than smoking/chewing. In patients where nicotine is associated with increased risk, such as following an MI or stroke, non-pharmacological methods of smoking cessation are preferred.

Side effects vary with preparations and may, in some cases, be confused with nicotine withdrawal symptoms, i.e. headaches, irritation, sleep disturbances, increased appetite, etc. Short-acting preparations are more likely to cause palpitations, whereas oral preparations tend to cause nausea and vomiting, as well as local irritation to the mouth and gums.

Bupropion

Bupropion is a weak inhibitor of dopamine and noradrenaline re-uptake, which can also antagonize nicotinic acetylcholine receptor function, and thus provides a multitarget approach.

Mechanism of action

Bupropion and its metabolites weakly inhibit dopamine re-uptake, and chronic treatment appears to increase extracellular dopamine in the nucleus accumbens, part of the dopaminergic system primarily implicated in nicotine dependence. This could reduce the dopamine deficit and brain reward function after nicotine withdrawal.

Although the weak inhibition of noradrenaline re-uptake causes only a small increase in extracellular noradrenaline, an observed dose-dependent reduction in the firing rate of noradrenergic neurons could have a significant contribution. Bupropion could also non-competitively antagonize the actions of nicotine at nicotinic acetylcholine receptors, which could attenuate the acute effects of nicotine and thus decrease the reinforcing effects.

Prescribing

Bupropion is administered orally, while the patient is still smoking, and a smoking stop-date set for the second week of treatment. Tablets must be swallowed whole, as crushing or breaking tablets can alter the release profile, increasing the risk of toxicity, including seizures. Doses are started low and doubled to a BD dose after 6 days. Treatment is continued for 7–9 weeks and ideally tapered to reduce the risk of withdrawal on discontinuation.

Unwanted effects

Due to its mechanism of action, the side effect profile to **bupropion** mirrors that of other anti-depressants, in particular neurological toxicity. Some of the most widely reported side effects include insomnia, dry mouth, rash, agitation, and constipation. Toxicity such as headaches and irritability, which are also widely reported, may be accounted for by symptoms of withdrawal. As bupropion can lower the seizure threshold, it should be avoided in patients with underlying risk factors.

Bupropion is contraindicated in severe renal or hepatic impairment. In patients with mild to moderate impairment, doses should be held at the OD dose.

Drug interactions

Although both a substrate and inhibitor of cytochrome P450 enzyme sub-groups, the incidence of clinically significant interactions with **bupropion** is small. It should, however, not be used in combination with MAOIs, and caution is recommended when co-prescribed with other drugs known to lower the seizure threshold.

Varenicline

Varenicline is a partial agonist of the α4β2 subtype of nicotinic acetylcholine receptors that has shown to triple abstinence rates. In addition, the capacity to act as an antagonist can reduce the reward from smoking and can thus be useful in preparation for cessation.

Mechanism of action

The *agonist* effects are hypothesized to reduce nicotine cravings as they can increase the dopaminergic tonus in relevant brain areas, while blocking nicotine's binding to these receptors (*antagonist* effects) can reduce its rewarding/reinforcing actions.

Prescribing

Like with **bupropion**, treatment with **varenicline** is initiated 1–2 weeks before the intended stop date. Doses are administered orally and titrated up over a week to a maintenance dose. Treatment is continued for a 12-week period.

Unwanted effects

Common side effects to **varenicline** include GI disturbances, headaches, and sleep disturbances. Patients should also be advised of the potential/controversial risk of an increase in suicidal ideation and to seek help should they experience this.

Cardiovascular toxicity has been reported with varenicline therapy, in particular hypertension, palpitations, and in some cases MI.

Varenicline is excreted via the kidneys, so dose reductions are recommended in severe renal impairment, as well as those with moderate impairment that fail to tolerate therapy.

Further reading

Bart G (2012) Maintenance medication for opiate addiction, the foundation of recovery. *Journal of Addictive Disorders* 31(3), 207–25.
Koob GF, Volkow ND (2010) Neurocircuitry of addiction. *Neuropsychopharmacology* 35(1), 217–38.
McKeon A, Frye MA, Delanty N (2008) The alcohol withdrawal syndrome. *Journal of Neurology, Neurosurgery and Psychiatry* 79(8), 854–62.
Olive MF (2009) Metabotropic glutamate receptor ligands as potential therapeutics for addiction. *Current Drug Abuse Reviews* 2(1), 83–98.

Guidelines

NICE CG52 (2007) Drug misuse in over 16s: opioid detoxification. https://www.nice.org.uk/guidance/cg52
NICE CG100 (June 2010) Alcohol-use disorders: Diagnosis and clinical management of alcohol-related physical complications. https://www.nice.org.uk/guidance/cg100 [accessed 11 April 2019].
NICE CG115 (2011) Alcohol-use disorders: diagnosis, assessment and management of harmful drinking and alcohol dependence. https://www.nice.org.uk/guidance/cg115?unlid=1275530362015121015426 [accessed 11 April 2019].
NICE Pathways (2014) Acute Alcohol Withdrawal. http://pathways.nice.org.uk/pathways/alcohol-use-disorders [accessed 11 April 2019].
NICE Pathways (2019) Alcohol-use disorders. https://pathways.nice.org.uk/pathways/alcohol-use-disorders [accessed 11 April 2019].
NICE TA114 (2007) Methadone and buprenorphine for the management of opioid dependence. https://www.nice.org.uk/guidance/ta114/chapter/1-guidance
NICE TA115 (2007) Naltrexone for the management of opioid dependence. https://www.nice.org.uk/guidance/ta115
NICE TA325 (Nov 2014) Nalmefene for reducing alcohol consumption in people with alcohol dependence. NICE Technical Appraisal guidance TA325. https://www.nice.org.uk/guidance/ta325 [accessed 11 April 2019].
SIGN 74 (Sept 2003) The management of harmful drinking and alcohol dependence in primary care: A national clinical guideline. http://www.careinspectorate.com/images/documents/3210/SIGN_74_The_management_of_harmful_drinking_and_alcohol_dependence_in_primary_care_-_Amended.pdf
Thomas F, Babor TF, Higgins-Biddle JC, et al. (2001) *AUDIT: The Alcohol Use Disorders Identification Test: Guidelines for Use in Primary Care*. 2nd edn. Geneva: World Health Organisation. https://apps.who.int/iris/handle/10665/67205 [accessed 23 April 2019].
WHO (2009) Guidelines for the Psychosocially Assisted Pharmacological Treatment of Opioid Dependence. Geneva: WHO.

11 Infectious disease

11.1 Bacterial infection

Antibiotics include an extensive range of agents able to kill or prevent reproduction of bacteria in the body, without being overly toxic to the patient. Traditionally derived from living organisms, most are now chemically synthesized and act to disrupt the integrity of the bacterial cell wall, or penetrate the cell and disrupt protein synthesis or nucleic acid replication.

Typically, bacteria are identified according to their appearance under the microscope depending on shape and response to the Gram stain test. Further identification is obtained by growth characteristics on various types of culture media, based on broth or agar, biochemical and immunological profiles. Further testing on broth or agar determines antibiotic sensitivity to guide on antibiotic therapy in individual patients. This process can take 24–48 hours to culture and a further 24–48 hours to measure sensitivities. Increasingly, new technology, e.g. Matrix Assisted Laser Desorption Ionization—Time of Flight (MALDI-TOF) and nucleic acid amplification assays, are being used to provide more rapid identification. The Gram classification, however, is still widely referred to as it differentiates bacteria by the presence or absence of the outer lipid membrane (see Figure 11.1), a fundamental characteristic that influences antibiotic management.

Antibiotic targets

Antimicrobial agents rely on selective action exploiting genetic differences between bacterial and eukaryotic cells. They target bacterial cell wall synthesis, bacterial protein synthesis, microbial DNA or RNA synthesis, by acting on bacterial cell metabolic pathways or by inhibiting the action of a bacterial toxin (see Table 11.1).

Cell wall synthesis

Both Gram-positive and Gram-negative bacteria possess a rigid cell wall able to protect the bacteria from varying osmotic pressures (Figure 11.1). Peptidoglycan gives the cell wall its rigidity and is composed of a glycan chain of complex alternating carbohydrates, N-acetylglucosamide (N-ATG), and N-acetylmurcarinic acid (N-ATM), that are cross-linked by peptide (or glycine) chains. In Gram-positive bacteria, the cell wall contains multiple peptidoglycan layers, interspersed with teichoic acids, whereas Gram-negative bacteria contain only one or two peptidoglycan layers that are surrounded by an outer membrane attached by lipoproteins. The outer membrane contains porins (which regulate transport of substances into and out of the cell), lipopolysaccharides, and outer proteins in a phospholipid bilayer. For both Gram-negative and Gram-positive bacteria, peptidoglycan synthesis involves about 30 bacterial enzymes acting over three stages. Since the cell wall is unique to bacteria, it makes a suitable target for antibiotic therapy.

Protein synthesis

Ribosomes are large molecular complexes that serve as the site for protein translation (synthesis) from messenger RNA (mRNA) templates. They differ between mammalian and bacterial cells in terms of subunits, i.e. bacteria have 50s and 30s subunits, whereas mammalian ribosomes consist of 60s and 40s subunits, this ensures that antibiotics that disrupt protein synthesis are more selective against the bacterial cells. Protein synthesis can be broken down into the following steps:

- *Initiation*: ribosomes attach to the 5' end of the mRNA and the first tRNA attaches at the start codon.
- *Elongation and translocation*: cyclic process in which a new aminoacyl tRNA is placed in the ribosome and transferred to the growing polypeptide chain.
- *Termination*: there are three termination codons that are not recognized by any tRNA. Instead, one of several release factors bind and facilitate the release of the mRNA from the ribosome.

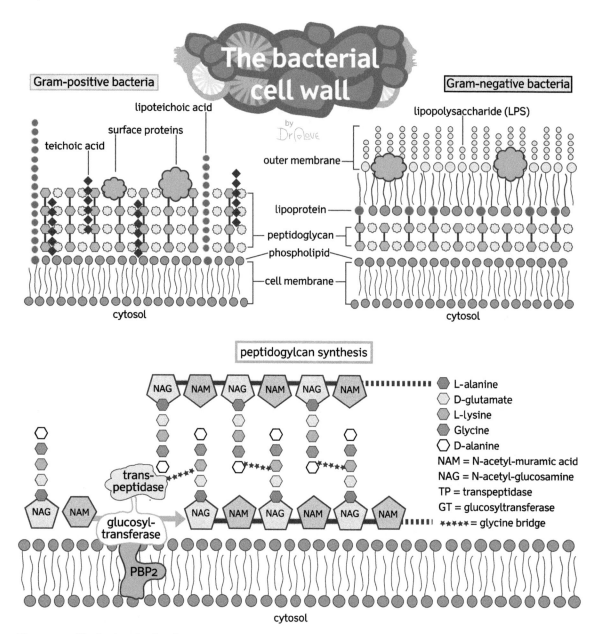

Figure 11.1 The bacterial cell wall.

Nucleic acid synthesis

Nucleic acids (DNA/RNA) are made up of nucleotides consisting of a purine or pyrimidine base, a phosphate group, and a pentose sugar (deoxyribose in the case of DNA and ribose for RNA). These nucleotides are bound together in a biopolymer, which is supercoiled to form a helical structure. Polymerase, gyrase, and topoisomerase enzymes are involved in DNA replication and transcription, and being

sufficiently different between eukaryotic and prokaryotic cells, make good targets for anti-bacterial therapy.

Folate synthesis

Folic acid is essential for the production and maintenance of new cells, and DNA and RNA synthesis, especially during periods of frequent cell division and growth. Bacteria can synthesize folic acid, although humans must obtain it

Table 11.1 Antibiotic classes and their mechanisms of action

Antibiotic class	Summary of mechanism	Examples
Beta-lactams	Inhibit cell wall synthesis	Penicillins, cephalosporins, carbapenems
Tetracyclines	Inhibit protein synthesis	Doxycycline, oxytetracycline
Aminoglycosides	Inhibit protein synthesis	Gentamicin, amikacin, tobramycin
Macrolides	Inhibit bacterial protein synthesis by effecting translocation	Erythromycin, clarithromycin, azithromycin
Glycopeptides	Inhibit cell wall synthesis	Vancomycin, teicoplanin
Lincosamides	Inhibit protein synthesis	Clindamycin
Sulfonamides and trimethoprim	Effects folate synthesis	Trimethoprim, co-trimoxazole
Metronidazole/tinidazole	Inhibits nucleic acid synthesis	Metronidazole, tinidazole
Quinolones	Inhibit DNA gyrase	Ciprofloxacin, moxifloxacin, levofloxacin

through diet. In both cases, enzymatic metabolism leads to the production of folate derivatives, in the form of a series of tetrahydrofolate (THF) compounds. These are substrates in a number of single carbon transfer reactions and are also involved in the synthesis of dTMP (2'-deoxythyminidine-5'phosphate) from dUMP (2'-deoxyuridine-5'phosphate). This is an essential substrate that works with vitamin B12 in the synthesis of DNA, so required by all living cells. All biological functions of folic acid are performed by THF and other derivatives. Antibiotics that interfere with folic acid and THF biosynthesis either inhibit enzymes absent from humans (e.g. sulfonamide inhibition of bacterial dihydropteroate synthase, which is not expressed in eukaryotes) or inhibit bacterial enzymatic pathways with greater affinity (e.g. **trimethoprim** inhibits dihydrofolate reductase essential for THF production).

Bacterial cell cycle

The cell cycle of bacteria is traditionally divided into three stages:

- *B period*: the period between division (cell birth) and the initiation of chromosome.
- *C period*: the period needed for replication.
- *D period*: the phase between the end of replication and completion of division.

Studies of *B. subtilis* and *E. coli* under different growth conditions identified that, at constant temperature, mass doubling time decreases in response to increase in nutrient availability, although the C period and D period remain fundamentally constant. Therefore, under nutrient-rich conditions bacteria can reach growth rates at which the period required for chromosome replication and segregation is greater than the mass doubling time. To overcome this, cells can initiate new rounds of chromosome replication before completing the previous round, so that several rounds of replication happen simultaneously. This process is known as 'multifork replication'.

Antibacterial resistance

Resistance to antimicrobials is becoming increasingly prevalent, with global implications on health care. Resistance can be defined as inherent or acquired, the latter determined by transfer or mutations of genes that code for resistant mechanisms. Resistant genes can be transferred via plasmids (circular molecule of double-stranded DNA that is independent of the chromosome), or transposons (jumping genes), by a number of methods:

- *Conjugation*: plasmid transfer with direct cell to cell contact.
- *Transduction*: bacteriophage (bacterial virus) that replicates in the bacterial cell and incorporates a piece of bacterial DNA into its assembly, this is subsequently transferred when it affects a further bacterial cell.
- *Transformation*: naked DNA taken from the environment.

Resistance to an antimicrobial can develop through several mechanisms:

- Inactivating enzymes, e.g. β-lactamases, carbapenemases.
- Altered drug target, e.g. alterations in penicillin-binding proteins (PBP).
- Increased drug efflux out of cell, e.g. tetracyclines.
- Decreased drug permeability, e.g. loss of porin channels in *Enterobacteriaceae*.

Increasing antibacterial resistance, coupled with the limited supply of new antimicrobials, means some older antibiotics that had fallen out of favour (e.g. **colistimethate sodium**), are now increasingly used. More investment in basic research is required in order to develop newer antibiotics to treat infections caused by resistant organisms, in conjunction with effective antimicrobial stewardship to impede resistance rates (see Figure 11.2). Bacteria that are showing an increase in resistance and are a cause of global concern to human health, include:

- *Staphylococcus aureus* especially meticillin-resistant *Staphylococcus aureus* (MRSA).
- Enterococci especially vancomycin-resistant *Enterococcus faecium* (VRE).
- *Enterobacteriaceae* with extended-spectrum beta-lactamases (ESBL).
- Carbapenemase-producing Enterobacteriaceae (CPE).
- Resistant *Pseudomonas aeruginosa*.

Management of infection

Empirical antimicrobial treatment is initiated following recognition that a patient has an infection or an infection is suspected. Choice is determined by a thorough clinical history and examination, to provide a working diagnosis and is, therefore, the most likely source of infection and possible pathogen (Figure 11.3). Investigations including blood tests, cultures and radiological tests help confirm the likely diagnosis. All cultures of suspected infected sites (i.e. blood, wounds, sputum, urine, CSF and tissue) should be taken prior to initiating empirical antimicrobial treatment.

Antimicrobial stewardship

Antimicrobial stewardship is an approach adopted to help slow the emergence and progression of antimicrobial resistance, through better prescribing and monitoring of treatment. The 'start smart—then focus' has been rolled out in the UK to promote stewardship (see 'Practical prescribing: start smart—then focus').

PRACTICAL PRESCRIBING

Start smart—then focus

Start smart

- Only start antimicrobial therapy where there is clear evidence of infection.
- Take a thorough drug allergy history.
- Initiate prompt effective treatment within an hour of diagnosis (or ASAP) in severe sepsis/life-threatening infections, avoid inappropriate broad-spectrum antibiotic use.
- Follow local antibiotic prescribing guidance.
- Document indication (and severity if appropriate), drug name/dose/route in patients notes and on drug chart.
- Include review/stop dates.
- Obtain cultures before starting treatment where possible, although do not delay treatment.
- Use single dose antibiotics for surgical prophylaxis where they are known to be effective.
- Document precise indication for prophylaxis on drug charts.

Then focus

- Review clinical diagnosis and ongoing need for antibiotics at 48–72 hours, document a clear plan of action in clinical notes and on the drug chart.
- Five antimicrobial stopping options are:
  1. Stop antibiotics if there is no evidence of infection.
  2. Switch antibiotics from intravenous to oral.
  3. Change antibiotics to narrower (ideally) or broader spectrum.
  4. Continue and document next review/stop date.
  5. Outpatient parenteral antibiotic therapy (OPAT).

Adapted from Start Smart - Then Focus Antimicrobial Stewardship Toolkit for English Hospitals. © Crown copyright 2015. Contains public sector information licensed under the Open Government Licence v2.0 (https://www.nationalarchives.gov.uk/doc/open-government-licence/version/2/).

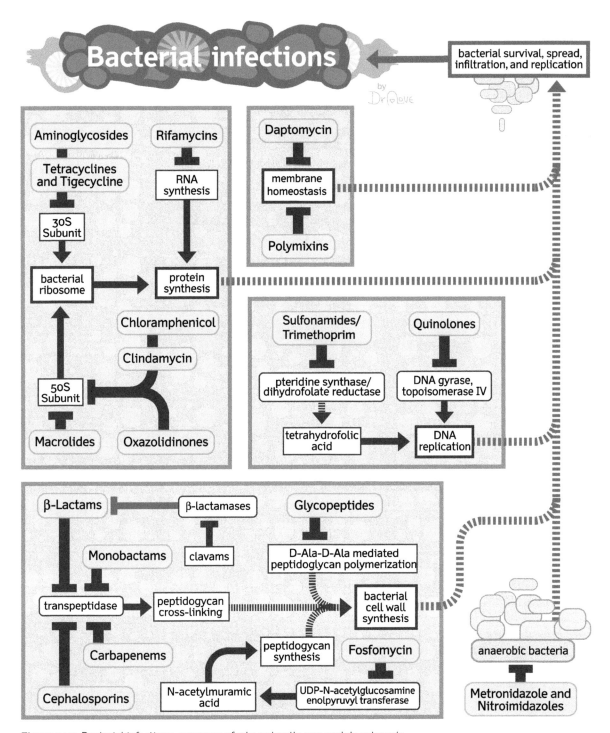

Figure 11.2 Bacterial infections: summary of relevant pathways and drug targets.

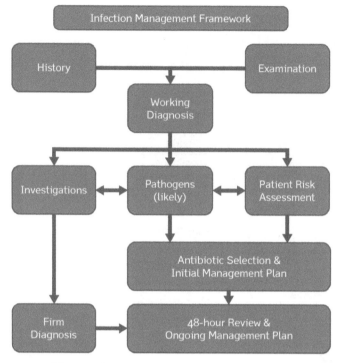

Figure 11.3 Infection management framework.

Sepsis

Sepsis is a systemic inflammatory response to infection, classified according to severity taking into account—patient's mental status, temperature, pulse rate, respiratory rate, BP, urine output, and skin changes (e.g. mottled colour or rash). Any patient with suspected sepsis requires rapid intervention to reduce the risk of mortality (see Box 11.1).

Box 11.1 The sepsis six

- The sepsis six was developed as part of the survive sepsis campaign to reduce mortality, with the aim of saving 1000 lives
- It includes three diagnostic and three therapeutic measures to be initiated within an hour of diagnosis:
  1. Oxygen at high flow
  2. IV fluid bolus
  3. Blood cultures, plus cultures from other possible infection sites, e.g. urine, sputum, wound swabs
  4. Empiric IV antibiotics
  5. Serum lactate and bloods (FBC, U&Es)
  6. Urine output monitoring

This includes administration of empirical antimicrobial treatment commenced within an hour of recognition, as per local treatment guidelines, informed by local epidemiology (Box 11.1).

The empirical antimicrobial chosen needs to be reviewed regularly, taking into consideration the patient's ongoing clinical state and any culture results obtained as per Figure 11.3.

Drugs used in management: inhibition of cell wall synthesis by β-lactams

β-lactams

β-lactams act to inhibit cell wall synthesis and despite being one of the first to be discovered, remain one of the most important antibiotics, especially in streptococcal infections. Examples include penicillins, cephalosporins, carbapenems, and monobactams (see specific sections).

Mechanism of action

β-lactams are a large class of antibacterials that share a common beta-lactam ring within their structure and therefore a common mode of action against bacteria. Within the class, however, there are distinct groups that differ in their spectrum of activity and pharmacokinetic properties.

Although their precise mechanism of action remains unclear, it is widely accepted that β-lactams inhibit bacterial cell wall synthesis, probably through inhibition of transpeptidase (also known as penicillin binding protein—PBP), responsible for cross-linking peptidoglycan chains. Its inhibition prevents the formation of the glycine bridge chain necessary in the formation of a rigid cell wall. With Gram-negative bacteria, β-lactams pass through the porin channels to reach the PBP, whereas in Gram-positive bacteria they can pass directly through the cell wall. Although bactericidal, effective destruction only works when bacteria are actively replicating, so that static or stationary phase bacteria are not killed by β-lactams.

Mechanisms of resistance

The most common resistance mechanism to β-lactams is the secretion of β-lactamases that hydrolyse the β-lactam ring by opening the amide bond. Some agents are designed to overcome this enzyme activity, e.g. the clavulates can bind tightly to β-lactamases to prevent resistance. Over time, however, bacteria can develop additional resistance mutations e.g. over-producing hydrolysing enzymes or increasing the size of the cell wall, thus reducing permeability.

β-lactamase is produced by both Gram-negative and Gram-positive bacteria. Gram-positive bacteria secrete β-lactamases in the extracellular environment, whereas Gram-negative organisms secrete into the periplasmic space, leading to high concentrations adjacent to the PBPs. *St. aureus* has acquired plasmids that produce β-lactamase, leading to innate penicillin resistance.

Further resistance mechanisms include alterations to PBPs or, in Gram-negative bacteria, impaired access to PBPs by altering the porins through which the β-lactams pass. Alteration to PBP sites is the mechanism responsible for resistance to most beta-lactam antibiotics (e.g. MRSA) so newer antibiotics have been designed to overcome this, e.g. **ceftaroline** and **daptomycin**.

β-lactams penicillins

Penicillins are natural or semi-synthetic antibiotics produced by or derived from the fungus Penicillium. Examples include phenoxymethylpenicillin, benzylpenicillin, amoxicillin, co-amoxiclav, flucloxacillin, pipercillin (+ tazobactam), and temocillin.

Mechanism of action

Penicillins contain a 6-aminopenicillanic acid (6-APA) nucleus, composed of a β-lactam ring fused to a 5-membered thiazolidine ring. Although the 6-APA nucleus has little antibacterial activity itself, it is a major structural requirement for the antibacterial activity of penicillins and cleavage at any point in the penicillin nucleus, including the β-lactam ring, results in complete loss of antibacterial activity. Addition of different side chains on the penicillin nucleus, results in derivatives which vary in spectra of activity, stability against hydrolysis by β-lactamases, acid stability, GI absorption, and protein binding.

Penicillins are widely distributed to most body tissues, with potentially therapeutic concentrations generally found in the liver, bile, kidneys, intestines, muscle, and lungs, but low concentrations in bronchial secretions, cartilage, and poorly vascularized areas such as the cornea. Being acidic, concentrations may be significantly reduced in a basic environment, such as prostatic fluid. Only about 10% crosses the blood–brain barrier into the CSF in healthy subjects, although this increases to about 40% when the meninges are inflamed, which is sufficient to kill bacteria. Penicillins are primarily excreted by tubular excretion in the kidneys, but some are lipophilic and excreted by biliary means (e.g. **flucloxacillin**).

Prescribing

Penicillins are widely used to manage numerous infections in primary and secondary care, according to spectrum and probable organisms (Table 11.2). For example, **phenoxymethylpenicillin** has a narrow spectrum, but is effective in tonsillitis caused by *Streptococcus pyogenes* (group A Strep.). However, **co-amoxiclav** has a broader spectrum of activity and is useful where multiple bacterial species may be in the differential diagnosis (e.g. urosepsis), or when anaerobic cover is indicated (e.g. animal bites).

Unwanted effects

The most common side effect to penicillins and most β-lactam antibiotics are hypersensitivity reactions, with approximately 10% of patients believed to have some degree of penicillin hypersensitivity. It is thought to be caused when degradation products of penicillin combine with the host's protein and become antigenic. Reactions range from mild skin rashes and fever, to more severe anaphylactic reactions. Other common side effects include GI effects, in particular diarrhoea and nausea. Where

Table 11.2 General spectrum of activity and pharmacokinetics of penicillins

Drug class	Drug	General spectrum of activity	Pharmacokinetics
Penicillins	Benzylpenicillin (IV) Phenoxymethylpenicillin (oral)	Streptococci, e.g. *Streptococcus pyogenes* (e.g. in tonsillitis, cellulitis, acute otitis media, vaginitis and occasionally bacteraemia associated with sepsis)	Benzylpenicillin Poor oral absorption, unstable in acid environment Phenoxymethylpenicillin (penicillin V) Poor oral absorption, affected by food, avoid in serious infections
	Amoxicillin (oral, IV)	Gram +ve Enterococci Similar to penicillins plus some Gram –ve, e.g. *Haemophilus influenza* *Moraxella catarrhalis* seen in community-acquired pneumonia Sometimes active against *E. coli* but increasing resistance *Salmonella* spp. High IV doses used in infective endocarditis and meningitis especially *Listeria* meningitis	Good oral absorption (~ 90%) unaffected by food Widely distributed in body tissues and fluids
	Flucloxacillin (oral, IV)	Gram +ve Staphylococci (except MRSA). Active against streptococci except enterococci. Skin and soft tissue infection, e.g. cellulitis and wound infection. High IV doses used in deeper staphylococcal infection, e.g. septic arthritis, osteomyelitis, and endocarditis	Oral absorption reduced by food, 95% plasma protein bound Widely distributed in body tissues and fluids
	Co-amoxiclav (amoxicillin + clavulanic acid) (oral, IV)	Gram +ve & Gram –ve. Similar to amoxicillin, less Gram -ve resistance. Anaerobic activity useful in GI infection, e.g. appendicitis	See amoxicillin
	Piperacillin/ Tazobactam (IV)	Gram +ve & Gram –ve (no MRSA cover) Broad spectrum cover, inc. anaerobic bacteria and *Pseudomonas aeruginosa* Empirical treatment in neutropenic sepsis, intra-abdominal sepsis and severe hospital acquired pneumonia in active ESBL or atypical intracellular bacteria	Not absorbed orally Widely distributed in body tissues and fluid
	Temocillin (IV)	Gram –ve only Active against ESBLs especially AmpC producers seen in severe urosepsis Inactive pseudomonas	Not absorbed orally Widely distributed in body tissues and fluid

penicillin absorption is unaffected by food, e.g. **amoxicillin**, GI toxicity may be partially alleviated by taking with food. The broader spectrum penicillins, especially **co-amoxiclav** and **piperacillin-tazobactam**, are associated with an increased risk of *C. difficile* infection so require strict monitoring.

Penicillins are primarily cleared by renal excretion so often dose requires adjustments in renal impairment. Co-administration with drugs that affect renal excretion (e.g. **probenecid**) can lead to increased levels. Similarly, penicillins can increase serum levels of other renally cleared drugs, e.g. **methotrexate**.

β-lactams cephalosporins

Cephalosporins are a group of broad-spectrum β-lactam antibiotics derived from the cephalosporium mould. For example:

- *first generation*: cefalexin, cefadroxil, cefradine;
- *second generation*: cefuroxime, cefaclor;
- *third generation*: ceftriaxone, ceftazidime, cefotaxime, cefixime;
- *fourth generation*: cefepime;
- *fifth generation*: ceftaroline.

Mechanism of action

Cephalosporins have a similar mechanism of action to penicillin, inhibiting bacterial cell wall synthesis. However, the β-lactam ring in cephalosporins fused to a dihydrothiazine ring makes them less susceptible to hydrolysis by β lactamase. The class is subdivided according to chronological order of production, as first, second, third, fourth, and fifth generation, each with a characteristic spectrum of action, successively demonstrating increasing activity against Gram-negative bacteria at the expense of Gram-positive activity (Table 11.3).

- *First generation*: good activity against staphylococci and streptococci, but not enterococci, which are resistant to all cephalosporins (except possibly **ceftaroline** see 'Fourth and fifth generation').
- *Second generation*: greater Gram-negative activity, for example, against *E. coli*, *Klebsiella* spp., and *H. influenza*, with slightly reduced Gram-positive activity. Good CNS penetration, but inferior to third generation cephalosporins which are preferred in meningitis.
- *Third generation*: Gram-positive and Gram-negative activity, with greater Gram-negative activity. Only

ceftazidime has sufficient anti-pseudomonal activity. Good CNS penetration and more stable against β-lactamase, so less prone to resistance.
- *Fourth and fifth generation*: extended activity, with increased beta-lactamase resistance. Fifth generation agents (**ceftaroline**), are effective against MRSA. The only fourth generation **cefepime** is widely available worldwide but not in the UK.

Prescribing

In general, the older agents have greater oral bioavailability, whereas the second and third generation cephalosporins tend to be more acid-labile so more commonly given via the parenteral route (IV, IM). The third generation drugs **ceftriaxone** and **cefotaxime** are widely used as empirical treatment for meningitis, due to their reliable CNS penetration. Ceftriaxone has the added advantage of being administered OD. Like the penicillins, cephalosporins are primarily cleared by renal excretion so may require dose alterations in severe impairment.

First-generation agents are generally used for non-severe infections in mild penicillin allergy e.g. cefalexin in uncomplicated UTI.

Unwanted effects

Cephalosporins are generally well tolerated, oral agents most commonly causing GI upset (diarrhoea, nausea, and vomiting). Due to their relatively broad spectrum of action, cephalosporins are also associated with *C. difficile*. Like the penicillins, there is a risk of hypersensitivity and cross-sensitivity in some patients known to react to penicillins; patients with a previous anaphylactic reaction to penicillin should not therefore be prescribed a cephalosporin.

β-lactams carbapenems

Unlike other β-lactams, carbapenems are relatively resistant to hydrolysis by most β-lactamases, and have a broad spectrum of activity and great potency against Gram-positive and Gram-negative bacteria. For example, ertapenem, imipenem, and meropenem.

Mechanism of action

Imipenem demonstrates a high affinity for PBPs and a bactericidal action similar to other β-lactams, inhibiting bacterial cell wall synthesis. It has a very broad spectrum of activity *in vitro*, against Gram-positive and Gram-negative aerobic and anaerobic organisms, and is stable

Table 11.3 General spectrum of activity and pharmacokinetics of cephalosporins

Drug class	Drug	General spectrum of activity	Pharmacokinetics
Cephalosporins	Cefalexin Cefradine (first generation) (oral)	Gram +ve and some Gram −ve *Staph.*, *Strep.*, coliforms (but increasing resistance)	Good oral absorption, delayed by food Widely distributed in the body, but insufficient CSF levels
	Cefaclor Cefuroxime (second generation) (oral), cefuroxime also IV)	Gram +ve and Gram −ve *Staph.*, *Strep.*, coliforms, *Haemophilus influenzae* (no pseudomonas cover) *Escherichia coli, Klebsiella pneumoniae, Neisseria gonorrhoeae*, and *Proteus mirabilis.*	Cefaclor Good oral absorption Widely distributed in the body Cefuroxime axetil Good oral absorption enhanced by food, rapidly hydrolysed in intestinal mucosa and blood to cefuroxime Widely distributed in the body
	Cefotaxime (third generation) (IV)	Gram +ve and Gram −ve. Bacterial meningitis, cerebral abscess or spinal infections.	Not orally absorbed Active metabolite desacetylcefotaxime has possible additive/synergistic effects against some species About 40% plasma protein bound Widely distributed in body tissues and fluids Good CNS penetration, particularly when meninges are inflamed
	Ceftriaxone (third generation) (IV)	Gram +ve and Gram −ve. Same as cefotaxime	Not orally absorbed 85 to 95% bound to plasma proteins depending on ceftriaxone concentration Non-linear pharmacokinetics Widely distributed in body tissues and fluids Good CNS penetration in inflamed/non-inflamed meninges
	Ceftazidime (third generation) (IV)	Gram −ve and some Gram +ve activity, especially against *Pseudomonas aeruginosa Burkholderia pseudomallei*, and *Enterobacteriaceae*, including *Citrobacter* and *Enterobacter* spp., *E. coli, Klebsiella* spp.	Widely distributed in body tissues and fluids Good CNS penetration in inflamed meninges

to hydrolysis by β-lactamases produced by most bacterial species (Table 11.4). Cilastatin, the enzyme inhibitor combined with imipenem, appears to have no antibacterial activity, but protects imipenem from enzymatic breakdown in the kidney by dehydropeptidase.

Meropenem is slightly more active than imipenem against *Enterobacteriaceae* and slightly less active against Gram-positive organisms. It is unaffected by dehydropeptidase thus not combined with cilastatin. **Ertapenem**, structurally very similar to meropenem, has

Table 11.4 General spectrum of activity and pharmacokinetics of carbapenems

Drug class	Drug	General spectrum of activity	Absorption and distribution
Carbapenems	Imipenem+ cilastatin (IV)	Gram +ve and Gram –ve Staph. (not MRSA)	Widely distributed into body tissue and fluids
	Meropenem (IV)	Gram +ve and Gram –ve Including some enterococci, most anaerobes, and *Pseudomonas aeruginosa*	Widely distributed into body tissues and fluids, including CSF and bile About 2% plasma proteins bound
	Ertapenem (IV)	Gram +ve and Gram –ve Similar to meropenem, but inactive against *Acinetobacter* spp., *Pseudomonas aeruginosa*, and enterococci	Over 90% plasma protein bound Poor CSF penetration

a more limited spectrum of action and no activity against *Pseudomonas aeruginosa*. Its OD IV dosing enables outpatient use when there is no oral alternative.

Prescribing

All carbapenems are administered IV and best reserved for use in severe infections or as second/third line treatment where initial empirical treatment has failed, although increasing resistance is limiting their value (see 'Prescribing warning: carbapenem resistance').

PRESCRIBING WARNING

Carbapenem resistance

- The broad spectrum of activity of carbapenems means they are relied on as last resort treatment. Growing resistance particularly against Gram-negative pathogens, is therefore of global concern.
- Resistance can be intrinsic, e.g. *Stenotrophomonas maltophilia*, or more commonly acquired.
- Acquired resistance involves horizontal gene transfer, e.g. mutations in PBPs seen in Gram-positive bacteria; in Gram-negative bacteria, diminished expression of the outer membrane porin OprD, through which carbapenems enter the periplasmic space in *Ps aeruginosa*.
- Enzyme-mediated resistance is mainly through carbapenemase production, which inactivates carbapenems and other β-lactams. Genes can be transferred horizontally by plasmids or transposons.

Unwanted effects

Carbapenems are generally well tolerated, although hypersensitivity reactions can occur, including cross-sensitivity with penicillins so caution advised with severe penicillin allergy. GI toxicity and deranged LFTs are relatively common. As with other broad-spectrum antibiotics, carbapenems are associated with *C. difficile*.

β-lactams monobactams

Monobactams are monocyclic β-lactam compounds resistant to β-lactamases, used in Gram-negative infections, especially of the meninges, bladder and kidneys. For example, aztreonam.

Mechanism of action

Aztreonam has a similar mechanism of action to penicillins, inhibiting bacterial cell wall synthesis, with a particularly high affinity for the penicillin-binding protein 3 (PBP-3) of Gram-negative bacteria (Table 11.5). Activity is therefore predominantly against Gram-negative bacteria. Structurally it differs from the other β-lactams, possessing only a single ring.

Prescribing

Aztreonam is effective in multiple infections caused by susceptible aerobic Gram-negative bacteria, including UTIs, gonorrhoea, sepsis, meningitis, skin/soft tissues infections, and intra-abdominal infections. As it provides only Gram-negative cover, empirical treatment may

Table 11.5 General spectrum of activity and pharmacokinetics of monobactams

Drug class	Drug	General spectrum of activity	Absorption and distribution
Monobactams	Aztreonam (IV)	Gram –ve only	Poor oral absorption
		Pseudomonas aeruginosa	About 56% plasma protein bound
		Haemophilus influenzae and *Neisseria* spp., including beta-lactamase-producing strains	Widely distributed in body tissues and fluids, including bile
		Active against most Enterobacteriaceae	Poor CSF penetration unless meninges are inflamed

require combination therapy with an antibiotic effective against Gram-positive infections, e.g. glycopeptides.

Unwanted effects

Common side effects include diarrhoea, nausea and vomiting, and rashes; as well as local injection site reactions, e.g. phlebitis. Monobactams are renally cleared so require dose adjustments in moderate to severe renal failure. As with all broad-spectrum antibacterial agents, there is a risk of *C. difficile* with treatment. Due to its distinctly different structure, the risk of cross-sensitivity to other β-lactams is minimal and so can be safely given in known penicillin allergy.

Inhibition of bacterial cell wall synthesis by non β-lactams

Glycopeptides

Glycopeptide antibiotics are large, rigid molecules capable of inhibiting a late stage in bacterial cell wall peptidoglycan synthesis. Useful in the treatment of Gram-positive bacterial infections. For example, teicoplanin and vancomycin.

Mechanism of action

Vancomycin inhibits cell wall synthesis, by inhibiting the formation of the peptidoglycan polymers of the bacterial cell wall, rather than preventing cross-linking as seen with penicillins. It prevents the transfer and addition of the muramylpentapeptides that make up the peptidoglycan molecule, and may also act to damage the cytoplasmic membrane of the protoplast, by inhibiting bacterial RNA synthesis (Table 11.6).

Teicoplanin has a similar mode of action to vancomycin but a significantly longer duration of action.

Prescribing

Vancomycin is administered by slow IV infusion, dosed according to patient's weight, age, and renal function. Due to its narrow therapeutic index serum monitoring is required (see 'Practical prescribing: vancomycin—therapeutic drug monitoring'). Oral vancomycin is generally reserved for localized treatment of *Clostridium difficile*, as oral absorption is unnecessary.

Teicoplanin is administered as a slow bolus injection and although levels are not routinely monitored, it may be required to optimize efficacy in some patients or against resistant organisms.

PRACTICAL PRESCRIBING

Vancomycin—therapeutic drug monitoring

- Vancomycin has a narrow therapeutic index.
- Take trough level after 3–4 doses, when concentrations reach steady state.
- Levels of 5–15 mg/L are necessary for most organisms and 15–20 mg/L in resistant organisms, doses should be adjusted accordingly.
- More frequent monitoring will be required in the elderly or in renal impairment where clearance is impaired.
- Vancomycin clearance is increased in burns patients

Unwanted effects

Vancomycin is associated with significant infusion-related reactions, including red man syndrome (see 'Prescribing warning: red man syndrome'). Hypersensitivity reactions

Table 11.6 General spectrum of activity and pharmacokinetics of glycopeptides

Drug class	Drug	General spectrum of activity	Pharmacokinetics
Glycopeptides	Vancomycin (IV, oral)	Gram +ve *Staph. aureus* Streptococci including *Streptococcus pneumoniae, Str. pyogenes* and other beta-haemolytic streptococci, the viridans *Streptococci* and *Enterococcus faecalis* and most *Ent. faecium*	Poor oral absorption (some in GI inflammation) Given orally for local effect (*C. difficile*) Widely distributed in extracellular fluid, small amounts in bile and lung Poor CSF penetration unless meninges inflamed
	Teicoplanin (IV)	As above	Poor oral absorption

can occur with either drug, including rare cases of Stevens–Johnsons syndrome or toxic epidermal necrolysis; affected patients should not be switched between vancomycin and teicoplanin, as there is risk of cross-sensitivity.

PRESCRIBING WARNING

Red man syndrome

- Red man syndrome is associated with rapid administration of vancomycin, presenting as flushing with or without an erythematous rash over the face, neck, and upper body.
- The risk is reduced by slow administration at a maximum rate of 10mg/minute and can be reversed by slowing or stopping the infusion.
- In extreme cases (e.g. bolus administration) this can lead to profound hypotension, shock, and rarely cardiac arrest.
- The risk of infusion-related reactions is considerably lower with teicoplanin.

Nephrotoxicity is a significant potential side effect of vancomycin, particularly in combination with other nephrotoxic drugs, e.g. aminoglycosides and diuretics, affecting 5–7% of patients. Ototoxicity has been associated with serum drug levels of 80–100 mg/L, but is rarely seen when serum levels are kept at or below 30 mg/L. The risk of toxicity is appreciably increased with high blood concentrations and prolonged therapy, although close monitoring of serum levels significantly reduces the risk of both nephro- and ototoxicity. The risk of ototoxicity and nephrotoxicity is lower with **teicoplanin**, although being renally excreted, dose alterations are required in severe renal impairment.

As oral bioavailability of vancomycin is poor, systemic effects with oral therapy are unlikely; however, absorption may be increased after multiple oral doses, or in patients with inflammatory disorders of the intestinal mucosa being treated for active *C. difficile*.

Fosfomycin

Fosfomycin is a broad-spectrum antibiotic that prevents the formation of *N*-acetylmuramic acid, an essential component of the peptidoglycan bacterial cell wall.

Mechanism of action

Fosfomycin is a phosphoenolpyruvate analogue that acts on proliferating pathogens, by preventing the enzymatic synthesis of the bacterial cell wall (Table 11.7). It inhibits the first stage of intracellular bacterial cell wall synthesis, blocking peptidoglycan synthesis by binding to the enzyme UDP-*N*-acetylglucosamine enolpyruvyl transferase. It is actively transported into the bacterial cell via two different transport systems (sn-glycerol-3-phosphate and hexose-6 transport).

Prescribing

Oral **fosfomycin** is used to treat uncomplicated UTI, either as a single dose of 3 g or as two doses 48–72 hours apart. IV (infusion), however, it is licensed in acute osteomyelitis, complicated UTIs, nosocomial lower respiratory tract infections and bacterial meningitis, typically, where first line treatment has failed due to resistance.

Unwanted effects

Fosfomycin commonly causes injection site phlebitis and mild gastrointestinal disturbances. It is excreted primarily

Table 11.7 General spectrum of activity and pharmacokinetics of fosfomycin

Drug	General spectrum of activity	Pharmacokinetics
Fosfomycin (oral, IV)	*Gram-positive and Gram-negative bacteria*: including *Staphylococcus aureus*, some streptococci, most *Enterobacteriaceae*, *Haemophilus influenzae*, *Neisseria* spp., and some *Pseudomonas aeruginosa* Inactive: *Bacteroides* spp.	Fosfomycin trometamol well absorbed salt of fosfomycin. Excreted unchanged in high concentrations in urine, hence use for UTI.

by the kidneys so requires dose modifications in renal impairment.

Daptomycin

> Although active on the cell wall, daptomycin has a unique mechanism of action that disrupts bacterial membrane potential. It is useful in severe Gram-positive infections.

Mechanism of action

Daptomycin is a naturally occurring cyclic lipopeptide compound, first discovered in the soil bacterium *Streptomyces roseosporus* in the late 1980s, but only approved by the FDA in 2003. It demonstrates concentration-dependant activity against Gram-positive bacteria only, by binding to bacterial membranes of both growing and stationary phase bacterial cells (Table 11.8). Binding and integration into the membranes are dependent on the presence of Ca^{2+}, which causes a conformational change that increases daptomycin's amphiphathicity. Insertion of the lipophilic tail into the membrane leads to rapid membrane depolarization and an efflux of potassium ions. The subsequent loss of membrane potential inhibits

protein, DNA, and RNA synthesis, and results in bacterial cell death.

Prescribing

Daptomycin is used mainly for complicated skin and soft tissue infections, and right-sided endocarditis for its specific action against *Staphylococcus aureus* bacteria. If mixed infections are suspected, it should be co-administered with antibiotics that possess Gram-negative activity.

Unwanted effects

Daptomycin is well tolerated, although patients receiving prolonged courses, higher doses, or with pre-existing renal impairment, are at increased risk of myopathy and rhabdomyolysis. CK should therefore be monitored weekly and treatment discontinued if raised. Patients are advised to report muscle symptoms.

Polymyxins

> Polymyxins bind to bacterial cell membrane phospholipids, thereby altering their permeability to K^+ and Na^+. For example, colisitin sulphate and colistimethate sodium.

Mechanism of action

Colistin is a cationic agent that works by damaging the cell membrane through the displacement of bacterial counter ions in the lipopolysaccharides, which is lethal to the bacteria. There is also evidence that polymyxins can precipitate ribosomes and other cytoplasmic components after entering the cell. Its hydrophobic outer surface makes it more selective for Gram-negative bacteria. Colistin is available in two forms—**colistin sulfate** (cationic) and **colistimethate sodium** (anionic).

Table 11.8 General spectrum of activity and pharmacokinetics of daptomycin

Drug	General spectrum of activity	Pharmacokinetics
Daptomycin (IV)	Gram positive activity only	Good tissue penetration, not lung tissue Minimal penetration into CNS or across placenta

Table 11.9 General spectrum of activity and pharmacokinetics of polymyxin

Drug class	Drug	General spectrum of activity	Pharmacokinetics
Polymyxin	Colistimethate sodium (IV, nebulized)	*Gram negative activity*: especially *E. coli*, *Klebsiella* spp. and *Pseudomonas aeruginosa*. Activity against some *Acinetobacter* spp.	Poor oral absorption Nebulized use in pulmonary infection Predominantly renal clearance

Use of colistin had reduced due to its nephrotoxicity, although being effective against multi-resistant Gram-negative bacilli (Table 11.9), especially carbapenemase-producing organisms, its use has increased again, at lower doses to reduce the risk of nephrotoxicity.

Prescribing

Colistin is indicated against susceptible bacteria following sensitivity testing, but rarely as empirical treatment. **Colistimethate sodium** is mainly used for the treatment of *Pseudomonas aeruginosa* in cystic fibrosis patients and increasingly in bronchiectasis patients colonized with *Pseudomonas*. It can also be used for multiresistant Enterobacteriaceae and multiresistant *Acinetobacter* where sensitivity has been confirmed.

Unwanted effects

The most significant toxicities associated with **colistin** are nephrotoxicity and neurotoxicity, both of which appear to be dose dependant. Treatment at standard doses is usually safe, but ensuring adequate hydration can further reduce the risk of toxicity. Colistin should be used cautiously in combination with other nephrotoxic drugs, e.g. aminoglycosides, glycopeptides, and **furosemide**.

The risk of systemic toxicity with nebulized therapy is reduced, but as it can cause bronchospasm, the first doses should always be given under supervision. The risk of bronchospasm can be reduced by pretreatment with a β-agonist therapy, e.g. **salbutamol**.

Drugs that inhibit protein synthesis

Tetracyclines and tigecycline

Tetracyclines cross the bacterial cell wall and outer membrane to accumulate in the periplasm, where they inhibit protein synthesis. Examples include first generation; oxytetracycline, second generation; doxycycline, lymecycline, minocycline, and third generation; tigecycline.

Mechanism of action

Tetracyclines inhibit protein translation in bacteria by binding to a high affinity site on the 30S ribosomal subunit, thus blocking the access of amino-acyl tRNA molecules to the A site of the ribosome. In this way, it prevents incorporation of amino acid residues into elongating peptide chains.

Tigecycline, a third generation tetracycline and first in class glycylcycline, is an antibacterial structurally similar to the tetracyclines, developed to overcome some resistance problems associated with first- and second-generation tetracyclines.

Prescribing

Tetracyclines although broad-spectrum antibiotics (Table 11.10), are used less frequently due to increased resistance. However, they remain the drug of choice for infections caused by chlamydia, rickettsia, *Coxiella burnettii*, brucella, and the spirochaetes. **Doxycycline**, a long-acting tetracycline derived from **oxytetracycline**, is especially effective in lower respiratory tract infection, being active against *Haemophilius influenza* and *Mycoplasma pneumoniae*.

Tigecycline is reserved for the treatment of complicated skin and soft tissue infections, or complicated abdominal infections caused by resistant organisms. It is not recommended for the treatment of foot infections in diabetics, due to lack of clinical effectiveness against *Pseudomonas aeruginosa*.

Tetracyclines are bacteriostatic so not recommended as treatment for bacteraemia or systemically septic patients. Doses should be taken apart from dairy products or some antacids as the calcium binds to the drug preventing absorption.

Unwanted effects

Most common side effect are GI intolerance and oesophagitis, which is usually dose dependent. Photosensitivity is a class effect for tetracyclines, most commonly seen with **demeclocycline** (more commonly used in SIADH). Tetracycline should be avoided in young children,

Table 11.10 General spectrum of activity and pharmacokinetics of drugs that inhibit protein synthesis

Drug Class	Drug	General spectrum of activity	Pharmacokinetics
Tetracyclines	Doxycycline (oral)	Gram +ve bacteria, (including MRSA), atypical intra-cellular bacteria (e.g. *Mycoplasma* spp.) Resistant against Gram –ve bacteria (except *Haemophilus influenzae)*	Rapid oral absorption, reduced by food (20%) and alcohol Distributes extensively into liver, biliary system, kidneys and digestive tract
	Minocycline (oral)	Similar to doxycycline, slightly more active against streptococci	Absorption unaffected by food, but reduced by milk
	Oxytetracycline/ tetracycline (oral)	Similar spectrum to doxycycline, although infrequently used due to resistance	Moderately well absorbed Absorption reduced by food (50%)
	Tigecycline (IV)	MRSA and VRE, but *Pseudomonas aeruginosa* and many strains of *Proteus* spp. are resistant	Distributed to most tissues, especially bone marrow, salivary glands, thyroid gland, spleen, and kidney
Aminoglycosides	Gentamicin (IV)	Aerobic Gram –ve bacilli (e.g. *Pseudomonas* spp., *Enterobacteriaceae*) some Gram +ve (e.g. S*taph aureus*) Limited activity against streptococci. *Actinomyces* and L*isteria* spp. moderately susceptible *Inactive*: anaerobic bacteria	Wide inter-individual variation in peak concentrations and half-lives, monitoring highly recommended
	Amikacin (IV)	Similar to gentamicin, more active against *Mycobacterium* species	Widely distributed in cerebrospinal fluid, pleural fluid, amniotic fluid and in the peritoneal cavity
	Neomycin (iv)	Similar to amikacin including streptomycin resistant strains of mycobacterium	Similar to gentamicin
	Tobramycin (IV)	Similar to gentamicin	Similar to gentamicin
Macrolides	Erythromycin (oral, IV)	Similar to penicillin. Effective against Gram +ve bacteria and spirochaetes. Less active against Gram –ve except *N. gonorrhoeae*	Rapid oral absorption, but variable affected by erythromycin salt and food
	Azithromycin (oral, IV)	Less active than erythromycin against Gram +ve, more active against Gram –ve organisms (e.g. *H influenza)* and legionella	Rapid oral absorption Long half-life (11–40 hours) Rapid tissue penetration, remains at therapeutic levels for 2–3 days

Table 11.10 Continued

Drug Class	Drug	General spectrum of activity	Pharmacokinetics
	Clarithromycin (oral, IV)	Similar to erythromycin, but twice as active against *H. influenza*, (not recommended for this) *Mycobacterium avium*	Rapid oral absorption, unaffected by food
Clindamycin	Clindamycin (oral, IV)	Good activity against anaerobic and aerobic Gram +ve bacteria, e.g. in osteomyelitis, discitis and maxillo-facial bone infection especially in penicillin allergy	Widely distributed especially in bone and soft tissues
Chloramphenicol	Chloramphenicol (IV, oral, topical—eye)	Active against *Neisseria meningitides, Streptococcus pneumoniae, Haemophilus influenzae* (all implicated in meningitis) *Escherichia coli, Staphylococcus aureus* and *Enterococcus faecium*	Orally absorbed Widely distributed into most tissue, excellent CNS penetration Inactivated in the liver
Oxazolidinone	Linezolid (oral, IV)	Gram +ve, particularly bacteria resistant to conventional treatment, including MRSA and VRE	Rapid oral absorption (~100% bioavailability), possibly delayed by food Good distribution to most tissues apart from bone matrix and white adipose tissue. CSF concentrations variable and lower than serum

pregnancy, and breastfeeding, as they are deposited in growing bones and causes bone staining.

Aminoglycosides

Aminoglycosides inhibit bacterial protein synthesis by binding irreversibly to the 30S ribosomal subunit, causing misreading of the amynoacil t-RNA. Examples include amikacin, gentamicin, kanamycin, neomycin, netilmicin, streptomycin, and tobramycin.

Mechanism of action

Aminoglycosides can be categorized into four main family groups:

1. *Neomycin group*: neomycin.
2. *Kanamycin group*: amikacin, kanamycin, tobramycin.
3. *Gentamicin group*: gentamicin, netilmicin.
4. *Other aminoglycosides*: streptomycin.

Aminoglycosides display concentration-dependant bactericidal activity against most Gram-negative aerobic bacilli and some Gram-positive bacteria, such as *Staphylococcus aureus*, but not against Gram-negative anaerobes (Table 11.10). **Gentamicin** is a mixture of three different, but closely related aminoglycoside sulfate antibiotics (gentamicins C1, C2, and C1a) produced by the growth of *Micromonospora purpurea* and related species. It has broad-spectrum action, with greater antibacterial capacity than **streptomycin, neomycin**, or **kanamycin**. Gentamicin acts to inhibit protein synthesis at the level of the 30s ribosomal subunit, causing the incorrect incorporation of amino acids into the polypeptide chain. It also acts on susceptible bacteria cells, affecting the integrity of the plasma membrane and RNA metabolism.

Prescribing

Aminoglycosides require close monitoring due to their narrow therapeutic index (see 'Practical prescribing: monitoring aminoglycosides'). **Gentamicin** is administered by IV infusion, usually OD.

PRACTICAL PRESCRIBING

Monitoring aminoglycosides

- Aminoglycoside are concentration-dependant antibiotics, requiring high doses for optimal effects.
- Toxic levels, however, are associated with renal and ototoxicity.
- Patients on treatment require monitoring of serum levels, measured at intervals determined by local guidelines.

Unwanted effects

The main side effects to aminoglycosides are ototoxicity and nephrotoxicity, due to tissue accumulation in the ears and kidneys. Ototoxicity manifests as either hearing loss and/or vertigo, secondary to cochlear or vestibular damage, presenting initially as tinnitus, which can be reversible if detected early and the drug stopped. Delays in cessation can lead to irreversible damage and permanent hearing loss. Aminoglycosides vary in their effects on the vestibular and cochlear systems, i.e. **kanamycin**, **amikacin**, and **neomycin** are preferentially cochleotoxic, whereas **gentamicin**, **tobramycin**, **streptomycin**, and **netilmicin** affect both, but are primarily vestibulotoxic. Patients should be advised to report any signs of hearing impairment and treatment avoided in those that are partially-sighted or blind.

Nephrotoxicity with aminoglycosides, of which gentamicin is the most toxic, is dose related and usually reversible if kidney damage is not too severe. Co-administration with other nephrotoxic drugs can potentiate the damage, e.g. **furosemide** and **cisplatin**, whereas adequate hydration reduces the risk.

Macrolides

Macrolides bind reversibly to the 50S ribosomal subunit and inhibit protein synthesis during the translation process. For example, azithromycin, clarithromycin, and erythromycin.

Mechanism of action

Macrolides bind within the nascent peptide exit tunnel near to the peptidyltransferase centre of the 50S subunit of the bacterial ribosome, where polypeptides are assembled from amino acids. This prevents passage of the polypeptide through the tunnel, essential for translation to proceed. Their action may be bactericidal or bacteriostatic, depending on concentration and micro-organism. They are actively concentrated within leukocytes and can therefore be transported to the site of infection.

Prescribing

Macrolides are typically used as an alternative to penicillins for respiratory infections in penicillin allergy and have good activity against atypical bacteria, e.g. *Mycoplasma* spp. Being bacteriostatic, however, they should not be used for life-threatening infections. Macrolides can all be administered orally, or IV, albeit as a long infusion due to the risk of thrombophlebitis. **Azithromycin** has a prolonged elimination half-life (2–4 days) so that 3 days of oral dosing provides the equivalent of 7 days of treatment, thus advantageous where compliance is likely to be poor.

Unwanted effects

The most common side effect of macrolides is GI disturbance, including nausea, vomiting, diarrhoea, and abdominal discomfort, which is usually reduced if taken with food. For some preparations, however, absorption can be affected by food. Due to its gastric motility properties **erythromycin** has been used off-label in the management of gastroparesis.

Macrolides, mainly erythromycin and **clarithromycin**, can also cause QT prolongation, and *torsade's de pointes*, thus care is required in at risk patients and in combination with other drugs known to have this effect.

Drug interactions

Erythromycin and **clarithromycin** are potent inhibitors of CYP 3A4 and can lead to toxic levels of an extensive list of drugs that are metabolized by this pathway, e.g. **simvastatin**, **phenytoin**, **sodium valproate**, **digoxin**, **tacrolimus**, **ciclosporin**, **theophylline**, and the azole antifungals. Patients on these will require close monitoring and possible dose alterations. Those on affected statins, are advised to stop the statin while taking clarithromycin/erythromycin and resume once the course is complete. **Azithromycin** does not interact with cytochrome P450.

Clindamycin

> Clindamycin inhibits protein synthesis by binding to the 50S ribosomal subunit, and although it shares this mechanism with macrolides, it is neither structurally nor chemically related to them.

Mechanism of action

Clindamycin belongs to a class of antibiotics known as the lincosamides, and like the macrolides and **chloramphenicol**, acts to inhibit protein synthesis, mainly by binding to the 50S ribosomal subunit of bacteria. In this way, it interferes with the transpeptidation reaction and inhibits early chain elongation. Impaired protein synthesis alters the surface of the cell wall, thereby decreasing adherence of bacteria to host cells and increasing intracellular killing of organisms. Clindamycin also demonstrates an extended post-antibiotic effect against some bacterial strains, possibly due to persistence of the drug at the 50S binding site (Table 11.10).

The killing activity of clindamycin likely varies with bacterial species and drug concentration; however, it is predominantly bacteriostatic, with bactericidal activity against some strains of streptococci, staphylococci, and anaerobes. Although penicillins are more rapidly bactericidal against *Staphylococcus aureus*, clindamycin inhibits production of staphylococcal and streptococcal toxins, so makes a useful adjunct in staphylococcal and streptococcal toxic shock syndrome.

Prescribing

Clindamycin is primarily used to treat skin and soft tissue infection such as severe cellulitis, dental and bone infections, due to its extensive tissue distribution including bone. It can be used as an alternative to **phenoxymethylpenicillin** or **flucloxacillin** in penicillin-allergic patients. Many strains of MRSA remain susceptible to clindamycin, although with increasing resistance, use should be reserved for confirmed sensitivity. Doses can be administered IV as an infusion, but preferably orally, being well absorbed and the risk of thrombophlebitis with IV therapy high.

Unwanted effects

Clindamycin is associated with a significant risk of *Clostridium difficile* overgrowth and pseudomembranous colitis (see 'Prescribing warning: pseudomembranous colitis with clindamycin'). Other side effects include jaundice and abnormal LFTs, which should be monitored during prolonged treatment. Approximately 10% of patients

taking clindamycin are reported to develop a rash. Drug interactions with clindamycin are infrequent, although it may increase the effects of **suxamethonium** and non-depolarizing muscle relaxants.

> **PRESCRIBING WARNING**
>
> **Pseudomembranous colitis with clindamycin**
> - Clindamycin kills normal GI flora leading to *C. difficile* overgrowth and pseudomembranous colitis, which presents as severe diarrhoea.
> - Patients that develop severe diarrhoea are advised to seek urgent medical advice and treatment stopped.
> - Delays in action can be life-threatening in susceptible patients.

Chloramphenicol

> Chloramphenicol is a broad-spectrum antibiotic that acts to inhibit protein synthesis, without the high risk of causing *C. difficile*.

Mechanism of action

Chloramphenicol, first discovered in 1947, is a bacteriostatic antibiotic that binds to the 50S ribosomal subunit of susceptible species and inhibits the peptidyl transferase enzyme, preventing peptide bond formation.

Prescribing

Chloramphenicol is effective against many bacterial infections, although its use has largely fallen out of favour due to the risk of bone marrow suppression and aplastic anaemia (see 'Prescribing warning: aplastic anaemia and bone marrow suppression with chloramphenicol'). It continues to be used as an eye preparation (ointment, drops), where the risk is significantly lower. More recently, IV chloramphenicol has been used short term in some hospitals, due to its relatively low risk of hospital acquired infections (e.g. *Clostridium difficile*) compared with other newer broad spectrum agents. Furthermore, due to its efficacy against the three main causes of meningitis (*Neisseria meningitides, Streptococcus pneumoniae,* and *Haemophilus influenza*) and its excellent CNS penetration, it is used to treat meningitis in penicillin allergy. Other indications include cholera, typhoid fever, pneumonias, and abdominal infections.

Unwanted effects

In addition to haematological toxicity with **chloramphenicol**, other reported side effects include Grey baby syndrome, hypersensitivity reactions, neurotoxic reactions (headache, mild depression, mental confusion, and delirium), and leukaemia.

> ### PRESCRIBING WARNING
>
> **Aplastic anaemia and bone marrow suppression with chloramphenicol**
> - Aplastic anaemia albeit rare, is a serious and potentially fatal side effect of chloramphenicol.
> - Cumulative doses (>20 g) have a toxic effect on human mitochondria protein synthesis leading to bone marrow suppression, which is usually reversible on cessation.
> - Patients on prolonged treatment will require FBC monitoring and treatment discontinued in the event of a falling count.
> - Avoid concomitant treatment with other drugs that cause bone marrow suppression.

Drug interactions

Chloramphenicol is a potent inhibitor of the cytochrome P450 enzymes in the liver, potentially leading to increased levels of numerous agents, including antidepressants, anti-epileptics, proton pump inhibitors, anticoagulants, CCBs, immunosuppressants, chemotherapy, benzodiazepines, azole antifungals, macrolides, statins, antiarrhythmics, and PDE5 inhibitors. Prescribers should be cautious when co-prescribing with any other medication.

Oxazolidinones

> Oxazolidinones inhibit protein synthesis by binding to the 50S ribosomal subunit of bacteria, and preventing the initiation of protein synthesis. For example, linezolid.

Mechanism of action

Linezolid, is a synthetic antibiotic that acts by binding to a site on the bacterial ribosome (23S of the 50S subunit) to prevent the formation of a functional 70S initiation complex, an essential component of the translation process. Resistance to other protein synthesis inhibitors does not affect linezolid activity, although rare resistance cases linked with 23S ribosomal alterations have been reported. It is mainly effective against aerobic Gram-positive infections, although as a bacteriostatic antibiotic it should not be used first line to treat serious infections.

Prescribing

Linezolid is primarily used in the treatment of infections caused by resistant Gram-positive bacteria (e.g. MRSA or VRE), where standard therapy with β-lactams cannot be used due to resistance or hypersensitivity. This includes pneumonia (community acquired and nosocomial) with known or suspected Gram-positive bacteria, or complicated skin and soft tissue infections. Treatment with linezolid should only be initiated in a hospital environment under specialist supervision.

Unwanted effects

Short courses of **linezolid** are relatively safe with mild side effects that commonly include diarrhoea, headache, nausea, vomiting, rash, constipation, taste/visual disturbance, and discolouration of the tongue. Disturbance of normal flora can also lead to oral thrush and vaginal candidiasis. Less common and potentially more severe reactions include pancreatitis and elevated transaminases, which may be indicative of liver damage. With longer-term use, bone marrow suppression, particularly thrombocytopenia may occur, so monitoring during treatment is necessary.

Drug interactions

Linezolid is a weak monoamine oxidase inhibitor (MAOI), so should not be used with other MAOIs or large amounts of tyramine-rich foods (such as aged cheeses, alcohol, smoked, or pickled foods). Co-administration with other serotonergic drugs like SSRIs or **pethidine** should be avoided where possible as it increases the risk of serotonin syndrome.

Drugs that inhibit folate synthesis

Sulfonamides/trimethoprim

> Sulfonamides and trimethoprim act to reduce the production of folic acid in bacteria, although they inhibit different steps in the folic acid pathway. Examples include trimethoprim and co-trimoxazole.

Mechanism of action

As most bacteria synthesize folic acid, whereas mammalian cells require exogenous sources, bacterial folate synthesis a useful selective target for drug therapy.

Sulfonamides are analogues of p-aminobenzoic acid that act by competitively inhibiting dihydrofolate synthetase, the enzyme that converts p-aminobenzoic acid to dihydropteroic acid in the early stages of folic acid synthesis. As the existing pool of folate can meet the needs of bacterial cells for generations, its onset of action is slow. Conversely, **trimethoprim** (diaminopyrimidines) acts later in the folic acid pathway, preventing the conversion of dihydrofolic acid to tetrahydrofolic acid through inhibition of dihydrofolate reductase. This, in turn, prevents the rapid production of bacterial growth, with a relatively fast onset of action. In combination, therefore, using a sulfonamide with trimethoprim increases overall antibacterial effect.

Prescribing

Trimethoprim is primarily used orally in uncomplicated UTI (Table 11.11), although resistance is an increasing problem. Similarly, increasing resistance has affected **co-trimoxazole** use over the years, although the associated risks of haematological reactions has limited its use to prevention and treatment of PJP, or for infections resistant to safer alternatives.

Unwanted effects

The most common side effects to **trimethoprim** are GI disturbance and rash. Thrombocytopenia and megaloblastic anaemia may be associated with trimethoprim due to inhibition of dihydrofolate reductase, as high serum concentrations can inhibit the mammalian enzyme. If this occurs folic acid rescue agents can be used to reverse this without affecting bacterial kill.

Side effects to **co-trimoxazole** are more common and largely attributable to the **sulfamethoxazole** component. These include hypersensitivity reactions and haematological effects, with skin rashes being the most common.

Due to its mechanism of action on the folate pathway, trimethoprim is generally avoided in the first trimester of pregnancy due to the theoretical risk of neural tube defects.

Drugs that affect bacterial DNA

Nitroimidazoles

Metronidazole is only active against anaerobic bacteria and not aerobic aerobes. For example, metronidazole and tinidazole.

Mechanism of action

Metronidazole inhibits nucleic acid synthesis by disrupting the DNA of microbial cells. This function only occurs when metronidazole is partially reduced, and because this reduction usually happens only in anaerobic cells, it has relatively little effect upon human cells or aerobic bacteria. Its unique spectrum means it is on the World Health Organization's List of Essential Medicines, deemed necessary in a basic health system.

Prescribing

Metronidazole is used to treat a number of infections where anaerobic bacteria are implicated including deep wound infections, dental abscess, vaginitis (*Trichomonas vaginalis* cover) and pelvic inflammatory disease (Table 11.12). It is also first-line treatment in mild-to-moderate

Table 11.11 General spectrum of activity and pharmacokinetics of inhibitors of folate synthesis

Drug class	Drug	General spectrum of activity	Pharmacokinetics
Dihydrofolate reductase inhibitor	Trimethoprim (oral)	Gram +ve bacilli and cocci, including *S aureus*. Gram −ve bacteria, including *Haemophilus* spp., and Enterobacteriaceae. Most anaerobes are resistant	Excellent oral absorption (~100%). Widely distributed in most tissue. Primarily renally excreted
As above + sulfonamide	Co-trimoxazole (oral, IV)	*Acinetobacter* spp., *B cepacia*, *Stenotrophomonas maltophilia*, and PCP pneumonia caused by *Pneumocystis jirovecii*	As trimethoprim

Table 11.12 General spectrum of activity and pharmacokinetics of drugs that affect bacterial DNA

Drug class	Drug	General spectrum of activity	Pharmacokinetics
Nitroimidazoles	Metronidazole (oral, IV)	Anaerobic cocci activity Baceroides, Fusobacteria, Clostridia (including *C. difficile*) *Trichomonas vaginalis, Giardia lamblia, Balantidium coli, Helicobacter pylori*	Well absorbed orally Widely distributed in all body tissue, including CSF
	Tinidazole (oral)	As above	As above
Quinolones	Ciprofloxacin	*Good activity against: Enterobacteriaceae, Acinetobacter* spp., *Campylobacter jejuni, Pseudomonas aeruginosa* *Less susceptible: Staph. aureus*, MRSA, and enterococci *Poor activity against*: anaerobes, but good against *Mycobacterium* spp. and some atypical bacteria, e.g. *Legionella pneumophila*	Good oral absorption (oral bioavailability ~90%) Widely distributed to most tissues
	Levofloxacin	Similar to ciprofloxacin, but a higher affinity for Gram +ve bacteria	Good oral absorption
	Moxifloxacin	*Gram +ve and Gram –ve bacteria*: including *Moraxella catarrhalis, Acinetobacter* spp., *Stenotrophomonas,* *Less active against: Pseudomonas* spp. and other non-fermenting Gram –ve rods *Good activity against*: atypical bacteria, e.g. *Chlamydia, Mycoplasma*, and *Legionella* spp. Good anaerobic activity *Good activity against: Mycobacterium tuberculosis*, but less against other *Mycobacterium* spp.	Oral absorption approx. 90% Widely distributed to all tissues

Clostridium difficile colitis. Doses are administered orally, IV, and via the rectum.

PRESCRIBING WARNING

Alcohol and metronidazole
- Metronidazole can cause a disulfiram-like reaction in combination with alcohol.
- Patients should be warned of the risk and advised not to drink alcohol during treatment and for at least 48 hours after.

Unwanted effects

Common side effects to **metronidazole** include nausea, a metallic taste, loss of appetite, and headaches. Less commonly, seizures or allergic reactions may occur. Patients should be advised not to take alcohol during metronidazole therapy (see 'Prescribing warning: alcohol and metronidazole').

In some patients there have been reports of increased anticoagulation effects when metronidazole was used in combination with **warfarin**, so prothrombin times may need to be monitored.

Quinolones (fluoroquinolones)

The quinolones are synthetic broad-spectrum antibiotics, first developed in the 1960s, that act by inhibiting DNA replication. Examples include ciprofloxacin, levofloxacin, moxifloxacin, nalidixic acid, norfloxacin, and ofloxacin.

Mechanism of action

Fluoroquinolones, derivatives of quinolones, are bactericidal antibiotics that inhibit DNA gyrase (the originally recognized target) and topoisomerase IV (a related type II topoisomerase); both required for DNA replication, transcription, and repair. They differ in their effects on the two enzymes, leading to variations in efficacy against Gram-positive and Gram-negative bacteria, i.e. newer fluoroquinolones tend to have a higher affinity for topoisomerase IV associated with enhanced Gram-positive coverage, whereas those with greater efficacy against Gram-negative bacteria primarily target DNA gyrase.

Fluoroquinolones easily enter cells via porins and can therefore be used to treat intracellular pathogens such as *Mycoplasma pneumoniae*. They have a concentration-dependent killing of bacteria. There are classified into four different generations:

- *First generation*: **nalidixic acid.**
- *Second generation*: **ciprofloxacin**, **norfloxacin**, **ofloxacin.**
- *Third generation*: **levofloxacin.**
- *Fourth generation*: **moxifloxacin.**

Prescribing

Due to excellent oral bioavailability and broad spectrum of activity, quinolones became widely over-used leading to increased resistance and outbreaks of *Clostridium difficile*. As a result, quinolone prescribing (especially **ciprofloxacin**) is now more restricted, especially in the elderly. Use also predisposes patients to MRSA colonization since many health care-associated strains of MRSA are resistant to ciprofloxacin, especially in the UK. In the USA, the predominant strain of MRSA tends to be more sensitive and is susceptible to ciprofloxacin.

PRESCRIBING WARNING

Antibiotic associated diarrhoea with quinolones

- Quinolones are associated with a high risk of *C. difficile* infection.
- Risk is increased in GI surgery, contact with health care facilities, and according to local epidemiology.
- Patients should be warned about the risk of diarrhoea when starting treatment.

Unwanted effects

Fluoroquinolones, despite being widely prescribed and generally well tolerated, possess numerous potentially severe side effects, thus require caution in patients with co-morbidities. The most common side effect of fluoroquinolones are GI effects, which include nausea, anorexia, and dyspepsia. Other symptoms like abdominal pain, vomiting, and diarrhoea occur less frequently, but may be more severe. The risk of *C. difficile* associated colitis needs to be considered prior to prescribing (see 'Prescribing warning: antibiotic associated diarrhoea with quinolones').

Other less common, but potentially severe effects include tendonitis and tendon rupture, particularly in patients over the age of 60, concomitant steroid therapy, as well as kidney, heart, and lung transplant recipients. The MHRA have recently issued a warning that such reactions may be irreversible and use therefore restricted to complex/severe infections. Patients should also be advised to stop treatment immediately at the first sign of a serious adverse effect. Patients should be monitored for tendon pain and inflammation, and the antibiotic discontinued if affected. Neuropathy, neuritis, although infrequently associated with fluoroquinolone use, can be severe. Use is cautioned in patients with history of cardiac arrhythmias (can cause QTc prolongation), or epilepsy (may alter seizure threshold).

Rifamycins

The rifamycins are a family of antibiotics that inhibit bacterial RNA polymerase and thus DNA transcription. For example, rifampicin.

Mechanism of action

Rifamycins work by binding to bacterial DNA-dependant RNA polymerase, (the enzyme responsible for transcription of DNA into RNA) to prevent the chain of RNA from elongating.

Mycobacteria are obligate intracellular bacteria, which live within the host cells, and hence, are protected against many other antibiotics. **Rifampicin**, is one of the few antibiotics able to penetrate cells and tissues sufficiently to reach the mycobacteria, thus mainly used in combination with other antibacterials in treating mycobacterial disease, e.g. tuberculosis and leprosy. Since rifampicin resistance is common as bacteria can acquire mutations that alter RNA polymerase structure preventing binding, combination therapy is recommended.

Prescribing

Rifampicin is most widely used in tuberculosis treatment, although it can be used in combination with another active drug for the treatment of skin and soft tissue, joint, and deep prosthesis infections. It can also be used as an adjunct to therapy for the treatment of panton-valentine leukocidin (PVL) *Staphylococcus aureus* infections or against biofilm-associated bacteria in prosthesis-associated infection. It is also particularly useful in combination with another active agent in patients with penicillin hypersensitivity. Doses are administered orally as capsules or liquid, or by IV infusion in patients unable to take oral medication. Combination oral preparations are available for the treatment of TB in order to promote better compliance.

Unwanted effects

> **PRACTICAL PRESCRIBING**
>
> **Staining of bodily fluids with rifampicin— patient counselling**
>
> Use of rifampicin can lead to red/orange staining of urine, skin, sweat, saliva, and faeces. Patients should be advised in advance of the risk, particularly to those who use soft contact lenses, which may be irreversibly stained.

Adverse effects to **rifampicin** tend to be GI (nausea, vomiting, anorexia, diarrhoea) or hypersensitivity reactions, including rashes and haematological reactions. Less commonly rifampicin can cause hepatic toxicity, because of this and being primarily hepatically metabolized, baseline LFTs should be carried out prior to starting treatment. Repeat LFTs should be carried out for patients on extended treatment courses, i.e. for TB, with raised ALT/AST/bilirubin at baseline or with clinical symptoms of hepatic toxicity, e.g. itching, jaundice, etc.

Drug interactions

One of the greatest limitation to **rifampicin** use, is its potent enzyme-inducing effect on the CYP450 enzymes, CYP 3A4, 2C19, 2C9, and 2D6, responsible for the metabolism of numerous commonly used drugs. Drug interactions are therefore common and can lead to therapeutic failure, due to increased clearance of concomitant therapies, e.g. anti-epileptics, immunosuppressants, and anticoagulants. Prescribers are advised to check prior to initiating any concomitant therapy.

Further reading

MacGowan A, MacNaughton E (2013) Antibiotic resistance. *Medicine* 41(11), 643–8.

Wang JD, Levin PA. (2009) Metabolism, cell growth and the bacterial cell cycle *Nature Reviews Microbiology* 7(11), 822–7.

Guidelines

Department of Health Green Book. Immunisationization against infectious disease. www.dh.gov.uk [accessed 12 April 2019].

NICE CG69 (2008). Prescribing of antibiotics for self-limiting respiratory tract infections in adults and children in primary care. http://guidance.nice.org.uk/CG69 [accessed 12 April 2019].

NICE CG102 (2009) Bacterial meningitis and meningococcal septicaemia. National Collaborating Centre for Women's and Children's health 2009. http://guidance.nice.org.uk/CG102 [accessed 12 April 2019].

NICE CG102 (2010) Meningitis (bacterial) and meningococcal septicaemia in under 16s: recognition, diagnosis and management, can be referenced though if not done so already. https://www.nice.org.uk/guidance/CG102 [accessed 17 April 2019].

NICE NG51 (2016). Sepsis: recognition, diagnosis and early management. https://www.nice.org.uk/guidance/ng51 [accessed 12 April 2019].

Public Health England (2015) Start smart—then focus; antimicrobial stewardship toolkit for English hospitals. https://www.gov.uk/government/uploads/system/uploads/attachment_data/file/417032/Start_Smart_Then_Focus_FINAL.PDF [accessed 12 April 2019].

Public Health England guidelines. Management of infection guidance for primary care available at www.gov.uk/phe [accessed 12 April 2019].

SIGN 102 (May 2008) Management of invasive meningococcal disease in children and young people: A national clinical guideline. [archived].

11.2 Fungal infections

Fungi are eukaryotic organisms with a cell wall containing chitin (a long-chain polymer of N-acetylglucosamine), as well as other polysaccharides. The fungal kingdom consists of over 100 000 species, but only a few are pathogenic to humans. This chapter focuses on the pathogenic and opportunistic fungi that cause disease in humans.

Types of fungi

Fungi are divided into three groups based on their growth form:

1. *Moulds*: multicellular fungi that consist of branching filaments, called hyphae. They reproduce by spores or conidia, e.g. *Aspergillus*, *Fusarium*, and *Rhizomucor* spp.

2. *Yeasts*: unicellular fungi that have a round or oval shape, although some form pseudohyphae or hyphae. Yeasts reproduce by budding, e.g. *Candida*, *Cryptococcus*, and *Trichosporon* spp.

3. *Dimorphic fungi*: change growth to a mould or yeast phase depending on growth conditions, (e.g. temperature). Most grow as yeasts within the human body, but as moulds in the natural environment, e.g. *Histoplasma*, *Blastomyces*, and *Coccidioides* spp. Systemic infections caused by dimorphic fungi are mainly found in North, Central, and South America, although some are also endemic in Africa, India and Australia.

Fungal infections

Fungal infections, or mycosis, can be classified according to the extent of tissue involvement, i.e. superficial, SC, or systemic. While superficial infections rarely cause significant morbidity, systemic fungal infections are associated with a high mortality.

Superficial fungal infections

Superficial fungal infections include infections of the skin, hair, nail, and mucous membranes caused by moulds or yeasts.

Dermatophytes

Dermatophytes are a closely related group of fungi that include the genera *Trichophyton*, *Epidermophyton*, and *Microsporum*. They infect the skin, hair, and nails (dermatophytosis), as they require keratin to grow, and are responsible for infections such as tinea or ringworm. Classification is according to infection site; i.e. tinea capitis (scalp and hair), tinea pedis (foot, athlete's foot), tinea manuum (hand), tinea cruris (groin), tinea corporis (skin of the arms, legs and trunk), and tinea unguium (fingernail or toenail). They can lead to the breakdown of the skin barrier, which increases the risk of bacterial invasion, particularly in immunocompromised hosts.

Non-dermatophyte

Non-dermatophyte organisms that cause superficial infections, include *Candida* spp. and pityriasis versicolor due to *Malassezia* spp. Superficial candida infections are most commonly due to *Candida albicans*, although 20 other species may be responsible, including *C. glabrata*, *C. krusei*, and *C. parapsilosis*. They most commonly affect the mucosa (e.g. oropharyngeal candidiasis, vaginal candidiasis), but can also cause skin infection (e.g. candida nappy rash) and nail infections. Pityriasis versicolor is a relatively common superficial infection that leads to hyper- or hypopigmentation of the skin, usually affecting the trunk or upper proximal limbs, and less commonly the neck and face. It is caused by the lipid-dependent yeast *Malassezia*.

Onychomycosis (fungal nail infection) are predominantly caused by dermatophytes. However, *Candida* spp., as well as moulds such as *Scopulariopsis, Scytalidium, Fusarium*, and *Onychocola* spp. can be responsible, usually in immunocompromised patients.

Although typically associated with invasive disease, *Aspergillus* spp. can rarely cause *aspergillus* keratitis and endophthalmitis in the immunocompromised host (e.g. following eye trauma), or allergic bronchopulmonary aspergillosis (ABPA), a hypersensitivity reaction affecting patients with asthma or cystic fibrosis.

Subcutaneous fungal infections

SC fungal infections are rare, occurring predominantly in tropical and subtropical countries, where organisms enter the tissue through cuts and grazes on bare feet. Infections usually remain localized within the skin and SC tissue, but can disseminate into adjacent bones and into the lymphatic system.

Systemic fungal infections caused by opportunistic pathogens

Deep-seated fungal infections and fungaemia (fungi isolated from blood cultures), are predominantly seen in patients with impaired immunity or in the presence of intravascular catheters. With increasing use of immunosuppressive therapy (e.g. transplants, chemotherapy), number of people living with HIV and use of central venous catheters, the incidenced of invasive fungal infections has increased over the last decade. Invasive fungal infections can be challenging to diagnose and are associated with a high mortality rate. Clinicians should have a high index of suspicion, especially when predisposing factors are present.

Invasive candidiasis

Invasive candidiasis has a worldwide incidence of about 250 000 cases a year, most commonly affecting those at the extremes of age, with a mortality rate as high as 40%. Although *Candida albicans* is the most common cause, *C. krusei* and *C. glabatra* are increasingly seen, especially in intensive care settings. Infection is usually associated with central venous catheters or a deep-seated source of infection, but may occur following translocation from the GI tract. Other sites of infection include hepatosplenic, intra-abdominal, endocarditis, and endophthalmitis. Less commonly, *Candida* spp. cause CNS infections, UTIs, or osteomyelitis. Candida auris is an emerging fungus, which has caused outbreaks in healthcare settings. Special laboratory tests are required to identify *C. auris* and it is often multidrug-resistant.

Invasive aspergillosis

Invasive aspergillosis, although less common than candidiasis, is harder to treat and is associated with a higher mortality rate (greater than 50%). Infections are most often pulmonary, but can affect sinuses, or following haematogenous spread, involve multiple organs including the CNS, and cardiovascular system. Diagnosis is problematic with blood cultures having a low yield; tissue culture from affected sites is more accurate, but can be falsely negative and hard to obtain.

Cryptoccosis

Cryptococcosis is an invasive fungal infection caused by the encapsulated yeast *Cryptococcus neoformans*, which has four serotypes. *Cryptococcus neoformans* var. *grubii* (serotype A) and *Cryptococcus neoformans* var. *neoformans* (serotype D), cause disease in the immunocompromised host, particularly in transplant recipients, people living with advanced HIV infection, or with prolonged courses of corticosteroids. *Cryptococcus neoformans* var. *gattii* (serotype B and C) affects mostly immunocompetent people, particularly in tropical and subtropical regions. Cryptococcal meningitis is the most common cause of meningitis in patients living with advanced HIV infection, classically presenting with fever and chronic headache. Diagnosis is confirmed by a positive CSF cryptococcal antigen, Indian ink stain of CSF, or CSF cryptococcal culture. Cryptococcosis can also cause skin lesions, lung involvement, disseminated disease, or osteolytic bone lesions.

Mucormycosis

Mucormycosis (zygomycosis) is a rare opportunistic infection caused by moulds belonging to the Zygomycetes class, which includes *Mucor, Rhizomucor, Rhizopus*, and *Absidia* spp. DM (particularly diabetic ketoacidosis), haematologic malignancies, and solid organ or haematopoietic stem cell transplants are the most common risk factors for mucormycosis. It tends to invade blood vessels, resulting in tissue necrosis typically affecting the nasal mucosa and palate, or lungs. The apparent increasing incidence of mucormycosis is probably due to increasing numbers of severely immunosuppressed patients. Some antifungal agents used as prophylaxis (e.g. **fluconazole**, **voriconazole**, echinocandins) have no activity against mucormycosis resulting in breakthrough disease.

Pneumocystis jirovecii

Pneumocystis jirovecii, an organism known to cause severe respiratory disease (pneumocystis pneumonia, PCP) in immunocompromised patients, was once considered to be a protozoan, but is now classified as a fungus. PCP incidence was particularly high in patients living with advanced HIV infection when the HIV pandemic emerged, although the use of combination antiretroviral therapy (cART) and co-trimoxazole prophylaxis, has significantly reduced this. In people living with HIV, PCP typically has a more indolent presentation, although non-HIV immunosuppressed patients tend to present with fulminant respiratory failure. Risk factors include transplant recipients, haematological malignancies, chronic corticosteroid use and immunosuppressive therapy (see Figure 11.4).

Management of fungal infections

The choice of antifungal agent depends on a combination of patient factors, e.g. severity, co-morbidities, as well as fungal factors, e.g. species, site of infection.

Superficial fungal infections

Dermatophyte infections of the skin (Trichophyton, Epidermophyton, Microsporum spp.)

Topical antifungals are used to treat most dermatophyte skin infections (tinea corporis, tinea cruris, tinea pedis, and tinea manuum). Patients should receive topical antifungal treatment, such as imidazoles or **terbinafine** cream until 1 week after resolution of symptoms and signs of infection, in order to decrease the risk of relapse. Oral treatment with terbinafine, **itraconazole**, or less favourably **griseofulvin** may be required if there is extensive skin involvement, or no response to topical treatment.

Dermatophyte infections of the scalp and hair (Tricophyton, Epidermophyton, Microsporum spp.)

Dermatophyte infection of the scalp and hair (tinea capitis) should be treated with systemic antifungals. **Griseofulvin** is used in preference over **terbinafine**, as the latter may be ineffective against infections due to *Microsporum* spp.

Fluconazole and **itraconazole** have also been used for treating tinea capitis, albeit with less evidence for their use. Topical treatment with **ketoconazole** or **selenium sulfide** shampoo may reduce the spread of infection to other people.

Onychomycosis (Candida, Scopulariopsis, Scytalidium, Fusarium, Onychocola spp.)

Systemic treatment with oral **terbinafine** is more effective for most nail infections (tinea unguium), although topical treatment with **amorolfine** can be considered in mild/distal disease. **Itraconazole** may be used as an oral alternative, either as pulsed or continuous therapy, whereas **griseofulvin** is considered the least effective and associated with the highest rate of recurrence. Oral therapy should continue for at least 6 weeks for fingernail and 12 weeks for toe nail infections, although toe nail treatment may be required for up to 12 months to ensure complete clearance.

Mucosal or cutaneous infections due to Candida spp.

Superficial candida mucocutaneous infections are relatively common (vulvovaginitis) and are effectively treated topically. The choice of agent will depend on the site of infection and the licensed formulations available. For example, **nystatin** suspension is applied topically in oropharyngeal infection and **clotrimazole** cream is commonly used for vulvovaginal candidiasis.

Oral **fluconazole** is used for widespread superficial infections (e.g. extensive oropharyngeal) or infections that do not respond to topical treatment, although non-albican spp. can be resistant to fluconazole, and so identification and sensitivity should be carried out to prevent recurrent treatment failure. Extensive oropharyngeal candidiasis is usually an indicator of immunosuppression and is an AIDS-defining illness, and should be investigated on presentation.

Pityriasis versicolor (Malassezia spp.)

Although relatively easy to treat, pityriasis versicolor has a tendency to recur and maintenance treatment may be necessary. Patients should be advised that altered pigmentation may persist once the infection has cleared. In the absence of high-quality studies, there is little to select one agent over another in the treatment of pityriasis versicolor, although it is likely that higher strengths and extended course will give better cure rates. First-line treatment is generally with topical therapy, either as

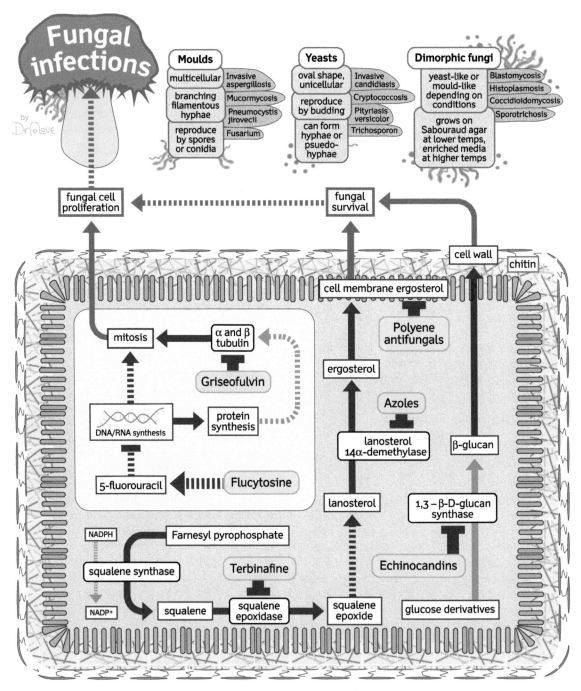

Figure 11.4 Fungal infections: summary of relevant pathways and drug targets.

shampoo (**ketoconazole** or **selenium sulfide**) or cream (ketoconazole, **terbinafine**, **clotrimazole**) used up to 4 weeks. In recurrence or resistance infections, oral therapy with **fluconazole** or **itraconazole** may be indicated.

Subcutaneous fungal infections

Management of SC mycoses will probably require antifungal treatment with or without surgical excision, although due to its rarity will require specialist referral. *Sporotrichosis* may be treated with IV lipid formulations of **amphotericin** or oral **itraconazole**.

Systemic fungal infections caused by opportunistic pathogens

Invasive fungal infections are often challenging to manage, especially in immunocompromised patients, and associated with high rates of mortality in spite of antifungal treatment. Management will require specialist involvement to identify species and sensitivities, and therefore optimize therapy.

Invasive candidiasis (e.g. C. albicans, C. glabrata, C. krusei, C. tropicalis, C. parapsilosis)

Diagnosis of invasive candidiasis can be made either directly through identification in blood or tissue cultures, or indirectly using surrogate markers, although due to limited accuracy more than one test is recommended. Antifungal therapy is often initiated as either prophylaxis in high risk patients, or as empiric therapy in suspected invasive candidiasis. Treatment options include echinocandins, **fluconazole**, **voriconazole**, and IV lipid formulations of **amphotericin**, which can be rationalized once the organism and respective sensitivities are known.

Lipid formulations of amphotericin B are the treatment of choice where CNS involvement is suspected, due to excellent CNS penetration and good efficacy against common pathogens (*C. albicans* and C. *glabrata*). Echinocandins are frequently favoured by clinicians as they have early fungicidal activity, minimal adverse effects and limited drug interactions. Treatment should be continued for a minimum of 2 weeks after the first negative blood culture, and intravascular catheters removed.

Invasive aspergillosis (e.g. A. fumigatus (most common), A. flavus, A. niger, A. terreus)

A diagnosis of invasive aspergillosis is defined by the level of certainty, i.e. possible, probable, or proven; the latter only made in the presence of a positive culture from a normally sterile site. To avoid unnecessary invasive procedures, a proven diagnosis is uncommon, instead a probable diagnosis is made based on clinical signs and symptoms. **Voriconazole** is the treatment of choice for invasive aspergillosis, with lipid formulation of **amphotericin**

a viable alternative if voriconazole is contraindicated. Echinocandins are generally reserved for use second-line, where first-line treatments are ineffective or poorly tolerated. In resistant disease, dual therapy may be advocated.

Cryptococcal meningitis and invasive cryptococcal disease (e.g. C. neoformans, C. gattii)

As an opportunistic infection, treatment options for cryptococcal meningitis are determined by host immunocompetency and any underlying predisposing factors, i.e. whether the patient is living with HIV, a transplant recipient, or neither. Due to the high mortality rate, rapid diagnosis and treatment is essential; the treatment of choice initially is with a lipid formulation of IV **amphotericin** plus IV **flucytosine**. In people living with HIV, these are given for 2 weeks as induction therapy, but longer in HIV-negative patients, as these patients are often harder to treat. **Fluconazole** is given as consolidation and maintenance therapy to treat disease and reduce the high risk of relapse associated with cryptococcal disease. Treatment duration is is determined by clinical signs and underlying risk factors.

Mucormycosis (zygomycosis) (e.g. Mucor, Rhizomucor, Rhizopus, and Absidia spp.)

Mucormycosis is associated with a high mortality; hence, early diagnosis with appropriate treatment is essential for a good outcome. Treatment of choice is with IV lipid formulation of **amphotericin** plus aggressive surgical debridement, plus treatment of the underlying metabolic or immunological disorder. **Posaconazole** is an alternative option and treatment continued for several months to years.

Pneumocystis jirovecii

Pneumocystis jirovecii causes a severe respiratory disease (Pneumocystis pneumonia, PCP) in people living with HIV and other severely immunocompromised patients. PCP is unresponsive to many antifungals. This is thought to be due to the absence of ergosterol in the cell membrane of *P. jirovecii*. Treatment of choice is therefore with the antibiotic **co-trimoxazole**, administered IV at high doses in moderate to severe disease, and orally in mild disease with adjunctive corticosteroids recommended in hypoxic patients. In patients with prolonged immunosuppression (e.g. ALL or where CD4 count <200 cells/uL) co-trimoxazole is given orally as primary prophylaxis.

Drug classes used in the management of fungal infection

Azoles

The triazole and imidazole antifungals contain a triazole or imidazole ring, respectively, and although they have the same mechanism of action, the triazoles have a broader spectrum of activity. Imidazoles are administered topically, while triazoles are administered orally or IV.

> Azoles inhibit the synthesis of ergosterol via their action on the enzyme lanosterol 14α-demethylase. Examples include fluconazole, itraconazole, voriconazole, and posaconazole.

Triazoles

Mechanism of action

The inhibition of cytochrome P450 dependent enzyme lanosterol 14 α-demethylase, impairs ergosterol synthesis, the main sterol in fungal cell membranes. It plays an important role in regulating fungal cell membrane fluidity and integrity. Insufficient ergosterol, as well as accumulation of toxic sterol intermediates, results in abnormal fungal cell membrane structure and function. **Fluconazole**

and **itraconazole** are considered fungistatic, whereas **voriconazole** and **posaconazole** are potentially fungicidal against moulds. New and emerging triazole antifungals include **ravuconazole, isavuconazole**, and **albaconazole**. As a class, the triazoles vary with regards to their spectrum of antifungal activity (see Table 11.13), pharmacokinetics, interactions, and side effects.

Prescribing

The azole antifungals are the most widely used antifungal agents indicated for the management and prevention of a broad spectrum of fungal disease (see Table 11.14). The triazoles vary in their pharmacokinetics influencing their use, route of administration, and need for monitoring blood levels.

Unwanted effects

Although **fluconazole** and **itraconazole** are generally well tolerated, significant side effects can occur with any of the triazole antifungals and vary with preparation, e.g. itraconazole solution is more likely to cause GI side effects than capsules.

Hepatotoxicity (transient-deranged LFTs, hepatitis, cholestasis and jaundice, and hepatic failure) can occur with any of the triazole antifungals. Treatment should be stopped immediately if significant dysfunction occurs and caution is required in at risk patients.

Table 11.13 Spectrum of antifungal activity of triazoles

Drug	Yeasts	Moulds	Other
Fluconazole	Most *Candida* spp. (except *C. krusei* and often *C. glabrata*) *Cryptococcus* spp.	Inactive against *Aspergillus* spp., *Fusarium* spp., and Zygomycetes	*Coccidioides immitis*—but less active against other dimorphic fungi Dermatophytes
Itraconazole	*Candida* spp. *Cryptococcus* spp.	*Aspergillus* spp. Less active against *Fusarium* spp. Inactive against Zygomycetes	Dimorphic fungi Dermatophytes Some dematiaceous fungi
Voriconazole	*Candida* spp. *Cryptococcus* spp. *Trichosporon* spp.	*Aspergillus* spp., *Fusarium* spp. *Scedosporium* spp. Inactive against Zygomycetes	Dimorphic fungi Dermatophytes Some dematiaceous fungi
Posaconazole	*Candida* spp. *Cryptococcus* spp. *Trichosporon* spp.	*Aspergillus* spp. *Fusarium* spp. Zygomycetes	Dimorphic fungi Dermatophytes Some dematiaceous fungi
Isavuconazole	*Candida* spp. *Cryptococcus* spp. *Trichosporon* spp.	*Aspergillus* spp, Zygomecetes, limited activity in vitro against *Fusarium* spp.	Dimorphic fungi Dermatophytes Some dematiaceous fungi

Table 11.14 Common clinical indications and pharmacokinetics of triazole antifungals

Antifungal	Common clinical indication	Pharmacokinetics
Fluconazole (oral, IV)	Superficial/invasive candidiasis Cryptococcal meningitis Dermtaophyte infection Pityriasis versicolor Candida prophylaxis in immunocompromised patients	Well absorbed orally Excellent CNS penetration Minimal hepatic metabolism, renally cleared Serum monitoring unnecessary
Itraconazole (oral, IV infusion)	Dermatophyte infections Pityriasis versicolor *Candida/Aspergillus* prophylaxis in high risk patients, e.g. BMT	Considerable interindividual variation in oral absorption. Capsules absorbed better with food/acidic drinks, liquid better on empty stomach Extensively metabolized by CYP 3A4 and saturable first pass metabolism Serum monitoring advisable
Voriconazole (oral, IV)	Invasive fluconazole resistant *Candida* spp. infections Invasive aspergillosis	Well absorbed orally (95%), IV route only when oral not possible Widely distributed, high concentrations in CSF and brain Extensively metabolized by CYP2C19, 2C9 and 3A4 Significant genetic variation in metabolism, serum monitoring may be necessary
Posaconazole (oral)	Invasive aspergillosis Fungal prophylaxis in high risk patients, e.g. BMT Fusarium infections when amphotericin not tolerated	Significant interindividual variation in absorption, increased by fatty foods Widely distributed Minimal CYP450 metabolism Monitoring may be necessary
Isavuconazole (oral, IV infusion)	Invasive aspergillosis Invasive mucormycosis	Well absorbed orally, Well tolerated and relatively safe. Widely distributed Hepatically metabolized by CYP3A4/3A5

Cardiovascular toxicity with the azoles includes arrhythmias, (including *torsades de pointes* and QT interval prolongation, particularly with **voriconazole** and **posaconazole**) and increased risk of heart failure, predominately attributed to itraconazole. Caution is advised in at risk patients or those on medication known to prolong the QT interval.

Renal impairment can develop during treatment with triazole antifungals, especially with voriconazole and renal function should be monitored on treatment. Furthermore, the IV preparation of voriconazole contains the cyclodextrin, sulfobutylether-β-cyclodextrin (SBECD), which can accumulate in renal insufficiency; subsequently, IV voriconazole is not recommended in moderate impairment, although oral voriconazole can be used.

Visual disturbances, such as blurred vision, altered colour perception and photophobia are frequently reported during voriconazole treatment, although effects tend to be transient and reversible, rarely necessitating discontinuation of treatment. Neurological symptoms, such as headache, confusion, and hallucination occur infrequently with voriconazole.

Skin reactions, including Stevens–Johnson syndrome, have been attributed to azole therapy. Notably, phototoxicity occurs frequently with voriconazole; patients should avoid significant exposure to direct sunlight or sunbeds, and ensure they use effective sunscreen. Premalignant skin lesions and squamous cell carcinoma have been reported with prolonged voriconazole use.

Drug interactions

Since the mechanism of action of triazoles involves binding to CYP450 enzymes, these antifungals inhibit the CYP 3A enzyme family (**itraconazole** and **posaconazole** more so than **fluconazole** or **voriconazole**) leading to significant interactions with substrates for these enzymes. Care is also advised when co-prescribing with potent inducers or inhibitors of CYP 3A4 as many of the triazoles are substrate for this enzyme thereby affecting efficacy or increasing the risk of toxicity.

Imidazoles

Mechanism of action

Like the triazole antifungals, the imidazoles interfere with the synthesis of ergosterol by inhibiting the CYP 450-dependent enzyme lanosterol 14 α-demethylase. This leads to abnormal fungal cell membrane structure and function.

Prescribing

The imidazoles are administered topically as a cream, solution, spray, pessary, etc. in the management of skin and mucosal infections due to *Candida* spp., as well as dermatophyte infections of the skin (see Table 11.15).

Unwanted effects

Local irritation can occur with any of the topical agents, although systemic absorption is minimal, making side effects unlikely, except for **miconazole** oral gel which can rarely cause hepatitis, allergic skin rashes, and drug interactions. As oral **ketoconazole** is associated with significant hepatotoxicity, its use is no longer recommended.

Echinocandins

> Echinocandins inhibit the synthesis of the polysaccharide glucan, an essential component of fungal cell walls, via their action on 1,3—β-D-glucan synthase. For example, caspofungin, micafungin, and anidulafungin.

Table 11.15 Common clinical indications of imidazole antifungals

Antifungal	Common clinical indications
Clotrimazole—cream, solution, spray, pessary	Fungal skin infections (including dermatophytes and *Candida* spp.)
	Vaginal candidiasis
	Otitis externa
Ketoconazole—cream, shampoo	Fungal skin infections (including dermatophytes and *Candida* spp.)
	Vulval candidiasis
	Seborrhoeic dermatitis of the scalp
Miconazole—cream, powder, gel, buccal tablet, vaginal capsule	Fungal skin infections (including dermatophytes and *Candida* spp.)
	Vaginal candidiasis
	Oropharyngeal candidiasis
Econazole—cream	Fungal skin infections (including dermatophytes and *Candida* spp.)
	Vaginal candidiasis
Tioconazole—topical solution	Mild onychomycosis

Mechanism of action

Inhibition of glucan synthesis affects fungal cell wall stability and results in fungal cell lysis. As glucan is not present in human cells, echinocandins are selectively toxic to fungi. All three echinocandins have a similar spectrum of antifungal activity, being fungicidal against all *Candida* spp., as well as fungistatic activity against *Aspergillus* spp. (see Table 11.16).

Prescribing

Caspofungin, **anidulafungin**, and **micafungin** vary with regards to their license, with all three licensed for the management of invasive candidiasis, but only caspofungin licensed for use as empirical treatment for systemic fungal infections in neutropenic patients. Caspofungin is also indicated for invasive aspergillosis in

Table 11.16 Spectrum of antifungal activity of echinocandins

Drug	Yeasts	Moulds	Other
Caspofungin, Micafungin, Anidulafungin	*Candida* spp.; *Inactive* against *Cryptococcus* spp.	*Aspergillus* spp.; *Inactive* against Zygomycetes, *Fusarium* spp.	Variable activity against dimorphic fungi in vitro; *Inactive* against dermatophytes

adults who have failed treatment with other antifungals, although as echinocandins are only fungistatic against aspergillus species, **voriconazole** or lipid formulations of **amphotericin** are preferred in suspected or proven aspergillus infections. Furthermore, echinocandins have minimal CNS penetration and are, therefore, not used in fungal meningitis or CNS disease.

As caspofungin and micafungin are metabolized by the liver, dose adjustment in moderate hepatic impairment is advised for caspofungin, while micafungin should only be used with caution. No dosage adjustment are required in renal impairment, although micafungin may worsen renal function (see Table 11.17).

Unwanted effects

Due to their selectivity for fungal cells, echinocandins are relatively safe antifungal agents, with few significant side effects. Histamine-mediated symptoms, such as pruritus, vasodilation, flushing, or rash are occasionally reported. Injection-site reactions, hepatitis, and cholestasis can also occur. Potentially life-threatening hepatotoxicity may occur with **micafungin**, see 'Prescribing warning: hepatotoxicity with micafungin'.

PRESCRIBING WARNING

Hepatotoxicity with micafungin

- Prolonged treatment with micafungin has been shown to cause liver tumours in mice.
- Manufacturers recommend it only be used when other agents are deemed inappropriate.
- While on treatment, patients should have LFTs, U&Es, and FBC monitored for signs of deteriorating hepatic or renal function, or haemolysis.
- Early discontinuation is recommended in the event of persistently elevated LFTs.
- Anybody initiated on micafungin requires a checklist to be completed and filed in their notes.

Drug interactions

As echinocandins neither inhibit nor induce the hepatic CYP450 enzymes, the risk of drug interactions is small. **Caspofungin** is, however, a poor substrate for CYP450 enzymes so could be affected by potent enzyme inducers (e.g. **rifampicin**, **dexamethasone**, **carbamazepine**, and **phenytoin**) and a higher caspofingin maintenance

Table 11.17 Common clinical indications and pharmacokinetics for the echinocandins

Antifungal	Common clinical indications	Pharmacokinetics
Caspofungin (IV infusion)	Invasive candidiasis / Invasive aspergillosis (second-line) / Empirical treatment in neutropenia	Poor oral bioavailability / Widely distributed, but negligible amounts in CSF/eye / Hepatic metabolism
Micafungin (IV infusion)	Invasive candidiasis	Poor oral bioavailability / Widely distributed, but negligible amounts in CSF/eye / Hepatic metabolism
Anidulafungin (IV infusion)	Invasive candidiasis / Candidiasis prophylaxis in prolonged neutropenia (second-line)	Poor oral bioavailability / Widely distributed, but negligible amounts in CSF/eye / Slow non-enzymatic degradation in blood

Table 11.18 Spectrum of antifungal activity of flucytosine

Drug	Yeasts	Moulds	Other
Flucytosine	*Candida* spp., except *Candida krusei, Cryptococcus neoformans*	*Aspergillus* spp. *Inactive* against *Zygomycetes, Fusarium* spp.	*Inactive* against dimorphic fungi

dose may be needed. It should not be given to patients on **ciclosporin** treatment, as it increases the risk of developing abnormal LFTs. Caspofungin also reduces serum levels of **tacrolimus**, while **micafungin** increases serum levels of **sirolimus** and **nifedipine**.

Flucytosine

Flucytosine is converted inside the fungal cell first to 5-fluorouracil and then to 5-fluorouridine triphosphate (5FUTP), preventing normal protein synthesis in fungal cells.

Mechanism of action

The conversion of **flucytosine** into 5-fluorouracil and then the active metabolite 5FUTP, leads to its incorporation into fungal RNA in place of uracil. This results in abnormal protein synthesis within the fungal cells. 5-fluorouracil is also converted to another active metabolite (5-fluorodeoxyuridine monophosphate, 5FdUMP), which inhibits thymidylate synthetase, leading to inhibition of DNA synthesis. Consequently, flucytosine metabolites inhibit both fungal RNA and DNA synthesis.

Prescribing

Flucytosine is predominantly used in combination with **amphotericin** in the management of cryptococcal meningitis and severe systemic candidiasis. To optimize efficacy and reduce the risk of toxicity, peak and trough serum concentrations of flucytosine should be monitored. Flucytosine is generally administered as an intermittent IV infusion, although unlicensed tablets are available (Tables 11.18 and 11.19).

Unwanted effects

At high serum concentrations, **flucytosine** is degraded to 5-fluorouracil and dihydrofluorouracil, resulting in bone marrow suppression (thrombocytopaenia, leucopaenia, and aplastic anaemia). It has a narrow therapeutic index and is minimally metabolized by the liver before being excreted via the kidney. The risk of toxicity is increased in renal/hepatic impairment (particularly in the elderly) and, while on treatment, close monitoring of renal and hepatic function, as well as FBC is recommended to reduce the risk of toxicity.

Other side effects include hepatitis, skin rashes, and neurological symptoms such as headache, confusion, and vertigo. Flucytosine is shown to be teratogenic in animal studies and must be avoided during pregnancy, unless the benefit outweighs the potential risk.

Drug interactions

Used in combination as it is with **amphotericin** the risk of renal toxicity is increased. Drugs that increase the risk of side-effects such as bone marrow suppression and hepatitis, should be used with care in combination with **flucytosine**.

Griseofulvin

Griseofulvin binds to α- and β-tubulin interfering with the function of spindle and cytoplasmic microtubules, and inhibiting fungal cell division.

Table 11.19 Common clinical indications and pharmacokinetics of flucytosine

Antifungal	Common clinical indications	Pharmacokinetics
Flucytosine (IV infusion, oral)	Cryptococcal meningitis Severe systemic candidiasis	Very good oral bioavailability Widely distributed, good CSF penetration Largely excreted unchanged in urine, minimal metabolism

Mechanism of action

Griseofulvin is a mycotoxic metabolic product of *Penicillium* spp. Its capacity to bind microtubular proteins disrupts formation of the spindle and prevents mitosis in fungal cells. Nucleic acid synthesis inhibition and disruption in the formation of hyphal cell wall material may also be involved. This leads to irregular swelling and spiral curling of the hyphae.

Prescribing

Griseofulvin is used to treat fungal infections of the skin, scalp, nails, and hair caused by dermatophytes (*Trichophyton* spp., *Epidermophyton floccosum*, *Microsporum* spp.), also referred to as ringworm and tinea; it is, however, ineffective against *Candida* spp. Doses are administered orally, ideally with a high-fat meal to increase drug absorption. Its use has been largely superseded by **terbinafine**, the latter being more effective and better tolerated with fewer drug interactions, and requiring shorter treatment courses (Table 11.20).

Unwanted effects

Griseofulvin can impair driving and other skilled tasks, as well as enhance the effects of alcohol. It is contraindicated in patients with SLE or acute porphyria, as it can exacerbate disease. Animal studies have shown this drug to be teratogenic, as well as fetotoxic and should not therefore be used in pregnancy. Due to its action on the mitotic spindle, it is also potentially tumorigenic and must be avoided in patients who are breastfeeding. Griseofulvin can cause liver dysfunction and is contraindicated in patients with severe liver disease. Severe skin reactions including Stevens–Johnson syndrome have also been reported.

Drug interactions

Griseofulvin is an inducer of CYP 3A4 and can therefore reduce the effectiveness of substrates such as coumarins and oral contraceptives. As griseofulvin is potentially teratogenic and foetotoxic effects; patients should

therefore be advised to use additional contraceptive methods, such as barrier contraception, during treatment and for at least 1 month after completion. Similarly, men should not father a child during treatment or for at least 6 months after completion.

Griseofulvin reduces **ciclosporin** blood levels, while **phenobarbital** reduces griseofulvin absorption.

Polyene antifungals

> Polyene antifungals bind to ergosterol in the fungal cell membrane, leading to increased membrane permeability, leakage of intracellular electrolytes, and molecules and cell death. For example, lipid formulations of amphotericin and nystatin.

Mechanism of action

In addition to binding to ergosterol, high concentrations of **amphotericin** molecules combine to form transmembrane channels (pores) in the fungal cell membrane and cause oxidative damage to fungal cells. Amphotericin also binds to the sterol cholesterol in human cells, leading to significant toxicity, especially with the use of the conventional formulations (e.g. amphotericin deoxycholate).

Nystatin is structurally related to amphotericin, although due to its poor oral absorption is limited to use topically in superficial fungal infections. Currently, the possibility of a liposomal nystatin is under investigation with the hope of showing efficacy against otherwise resistant fungal infections.

Prescribing

The use of the conventional formulation of **amphotericin**, amphotericin B deoxycholate, has been superseded by the use of lipid formulations, due to significant risk of nephrotoxicity and infusion-related reactions. As lipid formulations are considerably less toxic, higher doses may be administered safely. In all, three different lipid formulations were developed:

Table 11.20 Spectrum of antifungal activity of griseofulvin

Drug	Yeasts	Moulds	Other
Griseofulvin	*Inactive* against *Candida* spp. and *Cryptococcus* spp.	*Inactive* against *Aspergillus* spp., Zygomycetes, and *Fusarium* spp.	Dermatophytes *Inactive* against dimorphic fungi

Table 11.21 Spectrum of antifungal activity of the polyene antifungals

Drug	Yeasts	Moulds	Other
Amphotericin: lipid formulations deoxycholate formulation	*Candida* spp.; *Cryptococcus* spp.;	*Aspergillus* spp.[1] *Inactive* against some Zygomycetes, most *Fusarium* spp., and *Scedosporium* spp.	Dimorphic fungi[2] *Penicillium marneffei* Dermatophytes may be less susceptible
Nystatin: topical treatment	*Candida* spp.; *Inactive* against *Cryptococcus* spp.	*Inactive* against *Aspergillus* spp., Zygomycetes, and *Fusarium* spp.	*Inactive* against dimorphic fungi and dermatophytes

[1] *A. terreus* and *A. flavus* can be less susceptible.
[2] *Histoplasma capsulatum, Blastomyces dermatitidis, Coccidioides immitis, Sporothrix schenckii,* and *Paracoccidioides brasiliensis*

- *Liposomal amphotericin (Ambisome®):* amphotericin is encapsulated in phospholipid-containing liposomes.
- *Amphotericin lipid complex (Abelcet®):* amphotericin and two phospholipids, which form ribbon-like structures.
- *Amphotericin colloidal dispersion (Amphocil®):* amphotericin and cholesterol sulphate, which form small disc-like particles (no longer available in the UK).

Of the three, **liposomal amphotericin** is the most widely used and supported by the most evidence, including studies looking at extended dosing intervals (e.g. three times a week) due to its long half-life. Doses are administered by IV infusion to reduce the risk of toxicity (Table 11.21–22).

Unwanted effects

Amphotericin causes vasoconstriction of the renal arterioles, resulting in decreased glomerular and renal tubular blood flow, and impaired renal function. Risk can be reduced through adequate hydration and close monitoring of renal function, regardless of formulation. Although generally reversible, renal impairment can cause permanent destruction of renal tubular cells, the tubular basement membrane, and loss of functioning nephron units. As lipid formulations achieve lower concentrations within the renal tissue the risk of nephrotoxic effects are reduced.

Renal tubular damage and disruption of membrane transport commonly leads to renal wasting of potassium (hypokalaemia), magnesium (hypomagnesaemia), and bicarbonate (renal tubular acidosis), so electrolytes should be closely monitored and supplemented where necessary. Renal production of erythropoietin is also decreased potentially giving rise to mild normochromic, normocytic anaemia, thus FBC should be monitored on treatment. LFTs should also be monitored, due to the risk of deranged LFTs.

Infusion-related side effects include phlebitis, particularly where a peripheral vein is used and/or insufficient dilution is carried out; as well as fever, chills, and rigors,

Table 11.22 Common clinical indications and pharmacokinetics for the polyene antifungals

Antifungal	Common clinical infections	Pharmacokinetics
Amphotericin (IV infusion)	Invasive aspergillosis Invasive candidiasis Empirical treatment in neutropenia Cryptococcal meningitis and disseminated cryptococcosis Dimorphic infections Mucormycosis	Minimal oral absorption CSF levels 5% of serum levels Binds to tissue cell membranes and re-enters circulation prolonging action Liposomal formulations accumulates in higher levels in liver, spleen, and lung, but less in kidneys Predominantly excreted unchanged in bile and urine
Nystatin (topical)	Superficial *Candida* infections	Currently only available topically

Table 11.23 Spectrum of antifungal activity of terbinafine

Drug	Yeasts	Moulds	Other
Terbinafine	*Candida* spp. *Inactive* against *Cryptococcus* spp.	Activity against some *Aspergillus* spp. *Inactive* against Zygomycetes, *Fusarium* spp.	Dermatophytes Some dimorphic fungi *Inactive* against *Pityriasis versicolor*

which can last up to an hour. The risk of reactions are reduced through the use of liposomal formulations, slowing the rate of infusion or by premedicating with IV **hydrocortisone** and **paracetamol**. Rapid infusions can also increase the risk of cardiac arrhythmias.

Due to the risk of anaphylaxis, a test dose of 1 mg over 10 minutes is recommended prior to the first infusion, and the patient carefully observed for at least 30 minutes before giving a therapeutic dose.

Drug interactions

Concurrent treatment with other nephrotoxic drugs, such as aminoglycosides and **ciclosporin** increases the risk of renal impairment. Ventricular arrhythmias can occur with concomitant administration of some cytotoxic drugs. Risk of electrolyte disturbance and hypokalaemia is increased with concurrent treatment with corticosteroids, **digoxin**, and some diuretics.

Terbinafine

Terbinafine inhibits the enzyme squalene epoxidase, thereby impairing synthesis of ergosterol, which is the main sterol in fungal cell membranes

Mechanism of action

Inhibition of fungal ergosterol and accumulation of intracellular squalene, impairs fungal cell membrane function and cell wall synthesis (Table 11.23).

Prescribing

Terbinafine is administered orally or topically depending on extent of infection (see Table 11.24). Treatment should be continued beyond eradication of infection to reduce the risk of recurrence.

Unwanted effects

Terbinafine is generally well tolerated, although abnormal LFTs, exacerbation of psoriasis and allergic skin reactions may occur rarely. It can also trigger drug-induced lupus erythematosus, so caution is advised in autoimmune disease. Terbinafine should be avoided during pregnancy and when breastfeeding.

Drug interactions

Potent inducers of the hepatic CYP 2C9 and 3A4, such as **rifampicin**, reduce **terbinafine** levels by 100%, while inhibitors, such as **fluconazole**, can increase levels. Furthermore, terbinafine itself inhibits CYP2D6, leading to

Table 11.24 Common clinical conditions and pharmacokinetics of terbinafine

Antifungal	Common clinical conditions	Pharmacokinetics
Terbinafine (oral)	Dermatophyte infections of the skin Onychomycosis	Excellent oral absorption Widely distributed (lipophilic)
Terbinafine (topical)	Dermatophyte infections of the skin Cutaneous candidiasis *Pityriasis versicolor*	Accumulates in skin, nail and adipose tissue Metabolized by the liver

raised levels of substrates for this pathway, e.g. some tri-cyclic antidepressants, SSRIs and anti-arrhythmics.

Further reading

Andes D (2013) Optimizing antifungal choice and adminis-tration. *Current Medical Research Opinion* 29(Suppl. 4), 13–18.

Campion EW (2015) Invasive candidiasis. *New England Journal of Medicine* 373(15), 1445–56.

Chen SC, Slavin MA, Sorrell TC. (2011) Echinocandin antifungal drugs in fungal infections: a comparison. *Drugs* 71(1), 11–41.

Frothingham R (2002) Lipid formulations of amphotericin B for empirical treatment of fever and neutropenia. *Clinical Infectious Diseases* 35(7), 896–7.

Lipp HP (2010) Clinical pharmacodynamics and pharma-cokinetic of the antifungal extended-spectrum triazole posaconazole: an overview. *British Journal of Clinical Pharmacology* 70(4), 471–80.

Majoros L, Kardos G (2008) Fungicidal activity of azole antifungal agents. *Anti-Infective Agents in Medicinal Chemistry* 7(2), 118–25.

Purkins L, Wood N, Greenhalgh K, et al. (2003) The pharma-cokinetics and safety of intravenous voriconazole—a novel wide-spectrum antifungal agent. *British Journal of Clinical Pharmacology* 56(Suppl. 1), 2–9.

Rex JH, Stevens DA (2010) *Systemic Antifungal Agents*. In: Mandell GL, Bennett JE, Dolin R (Eds) *Principles and Practice of Infectious Diseases*, 7th edn, pp. 549–63. Philadelphia, PA: Churchill Livingstone.

Richardson MD, Warnock DW (2012) *Fungal infection: diag-nosis and management*, 4th edn. Oxford: Wiley-Blackwell Publishing.

Richardson MD (2005) Changing patterns and trends in systemic fungal infections. *Journal of Antimicrobial Chemotherapy* 56(Suppl. 1), i5–i11.

Vermes A, Guchelaar HJ, Dankert J (2000) Flucytosine: a re-view of its pharmacology, clinical indications, pharmacokin-etics, toxicity and drug interactions. *Journal of Antimicrobial Chemotherapy* 46(2) 171–9.

Warnock DW (2010) Antifungal agents. In: Finch RG, Greenwood D, Norrby SR, Whitley RJ (Eds) *Antibiotic and Chemotherapy*, 9th edn, pp. 366–82. Edinburgh: Elsevier Saunders.

Zonios DI, Bennett JE (2008) Update on azole antifungals. *Seminars in Respiratory Critical Care Medicine* 29(2), 198–210.

Guidelines

Nelson M, Dockrell D, Edwards S, et al. (2011) British HIV Association and British Infection Association guidelines for the treatment of opportunistic infection in HIV-seropositive individuals 2011. *HIV Medicine* 12(Suppl. 2), 1.

Pappas PG, Kauffman CA, Andes D, et al. (2015) Clinical prac-tice guidelines for the management of candidiasis: 2016 up-date by the Infectious Diseases Society of America. *Clinical Infectious Diseases* 48(5), 503–35.

Patterson TF, Thompson III GR, Denning DW, et al. (2016) Practice Guidelines for the Diagnosis and Management of Aspergillosis: 2016 Update by the Infectious Diseases Society of America. *Clinical Infectious Diseases* 63(4), e1-60.

Perfect JR, Dismukes WE, Dromer F, et al. (2010) Clinical prac-tice guidelines for the management of cryptococcal disease: 2010 update by the Infectious Diseases Society of America. *Clinical Infectious Diseases* 50(3), 291–322.

11.3 Viral infection

Viruses are small infectious agents that require the presence of intact host cells in order to replicate. Viral genomes exist in either DNA or RNA form. Unlike bacteria, they do not replicate by binary fission, but undergo a complex life cycle involving attachment and entrance into the target cell, disassembly, replication of their genomes and proteins, followed by assembly and release of viral particles. Antiviral drugs target essential steps in the viral life cycle.

The number of antiviral drugs in routine clinical use, although increasing in recent years, is small in comparison to other antimicrobial agents. This is largely due to the unique challenges in their development, such as targeting specific viral processes without unacceptable toxicity to human cells, and the relative difficulty in manipulating viruses experimentally.

HIV infection

Despite advances in knowledge on HIV/AIDS, the current global burden remains high, with an estimated 35 million people worldwide living with the disease in 2013, and 1.5 million AIDS-related deaths. Sub-Saharan Africa remains disproportionately affected by the HIV epidemic, accounting for nearly 71% of cases worldwide (WHO data). There are an estimated 107 800 people living with the disease in the UK (PHE data).

Human immunodeficiency virus (HIV) is a single-stranded, enveloped RNA virus of the family Retroviridae. Two types of HIV virus have been identified, HIV-1 and HIV-2, which share identical modes of transmission and clinical manifestations, although HIV-2 is more slowly progressive. The vast majority of infections world-wide are caused by HIV-1, with HIV-2 being largely confined to West Africa.

The HIV virus infects essential components of the cell-mediated immune system, particularly $CD4^+$ Helper T lymphocytes. Progressive destruction of these lymphocytes puts the host at risk of life-threatening opportunistic infections (e.g. PJP) and malignancies (e.g. Kaposi's sarcoma), leading to the condition known as acquired immunodeficiency syndrome (AIDS). AIDS was first described in 1981, in homosexual men and injection drug users, though the causative virus was not isolated until 1983, and named HIV in 1986. Initial treatment strategies centred on prevention and treatment of AIDS-related opportunistic infections or malignancies, until **zidovudine** was licensed in 1987. Monotherapy with zidovudine, however, led to rapid emergence of viral resistance; thus once the protease inhibitors were introduced in 1996, combination therapy became the accepted strategy and ultimately highly active antiretroviral therapy (HAART) was introduced, utilizing multiple classes, now referred to as combination antiretroviral therapy (cART).

HIV replication

A basic understanding of the steps in HIV replication is essential to appreciate the mechanism of action of antiretroviral agents and their potential targets (see also Figure 11.5):

- *Step 1—attachment*: proteins on the viral envelope (gp120) bind to the CD4 molecule on the surface of helper T lymphocytes. Co-receptors (either CCR5 or CXCR4) are required to facilitate binding and entry into the cell (*entry inhibitors*).

- *Step 2—membrane fusion*: the viral envelope fuses with the cell membrane, enabling viral particle contents, including the viral RNA genome and reverse transcriptase, integrase and protease enzymes, to enter the cell (*fusion inhibitors*).

- *Step 3—reverse transcriptase*: viral RNA is converted into DNA using reverse transcriptase (*nucleoside/ nucleotide reverse transcriptase inhibitors* and *non-nucleoside reverse transcriptase inhibitors*)

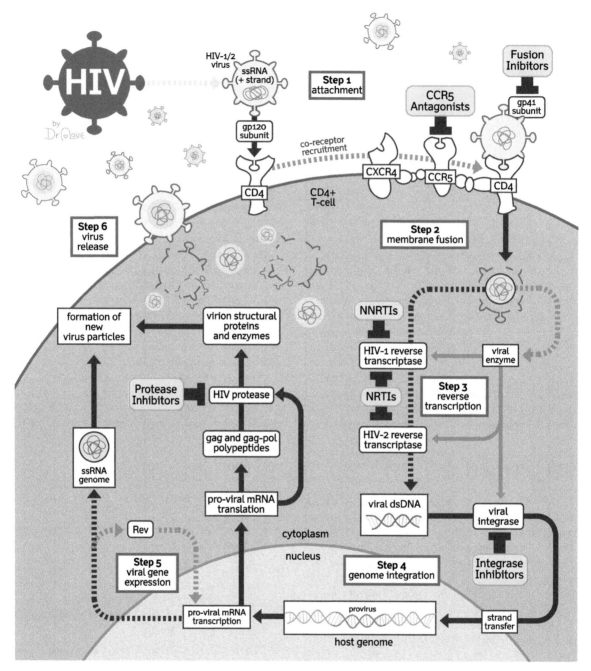

Figure 11.5 HIV: summary of relevant pathways and drug targets.

- *Step 4—genome transcription*: the transcribed DNA is transported into the cell nucleus, where the enzyme integrase facilitates integration into host cell DNA (*integrase inhibitors*). This integrated viral DNA is known as a provirus.

- *Step 5—viral gene expression*: using the host cell's own machinery, proviral DNA is transcribed into new viral RNA, which is then translated into viral polypeptide chains in the cytoplasm. These are then cleaved by protease enzymes to form smaller chains, necessary for the formation of mature virus particles (*protease inhibitors*).

- *Step 6—virus release*: these smaller chains combine with viral RNA at the cell's outer membrane to form new virus particles, which are released to infect other host cells and the viral life cycle is repeated.

Management of HIV

HIV management is complex and should always be led by a physician experienced in HIV medicine. The remarkable efficacy of combination antiretroviral therapy (cART), where available, has transformed HIV into a chronic disease; changing the focus from acute management of fatal complications, to managing non-HIV specific co-morbidities, such as cardiovascular disease or malignancy. It is therefore important for the non-HIV specialist to have a basic knowledge of HIV management, as patients living with HIV will be seen in a wide variety of clinical settings and specialties.

The six main classes of antiretroviral drugs (ARVs) in current use target different steps in the viral replication pathway (see Table 11.25). cART treatment is intended to suppress viral replication in order to maintain immunity and prevent HIV-related opportunistic infections and malignancies, although it does not eliminate the virus, so treatment is lifelong.

When to start treatment for HIV infection

The optimal time for initiating cART remains an area of active debate and research. The benefits of therapy such as preventing disease progression and maintaining cell-mediated immunity, must be balanced against the risk of drug toxicity and developing drug resistance. Historically numerous factors were taken into consideration, including patient's co-morbidities (both HIV-related and non-HIV related), CD4 count, and transmission risk, however now all patients are routinely offered therapy regardless of this. Patients starting treatment must be counselled on

Table 11.25 Main classes and target mechanism of anti-retroviral drugs

Class	Drugs
Nucleoside/nucleotide reverse transcriptase inhibitors (NRTIs)	Abacavir (ABC), didanosine (ddI), emtricitabine (FTC), lamivudine (3TC), stavudine (d4T), tenofovir (TDF), and zidovudine (AZT)
Non-nucleoside reverse transcriptase inhibitors (NNRTIs)	Efavirenz (EFV), etravirine (TMC-125), nevirapine (NVP), and rilpivirine (TMC-278)
Protease inhibitors (PIs)	Atazanavir (ATV), darunavir (DRV), fosamprenavir (FPV), indinavir (IDV), lopinavir with ritonavir (LPV/r), ritonavir (RTV), saquinavir (SQV), and tipranavir (TPV)
Integrase inhibitors	Dolutegravir (DTG), elvitegravir (EVG), and raltegravir (RAL)
Entry inhibitors	Maraviroc (MVC)
Fusion inhibitors	Enfuvirtide
Fixed-dose combinations	Abacavir/lamivudine (Kivexa®)
	Abacavir/lamivudine/zidovudine (Trizivir®)
	Emtricitabine/tenofovir (Truvada®)
	Lamivudine/zidovudine (Combivir®)
Single-tablet regimens	Dolutegravir/abacavir/lamivudine (Triumeq®)
	Efavirenz/emtricitabine/tenofovir (Atripla®)
	Elvitegravir/cobicistat/emtricitabine/tenofovir (Stribild®)
	Rilpivirine/emtricitabine/tenofovir (Eviplera®)

Box 11.2 Indications for initiation of treatment

- In all adults living with HIV regardless of WHO clinical stage and at any CD4 cell count
- Adults with severe or advanced HIV clinical disease (WHO clinical stage 3 or 4) and adults with CD4 count ≤350 cells/mm³
- In all pregnant and breastfeeding women living with HIV regardless of WHO clinical stage and at any CD4 cell count and continued lifelong
- In all TB patients living with HIV regardless of CD4 cell count

the consequences of poor adherence and be willing to commit, as missed doses and discontinuation can lead to rapid emergence of resistance.

Short courses of ARVs are sometimes used to prevent HIV infection, e.g. post-exposure prophylaxis (PEP) following needle-stick injury or high-risk sexual encounter, or in infants born to infected mothers to minimize the risk of vertical transmission. There is also ongoing research into 'pre-exposure prophylaxis' (PrEP), which involves giving ART to HIV-negative patients at high risk of HIV acquisition and transmission in order to protect them from infection.

Choice of regimen

The fundamental principle of cART is the use of three drugs with at least two separate sites of action given in combination. Generally, initial combinations include a nucleoside/nucleotide reverse transcriptase inhibitors (NRTI) 'backbone' of 2 NRTIs with a third agent, consisting of a non-nucleoside/nucleotide reverse transcriptase inhibitor (NNRTI), a protease inhibitor ('boosted' with **ritonavir**—see 'Protease inhibitors'), or an integrase inhibitor. Choice of regimen depends on multiple factors including patient preference, baseline viral resistance profile, comorbidities, and concurrent medications. With treatment failure due to resistance, regimens can become more complex, based broadly on sensitivities. Progress in treatment has seen significant reductions in pill burdens, with many treatments available in combination tablets (see 'Practical

Prescribing: examples of first-line cART combination tablet regimens').

PRACTICAL PRESCRIBING

Examples of HAART combination tablet regimens

- Atripla® (tenofovir + emtricitabine + efavirenz).
- Triumeq® (abacavir + lamivudine + dolutegravir).
- Truvada® (tenofovir + emtricitabine) + atazanavir + ritonavir.
- Kivexa® (abacavir + lamivudine) + darunavir + ritonavir.
- Truvada® (tenofovir + emtricitabine) + raltegravir.

Drug classes used in management of HIV

Nucleoside/nucleotide reverse transcriptase inhibitors

The NRTIs inhibit viral replication by binding to the HIV reverse transcriptase enzyme, preventing the addition of other nucleosides to the growing DNA chain. For example, abacavir, emtricitabine, lamivudine, stavudine, tenofovir, and zidovudine.

Mechanism of action

NRTIs are nucleoside or nucleotide analogues that inhibit reverse transcription, i.e. where viral RNA is transcribed into DNA. They are phosphorylated intracellularly to their active triphosphate forms, which compete with other nucleosides for binding sites on the viral reverse transcriptase enzyme. Once incorporated into viral DNA, they act as chain terminators, preventing the addition of other nucleosides, thereby inhibiting DNA synthesis and halting viral replication.

NRTIs also interfere with DNA synthesis in host cell mitochondriae. The enzyme polymerase-gamma is required for mitochondrial DNA replication. Like reverse transcriptase, this enzyme can incorporate nucleoside/nucleotide analogues into mitochondrial DNA chains, suppressing mitochondrial DNA synthesis, leading to mitochondrial dysfunction and cell death. It is believed this mechanism accounts for many of the side effects associated with NRTIs, such as lactic acidosis and lipoatrophy.

Prescribing

NRTIs in current use are usually prescribed as fixed dose combinations, such as Truvada® (**tenofovir** + **emtricitabine**) with its superior virological efficacy at high viral loads, or Kivexa® (**abacavir** + **lamivudine**) where baseline viral load is < 100 000 copies/mL. Truvada® is also the preferred backbone in patients with hepatitis B co-infection, as tenofovir and emtricitabine have good activity against both HIV and hepatitis B. More recently Triumeq® containing abacavir and lamivudine with the integrase inhibitor, dolutegravir has been introduced, and is increasingly being used first line, with its convenient one tablet OD formulation.

Both Truvada® and Kivexa® are also taken OD, with or without food. As all NRTIs apart from abacavir are predominantly renally excreted, dose-adjustment may be necessary in the case of renal impairment.

Zidovidine is now rarely used except in pregnancy or as prophylaxis in exposed neonates. Other early NRTIs such as **didanosine** and **stavudine** were associated with significant mitochondrial and hepatic toxicity, and are no longer widely used, except in low-income countries where there are fewer alternatives available.

Unwanted effects

GI disturbance is a common side effect to NRTI treatment, particularly in the first few weeks of treatment. They are also known to be hepatotoxic, thus LFT monitoring is recommended. NRTIs can also cause lactic acidosis, which may manifest as fatigue, muscle weakness, abdominal pain, and nausea and vomiting, and can be associated with hepatic steatosis with rapid deterioration in liver function. This rare, but potentially life-threatening complication is more common with the older NRTIs (i.e. **stavudine**, **didanosine**, and **zidovudine**) than the newer, favoured agents (**tenofovir**, **lamivudine**, **emtricitabine**, and **abacavir**), which abacavir also much better tolerated than the older agents are generally better tolerated.

Lipodystrophy, a syndrome of fat redistribution that may involve lipoatrophy, lipohypertrophy or a mixture of the two, has been associated with NRTIs, particularly stavudine and zidovudine. Didanosine and stavudine can also cause a severe peripheral neuropathy, and zidovudine is known to induce myelosuppression, most commonly manifesting as a macrocytic anaemia.

Abacavir treatment is specifically associated with hypersensitivity reactions (see 'Prescribing warning: hypersensitivity reaction to abacavir') and increased risk of myocardial infarction. Patients with a 10-year cardiovascular risk greater than 20% should not be treated with abacavir.

PRESCRIBING WARNING

Hypersensitivity reaction to abacavir

- Abacavir is associated with severe hypersensitivity reactions leading to fever, rash, GI disturbance, and respiratory symptoms.
- Reactions tend to occur in the first 6 weeks of treatment.
- Risk increased with HLA B*57:01 genotype, prescreening is therefore carried out and treatment avoided in patients shown to have the allele (about 5% of population).

Tenofovir has been associated with renal toxicity, including reports of acute and chronic renal failure, tubular dysfunction, and Fanconi syndrome, a rare complication of tenofovir therapy, especially in patients with normal renal function. As the risk of nephrotoxicity is increased in impaired renal function, baseline measurements are taken, and alternatives considered in impairment. Tenofovir should also be avoided in patients who are awaiting, or who have undergone renal transplantation.

Drug interactions

As NRTIs are neither metabolized by hepatic cytochrome P450 enzymes, nor inducers/inhibitors of these enzymes, the risk of clinically significant drug interactions with this class is low.

Non-nucleoside/nucleotide reverse transcriptase inhibitors

NNRTIs induce a conformational change in the HIV reverse transcriptase enzyme that prevents nucleosides from binding to it. For example, efavirenz, nevirapine, rilpivirine, and etravirine.

Mechanism of action

NNRTIs, although a chemically diverse group, share the same mechanism of action, binding non-competitively to a hydrophobic pocket (known as the NNRTI-binding pocket) near the catalytic site of the HIV-1 reverse transcriptase enzyme. This induces a conformational change in the enzyme, which prevents naturally occurring nucleosides from binding. As their site of action is distinct from NRTIs, they can be used in combination as part of a cART regimen.

First-generation agents include **nevirapine** and **efavirenz**, both of which are susceptible to resistance where a single mutation in viral reverse transcriptase alters the NNRTI-binding pocket. Second generation agents (**etravirine** and **rilpivirine**) were developed to overcome this and may retain their potency in the case of first generation resistance, although there is often cross resistance.

HIV-2 is innately resistant to NNRTIs as structural differences in the NNRTI-binding pocket of its reverse transcriptase enzyme, prevents NNRTIs from binding.

Prescribing

NNRTIs are usually prescribed as a 'third agent' in combination with two NRTIs. **Efavirenz** is currently the preferred first-line NNRTI, but **rilpivirine** is an acceptable alternative where viral loads are <100 000 copies/mL; as higher viral loads are associated with increased virological failure rates. **Nevirapine** is considered a second-line third agent because of CD4 count restrictions (see 'Prescribing warning: Nevirapine') and higher discontinuation rates due to poor tolerance.

NNRTIS are taken OD, except **etravirine**, which must be taken BD, and rilpivirine must be taken with a normal caloric meal (approximately 533 kcal) for adequate absorption.

NNRTIs have long half-lives, which should be taken into consideration when treatment is discontinued to avoid to a period of functional NNRTI monotherapy, where subtherapeutic drug levels increases the risk of developing class resistance.

Unwanted effects

As a class, NNRTIs are commonly associated with rash, particularly **nevirapine**, which can rarely manifest as Stevens–Johnson syndrome and toxic epidermal necrolysis. The risk of toxicity is lower with the second generation agents, although rilpivirine is associated with QT prolongation. **Efavirenz** is commonly associated with neuropsychiatric effects (see 'Prescribing warning: neuropsychiatric reactions with efavirenz') and although these usually only last for 2–4 weeks, this can limit its use.

PRESCRIBING WARNING

Nevirapine

- Severe, life-threatening hepatotoxicity and skin reactions can occur, particularly in the first 18 weeks of therapy.
- Risk is highest in women with a CD4 count >250 and in men with a CD4 >400, and should be avoided.
- Patients should be regularly monitored for severe reactions in the first 18 weeks of therapy.

Elevated liver enzymes are common with NNRTIs and hepatotoxicity a relatively frequent complication of **nevirapine** use, particularly in patients with more intact immunity (see 'Prescribing warning: nevirapine').

PRESCRIBING WARNING

Neuropsychiatric reactions with efavirenz

- Efavirenz has good CNS penetration, commonly leading to neuropsychiatric effects such as drowsiness, sleep disturbance, dizziness, impaired concentration, and aggravation of underlying psychiatric disorders.
- As food increases absorption, doses should be taken on an empty stomach at bedtime.
- Avoid in a history of mental illness.

Drug interactions

NNRTIs are metabolized by hepatic cytochrome (CYP450) 3A enzymes, therefore have the potential for numerous drug–drug interactions, which can lead to treatment failure and development of resistance to valuable treatment. It is therefore essential that any new therapy be checked prior to initiation and any potential interactions appropriately managed/avoided.

In particular, potent inducers of CYP3A4 e.g. **rifampicin** can reduce levels of **efavirenz** and **nevirapine** to sub-therapeutic levels. Concurrent use should ideally be avoided or, where rifampicin is deemed essential, patients closely monitored. Co-administration of nevirapine with rifampicin-containing TB regimens is associated with increased risk of hepatotoxicity so is not recommended. Conversely, potent inhibitors (e.g. azole antifungals) can lead to high NNRTI levels and increased toxicity.

As **rilpivirine** relies on an acidic gastric environment for adequate absorption, proton pump inhibitors should be avoided and other acid supressing drugs (e.g. histamine antagonists, antacids), spaced in time. Rilpivirine should not be co-administered with other drugs that cause QT prolongation.

Protease inhibitors

Protease inhibitors (PIs) prevent viral maturation by inhibiting the HIV protease enzyme, necessary for the formation of essential structural proteins and enzymes. Examples include atazanavir, darunavir, fosamprenavir, lopinavir, and ritonavir.

Mechanism of action

PIs are potent ARVs that bind to and inhibit the activity of HIV protease, which cleaves viral gag and gag-pol polypeptides into structural proteins and enzymes necessary for viral maturation. They are considered to have a higher genetic barrier to resistance than NNRTIs and integrase inhibitors, as multiple resistance mutations are usually required before activity is lost.

As a class, PIs undergo hepatic metabolism via the CYP 3A4 enzymes. **Ritonavir**, one of the earliest PIs, is no longer used for its antiviral effect, but given at sub-therapeutic dose (100 mg or 200 mg) to increase or 'boost' plasma levels of other PIs, enabling OD dosing.

Prescribing

The currently preferred first-line PIs are **atazanavir** and **darunavir**, both given with low-dose **ritonavir** to 'boost' levels. **Lopinavir** may be given as an alternative in treatment-naïve patients and is the only PI formulated in combination tablet with ritonavir (Kaletra®). Atazanavir, darunavir, and ritonavir (when used for boosting) can all be taken OD. Kaletra®, however, is usually taken as two tablets BD. PIs are generally given alongside two NRTIs in first-line regimens and are considered to have equivalent efficacy to **efavirenz** in terms of virological suppression and safety. The other PIs are rarely used due to inferior efficacy and tolerability.

Unwanted effects

The most notable side effects associated with the PIs are gastrointestinal disturbance and metabolic complications. Nausea, vomiting and diarrhoea are common and can be treatment limiting, particularly with the older PIs; the currently preferred PIs (**darunavir/ritonavir** and **atazanavir/ritonavir**) are associated with less GI disturbance.

Metabolic complications include hypercholesterolaemia, hypertriglyceridaemia, lipodystrophy, insulin resistance and type 2 diabetes mellitus. The aetiology of these sequelae is multifactorial, and thought to involve inhibition of apolipoprotein B degradation, inhibition of insulin receptor signalling pathways, glucocorticoid hypersensitivity, and interference with the GLUT-4 protein, which transports glucose into cells.

PIs are also associated with skin reactions ranging from a mild-moderate rash (usually appearing in the first 4 weeks of therapy, and resolving without stopping the medication) to less frequently, severe rashes, including Stevens–Johnson syndrome, requiring immediate discontinuation. Other side effects include increased bleeding risk in haemophiliacs and hepatic dysfunction, the latter more common in patients with chronic hepatitis B or C infection.

Cardiovascular toxicity to PIs include cardiac conduction abnormalities (e.g. PR prolongation with atazanavir and PR/QT interval prolongation with **lopinavir/ritonavir**) and increased risk of MI with lopinavir/ritonavir use. The latter should therefore be used with caution in patients with a 10-year cardiovascular risk greater than 20%.

Atazanavir commonly causes unconjugated hyperbilirubinaemia, which although not of clinical concern, the appearance of icteric skin and/or sclerae may be cosmetically unacceptable in some patients. Darunavir and **fosamprenavir** contain a sulfonamide moiety, so should be used with caution in patients with significant sulfonamide allergies. Lopinavir/ritonavir is also rarely associated with pancreatitis.

Drug interactions

All PIs have the potential for multiple drug interactions, primarily because of the potent CYP450 inhibiting properties of **ritonavir**, even at low boosting doses, which increases the levels of many drugs, e.g. **simvastatin**, **amiodarone**, corticosteroids, etc. Furthermore, drugs that induce CYP3A4 enzymes, e.g. **rifampicin** and **St. John's Wort**, can significantly reduce levels of PIs, leading to treatment failure and increase the risk of resistance. It is essential that prescribers check any concurrent therapy prior to initiation

Proton pump inhibitors should not be co-administered with **atazanavir**, as the increased gastric pH can significantly affect its solubility and absorption.

Integrase inhibitors

Integrase inhibitors (INIs) block integration of viral DNA into the host cell chromosome through inhibition of the HIV integrase enzyme. For example, elvitegravir, dolutegravir, and raltegravir.

Mechanism of action

Integrase combines with the newly formed viral DNA and cellular proteins to form a 'pre-integration complex' (PIC), which enters the host cell nucleus. Subsequent integration of viral DNA into the host cell chromosome is catalysed by the integrase enzyme, in a process known as 'strand transfer'. Integrase inhibitors block this process and, hence, are sometimes referred to as 'integrase strand transfer inhibitors'.

Prescribing

The INIs are a relatively new class of ARVs, used as an alternative third agents alongside two NRTIs in first-line therapy, as evidence demonstrates equivalent efficacy to currently preferred NNRTIs and boosted PIs. All INIs share the ability to achieve rapid reductions in HIV viral load.

Raltegravir, the first of the three INIs licensed for use if generally well-tolerated with few drug interactions, although due to its shorter terminal half-life, requires BD administration. **Elvitegravir** is formulated with **cobicistat**, a CYP3A4 inhibitor, essential for achieving therapeutic concentrations enabling OD administration, but with no anti-HIV activity of its own. Elvitegravir is currently only available in a single tablet formulation containing cobicistat, **tenofovir**, and **emtricitabine** (Stribild®). **Dolutegravir**, the newest INI, is used in combination therapy in both treatment-naïve and treatment-experienced patients. It is effective with Truvada® and **abacavir**, regardless of VL and can be given OD without boosting. It is also available in a combined tablet with abacavir and **lamivudine** (as Triumeq®).

Raltegravir and elvitegravir demonstrate a relatively low genetic barrier to resistance, with a high degree of cross-resistance between these two agents. Dolutegravir appears to have a higher barrier to resistance, and may retain activity against some viruses with mutations associated with raltegravir and elvitegravir resistance.

Unwanted effects

Raltegravir is generally well-tolerated, with GI side effects such as nausea and diarrhoea most commonly reported. Other side effects can include rash (rarely Stevens–Johnson syndrome) elevations in creatine phosphokinase levels and rarely, rhabdomyolysis. Hepatotoxicity can also occur, particularly in patients with underlying chronic liver disease.

As **elvitegravir** is currently only available in a combination tablet formulation with **cobicistat**, **tenofovir**, and **emtricitabine**, it is hard to attribute side effects to any one component. Elvitegravir can cause rash and insomnia, while cobicistat may induce GI upset such as nausea and diarrhoea.

Cobicistat can inhibit active tubular secretion of creatinine, without affecting glomerular function, which can lead to elevations in serum creatinine. That said, Stribild® should be avoided in patients with creatinine clearance of less than 70 mL/min as the cobicistat/tenofovir combination may increase the risk of nephrotoxicity.

The most common side effects to **dolutegravir** include nausea, diarrhoea, and headache. It has rarely been associated with hypersensitivity reactions manifesting as a rash with features that may include fever, eosinophilia, and hepatic dysfunction.

Drug interactions

Use of antacids with any of the current INIs, can significantly reduce their absorption, due to the chelating effect of the polyvalent cations magnesium and aluminium. Hence, co-administration should be avoided.

Cobicistat is a CYP450 inhibitor and has the potential for multiple drug interactions and similar contraindications to the **ritonavir**-boosted PIs, although **raltegravir** and **dolutegravir** are metabolized by hepatic glucoronidation.

CCR5 antagonists

CCR5 antagonists prevent HIV from binding to the CCR5 co-receptor, blocking viral entry into the host cell. For example, maraviroc.

Mechanism of action

The chemokine co-receptor 5 (CCR5) and the CXC chemokine receptor 4 (CXCR4) on the surface of CD4 cells act as co-receptors, in conjunction with the CD4 receptor, for HIV cell entry. Viruses that use the CCR5 receptor are known as 'M-tropic' or 'R5' viruses, while those that use the CXCR4 receptor are referred to as 'T-tropic' or 'X4' viruses. Some viruses use both co-receptors for cell entry, and are called 'dual/mixed tropic viruses'.

Maraviroc, the only drug in its class, binds to the CCR5 receptor, preventing attachment of the HIV envelope glycoprotein gp120, thus blocking viral entry into the cell. It is not effective against T-tropic or dual/mixed tropic viruses, therefore a 'tropism assay' is performed on blood plasma to determine which co-receptor is used by the virus prior to initiating treatment.

Prescribing

Maraviroc is used as a second-line agent in treatment-experienced patients, usually when virological failure has occurred due to multiple-resistance mutations. It is only used in patients with M-tropic viruses (see 'CCR5 antagonists, Mechanism of action', above), in combination with at least one other fully active agent. There is a relative absence of safety and efficacy data with maraviroc compared with current first-line agents and it requires BD administration.

Unwanted effects

Adverse effects include GI disturbance, fever, dizziness, skin rash, cough, and upper respiratory tract infections. Hepatotoxicity can also occur.

Drug interactions

Maraviroc is metabolized in the liver via CYP3A4 enzymes, so levels can be affected by inducers (e.g. **rifampicin**, **phenytoin**, etc.) and inhibitors (e.g. **clarithromycin**, PIs—except **tipranivir**) of this pathway, and dose alterations required.

Fusion inhibitors

Fusion inhibitors stop HIV from entering the host cell by preventing fusion of viral and cell membranes. For example, enfuvirtide.

Mechanism of action

The only licensed fusion inhibitor **enfuvirtide**, is a synthetic peptide that prevents viral entry into the host cell by binding to the gp41 subunit of the viral envelope glycoprotein, and preventing fusion of viral and cell membranes.

Prescribing

Enfuvirtide is administered BD as a SC injection, and reserved for treatment-experienced patients intolerant to other regimens, or those with resistant infection, in combination with other ARV agents.

Unwanted effects

Injection site reactions such as pain, induration, and erythema are common. Other potential side-effects include GI disturbance, fatigue, and insomnia, with hypersensitivity reactions also reported infrequently. There are no known clinically significant drug interactions with this agent; although the need for BD injections, combined with the high frequency of local adverse effects, has significantly limited its use in clinical practice.

Human herpes viruses

There are eight herpes viruses that naturally infect humans—herpes simplex virus types 1 and 2 (HSV-1 and HSV-2), cytomegalovirus (CMV), Epstein–Barr virus (EBV), and human herpes viruses 6, 7, and 8 (HHV-6, HHV-7, HHV-8). Collectively, they have a world-wide distribution, the majority of adults being infected with HSV-1, CMV, EBV, HHV-6, and HHV-7 during their lifetime. HSV-2 and HHV-8 have a more variable geographical distribution, with low seroprevalence in the UK.

All HHV remain latent in host cells following primary infection and have the potential for reactivation. Primary infections with HHVs tend to be more severe, and manifestations can be severe and life-threatening in neonates and immunocompromised patients, e.g. transplant recipients or in people living with HIV. Clinical manifestations are illustrated in Table 11.26.

Antiviral therapy is only clinically effective against HSV, VZV, and CMV, and all agents share the same general mechanism of action, i.e. inhibit viral DNA polymerase necessary for viral replication (Figure 11.6).

Drug classes used in management of human herpes viruses

Guanosine analogues

Guanosine analogues require phosphorylation to their active triphosphate forms by viral and cellular enzymes. They subsequently inhibit viral DNA polymerase by competing with guanosine triphosphate for incorporation into the growing DNA chain and causing premature termination. Examples include aciclovir, valaciclovir, penciclovir, famciclovir, ganciclovir, and valganciclovir.

Table 11.26 Clinical manifestations of human herpes viruses

Virus	Clinical manifestations	Antiviral treatment
HSV-1 and HSV-2	*Cutaneous*: vesicular rash, Herpetic whitlow *Orofacial*: pharyngitis, gingivostomatitis, herpes labialis ('cold sores') *Genital*: Painful vesicles and ulcers, inguinal lymphadenopathy, fever *Neurological*: Meningitis, Encephalitis, Transverse Myelitis *Ocular*: keratoconjunctivitis *Visceral*: oesophagitis, hepatitis, pneumonitis	Aciclovir, valaciclovir, famciclovir, ganciclovir, foscarnet, cidofovir
VZV	Chickenpox Herpes zoster (shingles)	Aciclovir, valaciclovir, famciclovir, ganciclovir, foscarnet
CMV	*Infectious mononucleosis*: fever, pharyngitis, lymphadenopathy, atypical lymphocytosis, hepatitis, rash *Immunocompromised patients*: retinitis, pneumonitis, colitis, encephalitis, thrombocytopenia, leucopaenia	Ganciclovir, valganciclovir, foscarnet, cidofovir
EBV	*Infectious mononucleosis*: *Post-infective complications*: haemolytic anaemia, splenic rupture, Guillan–Barré syndrome, encephalitis, malignancies (Burkitt's lymphoma, lymphoproliferative disease in the immunosuppressed)	None
HHV-6	*Sixth disease (roseola infantum)*: fever and maculopapular rash	None
HHV-7	Ubiquitous, role in human disease unclear	None
HHV-8	Associated with Kaposi's sarcoma	None

Mechanism of action

Aciclovir is an acyclic analogue of the nucleoside guanosine. It is phosphorylated to aciclovir monophosphate by viral thymidine kinase in host cells infected with HSV and VZV, and is subsequently converted to acyclovir triphosphate by cellular enzymes, which competes with guanosine triphosphate to ultimately induce termination of chain elongation, accumulation of mutations in viral progeny, or induction of apoptosis. As aciclovir phosphorylation is initiated by viral thymidine kinase, high concentrations are attained in infected cells, with minimal drug uptake in uninfected healthy cells. Furthermore, aciclovir triphosphate has a much higher affinity for viral DNA polymerase than its host cell counterpart, accounting for its high specificity of action and favourable side effect profile.

Valaciclovir is an oral prodrug of aciclovir that is readily absorbed and rapidly converted to aciclovir via intestinal and hepatic first pass metabolism, thus has the same mechanism of action and antiviral spectrum, with greater oral bioavailability.

Penciclovir also shares the same mechanism of action and spectrum of activity as aciclovir, although oral absorption is poor, so it is administered as the prodrug, **famciclovir** when given orally. Topical preparations of penciclovir are used in herpes labialis

Ganciclovir also a guanosine analogue, differs structurally from aciclovir by having an additional hydroxymethyl group on the acyclic side chain. It is a potent inhibitor of CMV replication, with clinically useful activity against HSV and VZV. In CMV-infected cells, ganciclovir is converted to its monophosphate form by a viral protein kinase encoded by the *UL97* gene. In HSV- and VZV-infected

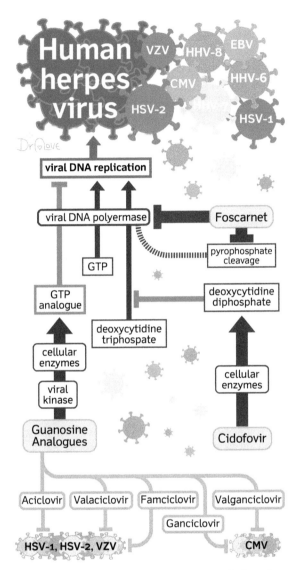

Figure 11.6 Human herpes virus: summary of relevant pathways and drug targets.

Prescribing

The only clinically useful antiviral spectrum of activity of **aciclovir** is against HSV-1, HSV-2, and to a lesser extent VZV. It is available in topical, oral, and IV formulations, with doses routes and durations dependent on indications. Due to modest oral bioavailability (approximately 20%), IV preparations are used in severe infections such as encephalitis.

Valaciclovir and **famciclovir** are generally used for the same indications as oral aciclovir, although improved oral bioavailability (50–70%) and extended half-life, allow for BD dosing.

Ganciclovir is primarily used for the prevention and treatment of CMV disease in immunocompromised patients, such as patients with AIDS and transplant recipients. Treatment is administered IV as oral bioavailability is poor (5–10%) and, due to significant toxicities, is reserved for use in life-threatening of sight-threatening infections. Treatment duration is typically guided by CMV viral load. CMV retinitis can be treated with a slow-release ocular ganciclovir implant.

Valganciclovir with its good oral bioavailability is commonly used as prophylaxis in CMV-negative solid organ transplant recipients in the first 100–200 days following transplantation and, increasingly, as an oral alternative in patients suitable for outpatient CMV treatment.

Unwanted effects

Side effects to guanosine analogues tend to vary with route of administration and the risk of severe toxicity increased in agents with improved oral bioavailability (e.g. **valaciclovir, famciclovir**) or following IV administration. Topical preparations can cause transient stinging and occasional irritation, such as erythema when applied to the skin or eye (eye ointment).

Systemic aciclovir is generally well-tolerated, but can cause GI disturbance, fatigue, headache, and rash. It is also associated with anaemia, leucopenia, and thrombocytopenia. Hypersensitivity reactions have very rarely been reported.

Severe toxicity includes neurotoxicity (e.g. lethargy, confusion, psychosis, involuntary movements, and seizures) and occurs in up to 4% of recipients of IV aciclovir, typically affecting those with renal dysfunction, so dose reductions are recommended even with mild impairment. Symptoms usually resolve within days of drug cessation.

IV aciclovir can also cause reversible renal dysfunction in approximately 5% of recipients, probably due to precipitation of aciclovir crystals in renal tubules, leading to

cells, this process is mediated by viral thymidine kinase. Like aciclovir, subsequent activation to ganciclovir triphosphate is mediated by cellular enzymes, leading to competitive inhibition of viral DNA polymerase. Unlike aciclovir, however, uptake by cellular DNA polymerase of ganciclovir triphosphate is greater accounting for its significant side effect profile.

Valganciclovir is a prodrug of ganciclovir that is rapidly absorbed with an oral bioavailability of over 60%, enabling oral administration.

an obstructive nephropathy. The risk is increased following rapid administration, and in patients with underlying renal disease, so doses are administered slowly and adequate hydration must be maintained.

In addition to the side effects seen with aciclovir, the most significant adverse reaction to **ganciclovir** and its prodrug, **valganciclovir**, is bone marrow suppression, usually leucopenia (up to 40% of patients), but thrombocytopenia and anaemia are also relatively common.

Drug interactions

Guanosine analogues are renally cleared, which may be impaired in the presence of drugs such as **probenecid** and **mycophenolate**. The risk of nephrotoxicity is increased in combination with other renally toxic agents such as **ciclosporin** or **amphotericin**, particularly where renal clearance is impaired.

Co-administration of **ganciclovir** (or **valganciclovir**) with **imipenem** (plus cilastatin) can increase the risk of seizures, while concomitant use with other agents can cause profound myelosuppression, e.g. **zidovudine** and should be avoided.

Foscarnet

Foscarnet inhibits viral DNA polymerase by preventing the cleavage of pyrophosphate from deoxynucleotide triphosphates, a key step in DNA chain elongation.

Mechanism of action

Foscarnet is a pyrophosphate analogue, and the only drug used in HHV infections that is not a nucleoside or nucleotide analogue. It blocks the pyrophosphate binding site of viral DNA polymerase, preventing the cleavage of pyrophosphate from deoxynucleotide triphosphates, necessary for DNA chain elongation. It has a much higher affinity (approximately 100-fold) for viral than cellular DNA polymerase.

Because it does not require activation by a viral protein kinase, it is active against many HSV/VZV and CMV strains, where thymidine kinase or UL97 mutations confer resistance to **aciclovir** and **ganciclovir**, respectively.

Prescribing

Foscarnet is licensed for CMV retinitis treatment in patients with AIDS, and for **aciclovir**-resistant mucocutaneous HSV infections; although due to its

unfavourable side effect profile, use is limited to patients intolerant of or resistant to **ganciclovir**. Doses are administered IV due to poor oral bioavailability, with dosing schedules dependant on diagnosis. Being renally cleared, dose modifications are required for small reductions in creatinine clearance and hydration necessary to reduce the risk of renal toxicity.

Unwanted effects

The principle treatment-limiting side effect of **foscarnet** is renal toxicity and electrolyte disturbances (see 'Prescribing warning: foscarnet nephrotoxicity'), probably due to direct tubular injury, although crystalline glomerulonephritis, interstitial nephritis, and nephrogenic diabetes insipidus have all been described.

> **PRESCRIBING WARNING**
>
> **Foscarnet nephrotoxicity**
> - Renal impairment is common (up to a third of patients) typically occurs in the second week of treatment and resolves over several weeks from cessation.
> - Electrolyte disturbances include hypocalcaemia, hypokalaemia, and hypomagnesaemia.
> - Monitor renal function and electrolytes at least 48-hourly during induction therapy, and weekly during maintenance therapy.
> - Avoid rapid infusions, ensure adequate hydration—500–1000 mL IV sodium chloride 0.9%.

Neurological disturbances, some of which may be related to electrolyte disturbances, have also been reported, such as paraesthesia, tremors, hallucinations, and seizures. Infusion-related nausea occurs in approximately 25% of patients, particularly with more rapid infusions. Genital ulceration has also been associated with foscarnet therapy, likely secondary to topical irritation from high urinary concentrations of the drug, thus managed in part by optimizing hydration during treatment. Other less common effects include bone marrow suppression, liver dysfunction, and cardiac conduction abnormalities.

Drug interactions

The risk of renal impairment may be increased when **foscarnet** is administered with other nephrotoxic agents, such as **amphotericin**, aminoglycosides, and calcineurin inhibitors. The risk of hypocalcaemia is increased with co-administration of IV **pentamidine**.

Cidofovir

> Cidofovir is phosphorylated to its active diphosphate form by host cell enzymes, competing with deoxycitidine triphosphate for incorporation into the growing DNA chain, where it acts as a chain terminator.

Mechanism of action

Cidofovir is a monophosphate nucleotide analogue of deoxycytidine that is phosphorylated to its active diphosphate form by cellular enzymes. This competitively inhibits deoxycitidine triphosphate, being incorporated into the DNA chain and impairing chain elongation.

Although cidofovir has demonstrated in vitro activity against a range of DNA viruses, (e.g. human herpes viruses, papillomavirus, and adenovirus), clinical efficacy is largely restricted to CMV treatment. Like **foscarnet**, it does not require activation by a viral protein kinase, so retains activity against strains of HSV and CMV with thymidine kinase and UL97 mutations, respectively.

Prescribing

Cidofovir is licensed for the treatment of CMV retinitis in patients with AIDS; however, due to its extensive toxicity profile, it is primarily used as a third-line agent for CMV disease in immunosuppressed patients, where **ganciclovir** or **foscarnet** are unsuitable due to intolerance or resistance.

With its poor oral bioavailability doses are generally administered IV, usually once a week as although plasma half life is short (3 hours) the intracellular half-life of cidofovir diphosphate is prolonged. Oral **probenecid** is administered with each dose, to inhibit renal tubular secretion, thereby increasing plasma levels and preventing accumulation in the renal cortex, which protects renal tubular cells from damage. Patients require prehydration with 1 L of sodium chloride 0.9% prior to each dose. Topical cidofovir has been used for the treatment of **aciclovir**-resistant mucocutaneous HSV infection.

Unwanted effects

Dose-dependent nephrotoxicity is the most clinically significant side effect of **cidofovir** therapy, (see 'Prescribing warning: cidofovir nephrotoxicity'), typically presenting with proteinuria, glycosuria, and raised serum creatinine. Metabolic acidosis with Fanconi's syndrome can also occur.

> **PRESCRIBING WARNING**
>
> **Cidofovir nephrotoxicity**
> - Renal impairment affects approximately 25% of patients.
> - Usually reversible but can lead to end-stage renal failure.
> - Contraindicated with CrCl < 55 mL/min or ≥ 2+ protein on urine dipstick.
> - Frequent monitoring of renal function and urine dipstick testing is required.
> - Co-administration of other nephrotoxic agents contraindicated.

Neutropenia occurs in 15–25% of patients, and regular monitoring of neutrophil count is required. Other adverse reactions associated with cidofovir include hepatic dysfunction, anaemia, and reduced intra-ocular pressure. Adverse features associated with co-administration of **probenecid,** include GI disturbance, fever, and rash.

Drug interactions

Administration of **cidofovir** with other nephrotoxic agents such as aminoglycosides, **foscarnet**, **amphotericin**, and contrast dye is contraindicated. Concurrent use of **probenecid** may also increase serum concentrations of other renally cleared drugs, e.g. **methotrexate**, **mycophenolate**, beta-lactams, and NSAIDs, which may necessitate dose reductions, or in the case of methotrexate, doses omitted.

Respiratory viruses

Despite the vast array of viruses causing clinically significant respiratory infections, in current clinical practice, antiviral therapy is only routinely available against the influenza viruses, and to a much lesser extent, respiratory syncitial virus (RSV).

Influenza

Influenza viruses are enveloped RNA viruses consisting of three distinct types that circulate in all parts of the world:

- *Influenza A*: infects humans, birds, and pigs.
- *Influenza B*: infects humans only.
- *Influenza C*: infects humans and pigs.

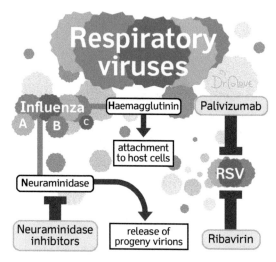

Figure 11.7 Respiratory viruses: summary of relevant pathways and drug targets.

Influenza A and B are of significant public health concern, (C causes only a mild upper respiratory tract infection) as they are easily transmitted from person to person, causing annual epidemics which peaks in winter months in temperate regions. Severe illness and death may occur, particularly in high-risk populations such as those who are pregnant, over 65 years or with co-morbidities, e.g. renal impairment, cardiac disease, diabetes mellitus, or immunosuppression.

The viral envelopes of Influenza A and B contain 2 important surface proteins which are used to classify strains of Influenza A (e.g. H1N1—'swine flu'):

- *Haemagglutinin (H)*: necessary for viral attachment to host cell surfaces.
- *Neuraminidase (N)*: cleaves progeny virions from infected host cells, releasing them to infect new cells.

Although influenza B is relatively stable, influenza A mutates constantly, so has the potential to cause global pandemics (e.g. H1N1 in 2009), as mutations can make the virus more infectious to humans (Figure 11.7).

Management of influenza

Vaccination is the primary management strategy for influenza, with all at risk patients and health care workers in the UK annually vaccinated. Vaccines, however, are developed against predicated strains, thus the predominant circulating influenza strains may be antigenically different to those contained in that season's influenza vaccine, limiting effectiveness.

The neuraminidase inhibitors **oseltamivir** and **zanamivir** are the only antiviral agents recommended for treatment and prophylaxis of influenza A and B in the UK. **Amantidine**, although licensed for treatment and prophylaxis of influenza A, is no longer recommended in the UK due to high levels of resistance and unfavourable side effect profile.

Respiratory syncitial virus

RSV is an RNA virus with a world-wide distribution. It causes annual epidemics that occur in winter in temperate regions, and is a major cause of bronchiolitis and pneumonia in young children. Almost all children have been infected with RSV by 2 years of age, although immunocompromised patients are at risk of severe disease.

Management of RSV

Palivizumab a monoclonal antibody licensed for the prevention of RSV in at risk patients, e.g. premature babies with chronic lung disease or congenital heart disease. In patients who go on to develop bronchiolitis secondary to RSV, treatment tends to be supportive management with oxygen, fluid, and nutritional support as required. **Ribavirin** is the only antiviral available against RSV, although it tends to be reserved for severe cases.

Drug classes used in management of respiratory viruses

Neuraminidase inhibitors

Neuraminidase inhibitors prevent the release of progeny virions from infected host cells by competitively inhibiting the influenza neuraminidase enzyme. For example, oseltamivir and zanamivir

Mechanism of action

Oseltamivir is a prodrug metabolized in the liver to its active form, oseltamivir carboxylate, a sialic acid analogue that potently inhibits the neuraminidase enzyme of influenza A and B. It acts by competitively inhibiting the cleavage activity of influenza neuraminidase upon sialic acid found on the surface of host cells, thus preventing release of viral progeny and spread through the respiratory tract.

Resistance to oseltamivir can develop rapidly, even during therapy, usually due to a point mutation in the viral neuraminidase gene which alters the enzyme binding site, thereby reducing affinity for oseltamivir carboxylate. H1N1 isolates are more likely to harbour resistance than other strains, especially in severely immunosuppressed patients.

Zanamivir is also a sialic acid analogue that potently inhibits the neuraminidase enzymes of influenza A and B, although unlike oseltamivir there are few reports of resistance

Prescribing

In the UK, **oseltamivir** is recommended first-line for treatment (or prophylaxis following contact) of patients with, or at risk of, complicated influenza infection, apart from severely immunosuppressed patients where the dominant circulating strain has a higher likelihood of resistance, e.g. H1N1. It is well absorbed orally (bioavailability of active metabolite approximately 80%), or when given via NG tube to critically ill patients. Treatment or prophylaxis is best started within 48 hours of symptom onset or contact. As oseltamivir is primarily eliminated renally, dose reductions are required in renal impairment.

In the UK, **zanamivir** is recommended for influenza treatment (or prophylaxis following contact) in severely immunosuppressed patients when the dominant circulating strain has a higher risk of oseltamivir resistance, e.g. H1N1; and considered where patients fail to respond to oseltamivir. Due to poor oral bioavailability, it is usually administered as an inhaled powder (Diskhaler®), but can also be given IV on a named patient basis (e.g. in intubated patients in a critical care setting). Being renally cleared, dose reductions may be required in renal impairment when given IV. Zanamivir should be administered within 36 hours of symptom onset or contact.

Unwanted effects

Oseltamivir is generally well tolerated, the most frequently reported adverse events being nausea, vomiting, dyspepsia, and headache, which tend to resolve with continued dosing. There have been rare reports of serious adverse events in patients with influenza taking neuraminidase inhibitors, although direct causal relationship with oseltamivir is yet to be established, e.g. neuropsychiatric disorders (hallucinations, abnormal behaviour, and convulsions) and severe skin reactions including Stevens–Johnson syndrome and toxic epidermal necrolysis. Children and adolescents appear to be at higher risk of these complications.

As inhaled **zanamivir** has minimal systemic absorption, it is generally well tolerated, but can cause local reactions such as throat discomfort and cough. More seriously, it can cause bronchospasm, so should be used with caution in patients with obstructive airways diseases including asthma and COPD, where treatment should be given under close observation, with a short-acting bronchodilator readily available. Reports of neuropsychiatric disorders and severe skin reactions in patients with influenza taking zanamivir are rare compared with **oseltamivir**, although probably increased when administered IV.

Drug interactions

Probenecid significantly reduces renal clearance of the active metabolite of **oseltamivir**, which may necessitate a dose reduction. No clinically significant drug–drug interactions have been reported to date with **zanamivir**.

Monoclonal antibody: palivizumab

> Palivizumab provides passive immunity against RSV by targeting the viral F protein, preventing its entry into host cells.

Mechanism of action

Palivizumab is a humanized monoclonal antibody that provides passive immunity against RSV. It targets the F protein of RSV that is critical for fusing the virus and host cell, thereby preventing its entry into the host cell. It has been shown to reduce rates of RSV-related complications and hospital admissions in children at high risk of severe disease.

Prescribing

In the UK, **palivizumab** is recommended for use in children under 2 years of age at increased risk of serious illness or death from RSV infection, i.e. with bronchopulmonary dysplasia, congenital heart disease and severe combined immunodeficiency syndrome (SCID). Doses are given monthly by IM injection from the start of the RSV season (beginning of October) to a maximum of five doses.

Unwanted effects

Treatment is generally well tolerated, although as a mono-clonal antibody, **palivizumab** is associated with a relatively high risk of hypersensitivity reactions, injections site reactions, and rash. Severe reactions preclude further use. Interactions are unlikely and palivizumab can be given alongside routine vaccinations.

Further reading

Dolin R (2009) *Mandell, Douglas and Bennett's Principles and Practice of Infectious Diseases*, 7th edn. London: Churchill Livingstone.

Kimberlin DW, Whitley RJ (2007) Antiviral therapy of HSV-1 and -2. In: Arvin A, Campitelli-Fiume G, Mocarski E, et al., (Eds) *Human Herpesviruses: Biology, Therapy, and Immunoprophylaxis*, Chapter 64. Cambridge: Cambridge University Press. https://www.ncbi.nlm.nih.gov/books/NBK47444/

Solomon T, Michael MD, Smith PE, et al. (2012) Management of suspected viral encephalitis in adults—Association of British Neurologists and British Infection Association National Guidelines. *Journal of Infection* 64(4), 347–73.

Guidelines

AIDS Info (2019) Current Guidelines. http://aidsinfo.nih.gov/guidelines [accessed 13 April 2019].

BHIVA (2014) BHIVA guidelines for the treatment of HIV-1 positive adults with antiretroviral therapy 2012 (2013). *HIV Medicine* 15(Suppl. 1), 1–85.

British HIV Association: Current Guidelines http://www.bhiva.org/guidelines.aspx [accessed 13 April 2019].

NICE TA168 (2009) Amantadine, oseltamivir and zanamivir for the treatment of influenza. https://www.nice.org.uk/guidance/ta168 [accessed 13 April 2019].

Panel on Antiretroviral Guidelines for Adults and Adolescents. Guidelines for the use of antiretroviral agents in HIV-1-infected adults and adolescents. Department of Health and Human Services. http://aidsinfo.nih.gov/contentfiles/lvguidelines/AdultandAdolescentGL.pdf [accessed 13 April 2019].

PHE guidance on use of antiviral agents for the treatment and prophylaxis of seasonal influenza. Version 9.1, January 2019. https://www.gov.uk/government/publications/influenza-treatment-and-prophylaxis-using-anti-viral-agents [accessed 23 April 2019].

11.4 Protozoal and helminth infections

Malaria

Malaria is a serious and potentially life-threatening illness caused by infection with the protozoan parasite, *Plasmodium*. It is transmitted by the bite of the female *Anopheles* mosquito and is seen predominantly in tropical parts of Africa, Asia, and Central and South America. World-wide efforts to control the mosquito vector, and identify and treat cases promptly, has led to a 25% global reduction in the number of deaths from malaria. In many African countries this has fallen by 50%. Despite these efforts, there were approximately 200 million cases worldwide in 2013 with 584 000 deaths, mostly occurring in children and in Africa.

Pathophysiology of malaria

There are five species of *Plasmodium* that cause clinical disease in humans; *Plasmodium falciparum, Plasmodium vivax, Plasmodium ovale, Plasmodium malariae*, and *Plasmodium knowlesi. P. falciparum* causes most severe disease and is responsible for the vast majority of malaria deaths. Red blood cells parasitized by *P. falciparum* can be sequestered (stick to the capillaries) in the brain and other organs causing cerebral malaria, renal failure, and respiratory distress, as well as severe anaemia. Vector control and bite protection, e.g. using bed nets and mosquito/insect repellents, helps prevent malaria transmission. Travellers to endemic countries can also take chemoprophylaxis to prevent malaria, with choice determined by the species and local drug-resistance pattern of the predominant forms of malaria. Drug resistance changes and develops over time, so accurate surveillance of antimalarial resistance patterns is crucial to inform chemoprophylaxis and treatment protocols around the world.

The life cycle of the malaria parasite is quite complex involving a sexual cycle in the female anopheline mosquito, and asexual reproduction in the vertebrate host, usually human (see Figure 11.8). Parasite multiplication occurs in hepatocytes, where the parasite is called a hypnozoite (*P. vivax* and *P. ovale*) or merozoite, a hepatic schizont (*P. falciparum*). The hypnozoites of *P. vivax* and *P. ovale* can remain dormant for months before reactivating.

Parasite multiplication also occurs in erythrocytes, the stage looked for by microscopy of thick and thin blood films, to enable speciation and quantification of the parasitaemia. Some erythrocytic forms of the parasite develop into sexual forms called gametocytes, which may be ingested by a female mosquito during a blood feed to complete the life cycle.

For a full summary of the relevant pathways and drug targets, see Figure 11.8.

Management of malaria

Management of malaria requires early diagnosis and prompt treatment to prevent rapid progression. Diagnosis must therefore include accurate identification of *Plasmodium* spp., either by examining blood films, or by means of rapid diagnostic tests, which detect parasite antigens, to ensure initiation of appropriate treatment. However, treatment should not be delayed in severe malaria (see Table 11.27) or high risk patients (e.g. with HIV) pending parasite identification.

A diagnosis of malaria requires a full clinical assessment to evaluate severity and therefore determine where

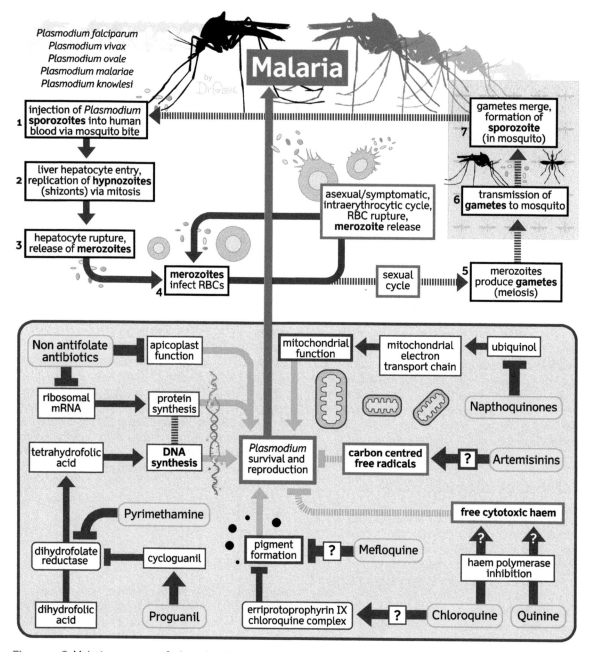

Figure 11.8 Malaria: summary of relevant pathways and drug targets.

the patient should be managed, i.e. at home, on a general hospital ward, or on an ICU with access to circulatory, respiratory, and renal support. Severe cases will require urgent hospital referral to ensure prompt initiation of highly effective therapy and supportive care, as death can occur within hours.

Drug therapy for malaria

Artemesin-based combination treatment has replaced **quinine** as the primary treatment for falciparum malaria in many countries around the world; although IV quinine remains a second-line recommendation for treatment of severe

Table 11.27 Major features of severe or complicated falciparum malaria in adults

Impaired consciousness or seizures	Acidosis (pH<7.3)
Renal impairment (oliguria <0.4 mL/kg/ hour or Cr >265 µmol/L	Hypoglycaemia (<2.2 mmol/L)
Pulmonary oedema/ acute respiratory distress syndrome	Haemoglobin (≤80 g/L)
Spontaneous bleeding/ disseminated intravascular coagulopathy	Shock
Haemoglobinuria (without G6PD deficiency)	Parasitaemia (>10%)

falciparum malaria in the USA, UK, and by WHO. Non-severe falciparum malaria can usually be treated with oral medications, unless the oral route is unavailable, e.g. with vomiting.

Artesunate is currently the drug of choice for all patients with severe malaria caused by *P. falciparum*. Patients are initially treated with IV therapy until there are signs of improvement and then switched to oral therapy with either:

- Riamet® (**artemether** /**lumefantrine**).
- **Doxycycline.**
- Malarone® (**atovaquone** /**proguanil**).
- **Clindamycin.**

In countries/areas with known resistance to artemisinin, combination therapies have been adopted, e.g. in Cambodia aretsunate-**mefloquine** is first line treatment in some provinces, with **dihydroartemisinin-piperaquine** as first-line treatment elsewhere. Resistance is closely monitored by the WHO with regular regional reports (see http://www.who.int/malaria/publications).

Malaria prophylaxis

Drug choice for malaria prophylaxis again depends primarily on local resistance patterns, and secondly on

patient preferences or the presence of co-morbidities that may exclude the use of some drugs. Options include **chloroquine/proguanil**, **mefloquine** and **atovaquone**/ proguanil. In all cases, courses are initiated prior to entering the endemic area and continued for 1–4 weeks after leaving.

Drug classes used in management

Quinine

Quinine acts on the blood form of the parasite (blood schizonticide) and although its precise mechanism of action is unknown, it is thought to inhibit haem-polymerase leading to build-up of cytotoxic haem.

Mechanism of action

Quinine occurs naturally in the bark of the cinchona plant and has been used since the 17th century for the treatment of malaria. It is a weak base and, as such, accumulates in the food vacuoles of *P. falciparum*. It is thought to kill the malaria parasite by interfering with its capacity to break down and digest haemoglobin, allowing a build-up of free cytotoxic haem.

Prescribing

Once the antimalarial drug of choice, **quinine** has been largely replaced by artemesin-based combination treatment due to widespread *P. falciparum* resistance. It is, however, recommended as IV second-line treatment of severe falciparum malaria in the USA, UK, and by WHO.

Quinine can be given orally (e.g. quinine sulfate) or by IV infusion (e.g. quinine hydrochloride) as various salts with different relevant potencies (see Table 11.28). The exceedingly bitter taste of oral quinine can make many patients vomit after ingestion, limiting its use. In the USA, **quinidine**, a dextroisomer of quinine is used for intravenous treatment.

For IV treatment quinine is administered by IV infusion over 4 hours at 8-hourly intervals, with the first dose given as a double-dose in order to 'load' patients. In patients who have received **mefloquine** in the preceding 3 days, a loading dose is not required. Treatment is continued IV until the patient shows sign of improvement and can reliably swallow tablets to complete a 7-day course with oral quinine. This is given together with 7 days of either **doxycycline** (not in children less than 12 years old or in pregnancy) or **clindamycin**.

Table 11.28 Potencies of quinine salts

Quinine salt	Dose equivalent to 100 mg of quinine base
Quinine bisulfate	169 mg
Quinine dihydrochloride	122 mg
Quinine hydrochloride	122 mg
Quinine sulfate	121 mg

Unwanted effects

The main side effect of **quinine** is cinchonism. Mild cinchonism manifests as flushing and sweating, with tinnitus, blurred vision, impaired hearing, confusion, headache, abdominal pain, rashes, dizziness, nausea and vomiting, and diarrhoea. Larger doses, however, may result in severe cinchonism, with symptoms of skin rashes, deafness (which is reversible), somnolence, diminished visual acuity/blindness, anaphylactic shock, or disturbances in cardiac rhythm. Most symptoms of cinchonism (except in severe cases) are reversible and disappear once quinine is withdrawn.

Quinine is a class 1a anti-arrhythmic agent and as such interferes with the Na^+ channels causing conduction disturbances. This anti-arrhythmic property manifests as QT interval prolongation ECG monitoring is recommended during parenteral treatment.

Patients treated with quinine can suffer from hypoglycaemia (especially if administered IV) as it acts to promote insulin secretion, and hypotension. In severe cases, this may be life-threatening so all patients should have serum glucose levels monitored while on treatment, particularly in children in whom falciparum malaria can cause hypoglycaemia.

Rarely quinine may trigger a hypersensitivity reaction in malaria patients called blackwater fever, which manifests as massive haemolysis, haemoglobinaemia, haemoglobinuria, and renal failure.

Chloroquine

As with quinine, the precise mechanism of action of chloroquine is yet to be determined, although it is also thought to inhibit haem-polymerase leading to accumulation of cytotoxic haem.

Mechanism of action

Chloroquine acts through interference with malaria pigment formation within the malaria parasite lysosome, producing a ferriprotoprophyrin (haem) IX-chloroquine complex which is highly toxic to the parasite. The toxic complex disrupts membrane function leading to cell lysis.

Prescribing

Chloroquine once first line treatment for falciparum malaria (1950–1990s), is no longer used due to high resistance rates. It remains, however, an effective treatment option for non-falciparum malaria and can also be used in combination with **proguanil** for prophylaxis against malaria in certain areas of the world, e.g. the Caribbean and Central and South America. Chloroquine is given in tablet form as chloroquine phosphate.

Unwanted effects

Chloroquine is well tolerated, the main side effects being GI disturbances. In patients of African origin, itching is a common side effect. As it can cause convulsions it is not recommended for use in people with a history of epilepsy and should be used with caution in other neurological disorders. Caution is also advised in patients with psoriasis (which may be exacerbated), severe GI disorders, G6PD deficiency, and myasthenia gravis, which it may exacerbate. Chloroquine is safe to use in pregnancy.

Primaquine

The 8-aminoquinolones have selective activity against hypnozoites, the liver stage of *P. ovale* and *P. vivax*, thus reducing the risk of relapse. For example, primaquine.

Mechanism of action

The precise mechanism of action of **primaquine** remains unknown, although it is believed to be a pro-drug whose active metabolites are responsible for its shizonticidal activity. These active metabolites are likely to interfere with parasitic DNA structure and mitochondrial membranes, as they accumulate within mitochondria causing swelling, leading to structural and functional change.

Prescribing

Primaquine as the only agent effective in eliminating the liver stages of *P. ovale* and *P. vivax*, is on the WHO list of essential medicines. It is used daily for 14 days in the treatment of non-falciparum malaria following **chloroquine** therapy, to ensure complete eradication, thereby preventing relapse. It is not licensed in the UK, but can be obtained through specialist importing companies.

Unwanted effects

Primaquine-induced haemolysis is a particular problem with treatment, attributed primarily to patients with G6PD deficiency, which should be excluded prior to starting treatment. Other common side effects include abdominal pain, dark urine, loss of appetite, and fatigue. Less commonly treatment is associated with QT interval prolongation and should therefore be avoided in patients with cardiac arrhythmias.

Mefloquine

> Mefloquine acts on the intra-erythrocytic asexual stages, although its mechanism of action is not fully understood. It does, however, have efficacy against some chloroquine-resistant strains of *P. falciparum*.

Mechanism of action

Like **chloroquine** the mechanism of action of **mefloquine** probably involves interference with malaria pigment formation. Mefloquine has rapid dose-related activity against the erythrocytic stages of *Plasmodium* spp.

Prescribing

Mefloquine hydrochloride is used primarily as prophylaxis in parts of the world where **chloroquine** resistance is high, e.g. sub-Saharan Africa. Tablets are taken orally once a week starting 2–3 weeks before entering the endemic area and continued for 4 weeks after leaving. It is approximately 95% effective, although significant resistance has been reported in some areas of south-east Asia and its use in non-falciparum malaria has been largely replaced due to its toxicity.

Unwanted effects

Mefloquine is generally well-tolerated, despite wide reports of neuropsychiatric reactions (see 'Prescribing warning: neuropsychiatric reactions with mefloquine'), which have been especially reported by women and may last months after stopping treatment. The main side effects, however, are dizziness, hence driving or performance of skilled tasks is not recommended while taking it. Mefloquine is not recommended for patients with epilepsy, since it antagonizes the anticonvulsant effect of anti-epileptics. Similarly, caution is advised in patients with cardiac conduction disorders as it interacts with a number of cardiac drugs.

PRESCRIBING WARNING

Neuropsychiatric reactions with mefloquine

- Mefloquine use is associated with psychiatric symptoms such as anxiety, depression, hallucinations, abnormal dreams, panic attacks, paranoia, and psychosis. In severe cases there have been reports of attempted suicides.

- If affected, patients should be advised to seek medical help immediately and an alternative antimalarial used.

- Mefloquine is not recommended for chemoprophylaxis in patients with a history of psychiatric illness.

Mefloquine is metabolized in the liver by CYP3A4. Caution is advised if it is administered with drugs that inhibit (e.g. **clarithromycin** and HIV protease-inhibitors), or induce this enzyme (e.g. some HIV non-nucleoside reverse-transcriptase inhibitors).

Artemisinins

> The mechanism of action of artemisinin remains somewhat controversial, but appears to involve the haem-mediated decomposition of the endoperoxide bridge, to produce carbon-centred free radicals, although is likely to involve more than one process. For example, artemether and artesunate.

Mechanism of action

Artesunate is a semi-synthetic derivative of artemisinin, an antimalarial lactone derived from the herb *Artemisia annua* used by Chinese herbalists for over 2000 years for the treatment of malaria; however, the active principle was only isolated in 1973. The exact mechanism of action is unknown, but artemisinins are considered pro-drugs that are activated to generate free radicals, which then cause cellular damage. Further proposed targets of artemisinin are intracellular proteins, including ATPases, in particular the Ca^{2+} pump PfATP6.

These drugs have also been shown to reduce gametocytogenesis, therefore reducing gametocyte carriage and the transmission of malaria.

Prescribing

Due to increasing drug resistance, the combined use of two or more drugs with different modes of action is recommended, to provide better cure rates and delay resistance development. Artemesin-based combination treatments use **artesunate**, **artemether**, or **dihydroartemesinin** as the rapid-acting component, in combination with a slower, longer-acting drug. Examples of ACTs in current use are:

- Artemether-**lumefantrine** (Co-artem®, Riamet®) used in south-central Africa.
- Aretesunate + **amodiaquine** used in West Africa.
- Artesunate + **sulfadoxine-pyrimethamine** (Fansidar®).
- **Dihydroartemisinin-piperaquine** (Artekin®) used in south-east Asia.
- Artemether + **mefloquine**.

Artesunate is currently the drug of choice for treatment of all patients with severe malaria caused by P falciparum, as it reduces mortality compared with **quinine** in both south-east Asia and Africa. Although WHO guidelines recommend avoiding artesunate in the first trimester of pregnancy, there is growing evidence that it is safe and effective. In pregnant patients returning from SE Asia with severe malaria, artesunate is the drug of choice in all stages of pregnancy due to the risk of quinine resistance. Doses are administered ideally IV, or failing that IM, until the patient shows signs of improvement, when a switch to an oral antimalarial can be considered.

Unwanted effects

Artesunate is generally safe and well-tolerated compared with other antimalarials, although artemesinins have been shown in animal studies to cause severe and irreversible neurological damage, in particular the more fat-soluble derivatives or following IM administration (as opposed to oral). This has not been seen in humans at clinically used doses.

Post-artesunate delayed haemolysis (PADH) can occur at the end of treatment in a phase of clinical improvement. It is not associated with a relapse of active malaria infection, and is distinct from the anaemia caused by P. falciparum during the blood stages of the parasite. Although many causes might contribute to this effect, the pitting of the infected erythrocytes is likely the main explanation. To avoid clinical complications, close follow-up of these patients is recommended with a haemoglobin level check at 14 days after completion of treatment.

Proguanil

> Proguanil inhibits the parasitic dihydrofolate reductase enzyme, thereby preventing folic acid metabolism.

Mechanism of action

Proguanil is a pro-drug that is converted to its active metabolite cycloguanil, which inhibits the enzyme dihydrofolate reductase.

Prescribing

Proguanil is used in combination with **atovaquone** (Malarone®), as both prophylaxis and treatment of malaria. As prophylaxis it is 90% effective against *P. falciparum* with doses administered OD initiated 24–48 hours prior to entering an endemic area and continued for 7 days after leaving. When used in treatment of malaria, doses are taken daily for 3 days. It is licensed for use as prophylaxis against malaria for up to 28 days, but can be taken for up to a year.

Proguanil is also available in combination with **chloroquine** for antimalarial prophylaxis.

Unwanted effects

The most frequent side effects are headache and GI upset, although in patients with renal impairment there have been reports of haematological toxicity, and doses should be adjusted accordingly. Malarone® should be avoided in severe renal impairment, and in pregnancy and breastfeeding unless there is no suitable alternative.

Drug interactions

Proguanil can enhance the anticoagulant effect of **warfarin**, and hence, if use is necessary increased monitoring is recommended.

Pyrimethamine

> Pyrimethamine is used in combination with sulfadoxine, as both target different enzymes in the folate pathway.

Mechanism of action

Pyrimethamine interferes with tetrahydrofolic acid synthesis from folic acid by inhibiting the enzyme dihydrofolate reductase (DHFR), with greater affinity for the protozoal than the human enzyme. It is used in combination with the sulfonamide, **sulfadoxine** (Fansidar®), which works synergistically on the folate pathway through inhibition of the enzyme dihydropteroate synthetase.

Prescribing

Pyrimethamine with **sulfadoxine** may be used as an adjunct to *quinine* in the treatment of falciparum malaria, although its use is limited due to widespread resistance. It is no longer available in the USA, in part due to resistance, but also because of the risk of severe adverse effects. Fansidar® is not recommended for chemoprophylaxis because of resistance.

Unwanted effects

Side effects to **pyrimethamine** include rash, GI, and neurological symptoms. It is contraindicated in patients with folate-deficiency anaemia, epilepsy, and pregnancy, especially during the first trimester.

More severe reactions, however, are attributable to **sulfadoxine**, which has been known to cause severe blood dyscrasias and skin reactions (see 'Prescribing warning: severe skin reactions and blood dyscrasias with sulfadoxine'). Other serious effects include crystalluria, which can in part be avoided by encouraging patients to drink plenty of fluids on treatment. Patients with a history of sulfonamide intolerance should not be prescribed Fansidar®.

As antifolates, **folinic acid** may be used to treat haematological toxicity in the case of overdose.

PRESCRIBING WARNING

Severe skin reactions and blood dyscrasias with sulfadoxine

- Pyrimethamine is always used in combination with a sulfonamide.
- As with other sulfonamides, sulfadoxine is associated with severe and, in some cases, fatal skin reactions (Stevens–Johnson Syndrome, toxic epidermal necrolysis) and blood dyscrasias.
- Fansidar® is contraindicated in patients with a history of sulfonamide hypersensitivity.
- Patients should be advised to stop treatment and seek help immediately if they develop a rash, sore throat, or shortness of breath.

Napthoquinones

The highly lipophilic drug atovaquone acts by affecting mitochondrial electron transport, ultimately affecting nucleic acid and ATP synthesis. For example, atovaquone.

Mechanism of action

Atovaquone (a hydoxy-1,4-naphthoquinone), is a competitive inhibitor of ubiquinol, causing inhibition of the mitochondrial electron transport chain, leading to loss of mitochondrial function.

Prescribing

See **'Proguanil'**.

Unwanted effects

Side effects include rashes, abdominal pain, nausea, vomiting, headache, dizziness, insomnia, abnormal dreams, anorexia, depression, coughing, and mouth ulcers.

Drug interactions

Plasma concentration of **atovaquone** is reduced by **rifabutin**, **rifampicin**, and **tetracycline** causing possible therapeutic failure of atovaquone, although the precise mechanism remains unknown.

Non-antifolate antibiotics

The antibiotics without antifolate actions that have also demonstrated antimalarial activity include those belonging to the lincosamides, tetracyclines, and macrolides classes. They predominantly target pathways within the parasite's apicoplast. For example, azithromycin, clindamycin, and doxycycline.

Mechanism of action

The apicoplast is a relict non-photosynthetic plastid found in most apicomplexan parasites, including *Plasmodium*. Since it is vital to the parasite's survival, it provides a good target for antimalarial drugs. Both **azithromycin** and **clindamycin** interfere with malarial parasite replication by targeting the unique apicoplast organelle of the parasite. Their slow onset of action means that they are clinically ineffective for treatment as monotherapy, but may be considered in combination with a fast-acting antimalarial such as **artesunate** or **quinine**.

Doxycycline inhibits protein synthesis by binding to ribosomal RNA and acts as a suppressive prophylaxis of comparable efficacy to **mefloquine**.

Prescribing

Doxycycline is one of the current recommendations for malaria prophylaxis in the UK and USA, although cannot be prescribed to children under the age of 12 and should be avoided in pregnant and breastfeeding women as it is affects tooth development. Doses are given orally for 2 days before entering the malarious area, and continued until 4 weeks after leaving. Its low cost makes it attractive to travellers on a low budget, although they should be advised of the risk of increased sun sensitivity and the heightened need for sun protection.

Clindamycin is used orally in combination with, or following treatment with, **quinine** to treat falciparum malaria as a cheaper alternative to the artemisinin-based combination treatments for 7 days. It is safe to use in pregnancy and breastfeeding.

Unwanted effects

See Topic 11.1, 'Bacterial infection'.

Helminth infections

Helminths are divided into three groups;

1. *Nematodes (roundworms)*: unsegmented worms that affect over a third of the world's population. They are rarely directly fatal, but cause huge morbidity and impaired development. Infection is by ingestion of eggs, or penetration of larvae through body surfaces, or arthropod borne, or ingestion of encysted larvae.

2. *Trematodes (flatworms or flukes)*: unsegmented leaf-like or cylindrical worms that can invade the liver, lungs, blood, or intestinal tract. Infection is mainly by larval stages entering the intestinal tract with subsequent migration to the target organ.

3. *Cesatodes (tapeworms)*: segmented worms.

Helminth infections cause symptoms as a direct result of either living in the intestine, or as they migrate around the body to the end organ (Figure 11.9). Intestinal infection may be asymptomatic, but may also contribute to malnutrition and anaemia (Table 11.29).

Management of helminth infections

Most helminth infections are problematic and endemic in tropical countries. The only clinically significant helminth infection in the UK is *Enterobius vermicularis* (pinworm/ threadworm). Infected patients are often asymptomatic, although some present with peri-anal itching, particularly at night when the female worm often emerges from the anus to lay their eggs. Treatment includes advice on hygienic measures (handwashing, clean sheets) and the use of **mebendazole** in all family members, to prevent the spread of infection.

Anthelmintics: benzimidazoles

> The benzimidazoles inhibit tubulin polymerization by binding to β-tubulin, causing subsequent defects in cellular transport and energy metabolism. For example, albendazole and mebendazole.

Mechanism of action

Of the drugs in this class only two are widely available for use in humans, **albendazole** and **mebendazole**; other benzimidazoles have been discontinued (e.g. tiabendazole) or only licensed for veterinary use (e.g. fenbendazole). Benzimidazoles act by binding to β-tubulin protein, which together with α-tubulin make up the microtubules. The microtubules are part of the cytoskeleton of the cell and as an intracellular structure in nematodes, are responsible for many functions including cellular transport, growth, and cell division. The observed inhibition of cellular transport and energy metabolism are ultimately a consequence of the depolymerization of microtubules. These effects progressively deplete energy reserves and inhibit excretion of waste products, essentially starving the parasite, rendering it immobile and inhibiting egg production. As a result onset of action is slower than other antihelminth agents and efficacy relies on prolonged contact time between drug and parasite.

Prescribing

Mebendazole is used to treat threadworm, roundworm, whipworm and hookworm. It is poorly absorbed from the GI tract so only acts on the intestinal forms of the helminth infection. It is given as a single dose for the treatment of

Table 11.29 Examples of common helminths

Group	Examples	Comments
Nematodes (roundworms)	*Ascaris lumbricoides* (large roundworm), *Ancylostoma duodenale* (hookworm), *Necator americanus* (hookworm), *Trichuris trichura* (whipworm), *Enterobius vermicularis* (pinworm or threadworm), *Strongyloides stercoralis*	Cause visceral larva migrins
	Zoonotic intestinal nematodes: *Trichostrongylus* spp., *Capillaria phillipensis* and *Anisakis* spp.,	
	Toxocara canis (dog roundworm), *T. cati* (cat roundworm), *Ancylostoma caninum* (dog hookworm), *Ancylostoma braziliense* (dog hookworm)	Cause cutaneous larva migrans Cause lymphatic filariasis
	Tissue nematodes: *Wucheria bancrofti*, *Brugia malayi*, *Brugia timori*, *Onchocerca volvulus*, *Loa*, *Trichinella spiralis*, *Angiostrongylus cantonensis*	Causes river blindness Causes eosinophilic meningitis
Trematode (flatworms/flukes)	*Clonarchis sinensis* (liver), *Fasciola hepatica* (liver), *Paragonimus* spp. (lung), *Schistosoma* spp. (blood)	
Cestatodes (tapeworms)	*Taenia saginta* (beef tapeworm)	Most common worldwide
	Taenia solium (pork tapeworm)	Causes cysticercosis
	Dog tapeworms: *Echinococcus granulosus*, *Echinococcus multilocularis*	Cause hydatid disease in sheep, cattle and humans

threadworms, with a second dose after 2 weeks required if re-infection occurs. For the treatment of whipworms, roundworms, and hookworms it is given BD for 3 days to adults and children over the age of 2 years.

Albendazole is used to treat strongyloidiasis, cutaneous larval migrans, lymphatic filariasis, giardiasis, hydatid disease, and cysticercosis in addition to being effective at treating nematode infections. It is better absorbed orally compared with other benzimidazole carbamates.

Unwanted effects

Mebendazole being poorly absorbed has low toxicity; however, it is associated with diarrhoea, abdominal pain, and elevated liver enzymes, although these adverse effects may also be due to the death of intestinal helminths. It is rarely associated with agranulocytosis, or Stevens–Johnson syndrome if prescribed with high doses of **metronidazole**.

Albendazole is relatively well tolerated, although prolonged use may cause hepatic and haematological abnormalities. It should not be given during pregnancy, since it may cause foetal harm and women should be advised not to become pregnant within a month of completing treatment.

Trichomonacides

Trichomonas vaginalis is a flagellated protozoon and the most common treatable sexually transmitted infection worldwide. Infection in women presents as vaginal discharge, vulval itching, dysuria, or offensive odour, and may be accompanied by the finding of a 'strawberry cervix'. In men, it presents as urethral discharge and/or dysuria. It is a significant cause of non-gonococcal urethritis and prostatitis. In both men and women, the infection may be asymptomatic.

Pathophysiology

T. vaginalis primarily infects the squamous epithelium of the genital tract and is transmitted through sexual intercourse. Infection is associated with cervical neoplasia in sexually active women.

Management

Metronidazole or *tinidazole*, 2 g, as a single dose is the recommended treatment regimen, although metronidazole can be given at lower doses for 7 days, e.g. in the first

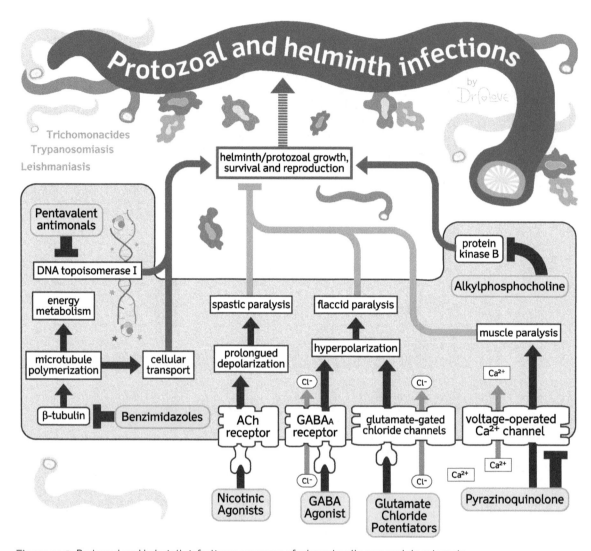

Figure 11.9 Protozoal and helminth infections: summary of relevant pathways and drug targets.

trimester of pregnancy or breastfeeding women. Sexual partners should be treated simultaneously and patients advised to avoid unprotected sexual intercourse including oral sex, until they have both completed treatment and follow-up. See Topic 11.1, 'Bacterial infection', for further drug information.

Further reading

Boillat O, Spechbach H, Chalandon Y, et al. (2015) Post-artesunate delayed haemolysis: report of four cases and review of the literature. *Swiss Medical Weekly* 145, 14181.

Dondorp AM, Fanello CI, Hendriksen ICE, et al. (2010) Artesunate versus quinine in the treatment of severe falciparum malaria in African children (AQUAMAT): an open-label, randomised trial. *Lancet* 376, 1647–57.

South East Asian Quinine Artesunate Malaria Trial (SEAQUAMAT) group (2005). Artesunate versus quinine for treatment of severe falciparum malaria: a randomised trial. *Lancet* 336, 717–25.

World Health Organisation reports including the World Malaria Report 2015 and antimalarial resistance reports available on the WHO website http://www.who.int/malaria/en/ [accessed 14 April 2019].

Guidelines

Chiodini PL, Patel D, Whitty CJM, et al. (2018) Guidelines for malaria prevention in travellers from the United Kingdom.

London: Public Health England. https://assets.publishing.service.gov.uk/government/uploads/system/uploads/attachment_data/file/774781/ACMP_guidelines_2018.pdf [accessed 23 April 2019].

Gothard P, et al. (2014) Malaria diagnosis and treatment guideline. The Hospital for Tropical Diseases. http://www.thehtd.org/Documents/Malaria%20Guideline_final_10_04_18.pdf [accessed 23 April 2019].

Lalloo DG, Shingadia D, Bell DJ, et al. (2016) UK malaria treatment guidelines 2016. *Journal of Infection* 72. 635–49. http://www.journalofinfection.com/article/S0163-4453(16)00047-5/pdf [accessed 14 April 2019].

World Health Organization (2015) *Guidelines for the treatment of malaria*, 3rd edn. http://apps.who.int/iris/bitstream/10665/162441/1/9789241549127_eng.pdf [accessed 14 April 2019].

12 Non-malignant haematology and allergy

12.1 Anaemia

Anaemia is very common, affecting over one-third of the world's population and can be defined as a reduction in the haemoglobin content of red blood cells (RBC). The normal range varies slightly according to the population being tested, but typically in the UK anaemia in males can be diagnosed if the haemoglobin falls to below 135 g/L and in females below 115 g/L. In addition to a reduction in the haemoglobin concentration there is usually an associated reduction in the number of circulating red cells and a low haematocrit. Anaemia is not a diagnosis, it is an abnormality that has an underlying cause and, therefore, a determination of that cause must be made before effective treatment can begin.

Pathophysiology

The production of red cells is termed 'haematopoiesis' and occurs in the bone marrow (liver and spleen in foetal life). The bones involved in production change as we age from almost all bones in neonates to long bones, pelvis, and thoracic cage when we reach our 4th decade.

As with all blood cells, production of RBCs begins with a pluripotent stem cell that is capable of forming many progenitor cells, including those of the erythroid (red cell) lineage (Figure 12.1).

It is estimated that a single pluripotent stem cell, following 18–20 successful divisions, is able to produce 10 million mature erythrocytes. For this process to occur a number of growth factors (GF) are required, which act in synergy and enable the process of haematopoiesis to follow a stepwise maturation process, ending in the release of mature erythrocytes into the blood stream. Examples of such factors include the interleukins (IL), i.e. IL-1, IL-3, IL-4, IL-5, and IL-6. Growth factors also act on the bone marrow stromal cells, enabling the correct environment for cell maturation and development. Tumour necrosis factor (TNF) and IL-1 are particularly important stromal acting growth factors and can stimulate the stromal cells to produce many of the IL factors described above. The GF erythropoietin (EPO) is required for successful red cell maturation.

Many of the growth factors work by binding to cell surface receptors. Activation of such receptors leads to targeted phosphorylation, usually involving the JAK-STAT pathway and resulting in a cascade of intracellular reactions. The cascade leads to the activation of transcription factors, which have their effect in the nucleus and can lead to gene transcription or inhibition therefore altering the function of the cell.

Haemoglobin

Although the production of RBCs is regulated in the bone marrow and dependent upon multiple rounds of cell division, the key to understanding the pathophysiology of anaemia relies on an understanding of the oxygen-carrying molecule found within the cell—haemoglobin. Haemoglobin is made up of four polypeptide globin chains, each of which contains a haem (iron) molecule, able to bind a single molecule of oxygen. Oxygen binds haem in the lungs, where the oxygen concentration is high and then dissociates in the lower oxygen concentrations found in the periphery. The oxygen dissociation curve illustrates this (See Topic 1.1, 'Principles of clinical pharmacology' and Figure 12.2).

Adults possess three different normal haemoglobin molecules, characterized by the type of globulin chain. The most common is haemoglobin A which is comprised of 2 α and 2 β chains ($\alpha_2\beta_2$) and makes up 95–98% of the haemoglobin concentration. Haemoglobin A_2 is made up of 2 α and 2 δ ($\alpha_2\delta_2$) molecules, while Foetal Haemoglobin of Haemoglobin F, found in the lowest concentration (0.5–1.0%) is comprised of 2 α and 2 γ ($\alpha_2\gamma_2$). There are other defective Hb molecules, such as HbS, found in sickle cell disease (see Topic 12.2, 'Haemoglobinopathies').

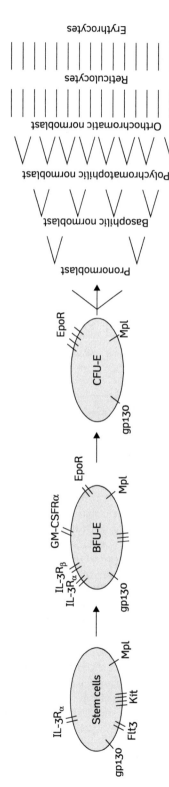

Figure 12.1 Erythropoiesis: erythropoiesis begins in the bone marrow from a pluripotent stem cell. Following successive divisions young RBCs leave the bone marrow as reticulocytes and complete maturation in the circulation into haemoglobin-packed mature erythrocytes. The number of bars on the cell surface is an estimate of the growth factor–receptor concentration/cell responsiveness during erythroid differentiation. A complex of IL–6 and its soluble receptor (or a fusion molecule called hyper IL–6) may induce growth of BFU-e and erythroid maturation in the absence of exogenously added EPO through activation of an autocrine EPO loop.

BFU-e, burst-forming units erythroid; EPO, erythropoietin; IL–6, interleukin-6.

Reproduced with permission from Warrell DA, Cox TM, & Firth JD, *Oxford Textbook of Medicine*. Figure 22.5.1.1, page 4368. Oxford, UK: Oxford University Press © 2013. Reproduced with permission of the Licensor through PLSclear.

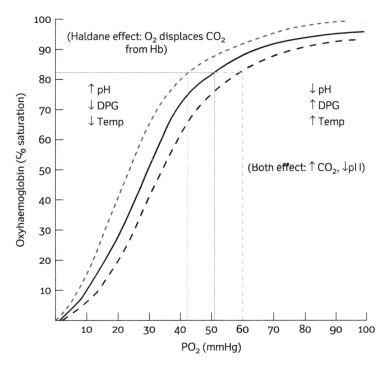

Figure 12.2 Oxygen dissociation curve. The oxygen dissociation curve and the effect of oxygen pressure on haemoglobin saturation (oxyhaemoglobin). The sigmoid nature of the curve means that small changes in pressure can cause marked changes in haemoglobin saturation (middle section). This is vital at ensuring tissues are adequately oxygenated, but also prevents dissociation at relatively high oxygen concentrations where extra oxygen is not required. Drugs, temperature, pH (the Bohr effect), and DPG concentration can all alter the angle of the curve (see learning point 1).

PRACTICAL PRESCRIBING

Oxygen dissociation curve

Many factors can alter the oxygen dissociation curve causing shifts to the left:

- resulting in oxygen dissociation at lower concentrations;

- allowing oxygen to be given up at higher concentrations if required.

Drugs can cause the generation of methaemoglobin, which shifts the oxygen dissociation curve to the left. This occurs because the iron molecules are changed from a ferrous state (Fe^{2+}) to ferric state (Fe^{3+}), which is unable to bind oxygen. Methaemoglobin can be converted back to haemoglobin by the enzyme methaemoglobin reductase. Examples of drugs that increase the production of methaemoglobin include chloroquine, dapsone, nitrates, quinolones, and sulfonamides.

Anaemia

The symptoms of anaemia are secondary to reduced oxygen perfusion of tissues and organs. The cause of anaemia may be obvious in the case of acute blood loss (e.g. trauma, GI bleed), but less easy to determine in chronic anaemia states. In such patients, the haemoglobin concentration may be very low (60–70 g/L) before symptoms are significant, as cardiovascular and other organ groups will have adapted to reduced oxygenation. The classic symptoms are of shortness of breath, lethargy, fatigue, palpitations, dizziness, and headache. In patients with cardiovascular disease intermittent claudication and angina may be a feature.

Pallor of the skin, mucus membranes and conjunctiva are often not seen until the haemoglobin level falls to below 90 g/L. Vital signs may be deranged with a resting tachycardia, tachypnoea, and hypotension. Features of heart failure may be evident in the elderly and include peripheral oedema, hyperdynamic apex beat,

Table 12.1 Causes of microcytic, normocytic and macrocytic anaemia

Microcytic anaemia (MCV <80 fL)	Normocytic anaemia (MCV 80–100fL)	Macrocytic anaemia (MCV >100fL)
Iron deficiency	Chronic renal failure	B12 deficiency
α and β thalassaemia	Haemolytic anaemia	Folate deficiency
Lead poisoning	Following acute blood loss (learning point 2)	Alcohol
Anaemia of chronic disease	Bone marrow failure	Liver disease
Sideroblastic anaemia	Anaemia of chronic disease	Myelodysplastic syndrome and myeloma
	Mixed deficiencies of iron + B12/folate deficiency	Drug therapy with antimetabolite, e.g. hydroxyurea

cardiomegaly, splenomegaly, and a systolic flow murmur. There may be signs that give further clues as to the aetiology of the anaemia. Koilonychia (spoon-shaped nails) is seen in patients with iron-deficiency anaemia, angular cheilitis in B12, and iron deficiency, jaundice, and splenomegaly with haemolytic anaemia, bone deformities may be evident in thalassaemia major and leg ulceration in sickle cell disease.

By using the red cell indices, it is possible to immediately draw up a differential diagnosis based on whether the cell is large (macrocytic, MCV >100 fL), within normal limits (normocytic, MCV 80–100 fL) or small (microcytic, MCV <80) (see Table 12.1). Iron deficiency anaemia, a form of microcytic anaemia, makes up the vast majority of cases world-wide.

Microcytic anaemia

Microcytic anaemia is characterized by a reduced mean cell volume, classically less than 80fL, although this will depend on the normal range of the population being tested. The most common cause of microcytosis is iron deficiency, and indeed this is the commonest cause of anaemia worldwide.

PRACTICAL PRESCRIBING

Clinical considerations in interpreting blood results

- *Acute blood loss*: blood samples taken immediately following acute blood loss may reveal an apparent normal haemoglobin and red cell mass/haematocrit. This is because the plasma volume and red cell mass ratio has remained the same. Over subsequent hours the intravascular volume will return to normal, thus diluting the red cell mass and revealing a new acute anaemia.
- *Dehydration*: may mask anaemia due to a concentration of red cell numbers creating a higher haematocrit.
- *Pregnancy*: apparent anaemia secondary to an increase in plasma volume.

Anaemia of chronic disease is secondary to inflammatory states such as rheumatoid arthritis or malignancy. The link between anaemia and chronic inflammation is due to the effect of cytokines (raised TNF, interferon-γ, and IL-1) and elevated levels of acute phase proteins, such as hepcidin, on iron absorption, bone marrow stromal cell function, and erythroid progenitor maturation. Both iron deficiency and anaemia of chronic disease are characterized by low iron, but in iron deficiency anaemia the ferritin is low and the total iron binding capacity (TIBC) is high whereas in anaemia of chronic disease the ferritin is high or normal and the TIBC is low, see 'Investigations of anaemia' section.

PRACTICAL PRESCRIBING

Association between microcytic anaemia and gastrointestinal blood loss

Microcytic anaemia must always raise a suspicion of GI blood loss. In most cases, and always in the elderly, referral should primarily be to the gastrointestinal team for consideration of GI investigations including OGD and colonoscopy +/– biopsies. Malignancy is the main concern.

Sideroblastic anaemia is characterized by the presence of ringed sideroblasts on bone marrow examination. These cells are immature erythroid cells identified by the presence of iron granules arranged around the nucleus and are usually seen in the context of myelodysplastic syndrome, although a congenital form is also known. Anaemia is a result of defective haem synthesis and therefore a reduction in haemoglobin concentration. Other causes of microcytic anaemia include thalassaemia and thalassaemia trait (see Topic 12.2, 'Haemoglobinopathies').

Macrocytic anaemia

The most common cause of macrocytic anaemia is B12 and folate deficiency, termed megaloblastic anaemia. In western countries, this is most probably secondary to autoimmune pernicious anaemia, in which antibodies bind intrinsic factor or gastric parietal cells, preventing B12 absorption.

The large RBCs seen in B12 and folate deficiency are secondary to ineffective erythropoiesis. Both B12 and folate are vital co-factors required for cell maturation, in particular, DNA synthesis and cell proliferation. Nuclear and cytoplasmic asynchrony occurs as a result, leading to the generation of larger cells. Large cells can be observed throughout the whole of the lineage with erythroblasts, visible on bone marrow aspirate as large oval cells with immature nuclei.

Alcohol and drugs are other common causes, but often the haemoglobin concentration is normal. Macrocytosis caused by haematological malignancy, such as myelodysplastic syndrome is secondary to defective bone marrow function and haemoglobin synthesis. Clues to macrocytosis in this context are the presence of abnormal white cell and platelet counts (high or low). Macrocytosis is not always clinically significant, for example, pregnancy and in infancy, although its presence should prompt a review for possible causes.

Haemolytic anaemia

Under normal circumstances, a RBC will survive in the circulation for approximately 120 days. Haemolytic processes result in a reduced lifespan and as a result, if the bone marrow is unable to compensate, anaemia will occur. Haemolysis can be classified into hereditary and acquired forms, and according to the site of red cell breakdown, i.e. intravascularly or extravascularly.

PRACTICAL PRESCRIBING

Direct antiglobulin test

The direct antiglobulin test (DAT) or Coombs test is used to determine if antibodies and/or complement, are coating RBCs. It is a way of determining the aetiology of haemolysis. In-order to conduct the test, red cells from the patient are washed and are then co-incubated with antihuman globulin, also known as the Coombs reagent. If the RBCs stick together (agglutination), then red cells must be coated with an antibody (IgG, M, or A) or complement (C3d). If no agglutination occurs then it is unlikely the red cells are coated and therefore an immune cause is not suspected.

The indirect antiglobulin test can also be performed, whereby the patient's serum is first incubated with red cells at 37°C followed by the DAT test as described. If the DAT is positive it indicates that there are antibodies present in the serum that have coated the red cells. The indirect antiglobulin test is mainly used to crossmatch blood for transfusion, ensuring that the recipient doesn't have antibodies present that may react with the donor cells.

Haemolysis can be classified into hereditary and acquired forms, and according to the site of red cell breakdown, i.e. intravascularly or extravascularly:

- *Hereditary haemolysis* is secondary to defects with the red cell membrane, red cell shape, haemoglobin molecule, defective enzymatic pathways (e.g. G6PD deficiency), or a combination of these. The consequence is early red cell breakdown and the development of anaemia.

- *Acquired haemolysis* occurs secondary to external factors, such as drug therapy or autoimmune haemolytic anaemia (AIHA). With the latter haemolysis is typically extravascular and will be DAT positive, indicating the present of antibodies or complement directed against RBC (see 'Practical prescribing: direct antiglobulin test (DAT)'). AIHA is typically classified as warm (w-AIHA) or cold (c-AIHA) agglutinin disease, distinguished by the presence of IgG (warm antibodies) or less commonly, IgM (cold antibodies). Microangiopathic haemolytic anaemias (MAHA) is a further acquired haemolysis that can be potentially life-threatening and requires immediate management. Thrombotic thrombocytopenia purpura (TTP) and haemolytic uraemic syndrome (HUS) overlap considerably in pathophysiology and clinical features. The two conditions are characterized by a triad of severe sudden haemolysis, thrombocytopenia and renal impairment, with TTP also presenting with neurological impairment and fever. Both conditions can be fatal if left untreated. In severe cases dialysis and plasmapheresis may be required. In many cases the aetiology is unknown but stool cultures may reveal *E.coli* 0157 positivity in HUS.

In patients with known G6PD deficiency it is important to note that certain drugs can precipitate haemolysis. Drugs to be cautious of include **dapsone**, **nitrofurantoin**, **primaquine**, quinolone antibiotics, **rasburicase**, and sulfonamides.

Anaemia secondary to chronic kidney disease

Anaemia in chronic kidney disease occurs as a failure of renal synthesis of erythropoietin. Management is therefore with erythropoietin stimulating agents (see Topic 5.2, 'Acute kidney injury').

Table 12.2 Full blood count indices and normal ranges

Red cell indices	Definition	Normal ranges	
		Male	Female
Haemoglobin (g/L)	Oxygen carrying molecule that fills the red cell	135–180	115–160
Haematocrit (HCT) (%)	Volume/space RBCs take up in the blood as a percentage. E.g. HCT of 45 means 45% of the total blood volume is made up of red blood cells	40–52	36–48
Red blood cell count (× 1012/L)	Absolute number of red blood cells	4.5–6.5	3.9–5.6
Mean cell height (MCH) (pg)	Amount of haemoglobin in the average red blood cell	27–34	
Mean cell volume (MCV) (fl)	Relates to the red cell size, used to classify anaemia into one of three groups: microcytic, normocytic or macrocytic.	80–95	
Mean haemoglobin concentration (MCHC) (g/dL)	Concentration of haemoglobin in the average RBC	30–35	
Reticulocyte count (× 109/L)	Number of immature RBC in the circulation. Release from the bone marrow increases in response to erythropoietin and severe anaemia to compensate for poor oxygenation	50–150	

Investigations of anaemia

The FBC is arguably the most frequently requested blood test and therefore being able to interpret the results is vital. The commonly tested red cell indices and the respective normal range are outlined in Table 12.2. The haemoglobin normal range is set for sex only, in a healthy individual there should be no impact of age on haemoglobin concentration.

A blood film is also a vital investigation that allows for direct visualization of red cells and other blood cells including the platelets and white blood cells; the presence of hypersegmented neutrophils can be seen in B12 deficiency, or pencil and target cells seen in iron deficiency.

Other laboratory tests include ferritin, B12, folate, iron, transferrin, transferrin saturation, and EPO. Ferritin is the storage form of iron and in the absence of inflammation, is an accurate method for monitoring iron stores. B12 deficiency is common and may be secondary to a dietary deficiency or malabsorption. B12 binds intrinsic factor in the stomach, which allows for it to be absorbed in the terminal ileum. Genuine dietary deficiency is rare in the developed world, but common in areas where malnutrition is a problem. Folate levels are also important to quantify. Folic acid is required for synthesis of the purine precursors of DNA and deficiency is thought to cause megaloblastic anaemia due

to inhibition of thymidylate synthesis. Supplementation is recommended during pregnancy to prevent foetal spinal cord and brain malformation (e.g. spina bifida). Serum iron and total iron binding capacity (TIBC) can be used to assess iron levels when the ferritin is not reliable or unhelpful e.g. in inflammatory states. In true iron deficiency the TIBC will be high and iron will be low, whereas in anaemia of chronic disease the TIBC is low or normal. Transferrin is produced by the liver and acts as an iron transporter, taking iron from the intestines to the bone marrow. Low levels may be seen in liver disease leading to increased renal excretion of absorbed free iron while low transferrin saturation means less iron is bound, due to poor iron absorption or a lack of dietary iron. EPO is required for effective erythropoiesis. It is produced by the kidneys thus may be reduced in chronic renal disease, thereby causing anaemia.

Haemolysis screen

Where haemolytic anaemia is suspected laboratory investigations should include lactate dehydrogenase (LDH), which is raised in high cell turnover states, including haemolytic anaemia, serum haptoglobin, very low or absent in haemolytic anaemia, reticulocyte count—the percentage and absolute number of immature RBCs will be high in haemolytic anaemia in the presence of normal bone marrow function. Unconjugated (indirect) bilirubin will be raised with haemolysis and the DAT positive in auto-immune aetiology (see box 'Practical prescribing: direct antiglobulin test').

For a full summary of the relevant pathways and drug targets, see Figure 12.3.

Management of anaemia

Management of anaemia is dependent upon aetiology and is often a consequence of systemic illness, inflammation, infection, or malignancy. As a result, control and reversal of anaemia is dependent on the successful management of the underlying cause, of which pharmacological intervention is just one aspect. A comprehensive drug history, including prescription, over the counter, and recreational drug and alcohol use should be taken, and excluded as a cause. Where haematinic (B12, folate, iron) or other deficiencies are found replacement should be initiated.

Microcytic anaemia

A detailed history and physical examination should be undertaken in all patients with anaemia, which should include identifying the possibility of chronic blood loss as a cause. Systems review, especially covering GI, genitourinary, and menstrual blood loss should be undertaken. Weight loss and other systemic symptoms such as tiredness, lethargy, and fever/sweats should be identified to help determine if malignancy, immune/inflammatory, and infective aetiology may be a cause. A review of medications, co-morbidities, and family history is also vital. Effective treatment of co-morbidities may be enough to resolve associated anaemias. Where no clear cause is identified, GI investigation is often required, especially in the elderly.

Iron preparations must only be used when iron deficiency anaemia is diagnosed and where the aetiology is determined, as its use may otherwise mask significant underlying pathology including GI malignancy, malabsorption, and renal insufficiency. It is thus vital to take a clear history and examination with consideration of referral for further investigation if appropriate prior to treatment. In female patients menorrhagia or pregnancy is a common cause, and in this group prophylactic treatment is often appropriate.

Macrocytic anaemia

Investigations in macrocytic anaemia should primarily be undertaken to exclude any underlying causes, e.g. medication, co-morbidity, liver disease, hypothyroidism, alcohol, and other states where deficiency of haematinics is not implicated. Such causes must be managed according to underlying aetiology. Malignant causes of macrocytosis include myelodysplastic syndrome and myeloma. Vitamin B12 and folate deficiency are the most common causes of macrocytic anaemia and must be managed with dietary and, in most cases, pharmaceutical replacement.

Haemolytic anaemia

Identification of the underlying aetiology in haemolytic anaemia may be difficult and, in many cases, never clearly determined. In the case of AIHA, the onset is usually sudden and requires urgent hospital admission with treatment determined by the class of AIHA, i.e. w-AIHA or c-AIHA. Warm AIHA is primarily managed with corticosteroids. Failing these thereapeutic options splenectomy may be required. Alternatively, immunosuppressants such as **azathioprine** or **ciclosporin** (see Topic 7.2, 'Inflammatory arthropathies'), or more recently, **rituximab** has been used in the case of corticosteroid failure. In cold AIHA as antibodies only react at cold temperatures, management includes keeping the patient warm (particularly extremities), as well as managing any underlying cause, e.g. lymphoma or infection.

Cases of MAHA, such as HUS or TTP, may require plasmapheresis or dialysis support, as well as blood replacement. Antimicrobials can be used to treat infective causes and cessation of culprit drugs may be required where no other cause is suspected.

Drug classes used in management

Oral iron

Oral iron therapy is traditionally prescribed for haemodynamically stable patients with iron-deficiency anaemia resultant from chronic blood loss from the gut. For example, ferrous sulfate, ferrous fumarate, and ferrous gluconate

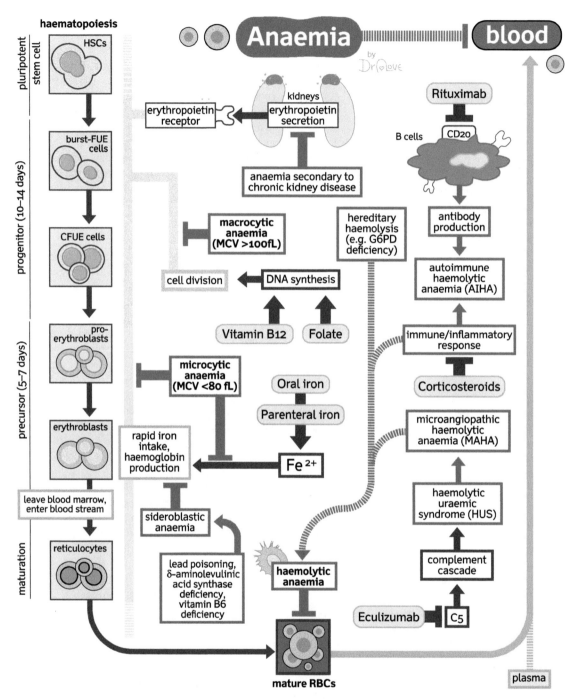

Figure 12.3 Anaemia: summary of relevant pathways and drug targets.

Mechanism of action

Oral iron is absorbed in the distal ilium, with bonding of vitamin C in the stomach and proximal duodenum aiding with absorption. Once in the plasma the iron is transported to the bone marrow, replenishing the stores that are required for haemoglobin synthesis and incorporation into the erythrocytes.

The two categories of iron supplements are those that contain the ferrous form of iron and those containing the ferric form of iron. Since the ferrous form of iron is better absorbed, it has become the most widely used.

Since GI side effects can be a limiting factor, enteric-coated and delayed-release iron supplements have been developed to increase compliance. However, they are not as well absorbed as the non-enteric-coated preparations.

Prescribing

Oral iron is equally effective as IV preparations and therefore should always be used first. There are a variety of oral iron salts available, with little difference in response rates between the various forms available; however, consideration should be given to the relevant elemental iron content when prescribing (see Table 12.3). Treatment of iron deficiency anaemia requires dietary supplementation with between 100–200 mg of elemental iron daily, given in 2–3 divided doses to give a typical response of 1 g/week if taken correctly and absorbed. As the body can only absorb a small amount of elemental iron at a time, a maximum of one tablet should be given at each dose.

Prophylactic requirements, for example, in pregnant females, are lower and usually administration of an OD regime is adequate. Monitoring of response including, FBC, ferritin, and possibly serum iron, TIBC and transferrin saturation should be conducted to check for recovery and ensure iron overload does not occur. The use of OD-modified release preparations to improve tolerance is not recommended, as absorption is poor. Patients should be advised

Table 12.3 Relative ferrous iron content of different ferrous salts

Salt	Dose/ tablet strength	Ferrous iron content
Ferrous fumarate	200 mg	65 mg
Ferrous gluconate	300 mg	35 mg
Ferrous sulfate	300 mg	60 mg
Ferrous sulfate (dried)	200 mg	65 mg

to avoid taking iron with food, in particular calcium containing foods (e.g. dairy) or caffeine can significantly impair absorption. Conversely, administration with vitamin C, e.g. orange juice can promote absorption.

Unwanted effects

GI irritation, including nausea, epigastric pain, constipation, and diarrhoea are reported with oral iron salts. Patients should also be advised that therapy is also likely to cause blackened tarry stools. Modified-release iron preparations can increase the risk of diarrhoea in people with a history of inflammatory bowel disease, strictures, or diverticular disease.

Parenteral iron

IV administered iron is used in patients where absorption is compromised, allowing the supplementation of 80–160 mg iron/day (compared with 40–60 mg iron/day in oral iron therapy). Examples include iron dextran, iron sucrose, iron isomaltoside 1000, and ferric carboxymaltose.

Mechanism of action

As with oral iron, parental iron replacement acts to replenish bone marrow iron stores (see above).

Prescribing

IV iron is indicated for those who have unacceptable side effects to oral therapy, malabsorption, ongoing blood loss, non-compliance issues, or require a more rapid correction e.g. pre-operatively or prior to delivery in pregnant women. Patients with chronic renal failure receiving haemodialysis or peritoneal dialysis may also require parental iron administration in addition to erythropoietin. Ferumoxytol, an iron oxide is specifically licenced for this indication.

Administration varies significantly between preparations from 6 hours (iron dextran) to 15 minutes (iron isomaltoside and ferric carboxymaltose) infusion/injection. Regimes also vary from three times a week schedules to single doses that may be repeated. Doses are calculated based on body weight and haemoglobin levels. Increasingly, the use of total daily dose schedules with agents that can be delivered over a short period are being used to alleviate pressures in day care settings.

Unwanted effects

Hypersensitivity reactions including anaphylaxis can occur in response to parental iron and, therefore, resuscitation equipment should be available during administration, and patients observed for a period of at least 30 minutes before a dose. Other side effects include GI disturbance (less frequent that with oral iron), headaches, dizziness, rash, and infusion site reactions.

Vitamin B12

Vitamin B12 plays an important role in DNA synthesis and neurological function, with deficiency leading to a wide spectrum of haematological and neuropsychiatric disorders. Supplementation with oral vitamin B12 is a safe and effective treatment for the deficiency state. For example, hydroxocobalamin and cyanocobalamin.

Mechanism of action

Vitamin B12 plays an essential role in nervous system functioning, including the brain and spinal cord. Therefore, neurological symptoms may be the first abnormality noted in vitamin B12 deficiency. In patients with folate deficit, vitamin B12 deficiency should be ruled out or addressed first, in order to prevent the development of spinal cord degeneration (see 'Prescribing warning: subacute combined degeneration secondary to B12 deficiency'). B12 is also required for DNA synthesis, amino acid formation, and normal red cell development.

In humans, only two enzymatic reactions are known to be dependent on vitamin B12. The first is methylmalonic conversion to succinyl-CoA using vitamin B12 as cofactor, thus deficiency can lead to increased serum levels of methylmalonic acid. In the second reaction, homocysteine is converted to methionine by using vitamin B12 and folic acid as cofactors, with deficiency potentially leading to increased homocysteine levels.

PRESCRIBING WARNING

Subacute combined degeneration secondary to B12 deficiency

Combined degeneration of the cord, brain, and peripheral nerves is a severe complication of B12 deficiency resulting in progressive nerve demyelination. Patients present with weakness of the limbs, altered sensation, proprioception dysfunction, and vibratory sensation loss. Prolonged deficiency results in irreversible neurological deficit, but early treatment may result in full recovery.

In cases of combined folate and B12 deficiency the B12 must be administered first to prevent cord degeneration from occurring. If folic acid is administered first the existing B12 stores are converted to methylcobalamin making the deficiency worse.

Prescribing

Hydroxocobalamin is given by IM injection, typically given as a loading regimen followed by a maintenance phase, e.g. 1 mg on alternate days for 5 doses followed by 1 mg every 3 months. If there is evidence of neurological involvement, the loading regime may be intensified, e.g. 1 mg on alternate days for 2 weeks.

Cyanocobalamin is an oral preparation again indicated for the treatment of B12 deficiency, although as effective as oral therapy is used less frequently due to the risk of poor compliance associated with its use.

Unwanted effects

Most patients will not notice any side effects, but nausea, headache, dizziness, and fever have been reported. Injection site reactions may occur as can hypersensitivity including rash and itch occasionally. In patients with low platelets should have a platelet count above 30 prior to giving as an IM injection.

Folate

Folate (vitamin B9) is an essential nutrient that is needed for DNA replication and as a substrate for a range of enzymatic reactions involved in amino acid synthesis and vitamin metabolism.

Mechanism of action

The term folate is typically employed as a generic name for the group of chemically related compounds based on the folic acid structure. Folate is one of the 13 essential vitamins and cannot be synthesized *de novo* by the body. It must thus be obtained from diet or supplementation. *Dietary folate* is a naturally occurring nutrient found in foods (leafy green vegetables, legumes, egg yolk, liver, and citrus fruit). Folic acid is a synthetic dietary supplement that is found in artificially enriched foods and pharmaceutical vitamins. However, neither folate nor folic acid are metabolically active, and must be reduced to participate in cellular metabolism.

To become metabolically active, folic acid must be converted first to dihydrofolate (DHF) and then to tetrahydrofolate (THF) through enzymatic reduction catalysed by the enzyme DHF reductase. The, THF can be converted to the biologically active l-methylfolate by the enzyme methylenetetrahydrofolate reductase (MTHFR). This conversion is needed to generate the L-methylfolate required for the one-carbon transfer reactions (methyl donations) used for purine/pyrimidine synthesis in DNA/

RNA assembly, DNA methylation, and homocysteine metabolism.

Considering its requirement for DNA and RNA synthesis, and DNA repair, folate deficiency can affect many physiological processes. In the context of haematopoiesis, deficiency slows cell division as a result of defective DNA synthesis. This results in clumping of cytoplasmic chromatin and a subsequent increase in RBC size and the presence of hypersegmented neutrophils. In pregnancy folate is required to enable the correct formation of the neural tube. Deficiency can, therefore, result in defects such as spina bifida.

Prescribing

Folic acid should never to be prescribed alone in the presence of B12 deficiency due to possible precipitation of subacute combined deficiency of the cord (see 'Prescribing warning: subacute combined degeneration secondary to B12 deficiency'). When prescribed as replacement therapy in deficiency states 5 mg orally daily is the usual initiation dose, although this may be increased to up to 15 mg daily in malabsorption states. In cases of chronic haemolytic anaemia 5 mg can be prescribed every 1–7 days depending on the severity of haemolysis.

Folic acid or folinic acid, is also prescribed for patients receiving the antifolate **methotrexate** to reduce toxicity. The dose of folic acid required and administration method depend on the dose and indication.

In pregnancy, lower doses of folic acid are required to prevent neural tube defects, typically 400 μg orally enough for the first trimester only, although 5 mg may be required in at-risk women, e.g. those on antifolate therapy such as **phenytoin**.

Unwanted effects

Folic acid is well tolerated with rare reports of GI disturbances.

Corticosteroids

Corticosteroids represent the first-line treatment for patients with warm antibody type AIHA, although their use is based on experience, rather than hard evidence, with effectiveness not yet supported by clinical trials. For example, prednisolone, hydrocortisone, and methylprednisolone

Mechanism of action

Corticosteroids inhibit inflammatory processes and work via binding of the glucocorticoid/glucocorticoid receptor complex to glucocorticoid responsive elements in the nucleus or cytoplasm resulting in alteration of gene expression and transcription factor activation. Many inflammatory cytokines and chemokines are down-regulated as a result, which can dampen immune activity in warm antibody AIHA (w-AIHA) and stop auto-immune antibody production.

Prescribing

Oral **prednisolone** is usually the first line steroid used in w-AIHA treatment with a starting dose of 1 mg/kg prescribed, increased to 2 mg/kg in severe or refractory cases, if tolerated.

Unwanted effects

See corticosteroids (Topic 6.6, 'Inflammatory bowel disease').

Monoclonal antibody therapies

Recent advances in the understanding of the mechanisms of autoimmunity and w-AIHA has led to the use of novel approaches to treating the disease. Monoclonal antibodies represent a major advance towards a targeted therapy that can improve treatment with reduction of toxicity. For example, eculizumab and rituximab.

Mechanism of action

Rituximab is an anti-CD20 chimeric murine/mouse monoclonal antibody, with some efficacy in the management of w-AIHA. Anti-CD20 therapy results in CD20 positive B cell destruction and results in reduced auto-antibody production and secondary effects via a reduction in pro-inflammatory cytokine production and T-cell activation.

Eculizumab is a recombinant humanized anti-C5 monoclonal antibody that has recently gained approval for use in HUS and is also used in paroxysmal nocturnal haemoglobinuria (PNH). By targeting C5 it inhibits the complement cascade and therefore hinders complement dependent cell lysis of RBCs.

Prescribing

Rituximab is administered IV at a standard dose of 375 mg/m² IV weekly for 4 weeks, and the patient then assessed for response.

Eculizumab is administered IV according to indication, initially weekly for the first 5 weeks, then every 2 weeks for life. Patients undergoing supplementary plasmapheresis or plasma exchange should have doses administered 60 minutes after.

Unwanted effects

Headache, hypertension, nausea, vomiting, diarrhoea, back pain, rhinorrhoea, and peripheral oedema have all been reported with **eculizumab**. There is also a risk of hypersensitivity, thus the need to give as a slow infusion and to observe patients for 1 hour after completion. In patients that react, treatment should be discontinued.

For **rituximab** see Topic 7.2, 'Inflammatory arthropathies'.

Further reading

Greenberg JA, Bell SJ, Guan Y, et al. (2011) Folic acid supplementation and pregnancy: more than just neural tube defect prevention. *Reviews of Obstetrics and Gynecology* 4 (2), 52–9.

Johnson-Wimbley TD (2011) Diagnosis and management of iron deficiency anaemia in the 21st century. *Therapy in Advanced Gastroenterology* 4(3), 177–84.

Liu B, Gu W (2013) Immunotherapy treatments of warm autoimmune haemolytic anaemia. *Clinical and Developmental Immunology* 2013, Article ID 561852.

Zanella A, Barcellini W (2014) Treatment of autoimmune haemolytic anaemias. *Haematologica* 99(10), 1547–54.

Guidelines

British Society of Gastroenterology (2011) Guidelines for the management of iron deficiency anaemia. https://www.bsg.org.uk/resource/guidelines-for-the-management-of-iron-deficiency-anaemia.html [accessed 14 April 2019].

British Society for Haematology (2015) Guidelines for the diagnosis and management of adult aplastic anaemia. https://onlinelibrary.wiley.com/doi/full/10.1111/bjh.13853 [accessed 14 April 2019].

British Society for Haematology (2016) The diagnosis and management of primary autoimmune haemolytic anaemia. https://onlinelibrary.wiley.com/doi/full/10.1111/bjh.14478 [accessed 14 April 2019].

British Society for Haematology (2017) Guidelines on the management of drug-induced immune and secondary autoimmune, haemolytic anaemia. https://onlinelibrary.wiley.com/doi/full/10.1111/bjh.14654 [accessed 14 April 2019].

Sickle cell anaemia, thalassaemia, and other genetic abnormalities associated with haemoglobin, are among the most common genetic abnormalities in the world. It is estimated that approximately 7% of the world's population are carriers.

In general, it is possible to divide haemoglobinopathies into two groups;

- *Thalassaemia*: α and β most common and clinically significant.
- *Structural haemoglobin variants*: HbS, HbE, and HbC.

The historic geographic distribution of the haemoglobinopathies corresponds to the historic geographic area affected by malaria, i.e. Mediterranean Europe, Asia, and Africa. With the advent of mass migration, distribution has become more global. Sickle RBCs are less likely to be infected by malaria and thus inheritance of sickle cell genes confers some protection to the potentially fatal infection.

Normal haemoglobin

During foetal development and, after birth, the dominant type of haemoglobin changes. The earliest haemoglobins—Gower I, II, and Hb Portland—are present at the highest concentrations during the first trimester. Towards the end of the first trimester, foetal haemoglobin (HbF) starts to take over and remains as the major haemoglobin molecule until birth. Adult haemoglobin (HbA) is detectable at low concentrations during the embryonic and foetal periods, but following birth quickly becomes the predominant oxygen-carrying molecule. In the adult, HbA makes up 98% of the haemoglobin with HbF being present only in trace amounts (<1%). The other component of the adult haemoglobin is HbA2, which makes up the remaining ~2%.

There are further forms of haemoglobin found in normal individuals, but these make up less than 1% of the total blood stream haemoglobins. The other adult 'minor haemoglobins' are again made up of heterodimers, but the β subunits are replaced by either γ chains (foetal haemoglobin) or δ chains (Hb A2).

The sole function of haemoglobin is to carry oxygen from the lungs to the tissues. For this to occur optimally, the structure of the globin chains must allow for correct folding and formation of the quaternary structure. In addition, there must be a vehicle to transport the haemoglobin and oxygen around the body, i.e. the RBC. Any condition that reduces the amount of red blood cells will have an impact on oxygenation (see Topic 12.1, 'Anaemia'). Finally, RBCs must be of optimal size in order to allow a good concentration of haemoglobin molecules to pack the cell (300×10^6 pg per erythrocyte).

HbA is composed of two alpha- and two beta-polypeptide chains, each containing a haem unit. The polypeptide chains are bound and folded to form a quaternary structure with the haem units located in clefts on the surface. The haem unit is created due to hydrophobic amino acid molecule orientated in the centre of the structure, and water-loving hydrophilic molecules lying on the surface. Within the centre of the haem unit, lies one atom of iron and just enough space for the addition of an oxygen molecule, which occurs at high oxygen concentrations in the lung. The complete haemoglobin molecule therefore has the capacity to bind four oxygen molecules, one haem ring/iron atom/oxygen molecule per α and β chain.

Once one haem molecule binds an oxygen atom it makes it easier for a second to bind and so on until all molecules are bound. The converse is true for the release of oxygen molecules in the lower oxygen tension environment of the tissues. This allosteric characteristic is the basis for the sigmoidal shape of the oxygen dissociation curve (see Topic 12.1, 'Anaemia').

Overall, the binding and release of oxygen means the entire haemoglobin tetramer is constantly shifting between two states, a relaxed 'R' conformation that follows oxygen binding in the lungs, and a tight 'T' conformation on the release of oxygen in the peripheries. The molecule 2,3-diphosphoglycerate (2,3-DPG) is involved in the facilitation of the release of oxygen and the formation of the T state, its concentration therefore varies according to the tissues requirement for oxygen, i.e. in tissues with a high oxygen demand the concentration is high. A variety of other factors also alter the likelihood of haemoglobin releasing its oxygen molecules.

Sickle cell disease

Pathophysiology

Sickle cell anaemia (SCD) is a phenotypically diverse condition arising from a common genotypic abnormality; the inheritance of the sickle β-globin gene (Figure 12.4). This

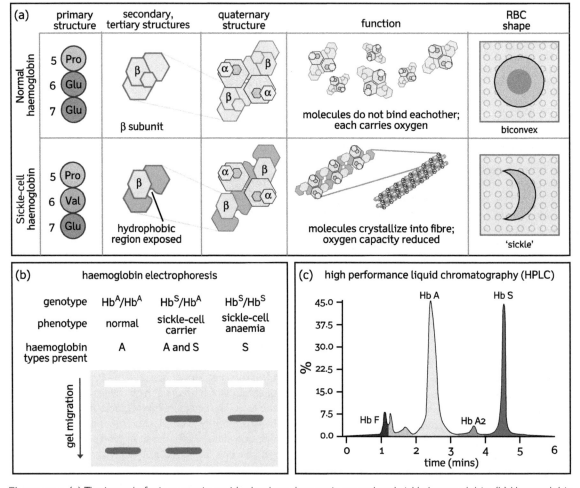

Figure 12.4 (a) The impact of primary amino acids structure changes in normal and sickle haemoglobin. (b) Haemoglobin electrophoresis for diagnosis: Haemoglobin electrophoresis showing the pattern seen in sickle cell disease, trait and normal. The position of the globin molecules. (c) High performance liquid chromatography for diagnosis; HPLC example of a sickle cell carrier showing two main haemoglobin peaks, Hb A and Hb S. Hb F and Hb A2 peaks are also evident.

(b) Reproduced from https://www.mun.ca/biology/scarr/Hemoglobin_Electrophoresis.html. All text material © 2014 by Steven M. Carr. (c) Reproduced with permission from Provan D (Ed). Oxford Handbook of Clinical and Laboratory Investigation, Third Edition. Figure 3.12. Oxford, UK: Oxford University Press © 2010. Reproduced with permission of the Licensor through PLSclear.

is evidenced by the vastly different symptoms displayed by individuals with the same underlying genetic abnormality. Typically, inheritance of a single βs gene, results in a carrier state which is a benign symptomatic condition. The full blood count indices may all be normal with no evidence of anaemia.

Pathophysiology is characterized by erythrocyte membrane instability and cell sickling. The sickle cells are prone to haemolysis which in turn leads to vaso-occlusion and organ damage including avascular necrosis of the bone.

The symptoms of sickle cell disease are similar to other haemolytic anaemia states (see Topic 12.1, 'Anaemia'), but during times of stress (dehydration, infection, surgery, etc.) can be accompanied by crises including;

- *Veno-occlusive crisis*: significant sickling within blood vessels can cause vessel occlusion. Prolonged vessel occlusion can result in infarction of the affected organ including the lungs, central nervous system (stroke and seizure), spleen, and bones. Bone pain may be severe and commonly affects the axial skeleton. Avascular necrosis of the femoral and humeral heads are common.

- *Visceral sequestration crisis*: accumulation of sickled cells in the spleen, liver, or lung leading to direct organ pathology, e.g. splenic infarction and acute chest syndrome.

- *Aplastic crisis*: bone marrow failure of erythropoiesis secondary to parvovirus B19 infection.

Chronic splenic micro-infarction secondary to sickling red cells can lead to marked hyposplenism and even autosplenectomy, which leads to immunocompromise and thus significantly increasing the risk of infection with encapsulated organisms. For this reason, all patients must keep up-to-date with vaccinations and receive prophylactic antibiotics. Other consequences include a higher incidence of gallstones, leg ulceration (haemosiderin deposition), cardiomyopathy, priapism (can be a medical emergency), retinopathy, and renal papillary necrosis.

Diagnosis is based on history (most patients will have a family history) and investigations including:

- *Full blood count*: Hb typically between 6 and 10 g/L, although patients will not display symptoms usually seen at this level of anaemia.

- *Reticulocyte count*: this should be raised. A low count should prompt investigation for infective agents responsible for an aplastic crises such as parvovirus.

- *Blood film*: this will show the classical sickle cells and features of hyposplenism with the presence of Howell jolly bodies and occasional nucleated RBC.

- *Haemoglobin electrophoresis*: this will provide a definitive answer to the type of haemoglobin present, (Figure 12.4B). Patients with sickle cell trait will have one HbA and one HbS, while those with homozygous disease will have no HbA present. The percentage of HbF is greater in individuals with homozygous disease and is typically between 3 and 15%. Furthermore, higher levels of HbF are associated with a reduction in the frequency and severity of crises, thus disease modifying therapy such as **hydroxycarbamide** and **azacitidine** are used to increase the percentage of HbF.

- *High performance liquid chromatography* (Figure 12.4C): this is similar to Hb electrophoresis, but is based on elute time and is becoming the most common diagnostic tool used to detect haemoglobinopathies.

For a full summary of the relevant pathways and drug targets, see Figure 12.5.

Management

Management of SCD involves patient education, avoidance of precipitating factors (e.g. dehydration, infection), prophylactic treatments, and acute management of crises. Dehydration is a significant cause of crises and, therefore, education regarding good fluid intake during the summer months and during exercise, can help reduce the frequency of acute episodes.

Chronic management

Prophylactic medications are used to:

- prevent folate deficiency;
- prevent infection;
- reduce frequency of crises.

Patients are therefore routinely prescribed folic acid and penicillin V as prophylaxis against pneumococcal infections. In addition, vaccination against pneumococcal, meningococcal, and haemophilus influenza type B (HIB) should be undertaken, together with an annual flu vaccine to help prevent infection.

Disease-modifying therapy with **hydroxycarbamide** is generally initiated to reduce the severity and frequency of sickle crises in patients that experience frequent (>3 per year), painful episodes, or where disease has resulted in severe complications, e.g. severe anaemia or vasoccluson. Efficacy is assessed through regular measurements of HbF, aiming for a level of at least twice baseline level after 6

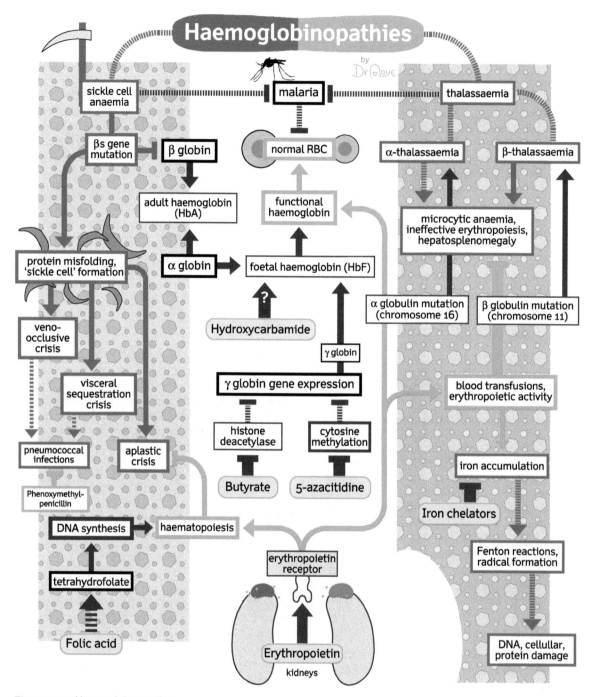

Figure 12.5 Haemoglobinopathies.

months of treatment. Where effective and tolerated treatment is continued long term. In severe disease or in the presence of deteriorating renal function, **erythropoietin** may be added in. Alternative agents such as **azacitidine** or **butyric acid** are less widely used off-label in SCD.

Management of acute crises

Management of sickle cell crisis is a haematological emergency that requires urgent hospital admission. IV fluids and oxygen therapy should be initiated during history and examination. If fever is present empiric IV antibiotics must be started, based on local guidelines, and the suspected site of infection, and a full septic screen including cultures obtained. Antibiotic choice will usually be with a broad spectrum agent, such as a third generation cephalosporin or pipercillin/tazobactam. IV or IM analgesics are required to alleviate pain; opiates are often required. As soon as safely possible, oral alternatives should be sought and weened to cessation. If hypoxia is a feature, chest crisis should be suspected and is managed with bronchodilators (e.g. salbutamol), red cell transfusion, and exchange transfusion considered to reduce the HbS concentration to <30%. ITU transfer may be required and continuous positive airway pressure (CPAP) administered to keep the arterial oxygen concentration above 70 mmHg. Mortality can be as high as 10%.

Drug classes used in management

Folic acid

> Folic acid administration replenishes the depleted folate stores observed in patients with SCD.

Mechanism of action

See Topic 12.1, 'Anaemia'.

Prescribing

Folic acid is administered orally at a dose of 5 mg OD in sickle cell disease for the prevention of folate deficiency.

Unwanted effects

See Topic 12.1, 'Anaemia'.

Hydroxycarbamide

> Hydroxycarbamide (hydroxyurea) prevents the complications of SCD by increasing HbF and total haemoglobin concentrations, by decreasing the adhesion of sickle cells to the endothelium in vitro, and by increasing polymerization time. Used for the prevention of crises and red cell transfusion.

Mechanism of action

The chemotherapy drug **hydroxycarbamide** is known to increase foetal haemoglobin (HbF) concentrations, although the precise mechanism by which it does this is poorly understood. It is thought to act through stimulation of nitrous oxide and other mediators, which in turn regulates the transcription and translation of HbF. Nitrous oxide stimulation may also be beneficial for its potent vasodilator properties through action on pulmonary vessels, thereby improving blood flow.

Prescribing

For almost three decades, hydroxycarbamide has been used as an effective prophylactic agent in SCD, where it has been shown to reduce the need for red cell transfusions and reduce the frequency of crises. Doses are taken orally, starting at a low dose and slowly increase as appropriate according to response. Treatment may take 2–3 months before a beneficial effect is noted.

Unwanted effects

As an antineoplastic agent **hydroxycarbamide** is associated with numerous side effects, in particular there is a significant risk of myelosuppression. A FBC should therefore be conducted prior to treatment initiation and repeated every 2 weeks for the first 2 months. As a general rule, the greater the level of foetal haemoglobin the greater the risk of myelosuppression. Patients on higher doses or with previous neutropenia, 2-weekly counts should continue for the duration of treatment. Renal and hepatic toxicity are also widely reported with its use so that renal and liver function should be monitored at regular intervals. Severe hepatic impairment is a contraindication to use.

Younger patients should be advised about the risk to fertility with a reduction in sperm count being observed in males, albeit infrequently. Pregnancy is an absolute contraindication to use. Female patients should be counselled about the risk to the developing foetus and a pregnancy test should be conducted prior to initiation.

Erythropoietin

> The glycoprotein hormone EPO, haematopoietin, or menopoietin, controls RBC production (erythropoiesis). It is used in SCD for the prevention of crises and red cell transfusion—erythropoietin.

Mechanism of action

Erythropoietin is a growth factor required for effective erythropoiesis. It binds to the erythropoietin receptors on the red cell progenitors surface and activates a JAK2 signalling cascade, which initiates the STAT5, PI3K, and Ras MAPK cellular second messenger signalling cascades. This causes the differentiation, survival, and proliferation of the erythroid cell. In the context of SCD, EPO causes an increase in Hb F levels and is often used in combination with **hydroxycarbamide**.

Prescribing

There is no agreed recommended dosing strategy, however the dose is usually higher than that used in chronic renal failure (Topic 5.1, 'The kidney, drugs, and chronic kidney disease'). If used in combination with **hydroxycarbamide**, it may be given on separate days, e.g. 3 days EPO and 4 days hydroxycarbamide in weekly cycles.

Unwanted effects

See Topic 5.1, 'The kidney, drugs, and chronic kidney disease'.

Azacitidine

The pyrimidine analogue azanucleoside azacitidine is an established molecular tool for the induction of DNA demethylation in cellular model systems. It is used for the prevention of crises and red cell transfusion.

Mechanism of action

Azacitidine has been used to treat sickle cell disease for over 30 years, acting to inhibit haemoglobin γ-chain cytosine methylation, which results in a beneficial rise in HbF concentrations. Following treatment, there is an increase in the percentage of reticulocytes and erythrocytes that contain HbF, and an increase in blood haemoglobin concentration.

Azacytosine-guanine dinucleotides can substitute for cytosine and are recognized by the DNA methyltransferases during the initiation of the methylation reaction. This reaction is blocked by azacytosine, where specifically carbon-5 is substituted by nitrogen, causing the covalent binding of the enzyme to DNA and subsequent blockade of its DNA methyltransferase function.

Prescribing

Azacitidine is administered SC in cycles, usually 5 days of treatment every 2 weeks. Use in SCD is currently off-license.

Unwanted effects

As with **hydroxycarbamide**, **azacitidine** is a chemotherapy agent and as such associated with significant haematological toxicity. Patients on treatment will require baseline blood counts carried out precycle and treatment delayed where counts are low. Caution is also required in hepatic or renal impairment and should not be used in pregnancy or during breastfeeding. Other common side effects include GI disturbance, hyper/hypotension, respiratory compromise including pneumonia and dyspnoea, insomnia, anxiety, headache, hypokalaemia, and arthralgia.

Butyrate

Butyrate is a short chain fatty acid derived from the microbial fermentation of dietary fibres in the colon. The mechanism of action involves an epigenetic regulation of gene expression via the inhibition of histone deacetylases.

Mechanism of action

Butyrate is part of a well-known class of epigenetic substances known as histone deacetylases inhibitors, which affect chromatin structures and regulate gene expression without changes in nucleotide sequence. Histone tail acetylation can enhance the accessibility of a gene to the transcription machinery, while deacetylated tails are highly charged and tightly associated with the DNA backbone, thus limiting accessibility of genes.

In the context of SCD, butyrate can increase the transcription of γ-globin genes leading to increased beneficial HbF concentrations.

Prescribing

The use of **butyrate** in SCD remains fairly experimental and as such it is not widely available. Pulsed therapy has resulted in the best results, with a typical regime being 250—500 mg/kg/day IV infused (6—12 hours) up to six times per month. The short half-life and long infusion times make this therapy difficult to administer due to non-adherence. The use may be limited to patients with leg ulceration, where butyrate therapy has been shown to be particularly effective.

Unwanted effects

Oral preparations have an unpleasant taste and odour, and are not used as a consequence. No other significant adverse effects have been noted.

Thalassaemia

Pathophysiology

The thalassaemia's are a group of autosomal recessive conditions of which α-thalassaemia and β-thalassaemia are the most common and clinically significant. As with SCD, thalassaemia provides some immunity to malaria and, therefore, the prevalence is highest in malarial regions such as the Mediterranean, Asia, and Africa. Prevalence of α-gene deletions may be as high as 25% in some regions.

As with SCD, diagnosis can be made in the presence of a positive family history and ethnic background, combined with laboratory tests to include;

- *Full blood count* may reveal a microcytic hypochromic picture, but the severity will depend on the type of thalassaemia and number of genes affected (see Tables 12.4 and 12.5).
- *Blood film* examination commonly shows the presence of nucleated red cells and target cells (codocytes).
- *Haemoglobin electrophoresis* is a way to measure the concentration of haemaoglobin molecules (based on charge) present and can therefore be used to determine the likely phonotype (see Figure 12.5B).
- *High performance liquid chromatography* is another way to determine the concentration of different haemoglobin molecules (Fig. 12.5C).
- *Genetic testing* will enable the detection of the exact mutations and deletions present.
- *Bone marrow* examination will be hypercellular for age, with marked erythroid series hyperplasia (not required for diagnosis).

α-Thalassaemia

α-Thalassaemia is caused by the deletion of one or more of the α globulin genes located on chromosome 16. In

Table 12.4 α-Thalassaemia syndromes

Genotype	Clinical significance
α-α- / α- α- (no α- chains produced)	*Hydrops foetalis*: no α genes are present thus the foetus is unable to make any foetal ($\alpha_2\gamma_2$) or adult haemoglobin ($\alpha_2\beta_2$) molecules. This syndrome is not compatible with life and death usually occurs in utero (0% of normal α globin levels)
α + α- / α- α-	*Haemoglobin H disease (Hb H)*: loss of three alleles results in a marked microcytic anaemia (Hb 60–100) with associated splenomegaly in most cases (20–25% of normal α globin concentration)
α+α- / α+ α- or α+α+ / α- α-	*Thalassaemia trait*: individuals with a loss of 2 α chain alleles results in the production of small pale red blood cells and subsequently a mild microcytic anaemia (50% of normal α globin concentration)
α+α+ / α+α-	*Silent carrier*: individuals carry one less copy of the α gene and have no signs or symptoms of thalassaemia (70–80% of normal α globin concentration)
α+α+ / α+α+	*Normal state*

normal individuals there will be four copies of each α gene, two inherited from each parent. The severity of α-thalassaemia will depend on how many alleles are mutated, (see Table 12.4) e.g. the loss of all four α alleles is the most severe form and commonly leads to death in utero. In contrast to β thalassaemia iron overload is not usually an issue unless frequent transfusions are required and bone abnormalities are rarely seen.

Management

Most patients with α-thalassaemia will be asymptomatic and in the case of silent carriers or thalassaemia trait, no therapy is required. Haemoglobin H disease may require supplementary folic acid support (see Topic 12.1, 'Anaemia') and infections must be treated promptly to prevent haemolysis and a worsening anaemia; for example, aplastic crisis can occur with parvovirus infection. Supportive therapy with fluids and blood products is required until immunity and clearance of the pathogen occurs.

Table 12.5 Thalassaemia syndromes

Genotype	Clinical significance
$\beta^\circ / \beta^\circ$ or β^+ / β°	**T**halassaemia major: compete (or almost complete (β-/β+) loss of β globin chain genes results in severe syndrome characterized by excess production of α chains leading to α: β chain imbalance. This imbalance results in marked microcytic anaemia (20–70 g/L), ineffective erythropoiesis (due to α chain deposition in erythroblasts) and extramedullary haematopoiesis. Hepatosplenomegaly is almost universal
β^+ / β^+ or β / β°	*Thalassaemia intermedia*: in this condition both β alleles are mutated or one copy of the gene is deleted. The phenotype displayed depends on the exact mutations acquired and the effect of these mutations on β globin function. Microcytic anaemia is generally much less severe (hb 50–100 g/L) compared with thalassaemia major because the imbalance of α to β and γ globin chains is less marked. Hepatosplenomegaly, extramedullary haematopoiesis and bone deformities still occur in many
β^+ / β or β° / β	*Thalassaemia minor/trait*: this results from a complete loss or mutation of only one copy of the β globin gene. Most individuals will not develop symptoms but a full blood count may show a mild microcytic, hypochromic anaemia with a raised red cell count. Haemoglobin A_2 ($\alpha_2\delta_2$) levels are also raised, typically between 3 and 5%
β / β	*Normal state*

β = Normal gene; β^+ = mutated gene; β°= deleted gene/completely ineffective.

Iron overload is uncommon, but can occur both in patients who have required frequent red cell transfusion and in the absence of transfusion. It is advisable to check iron stores by ferritin quantification at least once yearly in Hb H disease and if elevated, LFTs and an endocrine screen should be undertaken to assess end-organ damage. Liver imaging (MRI) to determine if liver iron is present may be undertaken. In some cases iron chelation therapy may be required, e.g. with **desferrioxamine**.

Historically, a number of patients receiving infected blood products contracted HIV, hepatitis B or C, although with screening such complications are now rare. Patients should also be vaccinated early against hepatitis B.

β-thalassaemia

β-thalassaemia results from either deletion or mutation of the β globin genes located on chromosome 11. There are two alleles, one present on each chromosome. Over 400 mutations and deletions have been identified meaning that β-thalassaemia presents with a very heterogeneous phenotype, (see Table 12.5).

In thalassaemia major the symptoms of anaemia manifest as failure to thrive, and pallor may begin as soon as the switch from γ to β globin occurs at about 3 months of age. Jaundice may be evident, especially during times of stress, such as infection, which is also common. Bone marrow hyperplasia developed in response to the anaemia can result in bone deformity and bone enlargement. The facial and skull bones are commonly affected with medullary expansion and a loss of cortical bone. For the same reason hepatosplenomegaly is common.

Regular transfusions are a feature of thalassaemia major leading to iron overload. Increased iron absorption from the gut also contributes. Complications of iron overload include organ failure (liver and heart) endocrinopathy (hypothyroidism, diabetes mellitus, and a failure of sexual development) and increased melanin pigmentation.

Management

The mainstay of thalassaemia major management, involves regular blood transfusion and iron chelation therapy to remove the excess iron that accumulates as a consequence of tissue deposition (siderosis). Iron chelation is achieved through the use of one of three commercially available iron chelator therapies (**desferrioxamine**, **deferasirox**, and **deferiprone**) used as monotherapy or with desferrioxamine and deferiprone in combination; see 'Iron chelators'. All three agents are considered to be as effective in controlling ferritin, liver, and cardiac iron, although there are differences with regards to administration and potentially adverse effects. Osteoporosis may also be an issue hence bisphosphonates in combination with calcium and vitamin D may be required for bone health (see Topic 7.4, 'Metabolic Bone Disease'). Management of other complications such as end-organ failure (e.g. heart failure, arrhythmias) and endocrinopathies is patient specific and will require standard treatment.

Splenectomy may be required in patients who require frequent transfusions and in whom splenomegaly and splenic infarction occurs. Allogeneic stem cell transplantation is also an option for some patients. As with a-thalassaemia a viral hepatitis screen and HIV test should be carried out.

Drug classes used in management

Unliganded or incompletely liganded iron ions can participate in 'Fenton-type' redox chemistry, reacting with hydrogen peroxide or lipid peroxides to generate highly reactive hydroxyl radical or lipid radicals, which can damage lipid membranes, proteins, and nucleic acids. As a result, iron chelators are needed to reduce this potentially toxic iron overload.

Examples include deferasirox, deferiprone, and desferrioxamine mesylate.

Iron chelators

Mechanism of action

In thalassemia, iron accumulation is the consequence of blood transfusions and of increased iron absorption caused by erythropoietic activity. The combined effects of iron overload and increased outpouring of catabolic iron from the reticuloendothelial system can overwhelm the capacity of transferrin to carry iron, resulting in toxic non-transferrin bound plasma iron.

Iron chelators bind serum iron so that iron is excreted in the faeces (e.g. **deferasirox**) or urine (e.g. **deferiprone**). There is evidence that deferasirox and deferiprone are also able to bind intracellular iron. Although iron chelators can be chemically diverse, they typically contain oxygen, nitrogen, or sulphur-donor atoms that form coordinate bonds with bound iron.

Prescribing

Desferrioxamine was the first iron-chelating agent to be launched for the treatment of iron overload. Doses are administered by SC infusion over 8–24 hours up to OD if required, though typically given for 10–12 hours 5–6 times a week. It is, therefore, usually supplied in an elastomeric pump to enable home administration and run overnight. Increasingly, however, the newer oral therapies **deferasirox** and **deferiprone** are being used in preference due to improved compliance, or where desferrioxamine therapy has failed or is contraindicated.

With all agents the dose is determined by weight and extent of iron overload, with doses adjusted according to ferritin. Liver and cardiac MRI may also be used to determine the extent of iron infiltration. Combination therapy with desferrioxamine and deferiprone may be required in resistant cases or in heart failure, where the two together have been shown to be of superior efficacy in improving cardiac function

Unwanted effects

Desferrioxamine tends to be better tolerated than oral therapy, although the rate of discontinuation is no higher, probably due to the inconvenience associated with SC infusion. The most common side effects to treatment varies with each agent, i.e. injection site reactions are most common with desferrioxamine, whereas joint pain, GI disturbance and cytopenias occur most commonly with **deferiprone**. Patients on the latter in particular require regular monitoring of white cell counts and counselling on what to do in the event of an infection. High doses and prolonged used of desferrioxamine have been known to cause visual and hearing impairment. This can be minimized through use of lower doses, close monitoring of ferritin levels, and also through the use of hearing and ophthalmologic assessments. The risk of renal toxicity is most pronounced with **deferasirox** and, although minimally renally cleared itself, may affect the clearance of other drugs excreted by the kidneys. Deferasirox has also been reported to cause GI ulceration and fatal haemorrhage.

Further reading

Canani RB, Costanzo MD, Leone L, et al. (2011) Potential beneficial effects of butyrate in intestinal and extraintestinal disease. *World Journal of Gastroenterology* 17(12), 1519–28.

Hankins J, Aygun B. (2011) Pharmacotherapy in sickle cell disease—state of the art and future prospects. *British Journal of Haematology* 145(3), 296–308.

Kohne E. (2011) Haemoglobinopathies, clinical manifestations, diagnosis and treatment. *Deutsches Ärzteblatt International* 108(31–32), 532–40.

Little JA, McGowan VR, Leone L, et al. (2006). Combination EPO-hydroxyurea therapy in sickle cell disease: experience from the National Institutes of Health and a literature review. *Haematologica*, 91(8), 1076–83.

Guidelines

Cappellini MD, Cohen A, Porter J, et al. (2014) *Guidelines for the management of transfusion dependent thalassaemia*, 3rd edn. Nicosia: Thalassaemia International Federation.

NICE CG143 (2012) Sickle cell disease: managing acute painful episodes in hospital. https://www.nice.org.uk/guidance/cg143 [accessed 14 April 2019].

12.3 Allergy

The term allergy was first used by the Austrian physician Clemens von Pirquet in 1906 who described a hypersensitivity reaction seen in patients injected with a second dose of a vaccine. Currently, the term encompasses a wide range of immune reactions, local or systemic, seen in susceptible individuals exposed on multiple occasions to an antigen (allergen, e.g. house dust mite, pollen, egg, peanut, drugs) exposure. A wide spectrum of clinical presentations are seen from localized rhinitis with hay fever through to full blow systemic anaphylactic reactions with shock following a bee sting or peanut exposure. The former is common where it is estimated that 26% of the population has allergic rhinitis, while the latter is rarely seen and occurs in the order of 1:3500.

The term atopy describes a genetic predisposition to allergy which can manifest clinically as rhinitis, eczema or asthma. Should both parents be atopic the risk of a child being atopic is 70–80%; this rate drops to 25–40% if a single atopic parent.

Pathophysiology

Hypersensitivity reactions are inappropriate immune responses of the body to stimuli and result in different clinical manifestations from four distinct mechanistic pathways. These mechanistic classifications were developed by Coombs and Gell where allergy, per se, is most often referred to as a type I hypersensitivity reaction. Type's I–III are antibody-mediated, while type IV reactions are T cell–mediated.

Herein, we concentrate on the type I reaction, which is an IgE-mediated process since this is a key player in allergic asthma, allergic rhinitis, and anaphylactic reaction. IgE is produced by plasma cells located in lymph nodes and located in high concentrations within tissues where it is strongly bound to a mast-cell surface receptor FcεRI. In population that suffer with allergy there are higher circulating levels of IgE, which result in an abnormal immune response. Exposure of IgE to an antigen results in FcεRI cross-linking of the receptors, which causes a large release of signalling molecules, such as histamine, cytokines, enzymes, and lipid mediators, from the mast cells. This mast cells are densely located in mucosal and epithelial tissue, and closely associated with blood vessels to help with the normal pathogen defensive mechanisms. However, the location of these cells and the degranulation process means disproportionate release of vasoactive compound like histamine that increase blood flow and vessel permeability can have significant clinical consequences in the form of inflammation, swelling and oedema. In addition to early release of histamine cytokines such as IL-4 and IL-13 are released, these stimulate and amplify a Th2 response, while released TNF-α can promote inflammation and enzymes, like tryptases, and carboxypeptidases may consequently cause local tissue damage. Th2 activation, via IL-5, also stimulates eosinophil production from bone marrow, which normally defend against micro-organisms or parasites, but such cells can also cause rarely inappropriate tissue destruction. Clinically, the immediate tissue changes are mediated via histamine and prostaglandins that increase vascular permeability and inflammation resulting in oedema and 'wheal and flare' reactions, but there is also a late-phase response, which occurs after ~8 hours resulting from the Th2 activation and recruitment of eosinophils, basophils, and lymphocytes, which can easily become a chronic inflammatory response; such as hyper-reactive airway in asthma (see Topic 3.1, 'Asthma').

Immunotherapy, in the form of allergen-specific vaccination has been shown in allergic asthmatics to reduce IgE levels and switch immune response from Th2-mediated toward a IL-10-mediated T-cell response, which reduces nasal, ocular and respiratory asthma symptoms by up to 80%.

The presentation of urticarial skin reaction, such as a round, macular pruritic rash, is common in drug, food, infective or contact causes (e.g. animal dander, grass, pollen) allergies but in ~20% the allergenic trigger may be elusive.

Patients who present with an anaphylactic reaction or a severe allergic reaction should have serum tryptase levels taken on arrival and again in <4 hours after exposure to the allergen as this can confirm evidence of a type I mast cell degranulation reaction; it is not always reliable in those <16 years old. These patients should be followed-up in a specialist allergy clinic where a third tryptase may be taken to establish a baseline. Allergen-specific IgE (SPT, RAST) tests taken outside of an active episode are useful to confirm antigen specificity.

For a full summary of the relevant pathways and drug targets, see Figure 12.6.

Management

Management of anaphylaxis

Anaphylaxis is a medical emergency requiring prompt recognition and intervention. Diagnosis, however, may be difficult, as signs and symptoms can be diverse. Criteria have therefore been developed to improve diagnostic certainty (see Box 12.1), thereby reducing the risk of inappropriate administration of **adrenaline**, or a missed diagnosis of anaphylaxis.

Reactions tend to occur within minutes of exposure to allergens (e.g. nuts, drugs, stings) and rapidly develop into a life-threatening condition that affects breathing and/or circulation, although onset will depend on the allergen itself; i.e. IV administered drugs and stings will probably have a faster onset than a food substance or orally administered agent. Treatment is therefore based on general life support principles using the airway, breathing, circulation, disability, exposure approach (see Table 12.6).

Where possible, initial management will include removal of the probable allergen, e.g. discontinuing potential drug causes, removal of bee sting. Inducing vomiting in patients that react to a food substance is **not** recommended.

Primary pharmacological management of anaphylaxis is with adrenaline, usually administered IM, to induce peripheral vasoconstriction, which reverses hypotension and oedema. Additional measures such as a fluid challenge with a crystalloid solution (20 mL/kg) may be required to manage hypovolaemic shock, and high-flow oxygen administered to maintain optimal oxygen saturations in respiratory distress.

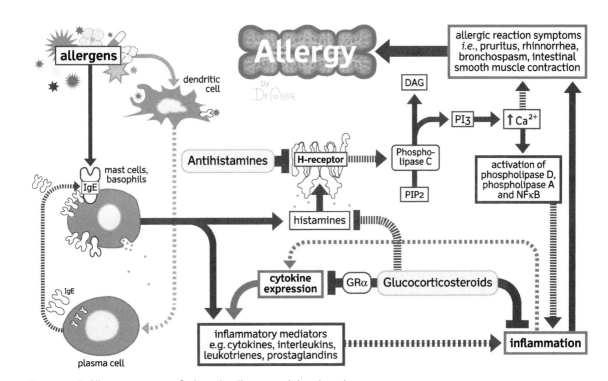

Figure 12.6 Allergy: summary of relevant pathways and drug targets.

Box 12.1 Criteria for anaphylaxis

Anaphylaxis is likely when all of the following three criteria are met:

- Sudden onset and rapid progression of symptoms
- Life-threatening airway and/or breathing and/or circulation problems
- Skin and/or mucosal changes (flushing, urticaria, angioedema)

The following supports the diagnosis: Exposure to a known allergen for the patient.
Remember:

- Skin or mucosal changes alone are not a sign of an anaphylactic reactions
- Skin and mucosal changes can be subtle or absent in up to 20% of reactions (some patients can have only a decrease in blood pressure, i.e. a circulation problem)
- There can also be GI symptoms (e.g. vomiting, abdominal pain, incontinence)

Second-line pharmacological measures include the administration of antihistamines, typically **chlorphenamine** IM, to manage histamine-mediated response, i.e. bronchoconstriction and vasodilation, although the evidence for their benefit is weak. **Hydrocortisone** IM, is also given to reduce the risk of a biphasic reaction and the duration of symptoms. Repeated doses of chlorphenamine and corticosteroids (prednisolone orally or hydrocortisone IV) may be necessary to manage ongoing symptoms.

Further treatment options may be required for specific symptoms such as the use of nebulized β_2 agonists (e.g. **salbutamol**) in patients with wheeze, or nebulized adrenaline for stridor. Vasopressors and inotropes (e.g. **noradrenaline**, **metaraminol**) may be necessary in severe cases of shock.

On discharge, patients will require advice on avoiding potential allergens and self-management strategies, as well as being provided with an adrenaline autoinjector and instructions on its use. For some patients, a second device may be required, e.g. for use at school.

Management of acute allergy (urticaria) and angioedema

Primary management of acute allergy is through avoidance of known allergens, however, following exposure, pharmacological therapy may be required depending on nature and severity of symptoms. Antihistamines (H_1 receptor antagonists) form the mainstay of treatment in the management of allergic symptoms and in mild disease or urticarial alone, they are used on their own. Antihistamines can be broadly classified into first generation agents (e.g. **chlorphenamine**, **promethazine**), which tend to be more sedating, and the less sedating second or third line agents (e.g. **cetirizine**, **loratadine**). In general, the first-generation agents are more commonly used in the management of an acute allergic reaction, with chlorphenamine typically the agent of choice and can be administered orally, IM, or by slow IV.

In mild-moderate allergic reactions, or in the case of angioedema, the addition of oral prednisolone may help reduce the duration of the reaction and relieve symptoms. In patients unable to tolerate oral therapy, or in more severe reactions, IV **hydrocortisone** may be administered in combination with IV chlorphenamine. Patients that fail to respond will likely require escalation to **adrenaline** (usually IM) and urgent management for anaphylaxis. Ongoing oral therapy with antihistamines and corticosteroids can help with symptom control, particularly in the case of urticaria.

Management of hereditary angioedema

As hereditary angioedema (HAE) occurs as a result of **C1 esterase inhibitor** deficiency, an exogenous source of C1 esterase inhibitor forms the mainstay of treatment. This acts to increase serum levels, thereby reducing the production of bradykinin by means of a C1 esterase inhibitor concentrate, a licensed product obtained from human donor blood. Treatment doses are based on body weight, or a single dose of 1000 units can be administered prophylactically preprocedure, e.g. medical, surgical, or dental procedure that is otherwise likely to precipitate an attack.

Alternative treatment options include the use of plasma kallikrein inhibitors (e.g. **ecallantide**), administered SC during an attack as a series of three 10 mg injections; or a bradykinin receptor antagonist (**icatibant**), again administered SC in the event of an attack. Neither of these agents are as widely available and C1 esterase inhibitors remain the on-demand treatment of choice.

Table 12.6 Management of anaphylaxis—ABCDE approach

Problem	Symptoms	Management
Airway	<ul><li>Airway swelling, i.e. difficulty breathing/swallowing</li><li>Hoarse voice</li><li>Stridor</li></ul>	Assess airways for obstruction Airway clearance, e.g. suction, airway opening manoeuvres, tracheal intubation. High concentration oxygen (>10 L/min) to achieve PaO_2 94–98%
Breathing	<ul><li>Shortness of breath</li><li>Wheeze</li><li>Fatigue</li><li>Confusion (secondary to hypoxia)</li><li>Cyanosis (late sign)</li><li>Respiratory arrest</li></ul>	Assess breathing, i.e. signs of respiratory distress, increased respiratory rate, reduced PaO_2, presence of wheeze/bronchospasm. Maintain saturations with high concentration oxygen Bag mask ventilation/tracheal intubation
Circulation	<ul><li>Shock (pale, clammy)</li><li>Tachycardia</li><li>Hypotension (dizziness, collapse)</li><li>Reduced consciousness</li><li>Myocardial ischaemia/EEG changes</li><li>Cardiac arrest</li></ul>	Assess for signs of shock, probably secondary to hypovolaemia, i.e. peripheral perfusion, capillary refill time, pulse, BP Manage with fluids—rapid infusion of a crystalloid solution, repeated as necessary Monitor CVP
Disability	<ul><li>Altered neurological state secondary to airway/breathing/circulation problems and reduced cerebral perfusion, i.e. confusion, agitation, loss of consciousness</li><li>*GI problems*: abdominal pain, vomiting, incontinence</li></ul>	Assess conscious levels, e.g. pupil response, response to stimuli Monitor blood sugars Manage hypoglycaemia with glucose 10% IV
Exposure	<ul><li>*Skin/mucosal changes*: diverse in presentation, e.g. generalized/patchy erythema, urticarial, angioedema (eyes, lips, throat)</li></ul>	Assess for skin/mucosal changes with a full body examination Full clinical history including potential allergen exposure Assessment of vital signs Ensure all prescribed medication is given

Reproduced with the kind permission of the Resuscitation Council (UK). Adapted from Emergency treatment of anaphylactic reactions: Guidelines for healthcare providers, pp.14–16. Copyright © Resuscitation Council (UK)

Management of chronic allergy

Symptoms of chronic allergy can be problematic, particularly as long-term use of systemic therapy can be associated with significant unwanted effects, e.g. drowsiness with antihistamines use or toxicity associated with chronic systemic steroids. For this reason, topical options are preferred, where possible, targeting specific symptoms to minimize systemic absorption and associated toxicity (see Table 12.7). As symptoms are often seasonal, therapy should be tailored accordingly.

Drug classes used in management

Antihistamines

The discovery in the early 20th century that injection of histamines results in physiological effects that closely match the symptoms observed in allergic reactions prompted the search for novel therapeutic drugs. At present, antihistamines are a molecularly diverse group of drugs able to prevent the effects of histamine in allergic reactions. Antihistamine examples include first-generation, e.g. chlorphenamine and promethazine; second-generation, e.g. acrivastine, bilastine, cetirizine, loratadine, mizolastine, and olopatadine; and third-generation, e.g. fexofenadine, levocetirizine, and desloratadine.

Mechanism of action

Histamine is a monoamine-signalling molecule with multiple physiological effects in both the central and peripheral nervous system. These actions are achieved by acting on four G protein–coupled histamine receptors (H_1, H_2, H_3, and H_4) that are expressed on a variety of target cells. The widespread distribution allows histamine to have crucial functions in immunomodulatory processes and allergic reactions, but also in wide ranging biological processes, including cell proliferation, differentiation, haematopoiesis, regeneration, wound healing, GI, and circulatory function and embryonic development.

H_1 histamine receptors are responsible for multiple symptoms observed in allergic reactions, including pruritus, rhinorrhoea, bronchospasm, and the contraction of the intestinal smooth muscle. The activation of this receptor leads to the stimulation of IP3 and diacylglycerol (DAG) pathways and subsequent increase in intracellular Ca^{2+} signalling. More recently it has been shown that H_1 receptors can activate other intracellular pathways, such as phospholipase D, phospholipase A and NFκB, also involved in the development of allergic diseases.

Classical (first-generation) H_1 antihistamines are lipophilic drugs classified into different groups depending on their chemical structure. Rapidly absorbed and metabolized, they need to be administered TDS–QDS. The lipophilic properties allow them to cross the blood–brain barrier and bind to cerebral H_1 receptors, generating their main adverse effect— sedation.

Second-generation H_1 antihistamines have been developed in the last 30 years, and although some have been derived from first generation drugs, a reduced anticholinergic or sedative effect affords their main advantage. They have higher specificity for H_1 receptors, lower affinity for non-histamine receptors and, being lipophobic, have poor penetration across the blood–brain barrier. As a result, they are less likely to have sedative effects compared with first-generation drugs. The longer half-lives also allow for OD or BD dosing.

Third generation H_1 antihistamines are active metabolites of first generation drugs and were generated with the aim of improving clinical efficacy, while diminishing side effects. The goal of third-generation antihistamines was to develop therapeutically active metabolites that lacked cardiac toxicity (as seen with **terfenadine** and **astemizole**).

Prescribing

Chlorphenamine is generally considered the treatment of choice in the management of allergy, although in chronic allergy or where prolonged courses are required, additional or alternative therapy with a non-sedating agent such as cetirizine should be considered.

Chlorphenamine can be administered orally, IM, or by slow IV injection depending on the severity of allergy and how quickly a response is required. IV treatment is, therefore, more commonly used in severe acute reactions, whereas oral therapy in milder prolonged cases.

Cetirizine and **loratadine** are more commonly used in the management of seasonal or perennial rhinitis, or in the management of chronic idiopathic urticarial. It is administered orally at a licensed dose of OD, although under specialist advice can be administered more frequently.

Topical preparations of antihistamines include the second generation agents, **azelastine** and **olopatadine**, formulated as eye drops for use in seasonal allergic conjunctivitis. Azelastine is also available in a nasal spray, either on its own or in combination with a corticosteroid (**fluticasone**) for the relief of perennial rhinitis.

Table 12.7 Localized treatment options for the management of allergy

Symptom	Preferred route	Treatment options
Rhinitis	Nasal drops, sprays	Corticosteroids, antihistamines
Allergic conjunctivitis	Eye drops	Sodium cromoglicate, corticosteroids (short term), antihistamines
Asthma	Inhalers / Oral	Corticosteroids / Leukotriene antagonists
Eczema	Topical/creams	Topical corticosteroids

Unwanted effects

Antihistamine can be broadly classified into sedating (first generation) and non-sedating (second and third generation) agents. The increased drowsiness associated with first generation agents is attributed to their lack of selectivity and ability to cross the blood–brain barrier. In particular, they tend to act on muscarinic receptors, giving rise to typical anticholinergic effects, i.e. sedation, dry eyes, blurred vision, dry mouth, and urinary retention.

The non-sedating agents such as **cetirizine** and **loratadine** being more selective for peripheral H_1 receptors, are not associated with anticholinergic effects. The first two second-generation, non-sedating antihistamines to be launched, **terfenadine** and **astemizole**, were withdrawn from the market due to the increased risk of cardiotoxicity associated with their use, such as ventricular tachycardia and *torsade de pointes*.

The third-generation antihistamines (**desloratadine**, **levocetirizine**, and **fexofenadine**) are enantiomers or metabolites of second-generation agents. Although fexofenadine demonstrates reduced cardiotoxicity compared with terfenadine, the advantages of levocetirizine and desloratadine over their second generation counterparts are largely unfounded.

Other less common neurological effects associated with antihistamine use include agitation and confusion.

Glucocorticosteroids

> Glucocorticosteroids are the most effective drugs for controlling the inflammation caused by allergic rhinitis, exerting anti-inflammatory actions and also induction of regulatory cytokines. Examples include prednisolone, hydrocortisone; while Topical agents include beclometasone, budesonide, fluticasone, and triamcinolone.

Mechanism of action

The effects of glucocorticosteroids at the molecular level occurs after crossing the cell membrane and binding to the intracellular glucocorticoid receptor (GR). Binding of glucocorticoids to the GR dissociates heat shock proteins that keep it inactive and allow the complex to translocate into the nucleus or interact with the cytoplasmic transcription factors.

The anti-inflammatory effects are achieved by at least two pathways—transactivation and transrepression. The first occurs when the receptor complex binds to gluococorticosteroid-response elements in the promoter regions of glucocorticosteroid-responsive genes, which encode anti-inflammatory genes, such as annexin, IκB and CD163. Alternatively, the receptor complex can also repress the transcription of pro-inflammatory genes via protein–protein interactions, such as GR-NFκB and GR-activator protein 1 (AP-1).

At the cellular level, glucocorticoids inhibit the functions of infiltrating inflammatory cells and their recruitment to the nasal mucosa. They also inhibit the maturation and cytokine production of mast cells and the histamine release from basophils, among other cellular mechanisms. Glucocorticoids also have anti-inflammatory effects on nasal constitutive cells (epithelial, fibroblasts, vascular endothelial cells, and glands).

Prescribing

Intranasal glucocorticoids are the most effective pharmacotherapy for seasonal allergic rhinitis, but their overall efficacy is moderate. Clinical effects appear within a day, but the maximum effect in cases of perennial rhinitis is not achieved for several weeks.

Corticosteroid nasal sprays or drops (e.g. beclo-beclometasone, budesonide, fluticasone, and triamcinolone) are primarily indicated for the relief of allergic and perennial rhinitis. With seasonal symptoms treatment should be started 2–3 weeks prior to the start of the season and continued for several months.

For information on systemic corticosteroids see Topic 6.6, 'Inflammatory bowel disease'.

Unwanted effects

Systemic absorption with nasal preparations is generally low, although with prolonged courses or high doses can be more significant, particularly with nasal drops where doses are more likely to be administered incorrectly. Use of nasal corticosteroids should be avoided in the presence of nasal infection or following nasal surgery as they have the potential to delay healing.

Further reading

Carson S, Lee N, Thakurta S (2010) Drug class review: newer antihistamines; Final Report Update 2. Portland, OR: Oregon Health and Sciences University. https://www.ncbi.nlm.nih.gov/books/NBK50554/ [accessed 16 April 2019].

Okano M (2009) Mechanisms and clinical implications of gluococorticoids in the treatment of allergic rhinitis. *Clin Exp Immunol* 158(2), 164–73.

Wheatley LM, Togias A (2015) Allergic rhinitis. *New England Journal of Medicine* 372(5), 456–63.

Guidelines

Doshi D, Foex B, Body R, et al. (2009) GEMNET: Guideline for the management of acute allergic reaction. CEM Guideline 5072. https://www.scribd.com/document/218554378/CEM5072-GEMNet-Guideline-for-the-Management-of-Acute-Allergic-Reaction-Dec-2009 [accessed 16 April 2019].

EAACI Anaphylaxis Guidelines (2013) Version 4.5 http://www.eaaci.org/attachments/Anaphylaxis%20guidelines%20Draft%204.5%202013%2006%20.pdf [accessed 16 April 2019].

Maurer M, Magerl, M, Ansotegui I, et al. (2018) The international WAO/EAACI guideline for the management of hereditary angioedema—the 2017 revision and update. *World Allergy Organization Journal* 11, 5.

NICE CG134 (2011) Anaphylaxis: assessment and referral after emergency treatment. https://www.nice.org.uk/guidance/cg134 [accessed 16 April 2019].

NICE CG183 (Sept 2014) Drug allergy: diagnosis and management. https://www.nice.org.uk/guidance/cg183 [accessed 16 April 2019].

NICE Pathway: Anaphylaxis https://pathways.nice.org.uk/pathways/anaphylaxis [accessed 16 April 2019].

NICE QS119 (March 2016) Anaphylaxis. NICE Quality Standard QS119. https://www.nice.org.uk/guidance/qs119 [accessed 16 April 2019].

Working group of the Resuscitation Council UK (2012) Emergency treatment of anaphylactic reactions: guidelines for healthcare professionals. https://www.resus.org.uk/anaphylaxis/emergency-treatment-of-anaphylactic-reactions/ [accessed 24 April 2019].

13 Haemato-oncology and malignancy

Cancer is a common cause of morbidity and mortality in the United Kingdom (UK), affecting approximately two out of every five people during their lifetime. In 2015 there was an estimated 2.5 million people in the UK who had had a cancer diagnosis, an increase of almost half a million in the previous 5 years. The proportion of people living longer after cancer is increasing, and the number of people alive more than 5 years from initial diagnosis is predicted to more than double between 2010 and 2030 to 2.7 million. By the end of 2020, more than a thousand people would have been diagnosed with cancer every day in the UK.

Most common cancers

Cancer can affect all organs of the body with over 200 types identified. However, only a small number of cancer types account for most cases. Over half of all new diagnoses are due to four cancers (in order of frequency)—breast, prostate, lung, and bowel. In 2011 there were approximately 50 000 new diagnoses of breast cancer in the UK. The incidence of cancer diagnosis is increasing year on year, in part due to improving diagnostic skills, but also because of an increasing elderly population. Cancer of unknown primary origin accounts for about 3% of total cancers.

Cancer prognosis

Although UK statistics show a general improvement in the 5-year survival rates for the majority of common cancers, some have not shown any notable improvement. Survival is not only determined by the type of cancer, but also the age at diagnosis, stage, and co-morbidities such as heart, pulmonary, and renal disease, which can affect the treatment regimen. As well as this, certain cancers carry a significantly worse prognosis than others. For example, 10-year survival for pancreatic and lung cancer are 1% and 5%, respectively. In comparison, the 10-year survival for testicular cancer is over 98% and almost 90% in skin confined melanoma. Newer diagnostic strategies are expected to detect all cancers early, allowing prompt intervention, and improving both morbidity and mortality rates further.

Pathophysiology

Cancer is a product of mutations in genes involved in controlling cell growth, differentiation, and death (apoptosis). There are two main classifications of mutations that induce cancer production—oncogenes and tumour suppressor genes. Oncogenes involve a mutated gene that results in over-production or over-activity of their transcribed protein product. This results in a dominant effect on cell growth and differentiation or inhibition of cell death. Examples of oncogenes include Ras, BCR-Abl, and Her2.

Conversely, genes that code for factors that slow or halt division, or induce apoptosis, are known as tumour suppressor genes (e.g. the retinoblastoma gene, Rb or BRCA1, and BRCA2 in breast cancer). Loss of tumour suppressor function can be conceptualized as a loss in quality control, allowing defective and harmful errors to progress through the cell replication process.

In certain cancers, activation of intracellular hormone receptors (e.g. oestrogen in breast cancer) is required to maintain progress through the cell cycle, which means that antagonists of these receptors may inhibit cell growth (e.g. **tamoxifen**).

As the cancerous cells replicate, they accumulate additional alterations, which can induce further properties that promote growth, such as development of appropriate blood supply through angiogenesis and changes in cell polarity and cell adhesion.

Cell polarity and cancer

Cell polarity is a property of a differentiated cell, when it is not a symmetrical uniform entity. In a normally functioning adult cell, different tasks are located in specific areas, while at the same time, different areas necessitate different functions and properties. Cells, for example, differ in their apical and basal functions. Cell polarity is demonstrated in epithelial cells through the different provision of transporters at apical and basolateral membranes. Furthermore, these spatial differences play a key role in cell migration.

The polarity of a cell appears to be guided through the actions of three different evolutionary conserved protein complexes—Par, Scribble, and Crumbs. The latter is associated with maintaining apical–basal polarity, with Scribble proteins located near the basolateral membrane and required to maintain basolateral membrane integrity. The Par protein complex is situated in the apical area of the cell and plays a key role in apical membrane integrity.

Loss of cell polarity is thought to contribute to initiation of *epithelial–mesenchymal transition* (EMT), which is a fundamental change in cell characteristics, from a differentiated epithelial cell to a less differentiated mesenchymal cell. This radical alteration is not only seen in cancer, but in non-pathological processes such as organogenesis and wound healing. EMT and the opposite process, *mesenchymal–epithelial transition* (MET), are key in the invasion and spread of cancer. While cell polarity plays an important role in EMT, it appears that changes in cell adhesion are required for initiation of this process.

Cell adhesion and cancer

Cell adhesion is fundamental to the formation of organized and integrated structures in the human body, and its disruption underlies tumorigenesis and cancer spread. Cell adhesion is governed by many proteins. The cadherin group of proteins E-cadherin, N-cadherin, and P-cadherin and a group of associated proteins called catenins, play a significant role in cell adhesion. The cadherins regulate cell–cell contact at specific sites of the cell, termed adhesion junctions. E-cadherin is particularly abundant in epithelial cells, N-cadherin in mesenchymal cells and

P-cadherin in placental cells, basal epithelia of the prostate, some skin cells, and cells in the mammary gland. Generally, changes in cadherin and particularly a reduction in E-cadherin levels, appear to be associated with induction of EMT and cancer invasion.

Cancer invasion

The ability of cancer cells to invade through tissues beyond the primary tumour site is a hallmark of the disease. Defects in cell adhesion through loss of E-cadherin have been shown to lead to earlier invasion and metastases. Mesenchymal cells produced through EMT are less well-differentiated and, in contrast to epithelial cells, do not have tight junctions binding them in place. These characteristics allow the cell to detach and mobilize. In addition, proteins such as the Rho family of GTPases play a key role in not only suppression of apoptosis, but also cellular motility across the extracellular matrix. Eventually, the cells invade local structures including the lymphatic and vascular system. At this stage, the tumour can stimulate macrophage production through tumour derived colony-stimulating factor 1, these macrophages in turn release growth factors (e.g. platelet-derived growth factor PDGF), proteases (matrix metallic proteases) and also stimulate other cells to produce cytokines that can induce production of further cancerous cells, such as the endothelial progenitor cell (EPC).

Cancer metastases

Metastatic disease in cancer is defined as a tumour that has developed in a site distant to the primary tumour. Essentially, this is the travel of cells and their seeding in another organ, which has been defined by the *seed and soil* hypothesis. As with all seeds there is a requirement of both a favourable external environment and the appropriate internal properties that allow growth. The EPC as mentioned above, is fundamental to metastatic disease since it has the ability to create new blood vessels (vasculogenesis) that facilitate tumour growth. Vasculogenesis is critical for tumour growth and animal studies have shown that depleting the bone marrow of EPCs results in decreased tumour cell growth. It is also possible that EPCs play a role in late recurrence after removal of a primary tumour.

Many cancers appear to have a predilection to metastasize in certain organs, with breast, bowel, prostate, renal, and thyroid cancers known to metastasize preferentially to the bone. Cancer of the bowel and pancreas most frequently metastasize to the liver. This may be due to not only the anatomy of blood and lymphatic flow, but also the genetic toolbox of the cancer cell itself. For example, it appears that breast cancer-derived metastases in bone are specially adapted to activate osteoclastic activity to stimulate cell proliferation factors that aid cancer growth. Much work and research is currently being conducted on understanding the metastatic process.

Carcinogenesis

Many hereditary cancer syndromes have been identified (Table 13.1), and most of these genetic defects relate to cell replication and are tumour suppressor genes.

However, although genetics plays a starting point, the majority of people who eventually develop a cancer have no defined familial or genetic predisposition. This would lead one to conclude that environmental factors must also play a role in the development of cancer. Many of these have been identified, and linked to the particular cancer they predispose (Table 13.2.). The most well-known being the strong link between smoking and cancer of the lung.

It is thought that these environmental agents produce damage to cellular DNA creating instability, which leads to an increased chance of aberrant cell replication. Cumulative exposure increases both the degree and likelihood of damage, thereby increasing chances of abnormal cell replication and, hence, cancer.

Cancer immunology

Cellular identification, being the differentiation between native cells, invaders, compromised native cells, and foreign substances, is the key principle that defines the immune system; a highly efficient, effective, and powerful agent. In relation to cancer, it is the recognition of compromised native cells that helps control cancer growth, but as cancer cells develop they appear to acquire the ability to subvert these normally robust mechanisms. Avoiding immune destruction is a newly emerging hallmark of cancer, but one that is being targeted with new drug therapies. **Pembrolizumab**, licensed in the treatment of metastatic melanoma, targets the 'programmed death receptor 1' (PD-1). It potentiates the immune response by blocking an inhibitory interaction between the PD-1 receptor on T cells and their ligands on tumour cells.

Cancer and cell surface receptors

Still, each cancer cell has characteristic antigens, including specific receptors or proteins that can be targeted therapeutically. The most widely known is the antibody **trastuzumab** (anti-HER2), used in the treatment of breast cancer and capable of binding HER2+ve cells and activating natural killer cells. Other agents include **rituximab** (anti-CD20) used in lymphoma, and **alemtuzumab** (anti-CD52), which is used in leukaemia treatment. These antibodies can be naked or combined with a drug to provide targeted chemotherapy, such as **brentuximab vedotin** used in the treatment of Hodgkin's lymphoma. Currently, vaccination targeted towards cancer antigens is not widely available, but is an area of intense investigation.

Targets of chemotherapeutic agents in cancer

In addition to immunological agents used in cancer therapy, several chemotherapeutic agents have been

Table 13.1 Hereditary cancer syndromes

Cancer syndrome	Gene	Predisposed cancer	
BRCA-1	BRCA1 (affects p53 activity)	Breast and ovarian cancer	Impaired DNA quality control and repair
BRCA -2	BRCA2 (effects on DNA repair)	Breast and ovarian cancer	Impaired DNA repair
Neurofibromatosis 1	NF1	Neurofibromatosis	Inability to inactivate ras oncogene.
Hereditary retinoblastoma	RB	Retinoblastoma	Impaired control of transition to S phase.

Table 13.2 Examples of environmental agents and associated type of cancer

Environmental exposure	Associated type of cancer
Smoking	Lung cancer, mouth cancer, oropharyngeal cancer, prostate cancer, pancreatic cancer, stomach cancer, bladder cancer
Alcohol use	Liver cancer, oropharyngeal cancer, oesophageal cancer, breast cancer
Asbestos exposure	Mesothelioma
Obesity	Colorectal cancer, breast cancer
Aniline dyes	Bladder cancer

developed in the treatment of the disease. In particular, since aberrant cell replication is the hallmark of cancer, much of the pharmacological factors affecting

cell replication will have an effect on cancer growth. Importantly, the proportion of cells in the M stage (mitosis) at any one point in time is the growth fraction, and this is an important aspect to consider in chemotherapy. Indeed, as cancer cells are actively requiring nutrients, blood supply, new DNA, and multiple growth factors, they are more susceptible to treatment than healthy cells. It is thus possible to predict that the higher the growth fraction, the more susceptible the cancer.

For a full summary of the relevant pathways and drug targets, see Figure 13.1.

Management of malignancy

Prevention of cancer

Cancer prevention is possible where predisposing factors have been identified (Table 13.2), so that reduced exposure to these can decrease the likelihood. As a result, significant public awareness campaigns have been developed to encourage behaviours that decrease the incidence

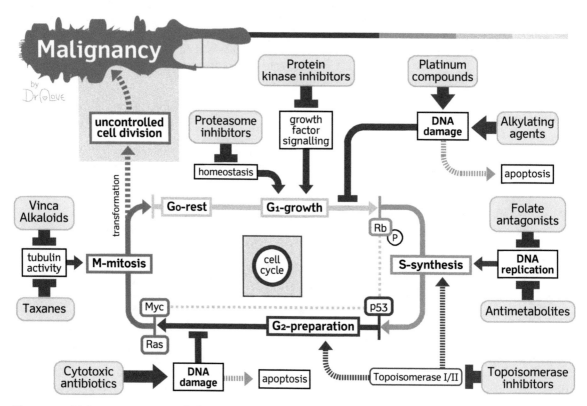

Figure 13.1 Malignancy: summary of relevant pathways and drug targets.

of cancer. In general terms, this means maintaining a healthy weight, regular physical activity, and high fruit and vegetable intake. In the case of smoking, an aetiological factor in many different cancers, smoking cessation significantly reduces the cumulative risk of lung cancer. Public awareness campaigns about the dangers of tobacco have included a legislative approach resulting in increased pricing, health warnings on packaging, and restrictions on sale and place of consumption. These restrictions appear to be making a significant impact on tobacco use in the UK.

Alcohol is another known carcinogen and abstinence from it may help prevent liver, oropharyngeal, and oesophageal cancer, among other neoplastic processes. Public awareness campaigns are the main strategies used to reduce consumption at present, but there is evidence to suggest that restrictions such as minimum pricing may also help.

In the case of some malignant diseases there is a strong link to communicable infections. Therefore, prevention, treatment, or vaccination against these diseases can reduce cancer incidence (Table 13.3).

Reducing the incidence of other environmental risks is equally important, including air pollution, dust (asbestos, silica, wood), carcinogenic chemicals, and ionizing radiation.

Treatment strategies in cancer

Overall, the cancer survival rate is improving due to early detection and treatment, as well as improved supportive care. Surgical intervention is often the first line treatment for many neoplastic processes, where it may be curative. In order to obtain the best possible outcome, surgical treatment is usually offered in combination with radiotherapy and/or chemotherapy. Surgery is also used as a screening and diagnostic tool, and due to advances in genetic testing, may also be preventative, e.g. mastectomy in patients with genetic mutation in *BRCA1* gene or the *BRCA2* gene. Surgical interventions may also be required in advanced malignancy for palliative reasons, helping to manage symptoms.

Radiotherapy causes irreversible damage to DNA via free radical production. It is estimated that radiotherapy is used in 50% of patients with cancer and may be offered as radical treatment or palliation. Chemotherapy may be offered as primary therapy with curative intent or adjuvant, aimed at reducing relapse of disease. Neoadjuvant therapy is mainly intended to shrink tumours prior to surgical intervention. Palliative care is a dedicated service provided by the specialist palliative care team to provide symptomatic relief predominantly, although not exclusively, aimed at terminal cancers.

Table 13.3 Communicable diseases linked to malignancy

Pathogen	Mode of transmission	Associated malignancy
Human papilloma virus	Sexual intercourse Saliva (head and neck)	Cervical cancer Anal cancer Head and neck cancers also
Hepatitis B virus	Sexual intercourse Sharing of contaminated needles Contaminated blood products	Hepatocellular carcinoma
Hepatitis C virus	Sexual intercourse Sharing of contaminated needles Contaminated blood products	Hepatocellular carcinoma
Epstein Barr virus	Saliva	Nasopharyngeal carcinoma
Human herpes virus -8	Sexual intercourse Saliva	Kaposi's sarcoma
HTLV -1	Sexual intercourse Sharing contaminated needles	Adult T lymphocytic Leukaemia/lymphoma

Principles of chemotherapy

In modern oncology practice, combination therapy regimes, including chemotherapy drugs, are often necessary, although for non-disseminated malignancy, surgical treatment and/or radiotherapy may be enough. The classification of cancer chemotherapy drugs is dependent on their mechanism of action or origin. Major drug classes used in cancer therapy include chemotherapeutic agents such as alkylating agents, antimetabolites, antitumour antibiotics, topoisomerase inhibitors, antimitotics, and platinum compounds.

Furthermore, biological agents such as protein kinase inhibitors, protein kinase receptor inhibitors, and proteasome inhibitors are also important.

The choice of therapy depends upon a number of tumour and patient factors, such as the underlying neoplastic process and tissue diagnosis, as well as staging and dissemination. Drugs are commonly used in combination to optimize efficacy, with regimens developed and accepted into practice following high quality clinical trials (see Table 13.4 for examples). The systemic delivery of these agents will almost always result in adverse drug reactions, which may vary from mild symptoms to severe and life-threatening events. The specific nature of these unwanted effects is described in detail below. In general, adverse drug reactions are class specific, although certain drugs in the same class may have different side effects.

Table 13.4 Examples of chemotherapy regimens

Cancer type	Commonly used regimens
Breast	*AC*: doxorubicin, cyclophosphamide
	CMF: cyclophosphamide, methotrexate, fluorouracil
	docetaxel
	FEC: fluorouracil, epirubicin, cyclophosphamide
	FEC-D/T: docetaxel
	GemCarbo/Cis: gemcitabine, carboplatin/cisplatin
	GemTaxol: gemcitabine, paclitaxel
	Paclitaxel
	Trastuzumab emtansine/trastuzumab containing regimens
Colorectal	fluorouracil/capecitabine
	CapOx: capecitabine, oxaliplatin
	FOLFIRI: fluorouracil, irinotecan
	FOLFOX: fluorouracil, oxaliplatin
	Irinotecan
Melanoma	Dabrafenib
	Dacarbazine
	Ipilimumab
	Pembrolizumab
	Vemurafinib

Management of acute leukaemias

Acute myeloid leukaemia

Acute myeloid leukaemia (AML) is the most common adult leukaemia, with a world-wide annual incidence of appropriately 250 000 people. Unfortunately, the overall prognosis from the condition remains poor with survival rates in the general population ranging between 10% and 40%. Incidence increases with age, with the median age of diagnosis being 64 years.

The aetiology of *de novo* AML is unclear, although viral infections, e.g. human T cell leukaemia virus and exposure to carcinogens such as benzene and cigarette smoke have all been implicated. Bone marrow failure is the most common cause for presentation, manifesting as bruising, bleeding, symptoms of anaemia and recurrent infection. Constitutional symptoms such as night sweats, weight loss, and lymphadenopathy may also occur (Figure 13.2).

Management

Treatment strategies

AML treatment is often a lengthy process undertaken over many months or even years, and can be classified as intensive and non-intensive (see Table 13.5).

Intensive therapy

This is reserved for younger and fitter patients, usually those < 70–75 years of age, with the aim of cure. It is usually administered as an inpatient regimen due to the high risk of complications, including bone marrow suppression, infection, and organ failure/impairment, particularly renal and liver toxicity.

Treatment is divided into two main phases, *remission induction therapy* and *consolidation therapy*, with allogeneic bone marrow transplant recommended following induction ± consolidation in young patients (<60 years), or in those with high risk disease as determined by

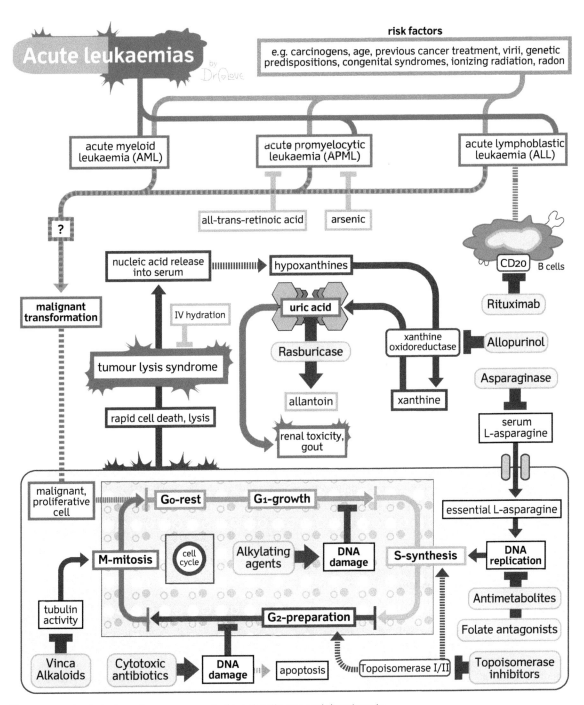

Figure 13.2 Acute leukaemias: summary of relevant pathways and drug targets.

adverse cytogenetic or molecular features. Transplant is usually undertaken at first remission.

Induction This is intensive chemotherapy, usually given over two cycles, to reduce disease burden and induce

morphological remission. The mainstay of induction treatment includes the combination of an anthracycline and an antimetabolite, typically, **daunorubicin** and **cytarabine** (DA), although many centres will also include **etoposide** (ADE). Some patients, however, may be treated with

Table 13.5 Summary of treatment regimes used in AML

Cycle	Regimen	Chemotherapy
Induction	DA	Daunorubicin, cytarabine
	ADE	Daunorubicin, cytarabine, etoposide
	FLAG-IDA	Fludarabine, cytarabine, GCSF, idarubicin
Consolidation	MACE	Amsacrine, cytarabine and etoposide
	MiDac	Mitoxantrone and cytarabine
Non-intensive/ palliative	LD-AraC	Low-dose cytarabine as a single agent
	Aza	Azacitidine as a single agent
	HU	Hydroxycarbamide as a single agent

high-dose cytarabine alone, or in those who are high risk or for refractory disease **fludarabine**, in combination with **cytarabine**, growth factors (**GFs**), and **idarubicin** (FLAG-IDA) may also be used as induction therapy. More recently, **amsacrine** has been used as an additional induction agent and can be added to any of the regimens described previously.

Allogenic bone marrow transplant Many patients will undergo a bone marrow biopsy during or after induction to determine the percentage of malignant blast cells that remain within the marrow. Peripheral blood flow cytometry will also be undertaken to look for circulating blast cells. If there is no evidence of residual malignant cells, transplant-eligible patients may continue to allogeneic stem cell transplant without the need for consolidation. Patients with low risk disease may progress to transplant if they relapse following initial treatment.

Consolidation Some patients, however, will undergo one or two courses of consolidation intensive therapy designed at eliminating the disease and inducing a molecular remission. This includes combination therapy with **amsacrine**, **cytarabine**, and **etoposide** (MACE), or

mitoxantrone and **cytarabine** (Midac), with the aim of reducing bone marrow disease burden prior to allogeneic stem cell transplant.

Targeted chemotherapy Several new targeted therapies are available via clinical trials for AML, often used alongside conventional agents, including:

- *Gemtuzumab*: a monoclonal antibody directed against CD33, which is found on the surface of myeloid cells (and some lymphoid cells).
- *Lestaurtinib*: a FLT3 kinase inhibitor used in FLT3 +ve AML only.
- *Everolimus*: an mTOR inhibitor (see malignancy Table 13.14).
- *Quizartinib*: a receptor tyrosine kinase targeting FLT3.

Maintenance Maintenance strategies are being trialled using a variety of agents including **nivolumab**, **quizartinib**, **azacitidine**, **sorafenib**, **lenalidomide**, **bortezomib** along with many others.

Non-intensive therapy

Older patients or those with significant co-morbidity may be offered lower dose regimens of those used in intensive therapy or fewer agents, many of which can be given in an outpatient setting. Such regimens are better tolerated and are aimed at controlling the disease, rather than cure it. In those able to tolerate the use of low dose **cytarabine** or **azacitidine** can be considered to slow disease progression. Alternatively, **hydroxycarbamide** may be used as a single agent with the added advantage of being given orally. In patients with advanced disease a palliative approach may be employed from the outset.

Acute lymphoblastic leukaemia

Acute lymphoblastic leukaemia (ALL) is more common during childhood with approximately five times as many cases diagnosed in comparison with AML and a median age at diagnosis of 3.5 years; the exact cause is unknown. Several predisposing factors have been identified, including congenital syndromes such as Down's, Fanconi, and Kleinfelter's syndromes. Exposure to ionizing radiation, radon, viruses, and pollution/chemicals has also been suggested.

Patients typically present acutely unwell with symptoms of bone marrow failure, in particular anaemia, with lethargy, dizziness, palpitations and light headedness, haemorrhage, and bruising are common. Lymphadenopathy is seen in most individuals. Neutropenia may manifest as sepsis, and is a medical emergency requiring administration of antibiotics and supportive therapy. Diagnosis and prognostication of ALL is by morphological assessment, immunophenotyping, cytogenetic, and molecular analysis.

Management

Treatment is tailored according to age, co-morbidities and patient 'risk', with eligible patients ideally entering into relevant clinical trials should they wish. Treatment consists of four phases (Table 13.6), with allogeneic stem cell transplantation considered for those with matched siblings, poor risk disease, or in relapse. The principles of therapy for ALL are the same as for AML, i.e. reduce the disease burden during induction and further enhance this with consolidation and allogeneic stem cell transplant in younger, fitter patients in whom cure is considered a possibility. Maintenance therapy can be used to slow or

prevent relapse in patients who do not progress to allogeneic stem cell transplant. Compared with treatment to AML, however, ALL regimens tend to be considerably longer, but involve less intensive chemotherapy.

In children and young adults where survival rates are typically higher, treatment strategies are designed to identify low risk patients in whom less intensive chemotherapy can be used, in order to minimize the risk of long term/late effects. Risk stratification is carried out by considering prognostic factors such as cytogenetics, rate of response, and MRD.

Supportive care

Although improvements in chemotherapy and risk stratification has contributed largely to improved survival rates in ALL, better supportive care has also had a significant part to play. In particular, comprehensive strategies for the management of neutropenic sepsis. Prophylaxis with co-trimoxazole to prevent PCP and, in some instances, antifungals (Topic 11.2, 'Fungal infection') is therefore paramount.

Table 13.6 Typical treatment phases for ALL

Treatment phase	Therapy
Induction	Commonly used therapy includes a combination of vincristine, dexamethasone/prednisolone, L-asparaginase, and either daunorubicin or cyclophosphamide (sometimes both, i.e. CALGB 8811 regimen).
	In Philadelphia-positive disease the addition of a tyrosine kinase inhibitor, e.g. imatinib can be considered which targets the BCR-ABL tyrosine kinase protein. Rituximab may also be added in CD20+ve disease
Consolidation	To reduce the burden of disease additional cycles of therapy are undertaken, which include many of the induction agents, but with alternating blocks of other high-dose regimens, including methotrexate (IV with folinic acid rescue), cytarabine, etoposide, amsacrine, mitoxantrone, idarubicin, and doxorubicin
CNS prophylaxis	CNS infiltration may occur in up to 6% of patients at presentation. CNS prophylaxis can reduce the incidence of CNS disease at relapse from 30% to 5%.
	Intrathecal methotrexate and/or high-dose IV methotrexate.
	Cranial radiation can be considered in adults with CNS disease, but not used in childhood due to the associated long-term morbidity
Maintenance	In patients who do not undergo allogeneic stem cell transplant maintenance with oral mercaptopurine (daily) and methotrexate (weekly) is often used.
	Vincristine and dexamethasone/prednisolone as monthly pulses ± IT methotrexate (usually every 3 months) may also be used.
	Maintenance, if tolerated is continued for 2–3 years

Management of chronic leukaemias

The chronic leukaemias tend to be indolent conditions, often picked up on routine blood tests as an incidental finding. They can be broadly divided into those affecting the myeloid or lymphoid (B or T) cell lineage, the most common being CLL and CML respectively (Figure 13.3).

Chronic lymphocytic leukaemia

Chronic lymphocytic leukaemia (CLL) is a B cell, non-curable malignancy that mainly affects the elderly

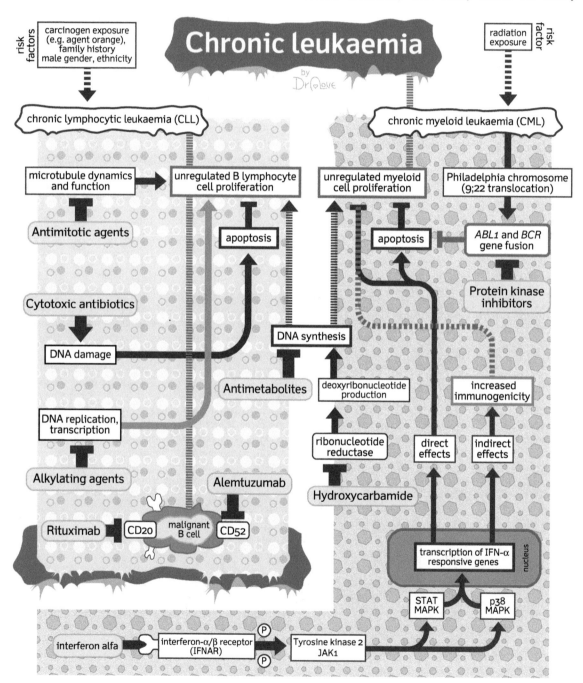

Figure 13.3 Chronic leukaemias: summary of relevant pathways and drug targets.

population. It has a median age at diagnosis and death (due to CLL), of 72 and 79, respectively; males:females (2:1). The aetiology remains unknown; although a family history of haematological malignancy is a strong risk factor with genetic anticipation. Failure of cellular apoptosis, with a high level of *BCL-2*, a gene known to enhance cell survival by blocking apoptosis, is seen in most cases.

The disease is heterogeneous, with a significant proportion of patients requiring no treatment, and a simple 'watch and wait' approach being sufficient. Others, however, develop an aggressive disease type with rapid progression and in many cases transformation to non-Hodgkin or Hodgkin's lymphoma (Richter's transformation). As with many malignancies the stage or extent of disease at diagnosis correlates with prognosis (BINET & RAI staging systems) and diagnosis is made by clonal and unique phenotyping of cells present on blood analysis by flow cytometry.

Management
Treatment strategies

The majority of patients with CLL are managed in the clinic using a watch and wait strategy. CLL can, however, transform (Richter's transformation) to aggressive non-Hodgkin lymphoma (or Hodgkin like disease in 10%) and it is therefore important to ask if the patient has developed 'B symptoms', i.e. night sweats, weight loss, and lymphadenopathy as treatment should be initiated. The use of combination chemotherapy is associated with both improved treatment success and can be further improved with immunomodulatory agent use (Table 13.7).

Table 13.7 Summary of treatment regimes used in CLL

Cycle	Regimen	Chemotherapy
Induction	R-FC	Rituximab, cyclophosphamide, fludarabine
Aggressive disease/Richter's transformation	ABVD	Doxorubicin (Adriamycin®), bleomycin, vinblastine, dacarbazine
	CHOP	Cyclophosphamide, doxorubicin, vincristine, prednisolone

Adapted from Swerdlow, SH, Campo, E, Harris, NL, Jaffe, ES, Pileri, SA, Stein, H, Thiele, J, Vardiman, JW. World Health Organization Classification of Tumours of Haematopoietic and Lymphoid Tissues. IARC, Lyon, 2008.

Primary treatment strategies

Good performance status (0–1) In the absence of a suitable clinical trials standard combination therapy is advised with **cyclophosphamide** I, **fludarabine** (F), **rituximab** I, **chlorambucil** (Cl), and **alemtuzumab** (A), i.e.:

- *R-FC*: studies have shown this the most affective combination in terms of percentage of patients achieving a CR and improvements in PS.
- FC dual therapy.
- C-A dual therapy.
- Chlorambucil, fludarabine, or alemtuzumab monotherapy.

Poor performance status (2–3) In this patient group, single agent **chlorambucil** is effective and has a favourable side effect profile, with **rituximab** potentially used second line.

Second line/relapse therapies

Patients who fail to respond adequately to treatment, in refractory disease or in Richter's transformation, e.g. CHOP or ABVD (see Table 13.7) or relapse will require second line treatment.

Newer targeted therapies may also be available for some who relapse early (<2 year) following initial therapy, e.g. ibrutinib, idelalisib, and venetoclax, where venetoclax is a potent BCL-2 protein inhibitor while ibrutinib and idelalisib are tyrosine kinase inhibitors.

Chronic myeloid leukaemia

Chronic myeloid leukaemia (CML) is a rare disease with an annual incidence of approximately 5 cases per 1 million people. The aetiology is unknown, but exposure to radiation is a known risk factor with median age at diagnosis of 50.

The disease is characterized by the presence of the Philadelphia chromosome, formed by a translocation that results in the fusion of two genes; *ABL1* on chromosome 9 and *BCR* on chromosome 22 (t(9;22)). The gene encodes for a 210 kDa protein that is thought to play a role in the pathogenesis. The protein appears to increase proliferation and prevent apoptosis of malignant cells.

Up to a third of those diagnosed have no symptoms, with the diagnosis being an incidental finding on routine blood testing. Lethargy, fatigue, sweats, and weight loss are reported by some. Diagnosis is made on FBC and blood film revealing raised white cell count (usually >25 × 10^9/L) comprised mainly of neutrophils and myelocytes ± blasts.

Management

Most patients remain symptom-free throughout the chronic phase which typically lasts for 3–6 years following diagnosis. Mortality is mainly associated with blast crisis and transformation to AML or ALL. The development and use of tyrosine kinase inhibitors has improved the prognosis significantly with 90% of patients alive at 7 years following diagnosis.

Treatment strategies

The treatment depends upon symptoms and the disease phase (Table 13.8). If treatment is commenced prophylactic therapy to prevent gout (e.g. **allopurinol**) and infection (antiviral, antifungal, and antibiotic) are required. The disease has a number of distinct phases (Figure 13.4).

Management of lymphomas

Classified as a disease of abnormal clonal B or T cell production, lymphomas are divided into Hodgkin's

Table 13.8 CML disease phases

Phase	Description
• Chronic phase	The majority of patients are diagnosed in the chronic phase. The white blood cell count remains stable or increases slowly, without the development of significant symptoms over a period of years.
• Accelerated phase	WHO criteria; • Blasts 10–19% in the peripheral blood or bone marrow • Peripheral blood basophils ≥20% • Platelet count <100 × 10⁹/L or >1000 × 10⁹/L unresponsive to therapy • Splenomegaly and raised white cell count unresponsive to therapy • Cytogenetic evidence of clonal evolution
• Blast crisis (rapidly fatal if not treated)	WHO criteria • >20% blasts in the peripheral blood or bone marrow • Extramedullary blast proliferation • Clusters of blasts identified on bone marrow

and Non-Hodgkin's. Lymphomas develop within the lymphoid tissues of the lymphatic system and are considered solid tumours. They comprise both indolent and more aggressive forms of disease and have an array of treatment options, which more recently includes novel agents beyond cytotoxic chemotherapy, in addition to radiotherapy and stem cell transplantation (Figure 13.4).

Hodgkin's lymphoma

Incidence is in the order of 2.7–2.8 per 100 000; ~1700 cases in the UK every year. Peaks of incidence are seen in both young adults and those over 60 years.

Classically, the malignant cell in Hodgkin's lymphoma, the Reed–Sternberg cell, lacks typical B cell markers, which would normally render them an apoptotic target. However, these cells incorporate a number of mechanisms to evade apoptosis, including NFKb transcription factors and the incorporation of EBV membrane proteins. Histologically, Reed–Sternberg cells exhibit staining for CD15 and CD30, and rarely CD20; these can be potential targets for therapy (e.g. brentuximab, which is an antibody–drug conjugate that sticks to CD30 delivering the antimitotic drug monomethyl auristatin E to the cell). The malignant cell is a minority cell within the abnormal lymphoid tissue or lymph node. *Classical Hodgkin's lymphoma*: represents 95% of all cases (Table 13.9).

Patients classically present with painless lymphadenopathy, although 25% have systemic symptoms or 'B' symptoms comprising weight loss (>10% over 6 months), fevers, and night sweats (drenching). Staging assessment is categorized using the Ann Arbor system (www.cancer.org). Prognosis is excellent in early stage disease, with overall survival around 96–97%. In advanced stage disease patients should have prognosis determined using the IPSS scoring system (Townsend et al., 2012).

Management

Treatment strategies

Early stage disease Typically, patients are young and as survival rates are high, recent trials have been designed to reduce early and late toxicity from treatment. This is done by reducing exposure to cytotoxic treatments and radiotherapy, without compromising efficacy. Omissions of radiotherapy have been shown to affect progression free survival, but not overall survival.

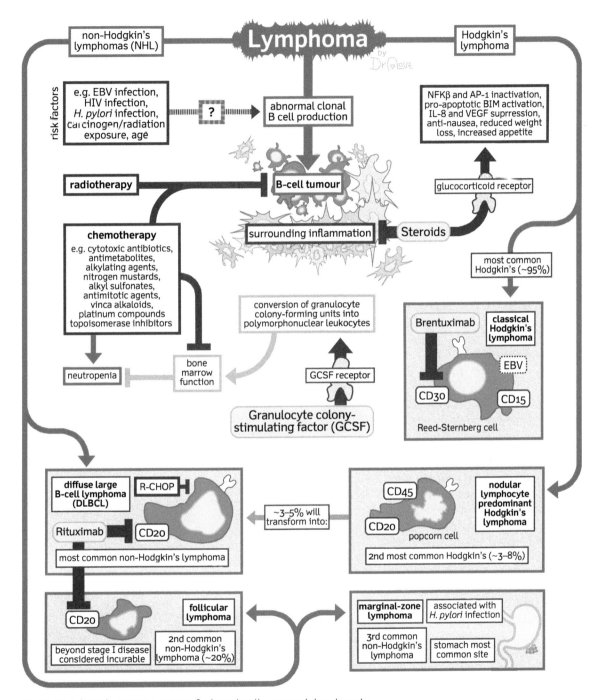

Figure 13.4 Lymphomas: summary of relevant pathways and drug targets.

In early stage favourable disease, the standard of care in adults' remains two cycles of ABVD (Table 13.10) followed by involved field radiotherapy (IFRT). Early stage unfavourable disease standard of care in adults involves four cycles of ABVD followed by IFRT. Sequential escalated BEACOPP (Table 13.10) followed by ABVD reduced early relapse, and although it showed no benefit of improved overall survival, it remains an option.

Table 13.9 Classification of Hodgkin's Lymphoma

	EBV association	Epidemiology	Clinical features
Classical Hodgkin's lymphoma			
Nodular sclerosis classical Hodgkin's lymphoma	Intermediate association; 10–40% of patients EBV positive	Accounts for 70% of classical Hodgkin's lymphoma	Prognosis better than other classical types; mediastinal mass very common
Mixed-cellularity classical Hodgkin's lymphoma	Up to 75% of patients EBV positive	Accounts for 25% of classical disease; prevalent in patients with HIV infection and developing countries	Peripheral and abdominal lymphadenopathy
Lymphocyte-rich classical Hodgkin's lymphoma	Intermediate association	Accounts for 5% of classical Hodgkin's lymphoma	Peripheral lymphadenopathy
Lymphocyte-depleted classical Hodgkin's lymphoma	Up to 75% of patients EBV positive	Rare subtype with less than 1%, but prevalent in patients with HIV	Present in advanced stage commonly

Adapted from Townsend W, Linch D (2012). Hodgkin's lymphoma in adults. *Lancet* 380, 836–47.

Young patients should be considered for fertility preservation options prior to starting systemic treatment.

Advanced stage disease The standard treatment is combination chemotherapy, with either six or eight cycles of ABVD or six cycles of escalated BEACOPP. Decision on either regimen can be guided by IPSS scores with higher scores suggesting escalated BEACOPP regimen.

The strategy for management of relapsed or refractory disease is to deliver salvage chemotherapy, followed by high-dose chemotherapy and autologous stem-cell transplantation in responding patients. **Brentuximab vedotin** is indicated for refractory or relapsed disease.

Children and young adults Hodgkin's lymphoma is typically a malignancy that affects younger patients, and with survival rates as high as they are, the emphasis on reducing long-term toxicity is even more pertinent; minimizing exposure to alkylating agents and restricting the use of radiotherapy. First line treatment is usually with two cycles of OEPA (see Table 13.10) followed by an FDG-PET, so that only those that are PET positive go on to receive radiotherapy. Higher risk individuals receive 2-4 cycles of COPDAC chemotherapy (Table 13.10).

In advanced stage or relapsed disease the use of targeted therapies such as **bortezomib**, **panobinostat**, **brentuximab** and **nivolumab** are current options under investigation.

Elderly patients Elderly patients account for up to a fifth of HL cases. They also suffer significantly higher toxicity compared to younger patients. Commonly used strategies include COPP or ChIVPP in an effort to reduce the anthracycline associated toxicity. However, outcomes are inferior to the 'gold standard' treatment regimens of ABVD/BEACOPP (see Table 13.10).

Non-Hodgkin's lymphomas

Non-Hodgkin's lymphoma encompasses an array of heterogeneous cancers predominantly B cell (85–90%) in origin in addition to T-cell lymphomas. Two-thirds of those diagnosed are >60 years. The male:female rate of incidence is 17.7 and 12.8/100 000, respectively.

Non-Hodgkin's lymphoma can present in a variety of different nodal patterns, and extra-nodal disease can be found in almost all organs. Common sites are gastric mucosa-associated lymphoid tissue (MALT), CNS, and testicular lymphoma. More aggressive lymphomas

Table 13.10 Treatment regimens used in HL

Regimen	Chemotherapy
ABVD	Doxorubicin (Adriamycin®), bleomycin, vincristine, dacarbazine
BEACOPP	Bleomycin, etoposide, doxorubicin (Adriamycin®), cyclophosphamide, vincristine (Oncovin®), procarbazine, prednisolone
COPP	Cyclophosphamide, vincristine (Oncovin®), procarbazine, prednisolone
ChIVPP	Chlorambucil, vinblastine, procarbazine, prednisolone
OEPA	Vincristine (Oncovin®), etoposide, prednisolone Adriamycin® (doxorubicin)
COPDAC	Cyclophosphamide, vincristine (Oncovin®), prednisolone, dacarbazine

present with B symptoms such as weight loss (>10%), fevers (>38°C), and drenching night sweats.

Normal B cell development occurs in three main stages:

1. B-cell progenitor development occurs in the bone marrow and thymus, termed the pregerminal centre. Once matured they migrate to the blood, spleen, lymph nodes, and mucosa-associated tissues. At this stage, they express an IgM molecule on their cell surface. B cells not exposed to antigens are termed antigen-naïve mature B cells.

2. B cells exposed to antigen and T cell activation then proliferates in lymph node germinal centres. Termed centroblasts they then become centrocytes in the light zone of the germinal centre. In the germinal centre, cells undergo genetic and somatic modification of immunoglobulin heavy and light chains to modify the affinity of a B cell population for a particular antigen.

3. In response to presentation of antigens by T cells and follicular dendritic cells, rapidly dividing B cells differentiate to memory B cells or plasma cells after the germinal centre reaction.

Non-Hodgkin's lymphomas that arise from the pre-germinal centre include *mantle cell lymphomas*. Those arising in the germinal centre, but yet to undergo immunoglobulin recombination, include *chronic lymphocytic lymphoma* or *small lymphocytic lymphomas*. Those having undergone immunoglobulin differentiation or post-germinal cells give rise to *Burkitt's lymphoma, follicular lymphoma, diffuse large B cell lymphoma*, and *mucosa- associated lymphoid tissue (MALT) lymphoma*.

The mechanisms responsible for the development of lymphomas exhibit some characteristics with other solid tumours; accumulation of genetic lesions affecting proto-oncogenes and tumour suppressor genes. In contrast to epithelial malignancies the genome is relatively stable in lymphomas, but does harbour chromosomal abnormalities such as chromosomal translocations

Management

Diffuse large B cell lymphoma

This is the most common sub-type presentation of NHL.

Early stage disease Patients with early stage disease can be offered single or combined modality chemotherapy/radiotherapy, both being equally efficacious. For stage IA with disease localized to the groin, neck, and axilla the recommended treatment is with R-CHOP (Table 13.11) followed by involved site radiotherapy. The addition of **rituximab** in the MabThera® trial gave an overall survival advantage to chemotherapy alone to 5-year survival 92–98%.

Bulky/advanced stage disease For those with bulky disease (>10 cm) six to eight cycles of R-CHOP followed by IFRT is recommended and prognosis is similar to those with advanced disease. Overall 5-year survival in advanced disease has benefitted from the addition of **rituximab** from 52% to 78%.

Table 13.11 Treatment regimens used in NHL

Regimen	Chemotherapy
R-CHOP/ R-miniCHOP	Rituximab, cyclophosphamide, doxorubicin, vincristine (Oncovin®), prednisolone
R-Bendamustine	Rituximab, bendamustine
R-ICE	Rituximab, ifosfamide (with mesna prophylaxis), carboplatin, etoposide
Gem-P	Gemcitabine, cisplatin (days 1, 8, and 15)

Elderly patients In the elderly over 80 years of age omission of **doxorubicin** from R-CHOP (R-CVP) is common to reduce cardiac toxicity. Other regimens such as R-miniCHOP have been shown to be efficacious and provide suitable prolonged survival (Table 13.11).

Salvage therapy Approximately 30–40% of early stage patients will relapse and require salvage chemotherapy such as platinum therapy with **gemcitabine** and R-ICE (Table 13.11).

Follicular lymphoma

Follicular lymphoma is the second most common non-Hodgkin's lymphoma, accounting for approximately 20% of cases.

- *Stage I disease*: defined by disease confined to one nodal group or one extra-nodal site and treated with radiotherapy, which is considered curative in up to 50% of patients. Observation is a considered an appropriate strategy in some and still associated with a long-term overall survival.
- *Stage II disease*: defined by more than one nodal group on the same side of the diaphragm. A decision to treat in this group should be guided by age and expected morbidity from treatment, and may include **rituximab** monotherapy or radiotherapy.
- *Advanced stage disease (stage III/IV):* defined as disease on both sides of the diaphragm. can be treated with a similar approach to diffuse large B cell lymphoma, i.e. with R-CHOP or other therapeutics such as **bendamustine** plus **rituximab**. There is a role for maintenance in delaying disease relapse, although it is unclear if this translates into a survival advantage.

Overall survival rates are measured in years with early stage disease having an overall survival greater than 10 years.

Marginal-zone lymphomas

This is the third most common lymphoma with stomach being the most frequent site of disease. Gastric MALT lymphomas are associated with *H. pylori* infection and all patients should be offered standard eradication therapy (Topic 6.2, 'Dyspepsia'). Those not responding should be offered second-line eradication followed by radiotherapy and chemotherapy if lymphoma is present on subsequent OGD surveillance.

Supportive care

As with other malignancies, supportive care plays a significant role in patients being treated for lymphoma. This will typically include the use of GFs, blood product support, antimicrobial therapy, and anti-emetics (Chapter 6, 'Gastroenterology'). There is a particularly high risk of tumour lysis in high-grade non-Hodgkin's lymphomas and Hodgkin's lymphomas, and high grade diffuse large B and T cell lymphomas. Management is with **allopurinol**, fluids, and in high risk patients, **rasburicase**.

Management of myeloma

Myeloma is a genetically diverse disease, characterized by malignant transformation of antibody-secreting plasma cells. It has an overall incidence of 6.3 persons per 100 000 of the population and median age 69 years. Patients typically present with signs and symptoms of bone marrow failure (e.g. bleeding, bruising, and lethargy), pathological fractures, and recurrent infections (Figure 13.5).

The cause of myeloma is unclear but initiating events include immunoglobulin heavy chain (IgH) translocations and hyperdiploidy (increase in the number of chromosomes). Such events result in the generation of an abnormal plasma cell clone which divides uncontrollably in the bone marrow, lymph nodes and occasionally at other distant sites. The resulting clonal plasma cell population secrets a single antibody type which is detected as a paraprotein in the plasma.

Although important in pathogenesis, translocations and hyperdiploidy are not alone sufficient to cause a pathological syndrome. This is evidenced by the presence of these abnormalities in the precursor conditions monoclonal gammopathy of unknown significance (MGUS) and smouldering myeloma (SMM). Patients with these conditions have no evidence of end-organ damage and transform to symptomatic myeloma at a rate of approximately 1% and 10% per year, respectively. The most aggressive disease state, plasma cell leukaemia (PCL) typically has a higher mutational load than the earlier disease phases. Some patients may present with a single focus of disease, called a plasmacytoma.

Patients with myeloma may present with back or other bone pain. Pathological fractures are often a feature at diagnosis, particularly crush fractures of the vertebral column. In patients with elevated light chains, renal failure

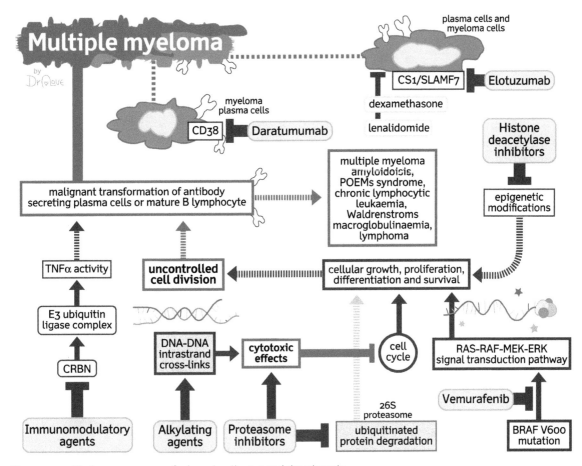

Figure 13.5 Myeloma: summary of relevant pathways and drug targets.

may be noted at presentation. Renal failure is, however, often multifactorial, secondary to hypercalcaemia, light chain, or paraprotein deposition within the kidney, infection, hyperuricaemia, or amyloid. Bone marrow failure can occur secondary to plasma cell infiltration causing bruising, bleeding, symptoms of anaemia, and infection.

To diagnose, there myeloma must be evidence of end-organ damage in addition to the presence of a detectable clonal plasma cell population and monoclonal paraprotein (PP) or light chain abnormality (see Box 13.1).

End-organ damage in myeloma is usually described by using the acronym CRAB;

- *Hyper**c**alcaemia*: corrected calcium >0.25 above the upper limit of normal or >2.75 mmol/ L.
- ***R**enal failure*: creatinine >173 mmol/L.
- ***A**naemia*: haemoglobin 2 g/dL below the lower limit of normal or Hb <10 g/dL.

Box 13.1 Diagnostic criteria for myeloma.

Myeloma

Clonal plasma cells of >10% identified on bone marrow or plasmacytoma biopsy and

1. Myeloma-related end organ damage (CRAB criteria).
   Or
2. Any one of the following if present is sufficient to diagnose myeloma.
   - >60% clonal plasma cells in the bone marrow;
   - more than one focal lesion on MRI that is at least 0.5 cm;
   - serum involved/uninvolved light chain ratio of 100 or greater provided the involved value is >100 mg/L.

- **B**one lesion: lytic lesions or osteoporosis with compression fractures.

Management

The treatment of myeloma has changed significantly over the past 20 years with median life expectancy improving from 3 to 9 years in that time. The disease is still, however, considered non-curable by most, although intensive therapy in combination with autologous stem cell transplantation in low risk individuals can lead to long-term remission.

Chemotherapy

Chemotherapy, immune-modulators, proteasome inhibitors, and targeted therapies ± autologous stem cell transplantation form the mainstay of myeloma treatment. It is, however, important to note that such agents are often associated with side effects, particularly anaemia, thrombocytopenia, leukopenia, infection (including neutropenic sepsis) and GI symptoms. These complications may require therapeutic intervention with blood product support, antibiotics, IV immunoglobulin and, in patients with anaemia contributed to by renal impairment, EPO may be of benefit. Additional complications of the disease and therapy include peripheral neuropathy and thromboembolism therefore requiring neuropathic analgesics and anticoagulation, respectively. Severe iatrogenic neuropathy, e.g. secondary to thalidomide or bortezomib should warrant a change in therapeutic approach.

Treatment of myeloma is divided into phases; induction, consolidation and maintenance:

- *Induction*: involves the use of multiple agents (see Table 13.13).
- **Consolidation**; in transplant eligible patients this involves bone marrow ablation with high dose **melphalan** followed by autologous stem cell return.
- Various **maintenance** regimes have been trialled and usually involve the use of one or two agents administered for 21 days of 28 day cycles e.g. **thalidomide** or **lenalidomide**. The overall aim of treatment is to reduce the burden of disease as much as possible and continue to suppress it.

Newer agents include monoclonal antibodies, histone deacetylase inhibitors, and oncogene targets, such as BRAF, are being trialled. Older agents such as **bendamustine** and **carmustine** may also be considered in patients who have progressed through multiple therapies.

Table 13.12 Summary of different drugs classes acting at different stages of the cell cycle to suppress cell replication

Drug class	Examples
Alkylating agents	Nitrogen mustards
	Nitrosoureas
	Busulfan
	Triazones
	Chlorambucil
Platinum compounds	Cisplatin, carboplatin
Antimetabolites	fluorouracil, mercaptopurine, capecitabine, methotrexate, fludarabine, gemcitabine, pemetrexed
Anti-tumour antibiotics (anthracyclines)	Daunorubicin, doxorubicin, epirubicin, idarubicin
Other anti-tumour antibiotics	Bleomycin, mitomycin-actinomycin, mitoxantrone
Topoisomerase inhibitors	Topotecan, irinotecan etoposide, tenisopide
Mitotic inhibitors	Taxanes, vinca alkaloids

In patients with aggressive disease or advanced disease combination therapy with 5, 6, or 7 agents may be considered (see Box 13.2). These regimes are associated with marked myelosuppression, GI toxicity, and infection risk so are given as an in-patient regimen. The drugs are commonly given over a 4-day period with a prolonged hospital stay until the neutrophil count recovers (usually to >1). Growth factor support with pegylated GSCF or daily SC GSCF is required to help blood count recovery and shorten hospital stay.

Supportive care

All patients initiating treatment with be prescribed a number of supportive medications to reduce the risk of complications. Examples include:

- *Bisphosphonates*: myeloma can cause bone damage, leading to a high risk of fracture (lytic skeletal lesions). Prevention and management of such complications include the use of bone-strengthening therapy by administration of bisphosphonates, i.e. **zolendronic acid** or, if

Table 13.13 Summary of treatment regimens used in myeloma

Regime	Example schedule
CTD(a)*	Daily thalidomide for 21/28 days, dexamethasone (40 mg 1–4 × per week) and cyclophosphamide 500 mg weekly.
CVD(a)*	Weekly or twice weekly bortezomib, dexamethasone 40 mg the day of and day after bortezomib, and weekly cyclophosphamide, 500 mg
VTD(a)*	Daily thalidomide for 21/28 days, weekly or twice weekly bortezomib, and dexamethasone 40 mg the day of and day after bortezomib.
RCD(a)**	Daily lenalidomide for 21/28 days, dexamethasone (40 mg 1–4 × per week) and cyclophosphamide, 500 mg weekly. Common regime at second relapse

* Can be used at presentation and following relapse.
** Can be used at first relapse in patients who have received bortezomib first line.

Abbreviations: C, cyclophosphamide; T, thalidomide; D, dexamethasone; V, bortezomib (Velcade)®; R, lenalidomide (Revlamid®); a, attenuated regime, i.e. lower doses for patients with significant comorbidity or advanced age in whom side effects are expected at higher doses, e.g. 20 mg dexamethasone and 250 mg cyclophosphamide.

contraindicated (e.g. renal impairment), **pamidronate** or **sodium clodronate** used (Topic 7.4, 'Metabolic bone disease').

- *Antimicrobial therapy.*
- *Gastric protection*: steroids form a component of most regimens so PPI protection is common.
- *Anticoagulation*: myeloma and many of its treatments increase the risk of thromboembolism, and therefore

Box 13.2 Intensive regimens: DT-PACE and VDT-PACE

DT-PACE is a combination chemotherapy regimen using dexamethasone, thalidomide, and a 4-day continuous infusion of cisplatin, doxorubicin, cyclophosphamide, and etoposide. Most recently, it has been combined with bortezomib as VDT-PACE.

aspirin or other anticoagulation medications are often indicated.

- *Growth factors*: low white blood cell counts including neutropenia are common, either due to disease infiltration of the bone marrow or as a side effect of treatment. **GF** injections are often prescribed.
- *Prevention of gout*: hyperuricaemia may be part of the presenting and require allopurinol.

Drug classes used in management

Prescribing chemotherapy

Considerable care and knowledge is required when it comes to prescribing and delivering chemotherapy in the management of both malignant and non-malignant conditions. In the absence of due care, treatment is associated with a high risk of toxicity to both the patient and the staff administering it. Patients require careful monitoring and baseline assessments must be carried out, prior to treatment cycles. Furthermore, treatment strategies are frequently complex in their delivery with regards to timing and practical administration, invariably given in cycles over periods of weeks to months or even years. For this reason, chemotherapy is generally prescribed and administered within a specialist service, by suitably trained staff who possess a sound knowledge of local and national policies, and treatment protocols.

The adverse effects from chemotherapy can be severe, both in the short- and long-term, and can give rise to late effects such as, cardiac toxicity, renal impairment, neurological toxicity, infertility, and endocrine dysfunction. The side effects covered within the following chapters should not be considered to be exhaustive. As chemotherapy agents are known to be mutagenic, teratogenic, and carcinogenic to patients, and to the staff handling them, it is essential that all staff involved in the dispensing and administration of these drugs are aware of these risks and adopt safe practices.

Chemotherapy agents can be administered via a number of routes, but are most frequently given IV, and where done so should always be administered in designated areas with access to appropriate emergency facilities including extravasation and spillage kits. With the emergence of targeted therapies, however, more agents are available for oral administration. It is essential that patients are instructed carefully on the administration, storage, and adverse effects of these medicines.

Chemotherapy agents may also be administered intrathecally for which extreme care is required and protocols in place, to ensure that certain chemotherapies are never administered by this route due to the potential for serious consequences. Vinca alkaloids administered intrathecally are associated with ascending myeloencephalopathy, which is invariably fatal.

PRACTICAL PRESCRIBING

Intrathecal chemotherapy

- *Intrathecal chemotherapy* (IT) is stringently regulated and only doctors who have undergone specific training are able to administer the agents. Administration must also be undertaken with an IT-trained nurse. The nurse, doctor, and patient must confirm the patient details and IT prescription are correct prior to administration.

- *IT chemotherapy* must not be released from the pharmacy at the same time systemic chemotherapy is released. All systemic chemotherapy must be completed before administration to ensure it is not administered intrathecally by mistake.

- *Methotrexate, cytarabine, and steroids* are the only agents administered intrathecally in the treatment of haematological malignancy.

- There have been cases of accidental death due to IT administration of agents meant for systemic use, such as vincristine.

Chemotherapeutic agents

Chemotherapeutic agents, although different in their specific mechanism of action, are unified in that all act to restrict cell replication or promote cell death, by acting at different stages in the cell cycle (Figure 13.1 and 13.12). Many agents also have a direct role on DNA synthesis and replication (seen in the Figure 13.2).

Targeted drug therapies

While conventional chemotherapy agents exert their effect by direct action on DNA replication, many of the newer agents are designed with specific molecular targets associated with cancer.

- Hormone therapies work by either interfering with hormone production or action, thus slowing or stopping the growth of hormone-sensitive tumours.

- Signal transduction inhibitors block the activity of molecules that are part of the signal transduction pathway (EGFR antagonists, BCR-ABL/C-Kit/PDGFR inhibition, FLT3 inhibitors, JAK2 inhibitors, RAS/MAP kinase pathway inhibitors, and mTOR inhibitors).

- Proteasome inhibitors induce growth inhibition and apoptosis of tumour cells (**bortezomib**, which is thought to act by suppression of nuclear factor kappa B).

- Angiogenesis inhibitors block the growth of new blood vessels required for tumour to grow (anti-VEGF antibodies, VEGFR inhibitors, **Thalidomide**, **lenalidomide** and **pomalidomide** are mainly immunomodulatory agents, although they do have some anti-angiogenic properties.

- Gene expression modulators modify the function of proteins involved in controlling gene expression (e.g. histone deacetylation inhibitors).

- Immunotherapies trigger the immune system to destroy cancer cells. Some immunotherapies are antibodies, which recognize surface molecules on cancer cells, while others bind to certain immune cells to enhance killing of cancer cells.

These classes of drugs are discussed in more detail below.

Cytotoxic antibiotics

The majority of antitumour antibiotics have been produced from bacterial and fungal cultures, and they affect the function and synthesis of nucleic acids in different ways. The mechanism of action is explained in detail for each drug. Examples include bleomycin, dactinomycin, anthracyclines (daunorubicin, doxorubicin, epirubicin, idarubicin), mitomycin, and anthraquinones (mitoxantrone, pixantrone). (See Figure 13.6.)

Bleomycin

Mechanism of action

The exact mechanism of action for **bleomycin** is unknown, although evidence suggests single-/double-stranded breaks in DNA as the main target site. In addition, there is some evidence of inhibition of RNA and protein synthesis.

Prescribing

Bleomycin uses include germ cell cancer and non-Hodgkin's lymphoma, Hodgkin's lymphoma, neoplastic

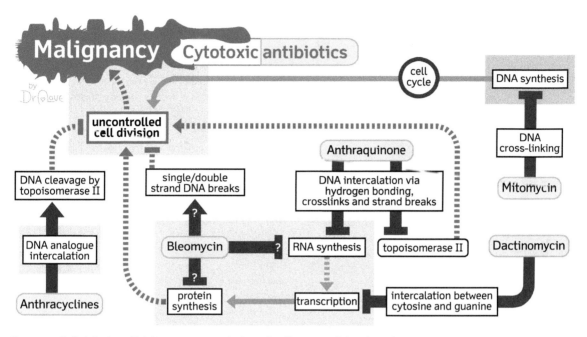

Figure 13.6 Cytotoxic antibiotics: summary of relevant pathways and drug targets.

pleural effusion, malignant pericardial effusion, and AIDS-related Kaposi sarcoma. It may be administered via parenteral route, intrapleural route, IM or SC, and is rapidly absorbed (peak plasma concentration reached within 30–60 minutes). Bioavailability of IM bleomycin is 100% compared with 70% following SC administration. The highest concentration of bleomycin is found in skin, lungs, peritoneum, and lymph.

Unwanted effects

Dermatological toxicity and GI symptoms are frequently experienced with **bleomycin**, although pulmonary fibrosis is the most severe side effect and the risk increased in patients that have had radiotherapy to the chest. It is dose-dependent, with elderly patients at higher risk. Anaphylactoid reaction secondary to bleomycin may be prevented through simultaneous administration of **hydrocortisone**.

Dactinomycin

Mechanism of action

Dactinomycin intercalates between guanine and cytosine base pairs, and interferes with transcription. At low doses DNA-directed RNA synthesis is blocked.

Prescribing

Dactinomycin is administered via the parenteral route and does not penetrate the blood–brain barrier. It has a terminal plasma half-life of approximately 36 hours and has been shown to be beneficial as a combination therapy in Wilm's tumour, childhood rhabdomyosarcoma, Ewing's sarcoma and metastatic, non-seminomatous testicular cancer. Dactinomycin is also indicated as monotherapy or combination chemotherapy in gestational trophoblastic neoplasm, and as palliative or adjunctive treatment for locally recurrent or locoregional solid tumours.

Unwanted effects

The combination of **dactinomycin** and radiation therapy may result in increased GI toxicity and bone marrow suppression, while potentiation of radiation effect is very likely with high dactinomycin dose. For this reason, doses of dactinomycin are often omitted during radiotherapy.

Primary hepatic sinusoidal obstruction syndrome (SOS), once termed veno-occlusive disease (VOD), is a rare, albeit serious adverse reaction associated with dactinomycin, with children less than 48 months old particularly at risk. There is also an increased risk of second primary tumours when dactinomycin is used in combination with radiation. Extravasation of this drug can result in severe soft tissue damage.

Anthracyclines (daunorubicin, epirubicin, doxorubicin, and idarubicin)

Mechanism of action

Anthracycline cytotoxic agents exhibits antitumour effects by intercalating between DNA nucleotide base pairs and triggering DNA cleavage by topoisomerase II. Anthracyclines are effective in the treatment of breast, ovarian, endometrial, bladder, and thyroid carcinomas. They are also used in several different combinations for the treatment of lymphomas, leukaemias, and Hodgkin's disease.

Prescribing

Daunorubicin is distributed widely after absorption, particularly in the liver, kidneys, lung, spleen, and heart, with a plasma half-life of 24–48 hours. It is primarily metabolized to daunorubicinol via hepatic metabolism. Doses are administered IV, diluted through a large vein to reduce the risk of extravasation.

Doxorubicin plasma clearance is predominately via metabolism and biliary excretion, with a terminal half-life of 20–48 hours. Dose adjustments may therefore be necessary in hepatic impairment and it is contraindicated in severe hepatic impairment. Doxorubicin is indicated as multi-agent adjuvant chemotherapy for breast cancer, as well as in metastatic solid tumours, leukaemia, or lymphoma. Due to its vesicant nature it must not be given IM or SC. It is also available in a liposomal formulation, developed to reduce the risk of toxicity, specifically cardiotoxicity.

Epirubicin is used as adjuvant therapy in breast cancer and has an elimination half-life of approximately 33 hours. As with daunorubicin, elimination is predominately via hepatic metabolism and biliary secretion, with dosing adjustment possibly required in hepatic impairment and bone marrow dysfunction. Renal dose adjustment is rarely required, although should be considered in severe renal impairment.

Idarubicin is highly lipophilic and extensively tissue bound, therefore has a high volume of distribution. The elimination half-life after oral intake is 14–35 hours and with IV administration 12–27 hours. Idarubicinol is the active metabolite, which also contributes towards its cytotoxic effects. It is mainly excreted via hepatic route and to lesser extent renally.

Unwanted effects

As a class, anthracyclines cause dose-limiting myelosuppression, primarily leukopenia. Chronic cardiomyopathies can occur with all agents and can manifest as congestive cardiac failure. The risk of cardiotoxicity increases with cumulative dose and, therefore, anthracyclines have a maximum cumulative lifetime dose that should not be exceeded, this may impact on treatment options in the case of relapse. All patients should have a baseline LVEF assessment performed and reassessed regularly.

Due to route of elimination dose reductions are required for anthracyclines in patients with hepatic impairment, based on bilirubin levels.

As a class anthracyclines are potent vesicants; extravasation may result in severe local tissue injury resulting in tissue necrosis and will require urgent management as dictated by local policies. Administration should, therefore, only be carried out in designated areas with access to an extravasation kit and care given in ensuring doses are administered adequately diluted through large veins.

Anthracyclines are also associated with an increased risk of secondary malignancies, including acute myelogenous leukaemia and myelodysplastic syndrome. Like many agents, **doxorubicin** may cause foetal harm in pregnancy and animal studies have shown teratogenicity and embryotoxicity.

Other more common adverse drug reactions include mild to moderate GI and dermatological reactions, and an increased risk of tumour lysis syndrome in the presence of a high tumour burden.

> ### PRESCRIBING WARNING
>
> **Doxorubicin: red urine**
> Doxorubicin will cause red discoloration of the urine and requires patient education.

Drug interactions

Although concomitant administration of anthracyclines with other drugs is unlikely to affect clearance or serum levels, care is advisable when they are coprescribed with other drugs known to be cardiotoxic.

Mitomycin

Mechanism of action

Mitomycin isolated from *Streptomycin* spp. exerts its effect via mitomycin-induced cross-linking, resulting in the inhibition of DNA synthesis. Mitomycin is unique in that it can produce both mono- and bifunctional alkylation.

Mono-alkylation is effective through the alkylation of the guanine base in the CpG (cytosine-phosphate-guanine) sequence in DNA strands. In the second stage of action, DNA cross-links are formed between CpG strands. It is these cross-links that account for a significant proportion of mitomycin's effects.

Prescribing

Mitomycin is used in combination therapy for disseminated adenocarcinoma of the stomach and pancreas. It should be given via slow IV injection to reduce the risk of extravasation, which may otherwise result in severe local soft tissue injury. Doses may also be administered intravesically in the treatment of bladder tumours.

Unwanted effects

As with most neoplastic agents, **mitomycin** is typically associated with bone marrow suppression, and nausea and vomiting (although classified as having low emetogenic potential). Toxicity will depend on the route of administration, with intervesical instillation in particular being associated with a risk of bladder toxicity. Another side effect reported with therapy is pulmonary toxicity, including, less commonly, pulmonary fibrosis. Use is contraindicated in patients with thrombocytopenia and coagulation disorders.

Anthraquinone (mitoxantrone, pixantrone)

Mechanism of action

Anthraquinones exert cytotoxic action via intercalation into DNA through hydrogen bonding, cross-links and strand breaks. Anthraquinones also inhibits topoisomerase II and interfere with RNA synthesis.

Prescribing

Mitoxantrone distributes widely in body tissues, resulting in a high volume of distribution, with excretion in urine and faeces either unchanged or as inactive metabolite. Due to its extended half-life (approximately 12 days) clearance is very slow. It is indicated in advanced hormone-refractory prostate cancer and multiple sclerosis, as well as combination therapy in acute non-lymphocytic leukaemia. Pre-existing myelosuppression is a contraindication for treatment with mitoxantrone, i.e. patients should have recovered their counts prior to starting a new cycle.

> **PATIENT WARNING**
>
> **Mitoxantrone: blue-green urine**
> Patient should be made aware that urine may turn blue-green for 1–2 days post-mitoxantrone infusion.

Pixantrone, an analogue of mitoxantrone, is licensed as monotherapy for treating multiple relapsed or refractory aggressive non-Hodgkin's B cell lymphoma. Like mitoxantrone it has large volume of distribution, but a considerably shorter terminal half-life that ranges from 14.5 to 44.8 hours.

Unwanted effects

Like the anthracyclines, the most clinically significant toxicities associated with **mitoxantrone** and **pixantrone** are bone marrow suppression (common), cardiotoxicity, the latter of which can have a delayed presentation and, in some cases, can be fatal, and urine discolouration (see 'Patient warning: mitoxantrone—blue-green urine'). Patients will require cardiac monitoring at baseline, while on treatment and on follow-up. Again, in common with anthracyclines the anthraquinones are vesicants, requiring urgent management in the case of extravasation.

Alkylating agents

> The alkylating agents are highly reactive compounds that produce their effect by covalently linking an alkyl group (R-CH2) to a chemical species in nucleic acids or proteins. The site and a number of cross-links is drug specific, with most compounds being bipolar, i.e. they contain two groups capable of reacting with DNA. The bridges formed interfere with the action of DNA replication enzymes. Examples include nitrogen mustards (chlorambucil, cyclophosphamide, ifosfamide, melphalan), nitrosureas (streptozocin, carmustine, lomustine), alkyl sulfonates (busulfan), and triozines (darcarbazine, temzolomide). (See Figure 13.7.)

Nitrogen mustard alkylating agents (cyclophosphamide, melphalan, ifosfamide)

Mechanism of action

Nitrogen mustard alkylating agents (NMAAs) have a long therapeutic pedigree and were first used

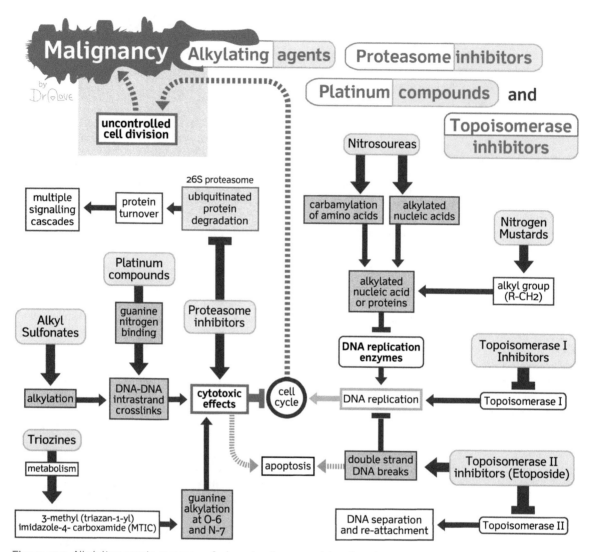

Figure 13.7 Alkylating agents: summary of relevant pathways and drug targets.

as chemotherapeutic agents in the early 1940s. **Cyclophosphamide**, **ifosfamide**, **chlorambucil**, and **melphalan** act by adding an alkyl group to guanine. The alkyl group attaches to the purine ring on the seventh nitrogen atom. This change results in cross-links in cellular DNA, which act as a barricade to progression of replication subsequently promoting cell senescence or death. Cellular resistance has been noted to NMAAs and this is most likely due to enhanced DNA repair mechanisms.

Prescribing

Cyclophosphamide is converted to its active form by the liver and is used extensively in the treatment of numerous malignant and non-malignant indications. It can be delivered IV or PO, with an oral bioavailability of greater than 75%. In malignant conditions, the oral route is often reserved for use where other treatment options have failed, in a palliative capacity. Cyclophosphamide is a pro-drug with several metabolites of unknown clinical efficacy or toxicity profile. Elimination half-live of unchanged drug is 3–12 hours.

Ifosfamide, also a pro-drug, is structurally similar to cyclophosphamide, but differs in terms of its efficacy and toxicity profile. It is only available for administration IV, despite being well absorbed orally, and it's use is limited to the management of malignant disease.

Melphalan can be administered IV or PO, although its oral bioavailability is highly variable ranging from 56% to

93%, making it an unfavourable route for curative treatment. It is used less frequently than cyclophosphamide or ifosfamide, and only in malignant conditions. Melphalan is also rarely administered by regional arterial perfusion for malignant melanoma of the extremities to help minimize systemic toxicity.

Unwanted effects

Although the nitrogen mustards vary in terms of their toxic side effects, the haematopoietic system is the most commonly affected organ. Other commonly experienced side effects are GI, nephrotoxicity, cardiotoxicity, neurotoxicity, hepatotoxicity, and pulmonary toxicity.

Cyclophosphamide and **ifosfomide** are associated with serious urotoxic side effects including haemorrhagic cystitis, which occurs as a result of the toxic by-product acrolein. Higher doses are therefore administered with concurrent hydration and **mesna**, which binds to acrolein and aids excretion. Cyclophosphamide may also potentiate **doxorubicin**-induced toxicity, whereas ifosamide can precipitate encephalopathy, which can be managed with **methylthioninium chloride**. Severe myelosuppression is observed where alkylating agents are used in combination with other chemotherapeutic drugs. In addition, alkylating agents are associated with an increased risk of secondary malignancies and infertility.

Drug interactions

Cyclophosphamide and **ifosfamide** are pro-drugs that are activated through metabolism via various cytochrome P450 enzyme subtypes. Drugs affecting CYP2B6 and CYP3A4 (e.g. **aprepitant**, azole anti-fungals, **rifampicin**, **grapefruit juice**, and **St John's Wort**) may alter cyclophosphamide metabolism, resulting in increased/decreased plasma concentrations and are generally best avoided. Similarly, metabolism of ifosfamide may be affected by changes in CYP3A4 metabolism.

Nitrosoureas (streptozocin, carmustine, lomustine)

Mechanism of action

As with other alkylating agents, nitrosoureas can alkylate DNA and RNA, but also exhibit the capacity to act via carbamylation of amino acids in proteins, thus disrupting enzymatic processes. Carbamylation is a post-translational modification, characterized by the formation of carbamyl groups through the binding of cyanate. It was first observed in high urea states such as renal failure as cyanate levels are proportional to urea levels.

Prescribing

Lomustine and **carmustine** are highly lipophilic and can therefore efficiently cross the blood–brain barrier, which makes them useful in the treatment of some brain tumours. Other indications include Hodgkin's disease and multiple myeloma. Carmustine is administered IV and also available as an implant for high-grade glioma. It is mainly excreted via the renal route, and its active metabolite may be responsible for its therapeutic and toxic effects. Lomustine is administered orally, and more commonly used second-line or as palliative treatment.

Streptozocin is infrequently used and not widely available. Unlike carmustine and lomustine, it does not cross the blood–brain barrier, although its metabolites do. It has a short half-life, and its highest concentration is found in the liver and kidneys. It can be used in metastatic pancreatic islet cell carcinoma.

Unwanted effects

Streptozocin is associated with severe dose-dependent, cumulative nephrotoxicity, which may be fatal; monitoring renal function is therefore mandatory. **Lomustine** and **carmustine** are associated with severe bone marrow suppression, which can delay subsequent cycles and require dose adjustment based on blood counts. Nausea and vomiting is also common with lomustine therapy (being administered orally), which can be, in part, managed by dividing up the daily dose or taking it on an empty stomach.

Carmustine is associated with an increased risk of pulmonary toxicity, particularly with cumulative doses >1400 mg/m². This can occur years after treatment, especially in patients treated in childhood, and can result in death.

Alkyl sulfonates (busulfan)

Mechanism of action

Busulfan is a bifunctional alkylating agent that can form DNA–DNA intra-strand cross-links to cause cytotoxic effects. These cross-links occur between adenine and guanine, and guanine and guanine.

Prescribing

Distribution of **busulfan** into the CSF is equivalent to serum levels. Terminal half-life is 2.8–3.9 hours, with approximately one-third of the drug being renally excreted. Doses can be administered PO or IV in the management of some haematological malignancies. It is also used in combination with **cyclophosphamide** as a conditioning agent pre-bone marrow transplant, due to its potent myelosuppressive properties.

Unwanted effects

Severe bone marrow suppression is the most common adverse drug effect associated with **busulfan** therapy, with dose adjustment/discontinuation sometimes being necessary. Plasma concentration versus time curve values (>1.500 µMCmin) increases the risk of hepatic sinusoidal obstruction syndrome, once referred to as veno-occlusive disease. As busulfan is predominantly hepatically cleared and associated with hepatic toxicity, LFTs should be carried out while on treatment and following transplant.

Triazines (dacarbazine, temozolomide)

Mechanism of action

The antitumour effects of the triazines are predominantly due to the alkylating properties of its active metabolite 3-methyl- (triazan-1-yl) imidazole-4-carboxamide (MTIC), which acts via alkylation of the DNA at the O-6 and N-7 positions of guanine. Both **dacarbazine** and **temozolomide** are metabolized via cytochromes P450 to the active metabolite MTIC, which is further metabolized to 5-aminoimidazole-4-carboxamide (AIC).

Prescribing

Temozolomide (TMZ) is only available as capsules for oral administration and is indicated for newly diagnosed glioblastoma multiforme, recurrent, or progressive malignant glioma and recurrent anaplastic astrocytoma. It is rapidly absorbed, achieving peak plasma levels within 1 hour. Doses are calculated on body surface area and rounded to the nearest capsule size. Although renally cleared, dose reductions are unlikely to be necessary in renal or hepatic impairment. As food can result in a 33% reduction in absorption, doses are best taken on an empty stomach.

Dacarbazine can be used in the treatment of metastatic melanoma and Hodgkin's disease

Unwanted effects

Haemopoietic toxicity is common with **dacarbazine**, while hepatic necrosis and hepatic vein thrombosis have also been reported, albeit rarely.

The longer dosing regimen of **temozolomide** is associated with *Pneumocystis jirovecii* pneumonia, for which suitable prophylaxis is recommended (especially in patients on concomitant steroid treatment). Temozolomide is also associated with serious hepatic injury, secondary malignancies, and myelodysplastic syndrome. It is genotoxic and men should seek advice regarding cryoconservation prior to starting treatment.

Antimetabolites

These compounds are defined by their structural similarity to naturally occurring substances such as vitamins, nucleosides, or amino acids. This allows them to compete with the natural substrate for the active site on essential enzymes or receptors. The main groups include folate antagonists, purine, and pyrimidine analogues and nucleobases. Examples include folate antagonists (methotrexate, pemetrexed, ralitrexed), purine nucleoside analogues (fludarabine, cladribine, clofarabine, nelarabine), nucleobases (mercaptopurine, tioguanine), and pyrimidine analogues (cytarabine, gemcitabine, fluorouracil, capecitabine, tegafur, azacitidine, decitabine). (See Figure 13.8.)

Mechanism of action

Folate antagonists or antifolates (**methotrexate**, **pemetrexed**, **ralitrexed**) are predominantly dihydrofolic acid reductase inhibitors, therefore, they prevent the reduction of inactive dihydrofolate to active tetrahydrofolate, blocking an essential step in DNA synthesis.

Purine nucleoside analogues

Purine nucleoside analogues such as **fludarabine**, **cladribine**, **clofarabine**, and **nelarabine** are incorporated into DNA synthesis resulting in synthesis inhibition and apoptosis. Fludarabine is an analogue of adenine and resistant to deamination by adenosine deaminase.

Nucleobases

Nucleobases (**mercaptopurine** and **tioguanine**) are purine antagonists that exhibit their cytotoxic effect via the metabolite tioguanine nucleotide, which is incorporated into DNA. The metabolites also inhibit purine synthesis and purine nucleotide interconversions.

Pyrimidine analogues

Pyrimidine analogues (**cytarabine**, **gemcitabine**, **fluorouracil**, **capecitabine**, **tegafur**, **azacitadine**, **decitabine**) achieve their cytotoxic effects via inhibition of DNA and RNA synthesis, through incorporation of these analogues into DNA and RNA.

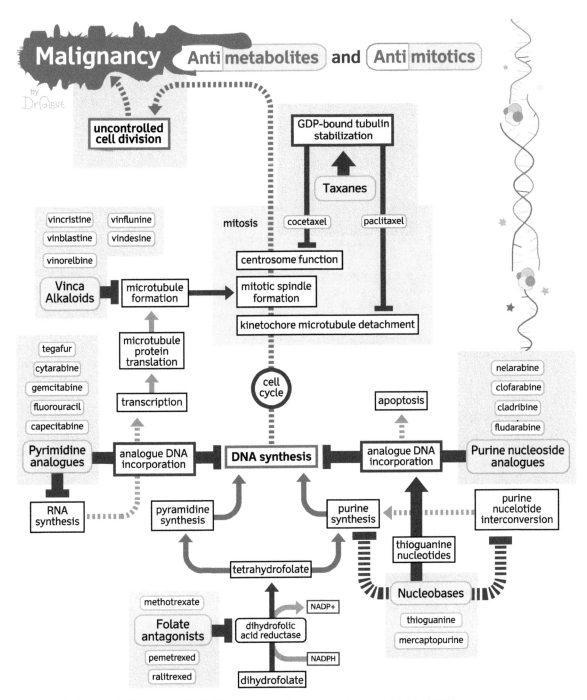

Figure 13.8 Antimetabolites and antimitotics: summary of relevant pathways and drug targets.

Prescribing

Of the *antifolates*, **methotrexate** is the most widely used. It may be administered orally or parenterally, either as antineoplastic chemotherapy, or for treatment of inflammatory diseases, such as rheumatoid arthritis or IBD. Doses can also be given intrathecally or IM (e.g. ectopic pregnancy). Doses vary considerably with indication, and folate rescue therapy is often indicated, particularly with higher doses (500–1000 mg/m²) to minimize toxicity. Rescue with **folinic acid** is required when very high doses of methotrexate are used in malignancy (high dose methotrexate is lethal otherwise), e.g. 12 g/m² in osteosarcoma. Particular care should be taken with the dosing interval of methotrexate where prescribed for repeated doses, as weekly doses have incorrectly been prescribed daily resulting in significant harm (see 'Prescribing warning: inappropriate frequency of oral methotrexate administration—never event').

> ### PRESCRIBING WARNING
>
> **Inappropriate frequency of oral methotrexate administration: never event**
>
> - A never event is a serious event that is completely avoidable, providing the necessary barriers in place are adhered to. Each year the DoH publishes an updated list of never events.
> - The inappropriate administration of methotrexate, so that the weekly dose is exceeded, is listed as a never event; this is more commonly seen in RA prescribing (Topic 7.2, 'Inflammatory arthropathies').
> - This follows reports of patients being administered daily doses of methotrexate instead of the intended weekly, leading to significant harm.
> - Prescribers should ensure they comply with local guidelines when prescribing methotrexate.

The *purine nucleoside analogue*, **fludarabine** is used in the treatment of B cell chronic lymphocytic leukaemia. Being renally cleared, dose adjustments are usually required in patients with renal impairment and use contraindicated in patients with creatinine clearance <30 mL/min/1.73 m². **Cladribine**, a further purine nucleoside analogue, is indicated for treatment of hairy cell leukaemia and also used in B cell CLL resistant to standard therapy. Both drugs doses are administered IV, although fludarabine may also be given orally in advanced disease.

The *nucleobases*, **mercaptopurine** and **tioguanine** are indicated for the treatment of leukaemias (ALL, AML, CLL, hairy cell). Mercaptopurine is also used as maintenance therapy in acute lymphoblastic and myelogenous leukaemia, with doses adjusted to maintain blood counts within a specified range. The oral bioavailability of mercaptopurine varies hugely between individuals, largely attributable to first pass metabolism by xanthine oxidase, which metabolizes the drug to an inactive metabolite.

Significant dose reductions (~75%) are required if given with **allopurinol**, which inhibits xanthine oxidase. Individuals with an inherited deficiency of the enzyme TMPT may be unusually sensitive to myelosuppression of 6-MP and prone to develop rapid bone marrow depression. For this reason, TMPT enzyme activity tests are recommended prior to starting treatment, to reduce the risk of unnecessary toxicity associated with accumulation seen in slow metabolizers. Outside of oncology, mercaptopurine is used off-label in inflammatory diseases, such as rheumatoid arthritis and Crohn's disease. Tioguanine is used less frequently in acute leukaemias and has no role in non-malignant conditions, as it is associated with a greater risk of hepatic toxicity.

The *pyrimidine analogue*, **fluorouracil** may be used as monotherapy or in combination for malignancies such as head and neck cancers, GI carcinomas, colon, and breast cancer. It is a pro-drug, which is converted intracellularly to the active form. The rate-limiting enzyme in 5-FU catabolism is dihydropyrimidine dehydrogenase, although rarely patients with an inherited deficiency of this enzyme, may be at risk of life-threatening toxicities (stomatitis, neutropenia, neurotoxicity). **Cytarabine** is used in acute leukaemia, and **gemcitabine** as combination chemotherapy to treat various malignant processes, including metastatic bladder cancer and metastatic adenocarcinoma of the pancreas. **Capecitabine** is used as adjuvant therapy in colon cancer and metastatic colorectal cancer, as well as other neoplastic processes such as metastatic breast cancer. It is a pro-drug of fluorouracil. With the exception of *capecitabine*, which is given orally, all the pyrimidine analogues are administered parenterally.

Unwanted effects

Adverse drug reactions to the *antifolates* (**methotrexate**, **pemetrexed**, **ralitrexed**) commonly arise from their inhibitory effect on folic acid, which leads to GI side effects, bone marrow suppression, hepatotoxicity, skin manifestations (including Stevens–Johnson syndrome), CNS disorder, and rarely, acute or chronic interstitial pneumonitis. The severity of adverse reactions appears to be dose dependent, and can be in part minimized with the concurrent use of folinic acid rescue, adequate hydration, and alkalinization of urine to promote renal clearance. Methotrexate is also associated with severe renal toxicity and treatment is contraindicated in significant hepatic and renal impairment. Baseline FBC, and renal and LFTs are necessary before initiating methotrexate therapy and should be repeated regularly throughout treatment. As with many other chemotherapeutic agents, effective contraception is required in child-bearing age females and males. Advice should be given not to father a child during therapy and for up to 6 months after discontinuation.

Purine nucleoside analogues

Purine nucleoside analogues are associated with severe bone marrow suppression, so that peripheral blood counts are necessary prior to, during and upon completion of treatment. They are also associated with severe neurological toxicity, albeit rarely within the licensed doses that can result in blindness, coma, and even death. Tumour lysis syndrome may occur in patients with a large tumour burden. Caution is recommended when using in patients with renal or hepatic impairment, where clearance may be affected.

Pyrimidine analogues

The **pyrimidine analogues** similarly cause significant bone marrow suppression requiring close monitoring before, during, and after treatment. GI toxicity, in particular diarrhoea, can be problematic with capecitabine, so that it is routinely co-prescribed with **loperamide** to offset this. In severe cases, however, dose modifications may be necessary as well as supportive management of dehydration. Fluorouracil is also associated with photosensitivity and skin discolouration, for which patients should be warned about.

Nucleobases

Nucleobases (**mercaptopurine** and **tioguanine**) are also associated with bone marrow suppression, which may be reversible if therapy is discontinued early. Other drugs that inhibit TMPT enzyme activity should be used with caution. Further side effects may include GI disorders and hepatobiliary disorders, such as biliary stasis and hepatotoxicity.

Drug interactions

Clinically significant drug interactions with **methotrexate** occur with drugs that inhibit renal clearance, e.g. penicillins, NSAIDs and **probenecid**. Concurrent use should be avoided while on treatment, particularly with high-dose therapy, as they are likely to lead to a significant increase in toxicity.

Antimitotics

Mitosis is a key part of the cell cycle where chromosomes are separated into two identical sets. Together with the division of the cytoplasm (cytokinesis) they define the mitotic phase of the cell cycle that leads to the formation of two genetically identical daughter cells. It is a strictly controlled

process and any agent that can stop this, will stop tumour growth. Antimitotic agents act at different stages and on differing components of mitosis. For example, taxanes [docetaxel, paclitaxel, vinca alkaloids (vincristine, vinblastine, vindesine, vinorelbine, and vinflunine].

Taxanes (docetaxel, paclitaxel, cabazitaxel)

Mechanism of action

Paclitaxel was initially synthesized in 1971 from an extract found in the bark of the Pacific yew tree (*Taxus brevifolia*). **Docetaxel** is a second-generation taxane and **cabazitaxel** a semi-synthetic taxane. They act by disrupting the function of microtubules, protein filaments that play a fundamental role in the cytoskeleton and the process of cell division.

In living cells, paclitaxel promotes microtubule polymerization and stabilization, inhibiting microtubule disassembly, essential in the process of cell division. Phenotypically, it arrests diverse cell types in mitosis due to the presence of unattached kinetochores, which have not made stable microtubule attachments. This leads to the activation of signal transduction pathways that delay mitotic progression. Although mitotic arrest was initially hypothesized as the cytotoxic mechanism, numerous studies have now shown that the length of time a cell spends in mitosis is not a reliable indicator of survival. This observation is further complicated by the fact that paclitaxel exhibits concentration-dependent effects, with high concentrations initially believed to be responsible for its efficacy.

There is a difficulty in determining the clinically relevant doses of paclitaxel as it has a capacity to accumulate intracellularly in cancer cells, with a concentration that is almost certainly higher in the tumour than the circulating plasma.

Docetaxel also interferes with the normal function of microtubules, preventing their disassembly, thus affecting cell division and survival.

Prescribing

Paclitaxel is highly hydrophobic and therefore administered IV in a solution of alcohol and purified castor oil, a preparation known to cause severe hypersensitivity reactions. It is metabolized by the liver and excreted in bile with non-linear kinetics and a half-life of 15–50 hours. **Docetaxel**, however, displays linear kinetics and has a short half-life of about 1 hour. Like paclitaxel it is metabolized

by the liver and excreted in bile. In the UK paclitaxel is licensed for the treatment of breast cancer, ovarian cancer,
and AIDS-related Kaposi's sarcoma. Docetaxel is licensed
in the UK for the treatment of breast cancer, lung cancer,
gastric cancer, and metastatic prostate cancer.

Paclitaxel is presently available in two different formulations with unique dosing. The traditional formulation
contains polyoxyl 35 castor oil and ethanol (Cremophor
EL), which can cause severe hypersensitivity reactions so
that patients are usually premedicated with dexamethasone and antihistamines. More recently, nab-paclitaxel, a
nanoparticle albumin bound paclitaxel product, has been
developed to reduce the risk of a hypersensitivity reactions
so that premedications are not required.

Unwanted effects

Side effects reported to the taxanes include neutropenia,
alopecia, vomiting, peripheral neuropathy, and cardiac
conduction abnormalities. **Docetaxel** can cause persistent fluid retention, predominantly in the legs, and may
cause ascites and pleural effusions. Premedication with
corticosteroid prior to administration of docetaxel can
help reduce the severity and incidence of fluid retention,
as well as the risk of hypersensitivity reactions more commonly associated with **paclitaxel** therapy (see 'Taxanes
(docetaxel, paclitaxel, cabazitaxel)').

Drug interactions

Neurotoxicity associated with taxanes can be aggravated if
co-administered with other neurotoxic agents. **Docetaxel**
is metabolized via the cytochrome P450 3A4 enzyme subgroup and therefore has the potential to be affected by
drugs that induce or inhibit this enzyme. Ideally, potent
inhibitors (**itraconazole**, **clarithromycin**) and inducers
(**phenytoin**, **rifampicin**, **carbamazepine**) should be
avoided, and where this is not possible, dose alterations
may be necessary to overcome the effects. **Paclitaxel** is
only in part cleared by the same enzyme system, so the
risk of clinically significant interactions is lower.

Vinca alkaloids (vincristine, vinblastine, vindesine, vinflunine, vinorelbine)

Mechanism of action

The vinca alkaloids are derived from a compound contained in the leaves of the periwinkle plant (*Catharanthus
roseus*) and, like taxanes, act on tubulin. However, unlike
taxanes, they counter microtubule formation leading to
the destruction of the mitotic spindle and failed mitosis.
This results in mitotic arrest or cell death.

Prescribing

There are five licensed vinca alkaloids in the UK, all of
which are administered IV, although **vinorelbine** can also
be administered orally. Vinca alkaloids should *never* be
given intrathecally (see 'Prescribing warning: neurotoxicity and intrathecal vinca alkaloids—never event'). They
have a large volume of distribution with a long and variable elimination half-life, being excreted primarily in the
faeces.

Vincristine, **vinblastine**, and **vindesine** are licensed
for the treatment of leukaemias, lymphomas, and breast
and lung cancer. **Vinorelbine** is licensed for the treatment of lung cancer, while **vinflunine** is licensed for the
treatment of advanced or metastatic transitional cell carcinoma. Collectively, however, they are used off-label in
the treatment of a wide number of malignancies.

Unwanted effects

Cautions and side effects

Peripheral and autonomic neuropathies are well-
recognized side effects, and although particularly related
to **vincristine**, they are associated with all vinca alkaloids.
Where symptoms are significant (e.g. severe constipation,
foot drop) doses can be reduced or omitted. Fortunately, it
appears that neurotoxicity can resolve, albeit slowly.

Although vincristine has minimal effect on the bone
marrow, this can be a dose-limiting side effect with the
other vinca alkaloids. All are extremely irritant to the skin
and extravasation should be avoided and, where evident,
recognized promptly. Hypersensitivity reactions have
been reported.

Drug interactions

Vinca alkaloids may affect the serum levels of some anticonvulsants and, although the exact causal link is unknown, caution is recommended.

PRESCRIBING WARNING

Neurotoxicity and intrathecal vinca alkaloids: never event

- The inadvertent administration of vinca alkaloids intrathecally has led to decerebration and death.
- Centres that administer intrathecal chemotherapy must have comprehensive policies in place to prevent this from happening.
- All personnel involved in prescribing, dispensing, and administering intrathecal therapy must be familiar with local policies.

Platinum compounds

> Platinum compounds produce cross-links in DNA that result in structural deformation, leading to cell stasis and apoptosis. For example, cisplatin, carboplatin, and oxaliplatin.

Mechanism of action

The effect of platinum compounds on tumour growth was first demonstrated in 1964. They act to bind the nitrogen atoms of guanine bases in cellular DNA to produce intrastrand cross-links, and cause inhibition of DNA repair or DNA synthesis. Mismatch repair proteins, such as hMSH2, appear to ameliorate some of the effects of platinum compounds and may play a role in resistance.

Prescribing

Cisplatin, **carboplatin,** and **oxaliplatin** are administered by IV infusion and, in the case of cisplatin, pre-hydration with IV fluids is essential to minimize nephrotoxicity. Platinum compounds should not be administered with aluminium-containing materials or compounds, as they form a precipitate. The terminal half-life of cisplatin is biphasic with half-lives of 10–20 minutes and 32–53 minutes, respectively. The terminal half-life of carboplatin is about 1.5 hours and that of oxaliplatin only 14.1 minutes. Platinum compounds are largely excreted renally, thus renal function can influence dosing.

Cisplatin is licensed for the treatment of metastatic non-seminatomous germ cell carcinoma, advanced and refractory ovarian cancer, metastatic testicular cancer, oesophagus, cervical, endometrial, head, and neck, all combined with radiotherapy. Carboplatin is licensed for the treatment of ovarian cancer and small cell lung cancer, while oxaliplatin is licensed as adjuvant treatment for resected colorectal cancer and metastatic colon cancer. That said, cisplatin and carboplatin are widely used off-label in a number of other cancer treatments.

Unwanted effects

Of the adverse effects associated with the platinum compounds, the most clinically significant are myelosuppression, nephrotoxicity, ototoxicity (particularly with **cisplatin**), and in the case of cisplatin, profound nausea and vomiting. Consequently, treatment is contraindicated in patients with pre-existing renal or hearing impairment. To reduce nephrotoxicity, patients require renal function monitoring, and cisplatin administered with adequate pre- and post-dose hydration.

All platinum compounds can cause peripheral neuropathy and, where evident, may require dose adjustment or cessation of treatment. **Oxaliplatin** may also cause reversible posterior leukoencephalopathy syndrome (RPLS), a rare reversible condition characterized by visual disturbance, headache, confusion, hypertension, and seizure. Diagnosis is clinical, but MRI typically shows cerebral white matter oedema. Acute laryngopharyngeal dysthaesia (ALPD) is also well recognized with oxaliplatin treatment, characterized by altered sensation in the throat with associated swallowing difficulties. In general, the peripheral neuropathies associated with platinum use are reversible, although not always. Symptoms are typically exacerbated by the cold.

As platinum compounds are emetogenic, pretreatment with anti-emetics is highly recommended, particularly with cisplatin where maximum anti-emetic prophylaxis should be considered, possibly to include the use of **aprepitant**. Cisplatin is particularly ototoxic so hearing tests must be performed prior to starting treatment, and intermittently, both during and after. All platinum compounds can cause myelosuppression, which can be severe, and in the case of cisplatin affects up to a third of patients treated.

Drug interactions

Drug interactions with **cisplatin** can occur as a result of augmented toxicity when co-administered with other renally toxic or ototoxic agents, such as aminoglycosides or loop diuretics.

Topoisomerase inhibitors

> The topisomerases are a group of enzymes that introduce and then repair strand breaks in DNA during the process of replication. Inhibition of these enzymes can thus stop DNA replication. For example, topoisomerase I inhibitors (irinotecan, topotecan) and topoisomerase II inhibitors (etoposide).

Topoisomerase I inhibitors

Mechanism of action

As the name implies, topoisomerases do not change the actual components of the DNA, but instead introduce a break that unwinds the DNA to allow reduction of tension and progression of the enzymes involved in DNA replication.

In the case of topoisomerase I enzymes, they introduce single-strand breaks in DNA that allow unwinding of one turn of DNA. The first topoisomerase inhibitor to be trialled was **camptotheticin**, obtained from the bark of the tree *Camptotheca acuminatum*, which has been used in traditional Chinese medicine as an anticancer agent. Although initial medical trials showed promising results, adverse effects offset these. Subsequently, more tolerable analogues were developed and both **irinotecan** and **topotecan** are currently widely licensed.

Prescribing

Irinotecan is administered as an infusion and has a half-life of about 12 hours. It has a large volume of distribution and over 50% is excreted unchanged in the faeces and urine. Irinotecan is indicated in the treatment of advanced colorectal cancer, either as mono- or combination therapy.

Topotecan can be administered as an IV infusion over 30 minutes or orally in capsule form. It has a short half-life of about 2–3 hours, a high volume of distribution, and low protein binding. It does not undergo significant metabolism and is primarily secreted unchanged in the urine and faeces. It is indicated IV in the treatment of metastatic ovarian cancer, relapsed small cell lung cancer, and advanced cervical cancer, although orally only for relapsed small cell lung cancer.

Unwanted effects

In addition to its antineoplastic effects, **irinotecan** is a potent inhibitor of acetylcholinesterase, which accounts for some of its more significant side effects, in particular severe diarrhoea, which can be delayed and life-threatening, especially in patients that have undergone abdominal radiotherapy. The risk of diarrhoea is lower with **topotecan**. Symptoms can be managed with antidiarrhoeals such as **loperamide**, although it is not recommended that they are given prophylactically. Irinotecan can also precipitate an acute cholinergic syndrome up to 24 hours after infusion, presenting as malaise, nausea, diarrhoea, hypersalivation, visual disturbances, lacrimation, and miosis. This syndrome resolves with administration of **atropine**. Due to its GI effects, irinotecan is contraindicated in chronic IBD and bowel obstruction. Significantly elevated bilirubin levels and severe bone marrow failure are also contraindications to its use. Bone marrow suppression is common with both irinotecan and topotecan, and less frequently, interstitial lung disease.

Drug interactions

As an acetylcholinesterase inhibitor, **irinotecan** has an increased risk of cholinergic-related toxicity and a cholinergic crisis when administered with other drugs known to have this effect. It is cleared via the cytochrome P450 enzyme system, specifically the 3A subgroup and is therefore affected by drugs that inhibit (e.g. **St John's Wort**) or induce (**phenytoin, carbamazepine**) this enzyme. No such interactions have been reported with **topotecan**.

Topoisomerase II inhibitors (etoposide)

Mechanism of action

Etoposide inhibits topoisomerase II, an enzyme involved in DNA separation and re-attachment. Through topoisomerase II inhibition, it prevents re-attachment of DNA leading to double-strand breaks. These double-strand breaks are incompatible with cell function and thus lead to cell senescence or death. Etoposide acts at the premitotic stage of cell division, is cell cycle dependent and phase specific, with maximum effect on S and G2 phases of cell division.

Prescribing

Etoposide can be administered IV or PO, although oral bioavailability varies depending on dose and formulation. It has a terminal half-life of between 5 and 11 hours, and is excreted in both urine and faeces. As levels are increased in low albumin states, such patients are at an increased risk of drug toxicity. Etoposide is licensed for the treatment of testicular cancer, lymphoma and lung cancer, although used frequently beyond these indications. In general, oral therapy is reserved for use where other treatment options have failed.

Unwanted effects

Etoposide causes alopecia, myelosuppression, and GI effects, such as nausea, vomiting, and diarrhoea. Severe hypersensitivity reactions as well as profound hypotension have also been reported, and may in part be avoided by slow dose administration. It is an irritant to the skin and extravasation should be avoided. Less commonly, etoposide use is associated with neurotoxicity, teratogenicity, and increased risk of secondary malignancies.

Drug interactions

Concomitant use of **etoposide** with **cisplatin** can reduce drug clearance, while concomitant use with **ciclosporin** can lead to markedly raised drug levels.

Targeted therapies

Targeted cancer therapies are drugs that target specific molecules to block cell growth or the spread of cancer, and are predominantly small molecules or monoclonal antibodies. Several targeted therapies have been approved for clinical use, which include hormone therapies, signal transduction inhibitors, gene expression modulators, apoptosis inducers, angiogenesis inhibitors, and immunotherapies.

The binding of ligands to receptors on cell surfaces, produces changes in conformation/function that results in the transmission of signals into the cell. When signals reach the nucleus, processes involved in DNA replication and cell division are triggered.

Ligands that bind to receptors can be a target for biological therapy, e.g. **bevacizumab** targets circulating vascular endothelial growth factor (VEGF). Receptors on the surface of the cells can also be inhibited directly by drugs. These will be discussed further in monoclonal antibodies.

Another way to block receptor function is by using small molecules that are able to inhibit protein kinases involved in intracellular signalling pathways. Two pathways implicated in cancer are the RAS-MAP kinase pathway, which is activated by multiple growth factor receptors, as well as several intracellular tyrosine kinases, such as SRC and ABL, and the PI3K/Akt/mTOR pathway.

Protein kinase inhibitors

Protein kinase inhibitors are a large class of chemotherapeutic agents that inhibit protein phosphorylation, affecting the activity, and function of cells. Thus, inhibition of these enzymes can have a direct impact on cell division and growth. Examples include afatinib, axitinib, bosutinib, crizotinib, dabrafenib, dasatanib, erlotinib, everolimus, gefitinib, imatinib, lapatinib, nilotinib, pazopanib, ponatinib, regorafenib, ruxolitinib, sorafenib, sunitinib, temsirolimus, vandetanib, and vemurafenib

Mechanism of action

Protein kinase inhibitors can be subdivided according to the amino acid whose phosphorylation is inhibited (e.g. serine, threonine, or tyrosine). Kinases mostly act on both serine and threonine amino acids, but tyrosine kinases act on tyrosine only and some dual-specificity kinases act on all three of these amino acid residues. Some protein kinases also phosphorylate other amino acids,

such as histidine kinases that act on histidine residues. Kinases are involved in various cell functions, including cell signalling, cell growth, and cell division, so that inhibition is important in arresting the growth of some cancers (Table 13.14).

Proteasome inhibitors

The ubiquitin-proteasome pathway plays an essential role in regulating the turnover of specific proteins, thereby maintaining homeostasis within cells. Inhibition of the 26S proteasome prevents this targeted proteolysis and affects multiple signalling cascades within the cell, ultimately resulting in cell death. For example, bortezomib.

The ubiquitin-proteasome pathway is the main pathway by which cellular proteins involved in the cell cycle, i.e. DNA synthesis, repair, transcription, translation, and apoptosis, are degraded, thereby controlling intracellular protein levels and cellular function. Malfunction of this system is implicated in cancer, as well as neurodegenerative and cardiovascular disease.

Enzymes called ubiquitin ligases catalyse ubiquitination, whereby ubiquitin acts as a tag, forming chains with proteins identified for degradation. The proteasome responsible for proteolytic degradation is the 26S proteasome, composed of a 20S core particle with a 19S regulatory particle at either end. Polyubiquitin chains are recruited by the regulatory particle within the 26S proteasome. The ubiquitin chain is subsequently cleaved and the protein unfolded, before being translocated to the 20S core. Here, it is degraded to peptides using three main catalytic activities: chymotrypsin-like (CT-L), trypsin-like (T-L), and caspase-like (C-L).

As cancer cells have a higher proteasome activity compared with normal cells, and a greater susceptibility to apoptosis, proteasome inhibition has become a target for anticancer treatment.

Bortezomib
Mechanism of action

The proteasome inhibitors were initially developed to prevent muscle breakdown in cachectic states, although it was found that they also block the activation of the nuclear factor kappa B (NF-κB) pathway, essential for cell growth, survival, metastases, and angiogenesis in tumorigenesis.

Table 13.14 Summary of protein kinase inhibitors

Drug	Kinases inhibited	Mechanism of action	Indications	Prescribing	Adverse effects	Drug interactions
Afatinib	ErbB1 (EGFR), ErbB2 (HER2), ErbbB4 (HER4)	Potent, selective, irreversible inhibitor of ErbB family (EGFR, HER2, HER4), implicated in epithelial cancers. Inhibits tumour growth or causes regression. Effective against EGFR mutations resistant to reversible inhibitors	NSCLC (adenocarcinomas)—metastatic and locally advanced	Orally OD adjusted to tolerance. Taken on an empty stomach as food (especially high fat content) can impair absorption	*Common:* paronychia, decreased appetite, epistaxis, diarrhoea, stomatitis, cheilitis, dry skin, and rash. Diarrhoea can be severe and require loperamide/hydration	Substrate for p-glycoprotein—avoid potent inhibitors for 6–12 hours after dose, e.g. ritonavir, ciclosporin, erythromycin, and ketoconazole
Axitinib	VEGFR 1–3	Potent selective inhibitor of VEGFR1–3, blocks cell angiogenesis/proliferation leading to apoptosis. Limited activity against PDGFRs, B-RAF, cKIT, Flt3	2nd line treatment for advanced renal cell carcinoma	Orally BD, adjusted to tolerance	*Severe:* cardiovascular (cardiac failure, hypertensive crisis, VTE/ATE), haemorrhagic (GI, cerebral) GI perforation, fistula formation. *Common:* diarrhoea, hypertension, fatigue, hand–foot syndrome, nausea, dysphonia	Substrate for CYP3A4/5—levels affected by potent inhibitors, e.g. ketoconazole, or inducers, e.g. rifampicin
Bosutinib	Bcr-Abl; also SRC family kinases	Dual inhibitor of Abl/ Src designed to overcome resistance problem with imatinib. Src, Lyn, Hck implicated in tumour cell growth, migration, proliferation and angiogenesis. Minimally inhibits PDGFR and c-Kit	Ph +ve CML in chronic, accelerated and blast phase—usually 2nd line	Orally OD adjusted to tolerance. Dose escalated in patients not achieving CHR by week 8 or CCyR by week 12	Toxicity common, grade 3/4 reactions affecting >60% of patients. *Most frequent* diarrhoea (4/5). *Others inc:* N&V, abdo pain, thrombocytopenia, anaemia, rash, deranged LFTs	Substrate for CYP3A4 levels affected by potent inhibitors, e.g. ketoconazole, or inducers, e.g. rifampicin

Drug	Target	Mechanism	Indication	Dosing	Adverse effects	Interactions
Everolimus	mTOR (serine threonine kinase)	Synthetic analogue of rapamycin. Selective inhibitor of mTOR—normally promotes cell survival/proliferation in optimal conditions. Up-regulated mTOR leads to growth/proliferation in suboptimal conditions. Reduces VEGF and angiogensis	Post-menopausal breast cancer (with exemestane), hormone receptor positive, HER2/neu negative. Not recommended by NICE. Also used in metastatic renal cancer 2nd line	Orally OD, based on BSA adjusted to tolerance	*Common:* bone marrow suppression (pancytopaenia), upper respiratory tract infections, hyperlipidaemia, hypertension, headache, increased creatinine kinase, GI toxicity (nausea, vomiting, stomatitis)	Substrate for CYP3A4 levels affected by potent inhibitors, e.g. ketoconazole or inducers, e.g. rifampicin. Moderate inhibitor of P-gly
Crizotinib	ALK, RTK, HGFR, c-Met	Selective, potent small molecule inhibitor of ALK, RTK and oncogenic variants. Inhibits growth and induces apoptosis in ALK positive tumours. Also inhibitor of HGFR, c-Met	ALK positive anaplastic NSCLC. Not approved by NICE	Orally BD, adjusted to tolerance	*Common:* GI (diarrhoea, nausea, vomiting), haematological (neutropenia, anaemia) elevated transaminases. *Severe/rare:* hepatotoxicity—monitor LFTs	Substrate for and moderate inhibitor of CYP3A levels affected by potent inhibitors, e.g. ketoconazole, or inducers, e.g. rifampicin
Dabrafenib	RAF	Reversible ATP-competitive inhibitor of RAF. Effective where mutations in B-RAF, e.g. BRAF V600, BRAF WT, activates RAS/RAF/MEK/ERK pathway to stimulate tumour cell growth	Melanoma—unresectable/metastatic with B-RAF V600 mutation	Orally BD until no further benefit or unacceptable toxicity	*Common:* hyperkeratosis, headache, pyrexia, arthralgia, fatigue, nausea, papilloma, alopecia, rash, vomiting. *Severe/rare:* haematological toxicity, raised LFTs, QT interval prolongation, renal failure	Substrate for CYP3A4 levels affected by potent inhibitors, e.g. ketoconazole or inducers, e.g. rifampicin. Inducer of CYP 3A4, 2B6, 2C9 can affect substrates of these enzymes
Dasatinib	Bcr-Abl1, Src family, c-Kit, ephrin receptor, PDGFR	Potent 2nd generation inhibitor of Bcr-Abl, effective against Bcr-Abl mutations (except T315I). Also inhibitor of Src, c-Kit, ephrin, PDGFβ	CML—accelerated, chronic and blast phase, Ph +ve ALL and lymphoid blast CML	Orally OD—until disease progression or intolerance	*Common:* fluid retention including, pleural effusion (may require steroids/diuretics), diarrhoea, haematological toxicity (myelosuppression, thrombocytopenia). *Less common:* increased risk of MI, QT interval prolongation	Substrate for CYP3A4 levels affected by potent inhibitors, e.g. ketoconazole, or inducers, e.g. rifampicin

(continued)

Table 13.14 Continued

Drug	Kinases inhibited	Mechanism of action	Indications	Prescribing	Adverse effects	Drug interactions
Erlotinib	ErbB1 (EGFR)	Selective, potent reversible inhibitor of ErbB-1/HER1. Inhibits cell proliferation, invasion and metastasis in epithelial cancers where EGFR is over-expressed	1st line treatment for NSCLC (locally advanced metastatic), NICE approved	Orally OD, adjusted to tolerance. Best taken on empty stomach as food affects absorption	*Common:* rash, diarrhoea, deranged LFTs, ocular toxicity. *Less common/severe:* interstitial lung disease, hepatic failure, gastric perforation	Substrate for CYP3A4 levels affected by potent inhibitors, e.g. ketoconazole, or inducers, e.g. rifampicin. Potent inhibitor of CYP1A1. Moderate inhibitor of CYP3A4, 2C8. Smoking can reduce levels by 50–60%
Gefitinib	Bcr-ABL, c-Kit, PDGFR	Selective reversible inhibitor—binds to ATP site of EGFR. Inhibits cell growth and proliferation in presence of EGFR activating mutation	NSCLC (locally advanced or metastatic) with activating EGFR mutations	Orally OD. Only one tablet formulation so treatment held in case of intolerance	*Common:* rashes, diarrhoea (>20%), deranged LFTs. *Uncommon/severe:* interstitial lung disease, hepatotoxicity incl. hepatic failure	Substrate for CYP3A4 levels affected by potent inhibitors, e.g. ketoconazole, or inducers, e.g. rifampicin. Also 2D6 to a lesser extent
Imatinib	Bcr-ABL, c-Kit, PDGFR	Potent inhibitor of Bcr-Abl. Inhibits proliferation and induces apoptosis in Bcr-Abl positive cells. Also inhibits PDGF and c-Kit. Use limited by amplifications of Bcr-Abl leading to mutations	Ph +ve CML accelerated, chronic and blast phase. Ph +ve ALL. MDS/MPD with PDGFR gene re-arrangement. Also used in GIST	Orally OD, adjusted according to phase/indication. Taken with a large glass of water to reduce the risk of gastric irritation	Common: haematological, e.g. neutropenia, thrombocytopenia, gastrointestinal, e.g. diarrhoea, rashes, fluid retention. *Less common/severe:* hepatic toxicity (including hepatic failure), cardiac toxicity, GI haemorrhage	Substrate for CYP3A4 levels affected by potent inhibitors, e.g. ketoconazole, or inducers, e.g. rifampicin, Potent inhibitor of CYP3A4, 2D6—caution with simvastatin, ciclosporin, tacrolimus

Drug	Targets	Mechanism	Indication	Dosing	Side effects	Interactions
Lapatinib	ErbB1 (HER1), ErbB2 (HER2)	Dual receptor reversible inhibitor of EGFR (ErbB1), HER2 (ErbB2). Prevents phosphorylation and activation. Designed to overcome trastuzumab resistance in HER-2 positive breast cancer	Breast cancer that over-expresses HER2 (ErbB2). Not recommended by NICE	Orally OD, adjusted according to concomitant therapy and intolerance	Common: diarrhoea, rashes Less common/severe: cardiac/ pulmonary toxicity, e.g. interstitial lung disease	Substrate for CYP3A4 levels affected by potent inhibitors, e.g. ketoconazole, or inducers, e.g. rifampicin, Inhibitor of CYP3A4, 2C8
Nilotinib	BCR-ABL1, c-Kit, ephrin receptor, PDGFR	Potent, selective inhibitor of Bcr-Abl. Higher affinity than imatinib hence active against imatinib resistant disease. Inhibits proliferation and induces apoptosis is Bcr-Abl positive cell lines	Ph +ve CML (chronic phase)—NICE approved	Orally BD adjusted to tolerance Taken on an empty stomach as food can considerably increase levels	Common: myelosuppression, rashes, GI toxicity Less common/severe: cardiac toxicity, e.g. QT interval prolongation, fluid retention	Substrate for CYP3A4 levels affected by potent inhibitors, e.g. ketoconazole, or inducers, e.g. rifampicin, Caution with other drugs known to cause QT interval prolongation
Pazopanib	VEGFR 1–3, PDGFR, c-Kit	Potent multi-active inhibitor of VEGFR therefore inhibiting angiogenesis Also inhibits PDGFR and c-Kit	1st line for RCC and some subtypes of STS Only NICE approved for RCC	Orally OD, according to hepatic function (monitor LFTs) Taken on empty stomach as food (particularly with high fat content) can significantly increase levels	Common: diarrhoea, rash, hypertension, nausea, vomiting Less common/severe: hepatic (including hepatic failure and death), cardiovascular (heart failure, stroke, MI) toxicity	Substrate for CYP3A4 levels affected by potent inhibitors, e.g. ketoconazole, or inducers, e.g. rifampicin, Inhibits multiple CYP isoenzymes e.g. 1A2, 3A4, 2C8, 2C9, 2C19, 2E1. Avoid simvastatin
Ponatinib	BCR-ABL1, c-Kit, FLT-3, some isoforms of VEGFR, PDGFR, FGFR	Potent inhibitor of Bcr-Abl effective against mutations (including T315I) Also inhibits FLT3, KIT, some isoforms of VEGFR, PDGFR, FGFR Inhibits proliferation and induces apoptosis	Ph +ve CML (accelerated, blast and chronic phase)—3rd/4th line	Orally OD, adjusted to response and toxicity. Taken without food	Common: thrombocytopenia, rash. Less common/ severe: pancreatitis, myelosuppression, cardiovascular toxicity (MI, AF). Assess cardiovascular status pretreatment	Substrate for CYP3A4 levels affected by potent inhibitors, e.g. ketoconazole, or inducers, e.g. rifampicin

(continued)

Table 13.14 Continued

Drug	Kinases inhibited	Mechanism of action	Indications	Prescribing	Adverse effects	Drug interactions
Regorafenib	VEGFR 1-3, TIE2, KIT, RET, RAF-1, BRAF, BRAF v600E, PDGFR, FGFR	Potent, multi-active inhibitor of VEGFR, TIE2 (involved in angiogenesis), KIT, RET, RAF-1, BRAF (involved in oncogenesis) and PDGFR, FGFR (maintain tumour microenvironment)	CRC (metastatic) and GIST (unresectable/metastatic)—3rd line treatment.	Orally OD on 4-weekly cycle (3 weeks on/1 week off)—until absence of benefit or unacceptable toxicity. Taken with food low in fat to optimize absorption	*Common:* fatigue, hand-foot skin reactions, diarrhoea, decreased appetite, hypertension, infection *Less common/severe:* severe hepatic injury (check base line LFTs), haemorrhage, GI perforation	Substrate for1CYP3A4 and UGT1A9. Inhibits UGT1A9 and UGT1A1. Caution in combination with irinotecan (substrate tor UGT1A9/ UGT1A1)
Ruxolitinib	JAK1, JAK2	Selective inhibitor of JAK1/JAK2, interrupts JAK-STAT pathway reducing splenomegaly and associated symptoms. Is not curative	Treatment of splenomegaly in myelofibrosis and polycythaemia vera. Not advocated by NICE	Orally BD adjusted to platelet count. Modified in renal/hepatic dysfunction. Discontinued if risks outweigh benefits or no further reduction in spleen size	*Common:* haematological/dose-related (thrombocytopenia, anaemia), infection (including activation of latent TB)—pre-screening for TB	Substrate for CYP3A4 and CYP 2C9—reduce dose by 50% with potent inhibitors of these enzymes
Sorafenib	VEGRF 2-3, PDGFR, c-KIT, FLT-3, RAF	Multi-active inhibitor of kinases involved in tumour vasculature (e.g. CRAF, VEGFR, PDGFR) and tumour cell growth (e.g. CRAF, BRAF, c-KIT, FLT-3)	Hepatocellular carcinoma, RCC (2nd line), differentiated (iodine refractory) thyroid cancer (advanced/metastatic) Not approved by NICE	Orally BD until benefit ceases or unacceptable toxicity	*Common:* diarrhoea, fatigue, alopecia, infection, hand-foot skin reactions, rash. *Less common/severe:* cardiovascular toxicity (MI, hypertension, QT interval prolongation), haemorrhage (including GI perforation)	Substrate for CYP3A4 levels affected by potent inhibitors, e.g. ketoconazole, or inducers, e.g. rifampicin, Inhibitor of CYP2B6, 2C8 and 2C9—minimal clinical significance

Sunitinib	VEGRF 1-3, PDGFR, c-KIT, FLT-3, CSF-1R, RET	Multi-active inhibitor of PDGFR, VEGFR, c-KIT, FLT-3, CSF-1R and RET—thus inhibiting tumour growth, angiogenesis, and metastatic progression	RCC (advanced/metastatic, GIST (2nd line unresectable/metastatic), pNET	Orally OD on a cycle basis with rest periods—adjusted to tolerance. Can be given with/without food	Common: GI (diarrhoea, taste disturbances), dermatological (skin discolouration, hand–foot reactions), haematological (neutropenia, thrombocytopenia), hypertension. *Less common/severe:* cardiovascular toxicity (MI, QT interval prolongation, cardiac failure), renal failure	Substrate for CYP3A4 levels affected by potent inhibitors, e.g. ketoconazole, or inducers, e.g. rifampicin
Temsirolimus	mTOR	Inhibitor of mTOR by binding to FKBP-12. Affects cell division and ability of tumour to survive/grow in unfavourable micro-environments. Inhibitor of HIF, VEGF and thus angiogenesis	RCC, (advanced), MCL (relapsed/refractory)	IV infusion over 30–60 minutes, once a week. Pre-medicate with anti-histamine to reduce risk of hypersensitivity reaction	*Common:* hypersensitivity/infusion-related reactions, e.g. flushing/rash to severe anaphylaxis. Infusion should be stopped/slowed as appropriate. Glucose intolerance, GI and haematological toxicity also common. *Less common/severe:* interstitial lung disease, intracranial haemorrhage, renal failure	CYP3A4 inhibited by active metabolite sirolimus
Vandetanib	ErbB1, VEGFR, RET	Potent inhibitor of VEGF (2, 3), RET including some RET mutations e.g. MEN2B. RET implicated in MTC At higher doses also inhibits EGFR	MTC (locally advance, metastatic)—especially in presence of RET mutations, thus pre-screening carried out	Orally OD until benefit ceases Can be taken with/without food and dispersed in water for patients with swallowing difficulties	*Common:* diarrhoea, rash, nausea, headaches, hypertension *Less common/severe:* risk of potentially fatal reactions incl. QT prolongation, *Torsade de pointes* (especially with electrolyte disturbance) and PRES (can cause permanent neurological toxicity and death)—patients should be advised to seek help immediately if they develop signs, e.g. confusion, headache, seizures, visual disturbance	Substrate for CYP3A4—however, clinically no evidence of increased levels with potent inhibitors. Avoid potent inducers, e.g. rifampicin. Avoid with drugs known to prolong QT interval, e.g. erythromycin, moxifloxacin, and class I and II anti-arrhythmics. Caution with drugs that can cause electrolyte disturbances, e.g. diuretics

(continued)

Table 13.14 Continued

Drug	Kinases inhibited	Mechanism of action	Indications	Prescribing	Adverse effects	Drug interactions
Vemurafenib	B-RAF V600 E	Inhibitor of mutated B-RAF V600E. B-RAF normally regulates MAPK/ERK pathway responsible for cell differentiation, proliferation and apoptosis. Mutation leads to uncontrolled growth	Melanoma (metastatic/ unresectable) that is B-RAF V600 positive	Orally BD until disease progression or unacceptable toxicity. Taken with/ without food, although high fat food will increase absorption and is preferred	*Common*: fatigue, nausea, rash, photosensitivity. Patients should be advised to wear sunscreen and protective clothing. Causes cuSCC in 20% of patients and less commonly non-cuSCC. dermatological screen pre-treatment *Less common/severe*: QT interval prolongation	Substrate for CYP3A4 levels affected by potent inhibitors, e.g. ketoconazole, or inducers, e.g. rifampicin, Induces/inhibits numerous isoenzymes, e.g. induces CYP3A4 and inhibits CYP1A2

CHR, complete haematological response; CCyR, complete cytogenetic response; CML, chronic myeloid leukaemia; Ph +ve, Philadelphia positive; mTOR, mammalian target of rapamycin; VEGF, vascular endothelial growth factor; NSCLC, non-small cell lung cancer; RCC, renal cell carcinoma; STS, soft tissue sarcoma; CRC, colorectal carcinoma; GIST, GI stromal tumour; CSF-R, colony-stimulating factor; MCL, mantle cell lymphoma; EGFR, epithelial growth factor; MTC, medullary thyroid cancer; PRES, posterior reversible encephalopathy syndrome; cuSCC, cutaneous squamous cell carcinoma.

Bortezomib is an irreversible inhibitor of the chymotrypsin-like activity of the 26S proteasome, leading to tumour cell death. It demonstrates activity in a number of cancer types, in particular multiple myeloma where NF-κB activity levels are high. Furthermore, NF-κB is implicated in osteoclast differentiation too, so bortezomib also acts to reduce osteoclast activity and bone resorption, thereby reducing the risk of osteolytic bone disease associated with multiple myeloma. In combination with other chemotherapeutic agents (e.g. **doxorubicin**, **melphalan**, **mitoxantrone**), bortezomib has been shown to increase sensitivity in otherwise resistant disease.

Prescribing

Bortezomib is used as monotherapy or in combination with other drugs in the treatment of multiple myeloma and mantle cell lymphoma. Doses can be administered by IV or SC injection, twice weekly for 2 out of 3 weeks, for a maximum of nine cycles if tolerated. Dose alterations are required in moderate to severe hepatic impairment, and also in patients that develop peripheral neuropathy or haematological toxicity.

Unwanted effects

Adverse effects to **bortezomib** commonly include GI and haematological toxicity. Constipation induced by therapy can be severe and has been known to cause ileus, so that patients should have their bowel habit monitored on treatment. Haematological toxicity (thrombocytopenia, neutropenia, and anaemia) can, in some instances, lead to reactivation of herpes zoster virus, and while on treatment patients should receive antiviral prophylaxis.

Bortezomib is commonly associated with peripheral neuropathy and, although this is predominantly sensory, can also include severe motor neuropathy. Incidence peaks at cycle 5, although patients should be closely monitored throughout for symptoms such as a burning sensation, neuropathic pain, or weakness.

Other side effects include renal impairment and cardiovascular toxicity, including hypotension and, less commonly, heart failure, particularly in high-risk patients who will require monitoring while on treatment.

Drug interactions

Bortezomib is primarily metabolized via CYP3A4 and is itself a weak inhibitor of 1A2, 2C9, 2C19, 2D6, and 3A4. Interactions of clinical significance are most likely to occur in combination with potent inhibitors or inducers of the CYP3A4 enzyme such as **itraconazole** or **rifampicin**,

respectively. Co-administration should be avoided if possible.

Monoclonal antibodies

Monoclonal antibodies can be used in cancer therapy to target proteins involved in tumour cell growth. Selective death of cancer cells is achieved by either stimulating the immune system to respond, or by carrying the therapeutic chemical, or radiation to the cancer cells, thus inducing selective cancer cell death. Examples include bevacizumab, cetuximab, panitumumab, rituximab, and trastuzumab.

Mechanism of action

Monoclonal antibodies (mAbs) in cancer therapy act in one of three different ways, and include naked monoclonal antibodies and conjugated monoclonal antibodies. Naked mAbs work by themselves, while conjugated mAbs are joined to a chemotherapy drug or a radioactive particle. For example, **ibritumomab tiuxetan** is a radiolabelled antibody, whereas **brentuximab vedotin** is an example of a chemolabelled antibody. There are also bispecific monoclonal antibodies such as **blinatumomab**, which can attach to two different proteins.

The development of antibodies for cancer therapy requires the identification of suitable targets. In essence, a desirable target for monoclonal therapy in cancer needs to have wide distribution on tumour cells, high level of expression, and relative absence from normal cell tissues. In recent years, monoclonal antibody technology has targeted epithelial growth factor receptors (EGFR), since over-expression of this receptor is linked with increased proliferation and metastatic potential. The blockade of EGFR pathway inhibits proliferation of malignant cells and appears to influence angiogenesis, motility, and invasion.

The therapeutic actions of monoclonal antibody can be varied, including direct induction of apoptosis, inhibition of receptor signalling needed for cell proliferation and amplification of immune response. Indirect effects also include antibody-dependent cellular cytotoxicity and complement-mediated cellular cytotoxicity.

Bevacizumab
Mechanism of action

Bevacizumab inhibits the formation of new blood vessels by binding to VEGF, which is involved in the

Table 13.15 Licensed indications of bevacizumab

Malignancy	In combination with	Indication specifics	NICE recommended
Breast	Paclitaxel	First-line for metastatic HER2-positive disease	No
	Capecitabine	First-line for metastatic HER2-positive disease unsuitable for taxanes or anthracyclines	No
Colon/rectal	Fluoropyrimdine-based chemotherapy	Metastatic disease	No
Non-small cell lung	Platinum-based chemotherapy	First-line for unresectable, advanced, metastatic or recurrent disease (except squamous cell)	No (nothing submitted from manufacturer)
Renal cell	Interferon alfa-2a	First-line for advanced and/or metastatic disease	No
Ovarian, fallopian tube, primary peritoneal	Carboplatin and paclitaxel	First-line for advanced disease (stages III B, III C and IV)	No
	Carboplatin and gemcitabine	First recurrence in platinum-resistant disease not previously treated with a VEGF inhibitor	No
	Paclitaxel, topotecan, pegylated doxorubicin	Platinum-resistant recurrent disease treated with 2 or less previous regimens and not with a VEGF inhibitor	Suspended
Cervical	Paclitaxel and cisplatin/topotecan	Persistent, recurrent of metastatic disease unable to receive platinum therapy	Not appraised

important step of vasculogenesis and angiogenesis. It thereby inhibits the binding of VEGF to its receptors, Flt-1 (VEGFR-1) and KDR (VEGFR-2), on the surface of endothelial cells. By inhibiting the biological activity of VEGF, tumour vascularization is reduced and the formation of new tumour vasculature inhibited, thereby inhibiting tumour growth.

Prescribing

Bevacizumab is licensed for use in combination therapy with various neoplastic agents and in the treatment of numerous advanced or metastatic malignancies. These include cancers of the breast, colon, rectum, kidney, cervix, lungs, and ovaries (see Table 13.15). Doses are administered by intravenous infusion every 2–3 weeks.

More controversially, bevacizumab has been used off-label for its antiangiogenic properties in the treatment of age-related macular degeneration (AMD) and retinal vein occlusion (RVO) as an intravitreal injection. Although this practice has been largely superseded with the use of mAb therapy licensed for these indications—**ranibizumab** and **aflibercept**.

Unwanted effects

As **bevacizumab** acts to inhibit angiogenesis, unwanted effects include impaired wound healing, GI perforation, haemorrhage, and the formation of fistulae. Other common side effects include hypertension, pancytopenia, fatigue, peripheral neuropathy, GI toxicity, and VTE. Less commonly, treatment has been associated with heart failure and, therefore, caution is advised in patients with pre-existing disease or in the presence of risk factors.

The clearance of bevacizumab is thought to mirror that of endogenous IgG, and is therefore largely done by proteolytic catabolism, relying on neither renal nor hepatic clearance. Dose modifications are therefore unnecessary in renal or hepatic impairment, and clinically significant drug interactions unlikely.

Cetuximab

Mechanism of action

Cetuximab is a chimeric monoclonal IgG1 (half-murine, half-human) antibody with specific activity against the

EGFR. EGFR is a member of a subfamily of type I receptor tyrosine kinases, including EGFR (HER1/c-ErbB-1), HER2, HER3, and HER4, that is over-expressed in many cancers, including colorectal, and head and neck. Cetuximab binds to the extracellular domain of the EGFR with an affinity that is approximately 5–10-fold higher than that of endogenous ligands, resulting in inhibition of the receptor function. It further induces the internalization of EGFR, which can lead to down-regulation of EGFR. Cetuximab also targets cytotoxic immune effector cells towards EGFR-expressing tumour cells [antibody dependent cell-mediated cytotoxicity (ADCC)].

Prescribing

Cetuximab is licensed for first line for the treatment of KRAS wild-type metastatic colorectal cancer that expresses EGFR in combination with oxaliplatin- or irinotecan-based chemotherapy. It is also licensed for use in squamous cell cancer of the head and neck, in combination with radiotherapy in those patients deemed inappropriate for platinum-based chemoradiotherapy. It is administered by IV infusion, usually once a week, over an hour. Premedication with an antihistamine and corticosteroid administered 1 hour prior helps reduce the risk of a hypersensitivity reaction including anaphylaxis. NICE recommend its use in metastatic colorectal cancer, although only in specific patient groups. Treatment is continued until disease progression or until unacceptable toxicity develops.

Unwanted effects

Hypersensitivity and infusion-related reactions are commonly reported with **cetuximab** treatment, ranging from a rash to anaphylaxis. Where reactions are mild this can be managed by slowing the rate of infusion; however, in severe cases treatment should be discontinued immediately and future use is contraindicated. Other significant reactions include cardiovascular toxicity (which can rarely be fatal), electrolyte disturbances (in particular hypomagnesaemia, which may be aggravated by severe diarrhoea) and interstitial lung disease. Drug interactions are infrequent, but can result when combined with drugs that induce similar adverse effects.

Panitumumab

Mechanism of action

Panitumumab is a recombinant, fully human IgG2 monoclonal antibody directed against human EGFR. Like **cetuximab** it binds with high affinity to the extracellular domain of the EGFR, thereby preventing its activation. This leads to internalization of the receptor, inhibition of cell growth and induction of apoptosis, and decreased interleukin 8 and vascular endothelial growth factor production.

Prescribing

Panitumumab is used to treat wild-type *RAS* metastatic colorectal cancer (mCRC), and like **cetuximab** can be used first-line in combination with **oxaliplatin**- or **irinotecan**-based chemotherapy. Doses are infused every 2 weeks based on body weight, with dose adjustments necessary in the case of severe dermatological reactions.

Unwanted effects

In common with other monoclonal antibodies, common adverse effects include infusion-related reactions and rash that can occur at the time of infusion or be delayed by more than 24 hours. Initial doses are therefore administered more cautiously and then more rapidly for subsequent infusions, if tolerated. In the case of severe hypersensitivity reactions, subsequent treatment is contraindicated. Other common side effects include diarrhoea, nausea and vomiting, electrolyte disturbances (in particular hypomagnesaemia), and conjunctivitis. More seriously, treatment has been associated with interstitial lung disease.

As an IgG molecule, elimination is likely through intracellular catabolism and therefore unlikely to be affected by hepatic or renal impairment, although studies have not been carried in these patient groups. Drug interactions are unlikely to be of clinical significance.

Rituximab

Mechanism of action

Rituximab, one of the first monoclonal antibodies to be introduced to the market, is a chimeric murine/human antibody that targets CD20 surface antigens present on pre-B and mature B lymphocytes. See Topic 7.2, 'Inflammatory arthropathies'.

Prescribing

Rituximab is indicated in numerous B-cell malignancies including CLL and non-Hodgkin's lymphoma, as well as in the management of severe rheumatoid arthritis. Doses are administered by IV infusion in cycles determined by indication.

Unwanted effects

See Topic 7.2, 'Inflammatory arthropathies'.

Trastuzumab

Mechanism of action

Trastuzumab is a recombinant humanized IgG1 monoclonal antibody against the human epidermal growth factor receptor subtype 2 (HER2), which is frequently over-expressed in breast cancer and associated with poor prognosis. It binds with high affinity to the extracellular domain IV on HER2, preventing its activation and thereby inhibiting the MAPK pathway. Consequently, trastuzumab inhibits the proliferation of human tumour cells that over-express HER2, and is a potent mediator of ADCC.

Trastuzumab emtasine has recently been developed and licensed for use in metastatic HER2-positive breast cancer. It is an antibody–drug conjugate combining trastuzumab with emtasine, a microtubule inhibitor.

Prescribing

Trastuzumab is licensed for the treatment of HER2-positive early breast cancer, metastatic breast cancer, and metastatic gastric cancer, with NICE recommending its use in patient groups extending beyond the license. It is available in two distinct formulations, the first solely for administration by IV infusion, and the second only by SC injection. The IV infusion is initially given over 90 minutes, then subsequently over 30 minutes if tolerated. Doses are repeated every 1 week or 3 weeks, depending on diagnosis. While on treatment, patients should be closely monitored for chemotherapy-induced myelosuppression and deterioration in left ventricular ejection fraction (LVEF). A significant fall in LVEF would require discontinuation of treatment.

Unwanted effects

Amongst the most serious and/or common adverse reactions reported with **trastuzumab** treatment (IV and SC formulations) are cardiac dysfunction, administration-related reactions, haematological toxicity (in particular neutropenia), infections, and pulmonary adverse reactions. As there is increased risk of developing heart failure on treatment, patients with pre-existing risk factors should be carefully monitored. Although the toxicity

profile is comparable between the two formulations, the incidence of adverse effects is increased when given SC. Clearance occurs independent of age or renal function, and as with other monoclonal antibodies, drug interactions are unlikely.

Monoclonal antibodies and immunotherapy

One of the emerging hallmarks in cancer research has been the investigation of the ability of cancer cells to evade immune destruction.

Mechanism of action

The human immune system responds against immunogenic cancer cells via a complex series of steps involving the presentation of antigens to T-cells via major histocompatibility complex (MHC) class-I antigen presenting cells (APCs), which leads to a cytotoxic response. The stability of the MHC/T cell receptor (TCR) interaction modulates the immune response as do other factors within the tumour microenvironment.

Cytotoxic T lymphocyte-associated protein 4 (CTLA4) is a negative regulator of T cell activation and works as an immune checkpoint preventing uncontrolled immune responses. It binds B7 on antigen-presenting cells, which results in an inhibitory response being generated within the T cell. In a normal immune response this prevents chronic autoimmune inflammation, but in antitumour responses, CTLA4, becomes an inhibitor of the immune response. **Ipilimumab** became the first anti-CTLA4 therapy developed and approved for treatment of metastatic melanoma. It is a monoclonal antibody which binds to the CTLA-4 receptor blocking the inhibitory signal and resulting in activation of the immune response.

Other areas of interest within the field of cancer immunology are centred around the so-called programmed death-1 (PD1) receptor which is expressed on T-cells, B-cells and natural killer cells. It binds to programmed death ligand-1 and 2 (PDL1/2), which is expressed on a multitude of cells but can be upregulated on cancer cells, resulting in inhibition of apoptosis and T cell proliferation, while promoting the conversion of T effector cells to regulatory T cells. This results in cessation of the cancer-immune response and is associated with poor prognosis in a number of tumour types including gastric, ovarian, lung, and renal carcinomas.

Both **pemobrolizumab** and **nivolumab** have been developed as PD-1 inhibitors, which prevent this interaction taking place resulting in activation of an immune response against the cancer.

Prescribing

In two large phase III trials, **ipilimumab** significantly prolonged overall survival and is approved for first-line therapy in BRAF wild type patients. Doses are administered by IV infusion over 90 minutes every 3 weeks.

Nivolumab is approved for use in metastatic melanoma, as monotherapy or in combination with ipilumumab. It is also available in the treatment of metastatic renal cell cancer and several studies have demonstrated benefit in non-small cell lung cancer and recently in head and neck cancers. **Pembrolizumab** is also approved for use in metastatic melanoma in those patients progressing after first line therapy. Both agents are administered again by IV infusion.

Unwanted effects

Side effects of **ipilimumab** are often related to unregulated immune-mediated reactions and can affect any organ system. Most reactions occur within the first few weeks of treatment and early diagnosis and treatment, often with high dose corticosteroids, are required to prevent serious complications. Immune-mediated dermatitis, which can include a spectrum of conditions such as Stevens–Johnson syndrome, toxic epidermal necrolysis, and complicated haemorrhagic, bullous, or necrotic rashes, have been documented. For moderate/severe cases ipilimumab must be discontinued permanently.

Immune-mediated endocrinopathies have also been identified, which can range from life-threatening hypophysitis and adrenal insufficiency, to hypo or hyperthyroidism. Patients may present with non-specific symptoms (headache, fatigue, confusion, and change in bowel habit), and thyroid function and blood sugars should be monitored prior to each treatment cycle. Other immune-mediated reactions include enterocolitis, which can range from a mild slight increase in bowel habit to severe, life-threatening colitis with risk of perforation. Management depends on the severity of symptoms and ranges from anti-diarrhoeal medication to systemic corticosteroids in severe cases. In addition, hepatotoxicity has been noted in 1–4% of patients and regular liver function tests are recommended prior to each treatment cycle. Finally, cases of immune-mediated neuropathies, which include Guillain–Barré syndrome, myasthenia gravis, and motor neuropathy have been documented although the risk of this is low (<1%).

Nivolumab and **pembrolizumab** have immune-mediated side effects similar to those seen with CTLA-4 inhibitors. While these side effects are generally rare, they can range from mild to life-threatening severe reactions, and must be treated quickly and effectively.

There are a number of new novel immunotherapies currently being utilized in clinical trial settings. Clinicians must be aware of the possible side effects related to these novel therapies and prompt assessment and treatment with high dose corticosteroids should be instigated. There is an ongoing trend in oncology that is moving away from traditional chemotherapeutic agents and utilizing a more targeted approach. These agents have shown, in a number of patients, long-term durable disease response and, as they begin to be used more readily by oncologists, clinicians have to be aware of the possible side effects related to these therapies.

Hormone therapy

Hormones are implicated in the growth of multiple cancers, including breast, prostate, and endometrial cancer, with hormonal therapy being one of the oldest systemic anti-cancer therapies, still utilized effectively today. The aim of hormone therapy is to restrict either the production of the hormone implicated in tumour growth or prevent its binding to requisite receptors on the cancer cell, leading to inhibition of cell growth and proliferation resulting in apoptosis. Examples include SERMS (tamoxifen), aromatase inhibitors (exemestane, anastrozole, letrozole), luteinizing hormone-releasing hormone (LHRH) agonists (goserelin, buserelin), GnRH antagonists (degarelix), and anti-androgens (abiraterone, enzalutamide).

Hormones are classified into two groups:

- *Non-steroidal hormones* (which include peptides, polypeptides, or amino acids), which bind to extracellular receptors and mediate their action via secondary intracellular messengers.
- *Steroidal hormones* (such as oestrogens, androgens and progestins), which bind to intracellular receptors directly.

Breast cancer and hormones

Approximately 80% of breast cancers are oestrogen (ER) positive. In premenopausal women, oestrogen is formed from cholesterol in the granulosa cells of the ovaries. In post-menopausal women, the main site of oestrogen production is in the adipose tissue, via the enzyme aromatase.

Selective oestrogen receptor modulator

Mechanism of action

Tamoxifen has been utilized since the 1980's and is a selective oestrogen receptor modulator (SERM) that binds to oestrogen receptors in target organs, thus inhibiting its effects.

Prescribing

Tamoxifen has been shown to significantly reduce the risk of breast cancer recurrence and mortality, with beneficial effects in both pre- and post-menopausal women. It has both agonist and antagonist actions, and has a positive effect on bone mineral density, but can also result in endometrial proliferation and, rarely, endometrial carcinoma. Doses are administered orally for 5 years or longer.

Adverse effects

Predictably, the most common side effects to **tamoxifen** tend to be gynaecological in nature, i.e. vaginal discharge/bleeding or pruritus vulvae. Many women also experience hot flushes and headaches. With long-term use the risk of VTE is increased 2–3-fold, but can be higher in the presence of other risk factors such as concomitant chemotherapy or obesity. In some instances, patients will require thromboprophylaxis with low molecular weight heparins to offset the risk.

Aromatase inhibitors

Mechanism of action

The other group of drugs utilized in breast cancer are aromatase inhibitors. These can be split into steroidal inhibitors, which irreversibly inactivate aromatase (e.g. **exemestane**) and competitive non-steroidal inhibitors (e.g. **anastrozole** and **letrozole**). They are used specifically in post-menopausal women as they inhibit the key enzyme in oestrogen production aromatase, but have no effect on oestrogen production in the ovary.

Prescribing

Aromatase inhibitors are administered orally for between 2 and 5 years either as monotherapy or in combination with **tamoxifen**

Adverse effects

Their major long-term side effect is reduction in bone mineral density, and associated osteoporosis and increased

fracture risk. Bone mineral density assessment is recommended regularly during treatment and appropriate lifestyle advice, calcium supplements, and bisphosphonates in high risk patients should be used.

Prostate cancer and hormones

It has been known since the 18th century that the prostate gland relies upon testosterone for its function and growth. In the 1940s, experiments demonstrated that surgical castration in prostate cancer patients resulted in disease response, although today this is achieved using LHRH agonists, anti-androgens, and GnRH antagonists.

Luteinizing-releasing receptor hormone agonists

Mechanism of action

The LHRH agonists (**goserelin, buserelin**) act on the pituitary gland, and after an initial flare of FSH and LH, result in castrate levels of testosterone within patients. Often, this hormone flare, which can result in worsening symptoms in patients, is covered by a short course of anti-androgen therapy, such as **cyproterone** (see Topic 4.7, 'Androgens, steroids')

Prescribing

LHRH agonists are considered first line treatment in all metastatic prostate cancer patients and are often given alongside radiotherapy in moderate to high risk curative patients. **Goserelin** is administered by SC injection monthly, or 3-monthly where the depot injection is used in the treatment of metastatic or locally advanced prostate cancer. **Buserelin**, although initially administered SC, is subsequently given intranasally for the same indication.

Adverse effects

Side effects to LHRH agonists are largely predictable form their effects on testosterone and include hot flushes, reduced libido, erectile dysfunction, hair loss, breast tenderness, and weight gain. There can also be a metabolic effect with an increased risk of diabetes, raised cholesterol, and ischaemic heart disease. Continued use is known to lead to a reduction in bone mineral density, which can, in part, be managed through the use of concomitant bisphosphonates. Patients at risk of osteoporosis (e.g. smokers, family history, etc.) should be closely monitored.

Gonadotropin-releasing hormone antagonists

Mechanism of action

The new GnRH antagonist (**degarelix**) has recently been developed to achieve medical castration without hormone flare. These can be useful in patients with widespread metastatic disease, especially in those where immediate disease response is sought, i.e. impending cord compression.

Prescribing

Degarelix is licensed for the treatment of men with advanced hormone-dependent prostate cancer and has been approved for use by NICE in the presence of spinal metastases. Doses are administered SC once a month after an initial loading dose.

Adverse effects

As with the LHRH agonists, side effects typically occur as a result of reduced testosterone levels, and include hot flushes, weight gain, reduced libido, etc. Clearance may be affected in the case of severe renal impairment, but the main route of elimination is via the hepato-biliary system.

Anti-androgens

Mechanism of action

While LHRH agonists prevent the testicles from making testosterone, there are other cells in the body, including prostate cancer cells themselves, which can still make androgens, resulting in continued cancer cell growth. **Abiraterone** was developed by the institute of cancer research and blocks the enzyme CYP17 that is expressed in testicular, adrenal, and prostatic cancer cell tissue. As it also blocks steroid hormone production within the adrenal gland, steroid replacement is given alongside this therapy.

   Enzalutamide is a new type of anti-androgen and works by preventing the binding of the androgen receptor to DNA and co-activator proteins.

Prescribing

Like **abiraterone**, **enzalutamide** is licensed for castrate-resistant metastatic prostate cancer patients who have progressed following dual hormone blockade (LHRH agonist therapy and anti-androgen therapy). For further information see Topic 4.7, 'Androgens, steroids'.

Adverse effects

Side effects to the anti-androgens typically include hypokalaemia, hypertension, peripheral oedema, diarrhoea, deranged liver function, gynaecomastia, breast tenderness, hot flushes, fatigue, headaches, and sexual dysfunction. See Topic 4.7, 'Androgens, steroids', for more details.

Further reading

Chang, AC, Massague, J (2008) Molecular origins of cancer: molecular basis of metastasis. *New England Journal of Medicine* 359, 2814–23.

Cogliano VJ, Baan R, Straif K, et al. (2011). Preventable exposures associated with human cancers. *Journal of the National Cancer Institute* 103, 1827–39.

Desantis CE, Lin CC, Mariotto AB, et al. (2014) Cancer treatment and survivorship statistics. *Californian Cancer Journal for Clinicians*, 64(4), 252–71.

Doll R, Hill AB (1950) Smoking and carcinoma of the lung. *British Medical Journal* 2(4682), 739–48.

Ford ES, Bergmann MM, Kroger J, et al. (2009) Findings from the European Prospective Investigation into Cancer and Nutrition—Potsdam study. *Archives of Internal Medicine* 169, 1355–62.

Global Burden of Disease Cancer Collaboration, Fitzmaurice C, Dicker D, et al. (2015) The Global Burden of Cancer 2013. *Journal of the American Medical Association Oncology* 1(4), 505–27.

Kerbel R (2008) Tumor angiogenesis. *New England Journal of Medicine* 358(19), 2039–49.

Office for National Statistics. Cancer Incidence and Mortality in the United Kingdom, 2008–10 http://www.ons.gov.uk/ons/dcp171778_289890.pdf [accessed 18 April 2019].

Reeves G, Pirie K, Beral V, et al. (2007) Cancer incidence and mortality in relation to body mass index in the Million Women Study: cohort study. *British Medical Journal* 335(7630), 1134.

Townsend W, Linch D (2012). Hodgkin's lymphoma in adults. *Lancet* 380, 836–47.

Index